Pharmacology
for Nursing Practice

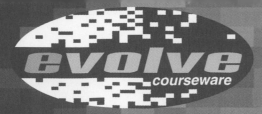

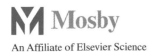

Pharmacology
for Nursing Practice

Kathleen Gutierrez, PhD, RN, ANP, CNS
Adult Nurse Practitioner
Private Practice;
Associate Professor
Regis University and
University of Colorado Health Sciences Center
Denver, Colorado

Sherry F. Queener, PhD
Professor of Pharmacology
Indiana University School of Medicine;
Associate Dean
Indiana University Graduate School;
and Director of the Graduate Office
Indiana University Purdue University Indianapolis (IUPUI)
Indianapolis, Indiana

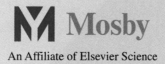 Mosby
An Affiliate of Elsevier Science

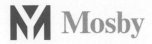

Mosby

An Affiliate of Elsevier Science

11830 Westline Industrial Drive
St. Louis, Missouri 63146

DEDICATION

*To my husband and soul mate, Pat, who stands beside me through thick and
thin, maintains our home, nourishes me, and helps me to keep my sanity—
I don't know what I would do without you.*

*To my daughter Pam and son-in-law Brad, whose abilities to be
forthright and honest keep my busy life in perspective. And to my son,
Michael, who remains the most compassionate, honest, devoted, and
nonjudgmental individual I have ever known.*

Kathleen Gutierrez

A NOTE TO THE READER

Pharmacology is an ever-changing field. Standard safety precautions must be followed, but as new research and clinical experience broaden our knowledge, changes in treatment and drug therapy may
become necessary or appropriate. Readers are advised to check the most current product information
provided by the manufacturer of each drug to be administered to verify the recommended dose, the
method and duration of administration, and contraindications. It is the responsibility of the licensed
health care provider, relying on experience and knowledge of the patient, to determine dosages and
the best treatment for each individual patient. Neither the publisher nor the author assumes any liability for any injury and/or damage to persons or property arising from this publication.

The Publisher

International Standard Book Number 0-323-01911-0

Vice President and Publishing Director, Nursing: Sally Schrefer
Associate Publisher: Barbara Cullen
Managing Editor: Lee Henderson
Developmental Editor: Celia Cruz
Publication Services Manager: Catherine Albright Jackson
Project Manager: Mary Stueck
Book Designer: Teresa Breckwoldt
Cover Designer: Paul Fry

Printed in the United States of America

Last digit is the print number: 9 8 7 6 5 4 3 2 1

Chapter Authors

Alan P. Agins, PhD, is currently an adjunct associate professor at Brown University in Rhode Island where he lectures and provides board review seminars to medical students. He is also an adjunct assistant professor in the Schools of Nursing at both Pennsylvania State University and Radford University in Virginia where he teaches graduate-level nursing pharmacology.

Joseph A. DiMicco, PhD, is professor of pharmacology and neurobiology and director of the course in medical pharmacology at the Indiana University School of Medicine in Indianapolis. He is a member of the American Society for Pharmacology and Experimental Therapeutics and the Society for Neuroscience and has served on advisory panels for the American Heart Association, National Aeronautics and Space Administration, and the National Institutes of Health.

Kathleen Gutierrez, PhD, RN, ANP, CNS, is a board-certified adult nurse practitioner and medical-surgical clinical nurse specialist in private practice in the Denver area. She is also an associate professor at Regis University and the University of Colorado Health Sciences Center in Denver. In addition to her work on *Real World Nursing Survival Guide: Pharmacology,* and *Real World Nursing Survival Guide: Pathophysiology* (Mosby), Dr. Gutierrez is the author and editor of *Pharmacotherapeutics: Clinical Decision-Making in Nursing* (Saunders).

Elizabeth Kissell, BSN, MSN, has been on the faculty of the University of Northern Colorado, University of South Dakota, and Regis University in Denver. She was a contributor to *Pharmacotherapeutics: Clinical Decision-Making in Nursing,* by Kathleen Gutierrez. Ms. Kissell is presently working part-time as a clinic nurse at the La Casa-Quigg Newton Family Health Care Clinic in northern Denver while caring for a growing family.

Sherry F. Queener, PhD, currently serves as professor of pharmacology at Indiana University School of Medicine in Indianapolis, as director of the Graduate Office at IUPUI, and as associate dean of Indiana University Graduate School. She has received several research awards from the National Institutes of Health, published over 125 scientific papers, and trained students at many levels. Dr. Queener was a founding author of *Pharmacologic Basis of Nursing Practice* (Mosby) and co-authored five subsequent editions.

Susan Sciacca, RN, BSN, is a contributor to the *Real World Survival Guide: Pathophysiology* (Saunders). She has worked as a staff nurse at Craig Hospital in Englewood, Colorado, and is currently employed as a staff nurse at Mount View Youth Services Center in Denver, and as a private duty nurse for Act for Health in Colorado Springs.

Michael R. Vasko, PhD, is the Paul Stark Professor of Pharmacology at Indiana University School of Medicine in Indianapolis and was recently named chairman of the Department of Pharmacology and Toxicology. He is a member of the American Society for Pharmacology and Experimental Therapeutics, the Society for Neuroscience, and the American Pain Society. Dr. Vasko serves as associate editor for *Pain, The Journal of Pain,* and *Sensory Neurons.*

Lynn Roger Willis, PhD, is Professor of Pharmacology and Medicine at the Indiana University School of Medicine in Indianapolis. He is a member of the American Society for Pharmacology and Experimental Therapeutics and the American Society of Nephrology and is a fellow of the Council for High Blood Pressure Research of the American Heart Association. He contributed to several editions of *Pharmacologic Basis of Nursing Practice* (Mosby) by Clark, Queener, and Korb.

Reviewers

Elizabeth Kupczyk, RN, MSN
Trinity Christian College
Palos Heights, Illinois

Natasha Leskovsek, RN, MBA, JD
Heller, Ehrman, White, & McAuliffe, LLP
Washington, DC

Dawn McKay, RN, BA, MSN, CCRN
Liberty University
Lynchburg, Virginia

Dorothy M. Obester, PhD, RN, BSNE, MSN
St. Francis University
Loretto, Pennsylvania

James J. Wojcik, BSN, MBA
Crestwood Medical Center
Huntsville, Alabama

Preface

Most contacts between health care providers and their patients end with a prescription for a drug or another kind of therapy. The dynamic nature of drug therapy and health care today presents constant challenges to both providers and patients. Direct-to-consumer advertising, managed health care, restricted drug formularies, and externally imposed time limitations increasingly complicate care and the choice of drug therapy. Moreover, pharmacology is a rapidly changing field. The role of the health care provider must become more sophisticated as new drugs and new strategies are applied to patient care.

GOAL

Our goal is to provide an up-to-date, scientifically based pharmacology text that enables students to gain pharmacologic knowledge, thereby empowering them to function in the changing health care environment. Successful, safe clinical practice is built on understanding the concepts and principles of pharmacology. We present the concepts of pharmacology that guide all drug use, discuss the major drug classes with an emphasis on the mechanisms of action, and apply this information to the multidisciplinary care of the patient across the lifespan. Our approach is to relate the physiologic and pathophysiologic factors of disease processes to drug mechanisms and subsequent nursing care.

Because students often express frustration about trying to remember the large number of drugs they must learn, we have adopted a *key drug* approach that highlights the most important drug or drugs in a particular class. We also strive to minimize students' difficulty by presenting drug classes first, followed by application of this information to nursing practice.

ORGANIZATION

Pharmacology for Nursing Practice is organized into two distinct content areas. The nine chapters of Parts I and II link pharmacology with professional nursing practice. These units ground the student in pharmacokinetics, pharmacodynamics, lifespan considerations, evidence-based practice and pharmacoeconomics, the legal implications of drug therapy, and the role of the nurse. The chapter on substance abuse discusses the use of both prescriptive and illicit drugs in a culture that sometimes promotes dependence.

The remaining units are organized around the influence of drugs on various body systems. The chapters of Parts III through XIV correlate physiology or pathophysiology with the pharmacology of various drug classes. Each clinical chapter is divided into three distinct sections: Pathophysiology, Drug Class, and Application to Practice.

DRUG CLASS

MECHANISM OF ACTION

The mechanism of action is related to both the desired effects of the drug and the potential adverse reactions. For example, by understanding that a drug acts on multiple receptor types, the student may more readily understand the mechanism not only for the desired effects but also for adverse reactions caused by actions on other receptors. Understanding these multiple effects also helps a student rationalize the importance of new drug classes with changed specificity for receptor types.

USES

Food and Drug Administration (FDA)–approved therapeutic uses for the drug or drug class are detailed in this section. Newer significant but unlabeled (non–FDA-approved) uses of specific drugs are also discussed here.

PHARMACOKINETICS

Pharmacokinetics describes what happens to a drug following administration (i.e., what the body does with the drug). For each drug class, key points concerning absorption, distribution, biotransformation, elimination, protein binding, and half-life are discussed, emphasizing those factors that most directly influence the clinical use of the class. Pharmacokinetic tables provide an overview of these variables when there is strong variation within the class and comparisons are useful.

ADVERSE REACTIONS AND CONTRAINDICATIONS

All drugs have the potential to produce undesirable effects. When considering the use of a specific drug, the potential for predictable and unpredictable reactions is taken into account. An effort has been made to include major adverse effects and contraindications, because it is nearly impossible to include all reported reactions in this section. Information regarding cautious use of the drugs is also included. This section is extremely important for nurses, who are often the first members of the health care team to observe adverse reactions and must be prepared to judge the significance of symptoms and to act appropriately to protect the patient from lasting harm.

INTERACTIONS

Drug interactions are the by-product of the concurrent administration of two or more drugs or of a combination of food or environmental chemicals and drugs. The number of potentially significant drug interactions increases as pharmacotherapy becomes more complex and drugs more potent. Some drug interactions are intentional and are seen as beneficial. However, most others are unintentional and have potentially harmful effects. Drug interactions often result in treatment delays and hospitalization or, in some cases, increase the length of a hospital stay. When drug classes have significant numbers of interactions, drug interaction tables are included in the chapter.

APPLICATION TO PRACTICE

HISTORY OF PRESENT ILLNESS

Information obtained here provides a chronologic account of how each of the patient's principal symptoms developed, as well as attributes and context (onset, duration, frequency, location, quality, quantity, severity, setting, aggravating and alleviating factors). This section also includes how the patient thinks and feels about the illness, what concerns led to seeking attention, and how the illness has affected activities of daily living.

Health History

Past health events may have residual effects on the current health state. This section explores pertinent childhood illnesses and any adult illnesses, surgeries, obstetric or gynecologic events, or psychiatric conditions that influence drug therapy. This section may also include information about family health history. Drug histories include information about a patient's experiences with over-the-counter, prescription, and illicit drugs.

Lifespan Considerations

Age is a significant variable determining how a patient responds to drug therapy. This section is adapted to include the changes of aging from the perinatal period to the older adult and how these changes influence how a drug acts in the body and how the patient responds.

Cultural/Social Considerations

Cultural dimensions are a vital consideration in drug therapy because the rich variety of cultural and ethnic backgrounds results in a wealth of folk practices. The health beliefs and practices of patients are integral to how health and illness are defined and to the success of drug therapy.

Physical Examination

This section helps identify and verify health-related concerns, explain signs and symptoms, and supply a database for future evaluation. This section identifies physical characteristics, body structure, mobility, behaviors, vital signs, and examination findings important to evaluate the patient for, and to monitor, drug therapy.

Laboratory Testing

Laboratory and diagnostic tests are tools that, in and of themselves, are almost useless. When these tools are used in combination with a history and physical examination, they help confirm a diagnosis or provide information necessary to monitor the patient's response to drug therapy.

GOALS OF THERAPY

Treatment goals are developed after the assessment is complete. Initial drug regimens are chosen from a variety of reasonable alternatives including drugs used to prevent, cure, restore, support, or palliate an illness.

INTERVENTION

This section identifies information needed to safely administer a drug or class of drugs. It includes information about drug formulations, administration routes and schedules, and documentation.

Poor understanding of verbal instructions and written materials remains a major factor in failure to achieve the goals of drug therapy. Thus this section also includes information about drug administration in the outpatient setting; drug storage, handling, and disposal; and patient variables to consider when teaching.

EVALUATION

Evaluation of patient response to drug therapy is organized around the following four areas: compliance, patient satisfaction, therapeutic response, and secondary or adverse effects of the prescribed therapy.

SPECIAL FEATURES

BODY SYSTEM ORGANIZATION

The body system approach in the clinical units helps the student make logical connections between major drug classes and the conditions for which drugs are commonly used. Each of the clinical units represents major body systems. Careful cross-referencing helps the student appreciate how a class of drugs may have several important clinical applications.

INTEGRATION OF PHYSIOLOGY, PATHOPHYSIOLOGY, AND PHARMACOLOGY

The integration of physiology and pathophysiology with the study of pharmacology provides students with an understanding of the drugs for specific disorders. Examples include pain and the use of opioids and nonsteroidal antiinflammatory drugs, multiple sclerosis and the role of skeletal muscle relaxants, the antimicrobial therapies used to treat infectious diseases, and the role of antiarrhythmic drugs in treating irregular heart rhythms.

PHARMACOKINETIC TABLES

Pharmacokinetic tables describe what happens to a drug following administration—what the body does with the drug. These tables appear in selected chapters and provide an overview of absorption, distribution, biotransformation, elimination, protein binding, and half-life.

EVIDENCE-BASED PRACTICE

Traditionally health care providers have favored experience, prevailing practice, professional education, and authority opinion as guides for day-to-day decisions about patient care. However, the continued rise of health care ex-

penses throughout the world has created an impetus to ground clinical decisions in a more critical examination of the benefits and costs of medical treatments. Knowledge of which treatments are most effective clinically and economically enables wiser decisions to be made about the distribution of limited health care resources.

CLINICAL CASE STUDIES

Fifty individual case studies highlight many of the variables influencing drug therapy. Each case study explores how factors such as age, economic status, comorbidity, and drug characteristics affect drug therapy.

PATIENT PROBLEM BOXES

Patient problem boxes discuss common clinical issues with suggestions for solutions. For example, there are discussions of the use of methylphenidate in the treatment of ADHD and the risk of dependency, and the problem of the correct use of metered-dose inhalers by patients who have a respiratory disease.

ALTERNATIVE THERAPIES

Nurses normally focus their attention on drugs ordered for patients by health care providers. However, because patients frequently self-treat with a wide array of over-the-counter drugs and, more recently, with an even wider array of herbal remedies, any of which may significantly influence the effects of prescribed drugs, nurses must also focus attention on these products. For example, St. John's wort is used as an alternative therapy for depression; saw palmetto is used as an adjunct in the treatment of prostatic hypertrophy. Alternative therapy boxes are thus included to address the more common alternative therapies. In addition, an entire chapter on herbal remedies gives the student a strong conceptual grounding in the uses and limitations of these agents.

INTERNET RESOURCES

Internet resources are included at the end of each chapter. These stable resources are included to provide the student with a starting point in searching for additional information on the use of a drug or class of drugs in patient care. A series of questions identified in Chapter 5 helps the student determine whether an online site is reliable.

ILLUSTRATIONS

The illustrations in this text show concepts and principles important to pharmacology. All were carefully chosen and designed to maximize visual communication and enable students to better understand how drugs work. Whether the illustrations depict pharmacokinetic phases, examine toxic range, outline anatomy, describe mechanisms of action, or follow the steps from an injured blood vessel to a fibrin-platelet plug, all become integral to the written text and enhance learning.

APPENDICES

The two appendices included in this text include dietary considerations and drugs with common adverse reactions. Dietary considerations include, for example, foods high in potassium or sodium and foods to be avoided for patients on tyramine-restricted diets. The summary of drugs with common adverse effects includes, for example, drugs that cause hearing loss, those that are hepatotoxic, nephrotoxic, or that cause peripheral neuropathy.

ADDITIONAL RESOURCES
For Faculty

The Instructor's Resource includes an Instructor's Manual consisting of objectives, content outlines, and a variety of teaching and learning activities. Learning activities include pharmflow diagrams, point-counterpoint discussions, thoughts-in-action, WYSIWYG exercises, case studies, and patient teaching scenarios. A Test Bank accompanies the Instructor's Manual.

For Students

Pharmacology is a demanding science. The companion *Study Guide for Pharmacology for Nursing Practice* provides students with a wealth of learning opportunities that reinforce pharmacology content. Clinical case studies assist students in applying pharmacology information to patients with common problems. Other learning activities such as crossword puzzles and anagrams, true and false, completion and matching exercises, mnemonics, point-counterpoint exercises, and thoughts-in-action expand student understanding of the importance of patient and family education. The puzzles are interjected for fun but are also designed to encourage critical thinking in a way that has previously been underused. Because suggested responses to exercises and case studies are provided in the back of this guide, students have an opportunity to check their understanding immediately.

ACKNOWLEDGMENTS

No author writes a book alone. A project of this size could not come to fruition without the collaboration of many people. We would like to acknowledge the support and encouragement of the Department of Pharmacology and Toxicology, Indiana University School of Medicine, and to the colleagues who saw the development of this book as part of our greater teaching mission.

Special thanks to a unique colleague who has encouraged this author (SFQ) through several book projects: Dr. Stephen W. Queener, Senior Research Scientist and Group Leader, Biochemical Systems, Eli Lilly & Company.

Thanks to educational and clinical colleagues who keep this author (KG) grounded in reality. Thanks also to Barbara Cicalese, Developmental Editor of Elsevier Science, who pushed, prodded, and persevered to keep us on schedule.

Table of Contents

PART III
AUTONOMIC NERVOUS SYSTEM DRUGS

CHAPTER

1

Drugs in the Body: Pharmacodynamics and Pharmacokinetics

SHERRY F. QUEENER

 Visit http://evolve.elsevier.com/Gutierrez/ for additional information.

KEY TERMS

OBJECTIVES

- Explain the concept of drug receptors.
- Identify and discuss the mechanisms that produce unwanted drug reactions.
- Describe the factors that can influence enteral absorption of drugs.
- Discuss the advantages and disadvantages of common routes of administration.
- Explain how the elimination half-life of a drug influences the time required to attain a steady-state concentration in the body when the drug is given on a regular schedule.

MECHANISMS OF DRUG ACTION: PHARMACODYNAMICS
Drug Action Is Determined by Where and How a Drug Interacts with the Body

Pharmacology is the study of how chemicals interact with living organisms to produce biologic effects. Chemicals that produce therapeutically useful effects are called *drugs*. Pharmacodynamics is the part of pharmacology that focuses on how drugs produce biologic effects by interacting with specific targets at the drug's site of action. The magnitude of the biologic effect produced by a drug is related to the effective concentration of the drug present at the site of action.

Sites of Drug Action. Where a drug acts may be determined by many factors. A few drugs are administered in such a way that they enter the body fluid where they are intended to act; for example, an antacid enters the stomach, dissolves, and neutralizes stomach acid. Alteration of gastric pH is the only intended action of this drug. Other examples are drugs that accumulate in urine and alter urinary pH. By acidifying the urine with ammonium chloride or alkalinizing the urine with sodium bicarbonate, ion flow in the kidneys is altered and drug excretion patterns are changed.

Certain classes of drugs are directed to their site of action because they are very lipid soluble and are thus able to interact with lipids and proteins in cell membranes. General anesthetic gases (see Chapter 16) may act in this way. These drugs alter properties of membranes by integrating into the lipid layers surrounding specific membrane proteins or by attaching to sites on membrane proteins that tend to attract lipid-like substances. Drugs of this type are chemically diverse, but they share the property of being very lipid soluble.

The biologic activity of many drugs is directed to specific types of cells. This localization is possible because each type of cell possesses a unique array of proteins called receptors.

Drug Receptors. A key concept in pharmacology involves specific proteins called drug receptors, which are natural components of the body intended to respond to some chemical normally present in blood or tissues (Table 1-1). For example, opioid receptors within the brain respond to morphine and related compounds from the opium poppy, but the natural function of these receptors is to bind to enkephalins and endorphins. These compounds produced in the brain are more potent than morphine in producing analgesia (see Chapter 13). The opioid effects are localized because only those cells that possess opioid receptors can respond to morphine.

The ability to bind to a specific receptor is determined by the chemical structure of the drug. This binding action resembles a lock-and-key fit. A critical portion of the drug usually determines its ability to bind (drugs *A* and *B* in Figure 1-1); drugs that differ in this critical region may not bind to the receptor at all (drug *C* in Figure 1-1).

Specificity is the property of the receptor that lets it discriminate among generally similar compounds and bind only to those with the critical features. Affinity is the property that determines the strength of the binding of a compound to a receptor. When receptors are highly specific and have high affinity for the compounds that bind to them, even very low concentrations of these compounds may show biologic activity. For example, hormones naturally present in the body act through specific receptors. Some of these hormones are found in

---

TABLE 1-1

Examples of Receptors

Receptor Type	Major Subtype*	Endogenous Agonists
Acetylcholine	Nicotinic Muscarinic	Acetylcholine Acetylcholine
ACTH	—	ACTH
Acidic amino acids	NMDA, kainate, quisqualate	Glutamate or aspartate
Purinergic	P_1, P_2	Adenosine, ATP, AMP
Adrenergic	Alpha, beta	Epinephrine and norepinephrine
Dopamine	D_1, D_2, D_3, D_4, D_5	Dopamine
GABA	A, B	GABA
Glucagon	—	Glucagon
Glycine	—	Glycine
Histamine	H_1, H_2, H_3	Histamine
Insulin	—	Insulin
Opioid	μ, μ_1, κ, δ, ϵ	Enkephalins or endorphins
Serotonin	5-HT_1, 5-HT_2, 5-HT_3, 5-HT_4	5-HT (serotonin)
Steroids	—	Several

5-HT, 5-hydroxytryptamine (serotonin); *ACTH*, adrenocorticotropic hormone; *GABA*, gamma-aminobutyric acid; *NMDA*, N-methyl-D-aspartate.
*Subclassifications may exist, based on selective drug binding and specific tissue localization.

the blood at concentrations of less than 1 picomole, or less than one part per trillion. Nevertheless, these tiny amounts are biologically effective because hormones are detected and bound by specific receptors.

Agonists and Antagonists. The abilities to bind to the receptor and to stimulate the receptor to action by the receptor are two different aspects of drug action. The ability to bind to the receptor is expressed as affinity. The ability to stimulate the receptor to some action is called efficacy.

Any compound, either natural or synthetic, that binds to a specific receptor and produces a biologic effect by stimulating that receptor is called an agonist. For example, norepinephrine produced in nerve terminals binds to specific proteins in the heart called *beta$_1$-adrenergic receptors*. Stimulation of these receptors causes the heart to beat faster. The synthetic drug isoproterenol acts on the same cardiac receptors and produces the same effects. Both norepinephrine and isoproterenol are therefore called agonists for the beta$_1$-adrenergic receptor (see Chapter 12). Agonists have both affinity for receptors and efficacy because they cause some action by the receptor (Figure 1-2).

Some drugs produce their action not by stimulating receptors but by preventing other, natural substances from stimulating receptors. These drugs are called antagonists (see Figure 1-2). For example, the drug propranolol blocks beta$_1$-adrenergic receptors and prevents agonists such as norepinephrine from stimulating the receptor normally. Propranolol is therefore classified as an antagonist of the action of norepinephrine. Antago-

nists have affinity for receptors but lack efficacy. When the receptor is occupied by an antagonist, the receptor cannot carry out its normal function.

Pharmacodynamic Drug Interactions. Combining agonists and antagonists may produce interactions that lower the response of both drugs. For example, consider the beta-receptor antagonist propranolol, often used to treat hypertension, and the adrenergic agonist epinephrine, a drug sometimes used to treat asthma. The therapeutic target for propranolol is the cardiovascular system, whereas epinephrine targets the bronchioles. However, if a patient were to take both drugs, they would antagonize each other because they both affect beta-adrenergic receptors. The bronchioles would fail to respond fully to epinephrine because propranolol would directly oppose it, and the cardiovascular system would fail to fully respond to propranolol because epinephrine would oppose the action. As a result, neither drug would give the desired therapeutic effect.

Pharmacodynamic drug interactions can also occur when the specific receptors involved may be different

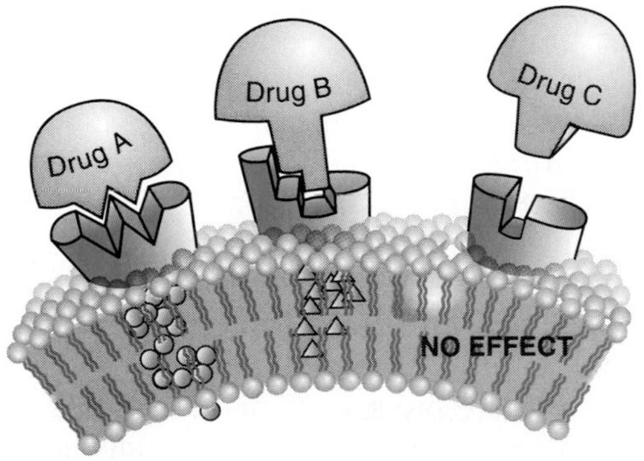

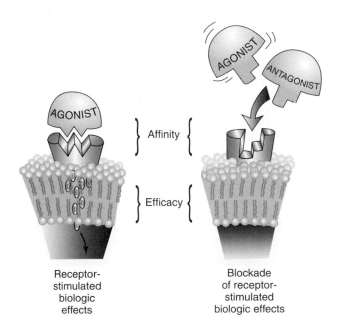

FIGURE 1-1 Lock-and-key fit between drugs and receptors. The site on the receptor that interacts with a drug has a definite shape. Drugs conforming to that shape can bind and produce a biologic response. Thus drug *A* interacts with a specific receptor that recognizes its critical features, but drug *B* binds to a different type of receptor. Drug *C* fails to bind because the specific receptor that would recognize it does not exist on the cell shown.

FIGURE 1-2 Biologic effects of agonists and antagonists. Agonists bind to the receptor and activate processes linked to it; thus they have both affinity and efficacy. Antagonists bind to receptors but fail to activate (i.e., they have no efficacy); thus the biologic effect of antagonists arises from blocking normal receptor activity.

BOX **1-1** **Drug Interactions**

Patients often have more than one condition for which they receive medical attention, and therefore they often take more than one medication at a time. This situation creates the possibility for drugs to interact. A **drug interaction** is any modification of the action of one drug by another drug. Interactions may either increase or decrease the action of the drugs involved.

- **Antagonism** arises when one drug interferes with the action of another. The mechanism may involve pharmacodynamics (i.e., one drug interferes with the action of another at its receptor target) or pharmacokinetics (i.e., one drug increases the metabolic inactivation of another drug or blocks its absorption). *Result for the patient: loss of therapeutic effect.*

- **Additivity** arises when two drugs seem to act completely independently of each other, and their combined effect is what would be expected by adding the effects of the two drugs alone. *Result for the patient: predictable combinations may be useful therapeutically.*

- **Synergy** occurs when the effect of two drugs combined is greater than the additive effect. Potentiation is a form of synergy in which a drug that produces a biologic effect has its effect increased by a second drug that has no activity alone. Synergy often arises from pharmacokinetic effects such as displacement of active drug from protein binding sites, which increases the effective concentration of the drug at the target; inhibition of metabolic inactivation of one drug by another; or inhibition of the elimination of one drug by another. *Result for the patient: unpredictable effect may lead to toxicity; occasionally used to achieve therapeutic goal.*

The negative aspects of drug interaction can be reduced if health care personnel (1) are aware of major drug interactions, (2) are thorough in determining which over-the-counter or prescription drugs a patient is taking, and (3) carefully instruct patients about drugs that interact with their prescribed medication.

---

but their actions lead to the same physiologic effects. For example, a vasodilator such as hydralazine might be part of a therapeutic program for control of hypertension. Nitroglycerin is another vasodilator, but it is used to relieve angina. A patient who takes hydralazine for hypertension and then takes nitroglycerin for angina will probably experience a severe hypotensive episode or faint as a result of the additive effects of the two drugs (Box 1-1).

Ethanol is a common cause of pharmacodynamic drug interactions. As a central nervous system depressant, ethanol acts synergistically with other drug classes that also depress the central nervous system, such as antihistamines, sedative-hypnotics, antianxiety drugs, antidepressants, antipsychotics, general anesthetics, and narcotic analgesics (see Box 1-1). At low dosages the drowsiness characteristic of these drug classes is exaggerated by ethanol, but at higher dosages respiration can be dangerously depressed.

Classification of Receptors. Receptors may be classified according to their affinities for agonists or antagonists (see Table 1-1). For example, receptors in the adrenergic nervous system have been divided into two categories, alpha and beta, based on differing affinities for two natural agonists, epinephrine and norepinephrine (see Chapter 12).

Receptors may also be classified by location within the cell or on the cell membrane. Receptors on the cell membrane are typically on the outside of the cell, allowing the receptor to interact with substances in the extracellular fluid. One class of membrane-bound receptors regulates function of ion channels, either opening or closing them as a result of binding to an agonist. This type of action produces a rapid change in cell function. An example of this type of ion channel–linked receptor is the acetylcholine receptor in the cholinergic system (see Chapter 11).

Another type of membrane-bound receptor gains enzymatic activity when it binds to an agonist. For example, the receptors for growth factors and for insulin (see Chapter 58) carry tyrosine kinase activity when agonists are present. The actions of tyrosine kinase change various intracellular processes, including gene transcription—thus changing the function of cells over a period of hours.

Many receptors that are important for pharmacology are linked to a system of membrane proteins called *G proteins*. These proteins are capable of stimulating or inhibiting a wide array of activities, including adenylate cyclase (see Chapter 12) and calcium channels (see Chapter 39).

The ion channels, protein kinases, and G-protein systems linked to receptors are called *transducers* because they convert a signal from receptors outside the cell into an action inside the cell. An important feature of these transduction cascades is that they can amplify the signal received (Figure 1-3). For example, for each molecule of agonist bound to one beta-adrenergic receptor, 10,000 molecules of the internal messenger cyclic adenosine monophosphate (cAMP) may be produced. Therefore a few molecules of agonist circulating in blood can have profound effects on target cells.

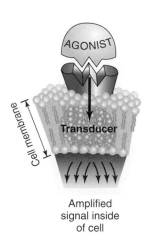

FIGURE 1-3 Amplification by transducers linked to receptors on the cell surface. One molecule of agonist bound to the receptor activates the transducer system, which generates an amplified signal involving many molecules inside the cell.

Receptors inside the cell require that the agonist either diffuse into or be transported into the cell to produce its biologic effect. Thyroid hormones (see Chapter 56) and corticosteroids (see Chapter 57) operate through receptors of this type. These receptors are activated in the cytoplasm by binding to agonists but then move into the nucleus, where they influence gene transcription. This mechanism requires hours to days for full effect.

Drugs Do Not Create Functions but Modify Existing Functions Within the Body

Drugs must always be considered in terms of the physiologic functions they alter in the body. In no case do drugs create a function in a tissue or organ. For example, the synthetic drug albuterol is used to promote dilation of the bronchioles (see Chapters 12 and 52). The drug produces this effect by interacting with beta$_2$-adrenergic receptors. Thus it does not create a new way for the bronchioles to dilate; it simply acts through the existing mechanisms normally regulating bronchodilation.

To emphasize this principle, subsequent chapters on drug families start with a brief description of the normal physiology or the pathophysiology influenced by the family discussed. This strategy simplifies the learning process for pharmacology. For example, physiology courses teach the function of beta-adrenergic receptors in regulating blood pressure, heart rate, and bronchodilation. Therefore when a drug is noted to stimulate beta-adrenergic receptors, the clinical result of that stimulation is predictable from the known physiologic functions of those receptors.

No Drug Has a Single Action

The desired action of a drug is an expected, predictable response. Ideally, each drug would have the desired effect on one physiologic process and produce no other effect. However, all drugs have the potential for altering more than one function in the body. These unintended actions are often called *side effects*. For example, the desired action of digoxin is to strengthen a failing heart, but at the same time it may cause erratic heartbeat, which is an undesirable side effect or **adverse reaction**.

Predictable reactions arising from known pharmacologic actions of drugs account for 70% to 80% of all drug reactions. For example, barbiturates put a patient to sleep because they depress the central nervous system, but excessive depression of the central nervous system is lethal because the brain centers that control breathing are also depressed. Respiratory depression would therefore be an expected adverse effect when barbiturates are used at dosages that allow the drug to accumulate in the body. Other predictable adverse effects may occur at normal therapeutic dosages and are related to the secondary actions of the drug. For example, at normal therapeutic dosages, barbiturates increase drug-biotransforming activity of the liver. This ability is unrelated to the desired clinical action of these drugs and actually leads to a number of interactions with other drugs.

Unpredictable reactions account for 20% to 30% of all drug reactions. Although experience shows that a certain percentage of the population may react to a drug in an unusual manner, it is often impossible to predict which individual will show the reaction. Unpredictable drug reactions are of two types: *idiosyncratic* and *allergic*. **Idiosyncratic reactions** have no obvious cause and may relate to an undetected genetic difference from most of the population. Allergic reactions account for 6% to 10% of all drug reactions. An allergic reaction may be triggered by the drug in its original form or by a metabolite of the drug formed in the body.

Drug allergies range from mild skin reactions to potentially fatal reactions involving the cardiovascular and respiratory systems (Table 1-2). **Anaphylaxis** is a severe, rare reaction marked by sudden contraction of the bronchioles, often including edema of the mouth and throat, which may completely cut off airflow to the lungs. In addition, blood pressure falls, and the patient may go into shock. These violent reactions may occur quickly, and aggressive therapy is required to save the patient's life.

Allergic reactions do not occur during the first exposure to a drug, because time is required for the immune system to develop antibodies that cause these reactions (see Chapter 35). Documenting prior exposure to a drug is helpful in preventing reactions but not always easy. Patients do not always know the

---

TABLE 1-2

Classification of Allergic Reactions*

Type	Synonyms	Antibody	Effector Cells	Mechanism	Example
I	Anaphylaxis	IgE	Mast cells	Antigen binds with basophils on surface of mast cells and basophils with release of histamine, leukotrienes, serotonin, and prostaglandins	Penicillin, pollens, insect venom, household cleaning agents
II	Cytotoxic	IgG, IgM	Polymorphonuclear leukocytes	Antigen binds to allergen on cell membranes; complement system activated with cell destruction	Penicillin, methyldopa, sulfonamides, hydralazine, procainamide, quinidine
III	Immune complex-mediated response	IgG, IgM	Polymorphonuclear leukocytes	Antigen binds to allergen in fluid phase and deposits in small blood vessels; complement system is activated with cell destruction	Penicillin, phenytoin, streptomycin, iodides, sulfonamides
IV	Cell-mediated response	Not involved	Not involved	Sensitized cells bind to allergen and release lymphokines	Tuberculosis skin tests, rabies vaccination, poison ivy, phenol, benzene products, halothane

Adapted with permission from McCance K, Huether S: *Pathophysiology: the biologic basis for disease in adults and children*, ed. 3, St. Louis, 1997, Mosby.
*Types I, II, and III allergic responses are immediately produced. Type IV has a delayed response.

---

names of drugs they have received and are not always reliable sources of information on previous reactions to drugs. Moreover, persons may have been unknowingly exposed to antibiotics or other drugs through food or milk if the drugs were improperly used in animal medicine.

HOW DRUG DOSAGE RELATES TO DRUG ACTION: PHARMACOKINETICS
The Role of Route of Administration and Elimination

Drugs differ in their intrinsic ability to produce an effect, in their ability to penetrate to the site of action, and in their rate of removal from that site. **Pharmacokinetics** is the study of how drugs enter the body, reach their site of action, and are removed from the body (Figure 1-4). Both the pharmacodynamics and the pharmacokinetics of a drug determine how a drug is administered, how often it is given, and at what dosage.

Factors Controlling Drug Absorption by Enteral Routes. To be systemically effective, a drug must be present in body fluids or tissues in a free or available form. For most medications, less than the total amount of administered drug is ultimately available to produce effects on target tissues. The term **bioavailability** describes what proportion of the administered drug is available to produce systemic effects. If a drug has low bioavailability, most of the administered dose of the drug is lost or destroyed, never reaching the blood in a form that can be effective. Drugs that are freely and rapidly absorbed have a high bioavailability. The many factors that can influence bioavailability are discussed in the following sections.

Drug Dissolution. About 80% of drugs used in clinical practice are administered orally, primarily because of the ease and convenience of administration by this route. The drug may be given in liquid form or in a solid form such as a tablet or capsule (Table 1-3). To make this solid form, the drug is usually mixed with other compounds that serve various functions. Starches and other compounds may be added as inert fillers, especially when the amount of drug required

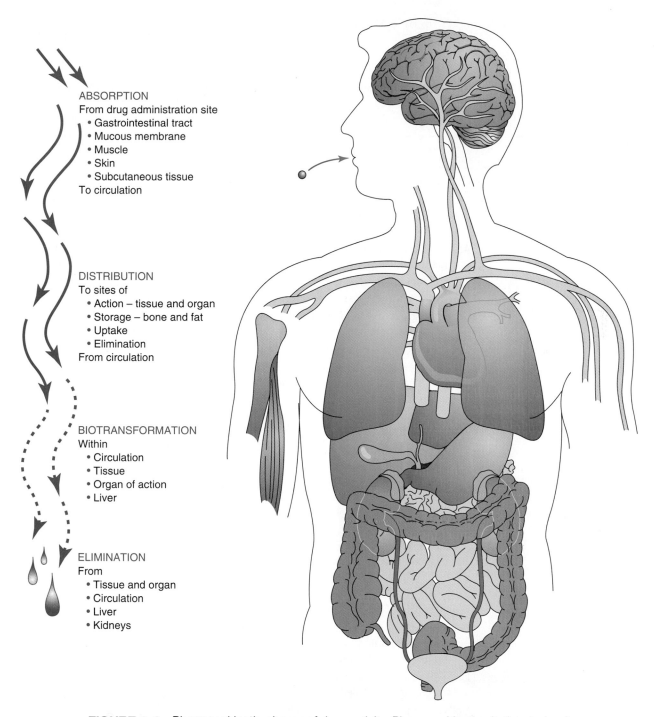

ABSORPTION
From drug administration site
• Gastrointestinal tract
• Mucous membrane
• Muscle
• Skin
• Subcutaneous tissue
To circulation

DISTRIBUTION
To sites of
• Action – tissue and organ
• Storage – bone and fat
• Uptake
• Elimination
From circulation

BIOTRANSFORMATION
Within
• Circulation
• Tissue
• Organ of action
• Liver

ELIMINATION
From
• Tissue and organ
• Circulation
• Liver
• Kidneys

FIGURE 1-4 Pharmacokinetic phases of drug activity. Pharmacokinetics is the study of how drugs enter the body (absorption), reach their site of action (distribution), and are removed from the body (biotransformation and excretion).

per dose is too small to be conveniently handled. Adhesive substances called *binders* may also be added to allow a tablet to hold together after it is compressed in manufacture. Other compounds called *disintegrators* may be required to allow a tablet to absorb water and to break apart in the body. Lubricants are often added to prevent tablets from sticking to machinery during manufacture. These additions may make up most of the tablet. For example, in tablets containing 100,000 units of penicillin, the active ingredient, potassium penicillin, makes up only 11% of the tablet mass.

To be effective, the solid dose of a drug must break apart in the gastrointestinal (GI) tract and allow the drug to go into solution. Only a dissolved drug can be absorbed from the GI tract into the blood. Because breakdown of the solid dosage form is required for absorption of a drug, any variability in this process can affect how rapidly and completely the drug is absorbed. The formulation of a tablet or capsule affects dissolu-

---

TABLE 1-3

Forms of Medication

Form	Description
Capsules	Solid dosage forms for oral use. Medication is enclosed in gelatin shell that dissolves in stomach or intestine. Gelatin shell is colored to aid in product identification. Manufacturers use distinctive shapes for identifying their capsules.
Douches	Aqueous solutions used as cleansing or antiseptic agent for part of body or body cavity. Usually sold as powder or liquid concentration to be dissolved or diluted before use.
Elixirs	Clear fluids for oral use. Contain water and alcohol with glycerin and sorbitol or another sweetener sometimes added. Alcohol content varies.
Enteric-coated drugs	Solid dosage forms for oral use. Drug in tablet form is coated with materials designed to pass through stomach and dissolve in intestine, where drug may be absorbed.
Glycerites	Solutions of drugs in glycerin for external use. Solution must be at least 50% glycerin.
Patches	Inner surface of the patch contacts skin and allows transdermal absorption of lipid-soluble drugs. The total amount of drug on the patch is very large, but typically only a small fraction is absorbed.
Pills	Solid dosage forms for oral use. Drug and various vehicles are formed into small globules or ovoids. True pills are rare; most have been replaced by compressed tablets.
Press-coated or layered drugs	Preformed tablets that have another layer of material pressed on or around it; thus incompatible ingredients may be separated and are dissolved at slightly different rates.
Solutions	Liquid preparations, usually in water, containing one or more dissolved compounds. Solutions for oral use may contain flavoring and coloring agents. Injectable solutions must be sterile; solutions for intravenous injection must also be particle free.
Suppositories	Solid dosage forms to be inserted into body cavity where medication is released as solid melts or dissolves. Often contain cocoa butter (theobroma oil), which is solid at room temperature but liquid at body temperature, or glycerin, gelatin, or polyethylene glycol, which dissolve in secretions from mucous membranes.
Suspensions	Finely divided drug particles that are suspended in suitable liquid mediums before being injected or taken orally. Must not be injected intravenously.
Sustained-action drugs	Form of drug altered so that dissolution is slow and continuous for extended time. Total dosage in sustained-action medication is greater than for regular formulations because drug is not all released at once.
Syrups	Drug dissolved in concentrated solutions of sugar such as sucrose. Flavors may be added to mask unpleasant taste.
Tablets	Solid dosage forms shaped like disks or cylinders that contain, in addition to drug, one or more of following ingredients: binder (adhesive that allows tablet to stick together), disintegrators (substances promoting tablet dissolution in body fluids), lubricants (required for efficient manufacturing), and fillers (inert ingredients to make tablet size convenient.
Tinctures	Alcoholic or water-alcohol solutions of drugs.
Transdermal creams	Relatively lipid-soluble drugs that may be absorbed transdermally. Dosage is usually measured in inches of cream extruded from tube.
Troches (also called *lozenges* or *pastilles*)	Solid dosage forms shaped like disks or cylinders that contain drug, flavor, sugar, and mucilage. Troches dissolve or disintegrate in mouth, releasing drug such as antiseptic or anesthetic for action in mouth or throat. Dissolve more slowly than tablets.

tion rates. Tablets from different manufacturers that contain the same amounts of active ingredients but different types and amounts of inert ingredients may not be identical in clinical action, because each formulation may dissolve differently. Tablets may also change with age and conditions of storage. Older tablets tend to dry out and are harder to disintegrate, which leads to reduced bioavailability of the drug.

Gastrointestinal Tract. The presence of food also influences the dissolution and absorption of drugs. For example, the antibiotic tetracycline should be given on an empty stomach because food blocks absorption of the drug. In contrast, the antifungal drug griseofulvin is best absorbed when taken with fatty foods (Table 1-4).

Stomach acidity also influences absorption. For example, penicillins are not stable in acid, and part of the dose is destroyed rather than absorbed. There is considerable variation from person to person in gastric emptying times and therefore in the length of time a drug spends in stomach acid. In addition, the amount of acid in the stomach varies with the individual and the time of day. Older adults and the very young have less stomach acid than middle-aged persons (see Chapters 3 and 4). Lower acidity may mean less drug is degraded and more is available to be absorbed.

Chemical Properties of the Drug. In addition to the physical state of the drug, its chemical nature determines

how suitable it is for oral administration. To pass through membranes lining the GI tract, a drug must be relatively lipid (fat) soluble, because the membranes themselves contain a high concentration of lipid. Ionic (charged) forms of drugs do not pass easily through these membranes. Many drugs can exist either in an ionic state or in an uncharged lipid-soluble state depending on the pH of the environment. This environment changes throughout the GI tract (Figure 1-5). Stomach fluid is highly acidic. A drug such as aspirin, a weak acid, is converted from a charged to an uncharged form by the strong acid in the stomach. Because the uncharged form of the drug can readily diffuse through the lipid membranes of the stomach cells, the drug is rapidly absorbed.

Enteric coatings on tablets or capsules protect some drugs that are sensitive to stomach acid (see Table 1-3). These coatings are inert at low (acidic) pH but soluble at higher (alkaline) pH. Therefore the drug passes through the stomach and is released in the intestine. Enteric coatings are also used for drugs that are highly irritating to the gastric mucosa.

Fluids in the small intestine are slightly alkaline. This higher pH favors absorption of weakly basic drugs, because at this pH range weak bases are uncharged (see Figure 1-5). The small intestine also has an enormous surface area, which makes it a major site of drug absorption. However, some drugs, particularly proteins such as insulin or growth hormone, are destroyed in the small intestine by the action of digestive enzymes from the pancreas.

First-Pass Effect. Drugs that are absorbed from the small intestine are transported by portal circulation directly to the liver before being circulated to the rest of the body (see Figure 1-5). The liver may biotransform much of the drug before it can enter general circulation. The term **first-pass effect** refers to this process. Liver biotransformation often inactivates drugs, thus reducing the amount of active drug released into systemic circulation. For example, morphine is rapidly extracted from the blood and biotransformed by the liver; therefore, to achieve the same level of pain relief, it is necessary to administer six times more morphine orally than intramuscularly. In contrast, the related drug codeine is much less susceptible to the first-pass effect; therefore it takes only twice as much codeine orally than intramuscularly to produce the same degree of pain relief. In these examples, the larger oral doses compensate for the drug lost through inactivation by the liver.

The first-pass effect may be avoided by using other routes of administration, such as sublingual (dissolved under the tongue), buccal (dissolved between the cheek

TABLE 1-4

Oral Administration of Selected Drugs

Normally Taken on Empty Stomach with Full Glass of Water	
acetaminophen	propantheline
aspirin	quinidine
cephalosporins	rifampin
erythromycin*	sulfonamides
isoniazid	tetracyclines*
penicillins	theophylline*

Normally Taken with Food to Improve Absorption	
carbamazepine	lithium
cimetidine	nitrofurantoin*
griseofulvin†	propranolol
hydralazine	spironolactone
indomethacin*	

*Gastric irritation may require that the drug be taken with food, but absorption is delayed or diminished.
†For best absorption this drug is taken with foods rich in fat.

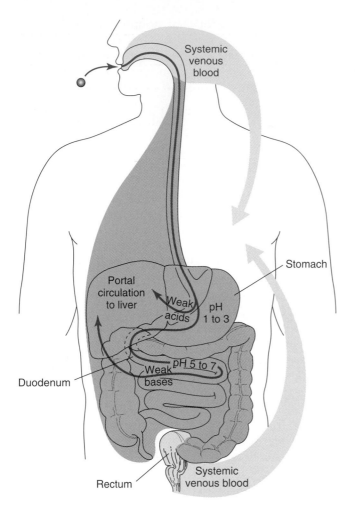

FIGURE 1-5 Absorption of drugs. Absorption through membranes lining the mouth or rectum delivers a drug directly to systemic circulation; drugs that are well absorbed at these sites are very lipid soluble. Drugs absorbed from the stomach, small intestine, or colon enter portal circulation carrying blood directly to the liver, thus exposing the drugs first to the action of liver microsomal enzymes before distribution to the rest of the body. The pH gradient through the GI tract influences drug absorption. Strong acid in the stomach (pH 1 to 3) maintains weak acids in more easily absorbed uncharged forms. Weak bases become charged in the stomach but lose charge as pH approaches neutrality (pH 7) or becomes slightly alkaline (pH 7 to 8) in the small bowel.

and gum), and rectal routes (see Figure 1-5). Drugs taken by these routes are absorbed directly across mucous membranes and rapidly enter the systemic circulation. The sublingual and buccal routes are useful when a palatable, highly lipid-soluble drug is involved. The rectal route is especially useful for administering med-

ication to an unconscious patient. The best physical form for rectal use is a suppository that will melt at body temperature and release the drug for absorption (see Table 1-3).

Factors Controlling Drug Absorption by Parenteral Routes. Parenteral drug administration requires injection into the skin, muscle, or blood (see Chapter 5). Injection necessarily involves breaking the skin; thus sterile techniques must be used to prevent pathogens from gaining entry (Table 1-5). Special precautions often must be taken to avoid producing undue tissue damage from irritating drugs. These precautions may involve preventing the drug from contacting the skin; some drugs require dilution before administration.

Subcutaneous Injection. Subcutaneous (under the skin) injection is appropriate for small drug volumes and for drugs intended to be slowly absorbed (e.g., insulin). When very slow absorption is desired, drugs may be formulated as solid inserts that release the drug over prolonged periods. An example is the insert that releases hormones and provides birth control for months (Chapter 59).

Intramuscular Injection. Intramuscular (into a muscle) injection is appropriate when large volumes of drugs must be injected. Absorption from intramuscular sites is faster than from subcutaneous sites because muscles have a better blood supply than skin. Absorption from subcutaneous or intramuscular sites can be hastened by applying heat or massage to the site to accelerate blood flow. Absorption can be slowed by decreasing blood flow to the injection site by applying ice packs or by simultaneously injecting a drug such as epinephrine, which constricts blood vessels.

The forms of drugs intended for intramuscular or subcutaneous injection may be relatively insoluble. Some drugs are formulated specifically to dissolve slowly and therefore to be absorbed slowly from injection sites. These dosage forms are called *depot injections.*

Intravenous Injection. Intravenous (directly into a vein) injection requires special precautions. Drugs for intravenous use must always be in solution and can contain no particulate matter. Some drugs irritate the veins and cause thrombophlebitis if administered at too high a concentration. Other drugs must be injected slowly to prevent toxic concentrations from reaching the heart or other vital organs. The intravenous route is valuable when drug concentrations must be maintained continuously, but potential harm to the patient is significant by this invasive route.

TABLE 1-5		
Summary of Major Routes for Administration of Drugs		
Description	*Advantages*	*Disadvantages*
Aerosol Fine particles or droplets are inhaled.	Direct delivery to lung. Action is usually restricted to lung.	Irritation of lung mucosa may occur. Special equipment is required. Patient must be conscious.
Buccal Drug is dissolved between cheek and gum and absorbed across oral mucous membrane.	Convenient. Sterility is not needed. Direct delivery to general circulation.	Not useful for drugs with unpleasant taste. Irritation to oral mucosa may occur. Patient must be conscious. Useful only for highly lipid-soluble drugs.
Inhalation Drug is inhaled as a gas.	Continuous dosing. Patient may be unconscious.	Useful only for drugs that are gases at room temperature. Irritation of mucosa may occur.
Intramuscular Drug is injected into muscle mass.	Rapid absorption. Soluble or insoluble drug forms. Patient may be conscious or unconscious.	Sterile procedures are necessary. Minor pain is common. Irritation and local reactions may occur.
Intravenous Drug is injected directly into vein.	Direct control of drug concentration in blood. Rapid attainment of effective blood levels.	Sterile procedures are necessary. Risk of transient high drug concentrations is possible if injected too rapidly.
Oral Drug is swallowed and absorbed from stomach or small intestine.	Convenient. Sterility not needed. Economical.	Unpleasant taste may cause noncompliance. Irritation to gastric mucosa may induce nausea. Patient must be conscious. Digestive juices may destroy drug. Absorbed drug enters portal circulation to liver, where it may be metabolized.
Subcutaneous Drug is injected under skin.	Patient may be conscious or unconscious.	Sterile procedures are necessary. Pain and irritation at site may occur.
Sublingual Drug is dissolved under tongue and absorbed across oral mucous membrane.	Convenient. Sterility not needed. Direct delivery to general circulation.	Not useful for drugs with unpleasant taste. Irritation to oral mucosa may occur. Patient must be conscious. Useful only for highly lipid-soluble drugs.
Transdermal Drug is absorbed directly through skin.	Continuous dosing. Sterility not needed. Direct delivery to general circulation.	Effective only for lipid-soluble drugs. Local irritation may occur. Discarded patches may pose danger of poisoning.

Special Injection Routes. A few drugs may be injected into very specific body sites. For example, local anesthetics may be injected into the spinal column to produce certain types of anesthesia, or steroids may be injected directly into joints. Such routes are used when conventional routes of injection do not allow high enough drug concentrations to be achieved at the desired site of action.

Factors Controlling Drug Persistence in Blood. After a drug has entered the blood, its fate is determined by the chemical properties of the drug and the way it is affected by blood and the tissues it contacts. Some drugs are biotransformed by enzymes in blood. An example is succinylcholine. Drugs that persist in blood are usually bound to blood proteins rather than being simply dissolved directly in plasma.

The most important carrier protein in blood is albumin, which is formed in the liver. Drugs bound to albumin or other carrier proteins remain in the blood because such proteins do not diffuse easily through capillary walls. Drug binding to albumin is a reversible process; thus an equilibrium can be established between drug that is bound to protein and drug that is free in solution. Only free drug is able to diffuse into tissues, interact with receptors, and produce biologic effects. The same proportion of bound and free drug is maintained in the blood at all times. Thus when free drug leaves the blood, some drug is released from protein binding to reestablish the proper ratio in blood between bound and free drug.

The anticoagulant warfarin is an example of a drug that binds to plasma protein. In blood, 99.5% of this drug is bound to plasma albumin. Therefore only 0.5% of the blood content of warfarin is free to diffuse to its site of action or to its sites of elimination. The net effect of binding to albumin is to create a reservoir of drug that is released to replenish free drug removed to other sites. In general, drugs that do not bind to plasma albumin remain in the body for shorter periods than drugs that are tightly bound. A drug such as warfarin, which is very strongly bound to albumin, remains in the body for several days. Thus drugs that bind to plasma proteins often have a long duration of action.

Factors Controlling Drug Distribution Throughout the Body. High lipid solubility and low protein binding favor diffusion of a drug through membranes. All transport into tissues involves passing through lipid-containing membranes, a process that is difficult for water-soluble compounds but easy for lipid-soluble drugs. High concentrations of free drug in blood also favor diffusion into tissues; high protein binding lowers free drug concentrations in blood and impedes diffusion into tissues.

Factors Controlling Drug Biotransformation in the Body. Biotransformation is the ability of living organisms to modify the chemical structure of compounds. Many types of chemical transformations are carried out, but these reactions generally create water-soluble compounds that are more easily excreted from the body by the kidneys. Biotransformation is sometimes divided into two phases: Phase I includes oxidation, hydrolysis, and reduction reactions, whereas Phase II reactions, also called *conjugations*, combine a drug or metabolite with other chemicals such as acetate, glucuronic acid, glutathione, or sulfate.

The liver is by far the most important site for biotransformation of drugs, but it is not the only one. For example, the kidneys are also capable of forming glucuronides and sulfates. Biotransformation may also be carried out by bacteria within the colon. This process may limit absorption of drugs from the bowel after oral administration, or they may diffuse from the blood into the bowel and be destroyed.

Biotransformation often inactivates drugs, but there are exceptions. For example, drugs such as codeine, diazepam, and amitriptyline are all converted by the liver into metabolites that are also active. A few drugs are not active until they are biotransformed by the liver. For example, the anticancer drug cyclophosphamide is inactive, but one of its metabolites produced in the liver is a highly reactive alkylating agent that is effective against cancer cells.

Phase I oxidation reactions are carried out by microsomal enzymes called cytochromes P-450. Three types of cytochromes P-450 carry out most of the oxidative reactions that inactivate drugs: CYP1, CYP2, and CYP3. Within each family there are subgroups designated by capital letters and individual enzymes identified by number; for example, CYP3A is the subgroup that performs more than half of the known drug oxidation reactions and CYP3A4 is an individual member of this subgroup. Examples of common drugs biotransformed by these enzymes are shown in Table 1-6.

These drug-biotransforming enzymes have two important features. First, they are rather nonspecific; therefore many drugs may be acted on by the same enzyme system. Second, the liver can synthesize more enzyme if it is chronically exposed to certain drugs. This property means that the liver can increase its capacity to destroy a drug over a few days. This increase in microsomal enzyme content in the liver is called *enzyme induction*.

Enzyme induction can give rise to drug interactions. As an example of this process, consider a patient who

---

TABLE 1-6

Cytochrome P-450 Subgroups

Enzyme Subgroup	Drugs Biotransformed
CYP1	acetaminophen caffeine theophylline
CYP2	codeine dextromethorphan naproxen
CYP3	acetaminophen cyclosporine estradiol theophylline

might receive both the anticonvulsant drug phenytoin and the antiasthmatic drug theophylline. Phenytoin induces CYP3A4, one of the liver enzymes that biotransforms theophylline. As a result, theophylline may be destroyed more quickly and its therapeutic action diminished. Other types of interactions can arise because a drug may inhibit specific enzymes, creating a deficiency in the body's ability to eliminate other drugs that require that enzyme for excretion. For example, the antifungal drug ketoconazole raises the blood levels of many other drugs because ketoconazole inhibits CYP3A4, the most common of the drug-biotransforming cytochromes P-450.

The activities of cytochromes P-450 can be influenced not only by drugs but also by environmental chemicals. For example, cigarette smoke is a potent inducer of CYP1A and chronic ethanol consumption induces CYP2E1.

Factors Controlling Drug Excretion. The three main routes by which drugs may be eliminated from the body involve the liver, kidneys, and bowel.

Excretion in Feces. This route involves uptake of drug by the liver, release into bile, and excretion in feces. For some drugs, such as erythromycin and penicillin, the concentration of drug in bile may be much higher than its concentration in blood. Because the liver forms 600 to 1000 mL of bile each day, this route of excretion may dispose of significant amounts of drug. However, drugs in bile enter the small intestine, where they may be reabsorbed into the blood, returned to the liver, and again secreted into bile. This secretion and reabsorption process is called **enterohepatic circulation**. Drugs that are extensively reabsorbed from the intestine after biliary secretion persist in the body much longer than drugs that remain inside the intestine and pass out with feces. If the reabsorbed drug is in an active form, the duration of action is prolonged.

Excretion in Urine after Biotransformation by the Liver. The second route of elimination involves both the liver and the kidneys. Common biotransformations of drugs by the liver and other organs tend to form polar compounds, which can be more efficiently excreted by the kidneys. For example, a drug such as morphine might enter glomerular fluid by passive diffusion but be reabsorbed from the tubules and reenter the blood. In the liver, however, morphine is transformed into at least two types of glucuronide. In this form the drug enters glomerular fluid, cannot be reabsorbed from the tubules, and hence is excreted in urine.

Various factors may influence the ability to biotransform drugs. For example, premature infants and neonates have immature livers that cannot perform certain biotransformations (see Chapter 3). Therefore these patients may accumulate drugs that must be biotransformed in the liver before they can be excreted renally. Patients who have experienced hepatic damage, such as those who have chronic alcoholism, may also accumulate drugs normally excreted by this route. In addition, hepatic damage may make a patient much more sensitive than normal to toxicity from specific drugs. For example, the antituberculosis drug isoniazid causes clinical hepatitis in about 0.3% of healthy young adults who receive it for prophylaxis. In contrast, the incidence of acute hepatitis is 2.6% in patients who drink alcohol daily or who have significant liver disease.

Excretion in Urine without Biotransformation by the Liver. Some drugs are not extensively biotransformed anywhere in the body and are excreted unchanged in urine. This excretion may take place in one of two ways: (1) by passive diffusion into glomerular fluid or (2) by active secretion in the renal tubule. These active processes lead to more rapid drug elimination and allow much higher urinary concentrations of drug to be achieved. The antibiotic penicillin G is a good example of a drug that is actively secreted by renal tubules. Half of an intravenous dose of penicillin G can be eliminated in about 20 minutes by active tubular secretion. In contrast, an antibiotic such as tetracycline, which is eliminated primarily by passive diffusion in the kidneys, persists in the body for several hours.

Drugs that are normally excreted unchanged in urine accumulate in the body when there is a loss of renal function. Renal function decreases with age, but it can also be diminished in younger people as a result of progressive hypertension, diabetes mellitus, or other causes. For many drugs excreted primarily through renal processes, dosages must be adjusted to compensate for reduced renal excretion. For example, cephalosporin antibiotics such as ceftazidime are excreted renally, and the blood level of the antibiotic is influenced by the degree of renal impairment. If reduced renal excretion is not taken into account, the drug may accumulate to a toxic level.

To adjust dosage to compensate for renal impairment, some measure of renal function must be made. A common measure of renal function is creatinine clearance, expressed in milliliters per minute (mL/min) or per second (mL/sec). Creatinine clearance is 100 to 120 mL/min when renal function is normal. Table 1-7 shows information from the package insert for the antibiotic ceftazidime. Note that if creatinine clearance is greater than 50 mL/min, no dosage adjustment is needed with this drug; the normal adult dose of 1 g every 8 hours can be given. If renal function is impaired, lower creatinine

TABLE 1-7	

Adjustment of Ceftazidime Dosage Based on Renal Function

Creatinine Clearance (mL/min)	Dosage
>50	Usual adult dose (1 g q8h)
31-50	1 g q12h
16-30	1 g q24h
6-15	500 mg q24h
<5	500 mg q48h
Hemodialysis patients:	1 g after each hemodialysis period

clearances are noted, and the dosage interval must be increased and/or the dose must be decreased. If renal function is lost and the patient is undergoing hemodialysis, the dose is given only once in the interval between hemodialyses. Without renal excretion, a high blood level of the drug persists for prolonged periods.

If direct measurement of creatinine clearance cannot be made, this value can be estimated from creatinine concentrations in the serum according to the following formula:

$$\text{Creatinine clearance (men)} = \frac{(140 - \text{Age}) \times (\text{Body weight in kg})}{(72 - \text{Serum creatinine})}$$

The creatinine clearance for women is 85% of the value calculated by this equation. This formula is not as accurate as a direct determination of clearance, but measuring serum creatinine is much easier than measuring clearances, and the accuracy of this calculation is adequate for most situations.

Genetic Factors Influencing Pharmacokinetics of Individuals

Gender. Men and women may respond differently to drugs. For example, metabolism of a drug such as propranolol occurs much more quickly in men than in women. As a result, when similar dosages are used, the level of drug in the blood is about twice as high in women. Similarly, the calcium channel blocker amlodipine lowers blood pressure more effectively in women. Whether such differences exist for most drugs is unknown, because specific trials to show differences based on gender have not been performed.

Men and women also respond differently to small amounts of ingested ethanol. In men a high level of the enzyme alcohol dehydrogenase exists in the stomach; this enzyme rapidly destroys significant amounts of the alcohol before it can be absorbed. In women the level of this enzyme is reduced, and as a result, more ethanol is absorbed, producing a higher blood level of the drug than the same dose produces in men.

Ethnicity and Drug-Biotransforming Enzymes. Various ethnic groups may respond differently to some drug classes. For example, blockers of the beta-adrenergic receptors are often used to control blood pressure, but African-American patients tend to respond less well to beta-blockers than do Caucasians. Chinese patients are much more sensitive to these drugs than either Caucasian or African-American patients. Asian populations in general also seem to respond to lower dosages of benzodiazepines and tricyclic antidepressants, two classes of drugs that are used extensively for mood disorders.

The causes of these differences are beginning to be understood. For example, Asian populations tend to have a lower activity of the drug-metabolizing enzyme CYP2D6, which acts on a variety of drugs, including the beta-blocker propranolol and the tricyclic amitriptyline (Table 1-8). Asian populations also have a higher proportion of persons with the slow variant form of CYP2C19, an enzyme also acting on benzodiazepines and tricyclics. Both of these changes lower drug-biotransforming capacity, an effect that tends to allow these drugs to accumulate unless dosages are reduced to accommodate the lowered metabolic capacity.

The rate of drug acetylation in liver is another genetically determined trait that may affect the incidence of certain drug reactions (see Table 1-8). About 50% of Americans, both African Americans and Caucasians, possess liver enzyme systems that acetylate drugs and other chemicals at rates less than half of those of the rest of the population. In contrast, slow acetylation occurs in about 20% of Chinese populations and is rare in Inuit and Japanese populations.

Isoniazid shows how the genetically determined ability to acetylate a drug can influence adverse reactions. This drug is inactivated primarily by acetylation and is excreted in urine entirely as metabolites. In slow acetylators its half-life is about 3 hours, but in rapid acetylators it is only about 1 hour. Liver damage may be more common in rapid acetylators because the concentration of a hepatotoxic acetylated metabolite is high. Slow acetylation may be more closely associated with dose-related toxicity (neuropathy, depression of liver biotransformation enzymes) because the untransformed drug may accumulate in persons with this trait. Therefore dosages may need to be lowered for slow acetylators.

Glucose-6-Phosphate Dehydrogenase Deficiency. Some drug reactions may be linked to a particular genetic trait that is more prevalent in certain ethnic groups. For example, the enzyme glucose-6-phosphate dehydrogenase (G6PD) is abundant in tissues of most people. In red blood cells this

TABLE 1-8

Drug Biotransforming Enzymes with Known Genetic Variants

Metabolic Reaction	Proportion of Variant in Populations of These Races		
	African/Black	*Asian*	*Caucasian*
Acetylation, slow variant	42%-65%	7%-22%	52%-62%
CYP2C19 oxidation, slow variant	Not established	12%-22%	3%-10%
CYP2D6			
Slow variant	1%-8%	1%	3%-10%
Intermediate activity		98%	
Normal activity	90%-98%		89%-96%
Super-fast variant	1%-2%	1%	1%

enzyme plays a role in forming reduced nicotinamide-adenine dinucleotide phosphate (NADPH), which is needed to maintain active hemoglobin. As a result of a genetic alteration, some people lack adequate concentrations of G6PD in their red blood cells. Therefore NADPH is generated slowly. Under normal circumstances this alteration would not be critical, but if a person with this trait is exposed to chemicals that enhance the conversion of hemoglobin to methemoglobin (a relatively inactive form of hemoglobin), serious problems can arise. A lower level of G6PD produces too little NADPH to fully reform active hemoglobin. When too much methemoglobin accumulates, red blood cells are destroyed.

G6PD deficiency is important in pharmacologic considerations because many drugs accelerate methemoglobin formation. Sulfonamides, antimalarial agents, and analgesic-antipyretic drugs (including aspirin) fall into this category. In a person lacking adequate G6PD activity, these drugs can cause life-threatening hemolysis (rupture of the red blood cells). The same drugs are relatively harmless in most people who possess adequate G6PD activity.

Certain populations have a high proportion of the gene that causes G6PD deficiency. For example, 13% of African-American men and 20% of African-American women may carry this gene. People of Sardinian, Iranian, Greek, or Sephardic Jewish ancestry have a high incidence of G6PD deficiencies. This genetic difference places patients from these groups at greater risk for serious reactions with certain drugs. When these patients receive medications, they should be observed carefully for signs of toxicity.

Pseudocholinesterase Deficiency. Not all differences in drug handling are related to observable traits such as gender or ethnicity. Unsuspected genetic differences can produce unexpected reactions to drugs. For example, a small percentage of the U.S. population lacks pseudo-cholinesterase, an enzyme usually found in blood. People lacking this enzyme show no signs of this difference until they are exposed to drugs such as succinylcholine, a paralyzing agent given before surgery to relax muscles and allow easy tracheal intubation. In most people the drug is very short-acting because it is destroyed by pseudocholinesterase. In people lacking this enzyme, succinylcholine stays in the blood, and the drug is very long-acting. These patients require artificial ventilation until the paralyzing effects of succinylcholine wear off, whereas most people recover within a minute and require no assistance.

Describing the Effects of Drugs in Patients

Dose-Response Curve. The relationship between the dose of drug and the response produced is described by an S-shaped (sigmoid) curve called the *dose-response curve* (Figure 1-6). This curve is created by plotting the observed response (on a linear scale) against the dose of the drug used to elicit that response (on a logarithmic scale).

The dose-response curve illustrates several important quantitative properties about drugs. First, there is a threshold for each drug-induced response. Doses of drug below that threshold will produce no observable effect. Second, the drug-induced response will reach a limit rather than increase indefinitely. For example, the drug shown in Figure 1-6 produces its maximum response at a dose of about 256 units. Doubling the dose produces no further therapeutic effect. Even at lower drug concentrations, doubling the dose still does not double the effect. In this example, the 50% maximum response is produced by a dose of 16 units, but twice that dose (32 units) produces only about 70%, not 100%, of the maximum response. In summary, the dose-response curve demonstrates that a finite dose is needed to cause a response and that doubling the dose does not double the response.

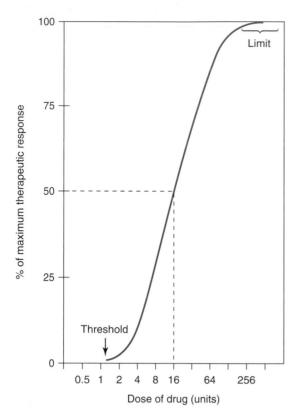

FIGURE 1-6   Log dose-response curve. Percent of maximum therapeutic response is plotted on a linear scale on the vertical axis. Dose of the given drug is plotted on a logarithmic scale on the horizontal axis. The *threshold* is the dose required to cause measurable response. The *limit* is the region of the curve where increasing the dose does not increase biologic response.

The dose-response curve in Figure 1-6 shows the magnitude of a drug's effect on an individual (or the average effect on several individuals). The same type of curve is produced when the drug response is instead defined as an all-or-none phenomenon (e.g., asleep versus awake) and the logarithm of the drug dose is plotted against the percentage of patients who show the drug effect at that given dose. This type of plot is called a *quantal dose-response curve.* The upper limit for this curve is the drug dose at which all patients respond, and the threshold is the drug dose below which no patients respond. The recommended therapeutic dose of the drug is one at which most patients respond. Figure 1-7 shows this second type of dose-response curve.

Drugs produce multiple predictable biologic effects, and for each of these effects, a dose-response curve may be drawn. For example, the drug digoxin increases the force of contraction of a failing heart (see Chapter 38), but it also causes nausea, headaches, visual disturbances, and arrhythmias, and ultimately it can trigger ventricular fibrillation. Each of these responses can be plotted as a dose-response curve (see Figure 1-7). The dose-response curve for nausea lies close to the dose-response curve for therapeutic effect; therefore, many patients receiving therapeutic doses of digoxin also experience nausea. With increasing doses, more patients experience visual disturbances and arrhythmias. At concentrations well above normal therapeutic doses, ventricular fibrillation occurs. These predictable drug reactions become an important part of patient care. For digoxin, the visual changes are a warning that the drug concentration in the patient is approaching a toxic level,

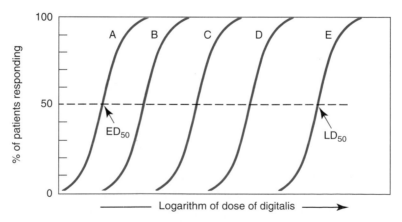

FIGURE 1-7   Log dose-response curves for effects of digoxin. Percent of patients responding to digoxin is plotted on the vertical axis, and the dose of digoxin is plotted on a logarithmic scale on the horizontal axis. These effects are all dose-related responses to digoxin. *Curve A*, strengthened force of heart contraction; *curve B*, nausea; *curve C*, visual disturbances; *curve D*, cardiac arrhythmias; *curve E*, ventricular fibrillation and death.

which can allow time for dosage adjustment before arrhythmias and ventricular fibrillation occur.

Each drug may be described as relatively safe or relatively dangerous, based on dose-response curves such as those in Figure 1-7. Doses of digoxin that produce serious reactions are only slightly higher than those that increase the force of contraction of the heart. Therefore digoxin is a drug with a narrow margin of safety; doses must be rigorously controlled, and great care must be taken to keep the blood level of the drug within a very narrow range. In contrast, a drug with a wide margin of safety, such as penicillin G, may be given in doses greatly exceeding normal therapeutic doses without much danger of producing direct toxic effects.

Therapeutic Index. The relative safety of drugs is also sometimes expressed as a therapeutic index. The **therapeutic index (TI)** is the ratio of the dose of the drug lethal in 50% of a tested population (LD_{50}) to the dose of the drug therapeutically effective in 50% of the tested population (ED_{50}), or $TI = LD_{50}/ED_{50}$. These figures come from tests conducted on animals. A drug with a high therapeutic index has a wide safety margin; the lethal dose greatly exceeds the therapeutic dose. A drug with a low therapeutic index is more dangerous for patients because small increases over normal doses may be sufficient to induce toxic reactions.

Time Course of Drug Action. Drugs may enter the body by several routes, and all except the intravenous route take time for the drug to enter the blood after administration. There is also a delay between the time the drug enters the blood and the time it reaches its site of action. If the response to a single dose of a drug is measured over time, the pattern shown in Figure 1-8 is seen. The time for the **onset** of drug action is the time it takes after the drug is administered to reach a concentration that produces a response. As the drug continues to be absorbed, higher concentrations reach the site of action and the response increases. The drug is also subject to influences that tend to eliminate it from the body. Ultimately, elimination dominates and the concentration of drug in the body begins to fall. As a result, the response will also begin to diminish. **Peak effect** is the

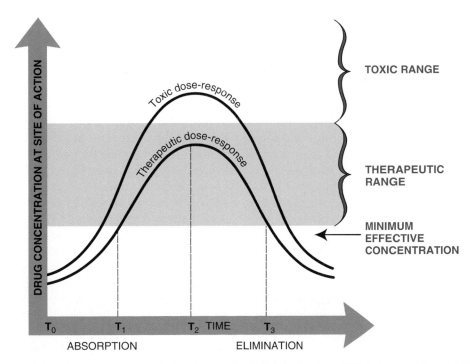

FIGURE 1-8 Time course of action of a single dose of a drug. The drug is given at T_0. The time interval between T_0 and T_1 is the time to onset of drug action. Peak action occurs at T_2. The time interval between T_0 and T_2 represents the time to peak effect. At T_3, drug response falls below minimum needed for clinical effectiveness. The time interval between T_1 and T_3 represents the duration of drug action. If the drug dose is increased so that drug concentration at the site of action exceeds the therapeutic range, the duration of effect is increased, but toxic as well as therapeutic effects are produced.

time it takes for the drug to reach its highest effective concentration. The duration of action of a drug is the time during which the drug is present in a concentration large enough to produce a response. Onset and duration are determined by the rates of absorption and elimination.

Insulins are good examples of drugs for which an understanding of onset and duration of action is critical for successful drug therapy. Insulin lowers the blood sugar level, and the peak drug action must be planned to coincide with the absorptive period after meals when blood sugar levels rise rapidly. If insulin is injected at the proper dose but at the wrong time, a serious hypoglycemic (low blood sugar) reaction may endanger the patient (see Chapter 58).

Half-Life. The **half-life** of a drug is how long it takes for excretion processes to reduce the blood concentration of the drug by half. For example, the peak concentration of penicillin G in the blood occurs a few moments after it is administered intravenously. Thereafter, it is rapidly excreted by the kidneys and disappears from the blood. The length of time required for these processes to decrease the blood concentration of penicillin by 50% is the drug half-life, which for penicillin G is about 20 minutes. After 40 minutes, only one quarter of the initial concentration remains, and after 60 minutes, only one eighth remains. During each succeeding 20-minute period, the remaining concentration decreases by half.

When drug absorption is not instantaneous, excretion competes with absorption, delaying the appearance of peak blood concentration. The drug shown in Figure 1-9 has a half-life of 1 hour. When it is given intravenously, the highest concentration is achieved on administration and decreases thereafter because of excretion processes. When the same dose is given orally, the drug is absorbed relatively slowly, such that drug elimination lowers the achievable peak concentration. Once in the general circulation, however, the drug is excreted in the same way, regardless of the initial route of administration.

Plateau Principle. When a drug is given repeatedly for therapy at fixed dosage intervals, its concentration in blood reaches a plateau and is maintained at that level until the dose or frequency of administration is changed. The blood concentration of the drug fluctuates around a mean value, which approaches a plateau after four half-lives have passed; this leveling off happens regardless of the dose or frequency of administration, as long as these factors are constant. The actual dose of drug and frequency of administration determine the plateau concentration of drug in the blood, but they do not determine how long it will take to reach that plateau.

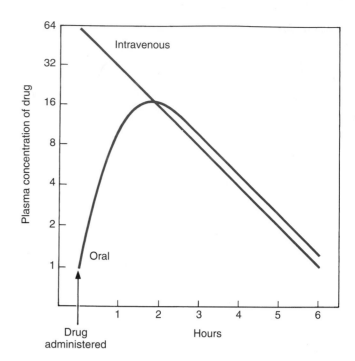

FIGURE 1-9 Absorption and excretion rates for a drug administered by oral or intravenous route. Plasma drug concentration is plotted on a logarithmic scale on the vertical axis.

An example of the plateau principle can be seen in a patient who is given a drug with a half-life of 24 hours (Figure 1-10). The patient takes one tablet at 8 AM every day. In 4 days the amount of drug being taken in each dose roughly equals the amount of drug excreted each day; the plateau has been reached. The dose in this case is sufficient to produce a clinically effective blood level but is below the level that produces toxicity. On day 6 the patient decides to take two tablets instead of one tablet each morning. As a result, the mean concentration of the drug in the blood rises, and after four half-lives (4 days for this drug) a new plateau concentration is reached. At this new higher level some drug toxicity is seen. When the patient returns to the old dosage schedule of one tablet daily, the mean drug concentration returns to the original plateau concentration after four half-lives and is maintained until the dosage amount or intervals change.

This example shows the importance of keeping regular dosage schedules and adhering to prescribed doses and dosage intervals. Timing and magnitude of the dose affect the peak and minimum (trough) blood concentrations of the drug. For many drugs these variations may not be critical, but for some the difference between safe and toxic doses is not great.

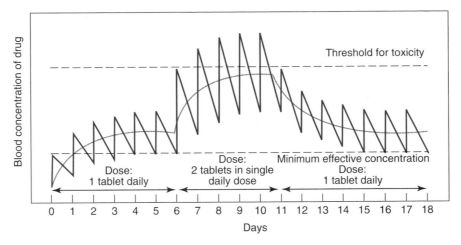

FIGURE 1-10   Plateau principle. A drug is given once each half-life (24 hours in this example). Plasma concentration of the drug rises and falls as doses are rapidly absorbed and slowly eliminated. The drug accumulates, but after four half-lives the average plasma concentration of the drug reaches a plateau. At day 6, the dose is doubled, which causes drug concentration to rise to a new plateau. At this higher dose the drug concentration crosses into the toxic range, and the dose is reduced to one tablet daily. Note that after any change in dose it takes four half-lives to achieve a new plateau.

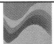

CASE STUDY   *Pharmacokinetics*

James, who is taking 2.68 mg of clemastine every 12 hours for allergies, begins to complain of dry mouth, drowsiness, and unsteadiness after taking the drug for 4 days. His dosage is then changed to one 2.68 mg tablet every 24 hours. After 1 week on the new regimen, James reports that the dry mouth and the other symptoms are less bothersome. However, he is concerned that 2 to 3 hours before it is time to take his next dose, he develops itchy eyes and congestion. In response, his dosing schedule is changed to one 1.34 mg tablet every 12 hours. On follow-up 3 weeks later, James reports good control of allergic symptoms and no recurrence of the original adverse effects.

1. How long would it take for a plateau concentration of clemastine to be achieved if the half-life of clemastine is 12 hours?
2. Why was James switched from the standard dose of 2.68 mg every 12 hours to 2.68 mg every 24 hours?
3. What happened to the plateau concentration of this drug after the first dose change?
4. Why was James switched from 2.68 mg once daily to 1.34 mg twice daily?
5. What happened to the plateau concentration after the second dose change? What happened to the fluctuation in blood levels after the second dose change?

Monitoring levels of certain drugs in blood is a routine part of patient care in many settings. Direct assays for drugs allow health care providers to adjust doses to ensure safe and effective blood levels of such drugs as gentamicin, amikacin, digoxin, and phenytoin, which have a low therapeutic index. The nurse's responsibility in dealing with patients being monitored in this way may include drawing blood samples, such as at the peak or trough concentrations (at specific times).

Bibliography

Rioux PP: Clinical trials in pharmacogenetics and pharmacogenomics: methods and applications, *Am J Health-Syst Pharm* 57(9):887-901, 2000.

Perinatal Pharmacotherapeutics

KATHLEEN GUTIERREZ

 Visit **http://evolve.elsevier.com/Gutierrez/** for additional information.

KEY TERMS

Lactation, p. 27
Organogenesis, p. 26
Perinatal, p. 29
Teratogen, p. 26
Teratogenicity, p. 26

OBJECTIVES

- Identify the changes of pregnancy that influence pharmacokinetics and pharmacodynamics.
- Explain teratogenicity.
- Explain the FDA drug categories.
- Discuss reasons for avoiding or minimizing drug therapy during pregnancy and lactation.
- Identify the goals of drug therapy for the perinatal patient.

Pregnancy causes striking changes in physiology. The changes are related to hormonal influences, growth of the fetus inside the uterus, and the mother's physical adaptation to the changes that are occurring (Figure 2-1; Table 2-1). To understand how pregnancy influences drug therapy, it is important to understand the changes that occur in the mother and fetus during pregnancy. Pharmacokinetic changes may require adjustment of some drug dosages. The hormones of pregnancy alter the pharmacodynamics and effectiveness of some drugs.

The drugs mentioned here are discussed in greater detail in later chapters.

MATERNAL PHARMACOKINETIC CONSIDERATIONS
Absorption

The absorption of orally administered drugs is influenced by gastric acidity, the presence of bile acids, mucus, and intestinal transit time. Slow gastric emptying and prolonged intestinal transit time induced by preg-

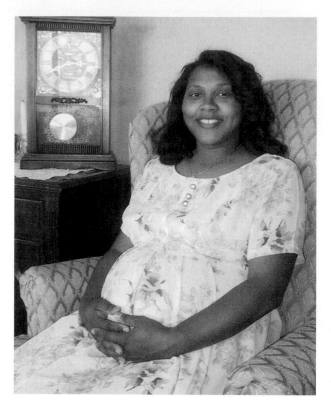

FIGURE 2-1

nancy delay the appearance of orally administered drugs in the plasma but also may enhance the absorption of lipid-soluble drugs. In addition, pH changes associated with heartburn and morning sickness, or the treatment of these symptoms with antacids, affects absorption of some orally administered drugs. Reduced gastric acidity slows the absorption of weakly acidic drugs (e.g., aspirin) but speeds the absorption of weakly basic drugs (e.g., opioids). Absorption of a drug given intramuscularly is increased because pregnancy increases tissue perfusion by inducing vasodilation.

Distribution

Weight gain in pregnancy results from increases in body fat, total body water, and the products of conception. These changes influence the distribution of fat-soluble drugs. For example, a higher percentage of body fat acts as a reservoir for fat-soluble drugs. Thus, drugs that are highly lipid soluble tend to concentrate in tissues and show a volume of distribution much higher than the blood volume. Generally, the impact of an increased volume of distribution reduces peak plasma drug concentrations, which decreases the amount of drug available to move to the site of action or to move to sites for elimination. The half-life of the drug would tend to be prolonged by these mechanisms.

TABLE 2-1

Changes of Pregnancy that Influence Pharmacokinetics

Physiologic Change	Pharmacokinetic Change
Total body water increases by 7-9 L (40%-50%) at 6 weeks gestation Aldosterone levels significantly increase by about 15 weeks gestation	Once in the circulation, a drug (particularly if it is water soluble) is distributed and "diluted" more than in the nonpregnant state. However, this change may be offset by other pharmacokinetic changes of pregnancy. Drug dosage requirements may increase in some instances.
Increased percentage of body fat and weight	Drugs (particularly fat-soluble ones) are more widely distributed and tend to linger in the body because they are slowly released from the fat storage sites into the circulation.
Dilutional decrease in serum albumin levels	Decreased capacity for drug binding results in greater unbound drug available to produce therapeutic or adverse effects on the mother and fetus. A given dose of a drug is likely to produce greater effects than it would in a nonpregnant state.
Increased levels of progesterone stimulates hepatic enzyme system	The hepatic enzyme system remains sensitive to inhibition as well as stimulation by certain drugs, just as in the nonpregnant state. Progesterone may be responsible for greater enzyme activity, leading to a measurable increase in liver clearance and the shortened half-life of a drug.
Cardiac output increases by 40% at 10 weeks gestation Renal blood flow and glomerular filtration rate increases in early pregnancy and decreases in late pregnancy because of the increased size and weight of the uterus	Renal excretion of drugs is increased early in pregnancy, particularly those excreted primarily unchanged in the urine. In late pregnancy, there may be decreased drug excretion and prolonged effects.

Drugs with low lipid solubility (i.e., water-soluble drugs) tend to be highly bound to plasma proteins. In pregnancy, the level of plasma albumin, to which most acidic drugs are bound, falls. Basic drugs (e.g., propranolol) tend to bind to alpha-1-acid glycoproteins. Endogenous ligands, such as free fatty acids, compete with drugs for binding sites on both albumin and alpha-1-acid glycoproteins. Both of these changes increase the concentration of free drug in plasma and favor increased distribution as well as elimination of the drug. These changes are greatest for drugs with relatively low lipid solubility and high protein binding (e.g., benzodiazepines, anticonvulsants).

Pregnancy causes many changes in addition to those noted above, and it is not necessarily easy to predict the overall outcome for a particular drug or patient. Therapeutic outcomes should be monitored closely during pregnancy. With certain drugs it may be necessary to monitor plasma concentrations to ensure that therapeutic blood levels are achieved and maintained.

Biotransformation

Drug biotransformation is heightened during pregnancy because elevated progesterone concentrations increase the level of drug-biotransforming enzymes in the liver. As a result, liver clearance of drugs is increased, excretion is accelerated, and the half-life is shortened. The hepatic microsomal enzyme system remains sensitive to inhibition as well as stimulation by certain drugs, just as in the nonpregnant state.

Drugs expected to have a shorter half-life in pregnancy (e.g., antibiotics, barbiturates) may have increased concentrations during labor, when the clearance of drugs is thought to decrease. Biotransformation during pregnancy also occurs in both the placenta and the fetal liver, although the contribution of the fetal-placental unit is thought to be very small.

Excretion

In the nonpregnant state, the kidneys receive 1000 to 1200 mL of blood per minute. Soon after conception, the glomerular filtration rate (GFR) rises. The GFR may peak at 150% of normal within 9 to 16 weeks. The rise in GFR increases excretion of amino acids, glucose, proteins, urea, uric acid, potassium, calcium, water-soluble vitamins, creatinine, and certain drugs. Dosage and frequency of administration of drugs may need to be altered. Pregnant women should also be evaluated for signs of toxicity as well as for evidence of subtherapeutic drug levels.

Drugs that are excreted unchanged (e.g., gentamicin, digoxin) are cleared in proportion to the creatinine clearance. Because blood flow through the liver is not appreciably changed in pregnancy, drugs that depend solely on hepatic blood flow for clearance are removed from the body at the same rate as in the nonpregnant state.

FETAL-PLACENTAL PHARMACOKINETIC CONSIDERATIONS

Absorption

The placenta allows transfer of substances between mother and fetus. It has a high basal metabolic rate, with energy needs supplied mostly by oxygen and glucose. The placenta transports oxygen and nutrients to the fetus and clears urea, carbon dioxide, and wastes produced by the fetus.

Gases and some drug molecules cross the placenta by simple diffusion. Transport depends on the concentration difference between the maternal side and the fetal side, the size of the molecule, and the surface area available for transfer. The highest rate of diffusion across placental membranes occurs with substances and drugs of low molecular weight, minimal ionic charge, and high lipid solubility.

Facilitated diffusion is accomplished by a carrier system. This transfer occurs more rapidly than simple diffusion, but in the same direction—that is, from high to low concentrations. Facilitated diffusion transports glucose, the major source of energy for the fetus.

Active transport requires energy, because movement of material may be from low to high concentrations, the opposite of what would occur by diffusion. Essential amino acids and water-soluble vitamins are transferred by active transport. These substances are maintained at higher concentrations in the fetus than in the placenta by this energy-requiring process.

Pinocytosis involves the ingestion of fluids and solute drug molecules through the formation of small sacs enclosed by pieces of pinched-off cell membrane. The particles are carried virtually intact from the outside to the inside of the cell, where they are released. Complex proteins, immune bodies, lipid, and viruses travel through the placenta in this way.

Distribution

The effect of drugs on the fetus depends on whether the drug is distributed throughout the body or selectively distributed (Figure 2-2).

The placenta is not an impermeable barrier. It actively transports molecules needed by the fetus and carries away wastes. The placenta does provide an effective immunologic barrier between mother and fetus. The physiochemical considerations that influence placental transfer of drugs are noted in Table 2-2 and described in more detail in the sections following.

Molecular Weight. The placenta permits transfer of drugs with molecular weights less than 600. The vast majority of drugs have molecular weights between 100 and 500. Some larger molecules with weights of up to 1000 may penetrate fetal tissues if the drugs are unbound and lipid soluble.

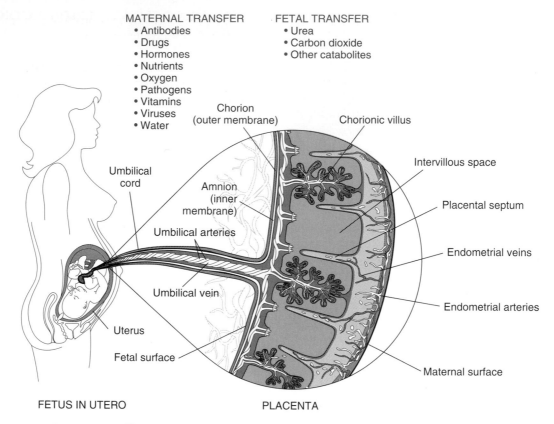

MATERNAL TRANSFER
• Antibodies
• Drugs
• Hormones
• Nutrients
• Oxygen
• Pathogens
• Vitamins
• Viruses
• Water

FETAL TRANSFER
• Urea
• Carbon dioxide
• Other catabolites

FETUS IN UTERO   PLACENTA

FIGURE 2-2   The maternal-fetal unit permits many substances to be transported from mother to fetus and back through the placenta. Maternal blood circulates through uterine arteries to intervillous spaces of the placenta and is returned to the maternal circulation through the uterine veins. Fetal blood flows through two umbilical arteries into the placenta and returns through the umbilical vein.

TABLE 2-2

Factors Affecting Placental Transfer of Drugs

Enhances Drug Transfer	*Inhibits Drug Transfer*
Lipid solubility	Increased diffusion distance
Non-ionized substances	High molecular charge
Molecular weight less than 600	High molecular weight
Lack of significant binding to albumin	Drug bound to maternal RBCs and/or proteins
Higher maternal-to-placental gradient*	Drug altered or bound by placental enzymes
Increased placental blood flow	Decreased placental blood flow
Increased fetal acidity, which retains basic drugs	Drugs highly biotransformed by the mother
Large placental surface area	

*The difference in concentration from maternal blood to fetal blood.

Acid-Base Balance. Drugs that are weak acids or weak bases produce an equilibrium between charged and uncharged forms of the drug, depending on the pH of the fluid in which they are dissolved. At a low pH, there is a high concentration of hydrogen ions. In this situation, the nitrogen ion of many weak bases will accept a proton and become charged. Conversely, at a high pH, there is a low concentration of hydrogen ions. In this case, the nitrogen molecule donates its proton to the solvent and becomes an uncharged molecule. The un-

TABLE 2-3	

Drugs with Affinity for Fetal Tissues

Drug	*Fetal Tissue*
tetracycline, warfarin	Teeth
Aminoglycosides	Middle ear
quinine, chlorpromazine	Retina
diethylstilbestrol	Mullerian duct
Corticosteroids, phenytoin	Adrenal gland
Iodides, propylthiouracil	Thyroid gland

charged forms cross the placenta more readily than ionized forms, and differences in pH can influence the distribution. For example, if a fetus becomes acidotic from prolonged cord compression, a weak base (e.g., amphetamine) diffusing into the fetal compartment with the lower pH becomes charged. The charged drug does not passively diffuse back into maternal circulation. The result is an accumulation of drug in the acidotic fetus.

Lipid Solubility. Lipid-soluble drugs passively diffuse across the placenta. Small molecules cross at rates dependent on their molecular weight, charge characteristics, and concentration in the maternal blood.

Tissue Binding. Lipid-soluble drugs are stored in adipose tissue, which increases during pregnancy. This condition leads to a slight decrease in the amount of unbound lipid-soluble drugs such as sedatives and hypnotics. When such a drug is discontinued, the tissue deposits of drugs may be slowly released, resulting in persistent drug effects. Just as drugs may bind to plasma proteins, they may also be removed from circulation and stored in tissue, such as bone, teeth, hair, and adipose tissue. Table 2-3 identifies examples of specific drugs that have an affinity for fetal tissues.

Protein Binding. Circulating plasma proteins act as a reservoir for drugs or as sites from which drugs are released. During pregnancy, plasma albumin levels are decreased, in part from the diluting effects of expanded plasma volumes. The decrease in albumin levels promotes an increase in unbound drug. It is important to remember that only unbound drug exerts a pharmacologic effect. In addition, only unbound drugs cross the placenta to the fetal compartment.

A second important concept related to protein binding is that many drugs bind to the same protein site. One drug therefore may displace another, resulting in a potentially dangerous increase in unbound drug concentration. During pregnancy, there is an elevation of free fatty acids, which may contribute to further competition for albumin binding sites.

Maternal-Fetal Blood Flow. Optimal uterine-placental blood flow is obtained with the patient in a right or left lateral recumbent or sitting position. Uterine blood flow is impeded by standing or by lying in a supine position. Any maternal position that does not optimize uterine blood flow decreases the potential for fetal drug exposure.

Blood flow through the umbilical cord is an important factor in the transfer of freely permeable drugs. Cord compression jeopardizes circulation and hence the delivery of oxygen to and removal of wastes from the fetus. Cord compression thus also affects the delivery of drugs to the fetus. Likewise, uterine contractions impair placental blood flow and reduce the transfer of intravenous drugs to the fetal compartment when bolus administration of a drug coincides with a uterine contraction.

Drug transfer via the placenta is greatest late in pregnancy. As pregnancy progresses, chorionic villi become more numerous, providing a greater surface area across which diffusion between the two circulations can occur. Near term, the membrane separating maternal and fetal circulations thins considerably, so that fetal capillary endothelium is separated from maternal circulation by a single layer of fetal chorionic tissue. Inflammation, hypoxia, vascular degeneration, or partial separation of the placenta affects drug transfer just as it affects transfer of oxygen and nutrients to the fetus. For example, a woman with diabetes tends to have a larger, thicker placenta, creating a greater distance for molecules to travel before arriving in fetal circulation.

Biotransformation

Biotransformation by the fetus is mainly an inactivation process whereby the fetal liver, adrenals, and placenta carry out oxidation, dealkylation, hydroxylation, and conjugation reactions. It is important to know that the metabolites and intermediate compounds from these processes may be harmful to the fetus.

Although the fetal liver contains the adult complement of enzymes, the activities of these enzymes at term are only about half those of an adult. Liver enzymes in the fetus are also poorly inducible compared with those of an adult. Therefore, the fetus must rely on maternal processes to clear drugs from fetal circulation.

Only unbound drugs in maternal circulation cross the placenta to reach the fetus. Therefore, the protein-bound component of plasma drug concentration is often discounted. The fetus, however, also possesses the ability to store drugs through plasma protein binding. The protein content of fetal plasma increases with gestational age. Fetal albumin levels usually exceed maternal levels at time of delivery. The high levels of bound drug in the fetus promote placental drug transfer as free drug continues to cross the placenta to replace drug bound to fetal proteins. The bound component also increases the overall fetal dose after a brief administration of a drug and thereby prolongs the fetal and, perhaps more important, the neonatal effects of a drug given to the mother. Following birth, the neonate is removed from the benefit of maternal biotransformation and must rely on its own limited ability to biotransform and remove a drug from its circulation. Hence, drug action following birth may be prolonged and may have adverse neonatal consequences (see Chapter 3).

Excretion

The presence of drug-biotransforming enzymes in fetal liver supports the notion that the fetus is capable of eliminating drugs. Drug metabolites have been found in fetal serum, but because metabolites can freely cross the placenta in both directions, it has been difficult to prove that they are of fetal origin.

A water-soluble drug crosses the placenta slowly to reach the fetus, but once there, it undergoes rapid excretion by the fetal kidneys. However, fetal urine voided into the amniotic cavity constitutes a substantial portion of the amniotic fluid. As the fetus goes through the normal process of swallowing amniotic fluid, it ingests the drug or its metabolites that have been excreted in fetal urine. The result is more prolonged fetal drug exposure.

Lipid-soluble drugs diffuse back across placental membranes to the mother, who provides the major route of excretion. Metabolites formed by the fetal liver are probably excreted in bile and deposited in meconium.

PHARMACODYNAMICS

A drug demonstrates the same mechanism of action in all individuals. If a drug normally inhibits the transfer of a substance into a cell, it will do so in persons of any age group. Nevertheless, the period of fetal development offers new and sensitive targets to both known and unexpected actions of drugs. The thalidomide crisis of the 1950s and 1960s showed health care providers and their patients just how profound the effects of a drug on a fetus can be. During that period, thousands of children with poorly formed limbs were born to mothers who took normal doses of thalidomide, a mild drug used as a sedative and to help control morning sickness. Prior to the crisis, the general rule of thumb was that a drug is safe until proven otherwise. Today, anyone who prescribes or administers drugs to a pregnant woman must assume that few, if any, drugs fail to cross the placenta. Thus it is prudent to consider the potential effects of any drug upon the fetus, as well as upon the mother.

Teratogenicity

A **teratogen** is any compound capable of interfering with embryonic and/or fetal development. The type and amount of drug, rate of elimination, extent of distribution to fetal tissue, gestational age, and fetal receptor function all influence the likelihood of a teratogenic effect. To prove that a drug is a teratogen, three criteria must be met: (1) the drug must cause a characteristic set of malformations; (2) it must act only during a specific period of time during gestation; and (3) the incidence of malformations should increase with increasing dosage and duration of exposure. In general, animal studies are of limited value in part because drugs that are teratogens in animals may not show those same effects in humans. More important, drugs that fail to cause malformation in animals may later prove to be teratogenic in humans. Thus, lack of **teratogenicity** in animals is not proof of safety in humans.

Some teratogens act quickly whereas others require prolonged exposure. Drugs that produce delayed effects are among the hardest to identify. The best example is diethylstilbestrol (DES), an estrogenic substance that causes vaginal cancer in females who were exposed in utero. The cancer usually appears in the late teen years. Teratogens that affect behavior may be nearly impossible to identify. Behavioral changes are often delayed, not becoming apparent until the child enters school. At this point it may be difficult to establish a correlation between drug use during pregnancy and the behavioral deficit.

The fetus is most vulnerable during the first trimester. During the preembryonic stage (conception to 14 days), there is little morphologic differentiation. Exposure to teratogens at this time generally has an all-or-nothing effect on the zygote: either the zygote is damaged so severely that it is aborted or there are no apparent effects.

The greatest risk for malformations in the fetus is during the period of **organogenesis** (15 to 60 days after conception). This is the time when the basic shape of internal organs and other structures is being established. Hence, it is not surprising that teratogen exposure at this stage results in conspicuous anatomic distortions (Table 2-4).

After the first trimester, drugs do not cause gross structural abnormalities but can have toxic effects or can affect growth and development. Immature fetal tissues also permit special tissue-specific accumulations of certain drugs. Drug exposure occurring after the first trimester may lead to brain damage, deafness, growth retardation, stillbirth, infant death, or malignancy.

Since 1984, the U.S. Food and Drug Administration (FDA) has required that new systemically administered drugs be assigned a risk category based on the level of known risk the drug presents to the fetus (Table 2-5).

Drugs put on the market before the introduction of current FDA categories generally do not have an FDA category

TABLE 2-4

Teratogenic and Other Effects of Drugs During Perinatal* Development

Effect	Drugs Known to Produce Effect in Humans
First Trimester	
Abortion	isotretinoin, quinine
Craniofacial anomalies	ethanol, isotretinoin, methotrexate, paramethadione, phenytoin, quinine, trimethadione
Neural tube defects	valproate
Goiter	iodide, methimazole, propylthiouracil
Abnormalities of reproductive organs	Androgens, diethylstilbestrol, estrogens, progestins
Inhibited growth	methotrexate, tetracycline, tobacco smoke
Second and Third Trimesters	
Abortion, mortality	heroin, isotretinoin, tobacco smoke
Mental retardation	ethanol
Altered cardiovascular function	Anticholinergic drugs, propranolol, terbutaline
Hearing loss and loss of balance	Aminoglycosides
Hyperbilirubinemia	nitrofurantoin, sulfonamides
Hemolytic anemia	nitrofurantoin
Goiter	iodide, methimazole, propylthiouracil
Abnormalities of reproductive organs	Androgens, diethylstilbestrol, estrogens, progestins
Inhibited growth	ethanol, heroin, methotrexate, tetracycline, tobacco smoke
Labor, Delivery, and Perinatal Period	
Increased mortality	cocaine, tobacco smoke
Altered cardiovascular function	Anticholinergic drugs, caffeine, heroin, lidocaine, meperidine, propranolol, terbutaline
Gray baby syndrome	chloramphenicol
Respiratory depression	diazepam, ethanol, meperidine, morphine, phenobarbital, tobacco smoke
Respiratory distress	reserpine
Bleeding	aspirin, indomethacin
Hypoglycemia	chlorpropamide, propranolol, tolbutamide
Hyperbilirubinemia	nitrofurantoin, sulfonamides
Hemolytic anemia	nitrofurantoin
Hyperirritability	cocaine

*Perinatal, the period before, during, and after labor and delivery.

listed in the patient package insert, but this information may be found in textbooks on drug use in pregnancy.

DRUGS AND LACTATION

Lactation, or breast-feeding, is the major form of neonatal nutrition. More than 60% of newborns are breast-fed. However, approximately 95% of lactating women are taking at least one drug during the first week after delivery. Drugs taken by lactating women can be excreted in breast milk. If drug concentrations in the breast milk rise high enough, a pharmacologic effect can occur in the infant, raising the question of possible harm.

The factors that determine entry of a drug into breast milk are the same factors that determine drug passage across other membranes. Accordingly, drugs that are lipid soluble readily enter breast milk, whereas drugs that are ionized, highly polar, or protein bound tend to be barred.

The Committee on Drugs of the American Academy of Pediatrics (1994) published a list of drugs and chemicals that transfer to breast milk. The list identifies drugs that are contraindicated during breast-feeding, drugs that require temporary cessation of breast-feeding, drugs that should be used with caution during breast-feeding, and drugs that are usually compatible with breast-feeding. Table 2-6 lists drugs that are contraindicated during breast-feeding, along with the reason for concern or the reported effect.

TABLE 2-5

FDA Pregnancy Drug Categories

Level of Risk with Drug Exposure	Drug
A *Remote risk of fetal harm:* Controlled studies in women fail to demonstrate fetal risk in the first trimester (and there is no evidence of risk in later trimesters). The risk to the fetus throughout pregnancy appears to be remote.	folic acid Thyroid hormones
B *Slightly more risk than A:* Animal studies have not demonstrated fetal risk, but there are no controlled studies in pregnant women. Animal studies have shown adverse effects that were not confirmed in controlled studies on women in the first trimester. There is no evidence of risk in later trimesters.	amoxicillin buspirone cimetidine fluoxetine hydrochlorothiazide metronidazole
C *Greater risk than B:* Animal studies have revealed adverse effects, but there are no controlled studies in women. Drugs in this category should be given only if potential benefits outweigh the risk to the fetus.	Recombinant plasminogen activator ciprofloxacin codeine isoproterenol morphine reserpine
D *Proven risk of fetal harm:* There is positive evidence of human risk, however, the benefits may be acceptable despite the risk, as in life-threatening diseases for which safer drugs cannot be used or are ineffective. A statement of risk will appear in the "contraindications" section of drug labeling.	amikacin captopril midazolam tobramycin
X *Proven risk of fetal harm:* Studies or experience in humans and animals have demonstrated evidence of fetal risk. The risk of using this drug during pregnancy far outweighs any potential benefit. The drug is contraindicated in women who are pregnant or who may become pregnant. A statement of risk will appear in the "contraindications" section of drug labeling.	isotretinoin lovastatin methotrexate

TABLE 2-6

Drugs Contraindicated During Breast-feeding

Drug	Reason(s) for Concern or Reported Effect(s)
Controlled Substances*	
amphetamine†	Irritability, poor sleeping pattern
cocaine	Cocaine intoxication
heroin	Tremors, restlessness, vomiting, poor feeding
marijuana	Only one report in literature; no effect mentioned
phencyclidine (PCP)	Potent hallucinogen
Antineoplastic/Immunosuppressants	
cyclophosphamide cyclosporine doxorubicin†	Possible immune suppression; neutropenia; unknown effect and growth or association with carcinogenesis
Others	
bromocriptine	Suppresses lactation; may be hazardous to mother
ergotamine	Vomiting, diarrhea, convulsions (in doses used for migraine headaches)
lithium	One-third to one-half therapeutic blood concentrations found in infant
methotrexate	Possible immune suppression; neutropenia; unknown effect on growth or association with carcinogenesis
nicotine*	

*The Committee on Drugs strongly believes that nursing mothers should not ingest any of these compounds. Not only are they hazardous to the nursing infant, but they are also detrimental to the physical and emotional health of the mother. This list is obviously not complete. No drug of abuse should be ingested by nursing mothers, even though adverse reports may not have been reported in the literature.
†Drug concentrates in human milk.

APPLICATION TO PRACTICE

ASSESSMENT

Although pregnancy is not considered an illness, it is important for the health care provider to gather a sufficient database with which to make drug administration safe. Nurses are assuming a more important role in **perinatal** care, especially in the area of assessment. The progression of a pregnancy depends on a number of factors, including the presence of disease states, emotional status, and past health care. Diagnosis of pregnancy and accurate dating are essential to reduce maternal and fetal risk during the early weeks of gestation. All risk factors do not threaten the pregnancy to the same extent.

History of Present Illness

The database for a perinatal patient should include a menstrual, contraceptive, gynecologic, and obstetric history. Amenorrhea is often the first sign of conception. However, a lack of menses can be due to other factors, such as anovulation, chronic disease, lactation, and stress. Other presumptive signs of pregnancy are breast tenderness/fullness, skin changes, nausea, vomiting, urinary frequency, and fatigue.

A known menstrual history is usually the most reliable predictor of delivery date. The mean duration of pregnancy, as calculated from the last menstrual period, is 280 days or 40 weeks. Include the date of the last menstrual period and course of previous pregnancies.

One area of concern is the substantial number of women of child-bearing age who have used illicit drugs or alcohol. Identification of these women depends on successful interview techniques. The reliability of drug testing via urinalysis depends on the pharmacokinetics of the abused substance and the time of the last exposure. Determining the woman's perception of her health and the effect of any drugs she is using will assist in gaining insights that may aid in effective intervention if necessary.

Health History

When a pregnant woman has a disease that predates her pregnancy, she may be taking medication for that condition when she becomes pregnant. It is important to establish the patient's past and present use of prescription, over-the-counter, and illicit drugs. If she is currently taking medication, identify whether the drug is a potential teratogen.

Once a pregnant woman has been exposed to a known teratogen, it is important to determine exactly when the pregnancy began and exactly when the exposure occurred, since the timing of drug exposure determines which organ system is affected. Teratogen exposure is of most concern during the first trimester. After 12 weeks gestation, teratogen exposure can result in decreased growth or function but generally not in a structural malformation. However, keep in mind that 3% of all infants have a noticeable defect, independent of teratogen exposure. This notion is important because otherwise the drug is sure to be blamed if the infant should turn out to have an anomaly.

The consequences of drug exposure during the period of organogenesis can be determined by consulting a reference book (e.g., Briggs et al.'s *Drugs in Pregnancy and Lactation*). At least two ultrasound scans should be done to determine the extent of injury. If the defect is severe, termination of the pregnancy may be considered. If the defect is less severe, it may be correctable by surgery after birth.

Lifespan Considerations

Pregnancy is a time of maternal psychologic adjustment and concern. It is a period with distinctive developmental tasks. Family dynamics, social support, cultural influences, and whether or not the pregnancy was planned distinctly influence the mother's as well as the family's adjustment to pregnancy. Thus, the woman's personal situation and support systems must be explored as the family prepares for a new member.

During the first trimester, the woman normally feels some ambivalence about the pregnancy, even if it was planned. These feelings should be discussed with the patient, because she may feel the need to hide the negative feelings, believing that they are abnormal. Helping her to understand the feelings will benefit her, especially if the baby should subsequently be aborted or be born with an anomaly. The ambivalence usually ends by the beginning of the second trimester.

When the pregnancy is well accepted, the woman will demonstrate feelings of happiness about it. On the other hand, failure to move toward maternal role attainment may be demonstrated through direct statements of dissatisfaction. Less directly, failure of role attainment may be demonstrated through excessive complaints of physical discomfort or illness, depression, expressions of feeling ugly, or failure to seek prenatal care or to comply with the plan of care. Other examples include missed appointments, refusal to take vitamins or other drugs that may be needed for concurrent medical conditions, and general noncompliance with recommended self-care activities such as diet, exercise, alcohol consumption, and drug use.

Cultural/Social Considerations

Other developmental considerations during pregnancy are related to cultural influences and beliefs. For example, awareness of a patient's use of indigenous healers or home remedies and adherence to folk beliefs are important for health professionals, because these factors influence health outcomes. Knowing the causes of non-compliance enables the health care provider to offer appropriate patient education or to incorporate the patient's cultural practices into perinatal care.

Nurses providing patient care must assess an awareness of potential cultural differences and individual knowledge. Determining a patient's needs and expectations helps bridge the cultural gap. Individual beliefs and values that are beneficial or harmless must be supported in order to promote the use of cultural systems. Practices that may be harmful can be modified through patient education. Flexibility, compromise, and respect for differences makes culturally appropriate nursing care an attainable goal. Some examples of such cultural value systems follow.

Many Mexican-American women believe that prenatal care is unnecessary because pregnancy is not an illness. Some women prefer to receive their care from parteras (lay midwives) or curanderas (folk healers). Motherhood is seen by many such women as the most important social role to be achieved. As a result, the times surrounding pregnancy and birth are especially rich in traditional beliefs and practices. Paradoxically, Mexican-American women who have not received prenatal care or who received care late in pregnancy have surprisingly healthy birth outcomes.

Women of Haitian background may believe that hot ginger tea should be taken during labor. During the postpartum period, the woman may sit in a hot, herbal bath containing added leaves and roots. Some Haitian women believe that hot, spicy food should be avoided during pregnancy and that the diet should consist of okra and tisane, a tea made from lettuce. After the baby is born, the woman and her family may massage the baby's head with palm oil, pinch the nose to give it shape, or press the cheeks to give the child dimples. Castor oil or lok (castor oil with nutmeg powder and mashed garlic) is sometimes used to speed the passage of meconium stool.

Many Southeast Asian women believe in the balance between yin (hot) and yang (cold). Childbirth is a precarious time, when a woman is in a cold state that may lead to illness. In Thailand, women have been seen lying on cots placed over smoldering charcoal fires on days when the air temperature is 90° to 100° F. In Cambodia, the women usually lie next to the fire with their heads covered by blankets or towels. When antibiotics are unavailable, this process of raising the body temperature may provide a way to kill some infectious organisms.

Women of Southeast Asian background often deal with illness through self-medication. Herbal preparations are widely used and facsimiles of Western prescription drugs are sold over the counter. A common belief in this culture is that if one pill is good, two are better. Traditional Southeast Asian healers will use herbal preparations, acupuncture, "coining" (rubbing the "sick" area with coins), or "cupping" (using small heated cups over the area). They believe that cutting into the body, such as occurs during an episiotomy, cesarean section, and circumcision, makes an exit point for a person's spirit, and should therefore be avoided. Many Southeast Asians may regard invasive treatments such as nasal oxygen or intravenous fluid administration as providing the means of exit for life's essence.

Physical Examination

A complete physical examination begins with assessment of vital signs. A decrease in blood pressure from baseline during the second trimester is expected because of normal physiologic changes of pregnancy. The examination continues with evaluation of body weight, skin, head and neck, cardiovascular and respiratory systems, breasts, musculoskeletal, and neurologic systems. Abdominal and pelvic measurements are taken.

If it has been determined that a woman has not started perinatal counseling, this is the perfect time to introduce patient education regarding the use of drugs, alcohol, tobacco, and environmental hazards. When a woman is required to take drugs during her pregnancy, the risks and benefits should be discussed, and the need to report adverse effects or lack of effectiveness of the drugs should be addressed.

Laboratory Testing

Laboratory testing of the pregnant woman includes a complete blood cell (CBC) count, ABO and Rh blood typing, a rubella titer, and screening for sexually transmitted diseases (e.g., gonorrhea, chlamydia, genital herpes, human immunodeficiency virus, syphilis) and sickle cell disease. A urinalysis and Papanicolaou (Pap) smear are also included in diagnostic testing. For some women, testing for illicit drug use may also be included.

GOALS OF THERAPY ▸▸▸

When drug therapy is required during pregnancy the goal is to use a drug that has been identified as safe for use in pregnancy or to substitute one drug for another suspected to be highly teratogenic. As a rule, some therapies are offered during the perinatal period simply to promote maternal comfort and, therefore, caution is required. The gestational age of the fetus is taken into consideration. Well-chosen therapies that provide relief from pregnancy-related symptoms make a significant difference in how a woman views her pregnancy.

INTERVENTION
Administration

Collaboration among and between members of the health care team is the best assurance that identification and appropriate interventions for a woman and fetus or infant at risk will occur. To minimize the risk of drug exposure to mother and fetus, the following administration principles should be used:

- Clearly identify the need for any drug used.
- Use the safest effective drug option available.
- Avoid use of the newest drugs on the market.
- Use the lowest effective dose for the shortest possible time.
- Use topical or local therapy whenever possible.

Minor Aches and Headaches. Minor muscle aches and headaches are common during pregnancy. Acetaminophen is often used short term during pregnancy. High doses, on the other hand, especially during the first trimester, may result in severe fetal liver damage. Pregnant women commonly use aspirin. However, use of aspirin has been associated with maternal anemia, antepartal and postpartal hemorrhage, and prolonged gestation and labor. Aspirin's effects on the fetus and neonate include intrauterine growth retardation, congenital salicylate intoxication, depressed albumin-binding capacity, and an increased perinatal mortality rate. Aspirin taken (even in low doses) during the week before delivery may affect the neonate's clotting abilities.

Opioids should be used cautiously, if at all, in a pregnant woman. When used on a regular basis, opiates induce an intense addiction in both mother and fetus. Pain relief during labor and delivery must be carefully coordinated with the time of delivery and the drug dose to protect the fetus from potentially harmful drug effects. Chapters 13 and 14 discuss analgesics further.

Heartburn. Antacids are used by approximately 50% of pregnant women for relief of heartburn (pyrosis). Heartburn often occurs in the later months of pregnancy, when increased intraabdominal pressure and a relaxed cardiac sphincter permit gastric acid to reflux into the esophagus. Nondrug interventions used to reduce the discomfort caused by reflux includes eating small, frequent meals; remaining in an upright position for 2 hours after eating; avoiding gas-producing and fatty foods; avoiding tight garments around the waist; and sleeping with the head of the bed slightly elevated.

Most antacids containing aluminum, magnesium, and calcium are safe in therapeutic dosages during the second and third trimesters. Because little systemic absorption occurs, the drugs are unlikely to harm the fetus when used in recommended dosages. Sucralfate and H_2 antagonists (e.g., cimetidine, ranitidine) are effective for nonpregnant patients, but their safety during pregnancy is not yet well established. Antacids and hyperacidity drugs are discussed further in Chapter 48.

Constipation. Constipation is a common problem during pregnancy, probably as the result of decreased peristalsis. The preferred nondrug treatment for constipation includes increases in fluids, high-fiber foods, and exercise. If a laxative is needed, a bulk-producing agent such as psyllium hydrophilic mucilloid or methylcellulose is the most physiologic for the mother and safest for the fetus. Bulk-producing laxatives are not absorbed systemically.

Certain laxatives are not safe for use during pregnancy. Castor oil can initiate premature uterine contractions. Saline laxatives (e.g., magnesium hydroxide) can lead to sodium retention in the mother. Furthermore, frequent use of lubricants such as mineral oil can lead to reduced absorption of fat-soluble vitamins, resulting in neonatal hypoprothrombinemia and hemorrhage. Stool softeners such as docusate sodium may be used occasionally. Laxatives are discussed further in Chapter 49.

Nausea and Vomiting. Nausea and vomiting may occur during pregnancy, especially during the first trimester. Nondrug therapy includes eating a few crackers when awakening and waiting a few minutes before arising; consuming liquid and dry foods separately; and avoiding fried, odorous, spicy, greasy, or gas-forming foods. It is important to maintain an adequate fluid and electrolyte balance.

Antiemetic drugs should be used only when the nausea and vomiting are severe enough to threaten the mother's nutritional or metabolic status. Meclizine and dimenhydrinate are thought to be low in teratogenic effects; however, many antiemetic drugs have been linked to an increased risk of fetal harm. Diphenhydramine may cause cleft palate. Trimethobenzamide may produce other congenital anomalies. Prochlorperazine has been linked to an increased risk of cardiovascular and other malformations. The best scheme for managing nausea and vomiting in pregnancy with antiemetics is to become familiar with two or three drugs. Antiemetics are discussed further in Chapter 50.

Anemia. There are three types of anemia common during pregnancy. Physiologic anemia results from the expanded blood volume and is to be expected during pregnancy. Physiologic anemia is not ordinarily treated. Iron-deficiency anemia is often related to long-term nutritional deficiencies but is managed prophylactically with iron supplements (e.g., ferrous gluconate or ferrous sulfate). Megaloblastic anemia is caused by folic acid deficiency but is manageable with the use of prophylactic folic acid.

Pregnancy-Induced Hypertension. Pregnancy-induced hypertension (i.e., preeclampsia and eclampsia), previously known as toxemia of pregnancy, is a serious complication that can endanger the lives of the mother and the fetus. Preeclampsia is characterized by edema, elevated blood pressure, and proteinuria in a patient without an underlying neurologic disease. The incidence is unclear but preeclampsia has been reported to complicate 5% of all pregnancies. Furthermore, 0.5% to 2% of preeclamptic patients will progress to eclampsia. Nondrug therapy for preeclampsia includes a high-protein, high-carbohydrate, low-salt, low-fat diet along with intravenous fluids and bed rest in a left lateral position. This position increases blood flow to the kidneys and placenta, promotes diuresis, and lowers blood pressure. When drugs are needed to control the blood pressure, intravenous hydralazine is often used because it does not cause adverse fetal effects.

Eclampsia is characterized by increased severity of the above symptoms and convulsions. It must be promptly and effectively treated to protect the life of mother and fetus. Intravenous magnesium sulfate is the drug of choice to prevent or treat convulsions. Delivery of the fetus is the only known cure for preeclampsia or eclampsia.

Infections. Sensitivity testing and considerations for maternal and fetal toxicity should guide the choice for an antibiotic. Penicillins and cephalosporins are generally considered safe in pregnancy. There is no known increase in maternal toxicity and no known teratogenicity. Tetracyclines are contraindicated during pregnancy since they cause staining and deformity of deciduous teeth and inhibition of fetal bone growth. Sulfonamides and nitrofurantoin can cause hemolysis in patients with glucose-6-phosphate dehydrogenase (G6PD) deficiency. Trimethoprim, a drug commonly seen in combination with sulfamethoxazole, is contraindicated.

Breast-feeding. The goal of the health care provider is to minimize the risk of potentially harmful drug exposure to the breast-fed infant. However, when a mother requires a drug that carries minimal hazards for the infant, the health care provider can make the following adjustments to diminish drug effects:

- Avoid sustained-release and long-acting drugs that have a long half-life. They are difficult for an infant to excrete, and drug accumulation in the infant is a significant concern.
- Identify the usual rate of absorption and peak blood levels of the drug, scheduling drug administration so the least amount possible gets into the milk. Having the mother take the drug immediately after breast-feeding is generally safest for the infant.
- Carefully schedule drug administration so a breast-feeding mother does not receive the drug within a short time before nursing. Breast milk contains higher amounts of fat at midday, so the breast-fed infant may be exposed to higher amounts of fat-soluble drugs at that feeding. Supplementing nursing with formula for the midday feedings may help reduce the amount of drug the infant receives.
- Once-daily doses may be taken by a breast-feeding mother before the infant's longest sleep period.

- Short-acting drugs may never fully equilibrate with milk if the drug is rapidly cleared. For this reason, expressing and discarding breast milk after drug administration may not be a useful alternative.
- When possible, a formulation that produces the lowest levels of drug in the milk should be used.
- Watch the infant for signs of drug reaction (e.g., changes in sleep or feeding patterns, fussiness, rashes).

Education

Patient teaching should include the names of the drugs that have been ordered and why. Special instructions about the timing of drug doses and drug-food interactions should be clarified. The patient should be told about which adverse effects should be reported as well as what to do if she forgets to take a dose. The patient should know the expected duration of the therapy and should be advised not to change the dosage or discontinue the drug without consulting the health care provider. The addition of any prescription or over-the-counter drugs should be approved before use. Written instructions are always helpful as a reference after the patient leaves the office, clinic, or hospital. Members of the health care team may access literature on drugs and pregnancy, or may use teratogen information resources or contact regional drug consultation centers.

EVALUATION

Meticulous, ongoing assessment is essential to achieve optimal perinatal outcomes. When drug exposure during pregnancy is inevitable, an awareness of the physiologic changes of pregnancy, attention to the pharmacokinetics and pharmacodynamics of the required drugs, and early recognition of potential complications are essential. Goals and outcomes center, in most cases, on prevention and alleviation of potential problems. Thus, the health care provider must maintain a current knowledge base to best respond to the health needs of the pregnant or lactating woman and her infant.

Bibliography

American Academy of Pediatrics Committee on Drugs: The transfer of drugs and other chemicals into human milk, *Pediatrics* 93(1):137-150, 1994.

Briggs GG, Freeman RK, Yaffe SJ: *Drugs in pregnancy and lactation*, ed 6, Philadelphia, 2001, Lippincott Williams & Wilkins.

Internet Resources

Fredericksen M: Physiologic changes in pregnancy: effect on drug disposition, 2001. Available online: http://www.fda/cder.

Merck Manual: Drug use during pregnancy. Available online: http://www.merck.com.

National Institute on Drug Abuse: National survey of drug use during pregnancy, January/February 1997. Available online: http://www.drugabuse.gov/NIDA.

Pediatric Pharmacotherapeutics

KATHLEEN GUTIERREZ

 Visit **http://evolve.elsevier.com/Gutierrez/** for additional information.

KEY TERMS

Adolescent, p. 34

Infant, p. 35

Neonates, p. 36

School-age child, p. 41

Toddlers, p. 40

OBJECTIVES

- Recognize the anatomic and physiologic differences in body systems of children that affect drug therapy.

- Explain the concept of body surface area as it relates to pediatric drug dosages.

- Discuss the responsibility of health care providers to recognize the biologic distinctions that affect pharmacokinetics in children.

- Discuss the developmental considerations that influence drug administration.

- Identify pediatric drug administration strategies.

In the last decade, an estimated 12% of all prescriptions written in the United States were for children under age 9. In spite of that fact, the term *therapeutic orphan* has been applied to pharmacotherapeutics in children because of the relative lack of information on drug safety and efficacy. The pharmaceutical industry has generated a wealth of data for adults, but similar studies in the pediatric population have generally not been done. Only a quarter of the drugs approved by the Food and Drug Administration (FDA) have specific indications in children.

Children differ from adults and from one another in regard to drug absorption, distribution, biotransformation, and excretion. The pharmacokinetic and pharmacodynamic components of pediatric drug therapy are a unique challenge because of differences in body composition and the maturation of various organ systems (Figure 3-1).

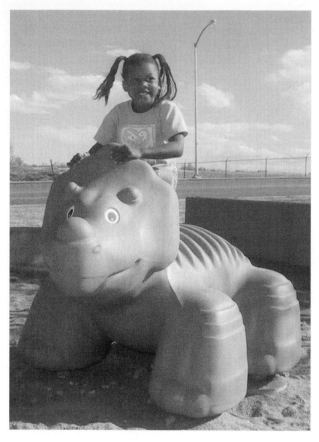

FIGURE 3-1

ANATOMIC AND PHYSIOLOGIC VARIABLES

Children are not small adults. Drug therapy for children requires an understanding of the anatomic and physiologic differences between children and adults. Assessment of the pediatric patient requires the health care provider to understand these characteristics and their clinical significance. Because children's body systems grow and develop at different rates, generalizations about the use of drugs in this population are not possible.

Body Composition and Size

Significant changes in body weight occur in infancy and childhood. The child is smaller in height and weight than an adult, and the proportions are also different. A child's weight increases about 20-fold between birth and adulthood, but height increases only 3.5-fold. A child's weight in kilograms may be estimated using the following formula:

$$\text{Weight (kg)} = 8 + 2 \text{ (Age in years)}$$

Approximate weight may be estimated according to age by using the following general rules:
- Two times the birth weight by age 5 months
- Three times the birth weight by age 12 months
- Seven times the birth weight by age 7 years
- Fourteen times the birth weight by age 14 years

Commercially available charts and devices have also been developed to assist in the estimation of weight in infants and children during an emergency, because accurate estimates of weight are essential for proper pharmacotherapy.

The concept of body surface area (BSA) is important in pediatrics because many physiologic functions are proportional to BSA (Figure 3-2). The child's proportionally large head accounts for much of the exposed surface area. The BSA, estimated as the relationship between height and weight, is about 7-fold greater in adulthood than at birth. Physiologic parameters influenced by BSA include the metabolic rate, extracellular fluid and plasma volumes, cardiac output, and glomerular filtration rate.

Fluid Balance

The amount and distribution of body water changes with age. Body water is important as the medium in which solutes, including drugs, are dissolved and as the medium in which all metabolic activities take place. Total body water, which in a newborn infant is approximately 70% to 80% of body weight (50% contained in extracellular fluid), decreases to about 67% during the first year of life. It reaches the adult level of 60% by 2 years of age. The body weight of the infant is composed of 45% intracellular fluid and 35% extracellular fluid (Table 3-1).

During adolescence, the percentage of body water approaches that of an adult, but gender differences begin to appear. Males develop a greater percentage of body water because of increasing muscle mass. Proportionally, females have more body fat and less muscle mass because of increases in estrogen; **adolescent** females thus have comparatively less body water than males of the same age.

Daily water turnover in children involves more than half of the extracellular fluid; in the adult, one fifth of the extracellular fluid is exchanged daily. Because of a child's greater proportion of body fluid, especially in the extracellular compartment, larger milligram-per-kilogram doses of certain drugs are required to achieve therapeutic drug levels.

Tissue Mass

Skeletal growth and muscle development in healthy children consists of two concurrent processes: the creation of new cells and tissues (growth) and the consolidation of the new tissues into a permanent form (mat-

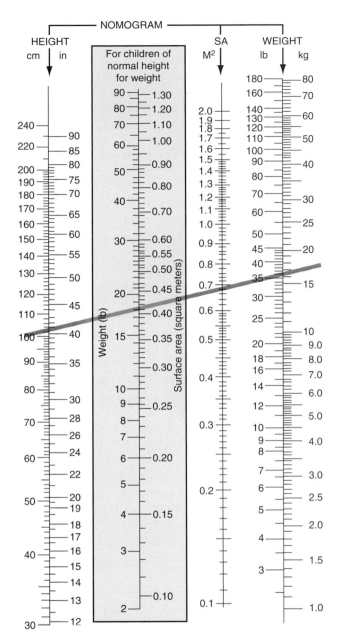

NOMOGRAM

FIGURE 3-2 West nomogram for estimating body surface area. Body surface area is indicated where shaded line connecting height and weight intersect surface area (SA) column or, if patient is of approximately normal proportion, from weight alone (see highlighted column). (Adapted from data of E. Boyd by CD West, presented in Behrman RE, Kliegman RM, Arvin AM: Nelson's textbook of pediatrics, ed. 15, Philadelphia, 1996, Saunders. Used with permission.)

TABLE 3-1

Body Weight Composition (in percentages)

	Body Weight (%)		
Body Fluid	*Infant*	*Adult Male*	*Adult Female*
Extracellular fluid			
Plasma	4	4	4
Interstitial fluid	26	15	10
Intracellular fluid	45	38	33
Total	75	57	47

Gender differences in muscle size and weight are minor during childhood but become considerable with the onset of puberty. Muscle growth during adolescence is a major factor in weight gain. Muscle fibers reach maximal size at about age 10 in females and age 14 in males. Therefore, the younger the child, the less muscle tissue is available for injections.

Body fat makes up approximately 16% of an infant's birth weight. Between the ages of 1 and 5 years, fat levels fall to between 8% and 12%. The levels increase again at about age 10, to 18% to 20% of body weight. Because drugs are water soluble or fat soluble, the percentage of body fat affects drug distribution. The relative mass of subcutaneous tissue in children also varies. Premature infants have very little fatty tissue. Fatty tissue development reaches a peak at 9 months and then decreases until about 6 years. In adolescence, subcutaneous fat tissue again increases.

Cardiovascular System

Cardiovascular dynamics of the young child change during the transition from fetus to newborn, from newborn to young child, and from child to adult. These dynamics affect the uptake and distribution of drugs. The heart rate and stroke volume (the amount of blood ejected during contraction of the ventricle) are greater in a child than in an adult. Like respiration and metabolism, the cardiac output of the newborn is about two times as much in relation to body weight compared with the adult, or approximately 550 mL/min. Further, peripheral circulation is poorly developed in the infant, so blood flow to various muscles changes a great deal during the first 2 weeks of life. The overall changes in cardiovascular dynamics ultimately affect the uptake and distribution of drugs.

Gastrointestinal System

Characteristics of the gastrointestinal (GI) system greatly influence the speed and efficiency with which drugs are absorbed into the body. For example, the gas-

uration). In the **infant**, muscle mass accounts for approximately 25% of total body weight, compared with 40% in the adult. The composition and size of muscles vary with age. In the fetus, muscle tissue contains large amounts of water and intracellular matrix. After birth, both are considerably reduced as muscle fibers enlarge.

tric emptying time in a newborn is 6 to 8 hours, compared with 2 hours in an adult. In addition, peristalsis may be irregular in young infants. Absorption of fats is somewhat less than in the older child. Consequently, milk with a high fat content (such as cow's milk) is often inadequately absorbed. The secretion of pancreatic amylase in the newborn infant is also low, so the infant uses starches less effectively.

The gastric pH in **neonates** ranges from 5 to 8. It drops to a more acidic pH of 1 to 3 within the first day of life. These changes may alter the solubility, ionization, stability, and absorption of a drug. Food may also interfere with drug therapy by altering the amount, type, and osmolality of GI secretions; pH; transit time; and motility.

Liver function develops considerably during infancy, so the greatest risk for drug toxicity is to the newborn. The ability to produce microsomal enzymes develops at varying rates in the young child. The immature liver of the newborn is unable to form plasma proteins, so their concentrations are 15% to 20% less than in older children. The lower plasma concentration of protein for binding with drugs makes children particularly vulnerable to the harmful effects of some drugs.

Renal System

Glomerular filtration is the most common mechanism by which drugs are excreted. The glomerular filtration rate in infants is 30% to 50% that of an adult. Therefore, drugs excreted through the kidneys have a half-life approximately 50% greater in infants than in adults.

Neurologic System

The mature brain is protected by the blood-brain barrier, which prevents substances from diffusing freely out of the circulatory system into brain cells. The processes that produce the blood-brain barrier are immature in children younger than 2 years, leading to unpredictable pharmacotherapeutic results. In certain pathologic conditions, such as hyperbilirubinemia, there is an increase in the permeability of the blood-brain barrier.

PHARMACOKINETIC CONSIDERATIONS

Data on the pharmacokinetics, pharmacodynamics, efficacy, and safety of drugs in infants and children are scarce. Thus, drug therapy in the pediatric patient presents a challenge to the health care provider. A poorly developed blood-brain barrier, weak microsomal enzyme activity, and immature mechanisms for elimination combine to make the fetus and neonate vulnerable to drug effects. Table 3-2 summarizes age-related physiologic factors related to pharmacokinetic drug action.

Absorption

Drug absorption depends on the route of administration, disintegration and dissociation of the drug, drug serum concentration, blood flow to the site, and absorptive surface area. Two factors affecting the absorption of drugs from the GI tract are pH-dependent diffusion and gastric emptying time. Both processes are strikingly different in a premature infant compared with older children and adults. Age-related variables such as delayed gastric emptying time and irregular intestinal

TABLE 3-2

Summary of Physiologic Factors that Alter Pharmacokinetic Variables

Pharmacokinetic Component	Age Group	Physiologic Change	Pharmacokinetic Change
Absorption	Neonates Infants Young children	Increased gastric pH	Increased bioavailability of basic drugs and reduced bioavailability of acidic drugs
	Neonates Infants	Reduced gastric and intestinal motility	
	Neonates	Decreased bile acids	Bioavailability is reduced
Distribution	Neonates Infants	Increased total body water and extracellular fluid	Volume of distribution is increased
		Reduced albumin concentration and protein binding	Concentration of unbound drug is increased
Biotransformation	Neonates Infants	Immature hepatic enzyme system	Half-life increases but clearance is reduced
	Young children	Increased enzyme capacity	Clearance increases but half-life is reduced
Excretion	Neonates Infants	Immature glomerular and tubular function	Half-life increases

motility are examples of mechanisms that affect absorption. The rate of absorption also depends on the specific characteristics of the drug and the child.

Oral Route. Absorption of orally administered drugs is often delayed in neonates and young infants, owing primarily to differences in the pH of the GI tract and reduced gastric motility. Immediately after birth, gastric pH is high. Acidic drugs, such as nalidixic acid, phenobarbital, and phenytoin, are less well absorbed. On the other hand, the absorption of acid-labile drugs (e.g., penicillin) may be enhanced.

Prolonged exposure of certain drugs to gastric contents increases the disintegration of unstable drugs and also delays drug entry into the lower GI tract, so drug absorption and attainment of peak serum levels are delayed.

Parenteral Routes. Intramuscular drug absorption may be uncertain because of unpredictable blood flow, decreased muscle tone, lower muscle oxygenation, and vasomotor instability. Repeated injections in the child's few available muscle sites may cause tissue breakdown and limited absorption of the drug. The absorption of drugs administered by the percutaneous route, however, is increased because of an underdeveloped epidermal barrier and greater permeability of the skin.

The intravenous route of administration is commonly used in pediatric therapy. For some drugs, it is the only effective route. When a drug is administered intravenously, the effect is almost instantaneous. Most drugs intended for intravenous administration require a specified minimum dilution and/or rate of infusion.

Intraosseous cannulation provides a reliable method for rapidly achieving venous access in emergencies, particularly in children younger than 6 years. In general, the intraosseous route can safely be used to administer any drug or fluid formulated for intravenous use. Reports of successful administration of catecholamines, calcium, antibiotics, digitalis, heparin, lidocaine, atropine, phenytoin, sodium bicarbonate, neuromuscular blocking drugs, crystalloids, colloids, and blood can be found in the literature. This route is used temporarily, until other venous access sites become available. The flat, anteromedial surface of the tibia, approximately 1 to 3 cm below the tibial tuberosity, is the preferred site.

Topical Routes. The absorption rate of a topically administered drug is the same in a child as in an adult. However, the relative dose absorbed in a child is larger because of the greater body surface area in relation to total body mass. When occlusive dressings are used, absorption of a topically administered drug is enhanced and the possibility of adverse reactions increased, particularly to steroid creams, salicylic acid, and silver sulfadiazine. Corticosteroids are used sparingly in children to prevent absorption that may lead to adrenal suppression. Growth retardation may occur if the adrenal glands are suppressed before bone epiphyses mature.

A few drugs are known for their bioavailability when given rectally, and this avenue provides an alternative to oral and parenteral routes. Rectal administration is generally disliked but may be preferred over intramuscular injection. Furthermore, acceptance of rectal administration may be culturally influenced. Examples of drugs available in suppository form include acetaminophen, sedatives, antiemetics, and analgesics such as morphine.

Distribution

Many age-related differences in drug distribution occur during the first 10 to 12 months of life. The distribution of a drug in children is affected by the changing percentage of body fat, total body water content, total blood volume, and blood flow to target tissues as well as by the ability of the drug to exit capillaries and move into cells.

Drug distribution and equilibration rates may be faster in children than in adults. Therefore, a larger average dose per kilogram of body weight is needed to reach desired serum concentration levels. The higher the percentage of body water, the greater the dilution of water-soluble drugs. The result is reduced serum concentration levels. As the percentage of body fat increases with age, so does the distribution of fat-soluble drugs. Therefore, the distribution of these drugs is more limited in children than in adults.

Decreased formation of plasma proteins in the immature liver also affects drug distribution and results in higher serum drug levels. The albumin in neonates and infants has a lower binding capacity for certain drugs (e.g., phenytoin, penicillin) compared with mature albumin. Thus, it is possible that unbound drug levels will be high enough to produce toxic effects. To minimize the possibility of toxicity and to compensate for the shorter duration of drug action, it is often necessary to decrease the amount of the drug given and/or lengthen the time between doses.

Adverse effects may also occur when drugs such as salicylates, penicillins, sulfonamides, phenytoin, phenobarbital, and imipramine compete with endogenous substances (e.g., free fatty acids, bilirubin) for the same protein binding sites. Competitive drug binding in the neonate increases the potential for adverse effects from increased concentrations of unbound, unconjugated bilirubin. Kernicterus (bilirubin encephalopathy) is a grave condition in which the basal ganglia and other areas of the brain and spinal cord are infiltrated with bilirubin. The greater permeability of the blood-brain barrier in children allows this to occur. Any drug that competes with bilirubin for protein binding sites or that inhibits the binding of bilirubin increases the risk. The signs of kernicterus are those of central nervous system depression or excitation, such as decreased activity, lethargy, irritability, loss of interest in feeding, seizures, and gastric or pulmonary hemorrhage.

Biotransformation

Hepatic enzyme activity is low in the neonate and premature infant, resulting in longer half-lives for some drugs (e.g., digoxin, indomethacin, acetaminophen, phenobarbital). However, the capacity of an infant's liver to biotransform drugs develops quickly during the first months after birth (Table 3-3). Altered biotransformation processes persist for approximately the first month of life and undergo a dramatic increase at about 6 months. Before these biotransforming enzymes increase to adult levels, neonates are more vulnerable than adults to chemicals requiring detoxification by the liver.

It is almost impossible to predict the effect of maturation on biotransformation solely on the basis of age. As a result, it may be necessary to monitor levels of certain critical drugs; it is always critical to monitor carefully for signs of inadequate therapy or drug toxicity.

Dosages and choice of drug may be altered for an infant with immature liver function or liver disease. For example, the antimicrobial drug chloramphenicol is inadequately biotransformed in infants, allowing toxic levels to be reached. Gray baby syndrome results. Tachypnea, ashen-gray cyanosis, vomiting, loose green stools, progressive abdominal distension, vasomotor collapse, and perhaps death characterize this disorder. Discontinuing the drug as soon as symptoms appear can reverse the progression of symptoms.

Body temperature regulation is unstable in children, creating implications for drug action. When infants and toddlers develop an infection, the sudden high temperature increases basal metabolic rates. For each degree Celsius rise in body temperature, the metabolic rate increases by approximately 12%. The higher metabolic rate reduces drug half-lives and duration of therapeutic effects. Antipyretic effects of drugs are short-lived because of this phenomenon.

Excretion

During the first 6 months of life, an infant has a small number of renal tubular cells, a shorter tubular length, and lower tubular blood flow. Dosages of drugs that depend on the kidneys for elimination must be adjusted to avoid toxicity from drug accumulation in the body. When renal blood flow increases in response to a rise in systemic arterial pressure, intrarenal vascular resistance decreases. This response allows the kidneys to receive a higher percentage of the cardiac output and the circulating drug.

Drug elimination is also affected by urinary pH, because some drugs are more readily eliminated in acid urine whereas others require more basic urine in order to be excreted. An infant's kidneys are less able to excrete hydrogen ions and reabsorb bicarbonate. As a result, the infant's urine is slightly less acidic than an adult's.

PHARMACODYNAMIC CONSIDERATIONS

Drugs use the same mechanism of action in all individuals, including children. The response to the drug, however, varies according to the maturity of the target organ and the maturity of the specific drug receptor. This area of pharmacology will receive more attention as less invasive methods are developed to help characterize the pharmacogenetics of individuals.

TABLE 3-3

Drug-Biotransforming Enzymes that Change During Development

Activity in Enzyme	Fetus/Neonate	Age Adult Level Achieved
Phase I		
CYP1A2	Nearly absent	4 months; may be higher than adult in children from 1 to 2 years of age
CYP2C	Nearly absent	6 months; may be higher than adult in children from 3 to 4 years of age
CYP2D6	Nearly absent	3 to 5 years
CYP3A4	Low	6 to 12 months; may be higher than adult in children 1 to 4 years of age
CYP3A7	High	Begins to decline in the first week of life; very low in adults
Phase II		
Acetylase	Low	1 to 3 years of age
Glucuronosyltransferase	Low	6 to 18 months of age

APPLICATION TO PRACTICE

ASSESSMENT
History of Present Illness

Except for the obvious age-related differences between children and adults, assessment of the child resembles that of the adult, with certain additions. Children 5 years of age or older are usually able to add to the history. They often describe more accurately than parents the severity of symptoms and their own levels of concern. Sometimes the accuracy of the information can be improved by interviewing the child without the parent in attendance. Further, it should be clearly determined whether the chief complaint is the problem of the patient, the parent(s), or both. It should be noted that the chief complaint gets the patient into the health care system—a sort of "admission ticket." However, once with the health care provider, the child or parent may bring up another problem that in and of itself was not viewed as a legitimate reason for seeking care.

Health History

A pediatric health history provides information about operations and injuries, hospitalizations, drug history, birth history (i.e., prenatal, natal, and neonatal history—particularly important during the first 2 years of life), feeding history, and childhood illnesses. Knowledge of the feeding history (i.e., breast, bottle, solid foods) helps the health care provider identify problems of under- and overnutrition. The use of vitamin and iron supplements and immunization history should also be noted.

Special attention should be paid to children who have immigrated, because they may have received immunizations that are not routinely administered in the United States. Specific dates of each vaccination should be noted so that an ongoing record can be maintained throughout childhood and adolescence. Any untoward reactions to specific vaccines should also be noted.

Information about existing or past conditions that are familial or hereditary in parents, grandparents, aunts, uncles, and siblings should be obtained. Drug regimens can be affected in a patient with a history of, or potential for, glaucoma, cataracts, tuberculosis, asthma, heart disease, hypertension, kidney disease, arthritis, epilepsy, diabetes, and sickle cell disease.

Lifespan Considerations

The developmental status of a child places him or her at greater risk than an adult for physical and psychologic trauma related to drug therapy. Taking the developmental aspects of a child into account can lead to a better understanding of the child's response to drug therapy. Considerations such as the developmental norms for fine motor skills, gross motor skills, feeding behavior, language, and social skills should be identified and used in the planning of appropriate drug administration techniques.

Cultural/Social Considerations

Sensitivity to the issues of culture is essential in the care of children. The detail and depth of the cultural assessment depend on the situation and the needs of the child and family. Cultural practices may involve the use of "protective devices" (strings, cords, beads, amulets) to keep the child from harm or illness or to help in the healing process. These devices should be removed only by the patient or family and only when absolutely necessary. Cultural acceptance of clinical medicine may become a compliance issue as well.

Physical Examination

Emphasis during the pediatric physical exam should be placed on the anticipated findings and the signs and symptoms that accompany common pathologic conditions. The health care provider may anticipate a child's cooperative ability by merely asking the child where the physical examination should take place—in the parent's lap or on the examination table. A systematic approach to the examination minimizes the possibility of missing parts of it because of distraction by the child's behavior or the parent's questions.

Laboratory Testing

Screening procedures may be done, such as evaluations of vision and hearing; measurements of hemoglobin and hematocrit; and testing for phenylketonuria, galactosemia, sickle cell anemia, lead toxicity, and alpha$_1$-antitrypsin deficiency. Because pediatric patients have a limited ability to communicate when they are experiencing adverse drug effects, monitoring of therapeutic serum levels may be especially useful. This is particularly true when the effects of a drug cannot be directly observed or when the drug has a narrow therapeutic index (e.g., anticonvulsants, antineoplastic drugs, theophylline, digoxin).

GOALS OF THERAPY

The primary treatment goal for the pediatric patient is to achieve appropriate outcomes while maintaining therapeutic drug levels and avoiding toxic effects. Treatment goals also include allaying fears and preventing injury associated with drug regimens. Principles relevant to pediatric pharmacotherapy are identified in Box 3-1.

Treatment goals may be accomplished by limiting the number of drugs prescribed (avoiding polypharmacy), avoiding inappropriate drug use (e.g., wanting

<table>
<tr><td>

BOX 3-1

</td><td>

Pediatric Pharmacotherapeutic Principles

</td></tr>
</table>

- Provide explanations using developmental, age-appropriate language.
- Keep the time between explanation and administration to a minimum.
- Prepare drugs in advance, keeping needles and syringes out of sight.
- Expect success with positive approaches. Act smoothly and quickly.
- Be honest, involving the child to gain cooperation (e.g., "it will hurt," "drugs are not candy").
- Solicit parent's help where appropriate.
- Provide distraction for a frightened or uncooperative child.
- Allow the child to express feelings. Assure the child that crying is okay.
- Praise the child for doing his or her best.
- Spend time with the child after medication administration.
- Let the child know he or she is accepted as a person of value.

to try out a new drug or choosing a particular drug because samples are available), and ensuring that the drugs are taken as directed. Although some drugs pose a significant hazard to the pediatric patient, caution should be used until the health care provider has absolutely determined that a drug is indicated and appropriate for the child. Specific end points of therapy should be determined so that dosage can be optimized, irrational combinations avoided, and adverse effects minimized. In general, the least toxic, least expensive drug that treats the underlying cause of the child's illness (in preference to symptoms) should be chosen.

INTERVENTION
Administration

Optimal tailoring of a drug dose to the neonate, infant, or child has long been a subject of discussion. Any method devised to calculate drug dosage for children (and adults) provides an estimate only, to be verified or corrected by clinical response and/or measurement of drug concentrations. No universal dosage rule can be recommended. Today, drug manufacturers usually recommend doses in milligrams per kilogram of body weight, which are generally expressed as ranges rather than fixed doses. There is ample evidence that dosage regimens cannot be based simply on information extrapolated from adult data.

Pediatric drug therapy requires that dosage regimens be designed to account for developmental changes and to optimize therapy at different stages of childhood. The fact that a pediatric dosage cannot be found in current publications and references should be carefully considered before any dose is calculated. If a pediatric dosage cannot be found in current drug references, the drug may not be suitable for pediatric use.

Table 3-4 is a summary of developmental considerations for each age group as they relate to drug administration. As is true for all procedures, parents and children require age-appropriate education about drug administration as well as information about the drug. Table 3-5 is a summary of nursing considerations for drug administration to infants and children. An explanation of why the drug is given, what is expected of the child, and how the parent can participate and support the child should be given.

Infant. Oral drugs are delivered in liquid form by means of nipple, dropper, or syringe. The tongue movements of sucking cause the infant to spit out materials other than the nipple. The infant should be positioned to avoid aspiration of a drug, which should be administered slowly to minimize choking, with the hands restrained if necessary. The infant younger than 3 to 4 months does not have a well-developed sense of taste. Drug administration requires feeding behavior that establishes an easy, comfortable situation to form a trusting relationship. A pacifier may be used to distract an infant before administration of an injection.

Toddler. Toddlers have a limited concept of time, and resistive behaviors peak in this age group. Games may be used effectively to gain cooperation. A toddler who displays negativism should be approached in a positive manner. The child's rituals should be followed as much as possible to allow for a sense of control and to decrease anxiety. Drugs should be administered promptly; the child should be restrained as necessary and rewarded for positive behavior. A favorite juice or other liquid should be given after an oral dose of drug. Caregivers should be taught procedures for proper storage and disposal of drugs and containers to prevent accidental ingestion and subsequent poisoning.

Preschooler. A preschool child benefits from the opportunity to play with equipment and responds positively to explanations and comforting measures. A child of this age fears bodily intrusion and mutilation, so the use of suppositories can be especially upsetting. The health care provider should be truthful with the child about painful sensations, should address the child by name, and should be aware of the preschooler's well-developed coordination and sense of taste. The loss of deciduous teeth occurs in this age group and may need

TABLE 3-4

Developmental Considerations in Drug Administration

Developmental Age	*Implications*
Infancy (1 Month to 1 Year)	
Period of most rapid growth	Poor head control requires support to minimize choking
Develops trust	Monitor hands to prevent interference
Limited sensory and motor experiences	Drug dosages require precise measurement
Enjoys sucking and eating	Physical comfort during administration calms infant
Attends to environment	
Toddler (1 Year to 2 Years)	
Growth rate decreases along with appetite	Allow child to choose a position to take the drug
Increased independence	Follow routine of home
Increased mobility	Taste of drug may be disguised
Enjoys exploration	Use single commands
Seeks parental reassurance	Allow child to become familiar with dosing device
Preschool (3 Years to 6 Years)	
Weight gain 2 kg/yr	Tablets and capsules should be placed near back of tongue
Height increases 6-8 cm/yr	Allow child to make decisions about dosage formulation and
Greater autonomy and initiative	place of administration
Age of discovery, curiosity	More cooperative since understands relationships between illness
Sense of self versus others	and treatment
Increased muscle coordination	
Uses language as a tool to express self	
Trial-and-error learning	
Fears mutilation, loss of control, dark, ghosts	
School Age (6 Years to 12 Years)	
Growth relatively latent	Can usually swallow capsules or tablets
Develops logic	Praise child after drug administration
Develops skills and talents	Drug taking may have long-term benefits
Age of industry and increased competence	
Needs parental support	
Fears separation from friends, physical disability	
Adolescent (12 Years to 18 Years)	
Growth spurt begins at 9½ years for females and 10½ years for males	Include child in therapeutic decision making to foster respect
Puberty at age 8-13 years for females and 10-14 years for males	Incorporate group or peer activities as appropriate
Can project consequences	Able to appreciate causal relationships
Transitions from childhood to adulthood	Minimize dependent-drug regimens where possible
Quest for independence	
Displays risk-taking behaviors	
Fears change in appearance or functioning, dependency	

to be considered in the selection of drug formulation. The health care provider should involve the preschooler in choices, wherever possible, so that the child experiences some control over his or her treatment and environment.

School-Age Child. The school-age child enjoys taking responsibility for him- or herself. A reward system is an effective feedback mechanism. The child should be given a means to express fears about injections. Play activities will assist with coping. Drawings can be used to explain the effects of drugs on the body. By age 9, the child can tell time and assume some responsibility for self-medication.

Adolescent. The adolescent gains an identity through group membership. An adolescent patient should be allowed to manage his or her drug regimen when possi-

---

TABLE 3-5

Strategies for Drug Administration

Route	*Implications*
Ophthalmic	Apply finger pressure to lacrimal punctum aspect of inner lid for 1 minute to prevent drainage of the drug into nasopharynx and unpleasant tasting of drug.
Otic	Children under 3 years of age: pull pinna down and back. Children over 3 years of age: pull pinna up and back. Warm drops to avoid causing pain of the tympanic membrane.
Nasal	Hold the infant in the cradle position, stabilizing the head and tilting it back. Give nose drops 20-30 minutes before feeding; infants are nose breathers and nasal congestion inhibits sucking.
Oral	Administer drug to infants using syringe, nipple, or dropper. Do not add drugs to formulas or other essential foods. Chewable tablets may be crushed and added to small amount of flavored syrup, jelly, or applesauce. Do not crush enteric-coated capsules. Do not open capsules if sustained-release formulation. In 1-month-old infants and children with neurologic impairments, blowing a small puff of air in the face elicits a swallow reflex.
Subcutaneous	Injections are made just below the skin at a 90-degree angle in the deltoid, anterior thigh, abdominal wall, or subscapular areas in volumes of 0.5-1 mL. Use 25 or 26 gauge $\frac{3}{8}$-inch needles for infants; use 25 or 26 gauge $\frac{5}{8}$-inch needles for larger children.
Intramuscular	Consider placing a wrapped ice cube on the site for 1 minute before injection to reduce discomfort. Select needle size appropriate to the volume to be administered, drug viscosity, muscle mass to be penetrated, and the child's age. Volume is limited to 0.5 mL for infants and 2.0 mL for older children. After drug is drawn into syringe, change the needle prior to giving the injection. Insertion of the needle through a rubber stopper dulls the tip. After injection, children should be comforted and given a reward. Injection sites include vastus lateralis (largest muscle group in children under 3 years); ventrogluteal muscle (for a child over 3 years—easily accessible; can tolerate large volumes); dorsogluteal (for children under 3 years—large mass in older children; danger of sciatic nerve injury); and deltoid (small muscle mass; rapid absorption rate).
Intravenous	Desired effect is rapidly achieved. Volumetric device and/or infusion pump should be used for infants and young children. Administer following guidelines for dilution and infusion time. Check drug-drug compatibilities.
Venous access device	Requires special procedures to access (i.e., Huber, Groshong, Broviac, Hickman catheters are above the skin; MediPort, Infus-a-Port are below the skin). Broviac and Hickman devices require clamping. Groshong devices do not because they contain a two-way valve. Broviac and Groshong devices require daily or weekly flush to maintain patency. Implanted ports such as the MediPort and Infus-a-Port are flushed monthly.
Rectal	Place the child in the side-lying position. Lubricate the suppository. Consult a pharmacist before cutting a suppository. If still appropriate, cut the suppository lengthwise since the drugs are not distributed evenly throughout.

ble. It helps to foster identity formation. However, close monitoring is essential to ensure compliance. Disorders and drugs affecting body appearance may be particularly stressful for an adolescent. Preparation for drug administration is important. A confident, matter-of-fact approach should be used, and the adolescent should be given an opportunity to express feelings or concerns about the treatment regimen.

Education

Children's and adolescents' reactions to drug regimens are affected by physical and cognitive abilities, developmental characteristics, environmental influences, past experiences, current relationship with the health care provider, and perception of the present situation. Helpful approaches and explanations can increase the potential for compliance.

Management of drug therapy requires of the caregiver or parent attention, coordination, and some understanding of the drug being given. Stress or fatigue from caring for a sick child may contribute to a drug administration error. In some cases, young or unseasoned parents do not have the experience to ask appropriate questions and thus clarify their understanding of the drug regimen. Drug misuse in pediatric patients has many common causes. The use of multiple medication dispensers (e.g., one each for father, mother, and day-care center personnel) may increase the risk of repeated or missed doses. Drugs prescribed for a previous illness or for a sibling with similar symptoms may be inappropriate for the present illness.

Considerable variation exists in the understanding of the term *teaspoon*, leading to errors in measurement. Misinterpretation of the route of administration may occur. For example, ear drops may be prescribed "for the ear" or prescribed to be placed "in the ear." The ability of the parent or caregiver to recognize adverse effects is complicated by the child's lack of language and inability to recognize, understand, and communicate symptoms. The belief that "if a little is good, more is better" can lead to accidental ingestion and possible overdose.

One solution to these potential problems is parent and caregiver education. Assessment of the parents' and caregivers' level of understanding is a must. Caregivers must know what the drug is. They must know the dosage, frequency, and route; the length of time the drug is to be administered; and the anticipated effects of the drug. Finally, they must be told whom to contact if they observe adverse reactions to the drug. The use of written instructions and a demonstration of administration techniques are appropriate to caregiver education. Following these general principles helps to ensure safe, accurate, and timely drug administration.

The issue of compliance with therapeutic regimens rests on the willingness of others to assist in the child's care. Follow-up by telephone or through a community health nurse may ensure that the pharmacotherapeutic regimen is accurately implemented.

EVALUATION

Application of the principles of normal growth and development and knowledge of what constitutes deviations from normal help to individualize care. Meticulous, ongoing assessment and evaluation is essential to optimal pediatric drug therapy. The approach chosen should facilitate a positive experience for the health care provider, the patient, and the family. Awareness of the physiologic and developmental changes, conscious attention to the pharmacokinetics and pharmacodynamics of the required drugs, and early recognition of potential complications is essential.

Bibliography

Bindler RM, Howry LB: *Pediatric drugs and nursing implications,* ed 2, Upper Saddle River, NJ, 1997, Prentice Hall.

Wong DL, Whaley LF, Wilson D, et al: *Nursing care of infants and children,* ed 6, St Louis, 1999, Mosby.

Yaffe SJ, Aranda JV: *Pediatric pharmacology: therapeutic principles in practice,* ed 2, Philadelphia, 1991, WB Saunders.

Internet Resources

Committee on Drugs, American Academy of Pediatrics: Guidelines for the ethical conduct of studies to evaluate drugs in pediatric populations, 1995. Available online: http://www.aap.org/policy/00655.html.

Committee on Drugs and Committee on Hospital Care, American Academy of Pediatrics: Prevention of medication errors in the pediatric inpatient setting. Pediatrics 102:2, 428-430, 1998. Available online: http://www.aap.org/policy/re9751.html.

School Nurse: Medications in school, 2001. Available online: http://www.schoolnurse.com.

CHAPTER

4

Older Adult Pharmacotherapeutics

KATHLEEN GUTIERREZ

 Visit http://evolve.elsevier.com/Gutierrez/ for additional information.

KEY TERMS

Aspiration, p. 47
Drug holiday, p. 51
Hypoalbuminemia, p. 49
Hypochlorhydria, p. 47
Polypharmacy, p. 50
Presbycusis, p. 47
Presbyopia, p. 47
Stroke volume, p. 47

OBJECTIVES

- Recognize the anatomic and physiologic differences in body systems of older adults that affect pharmacotherapeutics.
- Discuss the health care provider's responsibility in recognizing how aging affects pharmacokinetics and pharmacodynamics.
- Identify and discuss factors that promote polypharmacy in the older adult.
- Identify the management strategies associated with older adult pharmacotherapeutics.

In 1930, slightly more than 6 million persons were over age 65, and the average life expectancy was 59 years. At the beginning of the twenty-first century, life expectancy in the United States has reached 74.9 years, a record high. Those older than 65 years represent more than 12% of the population in the United States today, and by the year 2020 that number will increase to more than 20% (Figure 4-1). Advances in disease control and health care technologies, reduced infant mortality rates, improved sanitation, and better living conditions have helped to increase life expectancy for most Americans (Box 4-1).

Chronic illness contributes to self-care limitations in almost half of all older adults, and one fourth of this group has difficulty with the activities of daily living. The older the person is, the greater the likelihood he or she is undergoing drug therapy, and the greater the need for assistance with the tasks of daily living becomes,

45

FIGURE 4-1

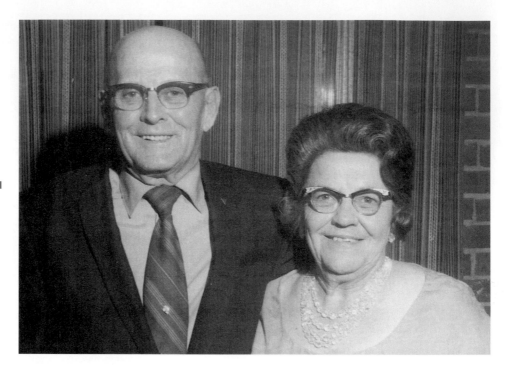

while the likelihood of remaining totally independent declines.

Persons over age 65 buy 35% of all prescription drugs and more than 40% of over-the-counter drugs sold in the United States at an annual cost exceeding $3 billion. The average older adult living at home has 11 different prescriptions filled annually; residents of extended care facilities average 8 prescriptions a year. The drugs most commonly prescribed include diuretics, potassium salts, histamine-2 antagonists, nitroglycerin, insulin, cardiac glycosides, beta-blockers, antianxiety drugs, and antihypertensives. The most common over-the-counter drugs purchased by older adults are analgesics, antiinflammatory drugs, laxatives, and antacids.

ANATOMIC AND PHYSIOLOGIC VARIABLES

As we age, a variety of physiologic changes increase the risk of drug sensitivity and drug-induced disease. It should be noted that chronologic age is not necessarily related to physiologic age. However, with aging there is a gradual decline in many body functions, with some

systems more affected than others. Indeed, the variations among people of the same age are so great that increased biologic variation is characteristic of this age group. This is particularly true of functions that affect drug disposition and response. Therefore, every older adult must be evaluated individually.

Body Composition

The age-related changes in body composition are best seen in the extracellular tissues. Elastin, found in tissues associated with body movement (e.g., walls of major blood vessels, heart, lungs, and skin), is reduced and replaced with pseudoelastin. Tissues become less pliable and ultimately less efficient. Double chins, elongated ears, and baggy eyelids are obvious manifestations of elastin loss. Aortic stenosis may also develop as elastin is replaced with pseudoelastin.

In men, there is a steady increase in lipids until age 60, after which there is a gradual decrease. As subcutaneous body fat atrophies, contours gain a bony appearance, with deepening of intercostal and supraclavicular spaces, orbits, and axillas. Skin-fold thickness is significantly reduced in the forearm and on the back of the hand with the loss of subcutaneous fat. This loss is also responsible for a decline in the body's natural insulation, making older adults sensitive to cold and putting them at risk for hypothermia. Many of the lipids are stored in endothelial tissues of arteries, contributing to atherosclerosis. In women, fat and lipids continue to accumulate.

Although the amount of extracellular fluids remains fairly constant, intracellular volume is decreased, resulting in less overall total body fluid. This change puts the older adult at risk for dehydration.

As with cells and tissues, there is a decrease in the functional capacity of body organs. Physiologic reserves begin declining at about age 30, especially in cardiac, respiratory, and renal function. As a result, maintenance of homeostasis becomes increasingly difficult. Although changes in these organ systems occur gradually and are generally insignificant, moderate or severe stressors can precipitate unexpected problems or organ failure.

Cardiovascular System

Various physiologic changes occur in the cardiovascular system. The efficiency and contractile strength of the myocardium decline, resulting in a 1% per year reduction in cardiac output. **Stroke volume**, the amount of blood ejected from the heart with each beat, decreases by 0.7% yearly, and systole and diastole are prolonged. Ordinarily, older adults adjust to these changes without much difficulty. However, when unusual demands are placed on the heart (e.g., shoveling snow, running to catch a bus, comorbid acute illness), the changes become more evident. Pulse rates may not reach the levels found in younger persons, and tachycardia lasts longer. In some older adults, blood pressure remains stable but tachycardia progresses to heart failure.

Resistance to peripheral blood flow increases by 1% each year. Reduced elasticity of the arteries is responsible for vascular changes to the heart, kidneys, and pituitary gland. The rigidity of vessel walls and narrowing of lumens require more force to move blood through the vessels. These changes lead to a higher diastolic blood pressure. There is also a decrease in the ability of the aorta to distend, in turn causing a rise in systolic pressure. Vagal tone increases as the heart becomes more sensitive to carotid sinus stimulation. Reduced sensitivity of baroreceptors potentiates orthostatic hypotension. The normal changes of aging do not usually influence venous circulation.

Gastrointestinal System

Although gastrointestinal (GI) problems are not seen as life threatening in most cases, older adults often have many GI complaints. Decreased activity of the salivary glands and drier mucous membranes contribute to difficulty swallowing. Lowered esophageal motility and relaxation of the lower esophageal sphincter may occur. **Aspiration** becomes a risk when these factors combine with a weaker gag reflex and delayed esophageal emptying.

Many indigestion problems are related to increases in gastric pH and reduced amounts of hydrochloric acid (**hypochlorhydria**), pepsin, lipase, and pancreatic enzymes. The aging pancreas produces normal amounts of bicarbonate and amylase, but there is a decrease in li-

pase, resulting in subclinical abnormalities in fat absorption. Reduced fat absorption is accompanied by reduced absorption of fat-soluble vitamins as well as faulty absorption of vitamins B_1 and B_{12}, calcium, and iron.

Liver cells change in size and character, and hepatic blood flow is altered. Hepatic protein synthesis is compromised, and there are changes in the microsomal enzyme systems involved in a variety of metabolic pathways. Thus biotransformation of drugs is altered.

Intestinal blood flow decreases, which may reduce the absorption of substances actively transported from the intestinal lumen (e.g., some sugars, minerals, and vitamins). The intestinal mucosa atrophies, decreasing in surface area, and the intestinal musculature weakens. Peristalsis slows, contributing to constipation.

Renal System

A 50% decrease in renal blood flow and glomerular filtration rate develops between the ages of 20 and 90 years. There is a possibility of protein loss because of decreased cardiac output, reduced renal blood flow, and lower glomerular filtration rates. Tubular reabsorption lessens, and a lower threshold for glucose and creatinine clearance develops. As a result, the kidneys are less effective in concentrating urine. At younger ages the urinary specific gravity is about 1.032, but at age 80 it may be as low as 1.024.

Sensory-Perceptual Function

The eyes of an older adult undergo a variety of changes that affect functional capacity as well as the ability to protect oneself from hazards and to enjoy a high quality of life. The aging eye loses the ability to accommodate and focus for near vision (**presbyopia**). As a result, many persons over 40 require corrective lenses. Lens opacity accompanied by a decreased tolerance for glare may develop. A gradual narrowing of the visual field also occurs.

Yellowing of the lens and altered color perception make the older adult less able to differentiate the low-tone colors of the blues, greens, and violets. Depth perception changes, causing problems in judging the height of steps or curbs; bifocals compound this problem. Adaptation to light and dark takes longer. Sclerosis of the pupillary sphincter and a decrease in pupil size make the pupil less responsive to light. Further, reabsorption of intraocular fluid is less efficient, increasing the risk for glaucoma. Reduced tear production leads to less lustrous eyes and complaints of dryness.

Deterioration of the cochlea and neurons of the higher auditory pathways leads to sensorineural hearing loss (**presbycusis**). High-pitched sounds such as *s, sh, f, ch,* and *ph* are initially impaired, followed by the middle and low frequencies. The change is so gradual and subtle that affected persons may not realize the magnitude of the hearing loss. Stiffening of the cilia combined with a higher keratin content causes cerumen to become easily impacted, further decreasing hearing.

PHARMACOKINETIC CONSIDERATIONS

Drug effects are different in older adults, owing either to pharmacokinetic or to pharmacodynamic factors. Comparatively speaking, older adults have less difficulty with drug absorption than with distribution, biotransformation, or elimination. A summary of the physiologic changes of aging that result in pharmacokinetic alterations is found in Table 4-1.

Absorption

A number of variables affect drug absorption in the older adult. Decreases in gastric motility and in the production of trypsin delay or impair drug absorption. Drugs affecting gastric acidity, motility, or trypsin production (e.g., laxatives, antacids, anticholinergics, levodopa) affect the absorption of other drugs. Conditions such as increased gastric pH alter the absorption of weak acids and bases. For example, weak acids (e.g., barbiturates) are more ionized in the GI tract at higher pH and therefore are less well absorbed. In contrast, at higher pH weak bases are less ionized and better absorbed. As a result, older adults may not respond as quickly to an oral dose of a drug as persons in other age groups.

In addition, the decrease in cardiac output results in a 40% to 50% reduction in perfusion of the GI tract because blood flow to the area must be sacrificed to maintain coronary and cerebral blood flow. The result is delayed, less thorough, and less reliable removal of drugs and other substances from the intestinal lumen.

Distribution

Changes in circulation and body composition affect drug distribution and equilibration rates because aging

---

TABLE 4-1

Pharmacokinetic Impact of the Changes of Aging

Normal Physiologic Changes	Pharmacokinetic Impact
Reduced long- and short-term memory in some patients	Increased risk of unintentional noncompliance
Reduced visual acuity	Increased risk of drug errors because of poor vision
Decreased cardiac output	Decreased biotransformation and excretion of drugs resulting in increased circulation time
Decreased blood flow to organs and tissues	Potentially decreased absorption of orally administered drugs; vaginal and rectal suppositories take longer to dissolve and may be prematurely expelled; decreased biotransformation and excretion of drugs
Altered peripheral vascular tone and reduced baroreceptor activity	Exaggerated effects of antihypertensives and diuretics
Decreased enzymatic activity in liver	Altered biotransformation and detoxification processes; biotransformation time is lengthened and both parent drug and active metabolites exert effects for extended periods; drug toxicity may occur more readily
Decreased serum albumin	Decreased availability of albumin for binding, leading to increased amounts of unbound drug and increased drug activity
Increased adipose tissue	Altered distribution and increased concentration of fat-soluble drugs in adipose tissue; some drugs reach greater peak concentrations with longer half-lives
Decreased tissue elasticity and reduced muscle mass	Poor absorption of drugs with poor healing of tissues after injection
Increased gastric pH and reduced gastric acid	Decreased absorption of drugs that are normally nonionized at low pH (weak acids)
Decreased body water	Drier mucous membranes may cause drugs to stick to the oral cavity and cause irritation; increased water-soluble drug concentration in bloodstream
Changes in sensitivity of drug receptor sites	Increased or decreased drug activity

alters many of the factors that influence protein binding, volume of distribution, the amount of body fat present, and regional perfusion patterns.

Body weight decreases, especially in those over 75, but the ratio of fat to lean body mass is usually greater. Adipose tissue levels increase from 18% to 30% in men and from 35% to 48% in women. The enlarged fat compartment increases the volume of distribution of lipid-soluble drugs. In other words, changes in adipose tissue raise tissue concentrations and the duration of drug action while lowering plasma concentrations. For example, a highly fat-soluble drug (e.g., diazepam) has a greater volume of distribution and a prolonged distribution phase, leading to an extended half-life.

The decline in total body water percentage with age means that highly water-soluble drugs will have a smaller volume of distribution. Drugs such as gentamicin may have elevated plasma concentrations in the aged. Because drugs in this class are almost exclusively excreted by the kidneys, and renal function falls with age, the end result can be a dangerous accumulation of drug.

Depressed plasma albumin levels (**hypoalbuminemia**) result in higher concentrations of unbound drug. The effect of this change is not always predictable. As the amount of unbound drug rises, the amount of drug available for producing an effect increases, but so does the amount available for biotransformation and excretion. For example, a highly protein-bound drug (e.g., phenytoin) undergoes greater biotransformation, decreasing serum drug levels and therapeutic effects. In contrast, another highly protein-bound drug such as the anticoagulant warfarin produces greater effects in patients with low serum albumin levels. Examples of highly protein-bound drugs that may require reduced dosages during states of dehydration and hypoalbuminemia are noted in Box 4-2.

Other factors altering drug distribution in the older adult include poor nutrition, extremes of body weight, electrolyte and mineral imbalances, inactivity, and prolonged bed rest.

BOX 4-2	**Examples of Highly Protein-Bound Drugs**

acetazolamine	digitoxin	propranolol
amitriptyline	furosemide	rifampin
cefazolin	hydralazine	Salicylates
chlordiazepoxide	nortriptyline	spironolactone
chlorpromazine	phenylbutazone	sulfisoxazole
cloxacillin	phenytoin	warfarin

Biotransformation

It is difficult to generalize the effect of advanced age on biotransformation. Because of wide differences in the decline of enzyme systems and organs of excretion, it is impossible to make blanket statements about drug biotransformation. Older adults are, in many ways, a more heterogeneous group than younger adults. Although biotransformation of some drugs decreases, there are no changes in the clearance of most drugs.

Although the liver remains functional in the older adult, the ability to biotransform drugs changes. A person who lives to be 100 has a 50% reduction in liver mass, with the greatest decrease occurring between the ages of 60 and 70. Drug biotransformation in the liver depends on two processes: hepatic blood flow and microsomal enzyme activity. With aging, blood flow to the liver is reduced such that less drug is delivered to the liver. The reduced blood flow and lower enzyme activity can be particularly significant with drugs for which metabolic rates depend on hepatic blood flow (e.g., propranolol).

The complex relationship between aging and hepatic enzyme function depends on the type of metabolic reaction and the patient's gender. Biotransformation of drugs occurs in two phases (see Chapter 1). Oxidation, reduction, and hydrolysis make up Phase I reactions. These processes lead to minor changes in drug molecules and typically produce active metabolites. Oxidative capacity declines with age, more so in men than in women. The effect on oxidative metabolism is consistent for drugs with low hepatic extraction rates. Data are less clear about drugs with high extraction ratios because their biotransformation rates depend on hepatic blood flow in addition to hepatic enzyme activity. Liver size is a significant determinant in the elimination of drugs with high extraction ratios, regardless of age.

Phase II reactions combine the drug or its metabolite with acetic, glucuronic, sulfuric, or amino acids, leading to the production of inactive compounds. Aging reduces the efficacy of both phases of biotransformation, but Phase I reactions are more affected than Phase II reactions. Although no significant effects have been reported, the smaller size and reduced function of the liver interferes with the formation of prothrombin, albumin, and vitamins A and D. Conditions such as dehydration, hyperthermia, immobility, and liver disease reduce drug biotransformation. As a consequence, drugs can accumulate to toxic levels. Additionally, the extended half-life of many drugs (e.g., morphine, meperidine, propoxyphene, propranolol, lidocaine, phenylbutazone, warfarin, amobarbital, and benzodiazepines) warrants close monitoring of drug clearance in older patients. Drugs that are normally subject to a considerable first-pass effect (e.g., propranolol) are especially prone to producing exaggerated effects in older adults.

Excretion

With aging, the number of functional nephrons falls by as much as 64% and the glomerular filtration rate by 46%. This normal decline in filtration rate is not reflected in the serum creatinine level, because the comparable loss in muscle mass reduces creatinine production. This means that an older patient may not have a higher serum creatinine level until the dysfunction is severe. These excretory changes are accompanied by a similar decrease in renal blood flow. Tubular secretory mechanisms decrease, and the ability to concentrate urine is diminished. In addition, cardiovascular disease, dehydration, and kidney disease commonly impair renal functioning. Thus the half-life of a drug may be increased by as much as 40%. Because drugs remain in the body longer, the risk of adverse effects increases.

PHARMACODYNAMIC CONSIDERATIONS

Many patient responses to a drug do not result from pharmacokinetic factors. Instead, they can be caused by drug-receptor or drug-organ interactions. Aging reduces tissue responsiveness to drugs in a number of ways. Drug-receptor response can be altered with age by the declining functional capacity of organs and thus the total number of receptors. Therefore any adverse effects are more keenly felt. The effects of drugs that impair liver, kidney, or cardiac function may go unnoticed in younger individuals with adequate reserves but can be dangerous in the older adult. In addition, the vitality of control mechanisms is reduced, the maintenance of homeostasis is less dynamic, and compensatory responses to primary drug effects are less profound; for example, drugs that raise blood pressure often do so in a more profound manner, because the vagal reflex is less efficient in generating a compensatory reduction in cardiac output.

Another age-related change in drug response is increased sensitivity of the myocardium to anesthetics. Inotropic drugs (see Chapter 38) are well known for their narrow therapeutic index in all patients, but older adults are particularly prone to toxicity. Older adults also exhibit reduced pharmacodynamic responsiveness to quinidine but a greater sensitivity to lidocaine. Vascular responses to norepinephrine and cardiac response to isoproterenol and other catecholamines are somewhat diminished (see Chapter 12).

Orthostatic hypotension caused by antihypertensive drugs (see Chapter 41), antidepressants (see Chapter 18), and antipsychotic drugs (see Chapter 19) is more common in older adults who are volume depleted as a result of diuretic therapy (see Chapter 46). In addition, potassium-wasting diuretics such as furosemide can cause hypokalemia, thereby potentiating the effects of cardiac gly-

cosides. The incidence of hyperkalemia in older patients taking potassium-sparing diuretics (e.g., spironolactone) is higher, possibly because renal function is impaired.

Older adults are also more susceptible to the effects of neuromuscular blocking drugs in that the blockade is more intense and prolonged. In general, patients of advanced age are more sensitive to drugs acting within the central nervous system. Thus barbiturates, benzodiazepines, lithium, opioid analgesics, tricyclic antidepressants, and phenothiazines demonstrate both therapeutic and toxic effects at lower doses.

In the autonomic nervous system, beta-adrenergic responses to both agonists and antagonists appear to be blunted. As a result, older adults show diminished response and increased toxicity to beta-blocking drugs. Aging causes a decline in parasympathetic control, which enhances the effects of anticholinergic drugs (see Chapter 11). Age also reduces the amount of neurotransmitters, particularly dopamine and acetylcholine. Reduced dopamine in the brain increases the older adult's susceptibility to the extrapyramidal effects of neuroleptics, metoclopramide, and other drugs.

Central nervous system effects of sedative-hypnotics and antianxiety drugs include paradoxical responses, characterized by restlessness, disorientation, and confusion. Balance disturbances are also of concern in that they often lead to falls and subsequent injury. In contrast, the effects of stimulants such as amphetamines on motor activity are diminished in the older adult, but their anorexic effects are enhanced.

Several endocrine changes influence drug response. For example, the age-related decline in glucose tolerance causes greater hyperglycemia than normal in response to a thiazide diuretic. Older adults do not seek treatment as early as a younger adult may, because their response to drug-induced hypoglycemia is reduced. In addition, diminished thyroid function decreases the metabolic rate, which in turn slows drug biotransformation.

Polypharmacy

Compounding the effect of physiologic aging on pharmacokinetics and pharmacodynamics is the presence of comorbid chronic disease. The higher incidence of chronic diseases generally results in greater use of prescriptive and over-the-counter drugs. **Polypharmacy** is the result not only of multiple disease processes but also of the prescribing behaviors of health care providers and of poorly coordinated patient management. Polypharmacy results in a higher risk of adverse effects, drug interactions, extended hospital stays, and reduced compliance. Ironically, drug reactions that mimic medical-physical complaints are often treated with yet another drug.

The rate of adverse effects is directly proportional to the number of drugs taken. Patients receiving two drugs have a 5.6% risk for a drug interaction, whereas those receiving five drugs have a 50% risk. Patients receiving eight different drugs have a 100% chance for a drug interaction. Adverse drug reactions in older adults are responsible for more than 243,000 hospitalizations, 32,000 hip fractures, 160,000 changes in mental status, and 2 million cases of drug dependence. Although polypharmacy is significant in older adults, it is commonly overlooked as a factor in patient symptoms. In addition, excessive drug use by the older adult inadvertently creates an economically, psychologically, and physiologically costly cycle of events from which he or she may never recover. One strategy that may be needed in sorting out drug interactions caused by polypharmacy is a **drug holiday**, that is, a period of time in which specific drugs are not taken and the patient responses are observed.

APPLICATION TO PRACTICE

ASSESSMENT

The health care provider must first establish a climate of reassurance and trust with the older adult. A warm greeting with an extended hand and good eye contact almost always results in acceptance of the hand. The health care provider should maintain the hand contact as long as the older adult shows an inclination to do so, but should be sensitive to painful, paralyzed, or traumatized hands.

Physical limitations the patient may have should be considered in the planning of the interview and physical examination. Sensory-perceptual impairments are often present. The patient who is hearing impaired should be faced directly, so that the interviewer's mouth and face are fully visible. Contrary to popular practice, it does not help to shout; shouting actually distorts speech.

In some cases, it may be necessary to break up the interview into more than one visit and collect the most important historical data first. Certain portions of the data such as health history or the review of systems can be provided on a form that the patient fills out at home. However, using a form assumes that the older patient has the capacity to complete it. The completed form should then be reviewed with the patient during the interview.

It is important to pace the assessment of older adults, who often have a great deal of background material to sort through. Furthermore, some older adults need more time to interpret questions and process answers. They should not be rushed—any indication of rushing may cause the patient to retreat with valuable data lost, leaving his or her needs unmet.

Touch is a nonverbal skill that is significant to older adults. Their other senses may be impaired, so touch helps ground the interviewer in reality. A hand on the patient's arm or shoulder is an empathic message communicating interest. It is important to keep a person's cultural background in mind, because certain cultures (e.g., Orthodox Jewish, Hindu Indians, Japanese, and upper class Vietnamese) avoid some types of touch.

Occasionally, an older adult asks personal questions about the interviewer's life or opinions. A brief response may be appropriate, but thought should be given to the motive behind the personal questions. Loneliness or anxiety may be directing them. Sexual innuendoes, flirtatious compliments, or advances occur on rare occasions. Some people perceive acute or chronic illness as threats to self-esteem and sexual adequacy. The interviewer should make sure to communicate acceptance of the older adult and understanding of the need to be self-assertive but should make clear that sexual advances will not be tolerated.

History of Present Illness

The patient should be carefully questioned about the problems for which he or she is seeking care. History of the present illness should include the onset of the problem, the setting in which it occurred, manifestations, and any self-treatment attempted. Principal complaints should be described in terms of location, quality, quantity or severity, timing, the setting in which they occur, aggravating and alleviating factors, and any associated symptoms.

The history of the present illness should also include the older adult's responses to symptoms and limitations. The interviewer should ask what the patient thinks caused the problem. What underlying worries might the patient have that led him or her to seek attention, and why are they worries? Any effects the illness has had on the activities of daily living should be noted. An older adult may shrug off a symptom as evidence of growing older and may be unsure that it is worth mentioning. Furthermore, some older adults maintain the philosophy that "if it ain't broken, don't fix it." These patients may seek care only when there is a blatant problem.

Health History

In addition to the history of the present illness, the general state of health as the patient perceives it over the past 5 years should be noted. The occurrences of adult illnesses, accidents, injuries, operations, and hospitalizations should be elicited. It is usually unnecessary to include obstetric history for a woman who has passed menopause and has no gynecologic symptoms. However, a perimenopausal history should be obtained, including any symptoms and whether or not estrogen replacement therapy is or was used.

Information on current use of prescribed and over-the-counter drugs, home remedies, herbals, and vitamins should also be elicited from the patient. Drug allergies should be documented, including the description of an allergic response, when it occurred, interventions used, and any sequelae. A listing of the name, strength, and directions for use of each drug should be noted. As-needed drugs should be included, especially if the patient reports taking them at least once a week. The prescriber of the drug(s) should also be identified during the interview, and the information elicited from the patient should be checked against prescription labels.

Ideally, older adults should be encouraged to bring to their appointments all drugs they are taking. Prescription bottles provide additional information, such as the name of the pharmacy that dispensed the drug. The reason for the use of more than one pharmacy should be elicited. Because the older adult tends to save leftover drugs, expiration dates should also be noted. Expired drugs should be destroyed because of the potential for ineffectiveness or toxicity; the patient's permission must be requested before disposal.

Additionally, older adults should be questioned about how they remember to take scheduled drugs, whether they ever forget to take a dose, and if so, what they do about it. Have they ever intentionally discontinued a drug, and if so, why? This information helps evaluate the patient's understanding of and compliance with the drug regimen as well as its safety. The interviewer should explore the possibility that physical impairments, memory loss, health or cultural beliefs, financial constraints, or lack of support systems are impairing safe self-administration of drugs.

Lifespan Considerations

The older adult has the potential for more personal losses than younger people. Losses of loved ones, job status and prestige, income, and an energetic and resilient body occur with time. The grief and despair surrounding these losses can affect mental status, leading to disorientation, disability, or depression.

The interviewer should attempt to learn the priorities and goals of the older adult as well as how he or she has handled crises in the past. Because the patient may pursue similar adaptive patterns in the present situation, this information can help with care planning. It is also helpful to determine the patient's perception of the sit-

uation. Such information can be elicited by asking questions such as the following:

- Can you tell me how you feel about getting older?
- What kinds of things do you find most satisfying?
- What kinds of things worry you?
- What would you like to change if you could?

It is normal for older adults to reminisce about the past and to reflect upon previous experiences, including joys, regrets, and conflicts. Listening to the life review process provides important insights into developmental conflicts.

Cultural/Social Considerations

Although variations exist, the typical older adult has at least one serious illness or limiting condition and is aware of the increasing frequency of death among his or her peers. These issues, coupled with society's generally negative view of aging, lead to a fear that all that remains of youth has been lost. The task, then, is not so much to look for new forms of youthfulness, but rather to seek forms of continued usefulness. The search may take the older adult toward new creative endeavors. He or she has often stepped offstage both in formal employment and in the family circle. This change can be traumatic, because it means a loss of recognition and authority. However, there is now an attempt to direct energy inward. When financially and socially secure, the older adult can pursue whatever activity is important. Spending more time at home also affects the marriage relationship. Some couples find that having one or both at home means invasion of previously held "turf," such as the kitchen, the garden, or the workshop.

The older adult has the task of finding the meaning of life, the purpose for his or her own existence, and adjusting to the inevitability of death. The majority of older adults possess self-assurance and a calm demeanor, providing satisfying answers to questions. However, the interviewer must watch for the occasional person who sounds hopeless and despairing about life at present and in the future. Requests for antianxiety drugs or sedative-hypnotics may help identify the person who has difficulty coping.

Physical Examination

When the history has been completed, the focus of the physical examination is established. The decision is made to perform either a baseline total examination or a limited but detailed examination of body systems related to the patient's complaint.

The approach to assessment must be tailored to the older person's needs. The standard method for physical examination may be quite appropriate for the young person or an alert, oriented older adult who is not acutely ill and has no sensory deficits. However, the examination may need to be modified for the older person who is acutely ill and who may not be able to accomplish or tolerate the usual positions for the examination. Rest periods may be required during the examination.

To organize the examination and to minimize omissions and patient fatigue, the examiner should follow three practices: (1) minimize changes of patient position (where possible), (2) organize the body into units for examination, and (3) integrate the information sought according to body systems. The entire body can be examined by placing the patient in a sequence of positions: standing, sitting, supine, sitting again, and the lithotomy, or side-lying, position (when needed).

Because older adults are often cold and at risk for hypothermia, it is necessary to limit exposure of body parts to a minimum. This is accomplished with the appropriate use of a patient gown and drapes, which also conveys to the patient the examiner's respect for privacy.

A major concern in working with the old-old is mobility and balance. The patient may need assistance getting into position for the examination because of limitations of sensory perception or physical mobility, confusion, agitation, or other problems. Assistance should be provided as indicated. Some physical examination techniques (e.g., deep knee bends) may not be appropriate. Other techniques need modification, such as testing the range of hip motion in a person who has had a total hip replacement or prosthesis. Care must be taken in performing any procedure that has the potential to result in injury or a fall.

Some patients have physical deformities that require modification in positioning. For example, the person with severe kyphosis may have difficulty maintaining a supine position. The person with hip contracture requires modifications in the lithotomy position. Patients who use wheelchairs or require walkers for balance cannot perform a Romberg test.

As the examination proceeds, each step should be prefaced with an explanation. Explanations help alleviate the fear, anger, and resistance that might occur if the patient were examined without explanation. For the hearing-impaired patient who can see, the demonstration of the instruments on the examiner before they are used on the patient improves understanding and increases cooperation.

For the patient who is both hearing and vision impaired, touch is the only means of communication. The examiner should gently guide the patient's hand to the examiner's face, shoulders, and hands. The patient should be allowed to feel the instruments before they are used in the examination. The investment of time and encouragement of touch communicate the examiner's goodwill and respect for the patient's identity.

Laboratory Testing

Laboratory testing of the older adult includes laboratory screening studies as well as hepatic and renal function testing to establish baselines and to monitor drug therapy. Because of the age-related decline in renal function and the use of potentially nephrotoxic drugs, monitoring of renal function is vital.

A variety of assessment instruments may also be used, such as the CADET, a self-care assessment tool. This tool addresses the patient's level of independence as it relates to Communication, Ambulation, activities of Daily living, Elimination, and Transfer abilities. The Comprehensive Older Person's Evaluation (COPE) instrument, similar to the CADET, uses cognition, social support, financial considerations, physical and psychologic health, and activities of daily living categories. A number of other instruments are available to help assess the patient's functional status. These assessments are vital, particularly for older adults who are living alone or who have multiple limitations. Not all older adults are in need of supervision.

GOALS OF THERAPY

The goal of drug therapy in the older adult is to maintain health status using the fewest drugs possible. Drug dosing should be individualized to decrease the likelihood of noncompliance, adverse drug reactions, or interactions. The purpose of and need for each drug should be weighed. The possibility of additive adverse effects from several drugs should be considered in the formulation of management objectives. Use of drugs that exacerbate disease states should be questioned. Although drug prescribing is in the hands of those with legal authority to do so, there are six basic principles that should be followed:

- Start low and go slow.
- Start one drug, stop two.
- Do not use a drug if the adverse effects are worse than the disease.
- Use as few drugs as possible, choosing nondrug therapies when possible.
- Assess the patient's response frequently.
- Consider drug holidays from time to time.

Ideally, drug regimens are kept simple with the least frequent administration schedule used. Keeping the number of drugs to a minimum reduces the potential for drug interactions and improves the patient's ability to comply with the drug regimen. Table 4-2 identifies selected reasons for noncompliance and possible solutions.

Although still somewhat controversial, drug holidays may also be considered from time to time. In addition to providing a cost savings and increasing mental alertness (in some cases), these breaks from medication reduce the likelihood that drugs will accumulate to toxic

---

TABLE 4-2

Reasons for Noncompliance with Drug Therapy Among Older Adults

Reason	Possible Solution
Inability to pay for prescribed drugs	Minimize number of drugs prescribed Use therapeutic alternatives where possible Refer to appropriate agency for assistance
Forgetfulness	Use calendars, diaries
Knowledge deficit regarding drug and/or disease state	Patient education
Confusion surrounding multiple drug regimens	Simplify drug regimen Be sure prescriptions are clearly labeled Provide written as well as verbal instruction
Misunderstanding of directions	Simplify directions
Inability to tolerate adverse effects of drugs	Closely monitor patient condition Consider changing to another drug Consider reducing dosage or frequency of administration
Interference with prescribed drug regimen because of use of self-treatment strategies	Patient education
Overdosage or underdosage based on patient's perception of need for the drug	Patient education
Expiration of prescription supplies prior to follow-up appointment with health care provider	Closely monitor patient profile
Fatigue or illness that prevents drug ingestion	Patient education Reevaluate patient condition

---

levels in the bloodstream. The health care provider may have overlooked this option and may need to be reminded of the length of time the patient has been using the drug. The use of drug holidays, however, requires interdisciplinary support, planning, and thorough assessment of the appropriateness of this strategy. Drugs that are usually not included in a drug holiday are antibiotics, anticoagulants, anticonvulsants, antidiabetic drugs, and ophthalmic drugs.

INTERVENTION
Administration

Alterations in the dosage forms of some drugs may be required for the older adult. Dry mucous membranes can cause tablets and capsules to stick to the roof or sides of the mouth and not be swallowed. If tablets and capsules dissolve in the mouth, they can be irritating. If they are spit out, they are of no value. Water should be offered before and after administering oral drugs if the patient's condition permits. The patient should be positioned upright so that gravity assists passage of the drug through the esophagus and minimizes the risk of aspiration. Because of diminished sensation, the older adult may be unaware that a tablet or capsule is stuck between the lip and the gum. The health care provider should examine the mouth to ensure that the drug has been swallowed. Further, dentures can mask where the tablet is in

the mouth. In some cases, a drug that is formulated as a liquid or suspension may be preferred to tablets.

In some cases, capsules can be opened and the contents placed in applesauce, ice cream, or other soft food. The exceptions to this practice are with enteric-coated, slow-release, and extended-release drug formulations specifically designed to begin action in the small intestine. Furthermore, caution should be used in mixing drugs with food, especially if the patient's appetite is already impaired.

Intramuscular and subcutaneous administration of drugs is necessary when immediate results are sought or when other routes are not available. Commonly, the older adult bleeds slightly or oozes after an injection because of decreased tissue elasticity or altered clotting mechanisms. Use of the Z-track technique facilitates sealing of the injection tract and reduces bleeding and leakage of the drug. (Blood dyscrasias are more common in the older adult.) A small bandage may be helpful. Injections should not be given in an immobile extremity, because inactivity reduces the rate of absorption. When frequent injections are required, the site of administration should be monitored for signs of irritation, inflammation, or infection. Reduction or absence of subcutaneous sensation in older persons may delay awareness of a complication at the injection site.

At times, intravenous administration is necessary. In addition to monitoring for drug effects, attention

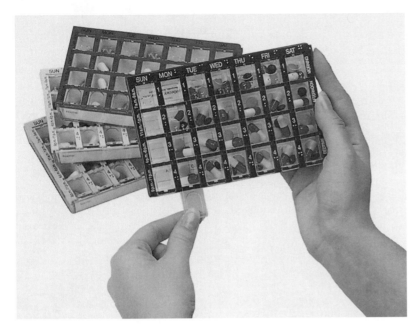

FIGURE 4-2 Commercially available drug boxes may contain a single compartment or multiple compartments. Some boxes contain just seven divisions, enough for a full week of medication. Others contain multiple compartments with space available for several doses throughout the day and the week. (Photo courtesy of Apothecary Products, Inc., Burnsville, Minn.)

should be paid to the amount of fluid in which the drug is administered. Declining cardiac and renal function makes the older person more susceptible not only to dehydration but also to overhydration. The patient should also be monitored for complications such as infiltration, air embolism, thrombophlebitis, and pyrogenic reactions. As with injection sites, decreased sensation may mask these potential complications.

The older adult may expel suppositories because circulation in the lower bowel and vagina is decreased and lower body temperature keeps the suppositories from melting. A special effort should be made to ensure that the suppository is not expelled. The suppository should be positioned above the rectal sphincter and away from any feces that may be present in the rectum. Having the patient remain in a supine or lateral recumbent position promotes retention of the suppository. More time should be given for the suppository to melt.

If the patient has a memory or sensory deficit, the use of prefilled syringes, prefilled envelopes, or containers labeled with the drug, day of the week, and time of administration may be helpful. Commercial medicine boxes are available that help organize the drugs and allow the patient and caregiver to check how much drug has been taken (Figure 4-2). A labeled egg carton can also serve the same compartmentalizing purpose at a much lower cost.

Education

The aging process leaves mental status intact. There is no decrease in knowledge and little or no loss of vocabulary with aging, although response time is slower than in younger persons. Slower responses affect new learn-

ing. The Patient Teaching Guidelines (see Chapter 5) are applicable to all who receive drug therapy and are particularly useful with the aging population.

The health care provider should review all drugs with the patient or caregiver, clarifying information as needed. In some cases, complex drug regimens can be simplified by discussing the possible alterations with the health care provider. A homebound, confused, or isolated older adult is less likely to follow a drug regimen properly. The functional assessment obtained during the history and physical exam helps determine whether the older adult needs a compliance aid or a memory cue to take the drugs. Additionally, if the older adult lives alone, the health care provider should determine whether a family member or a caregiver is available to assist as necessary. Furthermore, the ability of the patient to obtain the necessary drugs should be facilitated. If the patient is homebound, a pharmacy that delivers can be helpful. Referral to a social worker may be necessary to obtain financial or other forms of assistance.

EVALUATION

The purpose of evaluating drug therapy is to bring all parts of the regimen together. Evaluation involves looking at the overall drug regimen and answering the following questions:

- Were there any recent drug changes? Why were they made?
- Is cost or are the patient's physical limitations barriers to safe drug use?
- Are chronic symptoms improving? Are there new symptoms? Could the symptoms possibly be adverse drug effects?

- Is the older adult concurrently using nonprescription drugs, home remedies, or street drugs?
- Could there be information that has not been reported to the health care provider?
- Have plans for follow-up care been outlined and follow-up completed as necessary?

Furthermore, older adults who are managing drug regimens at home may misuse drugs in more than one way. They may share drugs with friends or family or save the drugs for use in self-treatment in the future. Additionally, they may not understand the purpose of the drug and, as a result, may increase their risk of taking duplicate drugs; this situation is a consequence not so much of the aging process as of poor prescribing practices. With the growing availability of generic drugs, the prescriber can choose drugs of different colors, sizes, and shapes to help the patient differentiate them. This possibility exists whether the patient uses the same pharmacy each time or has prescriptions filled at multiple pharmacies.

Some older adults maintain such strong beliefs in the efficacy of drugs and the wisdom of the health care provider that they continue to take drugs even after significant adverse effects appear. Others are reluctant to bother the health care provider with what they perceive as minor complaints. Still others attribute their symptoms to normal aging or may disregard signs and symptoms; these two factors cause a delay in calling or even mentioning the onset of drug-related adverse effects. The health care provider should reinforce the notion that adverse effects sometimes do occur and that the patient is expected to contact the health care provider promptly if they do.

Bibliography

Pearlman R: Development of a functional assessment questionnaire for geriatric patients: the Comprehensive Older Persons' Evaluation (COPE), *J Chron Dis* 40:85S-94S, 1987.

Rameizl P: CADET: a self-care assessment tool, *Geriatr Nurs* 4(12):377-378, 1983.

White P: Polypharmacy and the older adult, *J Am Acad Nurse Pract* 7(11):545-548, 1995.

Internet Resources

Dayer-Berenson L: Polypharmacy in the elderly. Available online: http://nsweb.nursingspectrum.com/ce/ce214.htm.

University of North Carolina at Chapel Hill: Polypharmacy in older adults. Available online: http://www.med.unc.edu/aging/polypharmacy.

CHAPTER

5

Role of the Nurse in Drug Therapy

KATHLEEN GUTIERREZ

 Visit http://evolve.elsevier.com/Gutierrez/ for additional information.

KEY TERMS

OBJECTIVES

- Discuss the collaborative nature of drug therapy.
- Explain the concept of chronotherapy and how it relates to drug therapy.
- Identify common health needs amenable to treatment with over-the-counter drugs.
- Compile a patient drug history.
- Identify the five rights of drug administration.
- Describe three drug administration systems.
- Give examples of information about drug administration that must be recorded on the patient's record.
- Discuss factors that influence patient compliance or noncompliance with drug therapy.
- Explain the two key nursing interventions related to drug therapy.
- Discuss the importance of evaluation as a component of drug therapy.

COLLABORATIVE NATURE OF DRUG THERAPY

Nursing practice at any level brings with it increasing responsibility for the appropriate use of drugs, identification of safe and appropriate dosages, and accurate monitoring and evaluation of drug effectiveness. Collaboration with physicians, advanced practice nurses, pharmacists, and other health care providers increases accountability for these actions. In turn, the quality of care is enhanced, and patient outcomes are improved. An awareness of each health care provider's role in drug therapy and the ability and willingness to interact with each other are vital safeguards to effective drug management.

The student of pharmacology is faced with an almost incomprehensible number and variety of drugs. This number can be greatly reduced by concentrating initial study on drug classification schemes, which functionally relate one drug to another in some fashion. For example, drug information can be organized by body system, therapeutic uses, or chemical characteristics. One of the more common ways to organize information is by drug classification, usually through the use of a **prototype drug**. A prototype drug represents all other drugs in a particular class. In many instances, it was the first drug developed and remains the best example of a drug in that class. For example, codeine was the first drug in the class of analgesics known as opioids.

SOURCES OF DRUG INFORMATION
Published Information

Official Sources. The only official book of drug standards in the United States is *The United States Pharmacopeia/National Formulary (USP-NF),* a privately issued compendium. The first edition of the USP-NF was published in 1820, and it is revised every 5 years by experts from nursing, pharmacy, pharmacology, and chemistry. Drugs included in the reference meet high standards of quality, purity, and strength and are identified by the letters USP-NF following the official name.

Clinical References. Two valuable, unbiased sources for clinical drug information are *USP Dispensing Information (USPDI)* and *American Hospital Formulary Service (AHFS) Drug Information.* The AHFS is a collection of monographs published by the American Society of Health-System Pharmacists (ASHP). The collection is updated annually. It frequently reviews the newer or investigational uses for drugs.

The *USPDI* is published annually, with regular updates issued during the year. It contains information for both the health care provider (Volumes I and III) and the patient (Volume II). The volumes for the health care provider offer information about approved drug products, drug indications, pharmacokinetics, dosing,

warnings, adverse effects, and precautions. Volume II is written for patients but is a valuable resource for patient teaching. Automatic permission is granted to health care providers who wish to copy a limited quantity of monographs to distribute free of charge to their patients.

Unofficial Sources. Goodman and Gilman's The Pharmacological Basis of Therapeutics is the classic reference on pharmacology. As the name implies, the primary focus is on the basic science information that underlies drug use and not on individual drugs. New editions are published approximately every 5 years.

Drug Evaluations is a comprehensive reference compiled by the American Medical Association. It discusses drugs from a therapeutic perspective and emphasizes clinical care rather than basic science information.

Drug Facts and Comparisons contains a comprehensive list of drugs with an index of the average wholesale price for equivalent quantities of similar or identical drugs. It is organized by drug classification and updated monthly.

The information contained in the *Physicians' Desk Reference (PDR)* is largely based on the results of Phase III clinical trials and is identical to that found in drug package inserts. The information is submitted and paid for by the drug companies. Its primary value is in identifying the clinical indications for an FDA-approved drug. It does not include nursing implications associated with a particular drug.

The *Medical Letter* is a biweekly publication of a nonprofit corporation. A typical issue provides summaries of scientific reports and consultant evaluations regarding the safety, efficacy, and rationale for the use of two or three specific drugs. This reference can be valuable to a health care provider when deciding whether or not to use a new drug.

The *Prescriber's Letter* is a monthly publication. Unlike the *Medical Letter* this newsletter briefly addresses most major drug-related developments, from new drugs to FDA warnings to new uses for older drugs. Additionally, subscribers can access an Internet site that provides expanded information on topics addressed in the newsletter.

Nurses' Drug Alert, a newsletter produced monthly, reviews other journal articles on the use of drugs for specific disorders. *The Nurse Practitioners' Prescribing Reference* is a quarterly publication that provides the advanced practice nurse with an up-to-date guide to commonly prescribed products available by prescription, as well as selected over-the-counter (OTC) drugs.

Textbooks. Depending on their purpose and scope, pharmacology textbooks offer basic pharmacologic principles and a discussion of drug categories and individual drugs. Administration techniques, patient assessment and monitoring, and patient teaching are included. The limitation to using textbooks is that they do not include information on recently introduced drugs.

Pocket reference books offer another resource. These references provide specific information regarding assessment, administration, dosage, evaluation of patient responses, and patient education considerations.

Online Databases. A number of online databases have been developed in recent years that provide drug and treatment information to health care providers and the public alike. A working knowledge of computer databases and resources will continue to be important to successful drug therapy.

The Internet can be a valuable source of drug information. However, drug information found on the Internet may not always be accurate, since anyone and everyone can post information. Accordingly, exercise discretion when searching for information. To determine if the online offering is reliable ask the following questions:

- Who maintains the site?
- Is there an editorial board or listing of names and credentials of those responsible for preparing and reviewing the contents of the site?
- Does the site link to other sources for pharmacology information?
- When was the site last updated?
- Are graphics and multimedia files, such as video or audio clips, available?
- Does the site charge an access fee?

People

Pharmacists/Pharmacies. Inevitably, clinical situations occur in which needed information is not contained in available resources. The health care provider is then wise to consult with a pharmacist. A pharmacist may be able to provide a package insert or other reference material on the drug. As an expert in the field of pharmacology, the pharmacist is a valuable member of the health care team and should be actively involved in drug regimen decisions.

The expansion and greater availability of OTC drugs and the likelihood of more sophisticated and technical products becoming available provide the impetus for the consumer and health care provider alike to use the services and expertise of community pharmacists (Box 5-1). Before the 1972 review of OTC drugs by the FDA, pharmacists avoided giving consumer advice or counseling about health care concerns. Now this practice is encouraged, however, and pharmacists' expertise uniquely qualifies them to participate in patient teaching as well as to provide advice about OTC drugs. Often the community pharmacist is the first contact the consumer has with a health care provider.

BOX 5-1	**Health Needs Amenable to Self-Treatment with OTC Drugs**

Acne
Allergic rhinitis, nasal congestion
Athlete's foot
Bacterial infections (superficial, uncomplicated, topical)
Boils
Burns (minor thermal burns, sunburn)
Calluses, corns, and warts
Cold and canker sores
Constipation, flatulence
Contact dermatitis (e.g., poison ivy, poison oak)
Contraception
Coughs and colds, sore throat
Dandruff
Diabetes mellitus (insulin, supplies)
Diaper rash
Diarrhea (e.g., traveler's diarrhea)
Dry skin, dry mouth
Dysmenorrhea, premenstrual syndrome
Fever
Halitosis
Head lice
Heartburn, dyspepsia
Hemorrhoids
Insect bites, stings
Insomnia
"Jock itch," prickly heat
Mineral and vitamin deficiencies
Minor aches and pains, headache
Motion sickness
Nausea and vomiting
Pinworms
Sprains and strains
"Swimmer's ear"
Vaginal yeast infection

Tracking drug regimens through computerized information networks helps provide a safety net, but only to the extent that appropriate information has been provided by the patient. According to the American Society for Automation in Pharmacy, more than 90% of U.S. pharmacies use computers to process prescriptions. Within a computerized system a patient's drug profile can be maintained for a defined number of years. Such systems are an avenue for checking food or drug allergies against each chemical contained in a drug preparation and for compatibilities with other drugs the patient is taking. When incompatibility information is found, the pharmacy can notify the health care provider and the patient before the drug is dispensed.

As more people engage in self-treatment, the importance of accurate, accessible information cannot be overstated. The patient must communicate information about food and drug allergies, the use of herbs and home remedies, prescription drugs that may have been dispensed by other health care providers, as well as OTC drugs that are used. Withholding such information places the patient at risk for harmful drug interactions and reactions and failure of the treatment plan.

Poison Control Centers. Poison control centers are located throughout the United States. These centers are accessible by telephone, permitting rapid access to information about drugs and toxic compounds. Obtain and post the number of your local poison control center where it can be found in the event of an accidental or intentional drug overdose.

Pharmaceutical Sales Representatives. Pharmaceutical sales representatives, otherwise known as "drug reps," can be useful sources of drug information. These individuals can provide authoritative, detailed information about the drugs they are selling, but keep in mind that the ultimate goal of the drug rep is to make a sale, not to educate. Because of this goal, the individual may not volunteer negative information about one of his or her drugs. Likewise, they may not identify the superior qualities of a competing drug. Since full disclosure is often inconsistent with success in sales, the drug rep may not always be the best source of information, particularly if the health care provider is searching for an unbiased comparison between drug products.

APPLICATION TO PRACTICE

ASSESSMENT
History of Present Illness

Assessment begins by identifying the patient's reason for the visit to the health care provider. Information obtained here provides a chronologic account of how each of the principal symptoms developed, their attributes and their context (onset, duration, frequency, location, quality, quantity, severity, setting, and aggravating and alleviating factors). This stage of treatment should also address how the patient thinks and feels about the illness, what concerns led to seeking attention, and how the illness has affected the patient's activities of daily living. Inquire if the patient is self-treating with either OTC drugs or alternative therapies before seeking medical assistance.

Health History

Questions about the health history should explore childhood illnesses and any history of adult illnesses, surgeries, obstetric or gynecologic events, and psychiatric conditions. Accidents and injuries as well as transfusions may also be included.

It is often difficult to ask about the patient's use of alcohol, tobacco, and drugs—illegal or prescription. Yet alcohol and drugs are often directly related to a patient's symptoms, and the use of or dependence on a substance may affect future care. Remember, it is not the role of the nurse to approve or disapprove of the use of substances; his or her role is to gather data, assess the impact on the patient's health, and plan a response. Certain drugs may interact with foods, so it is also important to assess dietary habits.

One significant component of the patient's health history is the drug history, which includes information

about a patient's experiences with drugs, although the scope of the drug history varies with the setting and patient situation. Any drug history should summon similar information each time the activity is undertaken (Box 5-2). Many patients are unaware of drug-drug interactions; therefore, it is appropriate to ask about the use of all types of drugs, including OTC and herbal remedies. Information about drug storage may not be as important a consideration in a health care environment, but it is important in the home.

Lifespan Considerations

Age is a significant variable in determining how a patient responds to drug therapy. The lifespan changes from the perinatal period to the older adult influence how a drug acts in the body and how the patient responds (see Chapters 2, 3, and 4).

Cultural/Social Considerations

The patient's health beliefs and practices are integral to how health and illness are defined. Health is usually viewed as a continuum. Wellness, located on one end of the continuum, is the optimal level of functioning; illness, at the other end, culminates in death. At any point along the continuum, a patient has both positive attributes of wellness and negative attributes of illness. In any group of people with the same attributes, some would seek medical care whereas others would ignore the symptoms, failing to associate them with illness. Except for gross abnormalities, signs that distinguish normal from abnormal are vague. The challenge is to determine at what point a change in structure and function becomes a sign or a symptom of disease requiring drug therapy.

BOX 5-2	**Components of a Drug History**

Drug Use, Past and Present (include purpose, dosages, duration of use)

- Prescription drugs used to treat illness/disease
- Self-prescribed drugs (OTC drugs, vitamins and minerals, borrowed prescriptions, home/folk/herbal remedies, use of obsolete prescriptions)
- Birth control
- Illicit or street drug use
- Caffeine intake and smoking history
- Drugs prescribed by other providers that may be unknown to current health care provider
- Who oversees or administers drugs if patient is unable to do so

Responses to Drug Use

- Therapeutic responses to drugs used in the past
- Adverse drug reactions
- Idiosyncratic and paradoxical reactions
- Allergic reactions
- Tolerance and dependence

Attitudes Toward Drug Use

- Cultural, social, and ethnic attitudes toward drugs and reasons for use and chosen route

- Compliance/noncompliance
- Any special monitoring required (e.g., blood glucose self-monitoring)
- Placebo effects that may have occurred
- Knowledge of drug-drug and drug-food interactions
- Educational level (impact on current health status and future planned drug regimens)

Storage of Drugs

- How long drugs are kept that are no longer in use
- Where drugs are stored in the home (e.g., bathroom medicine cabinet, bedside, kitchen)
- Measures taken to prevent inadvertent exposure of drugs to children

Identify

- Factors warranting cautious use or avoidance of a drug
- The patient's risk for adverse reactions
- Physiologic and psychologic response to previous drug use
- Potential problems with financial issues and adverse effects and when contact with the health care provider is appropriate
- Factors affecting administration, compliance, or both

Cultural dimensions are a vital consideration in drug therapy, because the rich variety of cultural and ethnic backgrounds results in a wealth of folk practices. Each of the four major ethnic subgroups in American society (i.e., African American, Hispanic, Asian, and Native American) has culturally diverse beliefs and practices that influence wellness and illness and ultimately drug therapy. The science of ethnopharmacology attempts to bridge the gap between traditional use of medicinal plants and their role in health care today.

Ethnopharmacology views the individual as a composite of psychologic, sociologic, cultural, spiritual, and physiologic forces that interact with the internal and external environments. This belief is in contrast to Western medicine, in which examining pathophysiologic deviations in body systems comprises the diagnosis of a disease. An exploration of folk beliefs and practices may reveal many cross-cultural differences and similarities and, as such, help explain differences in morbidity. The differences may be an indication of the culture-specific significance placed on certain disease-related problems. Societal differences in wellness- and illness-related practices influence both the degree to which a patient is aware of body symptoms and the decision to act on those symptoms. In most cases, drugs are generally more effective when the patient has a positive outlook and anticipates a therapeutic response.

All things being equal, consideration should also be given to the impact drug therapy has on a patient's financial resources, particularly for the older adult, who is often a victim of **polypharmacy**. Polypharmacy is the use of many drugs concurrently, which not only has an impact on the patient's finances but also increases the risk for drug-drug interactions. For example, 1 g of the antibiotic cefazolin given every 8 hours for 5 days costs between $42 and $110. On the other hand, ceftriaxone, a newer antibiotic, costs approximately $300 for a 2-g dose given every 12 hours for 7 days. Financial issues may lead to a patient "stretching out" their drugs to make them last or using drugs prescribed for another family member or friend. Box 5-3 identifies ways to help reduce the cost of drug therapy for all patients.

Physical Examination

The physical examination helps identify and verify health-related concerns, explain signs and symptoms, answer patient questions, provide an opportunity for patient teaching, supply a database for future evaluation, and increase both the credibility of and the patient's belief in the advice, recommendations, or reassurance pro-

---

| BOX 5-3 | **Reducing Drug Costs** |

Prescription drugs can be costly. Possible ways to reduce prescription costs include the following:

- Ask the health care provider if the prescribed drug is available in the generic form.
- Shop around (via telephone) for the best buy. Pharmacies vary in their prices.
- If the prescription is for a new drug, ask the health care provider for a few samples, or ask the pharmacist to fill part of the prescription (e.g., to give you 10 tablets of the 100 tablets ordered) until you see whether the drug causes serious adverse effects.
- Ask the health care provider if the tablet can be cut in half. Many drugs come scored permitting the tablet to be easily cut, thus extending the prescription for a longer period. For example, if the once daily dosage of a drug is 20 mg, 40-mg tablets may be cut in half, thus extending the prescription for another month.
- Ask the pharmacist how much the drug costs if the drug is paid for without using the pharmacy insurance plan. Some drugs are cheaper than the pharmacy co-pay. For example, the average retail price for one tablet of fluconazole (Diflucan) is approximately $14 whereas the pharmacy co-pay may be $20, a $6 difference.
- If a drug must be taken for an extended period, is there any organization through which drugs can be purchased at a reduced cost? For example, through the American Association of Retired Persons (AARP), members can buy 90 days of a prescribed drug at reduced cost. However, these drugs must be ordered through the mail, so this service is most economical for drugs needed on a long-term basis.

---

vided. Patients may be uneasy about what will be found but at the same time value and may even enjoy the detailed attention to their health care concerns.

Laboratory Testing

Laboratory and diagnostic tests are tools that, in and of themselves, are almost useless. When these tools are used in combination with a history and physical exam, they help confirm a diagnosis or provide information necessary to monitor the patient's response to drug therapy. Thus it is vital to know common laboratory reference values, particularly for drugs monitored by serum drug levels (e.g., cardiac glycosides, aminoglycoside antibiotics, anticonvulsants).

GOALS OF THERAPY

Treatment goals are developed after the assessment is complete. Initial drug regimens are then chosen from a variety of reasonable alternatives including drugs used to **prevent, cure,** or **palliate** an illness as well as those used to **restore** or support wellness. Complementary and adjunctive nondrug therapies may also be considered in the treatment plan (see Chapter 8). It is important to recognize that the final decision to accept drug therapy lies with the patient and their family.

Prevention. Preventive health behaviors are most commonly viewed as voluntary actions taken to decrease the threat of illness. Actions taken with this objective in mind are not curative or restorative because they occur before symptoms appear. Identifying and correcting precipitating factors, such as poor diet or lack of exercise, constitutes an important component of preventive regimens. Immunizations are a deliberate attempt to protect the individual against disease (see Chapter 35).

Cure. The degree to which signs and symptoms can be cured depends on the extent and severity of the illness or disease. For example, a patient who receives an antibiotic for a bacterial infection such as acute sinusitis may be cured of his or her illness.

Restoration. Restorative therapy may be short-term or lifelong and is appropriate when there is an identifiable deficiency of some type. For example, a patient who has a deficiency of thyroid hormone (hypothyroidism) requires lifelong supplements of thyroid hormone. In contrast, ferrous sulfate is an iron preparation most often used in the short-term treatment of iron deficiency anemia until the patient's own iron reserves are replenished.

Support. The purpose of supportive therapy is to maintain a patient's level of wellness while halting further progression of the disease and reducing its effects on other body systems. For example, hypertension is not curable; however, it can be effectively managed by lifestyle modification and drug therapy.

Palliation. The term *palliate* means to alleviate without curing. As used in common practice, palliative therapy is typically used for patients with an end-stage illness or disease. The purpose of treatment is to make the patient as comfortable as possible. For example, pain management for the patient with terminal cancer may be accomplished with the use of well-timed, around-the-clock administration of analgesics. Home oxygen therapy (oxygen is considered a drug) may be used for someone with end-stage pulmonary disease.

INTERVENTION
Administration

Drug Administration Systems. At least three drug administration systems are in use today. In the **unit-dose** system, the dose of a drug is individually wrapped, labeled, and supplied to the patient's unit in a quantity to last 24 hours. On the patient unit, each patient has a designated drawer, box, or container, and the exact number of drug doses for a 24-hour period is placed in that container daily by the pharmacy. The nurse prepares each patient's drugs as ordered from the supply in the patient's drug drawer. There are several advantages to this system, including the fact that the drug remains in a labeled container until the nurse is at the bedside, thus reducing the risk for mixing up drugs. Patients can be billed for the exact number of doses taken, and unauthorized use of drugs is decreased.

In the **stock drug system,** each nursing unit is supplied with large-quantity stock containers of the drugs commonly used in that setting or institution. The nurse administering a drug takes the order sheet, Kardex, or drug card to the drug room and prepares the dose of the drug from the stock supply, usually putting the drug into a small medicine cup. The advantages of this system are that the pharmacy need not restock the nursing unit daily, calculation and preparation of doses require fewer pharmacy personnel (because these duties are performed by the nurses), and stat and new orders can be filled immediately because the stock drugs are on the unit. A disadvantage of this system is that drug errors are more common.

The third drug administration system is the **computer-controlled dispensing system.** This system supplies drug to the unit in a locked cabinet or cart. To obtain a dose for the patient, the nurse enters the patient's name or hospital identification number along with the nurse's personal identification number or security code into the system. The system then delivers the dose of the drug, records it, and bills the patient's account. This system is especially useful in the management of controlled substances.

Most institutions combine the three systems. The nurse must learn as much as possible about the drug administration systems in use to be safe and efficient in preparing and administering drugs.

Drug Orders.   A drug order is a means for communicating drug treatment plans between the prescriber and other care providers (Box 5-4). There are several essential legal components to a **drug order:** patient name, date, drug name, dosage, frequency, route, and the signature of the care provider. If the drug ordered is for a controlled substance, the provider's Drug Enforcement Administration (DEA) number must be included on the prescription or be on record with the health care institution. The components are related in part to the **five rights of drug administration.** The *right drug* is given to the *right patient* in the *right dose* by the *right route* at the

---

BOX 5-4	Types of Drug Orders
Routine order*	enalapril maleate 10 mg po each AM
prn order	ibuprofen 400 mg po q4-6h prn pain
Single order	metoclopramide 10 mg po preoperatively at 9 AM
Stat order	furosemide 40 mg IV push now
Protocol order	Sliding scale insulin: If fingerstick glucose is:
	120-160 mg/dL, give 2 units regular insulin
	160-200 mg/dL, give 4 units regular insulin
	200-220 mg/dL, give 6 units regular insulin
	over 220 mg/dL, call health care provider

*An outpatient drug order would also include the quantity of drug to be dispensed (e.g., 30 tablets)

---

right time. These rights are put at risk if systems for oversight of drug administration are inadequate. Many institutions are now using computer systems to order drugs. The health care provider orders the drug, which goes directly to the pharmacy, thus eliminating the need to transcribe the drug order and reducing the potential for errors.

Although many nurses do not write drug orders, they do transcribe the orders from the patient's record into drug administration records. Caution should be taken when transcribing drug orders, since many drug names are too similar for comfort (Table 5-1). There are several strategies that can be used when transcribing or administering drugs that help prevent errors (Table 5-2).

Administration Schedules.   Body functions take their cue from the environment and the rhythms of the solar system that change night to day and lead us from one season to another. Biologic rhythms such as hormone production, blood pressure, blood clotting, sleep-wake cycles, and drug response are dictated by our genetic makeup. Biologic rhythms influence drug behavior and subsequently patient response. The rate of drug absorption, hepatic clearance, half-life, duration of action, and the magnitude of drug effect have all been shown to differ, depending on the time of day the drug is administered.

Ultracadian rhythms are shorter than a day. For example, a 90-minute sleep cycle and the millisecond it takes for a neuron to fire are considered ultracadian rhythms. Circadian rhythms last about 24 hours. A circadian rhythm exists for the sleep-wake cycle, suscepti-

---

TABLE 5-1

Drug Names Too Similar for Comfort

Instead of	For	The Patient Received	For
acetazolamide (Diamox)	Glaucoma	acetohexamide (Dymelor)	Diabetes
Anturane (sulfinpyrazone)	Gout	Antabuse (disulfiram)	Alcoholism
Celexa (citalopram)	Depression	Celebrex (celecoxib)	Osteoarthritis/pain
chlorpropamide (Diabinese)	Diabetes	chlorpromazine (Thorazine)	Psychoses
disopyramide (Norpace)	Arrhythmias	desipramine (Pertofrane)	Depression
Enduron (methylclothiazide)	Diuresis	Inderal (propranolol)	Arrhythmias
Feldene (terfenadine)	Inflammation	Seldane (piroxicam)	Allergies
hydroxyzine (Vistaril)	Anxiety	hydralazine (Apresoline)	Hypertension
Lamictal (lamotrigine)	Epilepsy	Lamisil (terbinafine)	Fungal infections
metolazone (Zaroxolyn)	Diuresis	metaxalone (Skelaxin)	Muscle relaxation
ritodrine (Yutopar)	Preterm labor	Ritalin (methylphenidate)	ADHD*
Sarafem (fluoxetine)	PMS* symptoms	Serophene (clomiphene)	Infertility
selegiline (Eldepryl)	Parkinson's disease	Stelazine (trifluoperazine)	Anxiety states
Zyprexa (olanzapine)	Bipolar disorder	Zyrtec (cetirizine)	Allergies

ADHD, Attention deficit–hyperactivity disorder; *PMS*, premenstrual syndrome.

TABLE 5-2

Selected Strategies for Preventing Drug Errors

Potential Problem	Recommended Action
Unusually large or excessive increase in dosage; drug form used in an unfamiliar fashion; a single order containing more than one drug; ambiguous, unclear orders; drug names that include numerals	Check order with health care provider, pharmacist, and/or the literature
Use of decimal figures (e.g., 0.125 mg versus 125 mcg)	Avoid as much as possible
Multiple tablets or several vials required to prepare a single dose	Check all dosage calculations with another professional nurse; contact pharmacist
Illegible, incomplete orders	Obtain clear copy of order; clarify order with health care provider
Familiar and unfamiliar (e.g., qd versus qid; U for units), apothecary abbreviations or symbols (e.g., the symbol for fluid dram [f℥] or the abbreviation for potassium [K+]); slang names, colloquialisms in notes or prescriptions	Avoid use as much as possible when transcribing orders
Telephone and verbal orders	Do not take or give a telephone or verbal order except in an emergency
First time drug has been ordered for the patient	Read package insert carefully; double-check patient allergies
A new drug is added to a patient's existing drug regimen	Check for drug-drug interactions; commit common interactions to memory
Use of erasable pens	Avoid, since the ink does not become permanent for about 3 days, increasing the risk of alteration without notice
Apothecary system	Use the metric system; when a decimal is required to denote less than one, a zero should precede the decimal (e.g., 0.5 mg rather than .5 mg)

bility to noxious stimuli, endotoxins, and drugs. Infracadian rhythms are cycles that are longer than 24 hours. A woman's menses usually cycle anywhere from 21 days to 5 weeks. Seasonal rhythms influence our reactions and behaviors during particular seasons of the year (e.g., late spring, early fall). For example, seasonal affective disorder causes depression in susceptible individuals during the short days of winter.

Coordinating these biologic rhythms with drug therapy is referred to as **chronotherapy** and is studied in relation to diseases such as asthma, arthritis, and cancer. Chronotherapy for asthma is directed at obtaining maximal effects from bronchodilator drugs during the early morning hours, when lung function normally undergoes circadian changes, reaching a low point. For example, the long-acting bronchodilator drug theophylline is taken once daily in the evening. Theophylline blood levels reach their peak during the early morning hours, thus improving lung function. In general, health care providers believe that unless asthma treatment improves nighttime symptoms, it is difficult to improve daytime manifestations. For patients with severe asthma who wake during the night gasping for breath, a good night's sleep can be a dream come true.

Chronobiologic patterns have also been noted in patients with pain from osteoarthritis. These patients tend to have less pain in the morning and more at night. For patients with rheumatoid arthritis, the pain is usually worse in the morning and decreases as the day goes on. In chronotherapy, drug dosing with corticosteroids and nonsteroidal antiinflammatory drugs is timed to ensure that the highest blood levels of the drug coincide with peak pain periods. For patients with osteoarthritis, the optimal time for administration of a nonsteroidal drug such as ibuprofen would be at lunch time or midafternoon. For the patient with rheumatoid arthritis, the best administration time would be after the evening meal.

Antineoplastic therapy may also be more effective and less toxic if the drugs are administered at carefully selected times. It is thought that there may be different chronobiologic cycles for normal cells and cancer cells. If this is indeed true, the treatment goal would be to time drug administration to coincide with the chronobiologic cycles of tumor cells, making them more effective against cancer and less toxic to normal tissues. Because some patients may be better served by receiving antineoplastic drugs in the late afternoon or even during the night, an implantable infusion pump might be appealing. Chronotherapy means that not all patients receive their antineoplastic drugs first thing in the morning, an otherwise common practice today. Furthermore, it is believed that timing breast cancer surgery to coincide with the last half of the menstrual cycle can increase the number of patients who are tumor free af-

ter 5 years. In the first half of the menstrual cycle, estrogen levels are high and progesterone is not produced. However, in the last half of the cycle, progesterone levels rise and estrogen falls. It is thought that progesterone may inhibit the production of some enzymes that help cancer to metastasize.

In other examples, patients undergoing skin testing for allergies experienced the mildest skin response at 11 AM. The most severe responses were noted to occur at 11 PM. Thus for example, administration of the antihistamine cyproheptadine provided 16 hours of relief when it was taken at 7 AM but only 7 hours of relief when it was taken at 7 PM.

The plasma cortisol level for daytime-active persons begins to rise in the latter part of the usual sleep cycle. These levels peak shortly before or just after awakening, then irregularly decline throughout the day and evening until minimal levels are reached early in the next sleep cycle. Transplant recipients, for example, are placed on lifetime steroid therapy to augment their endogenous cortisol levels and to prevent rejection of the donor organ. Under these conditions, the goal of treatment is to reinforce intrinsic adrenocortical activity with minimal suppression. To achieve this goal, a synthetic glucocorticoid such as prednisone is given after the peak secretion of endogenous cortisol on a daily or alternate-day midmorning schedule. On the other hand, when the treatment goal is replacement therapy for a person with adrenocortical insufficiency, the steroid may be given at a time that mimics natural endogenous rhythm. That is, approximately two thirds of the total daily dosage would be taken in the morning upon awakening, and the remaining one third prior to bedtime in the evening.

Patients are more likely to follow drug regimen schedules when the drugs are formulated for chronotherapy. That is, reformulating a drug so that absorption into the bloodstream is delayed, revising the dosing schedule, or using programmable pumps that deliver drugs to the patient at precise intervals not only optimizes a drug's desirable effects but also minimizes undesirable effects and promotes patient compliance. Although susceptible biologic rhythms are not as well documented in humans as in animals, research in this area is rapidly growing. The FDA regulates drugs that are reformulated to be chronotherapeutic agents.

Although drugs can be administered without a detailed understanding of pharmacology and chronotherapy, having such knowledge helps reduce medication errors. Unlike the ideal of chronotherapeutic schedules, drug administration schedules in many health care environments are dictated in part by agency policy, patient preference, laboratory testing, drug characteristics, and other treatment regimens. In the home the patient determines drug administration times. In the hospital or nursing home, however, the nurse usually determines drug administration times. For example, some nursing units routinely give drugs at 9 AM, 1 PM, 5 PM, and 9 PM when the drug is to be given four times a day; when the drug is to be administered every eight hours, it is usually at 6 AM, 2 PM, and 10 PM. On the other hand, specialty areas, such as intensive care, maternal-infant, or pediatric units, may have other administration times that better coincide with patient needs. However, dosing intervals for a given drug are seldom changed. For example, dosages of anticoagulants are based on the patient's partial thromboplastin time (PTT) or similar measure. In many cases, a drug is administered once daily in the afternoon to permit time for the test results to return. In another example, diuretics are usually taken early in the day to avoid interference with patient rest. Many antimicrobial drugs are usually administered every 4, 6, 8, or 12 hours to maintain a steady-state level of drug in the serum.

Drugs taken on a daily basis can usually be taken on a more flexible schedule; however, they should be taken as close to the same time each day as possible. Exempt from flexible schedules are one-time-only drug orders, such as those given before surgery or diagnostic procedures, and those that require more frequent administration schedules (e.g., every 2 hours, every 4 hours). Stat orders should be given when ordered. Scheduling can be difficult, but it requires application of the following principles:

- Multiple daily doses of the same drug ordinarily are evenly spaced over 24 hours to help maintain serum drug levels.
- Drugs with known interactions should not be administered at the same time (e.g., cholestyramine with digoxin).
- Drugs that interact with specific foods should not be given concurrently with those foods (e.g., tetracycline and dairy products).
- Some drugs are better absorbed when given before a meal; others are better absorbed after a meal.
- Some drug doses should be scheduled early in the day for appropriate effect (e.g., diuretics).
- The patient's sleep should not be interrupted any more than necessary. At home the patient may not get up during the night to take the drugs.
- In the hospital, drugs such as warfarin are arbitrarily scheduled at a time that permits the return of laboratory results prior to drug administration.

Patients with multiple health problems may need several drugs simultaneously. The number of drugs and the amount of fluid needed by the patient to swallow the drugs may be nauseating. If the patient refuses to take all the drugs, tires before they are taken, or becomes too nauseated, the nurse must ensure that the more important drugs are taken first and the less necessary ones left until last. Consider the patient who takes a cardiac glycoside, an antihypertensive, a diuretic, potassium replacement, vitamins, and an iron supplement each morning. All of these drugs are necessary; however, the nurse may decide that the cardiac glycoside, antihypertensive, diuretic, and potassium replacement are of greater priority. This is not to suggest that the nurse can simply decide not to administer certain drugs but that the nurse is often required to exercise judgment and make decisions on short notice. A better long-term solution to this problem might be to schedule the vitamin and the iron supplement at a time when the patient is taking fewer drugs. There is no evidence that the vitamins and iron supplement must be given in the morning.

When administering controlled substances, the nurse has legal and nursing responsibilities. The legal responsibilities include ensuring that controlled substances (United States Schedules II through IV) are kept under lock and key and made available only to authorized personnel. Because all of the controlled substances must be accounted for, records as to which patients received these substances must be kept. Unauthorized use of controlled substances must be reported to the proper authority.

The nurse must also be aware of institutional policies regarding these drugs. For example, for Schedule II drugs, the health care provider may need to renew the order for opioids every 48 hours; that is, a so-called *standing order* for an opioid is prohibited. The nurse who administers the drug after the 48-hour period without obtaining a renewal order is in violation of institutional policy. There are comparable national and institutional restrictions related to Canadian controlled substances.

Recording Drug Administration. Recording drug administration is an important responsibility of the nurse. The forms used vary among health care institutions, but some general points usually apply. The nurse should legibly record that a drug dose was given as soon as possible after administration. If a dose was omitted, the reason must be noted. Most institutions also require that doses given significantly earlier or later than the scheduled time be accompanied by a notation of the reason. Information related to the administration route, injection site (if appropriate), location of a topical application, or the blood pressure or pulse must also be recorded.

Assessment data might include the subjective and objective information that led the nurse to conclude that a prn drug was needed. Information related to the management of a patient, such as the patient's tolerating physical therapy better when a prn analgesic is administered 1 hour beforehand, becomes part of the care plan. Another kind of drug management information relates to the actual administration of the drug. For example, some patients may take a drug more easily if it is crushed and mixed with applesauce. The patient's response to the drug and the effectiveness should also be recorded.

Education

Patient education is vital to the successful outcome of drug therapy. By educating the patient about the drugs being taken, the health care provider can elicit the required level of participation. The void between a patient's understanding and the information needed for compliance with drug therapy is referred to as a **learn-**

ing deficit. To reduce the risk of serious damage resulting from adverse drug effects, the patient should be told about the expected drug effects, possible adverse reactions, and the time when these effects or reactions are likely to occur. Patients are thus more likely to call attention to the problem early. Patients should also be advised as to the proper drug storage techniques, drug handling, and disposal of old or outdated drugs.

A great deal of time can be spent in teaching-learning activities. Yet poor understanding of verbal instructions and written materials remains a major factor in failure to achieve treatment goals. Box 5-5 provides guidelines for patient teaching associated with drug therapy. Patients

---

BOX 5-5   Patient Teaching Guidelines for Drug Therapy

The following information should be provided for each drug taken:

1. All prescribed drugs should be taken until used up (e.g., antibiotics not taken as prescribed contribute to microbial resistance).
2. The name of the drug, both generic and brand name.
3. The purpose of the drug and what it does, and the disease or condition for which it is prescribed.
4. The color, size, and shape of the dosage form (e.g., tablet, capsule, liquid).
5. The route of administration (by mouth, inhalation, topical, etc.).
6. Develop a reasonable schedule for drug administration considering the patient's activities of daily living.
   a. Specify the times of day and associated meals or activities; for example: "Take one tablet at 7 am when you get up, one at noon with lunch, and one at 5 pm with your dinner."
   b. Do not assume the number of meals, timing of meals, or sleeping hours.
   c. Should the drug be taken on an empty stomach or with meals?
   d. Can the drug be taken at the same time as other drugs?
7. Are there any dietary or alcohol restrictions while taking the drug?
8. If the drug is prescribed on a prn basis, how often can it be taken? What signs or symptoms will be used to decide if it can or should be taken?
9. Indicate what to do if a dose is missed.
   a. Should the dose be skipped?
   b. Should two doses be taken at the same time?
10. When the dosage is to be changed, be specific about the instructions; for example, rather than telling the patient, "Take one tablet each day for the next 3 days, then increase to two tablets per day," instruct them as follows: "Take one tablet in the morning each day for

3 days, starting tomorrow, Tuesday, January 15. Then increase to one tablet in the morning and one tablet at night, starting Friday, January 19."
11. Indicate the length of time the drug should be taken—that is, a short time for an acute problem versus a prolonged time for a chronic one.
12. Indicate whether the new drug is intended to replace or to supplement current drug regimens.
13. Describe adverse effects so that they are recognizable and explain what action the patient should take if symptoms arise. Point out degree of urgency in reporting the adverse effects.
14. Identify any special precautions; for example, "Do not take this drug at the same time or within 2 hours of taking your antacid."
15. Provide storage instructions if this is an important consideration.
   a. Does the drug need to be refrigerated?
   b. Should it always be left in its original container?
   c. Does the drug have an especially short shelf life?
   d. Is it wise for the patient to request a non–child-proof cap, or is a child-proof cap warranted?
16. Give instructions on how to refill the prescription.
   a. Are the number of refills indicated on the container, and if so, where? This is particularly important for hospitalized patients preparing for discharge.
17. Give instructions in writing and review them orally with the patient.
   a. Have the patient repeat the information back to ensure accurate comprehension.
   b. Encourage the patient to call the health care provider if there are questions.
18. When and how should the patient follow up with the health care provider?
19. What is the procedure for disposing of noncurrent and expired drugs? Drugs should not be saved or shared with others.

vary greatly in their ability to hear, read, and translate verbal language and written instructions into a meaningful whole. Close attention should be given to the patient's attention span and reading and comprehension abilities. Drug compliance is most likely to be achieved when both verbal and written information are presented at the appropriate level of understanding. Most drug information provided to patients is written at the fifth- to eighth-grade level.

Drug Storage. Drugs stored in the home should be kept in their original containers to ensure availability of correct directions as well as to avoid misidentification and unknown expiration dates. Storage in a secure, locked cabinet is recommended. Storage of drugs in bathroom cabinets is not recommended because these cabinets rarely have a lock and are easily accessible to children. This principle holds true not only in homes where children live but also where they may visit.

Chemical deterioration of drugs is hastened by heat, moisture, and, in some cases, light. Light-sensitive drugs should be stored in their original amber-colored containers, and exposure to direct sunlight should be avoided. Moisture dissolves some solid dosage forms and heat melts away the waxy base of suppositories and ointments. To prevent changes caused by moisture, silica gel inserts are packaged with some drugs.

Not all drugs should be stored at room temperature. Some must be stored in refrigerators where temperatures range from 35° to 60° F (2° to 15° C), whereas other drugs are stored in a freezer. Multidose, injectable drugs (e.g., insulin) and suppositories in airtight containers are refrigerated to protect them from humidity and food residues. These containers should be placed where they are least accessible to children but away from freezer coils.

Drug Handling. Many drugs are dispensed in containers with childproof caps. Because the caps require complex manipulation, the time required for children to gain access to the drug is prolonged and the risk for accidental ingestion is reduced. Persons with impaired dexterity may request standard, easily opened containers at the time the drug is dispensed; however, special safeguards must be taken to prevent access by children. Containers should also be protected from soiling so that the label remains legible.

Drug Disposal. Expiration dates are printed on the label or package insert of each drug. Expiration dates are approximations and do not indicate that a drug is at once rendered useless or harmful on that date. Most drugs lose potency over time, although some can become

toxic (e.g., tetracycline, acetaminophen). The following situations mandate that the drug be discarded in an appropriate fashion:

- Aspirin products (e.g., Bufferin, Excedrin) or acetaminophen (Tylenol) that smells like vinegar has become toxic
- Any drugs in solid dosage form (i.e., pills, tablets, capsules) that are damaged, discolored, softened, or stuck together
- Liquids that have lost their original color, smell, or taste or that have developed gas formations may have deteriorated
- Ointments or creams that have changed in odor, color, or consistency
- Any oral drug that is past its expiration date or is more than 2 years old
- Any drug that has not been stored as directed

Oral drugs are best disposed of by flushing them down the toilet. In the absence of toilet facilities, tablets and capsules can be burned. Discarding drugs in a trash receptacle risks accidental poisoning of children or pets. The Centers for Disease Control and Prevention (CDC) recommends disposing of needles, syringes, and vials by placing them in a sturdy, preferably metal container (e.g., a metal coffee can) with a tightly fitting lid. The container should be taped closed, double bagged, and placed with the regular household trash for disposal. Commercially available containers may also be used for disposal. If the patient is not comfortable disposing of needles, syringes, and vials at home, the container can be taken to a hospital or clinic, where they will be disposed of with other medical waste.

Participation in Drug Research

The expanding roles in nursing often include drug research (see also Chapter 6). In fact, more nurses than ever before are conducting their own research, much of it clinical, even if not directly related to investigational drugs. Thus nurses involved in drug research projects that involve human subjects must be knowledgeable about the precepts of the Nuremberg Code and must protect human subjects by being alert to the possibility of subtle slip-ups in protocol or omissions in **adherence** to the tenets of the Code. The most important elements of the Code include the subject's rights to informed consent and participation that is done voluntarily and without coercion.

It is the nurse's obligation to ensure that the health care provider or researcher, not the nurse, gives a full explanation of the study and the expectations of the subject, and that he or she answers any questions. The information conveyed to the subject should be in lay terms and presented at a time when the subject is not sleepy or under the influence of mind-altering drugs. Informed consent to participate in a drug study must be obtained in writing.

Much like the subjects who are fully informed, nurses involved in clinical drug studies should also be knowledgeable about the study and the drug under investigation. All information available to the health care provider, researcher, or pharmacist should also be available to the nurse. Ethical and legal responsibilities require that a nurse's actions be based on adequate knowledge and skill and that subjects are protected from foreseeable harm. This means that the nurse must know and adhere to the study protocols and recommended dosage range as well as route of administration. An understanding of the desired therapeutic effects, adverse effects, and toxicities is vital to a successful, safe study. Documentation of all observations should be as precise as possible, because they have a direct influence on the study's outcomes.

EVALUATION

Like assessment and intervention, evaluation of patient response is an important aspect of drug therapy. After all, evaluation is the process that tells us if drug therapy was effective. Evaluation of patient response is organized around four areas: compliance, patient satisfaction, therapeutic response, and secondary or adverse effects of the prescribed therapy. Evaluating patient response to a drug that has more than one use requires that the health care provider know the specific purpose for which the drug was used.

Compliance versus Noncompliance

Compliance, how well the patient follows through with a drug regimen, has been a concern of health care providers for decades. Many assume that once a diagnosis is made and the prescription written, the patient complies with the plan of care. It should be noted, however, that **noncompliance** is a term generated by health care providers and defines the problem from their viewpoint only. The health care worker may regard **nonadherence** with the drug regimen as deviant behavior, but the patient may see the action as a cautious approach to self-administration of potentially harmful substances.

Patient Satisfaction

Satisfaction with the drug regimen is an important consideration often ignored or skimmed over. However, patient satisfaction is closely tied to compliance. Dissatisfaction may lead to noncompliance and failure of an otherwise appropriate drug regimen. Dissatisfaction can be reduced when therapy is designed around the pa-

tient's lifestyle, resources, preferences, health care needs, and knowledge of drug pharmacokinetics. Hence patient and family involvement is a necessity.

Techniques used to assess patient compliance and satisfaction with the drug regimen include pill counts, review of a drug diary, self-reports, direct observation, assessment of physiologic parameters, and input from other health care providers, family members, or friends. Combining several techniques allows for a more accurate assessment.

The complex medical problems of many patients and the varied drug regimens they are expected to follow lay the groundwork for intentional or unintentional noncompliance and drug interactions. One third to one half of prescription drugs are not taken as directed. In addition, some patients fail to have the prescription filled at all or fail to pick up the filled prescription. Still others stop taking the drug too early in the treatment regimen, leading to treatment failure. Compliance by older adults, for example, is reduced when five or more drugs are prescribed, when drug labels cannot be read, or when containers are difficult to open. Instead of investigating the cause of treatment failure, the health care provider often just increases the dosage of the same drug or changes to a new one. Table 5-3 provides examples of cues that may be predictive of noncompliance along with possible interventions.

Therapeutic Response

Evaluation of therapeutic response is accomplished by monitoring physiologic parameters (e.g., vital signs, absence of infection, serum or urine drug levels, body weight, and serum and urine chemistry values). For example, a reduction in systolic and diastolic pressures in a patient receiving nifedipine to treat hypertension should be noted. In contrast, when the same drug is used to treat angina, the patient should note decreased chest pain. When beneficial responses develop as hoped, ignorance of expected adverse effects might not be so bad. However, when desired responses do not occur, it is essential to identify the situation early because treatment with an alternative therapy may be needed.

Secondary Response

Evaluation of secondary or adverse effects is also conducted. The responses may be related to dose (which are predictable) or patient sensitivity (which are unpredictable). Dose-related responses result from unknown pharmacologic effects. An allergic reaction is an example of an unpredictable, sensitivity-related response unrelated to dosage. Secondary or adverse effects were discussed in Chapter 1.

TABLE 5-3			

Assessment and Interventions to Promote Compliance

Parameter or Problem Area	Factors Related to Noncompliance	Interview Questions	Possible Responses
Wellness-illness beliefs and practices	Illness not as severe as perceived by health care provider; denial of problem results in the patient ignoring information	"How would you describe the severity of your illness?" "Would you describe yourself as healthy or unhealthy?"	Be sure questions asked and information provided are relevant from the patient's perspective
Mistrust of Western health care	Patient does not believe Western health care is effective	"How would you describe the effectiveness of your care?" "Tell me about your beliefs."	Use nonjudgmental, active listening
Previous experiences with health care provider	Patient expresses dissatisfaction, lack of trust with care provider over past or present interactions	"How do you feel about the care you received?" "To what degree do you trust your health care provider?" "What can we do to foster your trust in us?"	Use nonjudgmental, active listening; take genuine concern in patient's concerns; avoid false reassurance
Complexity of treatment plan	Plan seems difficult to follow, vague, ambiguous, disruptive, or lengthy; patient is confused regarding multidrug regimens	"How does the plan of care affect your activities of daily living?"	Simplify regimen if possible; adapt it to the patient's lifestyle; make sure drug bottles are clearly marked; provide written and verbal instructions
Compliance/ noncompliance	Patient never intends to comply or has a history of noncompliance	"How do you plan to take your medications?" "How often did you take your medication for your other illness?"	Acknowledge difficulty with compliance. Explore strategies to improve compliance
Coping mechanisms	Patient uses denial, does not recognize need for treatment, exhibits repression, or is unable to mobilize energies to cope with treatment plan	Assess for cues such as "I'm not so ill."	Educate patient about disease, drugs, etc., and teach effective coping strategies
Patient self-esteem	Negative self-image	Assess for verbal and/or nonverbal cues such as "Don't bother with me. I'm not worth the effort."	Provide resources for counseling relative to the patient's underlying problem
Economic status	Patient is in lower socioeconomic group, is unemployed, lacks health insurance, or believes drugs are not worth the cost	"What resources do you have that help you with the cost of your treatment and medicine?"	Investigate situation and refer patient to appropriate resources for financial assistance; minimize number of drugs prescribed, if possible
Support systems	Patient lacks family or cultural support systems	"When you want to talk about a problem, to whom do you go?"	Enlist family and friends to assist patient; consider referral to appropriate counseling systems

Modified from Gutierrez K: *Pharmacotherapeutics: clinical decision-making in nursing,* Philadelphia, 1999, WB Saunders.

TABLE 5-3

Assessment and Interventions to Promote Compliance—cont'd

Parameter or Problem Area	Factors Related to Noncompliance	Interview Questions	Possible Responses
Reading and comprehension skills	Patient has limited reading and comprehension skills	Query patient about disease process, drug action, and adverse effects. "Can you tell me what you see on this prescription bottle?" "What directions are on this container?"	Increase sensory exposure with pictures, charts, demonstrations, verbal reinforcement Assess baseline knowledge and build on that foundation Use nonjudgmental behaviors; refer to literacy hotline, local literacy council, or other community service programs if appropriate
Physical capabilities to carry out plan of care	Patient physically unable to carry out plan of care	"What kind of problems do you have that make it difficult for you to take your medicine?" "Are you able to reach your medicines and open the containers?"	Assist patient in obtaining standard caps for drug bottles; explore alternative devices and methods of administration (e.g., automatic injection devices, magnifying glasses)
Memory	Patient forgets to take prescribed drugs or takes on irregular basis	"What strategies do you use so that you remember to take your medicine?"	Use calendars, diaries, drug boxes

Bibliography

Gutierrez K: *Pharmacotherapeutics: clinical decision-making in nursing,* Philadelphia, 1999, WB Saunders.

Hansen M, Fisher J: Patient-centered teaching from theory to practice, *Am J Nurs* 98(1):56, 58, 60, 1998.

CHAPTER

6

Evidence-Based Practice and Pharmacoeconomics

KATHLEEN GUTIERREZ

 Visit **http://evolve.elsevier.com/Gutierrez/** for additional information.

KEY TERMS

Cost-benefit analysis (CBA), p. 79

Cost-effectiveness analysis (CEA), p. 79

Cost-minimization analysis (CMA), p. 79

Cost-utility analysis (CUA), p. 79

Evidence hierarchy, p. 76

Evidence-based practice (EBP), p. 75

Open-label clinical trials, p. 81

Pharmacoeconomics, p. 78

Randomized controlled clinical trials, p. 76

Resource allocation, p. 78

OBJECTIVES

- Define the terms *pharmacoeconomics* and *evidence-based practice.*

- Discuss pharmacoeconomics analyses as they relate to resource allocation and increased efficiency.

- Summarize the four perspectives to be used when evaluating pharmacoeconomic claims.

- Compare and contrast the four models used for pharmacoeconomic analyses.

- Identify and explain three strategies that can be used to conduct pharmacoeconomic analyses.

- Identify the various proactive and reactive methods used for pharmacoeconomic analyses.

Traditionally, health care providers have favored past experience, prevailing practice, professional education, and authority opinion as guides for day-to-day decisions about patient care. The origins of medical and nursing myths and the reasons they persist are numerous and often murky. In our health care institutions and clinical experiences, unfounded beliefs of uncertain efficacy may be passed down as a kind of clinical lore from professors to students. Clinical practices can remain unexamined for decades because they stem from respected authorities. However, the continued progress of health care throughout the world has created an impetus to ground clinical decisions in a more critical examination of the benefits and costs of medical treatments. By knowing which treatments are most effective clinically and economically, wiser decisions

73

can be made about the distribution of limited health care resources.

Traditional beliefs have become less reliable as the volume and complexity of health care information has grown exponentially. The difficulties health care providers face in keeping abreast with the advances are obvious. Simply to keep up with advances in general practice, the health care provider would need to study many articles per day, 365 days per year. Obviously, most care providers have little time available to do so. However, studies have shown that busy health care providers who devote their scarce reading time to selective, efficient, searching methods as well as appraisal and incorporation of the best available evidence can successfully provide evidence-based care.

On any given day, many questions are asked about the outcomes of clinical practice questions (e.g., "Is this drug really the best treatment for this individual patient?" and "What happened after the patient took this drug?"). Clinical decisions are arrived at by an-

swering key questions about the outcomes of care and focus around four main areas: diagnosis, treatment, harm/etiology, and prognosis. Many questions cannot be answered by authority opinion, empirical evidence, or even the most current textbook. Journal articles may not answer clinical practice questions, because much of the information is not based on scientifically valid criteria. Even when a research article is found, health care providers must critically evaluate the study's scientific methodology and conclusions to determine the usefulness of its findings to their practice. In today's managed care environment it is particularly important to critically examine economic aspects of health care by explicitly delineating costs and benefits of various treatments. Yet how do health care providers know which methodologies best answer the questions?

Increasingly, the operating principle in health care has become "the best health care we can afford." Today's payors for health care services are demanding that

---

TABLE 6-1

Comparison of the Tenets of Evidence-Based Practice (EBP) and Research

Tenets	*EBP*	*Research*
Title	A strategy to change in the light of best evidence	An investigation into a particular topic
Abstract	Summarizes what was done, what was found, and what changes were brought about	Summarizes what was done and what was found No discussion about what changes were brought about
Introduction	Existing evidence from a variety of sources is used to set the context	Provides rationale for the selection of a research topic in light of existing gaps in knowledge
Problem	EBP question/hypothesis statement	Research question/hypothesis statement
Objectives	Conducts a systematic review of . . . Compares best evidence with current practice in . . . Devised a strategy to change practice . . . in light of the best evidence	Explores relationships between . . . and . . . in relation to . . . Develops predictive models of such relationships
Literature review	Systematic literature review includes inclusion/exclusion strategies Literature used as part of evidence on which to base clinical decision	Structured but exclusion/inclusion criteria less rigorous Literature used to justify the need for the study
Design	Strategy designed to establish other evidence (e.g., patient preferences) and determine current practice (e.g., audit data)	Identifies research approach used (e.g., quasi-experimental, experimental, ethnography, etc.)
Population	Focuses on specific patient groups about whom clinical decisions are to be made (e.g., all patients who have a specific condition and their relatives)	Concerned with generalizing results to a given population (e.g., all nurses in the United States)
Sampling	May involve sampling of audit data (e.g., every *n*th complaint about a specific area)	May involve random sampling to ensure high potential for generalization

Adapted from Carnwell R: Essential differences between research and evidence-based practice, *Nurse Res* 8(2):55-68, 2000.

new drugs demonstrate benefits that are worth the additional expense. However, this operating principle only confounds the question as to which methodologies best answer clinical practice questions while providing the best affordable health care. There are also essential differences between research and evidence-based practice, which further muddies the waters (Table 6-1). This chapter provides an overview of the key components of this paradigm that have particular importance for nursing.

EVIDENCE-BASED PRACTICE

Evidence-based practice (EBP) is a process of life-long, problem-based learning. It means integrating individual clinical expertise with the best available patient-centered evidence. Individual clinical expertise means using the proficiency and good judgment acquired through clinical experience and practice. The term *EBP* evolved from work done in *evidence-based medicine (EBM)*, defined by Sackett, Rosenberg, Muir Gray et al. as "the conscientious, explicit, and judicious use of current best evidence in medical decisions about the care of individual patients." The key here is to use research findings that are currently the best available. The EBP process involves six steps: (1) formally developing an answerable question to address a specific patient problem or situation; (2) systematically searching for research evidence that can be used to answer the question; (3) critically appraising that evidence for validity and clinical usefulness; (4) integrating the research evidence with information that may influence the management of the patient's problem (including clinical expertise, patient preference for alternative forms of care, and available resources); (5) applying the results to clinical practice; and (6) evaluating the outcomes of the evidence in clinical application. In other words, the best evidence, moderated by patient circumstances and preferences, is applied to improve the quality of clinical judgments. The Evidence-Based Practice box provides a listing of quality Internet resources on EBP.

TABLE 6-1

Comparison of the Tenets of Evidence-Based Practice (EBP) and Research—cont'd

Tenets	EBP	Research
Methods	Relies on existing data. New data collected only if there is an absence of available data	Uses interviews, observation, questionnaires, etc. Interviews could be analyzed through content analysis, questionnaires by statistical methods
Ethics	Applies the normal considerations of confidentiality and anonymity when accessing patient records or reviewing audit data	Addresses issues of consent, confidentiality, anonymity, freedom from harm, and benefits of the study Data collection tools often require approval from ethics committee
Presentation of findings	Evidence is presented from various sources (e.g., audit data, expert opinion, observation of local practices, clinical practice guidelines, etc.) Audit data may include descriptive statistical data Qualitative data may include quotations	Findings are presented as either field notes (e.g., from qualitative research) or as statistical results, depending on methodology used
Interpretation	Presents detailed interpretation of evidence from various sources Convergence or disagreement of data from different sources is discussed	Findings are presented and interpreted in light of the purpose of the study to make sense of them
Discussion	Compares evidence from current practice with best evidence from literature and clinical guidelines Deficiencies in current practice are explained	Findings are compared with those discussed in the literature Implications for practice are explained
Conclusion	Summary of main findings leads to an action plan Plan specifies specifically what changes are needed and how these will be brought about	Includes a summary of main findings and a list of recommendations for future research and practice

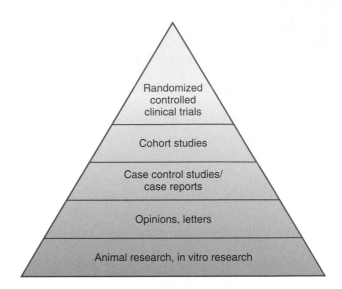

FIGURE 6-1 Evidence pyramid. Movement from the base of the pyramid decreases the amount of available literature but increases the best evidence and relevancy to clinical practice. Adapted from Schardt C, Mayer J: *Self-paced tutorial: evidence-based medicine,* Chapel Hill, NC, 1999, University of North Carolina. Copyright: Duke University Medical Center Library and Health Sciences Library, University of North Carolina at Chapel Hill.

Hierarchies of Evidence

EBP requires a new level of skill for the health care provider, including the ability to apply formal rules of evidence to effectively evaluate clinical literature. The notion that not all evidence is created equal and useful is not new. The literature reports the whole spectrum of the scientific research process, from in vitro studies to double-blind randomized controlled trials. According to the rules of evidence, **randomized controlled clinical trials** are located at the top of the **evidence hierarchy** because they represent the strongest form of support for clinical decisions. The evidence hierarchy identified in Figure 6-1 reflects the ever-increasing complexity of research activity and thus greater rigor. For example, a rigorously conducted quantitative research study, such as that found in randomized controlled clinical trials, has a tightly controlled study design, uses valid and reliable measurement tools, and takes a representative sample. When there is no evidence at the top of the hierarchy to support clinical decisions, health care providers should look for information from the next highest level of research studies available.

The base of the pyramid includes in vitro and animal research. This is usually where an idea or drug is first tested. Opinions or letters share anecdotal information based on strictly empirical data. Collections of case re-

ports have no control groups with which to compare outcomes; therefore the data have no statistical validity.

Case control studies compare a group of patients who already have a specific condition with those who do not have the condition. The problem with this type of study is that it is difficult to conclude reliably that a specific treatment or variable necessarily caused a specific outcome.

Cohort studies use a large population and follow patients over time who have a specific condition or who are using a certain drug treatment. Outcomes for these patients are then compared with those from another group not affected by the same condition. Cohort studies are best used for evidence of prognosis, cause, and prevention. However, because the variable under study may not be the only difference between the two groups, cohort studies are not as reliable as randomized controlled studies.

Randomized controlled clinical trials are considered the gold standard for determining the effect of treatments or tests on patients. These studies are more likely to be free of bias because patients are randomly assigned to treatment or control groups. By controlling for bias through randomization, characteristics such as ethnicity, gender, age, cultural beliefs, and health status are not considered. The limitation of the clinical trial is that

EVIDENCE-BASED PRACTICE
Skills

Necessary Background

- Understand what EBP is and is not and how it is different from what you are now doing
- Learn how to find and use EBP resources

When to Search for Evidence

- When a patient problem is bothering you
- When a patient presents with a common problem that you often encounter

How to Get Started

- Formally develop an answerable question to address your specific patient's problem
- Systematically search for research evidence that can be used to answer the question
- Critically appraise the evidence for validity, reliability, and clinical usefulness by considering the following questions

Assessment

- Describe the problem and why it is significant to clinical practice. Are the research variables and consequences of not solving the problem suggested?
- Include a literature review pertinent to the problem: Were the cited studies critically examined? Was reliability and validity of previous research discussed?
- Is the research design appropriate for studying the research question(s) or hypotheses?
- Are the sampling method(s) described and justified? Have proper controls been included? Is sample size sufficient to reduce Type II errors (i.e., something other than chance)? Have sources of sampling error been identified?

- Were biases, assumptions, and confounding, moderating, and/or extraneous variables identified?
- Are the methods of data collection sufficiently described to permit judgment of their appropriateness for the study? Were the validity and reliability of instruments pertinent to the study identified? Clearly identify assumptions made relevant to the measurement tools used?
- Were the statistical testing methods identified and obtained values reported?
- Were the statistical testing methods appropriate to the research questions or hypotheses?
- Are study conclusions clearly stated and substantiated by the evidence presented?
- Address their limitations and present information in an unbiased manner. Are methodologic problems identified and discussed?
- Present results that include all issues of concern: Are the results generalizable only to the population on which the study is based?

Planning

- USE YOUR COMMON SENSE!

Implementation

- Integrate the research evidence with information that influences the management of the patient's problem (including clinical expertise, patient preference for alternative forms of care, and available resources)
- Apply the results to clinical practice

Evaluation

---

it can only measure the variable it was designed to test; the effect of gender or age will not be assessed unless the trial is designed to do so. To test all the clinically relevant variables would be prohibitively expensive, which is a real limitation of the design and thus a frequent criticism of EBP. The skills needed for EBP are identified in the Evidence-Based Practice box.

The Future of EBP

The future of EBP lies in the outcome products that are produced. These products synthesize the primary research literature and include systematic reviews (i.e., meta-analyses); critically appraised topics (e.g., *ACP Journal Club*); clinical practice guidelines (e.g., AHRQ materials); evaluated bibliographic databases (e.g., Cochrane

Library); and consensus development reports. Dissemination and incorporation of valid research findings into clinical practice is the ultimate goal. These products help the health care provider and patient keep up with the literature while assessing the evidence for use in clinical practice.

EBP'S LINK TO PHARMACOECONOMICS

There is fear that EBP will be hijacked by purchasers and managers of health care insurance plans to cut the costs of health care. This would not only be a misuse of EBP but would also suggest a fundamental misunderstanding of its financial consequences. Health care providers who identify and apply the most effective treatments maximize the quality and quantity of life for individual patients, but this may either raise or lower the cost of care.

Pharmacoeconomics identifies, measures, and compares the costs and consequences of drug products and services. It is the means by which cost factors are incorporated into clinical decisions for drug therapy. In just a few years, pharmacoeconomics has grown from relative obscurity to a prominent role in the development and application of clinical pharmacology. This is because the provision for health care has dramatically changed in recent years. Health care's guiding principle was once "the best that money could buy," with little consideration given to cost. Furthermore, pharmaceutical companies developed new drugs on the belief that health care providers would use them even if the benefits were only marginal or the number of adverse effects decreased. However, as cost limitations increase and cost effectiveness becomes more critical in day-to-day patient care, health care providers must develop a basic understanding of pharmacoeconomics. The knowledge helps all to understand the rationale for choices made, to make the treatment decisions that will be cost-effective, and to help patients to become better health care consumers.

Pharmacoeconomics was initially concerned only with evaluating drug treatment; however, as the field matures, nondrug treatments are also being investigated. For example, a thorough evaluation of treatment for depression must consider not only the various antidepressant drugs but also psychotherapy. In keeping with that philosophy, this chapter discusses the evaluation of treatment options, not just drug therapy, though the vast majority of treatment options are pharmaceutical.

Philosophical Basis of Pharmacoeconomics

Pharmacoeconomics includes two related but separate philosophies—resource allocation and increased efficiency. Resource allocation is primarily concerned with allocating health care resources between broad treatment choices. Increased efficiency is concerned with increasing the effectiveness of medical care.

Resource Allocation. In a society with unlimited resources, it would be unnecessary to have methods that determine the best way to allocate resources. However, in today's health care environment, resources are limited. There are pressures on policymakers and the public as they begin to recognize that every dollar spent on health care is a dollar no longer available for education, crime prevention, or other vital community projects. Much of what we now spend goes for care that does not improve health and that yields small improvements at an exorbitant cost.

There has always been a basic question behind resource allocation: given a variety of treatment options and limited resources, which option should we choose? A common example is whether society is better off spending its limited resources on high-cost drugs that are marginally more effective or have fewer adverse effects, or whether the limited resources would be better spent on older, less expensive drugs that allow a greater number of people to be treated.

Resource allocation has been the main concern of governmental agencies such as the Centers for Medicare and Medicaid Services (formerly the Health Care Financing Agency [HCFA]) when determining what treatments to fund under Medicare, or the Agency for Healthcare Research and Quality (AHRQ) when developing EBP guidelines. Pharmaceutical companies have used a policy-making approach when conducting studies that evaluate the cost-effectiveness of drugs. Economic studies are done to meet FDA regulatory requirements and to convince managed care providers that their specific product is more cost-effective than a competitor's product.

Increased Efficiency. Resource allocation is helpful to a governmental agency trying to determine whether to fund an expensive new treatment. However, this philosophy provides little guidance to health care providers or managed care organizations trying to determine the most efficient means of treating a disease. Whereas general pharmacoeconomics helps determine the best allocation of resources throughout society, health care providers are concerned with choosing among competing treatment options to select the most effective course of action to treat a disease.

An example might provide a clearer understanding of the distinction between the philosophies of resource allocation and increased efficiency. It is generally agreed that when treating depression, there is little difference in the effectiveness of the available drugs. The differences that do exist are more related to the extent of adverse effects. One question facing an organization is whether it should pay the additional cost of newer antidepressants that appear to have fewer adverse effects or continue to pay for older drugs that are just as effective but have potentially more adverse effects. One way to answer this question would be to conduct a study to determine whether the marginal benefit to be gained from using a new drug is greater than the marginal savings from staying with an older drug. The answer suggests to the organization how to allocate its limited resources among the various antidepressant drugs.

At the same time, this information is of little benefit to the health care provider who must choose from 20 different drugs and psychotherapy to pick the option that will best treat the patient for the least cost. Instead, it is necessary to compare all reasonable treatment options to make the most efficient choice. Finally, it is possible that a new antidepressant can be cost-effective from a resource allocation perspective and still not be the best choice for the patient.

Perspectives

In attempting to understand pharmacoeconomic concepts (especially when evaluating pharmacoeconomic claims), the single most important issue is perspective. The analysis, treatment options, costs, and values chosen depend on perspective. For example, a societal perspective could use the average wholesale price of a drug in an analysis. On the other hand, a payor perspective could use the actual cost of a specific drug to that payor. Careful consideration of perspective is important because a real difference between the two costs dramatically changes the results and therefore the choice of the most cost-effective treatment. It is not uncommon for two separate analyses to reach different conclusions because of varying perspectives.

The following four perspectives are taken into account in pharmacoeconomic analyses. Each perspective has its own advantages and disadvantages. Thus it is important that the user of an analysis explicitly consider the perspective of that analysis when evaluating the results.

Society. The societal perspective is the most common because of the early influence of health economics research, which usually focused on society, and the interest of governmental policy making bodies to regulate and allocate resources across societal interests. From this perspective, the costs and values of treatment are based on the interest of society as a whole. A strong argument can be made that the societal perspective is the only one that should be used in pharmacoeconomic analyses, because it considers the well being of all members of society. However, society is made up of many different values and interests, and it is not always possible to determine which costs and values best reflect the interests of all members. In addition, the societal perspective does not take into account the particular interests and circumstances of individual organizations. In an effort to find a common denominator, the societal perspective can produce results that are not in the best interest of an organization or its patients.

Payor. From the payor's perspective, the costs and values chosen reflect those that apply to a specific payor or organization. Because this perspective begins with a specific organization and uses its costs, it can provide the most cost-effective and efficient treatment choice. But because the costs and values are specific to that organization, it is often difficult to generalize the results to other organizations. For example, the cost to a payor (e.g., Blue Cross/Blue Shield or Medicare) equals the charges that are allowed by that payor. This perspective has historically not been used to any great extent, although it is gaining favor, since payors demand pharmacoeconomic analyses relevant to their organizations.

Health Care Provider. From the perspective of the health care provider (e.g., a hospital), its own values and costs are chosen for the analysis. This perspective is often closely aligned with the payor perspective, especially when the values of the providers coincide with the interests of managed care organizations. To determine the provider's cost, it is often necessary to carry out cost-finding exercises using techniques that have been developed by accountants and industrial engineers (e.g., time and motion studies). For example, the savings to a hospital can be calculated by changing from a drug that requires multiple daily doses to one that requires once-daily dosing. This perspective has traditionally focused less on the cost differences between treatment options and more on the differences in effectiveness.

Patient. The patient's perspective is occasionally used in pharmacoeconomic analyses, and a persuasive argument can be made that it should be used more often. Unfortunately, this argument suffers from three major faults. First, there may be significant differences in perspective among various individuals or groups. Should the interests of patients whose diseases are uncommon be valued less because their disorders are not as prevalent as others? Second, thanks to insurance coverage, many patients do not pay directly for the health care resources they receive, which distorts true cost-benefit ratios. And finally, by its very nature, pharmacoeconomics is based on the population rather than on the individual. Thus there is an inherent conflict between what is in the best interest of the individual patient and what is in the best interest of a group of patients.

Pharmacoeconomic Models

There are four basic pharmacoeconomics models: cost-benefit analysis (CBA), cost-effectiveness analysis (CEA), cost-utility analysis (CUA), and cost-minimization analysis (CMA). Each of these approaches measures costs in dollars but measures outcomes (consequences) differently. Each also has its own advantages and disadvantages, degrees of usefulness, and value. Table 6-2 compares the four approaches to economic analysis.

Cost-Benefit Analysis. CBA has traditionally been the choice of economists. In CBA, all costs and benefits are measured in dollars. If the value is more than the cost, the option is cost-beneficial and should be undertaken. Be-

---

TABLE 6-2

Comparison of Approaches to Pharmacoeconomic Analysis (Costs in Dollars)

Approach	Outcomes (Consequences)	Formula
Cost-benefit analysis	Dollars	CB ratio = $ benefit − $ cost
Cost-effectiveness analysis	Natural units (e.g., blood pressure, lipid levels, lives saved, days of illness averted)	CE ratio = $\dfrac{\$ \text{ cost}}{\text{unit of effectiveness}}$
Cost-utility analysis	Quality adjusted life-years	CU ratio = (X years)(health state of patient)
Cost-minimization analysis	Equality of outcomes*	

*Assumes a constant outcome (consequence).

---

cause CBA measures everything in dollars, it allows analyses for different types of outcomes to be compared. For example, a decision maker with limited resources could choose between erecting a new administration building and funding a new treatment for Medicaid patients.

In most cases, a value can be assigned to the costs of treatment. However, trouble begins when we attempt to measure its benefit. The disadvantage of CBA is that it is difficult to place a dollar value on health benefits. How does one value the benefit of a few days of better health, much less the value of surviving an illness? Because answering this question is plagued with many problems, the CBA approach to pharmacoeconomic analysis is rarely used. There are occasional reports of research conducted using this approach, but those articles must be carefully scrutinized.

There are two methods commonly used to estimate a value for these types of questions—the human capital approach and the willingness-to-pay approach. The human capital approach presumes that the value of health benefits is equal to the economic productivity that they permit. The cost of a disease is related to the cost of productivity lost because of the disease. A person's expected income (before taxes) or an imputed value for nonemployment activities (e.g., housework or child care) is used as an estimate of the value of health benefits for that person. Then again, earnings may not reflect a person's true worth to society.

The willingness-to-pay method estimates the value of benefits by estimating how much people would pay to reduce their chance of an adverse health outcome. The difficulty with this approach is that what people say they are willing to pay may conflict with what they actually do. The willingness of third parties (i.e., insurers) to pay should also be taken into consideration.

Cost-Effectiveness Analysis. CEA measures the outcome of treatment in terms of natural health units such as reduction in blood pressure or lipid levels, the probability of cure, or days of illness averted. The choice of units is determined by what is most relevant to the disease

state or treatment in question. The benefit to this approach is that it is generally analogous to the logic used by health care providers when a clinical pharmacotherapeutic decision is made. Like the CBA model, the cost of providing treatment is valued in dollars. The worth of a CEA is in the ratio between a dollar amount and the unit of effectiveness.

The CEA ratio depends on the nonmonetary unit chosen, but the advantage is that the researcher is not responsible for assigning a monetary value to health. The disadvantage is that it becomes difficult to compare unrelated treatment options. The options to be compared must have similar outcomes that are measurable in the same units.

Cost-Utility Analysis. In CUA, the effectiveness unit is not a natural condition of the disease or treatment but rather an artificial measure designed to allow for comparisons among different diseases or populations. CUA takes patient preferences into account when measuring health outcomes. The most commonly used utility measure is that of quality life-years saved (QALY), the number of years of life a treatment option saves, adjusted to include a preference for quality of life. Although there is considerable debate about which dimensions should be used as QALY units, the most common are physical functioning, the ability to carry out prescribed roles, and mental health status. The concept of QALY is based on the notion that a year of being healthy is preferable to and worth more than a year of illness. For example, 1 year of perfect health has a score of 1.0 QALY. A disease that reduces the quality of life by one half takes away 0.5 QALY over the course of 1 year. If the disease affects five people, it will take away 5 times 0.5, or 2.5 QALY over a period of 1 year. A drug that improves the quality of life by 0.2 for each of the five people results in the equivalent of 1 QALY if the benefit is maintained over a period of 1 year.

Cost-Minimization and Cost-of-Illness Analyses. Cost-minimization analysis (CMA) is a variation of CEA in which the outcomes are assumed to be equivalent among possible options. Only the costs are evaluated. Although the costs are explicitly measured, the consequences are not. The measurement and comparison of costs for two equivalent generic drugs is an example of CMA. Another example is the measurement and comparison of total costs required for home intravenous antibiotic therapy with the total costs of providing this therapy in the hospital. The strength of CMA assumes that outcomes are the same. This evidence can be based on previous studies, publications, FDA data, or expert opinion.

Cost-of-illness analysis attempts to measure the cost factors associated with a particular disease, including direct costs such as medical services and indirect costs such as loss of productivity due to illness or premature death. The equality of outcomes assumes there is a constant, an unchanging consequence, in the equation.

Techniques for Conducting Pharmacoeconomic Analyses

Independent of the perspective or approach chosen, there are several strategies that can be used to conduct pharmacoeconomic analyses. The choice of strategy depends to some extent on the purpose of the analysis and the expectations of the audience.

Clinical Trials. The majority of pharmacoeconomic analyses are evaluations that have been piggybacked onto clinical trials evaluating the efficacy and safety of a specific treatment. The FDA requests that economic data be collected as part of the clinical trial and used to determine the cost-effectiveness of the treatment under study. However, most pharmacoeconomists are aware of the inherent limitation of a clinical trial—the results of experimental research do not accurately represent what occurs in the real world. Therefore the results of clinical trials are difficult to generalize to practice settings.

In an attempt to resolve these limitations, some researchers are using **open-label clinical trials.** An open-label clinical trial is done without control groups or the blinding of variables normally found in standard clinical drug trials. Patients and health care providers are allowed to participate, to take the drug of their choosing, and even to change drugs, if desired. Costs and effectiveness of the treatment is followed, and the results are evaluated to determine the most cost-effective treatment.

The assumption here is that an open-label trial more closely mimics what happens in real life. Many researchers and health care providers, however, are suspicious of the results of open-label trials because they lack control groups and blinding, the very components designed to produce unbiased results. Finally, the limitations of an open-label trial are similar to that of the randomized controlled clinical trial in that the expense restricts the number of treatment options that can be evaluated at any one time, making it difficult to evaluate more than just a few treatment options.

Retrospective Database Analysis. Retrospective database analysis analyzes clinical and economic information by using statistical and mathematical methods to determine the relationship between treatment options, outcomes, and costs. The advantage of this approach is that the data are usually readily available and reflect the historical experience of the particular organization.

This approach provides significant results and information to an organization, especially when external factors are properly controlled; however, three limitations must be kept in mind. Data analysis can be technically challenging, especially when there are large unrelated data sets. Also, the data may not be accurate—biases can and do distort the results of any analysis, regardless of the type of trial.

Finally, because of policies, circumstances, or changes in treatments over time, the data may not truly reflect a fair comparison of all treatment options. For example, some data sets may not include certain drugs, or there may be a perception among health care providers that a particular drug should be reserved for sicker patients, thereby distorting the cost experience of that drug. The limitations to data sets can often be controlled by statistical means, but there is a limit to these types of corrections, especially when subtle biases are not recognized. The net result is that retrospective database analyses can provide information with which to make accurate cost-effective determinations, but the user of the studies must carefully evaluate the analysis.

Mathematical Modeling. Mathematical modeling allows the researcher to predict a phenomenon that would otherwise be impossible to measure directly. For example, there are dozens of drugs available for the treatment of hypertension, any of which could be used singly or in many different combinations. Only a model can evaluate these treatment combinations.

The advantage of using a mathematical model is its ability to evaluate questions that cannot be directly analyzed because of complexity or cost. The disadvantage of modeling, especially as the model becomes more complex, is its underlying mathematical nature. A certain degree of comfort and familiarity with mathematical concepts and techniques is required. In addition, developing accurate models is as much an art as a science. Traditionally, mathematical models have not been the preferred means of conducting pharmacoeconomic analyses. However, this attitude may change as more people become familiar with the necessary techniques, managed care organizations begin to demand more applied pharmacoeconomic analyses, and health care providers realize that some pharmacoeconomic questions can be answered only by such models.

Methods for Pharmacoeconomic Analyses

A second way to understand pharmacoeconomic analyses is by the type of method or structure used. Ultimately, the data must be evaluated by using one of several methods. For example, during a clinical trial, economic data can be captured that could be used to determine the cost-effectiveness of the certain drug treatment options. Then, however, a pharmacoeconomic method must then be chosen to analyze those data. The following discussion includes some of the more commonly used methods.

Proactive Methods

Decision Analysis. A decision analysis is the most common method used. This method reduces the manage-

ment of a disease into a series of treatment choices made by the health care provider. Using this method, a decision tree is created that includes options from which the health care provider or health care system must choose. Costs and outcomes are assigned to these decisions, and ultimately, the cost-effectiveness of a particular decision is determined. This methodology can be used in conjunction with clinical trials, databases, or models.

Decision trees are easy to use, and several computer programs are available to create them. Unfortunately, as the number of treatment options increases, the number of decision points grows exponentially, causing a decision tree to quickly become a decision forest. This growth limits the usefulness of this method when more than a few drug choices must be evaluated. For example, consider the management of a sore throat. The treatment options include (1) giving antibiotics to all patients, (2) culturing for streptococcus and giving antibiotics to patients with positive cultures, or (3) giving antibiotics to none of the patients (Figure 6-2).

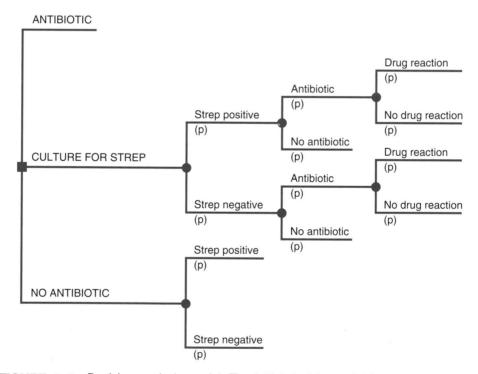

FIGURE 6-2 Decision analysis model. The initial decision point is represented by a square; subsequent decision points occur at each branch of the model. Only the beginning of the process is shown here. The upper branch represents the option of treating the patient empirically (i.e., giving an antibiotic without culturing for the streptococcus organism). The middle branch represents the option of culturing for the streptococcus organism and waiting for the results before determining the need for an antibiotic. The lower branch, no treatment, represents the option of not giving antibiotics nor culturing for the streptococcus organism. In analyses comparing various antibiotics, there would be a branch for each drug. There is an uncertain possibility of an allergic reaction, as represented in the branches for drug reaction and no reaction. At each decision point, a value *p* is assigned based on the probability of a reaction.

Simulation Modeling. Simulation modeling is a mathematical method that simulates real world events from inputs and choices made by health care providers. In many ways, this is directly analogous to mathematical modeling. When handled properly, this method can be easy to understand and provide tremendous insight into the choices and efficiencies of providers when making treatment decisions. At the same time, this approach can be difficult to implement. The results can also be difficult to understand and believe if the mathematics underlying the simulation are overly vague and complex. Despite this problem, simulation modeling remains the approach best able to answer complex questions of cost-effectiveness when the decision involves multiple treatment options.

Reactive Methods

Statistical Analysis. Statistical analysis is best used with large data sets. It can also be applied in clinical trials and models when sufficient data are available. Descriptive statistics (i.e., means, medians, standard deviations), inferential statistics (i.e., *t*-test, paired *t*-tests, chi-square analysis), and more advanced inferential techniques (i.e., regression analysis, factor analysis, and logistic regression) are used to evaluate both the costs and effectiveness of each drug option.

Statistical analysis works best when data already exist, either in the form of a database or as the results of a clinical trial or mathematical model. Statistical evaluation of alternative treatment regimens requires a thorough understanding of the process that generated the health care provider's and the patient's behaviors as well as the data collection effort. It is important to go beyond simple univariate statistical analysis to understand how much confidence can be placed in the results (i.e., estimated cost-effectiveness ratio). Sensitivity analysis shows which parametric variables will have a dramatic effect on the conclusions, but it fails to capture all of the variability resulting from estimating multiple parameter values.

Whereas other methods are predictive, statistical methods are descriptive, finding results already in the data. Such statistical analysis looks for relationships within a data set, whereas the other two methods begin with the data and predict (based on assumptions and an analytic framework) the cost-effectiveness. This means that statistical analysis is preferred when the data are extensive and complete.

FUTURE OF PHARMACOECONOMICS

The field of pharmacoeconomics and the data it evaluates change rapidly as the field evolves. Several themes will play increasing roles in the field and will be reflected in the published literature. These themes include increased pressure on health care providers to consider the economic impact of their decisions on individual patients and on the populations they serve; demands by managed care organizations for analyses that meet their specific needs rather than the needs of policymakers; and a push toward standardization and guidelines in conducting and reporting pharmacoeconomic evaluations. In addition, the philosophies, perspectives, models, and techniques used in pharmacoeconomics have influenced the movement of evidence-based practice.

SUMMARY

Although research and its analysis are becoming more and more complicated, all health care providers should understand some basic evaluation principles. From ethical and legal perspectives, and because of a desire for positive outcomes, health care providers today should strive to base their practice on the best evidence available. They should prescribe, encourage, or deliver treatment only when the evidence supports their actions. The empirical side of practice should be reserved for the art portion of health care delivery and not the science portion. Basing therapy on the best evidence available helps ensure that health care providers will be respected as safe, scientifically oriented practitioners.

Bibliography

Bootman J, Townsend R, McGhan, W (eds.): *Principles of pharmacoeconomics*, ed 2, Cincinnati, OH, 1996, Harvey Whitney Books.

Carnwell R: Essential differences between research and evidence-based practice, *Nurse Res* 8(2):55-68, 2000.

Davidoff F, Haynes B, Sackett D, et al: Evidence-based medicine: a new journal to help doctors identify the information they need, *Br Med J* 310:1085-1086, 1995.

Gerrish K, Clayton J: Improving clinical effectiveness through an evidenced-based approach: meeting the challenge for nursing in the United Kingdom, *Nurs Adm Q* 22(4):55-65, 1998.

Good CJ, Piedalue F: Evidenced-based clinical practice, *J Nurs Adm* 29(6):15-21, 1999.

Ingersoll GL: Evidence-based nursing: what it is and what it isn't, *Nurs Outlook* 48(4):151-152, 2000.

Jennings BM, Loan LA: Misconceptions among nurses about evidence-based practice, *J Nurs Scholarsh* 33(2):121-127, 2001.

Kessenich CR, Guyatt GH, DiCenso A: Teaching nursing students evidence-based nursing, *Nurse Educ* 22(6):25-29, 1997.

Michaud G, McGowan JL, van der Jagt R, et al: Are therapeutic decisions supported by evidence from health care research? *Arch Intern Med* 158:1665-1668, 1998.

Sloan F: *Valuing health care: cost, benefits, and effectiveness of pharmaceuticals and other medical technologies*, New York, 1995, Cambridge University Press.

Steinke DT, MacDonald TM, Davey PG: The doctor-patient relationship and prescribing patterns: a view from primary care, *Pharmacoeconomics* 16(6):559-603, 1999.

Stetler CB, Morsi D, Rucki S, et al: Utilization-focused integrative reviews in a nursing service, *Appl Nurs Res* 11(4):195-206, 1998.

Stevens KR, Pugh JA: Evidence-based practice and perioperative nursing, *Semin Perioper Nurs* 8(3):155-159, 1999.

Wilke R: What's all this about pharmacoeconomics? *Bus Econ* 30(2):26-31, 1995.

Internet Resources

Agency for Healthcare Research and Quality: Evidence-based practice, 2001. Available online: http://www.ahcpr.gov.

International Society for Pharmacoeconomics and Outcomes Research: Pharmacoeconomics: identifying the issues, 1998. Available online: http://www.ispor.org.

Sackett DL, Rosenberg WMC, Muir Gray JA, et al: Evidence-based medicine: What it is and what it isn't, 1996. Available online: http://cebm.warne.ox.ac.uk/ebmisisnt.html.

Legal Implications of Drug Therapy

LYNN ROGER WILLIS

 Visit **http://evolve.elsevier.com/Gutierrez/** for additional information.

KEY TERMS

Bioavailability, p. 86

Bioequivalence, p. 86

Brand name, p. 86

Carcinogenicity, p. 89

Clinical trials, p. 89

Double-blind study designs, p. 89

Efficacy, p. 86

Generic name, p. 86

Orphan drugs, p. 88

Potency, p. 86

Purity, p. 86

Teratogens, p. 89

Therapeutic index, p. 86

OBJECTIVES

- Explain how drugs are tested for safety.
- Explain how a drug is determined to be effective for use in patients.
- Explain what controlled substances are.
- Discuss the role of nurses in drug testing.

Patients who receive drugs always face certain risks, which include the possibility that the drug (1) will not produce the beneficial effect claimed by those who make and sell the drug, (2) may be directly harmful, or (3) may be improperly administered. Modern drug legislation is designed to reduce or eliminate these risks to patients and to outline the responsibilities of health care providers.

ESTABLISHMENT OF SAFETY AND EFFICACY OF DRUGS
History of Drug Development

The earliest medical practice depended on various natural products that, by trial and error, were discovered to have certain effects on the body. For example, ancient Egyptians knew that parts of the poppy plant could be used to relieve pain. This remedy was first recorded in the Ebers papyrus in 1500 BC. Equally ancient is the use of parts of the ephedra shrub by the Chinese, who called the preparation ma huang. In the New World, South American Indians used bark from the cinchona tree to relieve symptoms of malaria. Even in more recent times, natural products were used for medical practice. For example, in 1785 a British physician named Withering described the use of the leaf of the foxglove plant to relieve an edematous condition we now call heart failure ("the dropsy") that had previously resisted all therapy.

Until the mid-1800s, natural products were the only medicinal agents available. The most common drugs were made from plants and were called botanicals. Most botanicals have been replaced as chemists have identified the active ingredients in these crude products. The active ingredients are the chemicals in the crude preparation that are responsible for producing the biologic effect of the medicinal agent. For example, the poppy plant relieves pain because it contains opium. Ma huang affects the heart, lungs, and other organs because it contains ephedrine. Cinchona bark relieves the symptoms of malaria because it contains quinine, and the leaves of the foxglove plant relieve "the dropsy" (edema) because they contain digitalis.

Identification of the active ingredient in a crude medicinal agent has two benefits. First, the amount of active ingredient can be measured in the crude preparation, allowing effective standardization of dosage. For example, the digitalis content of foxglove leaves varies from plant to plant. Dosages based on the amount of leaf taken may actually contain variable amounts of digitalis and may therefore have variable biologic effects, whereas dosage based on the amount of digitalis contained in a batch of foxglove leaves should have a more predictable biologic effect. Wherever possible (i.e., if chemical analysis is possible), drug dosage should be based on chemical analysis of the drug itself.

The second benefit of identifying the active ingredient of a medicinal agent is that the chemical structure and properties of the active drug are revealed. This knowledge can lead to better ways of isolating the active material from natural sources. After the structure of an active agent is known, chemists may also be able to synthesize it. Ephedrine is an example of a drug that is now chemically synthesized in a simple process that has replaced the more complicated procedure of extracting the drug from plant materials.

Drug Standards

The United States Pharmacopeial Convention develops standards to ensure the uniform quality of drugs. These standards are published in the *United States Pharmacopeia/National Formulary (USP/NF)*. The Food and Drug Administration (FDA) enforces adherence to these stan-

dards for all drugs offered for sale in interstate commerce. The standards pertain to purity, bioavailability, potency, efficacy, safety, and toxicity. **Purity** refers to the uncontaminated state of a drug, but since additives are usually needed to facilitate the formulation of tablets, capsules, or other dosage forms, or to facilitate the absorption of a drug into the blood, the standards specified by the USP relate to the type and amount of such additives, too. These additives are called excipients.

Bioavailability is the degree to which a drug can be absorbed by the body and transported to its site of action (Chapter 1). Factors influencing bioavailability include solubility, polarity, crystalline structure, and particle size. Bioavailability is important for understanding drug laws because bioavailability is one way in which **bioequivalence** (biological equivalence) between two preparations can be evaluated.

Potency generally depends on the concentration of active drug in the preparation. Potency is determined by chemical assay when the active ingredient is known and assay methods exist, and by bioassay when the identity of the active ingredient is unknown or a chemical assay is not available.

Efficacy refers to the ability of a drug used in treatment of illness or disease to be effective. Objective measures are rarely available for determining efficacy; therefore, subjective data are cautiously interpreted. Double-blind studies (see below) are used to distinguish the greatest efficacy among alternative drugs.

The incidence and severity of adverse reactions determine the safety of a drug. As a general rule, no active chemical agent is free of toxic effects. The **therapeutic index** (margin of safety) of a drug is the difference between therapeutic and toxic doses.

Nomenclature

A drug generally has three names: its chemical name, based on the chemical structure of the drug, its **generic name** or common name, which is simpler than the chemical name and identifies the drug in the scientific literature, and its trade name or **brand name,** which identifies the drug as the product of a specific manufacturer. For example, 7-chloro-1,3-dihydro-1-methyl-5-phenyl-2*H*-1,4-benzodiazepin-2-one is the chemical name for the drug generically known as diazepam. Diazepam was first patented and produced by Roche Laboratories under the trade name Valium. Once patent protection for a drug has expired (see below), other companies may market the drug under other brand names.

Standards for medicinal agents vary among countries. In Canada, the current *Compendium of Pharmaceuticals and Specialties (CPS)* indexes available agents and contains monographs on specific drugs. The *British Pharmacopoeia* is the standard reference for the United

Kingdom. It also includes information from the *European Pharmacopoeia* and is updated yearly with published addenda. The *International Pharmacopoeia* published by the World Health Organization (WHO) includes drug methods and standardizations.

Legislation

Drug manufacturing and sales are regulated by state and federal agencies. For federal laws to apply, a drug must enter interstate commerce. A drug totally manufactured within a single state and sold only in that state would not be subject to the federal drug laws. Very few drugs fall into this category.

The first effective federal drug law in the United States was passed in 1906 (Table 7-1). This law was intended to protect citizens from adulterated drugs and drugs that contain harmful ingredients not listed on the label. Each new law or amendment adopted since that time has been intended to overcome unforeseen limitations of the existing law. For example, in the early 1900s, a certain patent drug was advertised as a cure for cancer. The federal government sought to force the manufacturer to stop using the false advertisement. However, the drug label on the bottle accurately named the contents. Under the 1906 law, accurate labeling of contents was all the government could require. When the Sherley Amendment was added in 1912, both advertising claims and contents of the drug label could be controlled.

The Food, Drug, and Cosmetics Act of 1938 added the requirement that a drug must be proven safe before it could be marketed. Before 1938, a company was not required to demonstrate that the drugs it manufactured and sold were safe. The situation changed

TABLE 7-1

Federal Drug Legislation in the United States

Date	Title of Law	Major Provisions
1906	Pure Food and Drug Act	USP and NF are established as official standards. Standards are set for proper drug labeling.
1912	Sherley Amendment	Fraudulent claims for therapeutic effects of drugs are prohibited.
1914	Harrison Narcotic Act	Importation, manufacture, sale, or use of opium, cocaine, marijuana, and other drugs likely to cause dependence was regulated.
1938	Food, Drug, and Cosmetic Act	A drug was required to be proven safe before it was marketed.
1941-1945	Amendments to Pure Food and Drug Act	Biologic products used as drugs (e.g., insulin) are required to be certified on a batch-by-batch basis by a government agency.
1952	Durham-Humphrey Amendment	Legend drugs are defined (must be marked "Caution: Federal Law prohibits dispensing without prescription"). The right of pharmacists to distribute legend drugs is restricted.
1962	Kefauver-Harris Amendment	Proof of efficacy was required for a drug to remain on the market. FDA authorized to establish official names for drugs.
1970	Comprehensive Drug Abuse Prevention and Control Act (or Controlled Substances Act)	Drugs are classified by abuse potential and medical usefulness. Manufacture, distribution, and sale of controlled substances were regulated.
1983	Orphan Drug Act	Companies are protected for 7 years against competition on non-patentable orphan drugs.
1984	Drug Price Competition and Patent Term Restoration Act	Drugs introduced after 1962 were eligible for shortened drug application. Generic drugs are more easily introduced. Guidelines were established for bioequivalence. Patent protection was restored up to 5 years for time used in drug development.
1986, 1988	National Childhood Vaccine Injury Act	Private health care providers are required to keep records of adverse events following immunization.
1987	Prescription Drug Marketing Act	Diversion of prescription drugs from legitimate channels was banned. Reimportation of drugs from other countries was restricted.
1988	Food and Drug Administration Act	FDA was established within Department of Health and Human Services. The mechanism for appointing Commissioner of Food and Drugs was set.

quickly, however, in 1937 when more than 100 people, many of them children, died after taking the new "elixir of sulfanilamide." The cause of death was not sulfanilamide but diethylene glycol, which had been used to dissolve the drug. Diethylene glycol is a common, and toxic, ingredient in antifreeze solutions. Tests of diethylene glycol toxicity had not been conducted before its use in this medicine because the law did not require such tests. Because the law did not address product safety, prosecutors could charge the company responsible for the disaster only with mislabeling their product, since an elixir is by definition a solution containing ethanol and not diethylene glycol. The 1938 revision of this law focused appropriate legal attention on product safety.

A later amendment to the 1938 law, adopted in 1962, requires that a drug must be effective in treating the medical condition for which it is recommended (see Table 7-1). This requirement for increased testing has increased the time and money spent to put new drugs on the market, but the trade-off is that the drugs that do enter the market now are much more reliable than new drugs introduced before this legislation.

The huge costs of developing and testing new drugs under the current laws quickly created an altogether new class of drugs, the so-called "orphan" drugs. Orphan drugs are drugs that have not been profitable to develop and market, either because the market is too small (e.g., drugs used to treat rare diseases) or because patent protection has expired on the drug. To promote the development of such drugs, Congress enacted the Orphan Drug Act of 1983 by which companies can recover much of their costs of developing these drugs. The law protects companies that develop and market non-patentable drugs by limiting approval for an orphan drug to one company for the first 7 years. Some examples of orphan drugs are listed in Table 7-2.

Legislation adopted in 1984 set guidelines for **bioequivalence** of drugs and streamlined application processes so that approval of generic drugs was facilitated. When a drug is first introduced under patent protection, it can be sold only by the company that developed it or by other companies licensed to sell it. Patent protection lasts for 17 years. After the patent expires, other companies can make the drug and sell it under its generic name (or a brand name of their choosing) if they have met FDA standards for chemical purity and bioequivalence. Bioequivalent drugs can be shown to be similar with respect to such pharmacokinetic parameters as dissolution within the gastric fluid and absorption into the bloodstream. The issue of bioequivalence among generic preparations of the same drug has been contentious over the past several decades, since reliable bioequivalence data were initially in short supply for many drugs. Today, however, ample bioequivalence data exists for most drugs being sold generically. Indeed, many companies that once owned the patent rights for a drug now sell the same drug generically.

TABLE 7-2

Examples of Orphan Drugs and Their Indications

Drug/Biologic (Trade Name)	*Proposed Use*	*Sponsor*
AIDS and AIDS-Related Disorders		
2'3'-dideoxyadenosine (DDA)	AIDS	Bristol-Myers, Squibb, National Cancer Institute
ganciclovir (Cytovene)	Cytomegalovirus, severe retinitis	Syntex (USA), Inc.
molgramostim (Leukomax)	Neutropenia	Schering Corp.
Cancers		
interferon alfa-2a (Roferon-A)	Metastatic renal cell cancer	Hoffman-La Roche, Inc.
monoclonal antibody 17-1A (Panorex)	Pancreatic cancer	Centocor, Inc.
filgrastim (Neupogen)	Neutropenia associated with bone marrow transplant	Amgen
Gastrointestional Disorders		
ethanolamine oleate (Ethamolin)	Esophageal varices	Block Drug Co.
somatostatin (Zecnil)	Secreting enterocutaneous fistulas	Ferring Laboratories, Inc.
Neurologic Disorders		
mazindol (Sanorex)	Duchenne muscular dystrophy	Platon J. Collipp, MD, Sandoz
baclofen, intrathecal (Lioresal)	Intractable spasticity related to multiple sclerosis or spinal cord injury	Medtronic, Inc.

DRUG TESTING

The development of new drugs and biologicals is a major industry in the United States. To meet the current standards set by drug legislation, a detailed format is followed to test drugs as they are developed for market. The testing begins in experimental animals and, if successful, proceeds through several phases of testing in human subjects (**clinical trials**). Nurses play an important role in the conduct of clinical trials (see Chapters 5 and 6).

Assessment of Safety of Drugs

All drugs intended for human use must undergo extensive toxicity testing in at least two species of animals. The toxicity tests must include acute and chronic studies.

Acute toxicity tests assess the short-term effects of extreme doses of the drug. The intent of these tests is to identify organs or tissues that may be sensitive to the drug.

Chronic toxicity tests assess the effects of prolonged dosage with the new drug. Several dosages are usually tested, with at least one group of animals receiving dosages far in excess of those expected to be used in humans. After prolonged exposure to the test drug (usually months to years), the animals undergo extensive pathologic and histologic examinations to detect any effects on organs or tissues. Significant toxicity observed in animals is usually sufficient cause for abandoning development of a drug.

Chronic toxicity tests are the stage at which a drug is usually tested for **carcinogenicity** or cancer-inducing effects. Carcinogenicity may also be assessed by the Ames test, which measures mutagenicity (the ability to cause mutations) in bacteria. Since many carcinogenic chemicals are also mutagens, this test can help predict carcinogenicity. The Ames test offers faster, less expensive carcinogenicity testing than chronic toxicity tests in animals.

Drugs are also tested for their effects on pregnant animals and fetuses. Drugs that cause fetal abnormalities are called **teratogens**. Some drugs are very dangerous to fetuses at certain stages of embryonic development but are relatively harmless to adult animals or more mature fetuses. The stage of fetal development in which the fetus is most sensitive to drugs or toxins is the first trimester of gestation. A tragic example of this sensitivity occurred with the drug thalidomide. Thalidomide is a sleep-inducing drug that was widely marketed in Europe during the late 1950s and early 1960s. The drug was not especially dangerous to adults, but when used by women in the early stages of pregnancy, it inhibited proper development of fetal limb buds. The result was the birth of several thousand babies with tiny nonfunctional limbs. This tragedy led Congress to adopt new requirements for teratogenicity testing, which had not previously been a part of the drug development process.

Efficacy of Drugs

After an experimental drug has been tested for toxicity in animals, the manufacturer may file with the FDA a "notice of claimed investigational exemption for a new drug (IND)." All the toxicity data in animals, data on drug absorption and biotransformation, and data on the expected biologic activity of the drug must be included in the IND. The manufacturer or licenser must justify the tests that will be conducted in human subjects.

Phase I, the first testing of a drug in humans, is carried out on a relatively small number of healthy volunteers (usually from 20 to 80 people). The purpose of these studies is not to examine the therapeutic efficacy of the drug, but rather to focus on absorption, distribution, biotransformation, elimination, the preferred route of administration, and the establishment of a safe dosage range. Unexpected adverse effects may appear at this stage of testing. For example, alterations of mood may not be easily recognized in experimental animals but are readily apparent in humans. The appearance of one or more severe adverse effects in Phase I tests may prevent further development of an experimental drug, thereby nullifying the previous years of intense investigation.

Phase II, the second stage of testing in humans, involves clinical trials on 100 to 300 patients who have the disease or condition for which the new drug is intended. This phase evaluates the same aspects as those in Phase I, with the emphasis shifted to compare the effects of the drug in healthy people with those in diseased people. Therapeutic dosages are refined during Phase II. As with Phase I testing, the appearance of serious adverse effects can stop the development of that drug.

Once an effective dosage range has been established (provided there is an absence of serious adverse effects), a more lengthy study of the drug in diseased people can be undertaken. The therapeutic effectiveness of the drug can now be verified with some confidence because larger numbers of individuals (1000 to 3000) will be studied in Phase III. To reduce bias from the evaluation, **double-blind study designs** are used. In this process, neither the patient nor the health care provider knows who received the investigational drug and who received an alternative therapy. The new drug is usually compared with a known effective treatment for the condition. Because the number of subjects exposed to the drug is substantially increased during Phase III, more (but not necessarily all) of the risks associated with taking the drug should become evident (see below).

After the first three phases of human testing have been completed, the drug company submits a report detailing the results of these studies to the FDA. After the report has been evaluated, the company developing the drug may submit a new drug application (NDA). Approval of the NDA means that the new drug has been accepted and therefore can be marketed exclusively by that company on a limited basis. This limited marketing constitutes Phase IV.

Phase IV testing involves monitoring all patients taking the drug for a period of 2 to 3 years, during which gradually more and more patients receive the drug. Controlled, limited release of the drug over this lengthy period is crucial. Before beginning Phase IV, fewer than 4000 people will have taken this drug. Accordingly, since some adverse drug effects occur only rarely (with an incidence, say, of 1 in 30,000), those effects will not likely have been seen during Phases I to III. Moreover, they may not become evident in sufficient numbers to associate them with the drug even during Phase IV testing until tens or possibly even hundreds of thousands of patients have taken the drug. For this reason, drug companies only slowly increase the distribution of new drugs into the population, hoping to be able to identify serious adverse effects in only a relatively small number of people. History shows that some drug companies—and more than a few patients—have paid a tragic price for new drugs that were released too quickly.

Streamlining New Drugs

The procedure for testing drugs as outlined in the preceding discussion entails a careful, conservative approach, taking many years to complete. In 1985, under pressure from interest groups (e.g., terminal cancer patients), the FDA streamlined procedures to bring new drugs into the marketplace more rapidly. The agency reduced the number of case reports required in the application but increased requirements for postmarketing surveillance. All serious adverse effects must be reported to the FDA within 15 days; all adverse effects must be reported every 3 months for the first 3 years and yearly thereafter. Forms for reporting these reactions are published regularly as part of the FDA Drug Bulletin and other publications.

Further pressure for more rapid movement of drugs into clinical tests arose as the acquired immunodeficiency syndrome (AIDS) epidemic began. Without treatment, AIDS patients live a very short time. For these patients and for others with conditions for which no effective therapy exists, a new procedure was created to allow experimental drugs to be used on a wider scale than was previously possible. This process releases drugs for use in patients who meet set criteria, even though the drug is not yet on the market. For example, while didanosine (DDI) was in trials against human immunodeficiency virus (HIV), it was available for use in AIDS patients who were more than 12 years of age, had symptomatic HIV infection, were intolerant to the standard drug zidovudine, and were un-

able to enroll in a phase II trial because of geographic location.

The goal of streamlining new drugs is worthwhile, but comes at the price of reduced safety for patients who would use the streamlined drugs. Of course, concerns about reduced safety often mean less to a patient facing certain death without the treatment than they do to healthy individuals, but the nurse needs to know issues and trade-offs associated with the use of streamlined drugs so that he or she can provide information that will enable a patient to make informed choices about using new drugs.

Drug Efficacy Study Implementation

All drugs introduced after the Kefauver-Harris Amendment in 1962 went through the extensive testing just described and were proved effective and safe before being marketed. Drugs already on the market in 1962 posed a special problem because they had been tested primarily for safety and not efficacy. The Drug Efficacy Study Implementation (DESI) was implemented to bring all drugs up to the same standard. Drugs were rated using the system shown in Table 7-3. Drugs rated as ineffective were removed from the market. Drugs listed as possibly effective or probably effective required reformulation or retesting to stay on the market.

TABLE 7-3

DESI Rating System

Rating	*Description*
Effective	Substantial evidence exists to show that the drug is an effective treatment for the defined medical condition.
Probably effective	Some evidence exists, but more is needed to prove the drug is effective.
Possibly effective	Minimum evidence exists to suggest that the drug may be effective.
Ineffective	Controlled trials failed to show that the drug is more effective than the placebo.
Ineffective as a fixed combination	Individual components of the drug might be effective along appropriate doses, but no evidence suggests that all components of the drug are necessary to effect.
Effective but . . .	A qualification to the use of the drug is made, which must be added to the labeling.

Rights of the Patient in Drug Testing

Anyone involved in assessing the clinical usefulness of a new drug is bound by certain moral and legal constraints. No one may be coerced into receiving a drug that is under investigation. All drug studies must be done on volunteers who have read, understood, and signed informed consent forms. The law requires that all potential hazards associated with use of the drug be explained clearly to the patient. The patient or volunteer must not be promised unrealistic benefits from therapy. The patient must also be free to withdraw from the study at any time without fear that his or her level of medical care will be compromised.

Although compliance with these constraints may seem a simple matter, there are complications in practice. For example, some people believe that experimental drugs are always better than currently used drugs. These people may not have realistic expectations, despite having been told the properties of the drug being tested. Another problem concerns patients who are intimidated by medical personnel and are afraid to refuse to participate in a drug study. These patients may confide their fears to an accessible and empathetic nurse. It is the duty of the nurse to assist such patients in making their true feelings known.

Nurses assist patients in many ways throughout drug testing, including acting as an advocate for the patient. The nurse assesses whether the patient understands the possible benefits and limitations of the drugs being tested and the testing protocol. During testing the nurse assesses the patient for benefits, fears, drug adverse effects, and changes in the underlying health problem. Finally, the nurse supports the patient's decisions about participation in drug testing. This may be a difficult process because the nurse may disagree with the patient's decision but must support it.

CONTROLLED SUBSTANCES
Dependency

Certain substances can alter normal functions of the human body so profoundly that the body becomes dependent on that substance and experiences physical discomfort or harm if it is withdrawn. This condition is physical addiction or dependence (see Chapter 9). Opioid analgesics and some general depressants may cause dependence. Substances such as cocaine and marijuana, although not producing clear evidence of physical dependence, cause psychologic dependence.

Regulation of Controlled Substances

Because substances that produce physical or psychologic dependence clearly have the capacity to harm their users, they have been extensively regulated. The Harrison Narcotic Act of 1914 was the first U.S. law to regulate addictive substances. This law restricted importation of addictive substances.

The Harrison Act did not eliminate the problem of illicit drug use and dependency. This legislation was replaced by a more comprehensive law, the Controlled Substances Act of 1970. In addition to supplying guidelines for defining drug dependence and establishing education and treatment programs, this law classified drugs based on their abuse potential and clinical usefulness, grouped them according to set "schedules," and specified the restrictions that apply to each scheduled group. The drug schedules are described in Table 7-4.

TABLE 7-4

United States Classification of Controlled Substances

Classification	Description	Specific Substances
I	Drugs that have high potential for abuse and no accepted medical use; containers marked C-I	Heroin, lysergic acid diethylamide (LSD), peyote, marijuana
II*	Drugs with high potential for abuse but accepted medical use (may include physical and psychologic dependence); containers marked C-II	Amobarbital, amphetamine, codeine, meperidine, methadone, hydromorphone, morphine, opium, methylphenidate, secobarbital
III†	Medically accepted drugs that may cause dependence but are less prone to abuse than drugs in schedules I and II; containers marked C-III	Codeine-containing medications, butabarbital, paragoric
IV†	Medically accepted drugs that may cause mild physical or psychologic dependence; containers marked C-IV	Chloral hydrate, chlordiazepoxide, diazepam, meprobamate, phenobarbital
V‡	Medically accepted drugs with very limited potential for causing mild physical or psychologic dependence; containers marked C-V	Drug mixtures containing small quantities of opioids such as over-the-counter cough syrups containing codeine

*Written prescriptions are required. Health care providers may prescribe these by phone in an emergency. No telephone renewals are allowed.
†Written prescriptions or verbal orders are required. No more than five refills are permitted within a 6-month period.
‡Written prescription may or may not be required; check the state law.

Drugs in each schedule defined by the Controlled Substances Act are regulated by rules appropriate to them. For example, schedule I substances have no approved medical use and are banned for all uses except research. Schedule II drugs are controlled at every stage from initial manufacture through distribution and final use by the patient. By law, no prescription for a schedule II drug may be refilled. Physicians or advanced practice nurses (i.e., nurse practitioners, clinical nurse specialists, nurse midwives, nurse anesthetists) must be licensed to prescribe these drugs and must keep accurate records to ensure that the drugs are used strictly for legitimate purposes. Likewise, pharmacies must be specially licensed to handle schedule II drugs and must keep accurate records to show how the drugs have been stored and dispensed. Some states have implemented centralized computer-based monitoring systems for drugs in schedules II to V to aid law enforcement in their efforts to control illicit drug use.

Drugs in schedules III, IV, and V are believed to have progressively lower abuse potential than drugs in schedule II. For the most part, this progression probably reflects the diminishing ability of such drugs to produce euphoria and positive reinforcement for people who would abuse them. Interestingly, however, some of these drugs, including drugs in schedule II, appear in more than one schedule. For example, codeine used alone as an antitussive is a schedule II drug, but the combination of codeine in the same tablets with aspirin, acetaminophen or other agents intended for pain relief is assigned to schedule III. The rationale behind the lower classification is that the possibility of unpleasant adverse effects occurring caused by high doses of the combination drugs will lessen the likelihood that a person would abuse that particular product. Codeine also appears in several cough syrups that are on schedule V. The recommended single dose of codeine for adults in schedule V medications is 5 or 10 mg, whereas the doses found in schedule II or III forms are 15 to 60 mg. This lower dose of codeine in cough syrups, and legal restrictions on quantities of the syrups that can be purchased without a prescription justify the schedule V classification.

CANADIAN DRUG LEGISLATION
Food and Drugs Act

Drug regulation is carried out through the Health Protection branch of the Canadian government. Under this branch the Drugs Directorate oversees the bureaus that deal with specific areas of regulation, such as prescription drugs, nonprescription drugs, biologicals, drug research, and control of drug quality. Updates and other current information can be obtained via the Health Canada web site (http://www.hc-sc.gc.ca/hpb-dgps/therapeut/htmleng).

Under the Food and Drugs Act of 1953, drugs are divided into categories (Table 7-5). When approved for sale, all Canadian drugs are assigned a six-digit number preceded by the letters GP (proprietary drug) or DIN (over-the-counter drug). In addition, each prescription drug must be well marked with a symbol to identify the schedule to which it belongs. Regulations covering the various schedules of drugs differ, making the clear identification system important. Drugs listed in schedule F are sold only by prescription, with refills limited to 6 months. Drugs in schedule G are called controlled drugs and have more stringent controls regulating the number and timing of refills for prescriptions. Certain controlled drugs are called designated drugs because their use is restricted to specific conditions described by law.

The Food and Drugs Act in Canada also protects citizens from contaminated, adulterated, and unsafe drugs. To ensure drug quality, the law requires inspection of manufacturing facilities, calls for analysis of drug samples by government laboratories, and maintains an active monitoring system to detect adverse effects to drugs. Drug labeling is also closely controlled so that false, misleading, and deceptive labels are prohibited. Just as in the United States, drugs may not be advertised to the general public as cures for alcoholism, cancer, heart disease, infectious diseases, and other specific conditions.

Narcotic Control Act

The Narcotic Control Act (1961) regulates the manufacture, distribution, and sale of narcotic drugs, establishing this group as separate from drugs regulated under the Food and Drugs Act. Regulations spell out specific provisions of this act and are often revised in response to changing needs.

All steps in the manufacture, distribution, and sale of narcotics are subject to stringent regulation. Possession of these drugs for any reason other than those related to medical use as described in the legislation is an offense subject to severe penalties. Dispensers of these drugs must be licensed by the government and must maintain extensive records documenting the sources of and recipients for all drugs and the amounts and dates for all transactions. As in the United States, nurses may possess opioids or controlled and restricted drugs only when authorized by a health care provider's order to administer the drug to a patient or when authorized to act as official custodian of drugs for a specific unit of a health care facility.

Development of New Drugs in Canada

New drugs are evaluated in Canada by a sequence of tests similar to those used in the United States. Promising drugs undergo preclinical testing in three mammalian species, including one nonrodent species, to de-

TABLE 7-5

Canadian Drug Classification

Classification	Description	Specific Substances
Nonprescription Drugs		
Proprietary drugs	Drugs that may be widely purchased for self-treatment of symptoms of minor limiting diseases; identified by six-digit code preceded by letters *GP*	Cough drops, medicated shampoos, minor pain self-relievers
Over-the-counter drugs	Drugs available in pharmacies, used on advice of health professional for control of minor self-limiting diseases; identified by six-digit code preceded by letters *DIN*	Laxatives, cough syrups, cold remedies, sinus preparations, certain vitamins
Prescription Drugs		
Schedule F	Drugs that may not be used except after professional consultation; identified by *Pr* on the label	Hormones, antibiotics, tranquilizers
Schedule G	Drugs that affect central nervous system(e.g., stimulants, sedatives); identified by C on label	Amphetamines, barbiturates
Narcotics	Drugs used mostly for relief of pain but have significant psychotropic activity; identified by *N* on label	Cannabis (marijuana), cocaine, morphine, opium, phencyclidine
Restricted Drugs		
Schedule H	Drugs with no recognized medical use and significant danger of physiologic and psychologic adverse effects; available only to institutions for research	Lysergic acid diethylamide (LSD), N,N-diethyltryptamine (DET), N,N-dimethyltryptamine (DMT), 4-methyl-2,5- dimethoxyamphetamine (STP, DOM)

termine threshold doses that produce toxicity or death. The next stage is a clinical pharmacology trial similar to Phase I trials in the United States. During clinical pharmacology trials, the drug is given to healthy human volunteers to establish safety for doses that might be used clinically. If the drug is proven safe and if manufacturing processes produce a pure and uniform preparation for human use, the manufacturer may apply for permission to distribute the drug to qualified investigators who will test it in patients. This stage of testing is similar to Phase II in the United States. Before the drug can be released for general use, extensive documentation concerning formulation, labeling, packaging, clinical data on humans, and test data on animals must be filed and evaluated. All new drugs are monitored after being placed on the market. The drug is released from controls required for a new drug only after extensive information has documented the safety of a new drug when used in normal medical practice.

Bibliography

Merrill RA: Modernizing the FDA: an incremental revolution, *Health Affairs,* 18(2):96-111, 1999.
Rusnak E: The Food and Drug Administration Modernization Act of 1997. *Research Nurse,* 4(2):1-6, 13-16, 1998.

Internet Resources

http://www.fda.gov/default.htm.
http://www.fda.gov/cder/handbook/orphan.htm.
http://www.hcfa.gov/medicaid/drugs/drug6.htm.
http://www.ceri.com/schedule.htm.

CHAPTER

8

Over-the-Counter Drugs and Herbal Remedies

LYNN ROGER WILLIS • KATHLEEN GUTIERREZ

 Visit http://evolve.elsevier.com/Gutierrez/ for additional information.

KEY TERMS

Dietary Supplement Health and Education Act of 1994 (DSHEA), p. 98

Drug interactions, p. 100

Efficacy, p. 96

Food and drug laws, p. 100

Poultice, p. 107

Pseudoscience, p. 98

Pure Food and Drug Act, p. 96

Safety, p. 96

Standardization, p. 99

OBJECTIVES

- Identify and explain the differences between FDA-approved drugs, herbal remedies, and dietary supplements.

- Identify and explain the differences in federal rules that govern the promotion and sale of herbal remedies and conventional over-the-counter (OTC) medications.

- Understand the distinction between claims of therapeutic benefit based on anecdotal information or scientifically derived data.

Nurses normally focus their attention on drugs ordered for patients by health care providers. However, patients frequently self-treat with a wide array of over-the-counter (102) drugs and, more recently, an even wider array of herbal remedies—any of which may significantly influence the effects of prescribed drugs. Nurses must therefore also focus attention on these products. This chapter examines the historical, legal, and practical dynamics of self-treatment with 102 and herbal remedies.

REGULATION OF OVER-THE-COUNTER DRUGS

Products intended for self-treatment have been sold in the United States since colonial times. Until the early twentieth century, no restrictions governed the contents, potency, purity, safety, efficacy, sale, or advertising of these products, which included a wide range of patent (secret recipe) drugs, tonics, and other remedies. The foundation for most of these remedies was botanical, because modern-day techniques for synthesizing

95

new drugs did not exist then (Figure 8-1). Because of the lack of approved standards for purity, **efficacy**, or **safety** in the nineteenth century, many of those products provided little if any therapeutic benefits and were of marginal safety at best. Indeed, they often contained alcohol, opioids, or other dangerous drugs in unspecified quantities, posing serious risks to an unsuspecting public.

Advertising and promotion of medicinal products were likewise unregulated in the nineteenth century. Ac-

cordingly, claims of therapeutic benefits covered literally all afflictions from carbuncles to cancer. A favorite promotional technique utilized published testimonials from supposedly satisfied customers, some of whom actually died from the very disease for which they were attesting a cure.

Some control of the patent medicine industry was achieved with passage of the first **Pure Food and Drug Act** of 1906 (see Chapter 7), which required that package labels accurately list the ingredients of medicinal

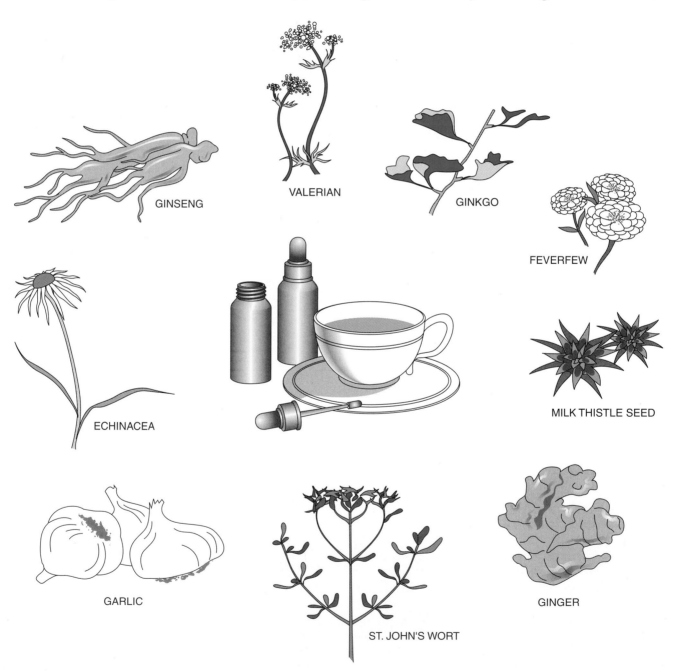

FIGURE 8-1 Phytomedicines are made from the extracts of a variety of flowers, seeds, stems, bark, and roots.

products. Any substance present in the product but not listed on the label was deemed an adulterant. A later amendment to the act, the Sherley Amendment of 1912, forbade false and fraudulent labeling claims. In 1938 a new Food, Drug, and Cosmetic Act was enacted, requiring proof of safety for all medicinal products intended for sale. In 1952 the Durham-Humphrey Amendment to the 1938 Act specified (1) which drugs were safe enough for sale without a prescription, and (2) which drugs were deemed dangerous or unsuitable for self-treatment that their sale was restricted to dispensing by prescription only. These laws forced many ineffective, unsafe products from the market.

Present control of 102 drugs stems from the Kefauver-Harris Amendment of 1962, which required proof of efficacy and safety as well as lack of teratogenicity (the ability to cause birth defects). This amendment affected all drugs introduced after 1962 and all drugs that had entered the market since 1938. To meet the conditions of this amendment, the Food and Drug Administration (FDA) convened several panels of experts to review the classes of 102 drugs and assign each such drug to one of the following categories:

- Category I: Recognized as safe and effective for the claimed therapeutic indication
- Category II: Not recognized as safe and effective
- Category III: Additional data needed to decide safety or effectiveness

Drugs assigned to Category I can be sold to the general public, whereas those in Category II cannot. Drugs in category III, if generally recognized as safe, may be sold even though the evaluation of their safety and effectiveness has not been completed. Since this review process began, many unsafe or ineffective 102 drugs and products have disappeared from the market. Others have undergone labeling changes or have had their formulations redesigned. This review has served the public interest well and established a sharp line of demarcation between 102 drugs and herbal remedies.

RESURGENCE OF HERBAL REMEDIES

Herbal remedies were all but absent from the U.S. marketplace throughout much of the twentieth century, but they have recently reemerged with astounding popularity. Current data estimates that one in three consumers of 102 and prescription drugs have used herbal remedies, and the herbal industry enjoys annual sales in the hundreds of millions of dollars. The skyrocketing expansion of this market in the space of a couple of decades has outpaced efforts to regulate the safety and efficacy of medicinal herbs and to provide reliable information for consumers. Legislative efforts initiated thus far to regulate the herbal industry and marketplace have focused more on opening this market and less on ensuring efficacy, safety, and truth in advertising.

REGULATION OF HERBAL REMEDIES

Herbal remedies receive far less rigorous legal scrutiny than 102 drugs. Indeed, current U.S. law actually views medicinal herbs more as foods (i.e., dietary supplements) than as drugs, because to sell an herbal remedy as a drug (i.e., with claims of efficacy in treating specific conditions), a manufacturer must provide the FDA with evidence that the remedy is safe and effective for the intended use. Most producers of herbal remedies have not provided such evidence, mostly because of the huge expense involved in doing so (through lengthy laboratory and clinical trials) and because herbal remedies, having been used for centuries, cannot be patented. Without patent protection there is no financial incentive for producers to invest in the rigorous and expensive studies needed to establish the safety and efficacy of their products. Moreover, many herbal remedies have had decades, even centuries, of accepted use in treating various disorders.

Foodstuffs must meet federal standards of purity and quality but are exempt from standards of therapeutic efficacy and safety applied to drugs, since foods are not drugs and are generally viewed as safe. Since herbs are edible plants, manufacturers and suppliers were quick to sell them under the legal definition of foods (i.e., as dietary supplements), by which strategy they could avoid the more stringent laws reserved for drugs. This strategy has been used to the great chagrin of those who believe that all claims of therapeutic efficacy for medicinal agents, foods or otherwise, should undergo the same scientific scrutiny currently required of drugs.

The problems inherent in allowing companies to market herbals as food when in reality they are drugs are obvious. If the law does not provide for objective evaluation of the therapeutic claims for such products, the door opens wide for promoters and manufacturers to make exaggerated, unfounded, even false therapeutic claims. Ironically, many of the claims made today for herbal remedies are disturbingly reminiscent of the dubious advertising claims made for these herbs by the manufacturers' nineteenth-century counterparts. Until recently, the promotion of herbal remedies was all but unregulated, occurring largely via word of mouth, mail-order catalogs, the popular press, televised infomercials, etc. In the early 1990s, in response to increasing complaints from the public and consumer-interest groups about promotional abuses for herbal remedies and other dietary supplements, the FDA appeared ready to remove these products from the market altogether. However, since there arose in response such a loud public outcry on behalf of open-market sales of dietary supplements, fueled in large part by the health food industry (with an obvious stake in the issue), the FDA did not act, and Congress passed the **Dietary Supplement Health and Education Act of 1994 (DSHEA).** Among other things, this law permits the sale of herbal remedies as dietary supplements, provided that therapeutic claims for the remedy do not appear on the product label. The label may contain a statement describing the product's *presumed* role in some aspect of human health as well as information presenting a balanced view of the available scientific information.

One troubling aspect of the DSHEA requires the FDA to prove a dietary supplement unsafe before removing it from the market for safety reasons. This requirement contrasts sharply with the laws regulating 102 and prescription drugs, which place the burden of proof of safety with the manufacturer. Accordingly, if the FDA has reason to suspect that a drug is unsafe, it can remove the drug from the market until the manufacturer provides proof of safety. This legislative difference severely limits the FDA's ability to protect the interests of consumers where herbal remedies are concerned.

The DSHEA effectively places a huge number of herbal remedies on a therapeutic par with conventional 102 remedies but without the same assurances of safety and effectiveness required for drugs. Accordingly, if nurses are to provide helpful information about herbal remedies to their patients, they must understand the differences between such remedies and conventional 102 drugs and be prepared to look beyond the information provided by manufacturers for the most credible information. Sadly, this information is not always easy to find, nor is it always reliable.

Authoritative information on the safety and effectiveness of herbal remedies, though accumulating, is still in short supply. Reports and reviews of clinical trials appear increasingly in the medical and scientific literature and can be obtained with the aid of reference librarians and such organizations as the American Pharmaceutical Association, the American Botanical Council, and the Herb Research Foundation.

Because herbal remedies for sale in the United States are not FDA-approved drugs, their labeling cannot be relied on to provide instructions for proper use and appropriate cautionary warnings. Additionally, no FDA-enforced standards of quality exist for herbal remedies; therefore products may contain subtherapeutic amounts of herbal constituents, and potential users can rely only on the good reputation of the manufacturer for reliability. The nurse should especially remind prospective users of herbal remedies that regardless of their classification as dietary supplements, they are in fact drugs of largely unproven safety. Potential users who are pregnant, nursing, or intending to administer these remedies to young children and infants should be especially advised against such use without qualified medical supervision.

HERBAL REMEDIES GO BEYOND THE SCOPE OF 102 DRUGS

By definition, 102 drugs are deemed safe enough for self-treatment of conditions not ordinarily requiring the attention of a health care provider. Some herbal remedies (e.g., laxatives for constipation) have a long history of reliability and safety in this regard and, in fact, are sold as drugs under FDA rules. Others, however, that are not subject to those rules, are widely promoted for use in treating potentially more serious, not-so-easily diagnosed conditions such as depression (St. John's wort), benign prostatic hyperplasia (saw palmetto), cirrhosis of the liver (milk thistle), and vascular insufficiency (*Ginkgo biloba*). Although evidence supports such uses for these and other remedies to some degree, the nurse should question the wisdom of self-medication to treat or prevent such conditions, all of which may have grave consequences for patients if not properly diagnosed and treated by qualified health professionals.

PSEUDOSCIENCE AND HERBAL REMEDIES

Myths and misinformation about herbal remedies abound in the vacuum created by **pseudoscience** and the lack of scientifically valid information. One such myth, for example, holds that herbal remedies, as so-called natural products, are safer than modern synthetic drugs. This myth relies upon centuries of safe use of herbal products by our forebears, but it ignores knowledge gained in past decades that dangerous chemicals (carcinogens, teratogens, mutagens, etc.) exist throughout the plant kingdom.

Another myth purports that so-called natural and organic herbs are superior to modern drugs that have been synthesized in the laboratory. Scientists have been discrediting this myth for more than 100 years by showing that natural chemicals synthesized in the laboratory (such as urea, vitamins A and C, ephedrine, and many others) are identical in all respects to their plant-derived counterparts. Nevertheless, the myth persists.

Still another myth promotes whole herbs as safer and more effective than extracts of isolated constituents of herbs. The rationale behind this myth is that plants may contain other substances that enhance the therapeutic action of the remedy by some synergistic process and that the lesser concentration of active constituents in the whole herb, as opposed to an isolated chemical, renders the remedy safer for the user. Neither of these notions stood the test of rational pharmacologic analysis. For one, dosage is easier to control with purified constituents of an herb than it is with the whole herb, especially where standardization of the whole herb may be difficult. For another, although synergistic interactions may well occur between the natural, possibly unidentified constituents of whole herbs, it is well known that toxic constituents also exist that have the potential to cause significant harm.

PHARMACOLOGY OF WIDELY USED HERBAL REMEDIES
Black Cohosh *(Cimicifuga racemosa)*

Black cohosh grows indigenously in North America and was prized long ago by Native Americans for its medicinal properties. The dried rhizome and roots of the plant were said to ease the pain of rheumatism, soothe sore throats, and relieve "diseases of women." Nineteenth-century physicians utilized black cohosh to treat menstrual disorders and symptoms of menopause, and the herb was one of the main ingredients in Lydia Pinkham's famous Vegetable Compound. The current popular use for black cohosh is in the relief of premenstrual syndrome (PMS) and symptoms of menopause.

The principal active ingredients of black cohosh are triterpene glycosides and isoflavones. While there are indications that black cohosh may influence the secretion of luteinizing hormone, follicle-stimulating hormone, and other estrogenic factors, there are also indications to the contrary. In short, the mechanism of action for black cohosh is unknown.

Recommended dosages of the herb may cause upset stomach. No interactions with other drugs have been reported. Pregnant and lactating women should not use black cohosh under any circumstances.

German Chamomile *(Matricaria recutita)*

Several varieties of chamomile exist, but German chamomile is by far the most widely used. Several classes of constituents have been isolated from chamomile and are used for specific medical applications (e.g., antiinflammatory, antispasmodic, and antimicrobial) and in cosmetics. The essential oil contains sesquiterpenes and flavonoids, the primary ingredients contributing to antiinflammatory and antispasmodic activity, perhaps by actions on local prostaglandin production.

The potential exists for chamomile to cause reactions in persons allergic to ragweed, asters, or chrysanthemums, since these plants are related, but reports of serious allergic reactions are rare.

Chamomile tea can be prepared by adding fresh or dried flower heads to a cup of boiling water and letting the mixture steep for 10 minutes. The resulting tea can be swallowed, used as a mouthwash, or applied to the skin as a poultice.

Cranberry *(Vaccinium macrocarpon)*

Cranberry grows indigenously from Alaska to the Carolinas. Early Americans fashioned dressings for wounds from the fruit of the cranberry and used the juice for treating stomach ailments, scurvy, and cancer. Juice and extracts of the berry are currently used to treat urinary tract infections. The results of clinical studies support this use.

Among the numerous constituents of the cranberry are fructose, tannins, and several organic acids. The acidic juice of the berry was initially believed to reduce urinary pH sufficiently to make the urinary tract undesirable for habitation by bacteria, notably *Escherichia coli* (which prefer a more alkaline environment), but studies on the effect of cranberry juice on urinary pH did not support this belief. Later studies identified compounds in cranberry juice that prevent bacteria from adhering to the walls of the bladder and urinary tract. It is currently believed that this action prevents and treats the infections.

No adverse effects or precautions have been reported for this use of cranberry juice. Cranberry juice cocktail is only about one-third cranberry juice. Commercial preparations normally contain relatively large amounts of sugar. Accordingly, daily doses of juice represent the addition of a substantial amount of calories to a person's diet. Artificial sweeteners have relieved these caloric pressures but raise for some the equally undesirable prospect of having to consume large quantities of the sweetener.

Echinacea *(Echinacea angustifolia, E. purpurea,* and *E. pallida)*

Echinacea (purple coneflower) is a prolific member of the daisy family *(Asteracea)* that grows wild throughout the midwestern United States. Native Americans recognized the medicinal properties of this plant long ago, and at least one American entrepreneur marketed the herb as a cure-all and tonic toward the end of the nineteenth century. Echinacea was also widely marketed as an antiinfective drug during the first half of the twentieth century, but its popularity and use faded with the discovery of sulfonamide and other antiinfective drugs, and it all but disappeared in the age of antibiotics. The recently rekindled interest in old herbal remedies has renewed public interest in echinacea.

Although several species exist, *E. purpurea* provides the largest source of the remedy in today's market. The medicinal properties of echinacea reside primarily in the parts of the plant that grow above ground, where cichoric acid, alkylamides, polysaccharides, and an essential oil are contained. It is not yet clear which, if any, of these constituents can be credited with the antiseptic and immunostimulant properties associated with the plant. Various constituents have been shown in vitro to stimulate and modulate immune function, but enhanced phagocytic activity stands as the only current evidence of an effect of the extract on immune function.

Clinical evidence supports the use of echinacea extract for the relief of cold symptoms, but the FDA has not approved any medicinal use for echinacea. Two independent clinical trials have shown that the extract was better than placebo at reducing the severity and duration of colds. There are as yet no reports of studies in which the effects of echinacea in cold sufferers were compared with conventional modes of symptomatic treatment.

Two clinical trials have also addressed the promotional claim that echinacea prevents colds. Neither of these studies demonstrated any significant reduction in the incidence of colds.

Echinacea may cause stomach upset, headache, and dizziness. Allergic reactions have been reported, but there are no known **drug interactions** with it.

Echinacea is not recommended for patients who have tuberculosis, multiple sclerosis, HIV infections, and other autoimmune diseases. Because the current **food and drug laws** cannot assure strict quality control of herbal remedies sold as nutritional supplements, potential users of echinacea should choose their remedy only after carefully evaluating the manufacturer's and supplier's reputations. In any case, a remedy containing echinacea should not be used for more than 8 weeks.

Tablets, capsules, and liquid formulations of echinacea (hydroalcoholic extract or pressed juice) are marketed for oral consumption.

Garlic *(Allium sativum)*

More therapeutic claims and folklore exist for garlic than for any other known herb. Garlic gets credit for virtually everything from lowering blood pressure, cholesterol, and fever to warding off bacterial infections, warts, atherosclerosis, and vampires. Most of these claims have no direct supporting evidence, and some, of course, are absurd. However, the results of clinical studies have supported several of the claims, foremost among them the herb's ability to lower blood pressure and cholesterol levels, inhibit platelet aggregation, and kill bacteria.

Much of the research on garlic has targeted allicin, the chemical responsible for garlic's characteristic odor. Allicin is produced when its chemical precursor, alliin, comes into contact with the enzyme alliinase, which likewise is a constituent of garlic. Chewing, chopping, or crushing a garlic clove puts alliin in contact with alliinase, thereby giving rise to the allicin. The evidence equating allicin with the purported antiplatelet, antihyperlipidemic, and antibiotic effects of garlic is more or less equivocal, since many different chemical agents are found in garlic, and it is far from clear which constituent is responsible. Even so, it is now generally

agreed that the therapeutic potency of garlic preparations relates directly to the ability of that preparation to generate allicin, believed by many to be the principal active ingredient in garlic. In that respect, preparations devoid of alliin (i.e., so-called deodorized garlic) appear to lack significant biologic activity and should be avoided.

Although crushing or chewing a garlic clove releases alliin and alliinase, stomach acid destroys the latter. Thus no additional allicin will be produced once the alliinase reaches the stomach. Recognizing this problem, makers of garlic-containing remedies have produced enteric-coated tablets containing garlic powder. The enteric coating remains intact while the tablet is in the stomach and dissolves only after the tablet passes into the less acidic fluid of the small intestine, where alliinase is less susceptible to degradation.

Alliinase is also destroyed by heat, so the method by which garlic powder is produced is also important. Properly freeze-dried garlic powder contained in enteric-coated tablets affords the highest likelihood for the systemic absorption of allicin.

The consumption of a moderate amount of garlic poses little risk under normal circumstances. Users may complain of nausea and gastrointestinal (GI) distress. Rarely, allergic reactions may occur. Since garlic inhibits platelet aggregation and has some antithrombin activity, patients who are taking anticoagulants (e.g., warfarin) or nonsteroidal antiinflammatory drugs (e.g., aspirin) should exercise caution when taking therapeutic doses of garlic.

Garlic is insufficiently potent to substitute for prescription drug therapy, but it holds promise as an adjuvant.

Ginger *(Zingiber officinale)*

Ginger is believed to have originated in Asia and has been grown in India and China for thousands of years. The underground rhizomes of the plant are used medically and as a cooking spice.

The most widespread and accepted medical use for ginger is as an antiemetic. Several clinical trials have established this action of ginger, particularly against motion sickness. One clinical study demonstrated that a 940-mg dose of powdered ginger was more effective than 100 mg of dimenhydrinate for motion sickness caused by sitting in a tilted, rotating chair. This effect appears to be the result of local actions of the ginger in the stomach and is not the result of an action in the CNS. Ginger may also prevent or relieve the nausea of pregnancy, but pregnant women are well advised to avoid this remedy because the possible effects of the drug on the fetus are unknown.

There have been no reports of significant adverse effects or toxicity associated with ginger. However, since there is evidence that ginger inhibits platelet aggregation, patients already taking anticoagulant or antiplatelet drugs should not use this remedy, nor should those who are about to undergo surgery.

Ginkgo *(Ginkgo biloba)*

The fossil record dates the ginkgo tree to some 200 million years ago from its origins in China. Chinese medicine has valued the fruits and seeds of this tree for nearly 3000 years. Western medicine, however, discovered a therapeutic use for the leaves of this tree only about 30 years ago, and its popularity has increased by leaps and bounds to the present time. Recent clinical studies of the extract of ginkgo biloba leaves (GBE) have supplied evidence supporting a therapeutic role for ginkgo in medicine.

Although traditional folklore views ginkgo as a uterine stimulant, an antibacterial, an antiinflammatory, and a vasodilator, GBE is most often used today in the treatment of conditions characterized by vascular insufficiency in the brain and legs. One area of particular clinical interest for the use of GBE is for memory loss associated with early symptoms of Alzheimer's disease, a disease characterized by cerebral changes associated with hypoxic injury. The recognized ability of GBE to dilate vascular smooth muscle and reduce oxidative stress by scavenging free radicals may be related to some of the perceived beneficial effects of GBE in affected individuals. Dilation of cerebral blood vessels increases cerebral blood flow, possibly preventing hypoxia and oxidative stress. GBE also appears to inhibit platelet aggregation, which may account for part of its effectiveness in treating circulatory disorders involving post-thrombotic events.

GBE typically contains a 50:1 concentrate of ginkgo leaves. The pharmacologically active constituents of the extract are believed to be a mixture of four ginkgolides (A, B, C, and M) and a sesquiterpene, bilobalide. The ginkgolides and bilobalide appear to impart the neuroprotective property of the extract, and ginkgolide B inhibits platelet-activating factor (PAF). GBE also contains bioflavonoids and flavone glycosides. The flavones are potent and effective scavengers of free radicals.

Adverse effects with ginkgo are uncommon but typically consist of upset stomach, headache, anxiety, insomnia and, rarely, allergy. Patients who are taking anticoagulants or inhibitors of platelet aggregation should avoid ginkgo because of the risk of an additive interaction.

GBE is commercially available as tablets or capsules.

It is a reflection of the current legislative disparity between the regulation of drugs and herbs that ginkgo is widely promoted as a memory-enhancing agent for the general population, although clinical evidence supports only such memory-enhancing effects in elderly patients with preexisting memory deficits. This disparity underscores the need for health professionals to be well informed on the subject of herbal medicine.

Ginseng *(Panax quinquefolium)*

Literally thousands of books, papers, essays, and articles about ginseng have been published since the mid-1600s, but to date only one well-controlled study of ginseng in human subjects has been reported, and the results of that study were inconclusive. Even so, the list of therapeutic benefits claimed for ginseng is enormous. From ancient times, ginseng has been viewed as a tonic for the body, helping to ward off illness and enhancing sexual prowess. In today's market, ginseng is promoted as an "adaptogen," which increases resistance to stress, builds one's general vitality, and strengthens normal body functions. The literature contains numerous reports attesting to these effects, but rigorous, objective clinical examination of these claims is lacking.

Much is known about the botany and chemistry of ginseng, which consists of several varieties in the family Araliaceae, but very little is known of the possible mechanisms by which it performs its various presumed effects. The constituents of the plant believed to be responsible for these effects are the triterpenoid saponins found in the roots.

High-quality ginseng is expensive and difficult to obtain. Accordingly, quality, standardization, and purity are not always assured in commercial products containing this plant. Moreover, some products sold as ginseng (e.g., Siberian ginseng), are not ginseng at all because they belong to an entirely different plant family.

Ginseng is generally considered safe, but potential users are cautioned not to combine it with drugs or beverages containing stimulants (including caffeine). Persons with hypertension, cardiac ailments or diabetes are likewise cautioned not to use ginseng.

Hawthorn *(Crataegus laevigata* and *C. monogyna)*

Extracts of hawthorn flowers, berries, and leaves have been recommended by herbalists for many years for the treatment of various heart and circulatory ailments. The extracts contain several potentially active constituents, including chlorgenic acid, quercin, vitexin, and triterpenoids, all of which have been shown to exert antiinflammatory and hypolipidemic actions.

Hawthorn is used in Europe to treat cardiac disorders. It has been shown to dilate coronary vessels and compares favorably with conventional inotropic drugs such as beta-adrenergic agonists and cardiac glycosides. The adverse effect and toxicity profile for this drug is favorable, with adverse effects normally evident only with high doses. The potential does exist, however, for hawthorn to interact with other cardioactive and vasoactive drugs. Accordingly, patients who may be taking conventional drugs for cardiac or circulatory conditions should not self-medicate with hawthorn. The consequences of doing so where cardiovascular drugs are concerned could be disastrous.

Kava Kava *(Piper methysticum)*

Kava kava (or simply kava) has a long history of use by the Polynesian inhabitants of Oceania. When the root of this pepper plant is chewed and mixed with saliva, an intoxicating, spicy substance is formed. This concoction is often mixed with coconut juice for use in ceremonies and rites of the South Sea islanders.

Extracts of kava root contain several substituted kavalactones that seem to produce primarily anxiolytic and sedative effects in the CNS. Commercial formulations of the extract are normally standardized to contain up to 70% kavalactones. The extracts are promoted and used to treat mild anxiety. Clinical trials in Germany demonstrated that kava extract is superior to placebo for the treatment of anxiety. The mechanism of action for this drug is unknown.

Stomach upset and allergic skin reactions occur at recommended doses of kava (200 to 300 mg daily provides 150 to 210 mg of kavalactones from a 70% standardized extract). Heavy use may precipitate development of a scaly skin rash that clears up when the drug is discontinued. There appear to be no signs of withdrawal after as many as 6 months of kava use, and tolerance to the anxiolytic action apparently does not develop. Alcohol and other CNS depressants intensify the sedating actions of kava and these drugs should not be taken simultaneously. The most dangerous adverse reaction to kava kava is liver toxicity. On the basis of reported liver toxicity in persons using dietary supplements containing kava kava, authorities in Switzerland have removed some of these supplements from the market. In the United States, the FDA has asked that health care providers report any cases of liver toxicity that may be linked to the use of dietary supplements containing kava kava, as a first step in evaluating the level of risk to the American public.

Milk Thistle *(Silybum marianum)*

Milk thistle is native to the Mediterranean region of Europe but has been transferred effectively to California and the eastern United States. The seeds, leaves, and stems of the milk thistle plant yield a mixture of compounds collectively referred to as silymarin.

Silymarin has been shown to exert hepatoprotective effects against a variety of toxins, including that of the deadly amanita mushroom, in experimental animals and human subjects. This protection extends to the hepatotoxic effects of hepatitis and cirrhosis. The mechanism for the protection appears related both to antioxidant and free-radical scavenging properties of silymarin and to its effect on the cell membrane to prevent or slow cellular entry of toxins.

Adverse effects of milk thistle are usually minor and infrequent. Diarrhea has been reported, and allergic reactions are possible.

Silymarin is poorly soluble in water and very poorly absorbed by the GI tract. Consequently, oral dosing with this herb is problematic. Teas made from it usually contain less than 10% silymarin, and oral bioavailability ranges from 20% to 50%. Injectable forms of silymarin are available in Europe, but since the FDA has not approved its use as a drug, it is available in the United States only in oral dosage forms as a dietary supplement. Capsules containing milk thistle that are sold in the United States usually contain 200 mg of the herb (standardized to contain 140 mg of silymarin). The recommended dosage for silymarin ranges from 200 to 400 mg per day.

St. John's Wort *(Hypericum perforatum)*

Extracts of the above-ground elements of St. John's wort have been widely used in Europe as a prescription and nonprescription treatment for mild to moderate depression. Recent clinical studies support the notion that the extract is more effective than placebo and about as effective as low doses of conventional tricyclic antidepressants (see Chapter 18). Clinical comparisons between this herb and newer antidepressant drugs have not yet been reported. The extract is not considered appropriate therapy for severe depression, especially if symptoms include suicidal tendencies. Nurses should be especially attentive to patients who express an interest in self-medicating their depression whether medically diagnosed or not.

The antidepressant effects of St. John's wort have long been ascribed to a group of naphthodianthrones contained in the herb. These include hypericin, pseudohypericin, protohypericin, and cyclopseudohypericin. Until recently, hypericin was thought to possess the greatest antidepressant activity among these compounds. Indeed, commercial remedies containing this herb are often standardized to contain at least 0.3% hypericin. More recently, however, attention has shifted to a phloroglucinol derivative, hyperforin, as the more likely constituent responsible for the antidepressant action. Hyperforin inhibits the neuronal reuptake of norepinephrine, dopamine, and serotonin in vitro. The mechanism of the antidepressant action of St. John's wort remains unclear at the present time; but standardization according to hypericin content may inadequately characterize the pharmacologic potency of the extracts.

The adverse effect profile for St. John's wort is generally favorable. At recommended doses patients may experience stomach upset, sedation, restlessness, headache, dizziness, and confusion. Photosensitivity has been reported in human subjects who have taken large doses (3600 mg, four times the recommended dose). Although this does not seem to occur at lower doses, patients are well advised to use a sunscreen with this product, particularly if they are taking other photosensitizing drugs. As is the case with conventional antidepressants, therapeutic effects do not appear for several weeks.

Saw Palmetto *(Serenoa repens)*

The volatile oils extracted from the berries of the saw palmetto plant were widely used during the nineteenth and early twentieth centuries in the treatment of cystitis and digestive disorders (and as an aphrodisiac). Even so, one textbook of pharmacology, published in 1926, rated the oils of the saw palmetto plant as being "of very doubtful value."* By 1950, physicians' faith in this remedy had waned to the point that saw palmetto was dropped from the *National Formulary (NF),* and clinical interest in this remedy faded away.

However, interest in saw palmetto has revived in recent years, particularly in Europe. The principal current use for extracts of saw palmetto berries is in the symptomatic treatment of benign prostatic hyperplasia (BPH). The historical record documenting the use of saw palmetto for male urinary problems goes back several centuries (before BPH was the known cause of those problems). In more recent years, as-yet-unidentified constituents of the berries have been found to have antiandrogenic properties, and it is this action that is believed may alleviate the urinary symptoms of BPH. (The conventional prescription drug, finasteride, likewise relieves the symptoms of BPH through an antiandrogenic mechanism.)

The antiandrogenic properties of saw palmetto appear to be associated with fat-soluble constituents of the berries. Accordingly, aqueous teas brewed from the berries do not extract these fat-soluble, water-insoluble molecules from the berries and do not exhibit detectable beneficial effects against BPH. Extracts of saw palmetto are widely used and prescribed in Europe for the treatment of BPH. German health authorities have approved such use for this herb but require that the commercial preparations contain these specific fat-soluble constituents.

The FDA has not approved saw palmetto for the treatment of BPH because sufficient evidence of safety and effectiveness has not been presented to the agency. Moreover, the FDA has specifically denied requests from manufacturers that package labels for the extract be permitted to include a statement that saw palmetto may improve the symptoms of BPH. The rationale for this denial stems from the view that it is not in the public's best interest for citizens to be self-diagnosing and treating the symptoms of BPH, because prostate cancer can cause the same symptoms.

Independent clinical trials conducted thus far with extracts of saw palmetto have shown the extracts to be more effective than placebo and just as effective as alpha-adrenergic receptor blockers or finasteride at relieving the symptoms of BPH, while at the same time less likely to cause adverse effects than finasteride.

Adverse effects are uncommon with extracts of saw palmetto, and there are no known drug interactions.

Valerian *(Valeriana officinalis)*

Concoctions prepared from the dried rhizomes and roots of valerian have been used for more than 1000 years to aid sleep and calm anxious nerves. Many varieties of the plant grow well in mild regions of North America, Asia, and Europe, which helps account for its widespread popularity as an herbal remedy. Although some of the constituents of valerian have been identified (several valepotriates and volatile oil), the substance responsible for causing the sedative effects of valerian is unknown. That other constituents may be active is suggested by the fact that aqueous extracts, which contain little, if any, of the lipophilic valepotriates and volatile oils of valerian, are effective sedatives.

Adverse effects are uncommon with valerian, but headache has been reported. Cytotoxic effects (alkylation) associated with some of the valepotriates have been identified in vitro, but concentrations of these substances in available extracts and other preparations of valerian are not present in high enough concentration to be of concern. Valerian may induce uterine contractions and should not be used by pregnant women. As with any CNS depressant, valerian should not be taken in combination with alcohol or other sedating agents.

Standardized extracts containing 0.8% valerenic acid are available.

POTENTIALLY DANGEROUS HERBAL REMEDIES

The currently unfocused legal environment in which herbal remedies and other dietary supplements are promoted and sold to a trusting public requires that some mention be made of herbal remedies—some of which are very popular—for which clear risks of danger exist.

Comfrey *(Symphytum officinale)*

Comfrey has been one of the most widely used herbs in folk medicine for many years. Concoctions of comfrey are applied as poultices, extracts are taken as teas, and the herb is promoted for ailments of the lungs, bowels, stomach, liver, and gallbladder.

The problem with comfrey is that every species examined to date has been found to contain pyrrolizidine alkaloids, which are hepatotoxic. The literature increasingly contains reports of liver injury and even death in persons who had been consuming herbal remedies containing comfrey.

Other herbs that can cause serious liver injury are chaparral *(Larrea tridentata)*, germander *(Teucrium chamaedrys)*, mistletoe *(Viscum album)*, pennyroyal *(Hedeoma pulegoides* or *Mentha pulegium)*, sassafras *(Sassafras albidum)*, senna *(Cassia angustifolia)*, and skullcap *(Scutellaria lateriflora)*.

Goldenseal *(Hydrastis canadensis)*

Goldenseal, like comfrey, also has long been used in folk medicine as a remedy for a long list of ailments, notably as a topical antiinfective for inflamed eyes and wounds. The herb is also promoted for internal use against colds and flu. Despite widespread promotion, there is no clinical evidence supporting its use for any therapeutic application. Moreover, large doses of the herb cause nausea, vomiting, diarrhea, seizures, and paralysis. This herb should be avoided.

Somehow, in recent years, the notion has been propagated that goldenseal, if taken as an herbal tea, will mask the detection of morphine in urine. This information was aimed, of course, at heroin users who may be subject to random urine screens. There is no truth whatsoever to this notion, but it persists and has even been extended through misinterpretation to include the masking of any drug's presence in urine. So popular has this myth become that it has been said that whole areas of wild goldenseal have been decimated by persons anxious to gather and process the herb as a means of foiling the urine screen. The latter notion may be more apocryphal than real, but it underscores the self-generating properties of misinformation in an arena where standards for controlling such information do not exist.

Ma Huang *(Ephedra sinica)*

Ma huang occupies an interesting place somewhere between conventional and alternative medicine. It contains ephedrine and pseudoephedrine, which have been isolated and synthesized for use in medicine for many years. Ephedrine actually is an FDA-approved drug for 102 asthma remedies and was prescribed for asthma for many years before safer, more effective drugs became available. Pseudoephedrine is the decongestant in virtually all FDA-approved 102 cold remedies (see Chapter 54).

The problem with the use of herbal extracts of ma huang sold as dietary supplements stems from the lack of enforced standards for standardization and promotion. Without proper standardization, the dosage of ephedrine and pseudoephedrine cannot be reliably controlled, thereby disproportionately increasing the risk of adverse reactions (see Chapter 12).

Other potentially dangerous herbs are aconite *(Aconitum napellus)*, which can cause arrhythmias and abdominal pain, and licorice root *(Glycyrrhiza glabra)*, which can produce full-blown symptoms of pseudohyperaldosteronism (hypertension, hypokalemia, metabolic alkalosis, sodium retention, edema, and reduced plasma renin activity).

NONHERBAL DIETARY SUPPLEMENTS

Although not herbal remedies per se, many other chemical agents are promoted and sold as drugs without FDA approval. Several such agents are discussed in this chapter to illustrate the problems that accompany the poorly controlled promotion of herbal remedies.

Chondroitin Sulfate

Chondroitin sulfate consists of repeating units of glucosamine (see below), and is promoted for use with glucosamine to treat symptoms of osteoarthritis. Promoters claim that chondroitin sulfate inhibits the action of enzymes that metabolize cartilage. This claim remains unproven, but evidence in support of it has accumulated. Clinical studies have demonstrated that chondroitin sulfate improves joint pain and function better than placebo, reducing symptoms by about 30%. One comparison with diclofenac, a nonsteroidal antiinflammatory drug (Chapter 14), showed that the effects of chondroitin lasted longer than those of diclofenac. This difference is due to the different pharmacokinetic profiles of these two agents, with the action of chondroitin being longer in onset and longer in duration than diclofenac.

Glucosamine

Glucosamine is a preferred substrate for the synthesis of proteoglycans, which incorporate into the structure of cartilage. It is presumed but not yet proven that a daily dose of glucosamine retards the degradation of cartilage (see Evidence-Based Practice box).

Adverse effects associated with glucosamine are considered minor and include peripheral edema, tachycardia, GI symptoms, drowsiness, headache, and skin rash. Promoters of glucosamine suggest that it be taken with chondroitin sulfate (see previous section).

Melatonin

Melatonin is a naturally occurring hormone in humans that is produced by the pineal gland and involved in the control of normal sleep-wake cycles. Several years ago melatonin was widely promoted as an aid in recovering from jet lag. That claim was not borne out by clinical investigation, and the popularity of melatonin has since substantially waned. More recently, interest in mela-

EVIDENCE-BASED PRACTICE
Glucosamine as a Treatment for Osteoarthritis

Setting

Osteoarthritis, also known as degenerative joint disease, involves the progressive loss of articular cartilage and reactive changes at joint margins and in subchondral bone. It is the most common form of arthritis; at any given time it affects approximately 60 million people more than 65 years old.

Objective of Literature Review

The objective was to review all randomized controlled trials that evaluated the effectiveness and toxicity of glucosamine. The search was carried out using Medline, Embase, Current Contents (to 1999), and the Cochrane Controlled Trials Register. In addition, letters were written to content experts and reference lists searched for additional potentially relevant citations.

Criteria for Inclusion of Studies in Review of Literature

Investigators included randomized controlled trials that evaluated the effectiveness and safety of glucosamine in the treatment of osteoarthritis. Single-blinded and double-blinded, and comparative and placebo-based studies were included.

Data Extraction and Analysis

Two reviewers independently performed the extraction and analysis of the data and the quality of the studies. Continuous and dichotomous outcome measures were pooled using inferential statistical techniques.

Results of Review

All 16 of the studies included in the review demonstrated glucosamine to be both safe and effective in the treatment of osteoarthritis. Glucosamine was found to be superior to placebo in 12 of 13 studies. In two out of four studies glucosamine was found to be superior to nonsteroidal antiinflammatory drugs (NSAIDs) and equivalent in the other two studies.

Investigators' Conclusions

Most of the studies reviewed evaluated the Rotta preparation of glucosamine. It is not known whether formulations from other manufacturers would be equally as effective. Additional research is necessary to confirm the long-term effectiveness and toxicity of glucosamine in the treatment of osteoarthritis.

Towheed TE, Anastassiades TP, Shea B, et al. Glucosamine therapy for treating osteoarthritis. In *The Cochrane Library*, Issue 2, Oxford, 2002, Update Software.

---

tonin has revived, this time as a sleep aid for insomnia. Research into this possible use for the hormone has proven fruitful for sleep-onset insomnia (difficulty falling asleep) but not for maintenance insomnia (difficulty staying asleep). Research in this area continues.

Doses of melatonin required for sleep-onset insomnia vary between individuals; therefore the lowest effective dosage should be used but for no more than 1 or 2 weeks.

S-adenosyl-L-methionine (SAMe)

SAMe occurs naturally in all body tissues and serves as a methyl donor for a variety of reactions necessary for amino acid, vitamin, and nucleotide biosynthesis, as well as a sulfhydryl donor in reactions necessary to produce essential amino acids. Though as yet unproven, SAMe is believed by some to be involved in preventing cartilage from breaking down. Exogenous supplements of SAMe presumably add to this protective action.

Shark Cartilage

Shark cartilage has been promoted as a cancer preventive for many years. Manufacturers claim that "sharks don't get cancer" and must therefore have something in their makeup or metabolism that protects them. That something, they say, is an inhibitor of angiogenesis in shark cartilage. Inhibitors of angiogenesis block the formation of new blood vessels in developing tumors, thereby depriving the tumor of vessels for the delivery of oxygen and nutrients needed for growth. Accordingly, so the notion goes, an existing tumor so treated dies, and new tumors fail to develop.

Inhibitors of angiogenesis do in fact exist and are the subject of much ongoing research. Unfortunately for the promoters of shark cartilage, however, sharks do develop cancer, endogenous inhibitors of angiogenesis notwithstanding, and no clinical evidence has yet been obtained to support the use of shark cartilage in treating or preventing cancer or solid tumors.

APPLICATION TO PRACTICE

ASSESSMENT
History of Present Illness

A directed history that includes questions about the use of herbal remedies is important. Ask the following: Why are you interested in taking this product? What allergies, if any, do you have to plant materials? Are you now pregnant or breast-feeding? What prescription or 102 drugs are you currently taking?

If the patient reports a symptom, it is important to identify the specific herb he or she is using. Many people are not sure what they are using, in part because many herbal preparations are combinations of plant products. Many foreign preparations include herbs about which little is known, particularly Asian and Indian herbs.

Health History

Patients should be asked about the existence of comorbid diseases or conditions and allergies.

Lifespan Considerations

Perinatal. Pregnant women generally like herbs because of their purported relative safety and lack of adverse effects, but no herbal remedy should be taken during pregnancy without first consulting a health care provider. Most herbs used for cooking are safe during pregnancy. The higher dosages typically found in dietary supplements should be avoided. Herbs to avoid during pregnancy include angelica, Chinese angelica, comfrey, dang gui, devil's claw, ginseng, lady's mantle, licorice, motherwort, peppermint, sage, thyme, uva ursi, vervain, wild yam, and yarrow. Pregnant women should also avoid any herbal laxatives except dandelion, yellow dock, and garlic. When a woman is breast-feeding, herbs that the infant should avoid should also be avoided by the mother. Lactating women should also avoid sage, which tends to dry up breast milk.

Pediatric. Children respond very well to herbal remedies, but children's illnesses can develop very quickly. An accurate diagnosis from a health care provider should be obtained before considering the use of an herbal remedy.

Older Adults. Herbal remedies should be used with caution in the older adult. The concern is related to the patient's comorbid conditions and the associated drug therapy used. Unknown dynamics of the remedy and adverse effects can complicate a patient's symptoms.

Cultural/Social Considerations

Factors that influence choices of cures are bound to cultural beliefs about the causes of illness. Herbal remedies are important aspects of the treatment process for many ethnic groups. Contemporary medical practices neither assimilate nor stamp out folk practices. Health care providers must therefore learn effective diplomacy to understand and deal responsibly with the cultural beliefs and practices of their patients.

Many people have turned away from conventional therapies because they believe that natural substances are safer than synthetic substances. Patients may not understand the dynamic properties of herbal remedies. The slogan "all-natural" may lead them to believe that all herbal products are safe because they do not think of these products as drugs.

Physical Examination

At a minimum, the physical examination should include height and weight, blood pressure, pulse, and breath sounds. Further examination should be system focused according to the patient's reports.

Laboratory Testing

Depending on the herbal remedy used, liver function and kidney function tests should be performed before and throughout therapy. Allergy skin testing may have to be performed for some patients before the use of herbal remedies.

GOALS OF THERAPY

Regardless of the herbal remedy or 102 product used, the two product types empower the patient to play an integral role in recovering and maintaining his or her health and wellness.

Herbs are usually chosen to work in unison with the inherent healing powers of the body. Despite obvious conflicts, herbalism and conventional medicine are not at odds with each other. What one does well, the other tends to do poorly, and vice versa. For example, contemporary medicine treats diseases using drugs that contain isolated compounds. The isolated compounds work well but are often potent and have serious adverse effects. However, for acute conditions, there is no substitute. On the other hand, traditional herbal therapy uses whole herbs, which contain hundreds of compounds with the hope for a better overall effect than one compound alone could deliver.

INTERVENTION
Administration

Herbal remedies should be taken exactly as identified on the package label. "If a little is good, more is better," does not apply here. For some herbal remedies, a fine line exists between safe dosages and toxicity. There are a number of ways herbs can be used. The formulation chosen depends on the herb to be used, the purpose for its use, and to some degree, personal preference.

Bulk herbs are sold loose to be used as teas; however, bulk herbs rapidly lose their potency. Herbs should have a vibrant color and a strong aroma. Leaves and flowers purchased should be as close as possible to whole. Herbs that have been shielded from light and stored in opaque containers to preserve their potency are preferred. The active ingredients of the herb must be water soluble to be effective in a tea formulation.

Pressing herbs, soaking them in alcohol or water, and allowing the excess alcohol or water to evaporate yields a concentrated extract. Extracts are the most effective form of herbs, particularly for people with severe illnesses or malabsorption syndromes. Herbal extracts are generally diluted in a small amount of water before ingestion. Alcohol-free extracts are best, if available.

Tinctures are liquid extracts of plants, often in an alcohol base, and are used internally or externally in gargles, douches, compresses, liniments, mouthwashes, and baths. These formulations are stable, convenient, and easy to take and digest. They are taken by the dropperful in a small amount of juice or water. Glycerine-based tinctures are available for those who want or need to avoid alcohol.

Capsules and tablets contain powdered or freeze-dried herbs or extracts. Freeze-drying preserves potency better than powdering, which exposes the herb to heat and oxygen. Both powdered and freeze-dried formulations may contain binders and fillers; thus they may not be fully absorbed. Capsules and tablet formulations are an option for herbs that have an unpleasant taste.

Water-based extractions include teas and decoctions, which can be used as skin washes, gargles, compresses, and lotions, or diluted as eye baths, douches, and baths. The herb is placed in a pot, the boiling water is poured over the herb, and the pot is covered. The herb should be brewed for 1 to 3 minutes if flowers are used, 2 to 4 minutes if the herb's leaves are used, and 4 to 10 minutes if the bark, roots, or hard seeds of the herb are used. Decoctions are brewed from seeds, bark, and roots using the same quantities as for a tea. The herb is placed in a pan, covered with water, and covered with a tight lid. The mixture is allowed to come to a boil and then simmered for 20 to 30 minutes. The mixture is strained, and water is added. Syrups are made from decoctions and reduced slowly over low heat to one third the original amount. Cane sugar or honey is added and the syrup poured into a clean, dark-glass bottle; labeled; and stored in a cool place.

Ointments are formulated from an extract, tea, pressed juice, or a powdered form of an herb. The herbal substance is added to a salve that is then applied to an affected area. A **poultice** is a hot, soft, moist mass of ground or granulated herbs spread on muslin or other loosely woven cloth and applied for up to 24 hours on a sore or inflamed area of the body to relieve pain and inflammation. The cloth is changed when it cools.

Education

Patients should be advised that herbs are not regulated in the United States at this time. Since there are no legal standards, formulations vary widely in potency and recommended dosages. Although most herbs are nontoxic when used at recommended dosages, toxic ingredients are found in herbs such as arnica, belladonna, hemlock, lily of the valley, and sassafras (Table 8-1). Patients should also be told of the resources that are available to them regarding herbal remedies.

Self-treatment with herbs is appropriate only for minor self-limiting conditions. When the decision is made to use an herbal remedy, a few cautionary tips should be given. The patient should learn about the therapy before engaging in its use. The more that is known about the efficacy of the remedy, the quality of the herb, and its adverse effects, the safer the remedy may be. Herbs should not be taken casually but rather only when the body has a specific need. They should not be used on a regular basis. Patients should be helped to understand that herbs take longer to work than conventional pharmaceuticals.

Teach the patient to buy from trusted manufacturers. If possible, ask how and where the herbs are grown and processed. The answer to this question provides the patient with a sense of the quality control used. Only standardized herbal remedies are recommended.

Have the patient start with a single herb and take less than the recommended dosage; carefully monitor the response. This is particularly important if the patient is an older adult or is of below average weight for height. Herbs should be avoided entirely if the patient is pregnant or lactating.

Information about potential drug-drug interactions or drug-food interactions should be obtained. The herbal remedy should be stopped immediately if the patient experiences adverse effects.

EVALUATION

The therapeutic effectiveness of many remedies has been based on patient self-reports. However, to date only a few herbs have been approved by the FDA for selected applications; therefore any lay press book or article touting the benefits of an herbal remedy must be considered in light of the scientific literature on safety. The Office of Alternative Medicine was established to support the studies of adjunctive therapies.

TABLE 8-1

Potential Adverse Reactions to Herbal Extracts

Herbal Remedy	Adverse Reactions
Black cohosh	Nausea, vomiting
Caraway	Nausea, vomiting, CNS depression
Cardamon	Nausea, vomiting, diarrhea
Castor bean	Nausea, vomiting, bleeding, protoplasmic toxin, phytotoxin
Chomper	Digoxin toxicity
Cinnamon	Local skin and eye irritation; vomiting, GU irritation
Coconut	Diarrhea
Cola nut	Insomnia, anxiety, tachycardia, worsening PUD
Darniana	GU irritation; may exacerbate pre-existing UTI
Dandelion	Vomiting
Foxglove	Vomiting, bradycardia, arrhythmia
Gentian	Nausea, vomiting
Goldenseal	Paresthesia, hypertension, CNS stimulation, respiratory failure
Grindelia	Drowsiness, bradycardia, mydriasis, increased blood pressure, nephrotoxicity, cardiotoxicity
Hellebore	Vomiting, hypotension, bradycardia
Hops	Possibility of hemolysis
Hydrangea	Dizziness, nausea, vomiting, chest pain
Jalap	Volume depletion, excessive catharsis, watery diarrhea
Jimsonweed	Hallucinations, anticholinergic syndrome, contact dermatitis
Kava kava	Hallucinations, yellowish skin (liver toxicity), drowsiness
Lobelia	Headache, nausea, vomiting, seizures, coma, hepatotoxicity possible
Maté	Hallucinations, diaphoresis, caffeinism, venous peripheral vascular disease
Mormon tea	Hypertension, tachycardia, nervousness, anxiety
Morning glory	Hallucinations, confusion, nausea, diarrhea, coma
Nutmeg, mace	Nausea, vomiting, hypothermia, chest pain, dizziness, headache
Oleander	Vomiting, diarrhea
Pennyroyal oil	Hepatotoxicity, seizures, GI bleeding
Periwinkle	Hallucinations, dry mouth, drowsiness, nausea, ataxia, hepatotoxicity, seizures, decreased bowel sounds, alopecia
Royal jelly	Severe bronchospasm
Scotch broom	Vomiting
Snakeroot	Bradycardia, diarrhea, dizziness, hypotension, miosis, nasal congestion, coma
Tobacco	Nicotine syndrome
Valerian	Vomiting, drowsiness
Wormwood	Seizures, coma
Yohimbe bark	Abdominal distress, fatigue, weakness, paralysis, elevated blood pressure, hallucinations

CNS, Central nervous system; *GI,* gastrointestinal; *GU,* genitourinary; *PUD,* peptic ulcer disease; *UTI,* urinary tract infection.

Bibliography

Gruenwald J, Brendler T, Jaenicke C (eds): *PDR for herbal medicines*, Montvale NJ, 1998, Medical Economics.

Miller LG, Murray WJ: *Herbal medicinals: a clinician's guide*, Binghamton, NY, 1998, Pharmaceutical Products Press.

Nemecz G, Combest WL: Herbal remedies. In Allen L, Berardi R (eds): *Handbook of nonprescription drugs*, ed 12, Washington, DC, 2000, American Pharmaceutical Association.

Tyler VE: *The honest herbal*, ed 3, Binghamton, NY, 1993, Pharmaceutical Products Press.

Internet Resources

Alternative Medicine Homepage. Available online: www.pitt.edu/~cbw/altm.html.

American Botanical Council. Available online: www.herbalgram.org.

Herb Research Foundation. Available online: www.herbs.org.

9

Substance Abuse

MICHAEL R. VASKO • KATHLEEN GUTIERREZ

 Visit http://evolve.elsevier.com/Gutierrez/ for additional information.

KEY TERMS

Abstinence syndrome, p. 112	**Drug dependence,** p. 112
Addiction, p. 112	**Physical dependence,** p. 112
CAGE, p. 123	**Polysubstance abuse,** p. 123
Cross-dependence, p. 112	**Psychologic dependence,** p. 112
Cross-tolerance, p. 112	**Tolerance,** p. 112
Drug abuse, p. 111	**Withdrawal,** p. 112

OBJECTIVES

- Define drug dependence and differentiate between physical and psychologic dependence to an individual drug.
- Identify the characteristics of drugs that may increase the potential for drug abuse.
- Describe the effects of dependence-producing drugs of a given class.
- Describe current drug dependence treatment modalities.
- Describe drugs that are used in withdrawal and treatment.
- Apply the nursing process to care for patients who abuse substances.

GENERAL CHARACTERISTICS OF DEPENDENCE-PRODUCING DRUGS

In modern society the term drug abuse has come to refer to the misuse of drugs to alter one's mood, to experience a "unique sensation," to alter one's perception of reality, or to attempt to improve one's physical or mental abilities. The use of the term is complicated, however, by legal issues and society's views of drug use, despite the fact that it is a diagnostic term defined by the American Psychiatric Association's Diagnostic and Statistical Manual (see later in the chapter). For example, a number of decades ago, it was common in the United States to smoke cigarettes in public. In contrast, today this action is seen by society as largely unacceptable behavior associated with drug abuse. For medical personnel, the term often used in place of drug abuse is **drug dependence**. Drug (or substance) dependence refers to a clinical syndrome of drug use that manifests itself as either psychologic or physical reliance on a drug and is associated with detrimental effects on the individual or society. A synonymous layman's term for drug dependence is **addiction**. Like drug abuse, drug dependence is a syndrome that has specific diagnostic criteria (see later in the chapter). Confusion may occur, however, when referring to the syndrome of drug dependence because chronic use of the drugs discussed in this chapter can result in psychologic or physical dependence. For the purpose of this chapter, we will use the terms *drug abuse* and *drug dependence* interchangeably to denote the misuse of drugs, rather than for the psychologic or physiologic states that occur as a result of chronic drug use.

Psychologic dependence is a condition in which the subject has an emotional and mental need to continue drug use to feel normal or to cope with reality. This complex set of feelings and behaviors is reinforced through use and experience with the drug, and these behaviors make giving up drug use more difficult. Psychologic dependence is often related to the use of the drug to reduce stress, which eventually becomes the only means of stress reduction for the user. **Physical dependence** is a condition in which chronic exposure to a drug alters the function of nerve cells (neurons) sufficiently so that a series of physiologic signs and symptoms occur upon diminishment or discontinuation of the drug. These signs and symptoms are referred to as the **abstinence syndrome**, or **withdrawal**. Withdrawal symptoms are characteristic of a given drug class and are often the opposite of the drug's action. For example, alcohol, a CNS depressant, produces withdrawal symptoms characterized by hyperactivity. Conversely, when cocaine, a CNS stimulant, is withdrawn, one of the effects is depression and a loss of pleasure. These withdrawal effects are a sort of neurologic rebound in that the neurons have adjusted their neurotransmitters to the presence of the drug. When this drug is withdrawn, the body lacks the drug's balancing effect. The withdrawal symptoms characteristic of alcohol, benzodiazepines, and barbiturates are the most dangerous and require careful monitoring. Individuals vary greatly in their potential for and range of withdrawal symptoms. Finally, it is important to point out that **cross-dependence** can occur with drugs of a given class (i.e., opioids or CNS depressants). With cross-dependence, one drug of a given class can substitute for another drug to prevent withdrawal. This phenomenon is clinically important and the reason for administering methadone to heroin addicts or for using a standard CNS depressant to detoxify someone physically dependent on these drugs.

In addition to dependence, chronic use of most of the drugs discussed in this chapter results in the devel-

opment of **tolerance** to the actions of the drugs. Tolerance is the loss of a drug's effectiveness at a given dosage, resulting from repeated use. This in turn increases the amount of the drug necessary to achieve the same physiologic or psychologic effect. It is important to point out that the development of tolerance is dependent on the characteristics of the drug, the amount administered, and the frequency of administration. In general, we define two types of tolerance: cellular and metabolic. Cellular tolerance refers to the adaptation of individual cells to chronic exposure to a given drug. In contrast, metabolic tolerance occurs when induction of metabolic enzymes results in a more rapid breakdown of a drug, thus decreasing the amount available at the site of action. **Cross-tolerance** is the development of a tolerance to one drug that also increases the tolerance to a related category of drugs. For example, tolerance to alcohol, a central nervous system (CNS) depressant, results in cross-tolerance to other CNS depressants such as benzodiazepines and barbiturates. Because of the potential for cross-tolerance, it is important to obtain a complete drug history for each patient, since a patient's tolerance to an illicitly used drug can result in cross-tolerance to a drug administered to him or her by a health care provider.

Although there is a correlation between the development of tolerance and physical dependence, they are not produced by the same cellular mechanisms. Furthermore, nurses should understand that tolerance and physical dependence can occur with long-term administration of certain drugs to patients. For example, chronic administration of morphine for pain results in a tolerance that renders the drug less useful. When the drug is discontinued, the patient will experience a mild withdrawal. These effects are part of the pharmacologic actions of the drug and do not mean that the patient has a drug abuse problem. Indeed, a common misconception that sometimes interferes with adequate drug therapy for pain is that long-term use of opioids will result in dependency. The development of a drug dependence syndrome after chronic therapeutic use of drugs is rare and usually associated with a preexisting drug dependence problem.

DIAGNOSIS OF DRUG DEPENDENCE

Drug use occurs on a continuum beginning with experimentation and leading to infrequent use, regular use, abuse with resulting health and social problems, and ultimately dependence characterized by loss of control. Both drug abuse and drug dependence are diagnostic terms defined by the American Psychiatric Association's Diagnostic and Statistical Manual (DSM). The current version, DSM-IV, identifies the abused drug of choice as part of the diagnosis. Drug abuse occurs when drug use becomes problematic, causing social and personal difficulties. Diagnostic criteria for drug abuse are evaluated during a 12-month period and must involve one or more of the following: (1) failure to fulfill major role obligations at work, school, or home; (2) use in physically hazardous situations; (3) recurrent substance-related legal problems; or (4) use despite persistent or recurrent social or interpersonal problems as a result of use. Drug dependence is diagnosed when physiologic effects appear or when loss of control over the drug and its use becomes increasingly apparent. Diagnostic criteria for drug dependence include the presence of at least three of the following factors within a 12-month period: (1) tolerance; (2) withdrawal; (3) a substance taken in larger amount or over longer period than intended; (4) persistent, unsuccessful efforts to reduce use; (5) an increased amount of time spent procuring, using, or recovering from the effects of the substance; (6) other previously important activities are avoided or reduced because of substance use; and (7) continued use despite knowledge of a problem.

Of the drugs that have abuse potential, some are legal, whereas others are illegal. Some drugs such as tobacco and alcohol are legal for persons who meet certain criteria, such as age. Illegality of a substance does not necessitate a diagnosis of abuse, but legal difficulties are one criterion for a diagnosis. In addition, legal problems can be an external condition that encourages the individual to recognize the problem and seek treatment. For example, repeatedly driving while under the influence of drugs, particularly alcohol, can result in legal difficulties such as a drunk-driving charge, and the individual may be given a choice between incarceration and treatment. A charge of possession of an illegal drug also can result in recognition of lack of control.

Variables Contributing to Drug Dependence

Not everyone who experiments with a drug develops personal and social complications or loses control of drug use. Why this happens to some individuals and not to others is a question not fully understood and is dependent on a number of factors, including the characteristics of the drug, the user, and the environment. Drugs that produce the strongest positive reinforcement, such as a pleasurable effect, elevated mood, euphoria, or a calming effect, are most likely to be abused. Drugs that do not produce a mood-altering effect are rarely intentionally abused. One exception is anabolic steroids, which are abused because of their muscle-building effects. In addition, the intensity and rapidity

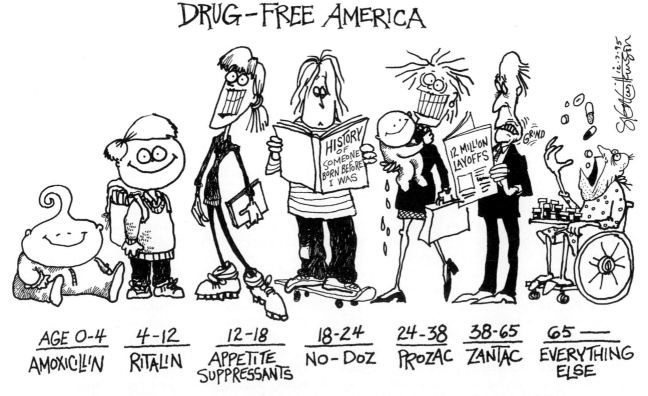

FIGURE 9-1 Drug use across American generations. How we view and use prescription and OTC drugs as a society has an impact on the issue of all drug use and abuse. ("Drug-Free America" by Signe Wilkinson, ©1997, *The Washington Post*. Reprinted with permission.)

of effect correlate with the likelihood of abuse. In general, the more rapidly a drug is delivered to the brain, the greater the effect and the higher the potential of the drug to produce dependence. For example, cocaine powder is usually taken intranasally (snorted), and crack cocaine is smoked. Although the nasal mucosa is highly vascular and snorting allows rapid transfer from blood to brain, inhalation is a faster route. This shorter time for delivery to the brain appears to be a factor in the highly addictive nature of nicotine in cigarettes.

Because the rapidity of drug delivery to the brain enhances the high, a number of drugs are self-administered by intravenous (IV) injection. The IV administration of drugs presents the nurse with a potential for a series of secondary problems associated with it. Of concern is infection at the site of injection and the danger of spreading such an infection, particularly hepatitis and human immunodeficiency virus (HIV)/acquired immunodeficiency syndrome (AIDS), when IV materials are shared. IV use also exposes the individual to cellulitis and scarred or sclerosed veins.

Ready access to drugs is another risk factor. Drug abuse by health care professionals is a source of professional and societal concern. Licensed health care professions have become increasingly active in identifying and addressing substance abuse among their members in recent years. For nurses in particular, some of the risk factors for substance abuse include a family history of substance abuse, a history of health problems, and a history of depression. The availability of drugs and a professional culture in which a drug is offered for every problem encourage nurses to self-medicate, thereby increasing the risk of abuse. Many professional organizations now sponsor peer assistance organizations that help identify substance abuse and resources for treatment as well as monitor the professional on return to employment.

Individual risk factors for drug dependence include genetic factors, psychiatric history, and prior experience with drug abuse. The genetic component of alcohol dependence, in particular, has been well documented with twin and adoption studies. For instance, a twin with alcoholism in the biologic family background is more likely to become alcohol dependent when adopted into a nondrinking environment than a twin with no alcoholism in the biologic family background adopted into a drinking environment. The family environment is, however, also a major risk factor for drug dependence. A child who grows up with a drug-abusing parent receives both role modeling and interpersonal experiences that may promote eventual drug abuse either during adolescence or adulthood. Family relationships are distorted to accommodate the drug-abusing parent.

Coping skills are another risk modifier. These skills reflect how an individual adapts his or her behavior in response to demands. Ineffective coping or coping strategies in times of overwhelming stress are a major risk factor for drug abuse. Drugs are often used as a temporary measure to decrease the psychologic discomfort caused by high stress or poor coping strategies. This situation is promoted in our society by advertisements featuring alcohol and nicotine as means of coping with stress. Individuals who model this behavior put themselves at risk for abuse by managing stress indirectly through drugs rather than directly through constructive action to decrease stress.

Personal crises are a risk factor. Coping skills are tested during situational or maturational crises. Situational crises are those that result from specific stressors such as job loss, divorce, and death. Maturational crises are a result of reaching new development stages such as adolescence or young adulthood. A desire to decrease the pressure, stress, or emotional pain during these personal crises increases the risk for drug use and abuse. Sometimes the health care system facilitates abuse. For example, stress may produce physiologic symptoms for which a health care provider prescribes a minor tranquilizer. This type of drug is subject to abuse when used over an extended period of time in place of learning new and more effective coping strategies.

Nurses encounter patients with a variety of conditions. Often the physical or mental condition is related, directly or indirectly, to drug abuse. It is important that nurses routinely assess drug use in an initial workup and continue to consider its possibility throughout their care of the patient. When drug abuse is part of the health care problem but is not addressed, care is incomplete, increasing the likelihood of recurrence. Underlying drug abuse may be a factor in as many as 40% of hospital admissions.

Characteristics of Specific Drugs

The drugs discussed in this chapter can be categorized into five groups: the opioids, the CNS depressants, the CNS stimulants, hallucinogens, and inhalants. Obviously these drugs have diverse pharmacologic and toxicologic effects, yet all have the capacity to produce dependence based on their euphoric and positive reinforcing actions. The major characteristics of commonly abused drugs are summarized in Table 9-1. Many of these drugs have prescribed clinical uses (e.g., opioids, CNS depressants, and some CNS stimulants), some are legally obtainable for recreational use (e.g., nicotine, alcohol), and others are illegal (e.g., LSD, cannabinoids). Regardless of their legal status, they all have the potential for chronic abuse resulting in substance dependence.

TABLE 9-1

Major Characteristics of Commonly Abused Drugs

Drug	Primary Route(s)	Dependence	Desired Effect	Withdrawal	Treatment of Overdose
Alcohol	Oral	Physical, psychologic*	Intoxication	Severe; convulsions	Support therapies†
Amphetamines	Oral, IV	Psychologic	Strong stimulation	Depression	Support therapies
Barbiturates	Oral	Physical, psychologic	Relaxation	Severe; convulsions	Support therapies
Benzodiazepines	Oral	Physical, psychologic	Relaxation	Severe; convulsions	Flumazenil
Caffeine	Oral	Psychologic	Mild stimulation	Minor; headaches	None
Cocaine	Nasal, inhalation	Psychologic*	Strong stimulation	Depression	Support therapies
Heroin	IV, inhalation	Physical, psychologic	Euphoria; coasting	Major; flu-like symptoms	Naloxone
Inhalants	Inhalation	Psychologic	Intoxication	Minor, if any	Support therapies
LSD	Oral	Psychologic	Distorted perception	Minor, if any	Environment; support
Marijuana	Inhalation	Psychologic	Distortion of senses	Minor, if any	None
Nicotine	Inhalation, buccal	Psychologic*	Mild stimulation	Minor; irritability	None
Phencyclidine	Inhalation, oral	Psychologic	Power, altered senses	Minor, if any	Support therapies

*Debate as to whether physical dependence occurs because withdrawal is observed but is not reproducible in all patients.
†These therapies include but are not limited to maintaining breathing, cardiovascular function, fluid balance, and body temperature.

OPIOIDS

Naturally occurring drugs, semisynthetic drugs, and synthetic derivatives are classified as opioids if they act at specific sites in the body called opioid receptors and have actions similar to the drug morphine. Morphine and codeine are produced from opium, which is harvested from the opium poppy. Opioids are used clinically to reduce pain perception and to treat cough, diarrhea, and dysentery (see Chapter 13). The most potent and highly abused opioid is the semisynthetic compound heroin (see Table 9-2 for street names), although a number of other opioids are also widely misused. Upon administration, heroin enters the CNS more rapidly than morphine, thereby producing a better high. This may account for its popularity. Recent trends also show an increase in the abuse of hydrocodone as indicated by a greater than twofold increase in emergency room encounters.

In general, opioids are self-administered intravenously, subcutaneously, or through smoking, and they produce feelings of peace and contentment. Most opioid-dependent individuals state that initial injection of heroin produces a rush, or thrilling sensation, followed by "coasting," or a drowsy state. In nontolerant subjects, opioids can produce sedation and sleep. Tolerance develops to these effects and to the euphoric actions of these drugs. Acute overdose of opioids produces CNS depression, respiratory depression, and pinpoint pupils. Death from overdose is usually secondary to respiratory arrest or pulmonary edema. Fatal overdose often occurs because the user does not know how much of the injected drug is actual opioid. Administration of naloxone (short-acting) or naltrexone (longer-acting), the pure opioid antagonists, to an overdosed patient rapidly reverses the coma and respiratory depression brought on by opioids (see Chapter 13). Since naloxone has little significant action on its own, it can be used to differentiate overdose with opioids from that of other CNS depressants, reversing toxicity of opioids but not of alcohol, barbiturates, or other CNS depressants. There are, however, two caveats with the use of naloxone. First, it is relatively short-acting, so more than one dose may be required. Second, caution should be exercised when administering pure antagonists to opioid-dependent individuals, since the drugs can precipitate withdrawal.

TABLE 9-2

Street Names of Commonly Abused Substances

Opioids	
Codeine	Captain Cody, cody, schoolboy, doors and fours, syrup
Heroin	H, horse, junk, noise, pee, skag, skunk, skid, smack, boy, white horse, brown sugar
Morphine	M, morph, white stuff, cube juice, emsel, hocus, Miss Emma, unkie, monkey
Opium	Black stuff, block, poppy, tar, hop, pin, yen, gum, wen shee, big O
Central Nervous System Depressants	
Amobarbital	Blue devils, blue angels, blue heavens, blues, bluebirds
Benzodiazepines	Candy, downers, tranks, sleeping pills, green and whites, libs, roaches
Methaqualone	Quaalude, ludes, mandrex, quad, quay
Pentobarbital	Yellow jackets, yellowbirds, nembies, yellows
Phenobarbital	Purple hearts
Secobarbital	Seccy, red birds, red devils, reds
Central Nervous System Stimulants	
Amphetamines	Dexies, oranges, hearts, Christmas trees, wedges, spots, uppers, bennies, black beauty, black Cadillacs
Cocaine	Blow, bump, coke, snow, lady, candy, rock, flake, crack, Charlie, dream, happy dust, heaven dust, joy powder, girl, nose candy, toot
Methamphetamine	Chalk, crank, fire, glass, Christine, speed, meth, crystal, ice
Methylenedioxymethamphetamine	Ecstasy, clarity, Eve, XTC, Adam, X, lover's speed, peace
Methylphenidate	JIF, Skippy, MPH, R-ball, the smart drug, vitamin R
Hallucinogens	
Cannabis (marijuana)	Ace, ashes, blunt, broccoli, dope, grass, hemp, jive, joint, Mary Jane, pot, THC, weed, herb, reefer, skunk, many others
Hashish	Boom, hash, black Russian, gangster, oil
Lysergic acid diethylamide (LSD)	Acid, cube, big D, blue dots, boomers, yellow sunshine, micro dots, purple haze, battery acid, sugar, window pane
Mescaline	Bad seed, big chief, buttons, peyote, mesc, cactus, white light, mescal
Phencyclidine (PCP)	Angel dust, dummy dust, boat, hog, mist, peace pill, tranq, whack
Psilocybin	Magic mushrooms, shrooms, purple passion

Both physical and psychologic dependence can develop during continuous use of opioids, with the degree of dependence varying with the individual as well as the amount and frequency of drug administered. When opioids are discontinued, a predictable set of withdrawal symptoms appears. Early on, individuals experience rhinorrhea, increased salivation, lacrimation, yawning, and stretching. Loss of appetite, dilated pupils, tremor, and gooseflesh ("cold turkey" symptoms) follow. At peak withdrawal, subjects are very restless, have nausea, diarrhea, muscle cramps, twitching, and tremors. This syndrome lasts 3 to 5 days but may be followed by extended periods of craving, insomnia, and weakness. Although the withdrawal syndrome is very uncomfortable, it is not life-threatening (as compared to withdrawal associated with other CNS depressants; see later in the chapter). It

is important to detoxify patients dependent on opioids as part of a treatment program to break the cycle of dependency.

Opioid withdrawal can be treated in several ways. Methadone is a long-acting, cross-dependence opioid that can be administered once daily to prevent withdrawal symptoms (see Chapter 13). The use of methadone as a replacement drug has long been the treatment of choice; however, recent data suggest that this approach may increase the likelihood of relapse to opioid use. Other alternatives are the use of the alpha-adrenergic agonist clonidine to relieve specific symptoms rather than to substitute for the opioid (see Chapter 41). Buprenorphine, the partial opioid agonist, may also be used for 5 to 8 days.

There are a number of clinical conditions that the nurse may need to address in patients chronically abus-

BOX 9-1	Medical Problems Associated with Opioid Abuse

- Acute overdose: respiratory depression, cardiovascular collapse; treat with naloxone
- Chronic user overdose: use caution with naloxone, may precipitate withdrawal; use support therapy
- Abstinence syndrome: treat with long-term detoxification (methadone); clonidine to treat autonomic symptoms
- Other complications (infection, etc.)
- Complications in pregnancy
- High recidivism rate (85%)

BOX 9-2	Medical Problems Associated with CNS Depressants

- Overdose: treat symptoms, no grandstanding; for benzodiazepine overdose, use flumazenil
- Withdrawal: if life threatening, get to maintenance dose and withdraw slowly
- Minimum tolerance to lethal actions
- Fetal alcohol syndrome
- Alcoholism: treat with disulfiram, naltrexone

ing opioids, especially heroin, that are not direct effects of the drugs. Use of communal or dirty needles to inject drugs results in secondary infections and the spread of diseases such as hepatitis and AIDS. Unknown additives mixed with street drugs can clog blood vessels and lead to embolism. Finally, nurses caring for newborns need to recognize that babies born to opioid-dependent mothers are also physically dependent on opioids and go into withdrawal soon after birth. A summary of the medical problems associated with opioid abuse and potential treatments is outlined in Box 9-1.

CNS DEPRESSANTS

A number of different drugs comprise this class, including alcohol, barbiturates, benzodiazepines, and nonbarbiturate sedatives (see Table 9-2 for street names). These drugs primarily are used to relieve anxiety, to produce sedation, and to induce or maintain sleep. For greater detail on their clinical uses and adverse reactions, see Chapter 17. These drugs are usually abused for the purpose of extending their clinical use, that is, to eliminate anxious feelings, to induce feelings of tranquility, relaxation, or disinhibition. Although patterns of abuse vary greatly, chronic long-term use causes adverse effects in the individual.

CNS depressants produce a decrease in mental ability and a loss of coordination. Slow speech and emotional imbalance are followed by ataxia, stupor, and sleep as the dose increases. An overdose produces respiratory depression or arrest, coma, and death (usually from hypoxia). In addition, although tolerance develops to the sedative and euphoric effects of these drugs, little tolerance develops to the lethal effects. Consequently, chronic users who increase their dosage to get high are at risk for poisoning. Finally, the fact that these drugs impair mental function and memory may lead individuals to forget how much they took and therefore to take more. Unlike opioids, there is no specific antago-

nist for the respiratory depression associated with most of these drugs, although flumazenil does reverse the effects of benzodiazepine overdose (see later this chapter and Chapter 17). A summary of the medical problems associated with CNS depressants is presented in Box 9-2.

Chronic use of these drugs can result in both psychologic and physical dependence. In the case of physically dependent individuals, the withdrawal is a potentially life-threatening event that needs to be taken seriously by the caregivers. The severity of withdrawal is dependent on the type of drug taken, the frequency of administration, and the dose; however, delirium tremors, convulsions, and even continuous seizures are common in patients who are not appropriately detoxified. Indeed, treatment requires the patient to be hospitalized and stabilized on a suitable CNS depressant. Since the drug produces cross-tolerance and cross-dependence, once stabilized on it, the patient's dosage can be slowly reduced over time without producing an abstinence syndrome. As with opioids, it is important to remember that babies born to mothers dependent on CNS depressants will also be physically dependent and experience a dangerous withdrawal after birth.

Barbiturates and Nonbarbiturate Sedatives

Most barbiturate abuse occurs with the use of short-acting drugs such as pentobarbital, secobarbital, or mephobarbital. Nonbarbiturate sedatives include methaqualone (quaaludes or ludes) and chloral hydrate (Mickey Finn or Finn). These drugs and other drugs of this class have additive or greater than additive effects, so mixing these agents can result in overdose. These drugs are abused for their ability to decrease anxiety, to produce relaxation, and to render the individual carefree and tranquil. Individuals ingesting barbiturates become sedate and drowsy. In addition, users have slow speech, slow reflexes, and decreased mental activity. As mentioned above, tolerance develops to the sedative effects of these drugs, and metabolic tolerance can develop, since some of these drugs induce their own metabolism in the liver. Chronic users develop both psychologic and physical dependence. Withdrawal can be life threatening and is characterized by weakness, insomnia, cramps, nausea, vomiting, hypotension, fever, delirium, and seizures.

Alcohol

Despite the fact that low to intermediate doses of alcohol sometimes appear to stimulate individuals by disinhibiting pathways in the CNS, this drug is a CNS depressant. It is widely available, relatively inexpensive, and comes in a variety of forms, such as beer, wine, wine coolers, and distilled spirits. In the United States, alcohol is commonly served in social settings, where it is thought to promote conviviality. Low doses produce a feeling of tranquility and decreased anxiety with impairment of motor skills. Higher doses produce exaggerated emotions, further impairment of motor skills and judgment, slurred speech, ataxia, stupor, memory loss, and loss of consciousness. Extremely high amounts can produce respiratory depression and coma. Note that a blood alcohol level of 0.08% is the legal limit for driving in many states. Chronic drinking can result in alcoholism, a dependence on the drug, particularly in those genetically predisposed. Physical damage most commonly appears in the liver and brain. The alcohol withdrawal syndrome can be serious, characterized by tremors, changes in level of consciousness, with progression to seizures and delirium tremors, which are life-threatening conditions. These withdrawal symptoms are treated with a decreasing dose of benzodiazepines, most often chlordiazepoxide or diazepam. As with opioids and other CNS depressants, babies born to alcohol-dependent mothers are also physically dependent. Furthermore, alcohol use by mothers during pregnancy can result in a syndrome of birth defects known as fetal alcohol syndrome. The child with fetal alcohol syndrome has craniofacial abnormalities, stunted growth, and CNS dysfunction.

Benzodiazepines

Benzodiazepines are antianxiety drugs widely prescribed for reducing stress and tension and for sleep disorders (see Chapter 17). As with other CNS depressants, acute overdose of benzodiazepines produces sedation, gait disturbances, stupor, and respiratory depression, but these drugs are less potent than barbiturates. Tolerance develops to the sedative actions of these drugs. Benzodiazepines act at specific receptor sites in the CNS; however, administering flumazenil can block the depressant action of these drugs. Although they are not as labile as the short-acting barbiturates, long-term use can result in physical and psychologic dependence. Withdrawal symptoms include tremors, anxiety, and

potential for seizures, symptoms which can be avoided by gradual reduction of the dosage over a relatively long period of time. Prescription benzodiazepines that are most often abused include diazepam, alprazolam, triazolam, and chlordiazepoxide. Recently, there have been increasing reports of drug dependence problems associated with the use of clonazepam.

CNS STIMULANTS

There are a number of CNS stimulants that produce drug dependence, including amphetamines and cocaine. Other drugs of abuse include methylphenidate, caffeine, and nicotine (see Table 9-2 for street names). These drugs are generally self-administered for positive reinforcement, for feelings of confidence, and for heightened energy. It is important to point out that these drugs produce a strong psychologic dependence in individuals and therefore represent a major concern for nurses. One only has to look at the number of individuals who smoke cigarettes and use other forms of tobacco and who have difficulty stopping to recognize the powerful addictive nature of these drugs. Adverse reactions to CNS stimulants include increased heart rate and blood pressure and, with the more potent stimulants such as amphetamines and cocaine, reduced appetite, arrhythmia, and heart failure. Interestingly, these drugs do not produce the characteristic set of physiologic withdrawal symptoms after chronic use, but the abstinence syndrome may vary (see later this chapter for individual drugs). The detailed pharmacology of most of these drugs is discussed in Chapter 20, but a brief summary of the medical problems associated with these drugs is outlined in Box 9-3.

Amphetamines and Cocaine

Although amphetamines (D-amphetamine, methamphetamine) and cocaine are different classes of drugs, they are discussed together, since the reinforcing and adverse effects are subjectively similar (see Table 9-2 for street names). Amphetamines are synthetic drugs used

---

BOX 9-3   **Medical Problems Associated with Abuse of CNS Stimulants**

- Cardiovascular difficulty, violent reaction, overdose
- Chronic use or "run": amphetamine psychosis, violent and paranoid behavior, exhaustion, convulsions
- Withdrawal: suicidal depression
- Nasal septal ulceration and perforation
- Eye damage
- High recidivism rate; for nicotine cessation, use replacement therapy

clinically for weight loss, narcolepsy, and attention deficit–hyperactivity disorder (ADHD). Cocaine is purified from the leaves of the coca plant and is used clinically as a local anesthetic (see Chapter 16); it is self-administered by snorting, smoking, or IV injection. Amphetamines are also taken orally. Cocaine hydrochloride can be processed with ammonia or bicarbonate to make a smokable form called crack. This drug got its name because of the crackling sound it makes when heated. Methamphetamine hydrochloride crystals (called ice or glass) are also smoked. Inhalation of these drugs usually produces a rush or high and increases the likelihood of the rapid development of drug dependence.

Acute administration of moderate amounts of these drugs produces a sense of well-being, whereas higher doses produce an intense, short-lived euphoric feeling. In general, subjects taking these drugs feel that they can perform physical and mental tasks better, but they also develop restlessness, insomnia, and irritability. These drugs also have dramatic effects on the cardiovascular system, increasing blood pressure and heart rate, causing arrhythmias, and enhancing the possibility of cerebrovascular accidents (stroke). Chronic use is associated with an increased likelihood of developing irrational behavior, including paranoia and delusions or hallucinations. Tolerance develops to the euphoric effects of these drugs, which can lead the user to increase the dosage. Strong psychologic dependence develops to these drugs, whereas the possibility of developing a physical dependence is unclear. However, with high dosages of these drugs, withdrawal is characterized by an initial dysphoric reaction followed by depression, craving, prolonged sleep, and the inability to experience pleasure. Overdosage produces a medical emergency consisting of increased body temperature, hypertension, tachycardia, seizures, dyspnea, and ventricular arrhythmia. The fatigue and depression associated with the end of the drug effect (often referred to as "crashing") produces a labile state where subjects may feel it necessary to take an additional drug that can result in a number of days of continuous use (referred to as a "run"), or they may be depressed to the point of attempting suicide.

Methylphenidate

Methylphenidate is a prescription drug useful in treating narcolepsy, a disorder where patients fall asleep frequently and at inappropriate times. The drug's major use, however, is in treating attention deficit–hyperactivity disorder (ADHD). Although therapeutic doses produce less dramatic effects than amphetamines and cocaine, the drug can cause excessive stimulation, loss of appetite, and insomnia. Caution should be exercised in obtaining a diagnosis of ADHD before giving these drugs to active children who may have some difficulty in concentrating,

since the adverse effects of the drug need to be weighed against the potential benefits.

Caffeine

Caffeine is one of the most widely abused drugs in the United States, although the effects of this abuse are much less obvious and usually less harmful than those produced by other abused drugs. Like other, more potent stimulants, acute administration elevates alertness and mood while decreasing fatigue. Caffeine dependence is often subtle, and the user frequently develops it unwittingly. Most people are aware of the caffeine content of coffee, which ranges from 80 to 150 mg per cup. Less well known is the fact that tea, cola, chocolate, and some nonprescription medications (e.g., Excedrin) also contain caffeine (Table 9-3).

Ingestion of more than 500 mg of caffeine daily produces a variety of CNS effects and cardiovascular reactions. Irritability or nervousness is a common complaint, along with sleep disturbances. Patients may report heart palpitations or say that their heart is "racing." These descriptions may suggest premature ventricular contractions and tachycardia, common symptoms of chronic caffeine toxicity. Diarrhea, gastrointestinal irritation, and increased urination often accompany chronic use and overdosage with caffeine. Patients complaining of symptoms such as these should be ques-

---

TABLE 9-3

Caffeine Content of Commonly Ingested Substances

Substance	Caffeine Content
Foods and Beverages	
Coffee	
Brewed	80-150 mg per 5-oz cup
Instant	85-100 mg per 5-oz cup
Decaffeinated	2-4 mg per 5-oz cup
Tea, brewed	30-75 mg per 5-oz cup
Cocoa	5-40 mg per 5-oz cup
Cola soft drinks*	35-60 mg per 12-oz bottle or can
Nonprescription Drugs	
Analgesics (Anacin and Vanquish)	32 mg per tablet
Excedrin	65 mg per tablet
Cold medications	
Dristan AF	16.2 mg per tablet
Korigesic	30 mg per tablet
Stimulants	
Nodoz	100 mg per tablet
Vivarin	200 mg per tablet

*Many soft drinks other than colas contain caffeine as an additive. The label reveals the presence of caffeine but not the amount.

tioned about their caffeine intake. The person taking the history should ask specifically about individual beverages, foods, and medications that contain caffeine to make an accurate estimate of intake.

Tolerance does develop to the stimulant effect of caffeine, as does psychologic dependence. Indeed, many people have great difficulty eliminating caffeine from their diet. Although the possibility of developing a physical dependence is questionable, persons withdrawing from the drug often experience headaches, nervousness, and irritability. There are few, if any, studies linking caffeine use to other diseases; however, patients with peptic ulcer disease or gastroesophageal reflux disease (GERD) should avoid caffeine, and pregnant women may wish to reduce or avoid caffeine because it freely passes to the fetus. Any person who ingests more than 200 mg of caffeine daily should be encouraged to reduce his or her caffeine intake to avoid the subtle onset of chronic toxicity.

Nicotine

Nicotine is the major active ingredient found in the tobacco plant and usually is self-administered by smoking tobacco products, including cigarettes, cigars, and pipe tobacco. The drug is also absorbed through the oral mucosa when subjects chew tobacco or use snuff. In addition, a number of OTC drugs containing nicotine are available to assist smokers in quitting, including nicotine patches and gum. When burned, tobacco products also release carbon monoxide, carcinogens, and tar, which are also inhaled and absorbed in the body. The stimulant properties of nicotine are less pronounced than those observed with amphetamines, yet the drug does increase alertness and improve mood. This latter action may account for the subtle but strong reinforcing properties of the drug. Acute use can produce nausea, vomiting, and dizziness. Nicotine also increases heart rate, blood pressure, and respiration and can cause tremors. Toxic doses of nicotine can cause twitching of muscles, loss of muscle control, or convulsions. Tolerance develops to the reinforcing effects of nicotine, so the user must keep increasing the amount of drug used to obtain the same effect. Nicotine produces a strong psychologic dependence, and the user finds it extremely difficult to abstain. As with other stimulants, physical dependence is hard to define, but withdrawal symptoms include craving, restlessness, decreased concentration, and hyperirritability.

Nicotine use contributes to a variety of serious health problems, including lung cancer, hypertension, and cardiovascular disease. It is estimated that 80% of American smokers have attempted to quit smoking at some time. There are organized programs to assist smokers in quitting, which have about a 20% to 30% success rate for 1 year of abstinence. Interestingly, more

than 90% of those who do quit do so without support programs. Both nicotine chewing gum and transdermal patches are available to use in combination with other forms of treatment. Additionally, the antidepressant drug bupropion (Wellbutrin) has recently been shown to help people quit smoking; however, many smokers "quit" several times before finally achieving long-term cessation.

HALLUCINOGENS

Although a number of different classes of drugs alter perception of reality and can produce hallucinations, for the purpose of this chapter we will subdivide them into (1) general hallucinogens, including D-lysergic acid diethylamide; mescaline; psilocybin; 3,4,methylenedioxymethamphetamine (MDMA), and cannabinoids (marijuana, hashish); and (2) dissociative anesthetics such as phencyclidine and ketamine. See Table 9-2 for common street names of these drugs. At the present time, these drugs have no medical uses, with the exception of cannabinoids, which can decrease nausea associated with antineoplastic therapy. It is important to note, however, that there are other, more promising drugs available for this use (see Chapter 50). In general, these drugs are abused for the desire to alter thought processes and induce unique experiences. They do not provide the opportunity for persons to gain insight or to better understand themselves or others. Indeed, high doses of these drugs produce altered sensations, disorientation, delusions, and frank hallucinations. As with other drugs, tolerance develops to the effects of these agents. In addition, persons taking these drugs chronically can develop a psychologic dependence. This is especially true for the cannabinoids, since they often are self-administered with much greater frequency than other drugs of this class. A brief summary of the medical problems associated with hallucinogens is outlined in Box 9-4.

BOX 9-4   Medical Problems Associated with Hallucinogen Abuse

- Depersonalization
- Emergence of underlying mental illness
- Bad trip (exercise caution using neuroleptics)
- Hallucinogen-persisting perception disorder (flashbacks)
- Apathy, impaired memory and judgment
- PCP psychosis; to treat:
  Prevent injury to patient or others
  Assure continued treatment
  Reduce external stimuli
  Ameliorate psychosis with neuroleptics

General Hallucinogens

The most potent hallucinogen is LSD (D-lysergic acid diethylamide); the single dose usually consists of only 20 to 200 mcg. Subjects taking this synthetic drug experience mixed senses (i.e., seeing sound and hearing colors), disorientation, emotional swings, delusions, and visual hallucinations. Physiologic effects include tachycardia, increased blood pressure, fever, sweating, dilated pupils, loss of sleep, and tremors. The drug experience, or "trip," lasts for hours and varies greatly depending on the environment, the mood of the subject, and the expectations. One clinical concern is the possibility that the drug experience will be adverse (a bad trip) and that the subject will have terrifying thoughts, panic attacks, fear, or despair. Although these can be treated with sedatives, nurses should exercise caution when attempting to use drugs to treat a bad trip. For example, administering antipsychotic medications to patients on some hallucinogens can cause convulsions. Since it is difficult to know which drug the patient is on, the decision to use drugs to reverse toxicity can be difficult. In the case of a bad trip, providing a safe, friendly environment while talking soothingly to the subject until the drug's effects subside is often successful. Another concern with LSD use is the potential for the user to experience so-called flashbacks days, months, or even years after the drug experience. This syndrome is called persisting perception disorder and is a recurrence of some part of the initial drug experience. It can occur unexpectedly months to years after using the drug. It is more often associated with long-term drug use but can also occur in infrequent users. Finally, the use of LSD and other potent hallucinogens can precipitate psychotic episodes in subjects with underlying mental or emotional illness.

Mescaline is a shorter-acting hallucinogen and is the major psychoactive ingredient found in the peyote cactus. Like LSD, it produces altered senses and visual hallucinations but is much less potent. Acute administration can produce nausea, sweating, and tremors. Other adverse effects are similar to LSD. Psilocybin is one of the active hallucinogens found in certain types of mushrooms. Its effects are similar to LSD but with a more rapid onset (15 minutes) and a much shorter duration.

Another hallucinogen that has gained popularity is 3,4,methylenedioxymethamphetamine (MDMA). This drug not only produces stimulant actions similar to amphetamines but also produces hallucinations. This drug has been shown to produce a selective neurotoxicity by damaging 5-hydroxytryptamine–containing neurons in the brain. Adverse effects of this drug include nausea, blurred vision, increased blood pressure and heart rate, confusion, sleep disturbances, anxiety, and paranoia. High doses could result in a syndrome called malignant hyperthermia, chronic high fever that can result in renal failure and cardiovascular collapse. As with other hallucinogens, subjects can develop psychologic dependence.

Cannabinoids

Marijuana is the most widely used illicit drug in the United States; approximately one third of the population 12 years or older report that they have tried the drug, and close to 9% used it in the past year. Marijuana is made mostly from the dried leaves of the cannabis plant, whereas the more potent hashish is a dried resin from the flowering parts of the plant. The active ingredients in the plant are cannabinoids, with the principle ingredient being (-)-delta(9)-trans-tetrahydrocannabinol (Δ 9-THC). Recent studies have demonstrated specific binding sites for cannabinoids in the CNS and on an endogenous substance called anandamide, which is an agonist at these receptors. This suggests a specific site of action for these drugs in the brain.

Low to moderate doses of marijuana produce euphoria, an increased sense of well-being, and altered perceptions of time, space, and sensation. While under the influence, subjects have problems with learning and memory, loss of coordination, difficulty thinking and solving problems—despite the subjective impression of the user that senses are augmented. Physiologic effects include an increase in heart rate, dry mouth, and reddening of the conjunctiva. Adverse reactions in the form of anxiety or panic attacks can occur. Although moderate doses of marijuana do not produce hallucinations, high doses can.

Tolerance develops to the physiologic and psychoactive effects of cannabinoids, and chronic users can develop a psychologic dependence. Long-term use can produce respiratory problems and is associated with a syndrome characterized by apathy and loss of motivation. Marijuana is stored in the fat cells of the body and released gradually; therefore, in heavy smokers such syndromes may be related to the presence and continuous slow release of the drug in the body. Withdrawal symptoms are mild and rarely require medical intervention.

Dissociative Anesthetics

Phencyclidine (PCP) and ketamine were developed as anesthetics, but the use of PCP caused agitation, delusions, and irrational thoughts and behaviors on emergence. Phencyclidine is a white powder that is snorted, smoked (often laced in marijuana), or eaten. Although abused for its ability to produce feelings of power and invulnerability, the drug can produce violent reactions. Subjects are often a danger to themselves and others and should not be left alone. At moderate doses, PCP produces an increase in heart rate and blood pressure, sweating, numbness of extremities, loss of motor coordination, and shallow respiration. In contrast, high doses decrease blood pressure, heart rate, and respiration and produce hallucinations. Higher doses cause blurred vision, loss of balance, dizziness, nausea, and vomiting,

TABLE 9-4

Types of Inhalants

Category	Active Chemical	Effects
Acrylic paint	Methylethyl ketone	Intoxicant
Adhesives	Hydrocarbons, aromatic hydrocarbons	Intoxicant
Aerosols	Fluorinated hydrocarbons, propane, isobutane, isopropanol, xylene, ethanol	Intoxicant
Amyl nitrite	Aliphatic nitrites	Intoxicant, enhanced orgasm
Anesthetics	Halothane, chloroform, ether	Intoxicant
Antifreeze	Ethyl glycol, methanol, isopropanol	Intoxicant
Butyl nitrite	Aliphatic nitrite	Intoxicant
Cement cleaners	Toluene and toluene mixtures	Intoxicant
Correction fluid	Trichloroethylene, trichloroethane, chloroform, methylchloroform, amyl acetate	Euphoriant, intoxicant
Degreasers	Isopropanol, benzene, ketones, N-butyl acetate, xylene, methylethyl ketone	Intoxicant
Dry cleaning solvents, spot removers	Trichloroethylene, trichloroethane petroleum distillates, perchloroethylene	Intoxicant
Fingernail polish remover	Acetone, alcohol, aliphatic acetates	Intoxicant
Fire extinguishers	Bromochlorodifluoromethane	Intoxicant
Foam dispensers	Nitrous oxide	Intoxicant, giddiness
Gasoline	Aliphatic and aromatic hydrocarbons	Intoxicant
Glue	Toluene, naphtha, petroleum distillates, acetone, polyvinyl chloride, benzene, hexane, heptanes	Intoxicant
Household cleaners	Chlorine, trichloroethane	Intoxicant
Lighter fluid	Butane, naphtha, aliphatic hydrocarbons	Intoxicant
Nitrous oxide	Nitrous oxide	Intoxicant, giddiness
Paint thinners, removers	Benzene, naphthalene	Intoxicant hallucinogen
Printing ink	Ketones	Intoxicant
Refrigerant	Freon	Intoxicant
Room deodorizers	Amyl nitrite, butyl nitrite, isobutyl nitrite	Orgasm enhancers, giddiness
Shoe polish, spray	Isopropanol	Intoxicant
Spray paint	Ketones	Euphoriant

and still higher, toxic amounts produce seizures, coma, and death. In a number of cases, subjects on PCP exhibit psychotic symptoms including delusions, paranoia, and catatonia. PCP-induced psychosis can be treated with antipsychotic medications (see Chapter 10). As with other hallucinogens, tolerance develops to the effects of PCP, and abuse can lead to psychologic dependence. Chronic use is also associated with memory loss, depression, and impaired mental abilities, which can persist for months after the drug is discontinued.

INHALANTS

There are a number of different types of inhalants that are abused for their intoxicating effects (Table 9-4). Inhalants include various types of solvents (e.g., glues, paint thinners, and gasoline), gases (nitrous oxide, ether, and propellants used in aerosol products), and various volatile nitrites (such as amyl nitrite). Inhalation of these substances produces rapid neurologic effects, and many of the inhalants are neurotoxic. In addition, inhalation allows little dose control. The substance is often kept in a plastic bag that is then placed over the face, and the vapors are inhaled, which creates a real potential for asphyxiation. Inhalant use is most common in children and adolescents who do not have ready access to alcohol and other intoxicating drugs. However, health care professionals such as dentists and anesthesia personnel may abuse nitrous oxide. These drugs are also quite toxic, and repeated use can severely damage the central nervous system, liver, kidneys, and bone marrow. As with previous classes of drugs, a summary of medical problems associated with inhalants is found in Box 9-5.

> **BOX 9-5**   **Medical Problems Associated with Inhalant Abuse**
>
> - Acute overdose: respiratory depression, death secondary to asphyxiation, which is secondary to route of administration
> - Severe toxicity to brain, liver, kidneys

APPLICATION TO PRACTICE

ASSESSMENT
History of Present Illness

Assessing for substance abuse or misuse should be done during the initial patient encounter, even though the patient may present a different problem to the health care provider. This approach is important so as to (1) avoid withdrawal symptoms, (2) identify underlying reasons for physical examination findings, (3) assist with appropriate drug or anesthetic choice for a patient, and (4) determine appropriate treatment and referral for the patient.

A factual drug history may be difficult to obtain when **polysubstance abuse** exists. Nonetheless, elicit information from the patient about the initial use of substances, the setting in which the substances are used, and how often. Inquire when the substances were last taken and the route of administration. Explore how the patient feels when the substance is used and what behavior changes occur. Ask about withdrawal symptoms and if the patient has had legal problems. Assume that the patient is a polysubstance abuser until convinced otherwise. Whenever possible, find an additional source of information to corroborate what the patient is saying. The patient often minimizes the amount of substances taken or may actually not know. A tool commonly used for screening of alcohol abuse is the **CAGE** (Box 9-6). This tool can be readily reworded for assessment of drug abuse. Other tools useful in assessing alcohol abuse include the Michigan Alcohol Screening Test (MAST) and the Alcohol Use Disorders Identification Test (AUDIT).

Health History

Has the patient been treated for substance abuse in the past? If so, where, when, for what, and how long? Was the treatment successful for a period of time? When was the last time an OTC drug was taken? For what conditions? Has the patient ever borrowed his or her spouse's or friend's drugs? Determine whether or not there is a family history of substance abuse.

> **BOX 9-6**   **Assessing Alcohol Abuse**
>
> Patients often deny alcohol abuse. CAGE is a series of four questions that can be easily inserted into any assessment. To help remember the questions, the first letter of a key word in each question is highlighted and spells CAGE. One "yes" response suggests possible alcohol abuse. More than one "yes" response makes it highly likely that a problem exists and indicates the need for a much deeper assessment, including a history of blackouts, legal problems involving alcohol, presence of alcohol-related diseases, and possibly other substance abuse. This tool can be readily reworded for drug abuse.
> "Have you felt you ought to **c**ut down on your drinking?"
> "Have people **a**nnoyed you by criticizing your drinking?"
> "Have you felt bad or **g**uilty about your drinking?"
> "Have you ever had a drink first thing in the morning to steady your nerves or get rid of a hangover?" (a so-called **e**ye-opener)

From Ewing JA: Detecting alcoholism: the CAGE questionaire, JAMA 252:1905, 1984. Copyright © 1984, The American Medical Association.

Be alert for conditions that suggest substance abuse, remembering that these conditions are only suggestive because they can be caused by factors other than substance abuse. Their presence does not prove substance abuse has occurred but may heighten suspicion of use.

Lifespan Considerations

The choice of substances appears to follow a progressive pattern. The pattern of abuse usually begins early with the individual abusing wine or beer and, in most cases, nicotine in the form of cigarettes. This practice is followed by marijuana use and finally use of other illegal drugs (e.g., cocaine). Initially, the period of substance abuse is short-term and without a defined pattern. During this experimental phase, the individual explores use of the substance, after which a decision is made to accept or reject continued use. During the recreational-social phase, the individual uses the substance in social contexts. A mood-altering experience is desired—no longer is experimentation the purpose for using the drug. Situational drug abuse follows, whereby the individual uses the drug to accomplish a specific task. In time, substance abuse becomes patterned, long-term, and intensive. Compulsive use ordinarily follows.

Perinatal. The effect of substance abuse on mothers and unborn infants has been studied intensely, although many questions remain unanswered. The fetus is exposed to virtually all substances the mother consumes. Which effects are the direct result of the substances themselves and which are related to indirect consequences such as the mother's general health, prenatal nutrition status, or her general lifestyle and living conditions are not known.

Pediatric. Substance abuse affects growth and development, contributes to school dropout rates and gang membership, can result in violence and death, and can be a catalyst for sexual promiscuity, teen pregnancy, and transmission of sexually transmitted diseases.

Preadolescent and adolescent males tend to abuse volatile substances and other inhalants. These, along with tobacco, marijuana, and alcohol may be associated with risky sexual behavior. Many substances break down inhibitions and increase desire so that the use of safe sex techniques and safe drug administration become secondary to immediate gratification.

Older Adults. Approximately 15% of community-based older adults are dependent on alcohol, but as many as 44% in inpatient medical and psychiatric facilities abuse alcohol. Individuals who have a dual diagnosis are more likely to become substance abusers than the rest of the population. A dual diagnosis is defined as a psychoactive substance use disorder and a coexisting psychologic disorder that require simultaneous treatment. Loneliness, depression, and isolation seen in many older adults who have not abused drugs in the past contribute to the potential for substance abuse.

Specific Populations at Risk. Health care providers over 40 years of age may abuse alcohol by itself, whereas providers younger than 40 years of age tend to use other drugs, either alone or in combination with alcohol. Common substances abused by health care providers include opioids, benzodiazepines, alcohol, and to-

bacco. However, the incidence is in line with that of the general population. Injectable drugs are more likely to be used by providers working in acute care settings. Pharmacists tend to abuse orally administered drugs, with central nervous system (CNS) stimulants being the most common. Nitrous oxide use by dentists is not uncommon. Anesthesiologists and nurse anesthetists may use fentanyl or its analogs.

For various reasons, Vietnam War veterans have had a much larger problem with substance abuse than Gulf War veterans or those of World War I, World War II, or the Korean War. Geographically, Vietnam neighbored the so-called Golden Triangle of opiate production and use; thus access to easily abused drugs was easy. Also, the Vietnam War was fought during a period when laws against these substances were not enforced as stringently as they are today. Alcohol remains the most commonly abused substance for veterans.

Individuals with chronic pain may not meet official diagnostic criteria for drug abuse or dependence, and as a consequence, the diagnosis of substance abuse is often overlooked. Few health care providers deny appropriate analgesia to patients with a terminal disease. However, they do not freely give analgesics to people they suspect are using a physical condition as an excuse to obtain drugs. Yet there is a large middle ground difficult for the health care provider to assess. These are individuals who have chronic headaches, back or neck pains, fibromyalgia, and so forth. On the one hand, pain relief is important and humane. On the other hand, the health care provider does not want to be an unwitting enabler to a potential drug abuse problem.

Cultural/Social Considerations

Whatever the basis for substance abuse, the effect on those who are abusers and those who depend on them is remarkable. When patients become substance dependent, they are held hostage by that substance, and rational thinking functions are subverted to focus on obtaining and using the drug. Commitments to other people or to responsibilities become secondary. Cognitively, the abuser develops impaired judgment, recall, and problem-solving abilities. Psychosocial manifestations include anger, denial, withdrawal, and loss of self-control. Feelings of anxiety, paranoia, depression, apathy, shame, and failure arise. The individual may experience a sense of powerlessness and destructiveness toward the self and his or her family. The patient may realize the need to stop and often feels guilty about the effect of abuse on family and self. People initially drink to feel good but then continue drinking to stop feeling bad.

Interpersonal relationships, particularly those with family, become impaired and disrupted. Communication, role performance, and sexual interactions become distorted. Family or friends may display behaviors consistent with codependence or coping strategies that contribute to the progression of illness. To protect the user, family and friends may act as if nothing is wrong or may terminate outside friendships and community activities. Children of dependent parents are often emotionally distant, perform poorly in school, and show withdrawal, anger, or aggressive behaviors.

Physical Examination

Physical manifestations of substance abuse depend on the type of substance, route of administration, frequency of use, and the individual's overall health status. The longer substance abuse persists, the more body systems become involved. Some substances promote impulsive or unprovoked and unpredictable violent behavior.

During the examination, observe the general appearance of the patient. Is he or she well kept? Observe hygiene and dress. Patients may have concealed drugs and weapons in body cavities as well as in clothing or other personal items. Be sure to note the patient's affect or the presence of confusion or agitation. Does the patient appear to be under- or overweight? Do you note any jaundice or skin discoloration? Does the patient have an unsteady gait? Is speech slurred? Inspect the skin for needle tracks or lesions over veins. Tracks or lesions are commonly found on the forearms, in the antecubital fossa, on the legs, or between the toes.

Examine the eyes and note if they are red or glassy. Note pupil size and reaction. Are the pupils dilated or constricted? Check the patient's nose and throat. Is the nose red and bulbous with broken blood vessels? This finding is often associated with excessive alcohol intake over a long period of time. Is the nasal mucosa edematous, reddened, or necrotic? Is the septum intact, or is there evidence of perforation? Swelling, necrosis, bleeding, or perforation are usually associated with cocaine snorting, or inhalation of the powder through a straw or rolled currency.

Assess for the presence of tachycardia and arrhythmia. Measure blood pressure carefully because long-term substance abuse contributes to the development of hypertension (see Case Study: Substance Abuse Masquerading as Hypertension). Observe for evidence of hyperventilation and cough and auscultate for abnormal breath sounds. Test deep tendon reflexes. The physical examination should also include palpation of the liver and spleen.

Laboratory Testing

The choice of laboratory tests depends on patient circumstances. For example, if inhalant use is suspected, tests that evaluate the respiratory tract are important. If the patient uses mind-altering drugs, tests of higher cortical functions may be warranted. If the patient shares needles, testing for hepatitis, HIV, and other sexually transmitted diseases may be warranted.

Gamma-glutamyl transferase (GGT) is the most common marker of alcohol use. It is often raised 75% to 80% above normal in alcoholics and heavy drinkers. The GGT correlates with the total amount of alcohol consumed, but the results should be interpreted cautiously because it takes weeks to reflect alcohol use. Furthermore, elevated GGT levels may be caused by liver disease, gallbladder disorders, liver cancer, and metastasis. Other liver function tests indicative of impaired functioning include alanine aminotransferase (ALT) and aspartate aminotransferase (AST), but they are nonspecific for alcohol. However, there is greater specificity for alcohol if the AST:ALT ratio is greater than 2. Obtaining levels of albumin and total proteins is also important for determining liver damage.

A complete blood cell (CBC) count, prothrombin time (PT), partial thromboplastin time (PTT), and blood chemistry tests evaluate the presence of blood dyscrasias as well as liver function. The mean corpuscular volume (MCV) is an important and reliable but nonspecific indicator of hematologic system damage. The MCV is elevated in many alcoholic patients but is slow to respond, so it is not a reliable indicator of abstinence and relapse.

Drug screens should be conducted on both blood and urine to determine what substances the patient has consumed and how much still remains in the body. In an acute care setting, drug screens should be conducted as soon as possible after admission. Many substances and their metabolites have very short half-lives and may be eliminated before they are detected. The health care provider cannot ensure the authenticity of the specimen unless the collection was witnessed. Here the patient's right to privacy must be weighed against the need to ensure authenticity of the specimen. Patients have done many things to foil the testing results, such as switching urine samples.

Sometimes a disparity is noted between the patient's clinical condition and the results of a drug screen. The patient appears to be under the influence of a substance or may even admit to being under its influence, but the laboratory results are inconclusive. The accuracy of test results depends not only on accurate specimen collection but also on the sophistication of the devices used to analyze it. Gas chromatography and mass spectrometry are often too expensive for smaller laboratories, but some of the metabolites are not easily detected without it.

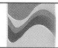

CASE STUDY   *Substance Abuse Masquerading as Hypertension*

ASSESSMENT

HISTORY OF PRESENT ILLNESS

CF is a 45-year-old white man returning for a follow-up visit for hypertension of 10 years' duration. Despite aggressive treatment, CF's blood pressure has been increasing during the past few months. He complains of heartburn, headaches, irritability, intermittent recent memory loss, and occasional night sweats. CF notes that he has been compliant with his drug therapy, follows a low-fat diet, and exercises regularly at the health club.

HEALTH HISTORY

CF has had two hospitalizations in the past 10 years for a broken right femur, a result of what he reported as skiing accidents. Later he admitted that these accidents occurred in the lodge after skiing when he lost his balance. He has a 5-year history of gastric ulcer, for which he takes ranitidine daily. His blood pressure has been treated with atenolol 50 mg bid and clonidine 0.2 mg qid prn. He admits to drinking "on occasion" to relax his nerves when his office work becomes too hectic. He has no known allergies. He is a 15 pack year smoker. CF has an adequate dietary intake.

LIFESPAN CONSIDERATIONS

CF is a successful stockbroker who works with a nationwide company. His history of a broken femur is not incompatible with his age and level of activity, but a repeat of the same accident is unusual.

CULTURAL/SOCIAL CONSIDERATIONS

CF has been married to the same woman for 20 years. They have three children—a son, 18, who is in college, and a daughter and son, 16 and 13, who live at home. He has recently become unpredictable, coming home late, missing meals and the children's school activities, which has in turn created problems at work and at home. As a result, he is spending more and more time away. He becomes angry easily, flying off the handle at his children. He also received a citation for driving under the influence. CF is the primary provider, but his wife teaches part-time at an elementary school while her children are in school. They have been fighting lately, and a separation is imminent. He admits to experimenting in the past with street drugs, specifically marijuana. He was charged twice during his "younger" years with illegal possession of cocaine. CF is upper-middle class in income. Although his salary is adequate for most of the family's needs, he worries about college expenses for his children. They do not qualify for public assistance programs.

PHYSICAL EXAMINATION

BP is 175/98. He is pleasant, cooperative, and articulate, although there is a slight odor of alcohol on his breath today. CAGE score 3. There are many spider telangiectasias over his nose and cheeks. His liver is enlarged and tender, but there are no masses.

LABORATORY TESTING

Upper GI series positive for healing ulcer. CBC, PT, and PTT results are all within normal limits. GGT elevated. AST:ALT ratio 2.5. BAC over 150 mmol/L, but no obvious signs of intoxication. MCV elevated. Albumin, total protein, calcium, magnesium, and phosphorus levels slightly depressed.

PATIENT PROBLEM(S)

Hypertension related to alcohol abuse.

GOALS OF THERAPY

Patient will acknowledge that alcohol is a problem and take positive steps to improve his situation.

CRITICAL THINKING QUESTIONS:

1. What are the criteria for diagnosing alcohol abuse?
2. Which psychosocial or developmental factors may have contributed to CF's alcohol abuse?
3. Which lab test results are suggestive of alcohol abuse?
4. Next to alcohol, which commonly abused substance has the highest abuse potential?
5. Describe the interrelationship between tolerance, dependence, and withdrawal.
6. Identify treatment modalities available for CF and his family.

GOALS OF THERAPY

The primary treatment goal for patients with a substance abuse problem is to stop the abuse and to correct the resulting health problems. The treatment goal for a patient with an overdose is primarily symptomatic and supportive, to maintain vital functions until the drug is biotransformed and eliminated from the body.

Treatment options vary, depending on the substance the patient is abusing, the extent of the dependence, the patient's incentive to stop the abuse, the depth of the commitment to stop, and the support structure available to the patient. Some patterns of substance abuse, such as weekly use of marijuana, do not require treatment any more than does occasional smoking of tobacco or the social use of alcohol. Furthermore, such patterns do not necessarily constitute a treatable disorder, though casual use is not without hazard. Changing views of substance abuse will continue to create gray areas where the justification for drug testing and the necessity for treatment are unclear.

INTERVENTION

Overall interventions for the substance abuser include maintenance of existing body system function along with adequate nutritional support. A multidisciplinary team approach assists the patient to make the necessary biologic and psychosocial adjustments to successfully eliminate the substance abuse habit.

It is important to know what substances the patient is withdrawing from to anticipate the characteristics of the withdrawal. During the acute phase of withdrawal, monitor the patient frequently for changes in vital functioning. Cardiovascular, respiratory, and neurologic functions along with mental status and behavior should be monitored regularly. Environmental stimuli should be reduced. Check laboratory reports, when available, for abnormal liver function tests, indications of anemia, and abnormal white blood cell or electrolyte counts. Hypocalcemia, hypomagnesemia, and acidosis are common in substance abusers. Drug and alcohol blood levels should be monitored.

Administration

Drug therapy for the substance-abusing patient is relatively controversial for several reasons. Specific antidotes are available only for benzodiazepines (i.e., flumazenil) and opioids (i.e., naloxone, naltrexone). There is a high risk of substituting one abused substance for another, and there are significant risks to giving CNS stimulants to reverse the effects of CNS depressants and vice versa. However, there are some clinical recommendations for drug therapy, including disulfiram as a deterrent for chronic alcohol abuse, methadone maintenance for opioid drug dependence, symptomatic treatment of acute drug toxicity or overdose, and treatment of withdrawal syndromes.

Benzodiazepines are the treatment of choice for many patients in need of assistance with substance abuse. It is a point of debate as to which benzodiazepine is most effective and yet carries the fewest adverse effects. Some are long-acting (diazepam, lorazepam, and clorazepate), and others are short-acting (oxazepam). The problem is that when the longer-acting drugs are used in a patient who has a compromised liver, the drug may remain in the system for extended periods and accumulate to excessive levels. Health care providers who prefer the longer-acting benzodiazepines assert that the effects remain in the system long enough to prevent breakthrough gaps in sedation. A positive effect of benzodiazepines is that they are known to cause an increased intake of food and water in the patient taking them. However, if benzodiazepines are used long-term and then stopped, they may produce symptoms of withdrawal.

Education

The patient bears the burden of stopping substance abuse. The patient who accepts responsibility for choices made and does not blame external situations for the abuse has a better chance of success. The likelihood for successful recovery after the acute withdrawal phase has passed is greater if the patient is willing to accept the discomfort of the emotional withdrawal from the substances without seeking or demanding immediate relief. The chance of success is also increased if the patient resists the temptation to think too soon that recovery has taken place. If the patient substitutes a comfortable support system for the previously abused substances, the chances for success are even greater.

Teach the patient about available substance abuse treatment programs and their rationales to help the patient decide on the type of treatment and the format that will be most helpful. Discuss the concept of substance abuse as a disease and the role of treatment and support groups. Self-help groups such as Alcoholics Anonymous (AA), Synanon, Alateen, Al-Anon, Narc-Anon, and others provide support and educate the public about the dangers of substance abuse. Behavioral approaches, marital and family counseling, and hypnosis have been tried with varying degrees of success. Educate family members and significant others so they can provide support and encourage the patient to continue treatment.

Because substance abuse is correlated with child abuse and neglect, it is important to educate parents not only about the effects of the substance abuse but also about successful parenting techniques. Parents can be encouraged to model appropriate behaviors by minimizing their own substance use and avoiding smoking. Children are more likely to abuse a substance if their parents have a permissive attitude about use or if either parent is a heavy drinker, smoker, or user of mind-altering drugs.

When disulfiram therapy is chosen, the patient needs to be taught about the physiologic effects of this drug and its restrictions. Teach the patient that various OTC substances (e.g., mouthwash, cough medicines, aerosol drugs used in the treatment of respiratory disorders, backrub lotions, aftershave lotions, and fermented vinegar and sauces) contain alcohol and will elicit adverse reactions.

EVALUATION

Evaluating the effectiveness of forms of treatment for substance abuse involves the patient's and family's responses to the treatment plans. The patient and family should be able to identify the signs and symptoms of withdrawal and their relationship to substance abuse, voice an understanding of how substance abuse is related to health care status, and plans for further treatment if warranted.

Some health care providers believe that treatment is successful when the patient is clean and sober. This means that the patient abstains from illegal drug use and alcohol completely. It also means that the patient uses prescription drugs according to directions and for the condition for which they were prescribed.

Bibliography

Coombs RH: Addicted health professionals, *J Subst Misuse Nurs Health Soc Care* 1(4):187-194, 1996.

D'Apolito K: Substance abuse: infant and childhood outcomes, *J Pediatr Nurs* 13:307-316, 1998.

Gawin FH, Ellinwood EH Jr: Cocaine and other stimulants: actions, abuse and treatment, *N Engl J Med* 318:1173, 1988.

Haack MR: Treating acute withdrawal from alcohol and other drugs, *Nurs Clin North Am* 33:75-92, 1998.

Kinney J: *Clinical manual of substance abuse*, ed 2, St Louis, 1996, Mosby.

Kowalski SD: Self-esteem and self-efficacy as predictors of success in smoking cessation, *J Holistic Nurs* 15(2):128-142, 1997.

Simmons DH: Caffeine and its effect on persons with mental disorders, *Arch Psychiatr Nurs* 10(2):116-122, 1996.

Smith DE, Seymour RB: Cannabis and cannabis withdrawal, *J Subst Misuse Nurs Health Soc Care* 2(1):49-53, 1997.

Tran JH: Treatment of neonatal abstinence syndrome, *J Pediatr Health Care* 13:295-300, 1999.

Wewers ME, Ahijevych KL: Smoking cessation interventions in chronic illness, *Ann Rev Nurs Res* 14:75-93, 1996.

Internet Resource

NIDA Website. Available online: http://www.nida.nih.gov/DrugsofAbuse.html.

CHAPTER

10

Introduction to Autonomic Nervous System Pharmacology

JOSEPH A. DiMICCO • KATHLEEN GUTIERREZ

 Visit http://evolve.elsevier.com/Gutierrez/ for additional information.

KEY TERMS

Acetylcholine, p. 130

Acetylcholinesterase, p. 133

Adrenergic, p. 130

Afferent neurons, p. 130

Alpha-adrenergic receptors, p. 136

Alpha blockers, p. 137

Antiadrenergic, p. 137

Anticholinergic, p. 137

Autonomic nervous system, p. 130

Beta-adrenergic receptors, p. 136

Beta blockers, p. 137

Catechol-O-methyltransferase (COMT), p. 136

Central nervous system, p. 130

Cholinergic, p. 130

Cholinomimetic, p. 137

Dopamine, p. 135

Efferent neurons, p. 130

Epinephrine, p. 133

"Fight or flight," p. 131

Isoproterenol, p. 136

Ligand-gated ion channel, p. 135

Monoamine oxidase (MAO), p. 136

Muscarine p. 133

Muscarinic receptors, p. 133

Neuroeffector junction, p. 130

Neuromuscular junction, p. 130

Neurotransmitters, p. 130

Nicotine, p. 135

Nicotinic ganglionic receptors, p. 133

Nicotinic neuromuscular receptors, p. 133

Norepinephrine, p. 130

Parasympathetic nervous system, p. 131

Peripheral nervous system, p. 130

Reuptake, p. 136

Somatic motor nervous system, p. 130

Sympathetic nervous system, p. 131

Sympathomimetic, p. 137

Synapse, p. 130

OBJECTIVES

- Differentiate between the somatic motor nervous system and the autonomic nervous system.
- Describe the divisions of the autonomic nervous system: sympathetic and parasympathetic.
- Distinguish among acetylcholine, norepinephrine, and epinephrine, and describe where and how each is used in the peripheral nervous system.
- Differentiate between muscarinic and nicotinic receptors and describe their locations in the peripheral nervous system.
- List the effects of sympathetic (adrenergic) stimulation and parasympathetic (cholinergic or muscarinic) stimulation on major tissues and organs and the specific receptors involved.
- Describe the "fight-or-flight" response.

Drugs that influence the autonomic nervous system play important roles in the treatment of many clinical disorders. Some of these drugs are specifically designed and used to alter the function of part of the nervous system, whereas others alter functions of the nervous system as an adverse effect. For this reason, a clear understanding of the basic physiology of the autonomic nervous system is key to understanding why and how these drugs produce their effects. Therefore this chapter presents a review of the anatomy and physiology of the peripheral nervous system, which includes the autonomic nervous system and the somatic motor nerves that innervate skeletal muscle. Chapter 11 provides an overview of **cholinergic** drugs that interact with mechanisms or receptors where the principal neurotransmitter is acetylcholine. Chapter 12 reviews drugs that interact with the sympathetic nervous system, often called **adrenergic** drugs. Many of these same drugs will be encountered again in later chapters in this book.

OVERVIEW OF THE AUTONOMIC NERVOUS SYSTEM

The nervous system is divided into the central nervous system and the peripheral nervous system. The **central nervous system** includes the brain and spinal cord. The central nervous system has three functions: (1) to monitor, convey, and process information from sensory receptors and systems; (2) to integrate this information in the context of hard-wired circuits and past or learned experience; and (3) to convey appropriate signals that initiate or modify actions or processes of the body.

The **peripheral nervous system** consists of afferent and efferent neurons. **Afferent neurons,** also called sensory nerves, transmit information from the entire body back to the central nervous system for processing. **Efferent neurons** relay signals from the central nervous system to the rest of the body and through these signals initiate and coordinate the body's responses. The efferent peripheral nervous system, the subject of this chapter, is further subdivided into the **somatic motor nervous system** and the **autonomic nervous system.**

Neurotransmitters and Receptors

All neurons use chemicals as messengers to contact neurons and other cells. These chemicals, called **neurotransmitters,** are synthesized in the nerve cell and stored in the nerve ending inside tiny membrane-bound structures called vesicles. When the neuron is stimulated, some of these vesicles merge with the nerve terminal membrane—a process called *exocytosis*—resulting in the release of the stored neurotransmitter. Transmitter molecules then diffuse across the space between the neuron and the cell with which it communicates. The space between two neurons is called the **synapse,** or the synaptic cleft; however, if the neuron is signaling any other cell type, the space is called the **neuroeffector junction.** The transmitter molecules then bind to specific receptors on the cell surface. The function of the receptor is to recognize a specific neurotransmitter and produce a response to that substance. The binding of the neurotransmitter to its receptor is reversible. When the neurotransmitter diffuses away from the receptor, the response is terminated.

Two neurotransmitters, **acetylcholine** and **norepinephrine,** are the principal neurotransmitters used by the peripheral nervous system. A given class of neurons will use only one of these neurotransmitters. The main features of the peripheral nervous system and its neurotransmitters are reviewed here in preparation for discussing drugs that act by modifying the actions of these neurotransmitters in the peripheral nervous system. The somatic motor nervous system is discussed first, then the more complex autonomic nervous system will be considered at length.

Somatic Motor Nervous System

The somatic motor nervous system can cause skeletal muscle contraction by both conscious and unconscious control (Figure 10-1). A motor neuron has a cell body in the spinal cord that sends one long nerve fiber to a specialized region of a striated muscle called the **neuromuscular junction.** Fibers from these motor neurons are found in several cranial nerves and in all spinal nerves. Stimulation of a motor neuron results in the release of acetylcholine at the neuromuscular junction, and the muscle cell reacts to acetylcholine by contracting. Stimulation of a motor neuron may arise either as a result of a willed impulse originating in the brain and transmitted to the appropriate neuron in the spinal cord or unconsciously as a spinal reflex. A spinal reflex is initiated by sensory input (i.e., heat, touch, pressure, or pain) that is transmitted to the spinal cord and then out to the motor neurons without being processed by the brain.

Autonomic Nervous System

The autonomic nervous system acts primarily below the level of consciousness to regulate internal body functions necessary for life. These vital functions include cardiac output, blood volume, blood composition, blood pressure, and digestive processes. The autonomic nervous system exerts control over all these functions by modifying the tone of smooth muscle and the quantity of glandular secretions in various tissues and organs (see Figure 10-1). Autonomic tone refers to the minimal but constant release of the autonomic neurotransmitters that occurs under normal conditions in most tissues.

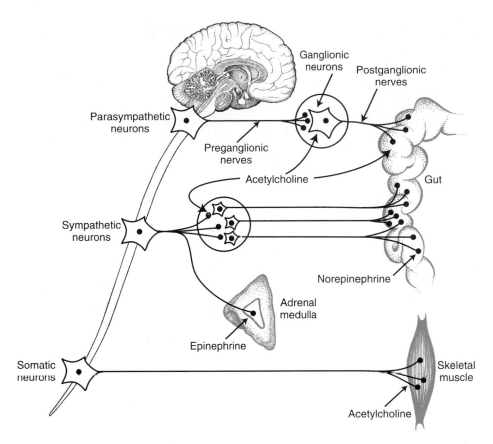

FIGURE 10-1 Neurotransmitters of autonomic nervous system. Acetylcholine and nor-epinephrine are released from neurons as indicated to act on adjacent cells. Note that only the gut is shown as representative of many different tissues and organs innervated by the autonomic nervous system (see Table 10-1). Epinephrine is released from the adrenal medulla into the bloodstream to act throughout the body. The parasympathetic pregan-glionic neurons originate mainly in the brainstem with axons in cranial nerves II, VII, IX, X, and XI, although a few neurons originate in the lower spinal cord with axons in sacral nerves II, III, and IV. The sympathetic preganglionic neurons originate in the thoracic and lumbar parts of the spinal cord. Somatic (motor) neurons arise from all parts of the spinal cord.

The autonomic nervous system has two distinct efferent divisions: the parasympathetic nervous system and the sympathetic nervous system. The effects of these two branches on different body systems are summarized in Table 10-1. Generally, one branch of the autonomic nervous system is dominant in a given tissue. For example, the sympathetic nervous system provides the dominant tone for the blood vessels; therefore blood pressure predominantly reflects the degree of sympathetic tone, which is itself determined and coordinated by the central nervous system (see Chapter 12). The parasympathetic effect on the cardiovascular system is primarily that of a reflex "brake" on the function of the heart to protect against rapid or extreme rises in blood pressure. In contrast, the parasympathetic nervous system provides the dominant tone responsible for coordinating visual, digestive, and excretory functions. Here, the sympathetic nervous system functions as an override mechanism to depress these functions in times of stress or emergency. Once again, certain centers in the brain regulate parasympathetic nerve activity to determine the intensity of these responses.

A general distinction can be made between the functions of the parasympathetic and the sympathetic nervous systems. The parasympathetic nervous system has dominant control over regulatory processes of the body that take place under resting or basal conditions, whereas the sympathetic nervous system provides immediate adaptation for an emergency, or "fight-or-flight." Indeed, the

TABLE 10-1

Autonomic Nervous System Actions

Tissue or Organ Affected	Parasympathetic Nervous System		Sympathetic Nervous System	
	Response	Receptor	Response	Receptor
Eyes	Pupillary constriction (miosis)	Muscarinic	Pupillary dilation (mydriasis)	Alpha$_1$
	Focusing of lens (accommodation)	Muscarinic		
Glands	Increased salivation	Muscarinic	Increased sweating*	Muscarinic*
	Increased lacrimation	Muscarinic		
	Increased secretions in airways and GI tract	Muscarinic		
Heart	Decreased rate (negative chronotropy)	Muscarinic	Increased rate (positive chronotropy)	Beta$_1$
	Slowed conduction through A-V node (negative dromotropy)	Muscarinic	Enhanced conduction through A-V node (positive dromotropy)	Beta$_1$
	Decreased strength of contraction (negative inotropy)	Muscarinic	Increased strength of contraction (positive inotropy)	Beta$_1$
Bronchioles	Constriction	Muscarinic	Relaxation (dilation)	Beta$_2$
Blood vessels			Constriction in skin, viscera, erectile tissue, kidney	Alpha$_1$
			Dilation in heart and skeletal muscle	Beta$_2$
			Dilation in kidney	DA, beta$_2$
GI smooth muscle	Contraction	Muscarinic	Relaxation	Alpha$_2$, beta$_1$, beta$_2$
GI sphincters	Relaxation	Muscarinic	Contraction	Alpha$_2$, beta$_1$, beta$_2$
Fundus of urinary bladder	Contraction	Muscarinic	Relaxation	Beta$_2$
Trigone and sphincter of urinary bladder	Relaxation	Muscarinic	Contraction	Alpha$_1$
Uterus			Contraction	Alpha$_1$
			Relaxation	Beta$_2$
Liver			Glycogenolysis and gluconeogenesis	Alpha$_1$, beta$_2$
Fat cells			Lipolysis	Beta$_3$

A-V, Atrioventricular; *DA,* dopamine; *GI,* gastrointestinal.
*Acetylcholine is the neurotransmitter responsible for this sympathetic response. This is an exception to the rule that norepinephrine is the postganglionic neurotransmitter at all sympathetic postganglionic nerve endings.

easiest way to remember the actions of the sympathetic nervous system (and by contrast the parasympathetic nervous system) is to review the fight-or-flight response: the pupils of the eyes dilate so that vision is improved even in dim light; the bronchioles dilate to let air flow to and from the lungs more readily; the heart beats faster and with greater strength to supply blood to the muscles; the visceral blood vessels are constricted, but blood vessels in muscles are dilated so that the increased blood flow can meet the demands of cardiac and skeletal muscle for oxygen and nutrients; digestive and excretory processes are slowed; and the liver breaks down stored glycogen to provide glucose for fuel. All these responses represent actions of the sympathetic nervous system, and in many cases, the parasympathetic nervous system produces effects that are opposite to these. In the heart, for example, whereas activating sympathetic nerves increases the heart rate, stimulating the parasympathetic innervation slows it. This dual antagonistic innervation is a hallmark of the autonomic nervous system; it allows a broad range of control of organ function according to body requirements. This antagonism is a result of two distinct kinds of receptors, adrenergic and cholinergic, coexisting on the same organ. Often, activation of the cholinergic receptor produces the opposite response from activation of the adrenergic receptor. Cholinergic and adrenergic receptors are discussed in detail below.

Preganglionic and Postganglionic Autonomic Nerve Fibers

For both parasympathetic and sympathetic nerves, the pathway from the central nervous system to the innervated tissue consists of two neurons. The cell body of the first neuron is located in the central nervous system and sends a projection out to interact with a second neuron. These second neurons are usually located in clusters in a specialized nervous structure called a *ganglion* (see Figure 10-1). Therefore the first neurons in this central nervous system pathway are called *preganglionic neurons,* and their projections to the secondary neurons found in the periphery are called *preganglionic fibers.* The neurotransmitter used at the synapse of preganglionic fibers in all autonomic ganglia—whether they are sympathetic or parasympathetic—is acetylcholine. The second (or ganglionic) neuron sends a fiber to innervate an internal organ or tissue, usually modifying the action of a gland or of involuntary muscle such as smooth muscle or cardiac muscle. Since this fiber makes up the pathway following the ganglion, it is termed a *postganglionic fiber.*

Preganglionic neurons of the two systems are found in different areas of the central nervous system. Most of the efferent neurons of the parasympathetic nervous system are found in the lower area of the brain, or brainstem. These parasympathetic cell bodies include centers in the medulla, pons, and midbrain that influence vision, cardiac and gastrointestinal (GI) processes, the smooth muscle of the airways, and glands of the head and neck. The remaining preganglionic neurons of the parasympathetic nervous system are located in the sacral portion of the spinal cord and allow parasympathetic control of digestive, excretory, and reproductive processes. In contrast, the preganglionic neurons of the sympathetic nervous system are found in the middle (thoracic and lumbar) regions of the spinal cord.

Roles of Neurotransmitters

The most important pharmacologic difference between the parasympathetic and the sympathetic nervous systems is that the final transmitter released by postganglionic fibers at innervated tissues is different for the two divisions. At the synapses within the ganglia, the preganglionic neurotransmitter is acetylcholine for both divisions. Acetylcholine is also the neurotransmitter used by all of the postganglionic fibers in the parasympathetic nervous system. Therefore the parasympathetic nervous system is sometimes called the cholinergic nervous system. In contrast, the vast majority of sympathetic postganglionic fibers release norepinephrine as their neurotransmitter. **Epinephrine,** which is closely related to norepinephrine, has a special role in the sympathetic nervous system that will be discussed later in this chapter.

Acetylcholine

Acetylcholine is synthesized in the nerve terminal by the enzyme choline acetyl transferase from choline and an acetate molecule activated by coenzyme A (Figure 10-2). This acetylcholine is packaged in vesicles. When the neuron is stimulated, some of the vesicles release their contents—including acetylcholine—into the synapse. There the acetylcholine diffuses to the opposing membrane and binds at the specific receptors that recognize its molecular structure. However, the opposing membrane also contains the enzyme **acetylcholinesterase,** which breaks down acetylcholine to inactive products, acetate and choline. Acetylcholinesterase is very active, so that most of the acetylcholine released is destroyed in a few milliseconds. Any remaining acetylcholine that diffuses from the synapse is almost instantly degraded by nonspecific cholinesterases in the blood or tissues. Thus, when released, acetylcholine produces a response in the next cell by way of acetylcholine (or cholinergic) receptors and is rapidly inactivated. Because the rapid breakdown of acetylcholine plays such an important role in normal cholinergic transmission, drugs that inhibit cholinesterase activity can have dramatic effects at sites where acetylcholine is used as a neurotransmitter (see Chapter 11).

Cholinergic Receptors. Wherever acetylcholine functions as a neurotransmitter, it produces its effect by interacting with cholinergic receptors. As we will see in Chapter 11, important cholinergic drugs are useful because they act selectively at one of three basic subtypes of cholinergic receptors: **muscarinic receptors, nicotinic ganglionic receptors,** and **nicotinic neuromuscular receptors.**

Muscarinic Receptors. Chemical differentiation of receptors for acetylcholine was first made with **muscarine,** a chemical found in certain mushrooms. Muscarine mimics acetylcholine only at those cholinergic receptors on tissues innervated by postganglionic cholinergic neurons of the autonomic nervous system. In fact, the

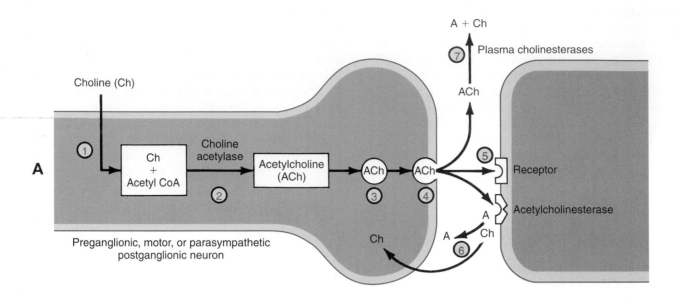

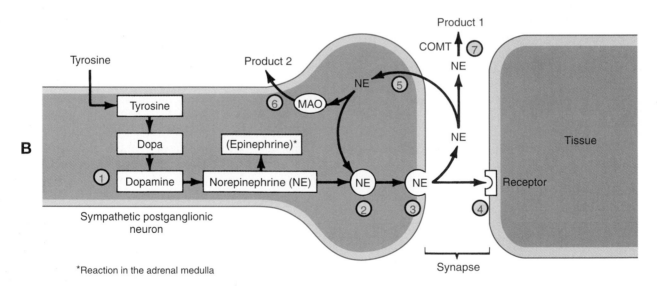

*Reaction in the adrenal medulla

FIGURE 10-2   Synthesis, release, and termination of principal neurotransmitters of the peripheral nervous system. **A,** Acetylcholine. *(1)* Choline is taken up by the neuron and *(2)* used to synthesize acetylcholine, which *(3)* is stored in vesicles. On stimulation of the neuron *(4),* some vesicles merge with membrane to discharge acetylcholine into the synapse or neuroeffector junction, where acetylcholine diffuses to *(5)* its receptor to activate the cell, or *(6)* is broken down by acetylcholinesterase, an enzyme that degrades acetylcholine. Plasma cholinesterases *(7)* can also degrade acetylcholine. **B,** Norepinephrine. *(1)* Tyrosine is taken into the neuron and converted first to dopamine and then to norepinephrine, which is *(2)* stored in vesicles. On stimulation of the neuron *(3),* some vesicles merge with the membrane to discharge norepinephrine into the synapse or neuroeffector junction, where it diffuses to *(4)* its receptor to produce some effect in the cell. Most of the norepinephrine is *(5)* taken up by the neuron through a membrane transporter and reused, but some norepinephrine is degraded by *(6)* the mitochondrial enzyme monoamine oxidase (MAO) or *(7)* the enzyme catechol-O-methyltransferase (COMT) found in most body tissues.

effects of fast mushroom poisoning, appearing within an hour or so of ingestion, result from muscarine stimulating these receptors. The symptoms therefore resemble generalized parasympathetic overstimulation and include glandular stimulation (sweating, tearing, salivation), an overactive GI system (nausea, vomiting, cramps, diarrhea), cardiovascular symptoms (flushed skin, slow heart rate), and excessive urination (see Table 10-1). Based on their susceptibility to stimulation by muscarine, the cholinergic receptors that mediate these effects are called **muscarinic receptors.** Muscarine produces no effect when applied to skeletal muscles or to ganglia. Note that muscarinic cholinergic receptors are also found in the brain, but because muscarine does not effectively penetrate the blood-brain barrier, stimulation of these receptors does not occur when muscarine is ingested. As a cholinergic agonist, muscarine is only useful as a laboratory tool.

Five subtypes of muscarinic receptors (M1 to M5) have been identified, and all are coupled to regulatory membrane proteins called G proteins. Although the specific subtype of muscarinic receptor mediating the effect of acetylcholine at different sites is known in many cases, clinically useful drugs that act through muscarinic receptors (see Chapter 11) do not distinguish among the different subtypes to any practical degree.

Nicotinic Receptors. **Nicotine,** a naturally occurring toxin found in tobacco, is not an effective agonist at muscarinic cholinergic receptors, but instead acts at those cholinergic receptors that are not stimulated by muscarine. Thus nicotine mimics the effects of acetylcholine at the skeletal muscle and ganglionic receptors in the peripheral nervous system and acts at certain acetylcholine receptors in the CNS. Therefore these receptors are called nicotinic receptors.

The molecular biology and function of nicotinic receptors differs from that of the muscarinic receptors. Nicotinic receptors are actually complexes made up of five protein subunits. When acetylcholine (or nicotine) binds to the receptor, the conformation of this complex changes to form an open pore through which sodium and potassium ions can move freely across the membrane. Such a receptor is called a **ligand-gated ion channel,** because binding of the ligand—in this case acetylcholine—to its recognition site on the receptor operates a sort of gate that permits the movement of ions. The subunits that make up a given nicotinic receptor determine various aspects of its function, including its pharmacology. Nicotinic receptors found on autonomic ganglia and at the neuromuscular junction are different, and therefore clinically useful drugs can distinguish between them. Thus drugs that selectively block ganglionic nicotinic receptors (called ganglionic blockers) can be used to shut off the entire autonomic nervous system without causing neuromuscular paralysis (see Chapter 11). On the other hand, drugs that act selectively at nicotinic neuromuscular receptors (or neuromuscular blockers) can be used to paralyze patients where movement must be avoided (for example, during surgery; see Chapter 16) without significantly impairing the autonomic nervous system.

Norepinephrine and Epinephrine

The vast majority of postganglionic fibers in the sympathetic nervous system use norepinephrine as the neurotransmitter. Norepinephrine is synthesized in the nerve terminal from the amino acid tyrosine (see Figure 10-2). Note that **dopamine,** the chemical precursor of norepinephrine, functions as a neurotransmitter itself in some neurons, primarily in the central nervous system. Dopamine and norepinephrine belong to a class of compounds called *catecholamines.*

Norepinephrine released from sympathetic nerves acts directly on an adjacent cell. However, the sympathetic nervous system includes a somewhat different component called the adrenal medulla. The cells in the adrenal medulla are similar to other sympathetic ganglionic neurons because they are innervated by a preganglionic fiber and on stimulation release their chemical messenger. However, they differ from other postganglionic neurons in the following two important ways:

1. Adrenal medullary postganglionic neurons do not send projections to a specific target tissue where a neurotransmitter is released to produce a specific and localized effect. Instead, these specialized quasi-neurons (called adrenal chromaffin cells) release their chemical messenger into the bloodstream where it can produce effects on a wide variety of tissues all over the body. Such a chemical messenger released from neurons into the bloodstream to act at distant sites is called a *neurohormone.*

2. These adrenal chromaffin cells synthesize norepinephrine like other sympathetic ganglionic neurons, but most of the norepinephrine made (80% to 85%) is biotransformed to epinephrine, another catecholamine. Thus the neurohormone released by the adrenal medulla under conditions of stress is primarily epinephrine (along with small amounts of norepinephrine). Epinephrine carried by the blood not only activates tissue receptors that respond to norepinephrine, but also stimulates other receptors more specific for epinephrine itself.

Unlike acetylcholine, most norepinephrine is not degraded after release. Instead, it is taken back up into the neuron from which it was released and stored again in granules. The process responsible for transporting norepinephrine back into the sympathetic terminal is called **reuptake.** Any norepinephrine that diffuses away from the synapse (or neuroeffector junction) or epinephrine in the blood is quickly degraded. Two enzymes can metabolize and thus inactivate norepinephrine and epinephrine. **Monoamine oxidase (MAO)** is located in the mitochondria of most cells, including nerve terminals that release norepinephrine. **Catechol-O-methyltransferase (COMT)** is found in the cytoplasm of most cells. Both MAO and COMT are found in large concentrations in the liver and kidney. No drugs that interfere with COMT are used clinically, but in later chapters we shall see that drugs that inhibit MAO are used for treating depression and Parkinson's disease.

The sympathetic nerves and adrenal medulla often work together and are sometimes called the sympathoadrenal system. Adrenergic pharmacology refers to drugs that act on receptors or mechanisms related to norepinephrine and epinephrine. The term *adrenergic* comes from *adrenaline,* the British term for epinephrine (norepinephrine is sometimes called noradrenaline). The sympathetic nervous system is sometimes called the adrenergic nervous system because of the dominant role of epinephrine and norepinephrine as the chemical messengers released by almost all sympathetic ganglionic neurons. However, there are two important exceptions to this general rule. First, sympathetic nerves found in sweat glands release acetylcholine as their postganglionic transmitter, making them cholinergic. Second, some of the sympathetic postganglionic fibers that innervate blood vessels in the kidney release dopamine. Norepinephrine released from most sympathetic nerves in blood vessels throughout the body acts at receptors to cause constriction of blood vessels. However, dopamine released from these special nerve endings acts on dopamine receptors to relax or dilate the blood vessels. The identity of the neurotransmitter at the various sites of the peripheral nervous system is diagrammed in Figure 10-1.

Adrenergic Receptors. As discussed above, norepinephrine and epinephrine exert their effects on tissues influenced by the sympathoadrenal system by acting at adrenergic receptors. The existence of two classes of adrenergic receptors was proposed in the late 1940s to explain the different physiologic effects elicited by norepinephrine, epinephrine, and a synthetic catecholamine called **isoproterenol. Alpha-adrenergic receptors,** or simply alpha receptors, are stimulated about equally by both norepinephrine and epinephrine, whereas isoproterenol is practically ineffective. **Beta-adrenergic receptors,** or beta receptors, are those receptors for which isoproterenol is more potent than or as potent as epinephrine or norepinephrine. Molecular cloning has shown that all adrenergic receptors are closely related proteins. There are two major subtypes of alpha receptors: $alpha_1$ and $alpha_2$ receptors, and three subtypes of beta receptors: $beta_1$, $beta_2$, and $beta_3$ receptors. Because only the $beta_1$ and $beta_2$ subtypes of beta receptors are therapeutic targets for clinically important drugs, only these receptors will be discussed further in this chapter.

Alpha- and beta-adrenergic receptors are all G protein–coupled receptors but are linked in different ways to second messenger systems in the cells. Beta receptors are positively coupled to adenylate cyclase. Thus occupation of beta receptors leads to activation of the enzyme, resulting in an increased level of cyclic adenosine monophosphate (cAMP) in the cell. In different tissues, this increase may result in different responses. $Alpha_2$ receptors are also linked to adenylate cyclase, but stimulation of $alpha_2$ receptors results in inhibition of the enzyme. Therefore, in many tissues the stimulation of beta receptors ($beta_1$ and $beta_2$) and the stimulation of $alpha_2$ receptors have opposite effects. Activation of $alpha_1$ receptors produces effects through a different second messenger. This activation also initiates interaction with a G protein called *Gq,* but the result is activation of mechanisms that elevate intracellular calcium. The increased concentration of calcium changes the activity of certain enzymes. The changes in enzymatic activities account for the actions produced by the activation of the $alpha_1$ receptor. A detailed overview of drugs acting at adrenergic receptors appears in Chapter 12.

Roles of Other Autonomic Neurotransmitters

An expanded view of the autonomic nervous system is evolving. First, the concept that a neuron makes only one kind of neurotransmitter has proven incorrect. Current evidence indicates that in addition to norepinephrine and acetylcholine, other chemical messengers, such as peptides, eicosanoids, or purines may be co-released from autonomic nerves. These messengers modulate the response to the neurotransmitter. For instance, vasoactive intestinal peptide (VIP) appears to be co-released with acetylcholine from parasympathetic fibers that innervate blood vessels and exocrine glands. In this case, VIP enhances the action of acetylcholine to cause vasodilation or secretion. A second evolving concept is that nonadrenergic, noncholinergic neurons control smooth muscle activity in many tissues. Purinergic nerves using adenosine triphosphate (ATP) as the neurotransmitter appear in the GI tract, the genitourinary tract, and some blood vessels. Endothelial cells of blood vessels act as modulators of autonomic and hormonal messengers. In particular, these cells release nitric oxide, which has emerged as the important agent causing vasodilation of vascular smooth muscle. In fact, sildenafil (Viagra) facilitates erection of the penis by enhancing this effect of nitric oxide. Thus emerging knowledge about these alternative modes of chemical signaling in the autonomic nervous system has already begun to make an impact on drug therapy.

CONFUSING TERMINOLOGY OF DRUGS ACTING THROUGH THE AUTONOMIC NERVOUS SYSTEM

Autonomic drugs act on mechanisms that involve either acetylcholine (cholinergic drugs) or the catecholamines norepinephrine or epinephrine (adrenergic drugs). The terminology used in connection with these drugs can sometimes be confusing, because different terms may be used to describe the same type of drug, or the same term may have more than one meaning.

Drugs that stimulate cholinergic receptors or enhance the action of acetylcholine are often referred to simply as cholinergic or occasionally **cholinomimetic** because they mimic the effect of acetylcholine. Drugs that interfere with cholinergic transmission in some way are called **anticholinergic,** or cholinergic blockers. As discussed in Chapter 11, the term anticholinergic is often used to describe drugs that interfere specifically with the muscarinic subtype of cholinergic receptors. Because acetylcholine is the dominant neurotransmitter in the parasympathetic nervous system, drugs that act directly or indirectly to cause increased stimulation of muscarinic cholinergic receptors are sometimes called parasympathomimetic, and drugs that block these receptors are termed parasympatholytic. All these types of drugs are discussed in Chapter 11.

Drugs that stimulate adrenergic receptors or enhance the action of norepinephrine or epinephrine are sometimes referred to as adrenergic or **sympathomimetic** because they mimic the effects of sympathetic nervous system activity. Drugs that interfere with transmission at sites where these catecholamines act are called **antiadrenergic,** or adrenergic blockers.

Drugs that antagonize specific subtypes of adrenergic receptors are commonly named for the receptor at which they act. Thus, alpha receptor blockers, often called simply **alpha blockers,** are antagonists at alpha-adrenergic receptors, and beta receptor blockers, or more commonly **beta blockers,** are antagonists at beta-adrenergic receptors. Adrenergic drugs are discussed in Chapter 12.

Bibliography

Blows W: Systems and diseases. Exploring normal anatomy and physiology, Nervous system 7, *Nurs Times* 97(10):41-44, 2001.

Internet Resources

National Dysautonomia Research Foundation. Available online: http://www.ndrf.org/ans.htm.

University of Washington: Autonomic Receptors. Available on-line: http://courses.washington.edu/chat543/cvans/ansrec.htm.

Parasympathetic Nervous System Drugs

JOSEPH A. DiMICCO • KATHLEEN GUTIERREZ

 Visit **http://evolve.elsevier.com/Gutierrez/** for additional information.

KEY TERMS

Asthma, p. 140

Cholinomimetics, p. 141

Cycloplegia, p. 143

Glaucoma, p. 140

Heart block, p. 140

Incontinence, p. 140

Irreversible cholinesterase inhibitors, p. 147

Miosis, p. 142

Myasthenia gravis, p. 145

Mydriasis, p. 143

Neuromuscular blockers, p. 145

Reversible cholinesterase inhibitors, p. 147

Sinus bradycardia, p. 140

Urinary retention, p. 140

Xerostomia, p. 142

OBJECTIVES

● Explain the difference between direct- and indirect-acting cholinomimetic drugs.

● Explain the difference between reversible and irreversible acetylcholinesterase inhibitors.

● List three therapeutic uses of cholinomimetic drugs.

● Identify and describe three kinds of cholinergic antagonists.

● Identify six therapeutic uses of muscarinic receptor antagonists (such as atropine).

● Describe six adverse effects that might be expected in a patient treated with a systemic cholinesterase inhibitor.

● Develop a nursing care plan for the patient receiving a parasympathetic nervous system drug.

Most cholinergic drugs achieve their effects through stimulation and inhibition of muscarinic cholinergic receptors. In fact, the term cholinergic is sometimes loosely used to describe effects that are mediated specifically through muscarinic receptors. In this regard, the organs and systems most prominently affected include glands, the eye, the gastrointestinal system, and smooth muscle. As discussed in Chapter 10, muscarinic cholinergic activity in the peripheral nervous system plays numerous important physiologic roles.

EYE

Acetylcholine released from parasympathetic nerve endings plays an important role in regulating the amount of light entering the eye by constricting the pupil. Through changes in parasympathetic activity, the pupil closes in bright light and opens wide in dim light or darkness. Acetylcholine acting at muscarinic receptors is also responsible for focusing the lens for near vision. Cholinergic stimulation in the eye has a beneficial effect in the treatment of **glaucoma,** a condition in which intraocular fluid secreted inside the eye is made at a rate faster than the normal drainage systems can handle. The result is an increase in intraocular pressure that can permanently damage the eye and cause blindness. Constriction of the pupil and contraction of the ciliary muscle make drainage of intraocular fluid easier and so reduce intraocular pressure (see Chapter 65).

EXOCRINE GLANDS

Cholinergic activity stimulates the secretory activity of exocrine glands to keep mucous membranes moist and lubricated, particularly in the upper airways, gastrointestinal tract, eyes (tear glands), and mouth (including salivary glands). Sweating is an important means of losing excessive body heat, especially in children, and is also caused by cholinergic activation of sweat glands (although recall from Chapter 10 that this is actually a sympathetic pathway).

SMOOTH MUSCLE OF GASTROINTESTINAL TRACT AND BLADDER

In addition to the secretory activity of glands, the tone and motility of the gastrointestinal tract is also maintained by cholinergic stimulation, and defecation involves sacral parasympathetic activity. Voiding the bladder (i.e., urination or micturition) occurs through reflex activation of cholinergic parasympathetic nerves to cause relaxation of the sphincter and contraction of the muscular wall of the bladder, or detrusor muscle. These functions of the parasympathetic nervous system are often disrupted after surgery or in older adults, resulting in chronic constipation or **urinary retention.** Conversely, hyperactive bladder reflexes can cause **incontinence** in some patients.

AIRWAYS

Although gastrointestinal and bladder reflexes are important for normal body functioning, other reflexes involving cholinergic mechanisms can be harmful and, in some cases, even life threatening. Irritation of the upper airways provokes a reflexive activation of parasympathetic innervation of the same region. The resulting bronchoconstriction (sometimes accompanied by glandular secretion) can significantly impair normal respiration. It is now believed that this reflex may contribute to attacks of **asthma** in susceptible patients and may become hyperactive in some. This reflex was once responsible for excessive secretion in the airways of patients undergoing surgery because of the irritating properties of certain gaseous anesthetics; however, this problem has been alleviated with the use of newer, nonirritating drugs.

HEART

Vagus (parasympathetic) nerve activity slows heart rate and conduction through the atrioventricular (A-V) node. In some patients, conduction through the A-V node may be slowed excessively so that some impulses die out before they reach the ventricles. This situation is called **heart block** and may require treatment. Similarly, an abnormally slow heart rate **(sinus bradycardia)** may result from excessive parasympathetic activity to the heart. This arrhythmia may require treatment in certain patients (see Chapter 40).

BLOOD VESSELS

An unusual situation is found in blood vessels. As discussed in Chapter 10, contraction of vascular smooth muscle is regulated under normal conditions by the sympathetic nervous system through activation of alpha-adrenergic receptors. Parasympathetic nerves are not generally found on blood vessels and so play little role in regulating arterial pressure. However, muscarinic receptors are found on almost all blood vessels. When stimulated, these receptors cause local release of nitric oxide, which relaxes vascular smooth muscle and thus provokes vasodilation. The reason for the presence of these receptors in the absence of parasympathetic innervation is unknown.

DRUG CLASS • Muscarinic Receptor Agonists or Cholinomimetics

acetylcholine (Miochol-E)

bethanechol (Duvoid, Urecholine, Duvoid, ❋ Urecholine ❋)

carbachol (Carbostat, Miostat, Miostat ❋)

methacoline (Provocholine)

△ pilocarpine (Ocusert Pilo, Salagen, Akarpine, Isopto Carpine, Pilocar, Pilopine HS, Pilocarpine ❋)

MECHANISM OF ACTION

Cholinomimetics, or drugs that mimic the action of acetylcholine, exert their therapeutic actions by stimulating muscarinic cholinergic receptors (Figure 11-1). Pilocarpine, the prototype drug in this class, is a naturally occurring compound that selectively stimulates these receptors. Bethanechol and methacholine are also more selective for muscarinic receptors. Acetylcholine and (to a lesser extent) carbachol both have activity at nicotinic receptors as well, but this additional activity plays no role in their clinical usefulness.

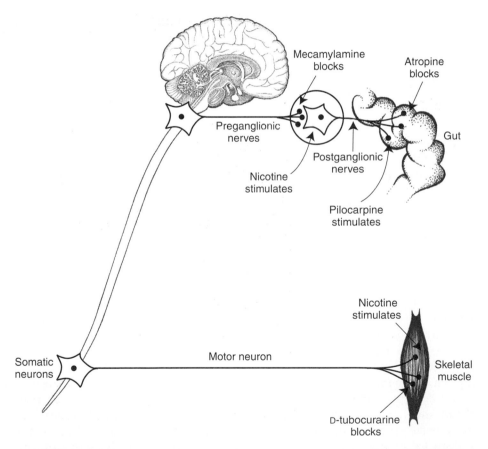

FIGURE 11-1 Acetylcholine acts as a peripheral neurotransmitter at three receptor populations. Each population is characterized by an agonist and an antagonist. Pilocarpine serves as an agonist at muscarinic cholinergic receptors in tissues innervated by all parasympathetic postganglionic nerves (and sympathetic postganglionic nerves, for sweat glands); atropine serves as an antagonist in these tissues. Nicotine serves as an agonist at nicotinic cholinergic receptors on parasympathetic and sympathetic ganglia; mecamylamine serves as an antagonist. Nicotine serves as an agonist at nicotinic cholinergic receptors at the neuromuscular junction; D-tubocurarine serves as an antagonist.

USES

Pilocarpine is used in the management of glaucoma (see Chapter 65). For unknown reasons, this drug has especially strong effects on the salivary glands and therefore is sometimes used in the treatment of xerostomia (dry mouth).

Acetylcholine itself is rarely used because of its rapid degradation by cholinesterases and its ability to produce effects at nicotinic receptors. It is occasionally employed in ocular surgery to produce miosis when a very short duration of action is required. A 1% solution can be applied directly to the eye without any danger of systemic absorption and effects.

Bethanechol is sometimes used in the treatment of urinary retention or to stimulate gastrointestinal motility. Carbachol is used in ocular surgery as described above and in the acute management of glaucoma. Methacholine is occasionally used to determine whether the airways are hyperreactive.

PHARMACOKINETICS

All of the synthetic cholinomimetic drugs (bethanechol, carbachol, methacholine) are, like acetylcholine, positively charged and so are poorly absorbed if given orally. Therefore bethanechol can be given by mouth to produce effects on the gastrointestinal tract itself, but it is generally administered by subcutaneous injection to treat urinary retention. In either case, the drug produces its effect quickly (5 to 15 minutes after injection and 30 to 90 minutes after oral administration), and complete recovery occurs within several hours. Methacholine is sometimes given by inhalation in order to test for airway hyperreactivity and produces its action almost immediately. Acetylcholine and carbachol are applied directly to the eye to cause miosis within minutes. Whereas the response to acetylcholine is relatively brief because of its rapid metabolism by local cholinesterases, the effects of carbachol may persist for up to 24 hours because of its relative resistance to these enzymes.

Because pilocarpine is not positively charged like the synthetic cholinomimetics, the drug can be absorbed systemically. When given orally for the treatment of xerostomia, the effect of pilocarpine appears in about 20 minutes. Because the plasma half-life of the drug is less than an hour, it must be taken several times a day. Pilocarpine can also be absorbed systemically when applied directly to the eye in the treatment of glaucoma. Again, effects on the eye are seen in about 20 minutes but may last for only a few hours as the pilocarpine diffuses

away. To provide a longer duration of action, tiny pill-like devices have been designed that are placed in the eye and slowly release pilocarpine to produce a therapeutic effect for up to a week.

ADVERSE REACTIONS AND CONTRAINDICATIONS

With the exception of pilocarpine in the treatment of glaucoma, cholinomimetic drugs are rarely used in patients because of the potential to cause life-threatening reactions, even in relatively healthy patients. All can cause bronchoconstriction and excessive secretion in the upper airways; therefore these drugs are not recommended for patients known or suspected to have asthmatic tendencies.

Cholinomimetic drugs can also cause death by affecting the cardiovascular system, either by acting directly on the heart or by stimulating muscarinic receptors on blood vessels to cause a sudden severe decrease in blood pressure. Therefore these drugs should never be used in patients with coronary artery disease or certain other heart problems.

Other effects of muscarinic receptor stimulation are possible with any of these drugs. These effects are predictable from knowledge of the autonomic nervous system as described in Chapter 10 and include nausea, vomiting, and diarrhea (from gastrointestinal stimulation), as well as increased sweating. Such adverse reactions are relatively common with the use of pilocarpine in the treatment of glaucoma.

TOXICITY

As described above, life-threatening reactions are always possible when administering cholinomimetic drugs, particularly by injection. Because these reactions are mediated through muscarinic receptors, it is common practice to have atropine, a muscarinic receptor antagonist (see next drug class), readily available when cholinomimetics are given in a clinical setting.

INTERACTIONS

Many drugs that are not usually considered cholinergics may cause some degree of muscarinic receptor blockade as an adverse reaction. These drugs interfere with the therapeutic action of cholinomimetics. On the other hand, administration of different drugs with cholinomimetic properties in combination or of any cholinomimetic with a cholinesterase inhibitor (see next drug class) greatly enhances the potential for adverse effects or toxicity.

DRUG CLASS • Muscarinic Receptor Antagonists or Anticholinergics

atropine (Atro-Pen)

glycopyrrolate (Robinul)

ipratropium (Atrovent)

oxybutynin (Ditropan)

propantheline (Pro-Banthine)

scopolamine (Transderm-Scop, Transderm-V✱)

tolterodine (Detrol)

tropicamide (Mydriacyl)

MECHANISM OF ACTION

As with other terms discussed above, anticholinergics usually refers more specifically to drugs that act as antagonists at muscarinic receptors, or muscarinic receptor antagonists. Thus these agents bind to muscarinic receptors but produce no effect. The effects of an antimuscarinic drug are usually a result of blocking the action of neurally released acetylcholine acting at muscarinic receptors (see Figure 11-1). Other terms for muscarinic receptor antagonists are parasympatholytic and cholinolytic.

USES

Atropine, the prototype drug in this category, is an alkaloid originally derived from the leaves of the deadly nightshade, *Atropa belladonna*, which is a member of the potato family. Several other plants also contain atropine and a related drug, scopolamine. These two drugs are often referred to as belladonna alkaloids. Many references to the use of these plants as medicinal agents are found in ancient medical literature. To this day, atropine remains the most versatile drug in this class.

Muscarinic receptor antagonists are often used in eye examinations to cause dilation of the pupil (mydriasis) and paralysis of accommodation (cycloplegia). Atropine is applied by drops to the eye to block the actions of acetylcholine released from parasympathetic nerve endings. The result of this antagonism is a relaxation of the circular muscles of the iris and blurred vision. Mydriasis and cycloplegia allow measurements of lens refraction and examination of the retina. Tropicamide is preferred over atropine for this purpose because it has a shorter duration of action. Drugs affecting the eye are discussed further in Chapter 65. Photophobia, or sensitivity to light, as a result of the pupillary dilation, and blurred vision caused by cycloplegia are common adverse reactions of oral administration of atropine and atropine-like drugs that can reach the eye.

A muscarinic receptor antagonist is often given as a preanesthetic agent before surgery in order to inhibit bronchial and salivary secretions. Excessive secretions are a particular problem with certain gaseous anesthetics that irritate the upper airways (see Chapter 16). The drying effect of an antimuscarinic drug reduces the possibility that secretions may be involuntarily aspirated when the patient is drowsy or unconscious. Glycopyrrolate is the drug most commonly administered for this effect.

Atropine or other antimuscarinic drugs are occasionally used to depress an overactive gastrointestinal tract. A prominent antimuscarinic effect of atropine is to inhibit gastrointestinal tone and motility. Atropine and related drugs are modestly effective in depressing gastric acid secretion in patients with peptic ulcers, and propantheline in particular has been used for this purpose. Today, however, more effective drugs are available. Drugs affecting gastrointestinal motility and secretion are discussed in Chapters 48, 49, and 50.

Atropine and related drugs are useful in the treatment of certain cardiac rate and rhythm problems. Atropine may be given to treat excessively slow heart rate (sinus bradycardia) by antagonizing the acetylcholine released by the vagus nerve at the sinoatrial node. These drugs may also be useful in the treatment of certain forms of heart block (see Chapter 40).

Muscarinic receptor antagonists can often block the contraction of bronchial smooth muscle, particularly in bronchospastic states. Ipratropium is an atropine-like drug that can be taken by inhalation to prevent asthmatic attacks and that produces a lower incidence of unwanted antimuscarinic effects (see Chapter 43).

Muscarinic receptor antagonists are useful in the treatment of overactive bladder reflexes. Oxybutinin has been popular for this purpose in the past. Tolterodine, a relatively new drug, may be superior because it appears to produce effects on the bladder at doses that cause fewer typical adverse reactions than are seen with other drugs. The reason for this apparent selectivity is unknown but does not appear to occur at the receptor level.

Muscarinic receptor antagonists can also be used to treat toxicity caused by cholinergic drugs, most commonly those involving acetylcholinesterase inhibitors. This topic is discussed later in the chapter.

Finally, muscarinic receptor antagonists have other uses unrelated to peripheral muscarinic receptors. Many also have effects in the CNS. Scopolamine, unlike atropine, is useful in preventing motion sickness. Some drugs have antitremor activity and are used to relieve extrapyramidal motor movements caused by Parkinson's disease, other diseases, and some drugs. Muscarinic receptor antagonists used in the treatment of parkinsonism are discussed in Chapter 23.

PHARMACOKINETICS

Differences in the pharmacokinetics of muscarinic receptor antagonists can have a dramatic effect on their usefulness in different clinical situations. For example, atropine and related alkaloids were once used in the treatment of asthma, but they produced adverse effects that made them hard to tolerate. Ipratropium is similar to atropine but has a positive charge that makes it difficult to cross membranes. Because of this, when taken by inhalation, ipratropium blocks cholinergic bronchoconstriction, but very little is absorbed into the systemic circulation to cause other, unwanted effects. Ipratropium has for this reason become a popular and useful drug in the management of asthma. Other positively charged muscarinic receptor antagonists are glycopyrrolate and propantheline.

Atropine and other muscarinic receptor antagonists that can enter the brain are effective in the treatment of motion sickness. Once again, however, the dose of atropine required produces blockade of almost all muscarinic receptors in the periphery, thereby causing many adverse effects that make the drug impractical for this purpose. In contrast, scopolamine generally produces greater effects on the CNS than other muscarinic receptor antagonists. Therefore scopolamine effectively treats motion sickness at doses that cause less blockade of muscarinic receptors in the periphery. The reason for this difference is probably not greater receptor selectivity but may be instead related to scopolamine's much higher degree of lipid solubility than atropine. In fact, scopolamine is so lipid soluble that the drug is easily absorbed through the skin in slow release patches that provide relief of nausea for up to 72 hours.

When administered at the usual doses, most anticholinergics have a duration of action of 4 to 8 hours and are eliminated primarily by hepatic biotransformation.

ADVERSE REACTIONS AND CONTRAINDICATIONS

With most of the anticholinergics, adverse reactions may and usually do occur in addition to therapeutic effects. These adverse reactions are extensions of the drug actions described above. One of the most common and bothersome adverse effects of anticholinergic drugs is xerostomia, but patients may also experience constipation. Urinary hesitancy or retention is also common, particularly in older adults. The expected cardiovascular effect is tachycardia, although bradycardia may be noted with small doses administered intravenously. Dilated pupils and blurred vision are accompanied by photophobia and sometimes ocular pain. The skin may become dry and flushed, and some patients may develop an increased body temperature from an inability to dissipate heat through sweating. This is especially true in children, where this effect can lead to life-threatening increases in body temperature (hyperthermia).

Anticholinergics are generally inadvisable for patients with glaucoma, cardiac rhythm disturbances or diseases where increased heart rate is undesirable, or in various gastrointestinal disorders.

Adverse reactions produced by anticholinergics acting in the CNS vary. Atropine, particularly in an overdose, produces generalized excitement, which at a toxic level may result in hallucinations. In contrast, although scopolamine can produce hallucinations and psychosis, it also produces sleepiness, sedation, and amnesia. Older adults may be especially sensitive to the CNS effects of anticholinergics.

TOXICITY

The characteristic signs of systemic overdose of atropine or another muscarinic receptor antagonists are confusion and delirium; hot, flushed dry skin; dilated pupils; and tachycardia. With the exception of the potential to cause hyperthermia in children, none of the peripheral actions of overdose of muscarinic receptor antagonists is likely to be life threatening in most patients. At very high doses, propantheline may produce ganglionic blockade, causing hypotension, or effects at the neuromuscular junction resulting in muscle weakness.

INTERACTIONS

Anticholinergics may increase gastrointestinal pH (by inhibiting the secretion of gastric acid), which may affect the absorption of certain drugs. Scopolamine should be used cautiously in patients who are taking other CNS depressants.

PHYSIOLOGY • **Nicotinic Cholinergic Mechanisms**

As discussed in Chapter 10, acetylcholine acts on nicotinic receptors in the periphery primarily in autonomic ganglia and at the neuromuscular junction in skeletal muscle. Once acetylcholine is released from a nerve ending in response to a nerve impulse, it is quickly destroyed by acetylcholinesterase—so quickly that the transmitter is completely gone from receptors before the next nerve impulse releases more acetylcholine. This is an important sequence for normal cholinergic transmission at nicotinic receptors, especially those at the neuromuscular junction in skeletal muscle, because the receptors trigger muscular contraction through a mechanism that involves ligand-gated sodium channels. These channels open briefly in response to changes in the membrane caused by stimulation of nicotinic receptors. Before they can open again, these channels need time to reset between stimulations, during which all of the released acetylcholine is destroyed between nerve impulses. Therefore what looks like a smooth contraction in skeletal muscle during movement of a limb or breathing is really the result of this cycle repeated at nicotinic receptors many times. Recall from Chapter 10 that nicotinic receptors at the autonomic ganglia are different from those at the neuromuscular junction.

Myasthenia gravis is a disorder of nicotinic receptors at the neuromuscular junction and is characterized by rapid development of fatigue and muscular weakness. In its later, severe stages, respiration becomes impaired and eventually fails. The cause of the disease is thought to be an autoimmune reaction by the body to nicotinic receptors on skeletal muscle. The immune system then sends antibodies to the receptors to destroy them. Because fewer receptors are present afterward, neuromuscular transmission becomes impaired, and muscle contraction cannot be sustained and therefore weakens. The specific treatment of myasthenia gravis is covered in Chapter 23.

The use of drugs that act at the nicotinic receptors at the neuromuscular junction in skeletal muscle is highly specialized and generally limited to surgical settings. These **neuromuscular blockers** (an example is curare, or D-tubocurarine) are discussed in Chapter 16.

There is no practical clinical use for drugs that stimulate nicotinic receptors in autonomic ganglia. Nicotine itself, usually administered by a skin patch, is used in smoking cessation programs, but the doses involved do not seem to produce any significant effects on the autonomic nervous system.

DRUG CLASS • **Ganglionic Nicotinic Receptor Antagonist (Ganglionic Blocker)**

mecamylamine (Inversine)

MECHANISM OF ACTION

Ganglionic blockers are antagonists at the specific subtype of nicotinic receptor responsible for excitatory transmission at all sympathetic and parasympathetic ganglia (see Figure 11-1). Therefore these drugs have the potential to paralyze the entire autonomic nervous system without affecting neuromuscular transmission to skeletal muscle. Ganglionic blockers are very effective in lowering blood pressure and thus were once important drugs in the treatment of hypertension. However, because of the many adverse reactions they produce, their uses today are extremely limited. Therefore, only one ganglionic blocker, mecamylamine, is currently available for use.

USES

The past and present uses of ganglionic blockers are all based on their ability to lower arterial pressure by blocking the sympathetic nervous system. Mecamylamine may be used in the management of essential hypertension, but this is extremely rare because of the many troublesome adverse effects also produced by blocking the activity of all parasympathetic and sympathetic pathways. The first ganglionic blocker, hexamethonium, was developed for the treatment of hypertension but is no longer in use. Other drugs are more useful than ganglionic blockers as antihypertensives, as discussed in Chapter 41.

PHARMACOKINETICS

Mecamylamine can be taken orally, is well absorbed from the gastrointestinal tract, and produces effects that last for 6 to 12 hours. The drug is eliminated unchanged by the kidneys.

ADVERSE REACTIONS AND CONTRAINDICATIONS

Most of the potential adverse reactions of ganglionic blockade reflect the loss of parasympathetic activity. These include dry mouth, constipation, cycloplegia, mydriasis, paralytic ileus, urinary retention, impotence, and tachycardia. Orthostatic hypotension and precipitation of angina may also occur. Mecamylamine may produce drowsiness and fatigue as well as uncontrolled movements of the extremities. Ganglionic blockers should be used with great caution in patients with impaired renal function.

INTERACTIONS

Ganglionic blockers should be used with caution in any patient being treated with another drug that lowers blood pressure.

 PHYSIOLOGY • Acetylcholinesterase

As described in Chapter 10, acetylcholinesterase is an active enzyme found at cholinergic nerve terminals. One molecule of acetylcholinesterase can destroy about 5000 molecules of acetylcholine in 1 second. Because of this, all of the acetylcholine released into the synaptic cleft by a nerve impulse is completely destroyed before the next nerve impulse releases another pulse of acetylcholine. Under normal circumstances, most of the acetylcholine released in these pulses is probably destroyed before it has a chance to bind to a receptor and cause an effect.

 DRUG CLASS • Acetylcholinesterase Inhibitors

Reversible

ambenonium (Mytelase)

donepezil (Aricept)

edrophonium (Tensilon)

galantamine (Reminyl)

neostigmine (Prostigmin, Prostigmin✴)

⚠ **physostigmine (Antilirium, Eserine, Isopto Eserine✴)**

pyridostigmine (Mestinon, Regonol, Mestinon,✴ Mestinon-SR,✴ Regonol✴)

rivastigmine (Exelon)

tacrine (Cognex)

Irreversible

demecarium (Humorsol)

echothiophate (Phospholine)

MECHANISM OF ACTION

As discussed above, many cholinergic drugs act directly at cholinergic receptors to produce effects. In contrast, inhibitors of acetylcholinesterase (cholinesterase inhibitors) influence cholinergic transmission indirectly by preventing the rapid degradation of synaptically released acetylcholine. These drugs allow the acetylcholine released from cholinergic nerve endings to remain intact longer because its degradation is inhibited. Therefore the acetylcholine that is released has more opportunity to act at cholinergic receptors, usually resulting in a greater effect. Drugs in this class can produce significant effects at both muscarinic and nicotinic receptors (see Figure 11-1).

Although all drugs in this class inhibit acetylcholinesterase, the exact manner in which they accomplish this inhibition of the enzyme varies. A few drugs simply bind to the enzyme reversibly just as many drugs bind to their receptors. While the drug occupies the enzyme, it is unavailable to biotransform acetylcholine. As the concentration of the drug in the area of the enzyme falls, the drug molecules dissociate from the binding site unchanged, and the enzyme is immediately available and active. Edrophonium and tacrine both act in this way.

In contrast to this simple mechanism, most cholinesterase inhibitors are actually substrates for the enzyme; that is, the enzyme interacts with the drug molecule in much the same way it interacts with acetylcholine and literally breaks it apart. However, biotransforming the drug molecule and cycling back to the active form of the enzyme takes much longer than degrading a molecule of acetylcholine. During most of this time, the enzyme is trapped in an inactive state in which part of the drug molecule remains bound to the enzyme. A key difference between the drugs is the exact nature of this inactive state they form. One group of drugs is called carbamates and includes all of the drugs ending in -*stigmine*—physostigmine, neostigmine, pyridostigmine, and rivastigmine. After interacting with carbamate substrate–type inhibitors, acetylcholinesterase eventually releases the bound fragment of the drug molecule (although it may take minutes to hours, depending on the specific drug). The enzyme is then active again. Therefore the carbamates as well as drugs such asedrophonium are called reversible cholinesterase inhibitors.

The other class of cholinesterase inhibitor is termed irreversible. The **irreversible cholinesterase inhibitors** form a permanent covalent bond with acetylcholinesterase so that the enzyme must be completely replaced before the drug effect wears off, a process requiring days to weeks. The most common examples of irreversible acetylcholinesterase inhibitors are the organophosphate compounds, which include potent drugs for constricting the pupil, called miotics: demecarium and echothiophate. This same mechanism is involved in the toxic effects of the insecticides parathion and malathion and several agents developed for chemical warfare, the so-called nerve gases (see later in the chapter).

Inhibiting acetylcholinesterase permits the released acetylcholine more time to interact with cholinergic receptors, allowing greater effects at muscarinic receptors. However, at nicotinic receptors under normal conditions, the opposite may and usually does occur. In fact, blockade of acetylcholinesterase at the neuromuscular junction may cause muscle weakness or even paralysis because nicotinic receptors act through a mechanism requiring resetting for a continuous effect, as described earlier. If the acetylcholine released by the nerve ending is not completely destroyed before the next nerve impulse, this mechanism cannot recover and transmission fails. The muscle weakness and paralysis that may be caused by inhibition of acetylcholinesterase is in part the basis for the use of irreversible inhibitors of the enzyme, such as insecticides and military nerve gas.

USES

Interestingly, the most important therapeutic use for acetylcholinesterase inhibitors is in the treatment of myasthenia gravis (discussed in detail in Chapter 23). Recall that in this disorder, functional cholinergic nicotinic receptors at the neuromuscular junction have been lost. As a result, the receptor stimulation caused by the normal amount of acetylcholine released from the nerve ending may not be sufficient to trigger muscle contraction. Under these conditions, inhibition of acetylcholinesterase means that released acetylcholine has more opportunity to interact with the greatly reduced number of receptors, thus improving muscle strength. Pyridostigmine, neostigmine, and ambenonium are commonly used for this purpose. Antimyasthenic drugs are discussed further in Chapter 23.

Inhibition of cholinesterase in the eye also has a therapeutic effect in patients with glaucoma by enhancing the activity of acetylcholine at muscarinic receptors. As discussed above, the resulting pupillary constriction and ciliary muscle contraction improve drainage of fluid from the eye and so reduce intraocular pressure. Demecarium and echothiophate are irreversible cholinesterase inhibitors commonly used for this purpose. Cholinomimetic drugs administered to act in the eye are described in Chapter 65.

More recently, cholinesterase inhibitors have been found to be of value in the treatment of Alzheimer's disease. Drugs used for this purpose are tacrine, donepezil, and rivastigmine. Drugs used in the treatment of Alzheimer's disease are discussed in Chapter 23.

Additionally, cholinesterase inhibitors are occasionally used to reverse the effects of neuromuscular blocking drugs (see Chapter 16).

PHARMACOKINETICS

As discussed above, the mechanism of action of many cholinesterase inhibitors involves their action as substrates for acetylcholinesterase and destruction by the enzyme. Lipid solubility also has an important effect on the pharmacology of these drugs. For example, neostigmine is positively charged and therefore has little effect on the brain. On the other hand, physostigmine is chemically similar to neostigmine but has no positive charge. Because of this, physostigmine is sometimes used to treat the CNS effects of overdose with centrally acting antimuscarinic drugs. Donepezil, rivastigmine, and tacrine are all relatively lipid soluble and therefore exert especially pronounced effects on the CNS.

Many irreversible cholinesterase inhibitors belonging to a class called organophosphates are extremely lipid soluble and can be quickly absorbed through the skin. This includes nerve gas such as sarin, tabun, and VX, which were specifically designed to be highly toxic.

Specific information about the pharmacokinetics of clinically used cholinesterase inhibitors appears where these drugs are discussed in later chapters.

ADVERSE REACTIONS AND CONTRAINDICATIONS

As explained above, inhibition of cholinesterase can produce overactivity at muscarinic receptors and failure of transmission at nicotinic receptors. Effects at muscarinic receptors resemble overstimulation and are the opposite of adverse reactions caused by muscarinic receptor antagonists. These effects of cholinesterase inhibitors include salivation, sweating, nausea, diarrhea, and bradycardia. Gastrointestinal effects may be especially pronounced with drugs taken orally. Excessive acetylcholine at nicotinic receptors may result in muscle fasciculation (twitching) and weakness.

TOXICITY

Cholinesterase inhibitors have the potential to be highly toxic and may cause death through a variety of mechanisms, among which are respiratory failure, convulsions, and cardiovascular collapse. As mentioned above, this potential for toxicity has been exploited in the development of nerve gases used in chemical warfare. However, insecticides such as malathion and parathion are also made with organophosphates, which inhibit acetylcholinesterase. Consequently, anticholinesterase intoxication is a significant potential problem, especially among agricultural workers. The treatment for organophosphate poisoning includes atropine to block the resulting overactivity at muscarinic receptors and pralidoxime (2-PAM, Protopam). Atropine will block the muscarinic effects in the periphery (i.e., salivation, tearing, diarrhea, bradycardia) as well as in the CNS (respiratory depression and convulsions) but will not reverse the neuromuscular paralysis. Pralidoxime, or 2-PAM, which regenerates acetylcholinesterase at all peripheral sites, must therefore be given as well. 2-PAM is able to compete with the enzyme for the phosphate group of the inhibitor, thereby eliminating itself and the inhibitor from the enzyme and reversing the otherwise irreversible inhibition.

INTERACTIONS

Any drug that interferes with the actions of acetylcholine at the neuromuscular junction is likely to interfere with the therapeutic action of a cholinesterase inhibitor in a patient with myasthenia gravis, and some of these are identified in Chapter 23. Similarly, drugs that block muscarinic receptors are likely to interfere with the therapeutic effect of these agents in the treatment of glaucoma (see Chapter 65). These drugs will also inhibit the enzymatic activity of esterases in the plasma as well as slow or prevent the metabolism of certain local anesthetics, increasing the likelihood of systemic toxicity (see Chapter 16).

 APPLICATION TO PRACTICE

Since the use of muscarinic agonists is somewhat limited in practice, and additional uses of antagonists are discussed elsewhere in other specific settings, this section focuses on the care of the patient receiving a cholinergic drug for treatment of urinary retention or an anticholinergic for treatment of an overactive bladder. Care of the patient receiving muscarinic agonists for treatment of glaucoma will be discussed in Chapter 65. The care of patients receiving anticholinesterase drugs for myasthenia gravis is discussed in Chapter 23.

ASSESSMENT
History of Present Illness

Elicit from the patient whether he or she has noticed any change in the usual pattern of voiding, including frequency, amounts, and the usual times of day and night. Ask if the patient has to rely on methods to stimulate urination, such as listening to running water, applying pressure over the bladder, or performing Valsalva maneuvers. Do they have trouble starting or maintaining the urine stream? Does the patient have feelings of urgency or difficulty controlling voiding? If so, is the urgency associated with consumption of caffeine or following pregnancy with vaginal delivery? Does the patient leak urine when coughing, sneezing, or lifting a heavy object? Determine in older men if there is a gradually diminishing force and hesitancy to the urinary stream. These findings may suggest an enlargement of the prostate gland known as benign prostatic hyperplasia (BPH). A good history helps to determine the type of urinary problem (Box 11-1).

BOX 11-1	Types of Urinary Problems
Urinary retention	Although production continues, urine is retained in bladder, but accumulated urine is not released
Stress incontinence	Increased intraabdominal pressure caused by coughing, laughing, sneezing, walking, or running leads to involuntary loss of urine
Urge incontinence	Inability to hold back urine flow when feeling urge to void
Overflow incontinence	Retention with overflow of small amounts of urine
Reflex incontinence	Caused by spinal cord injury or congenital conditions leading to loss of voluntary control of bladder
Psychologic incontinence	Aware of need to urinate but unable to respond appropriately because of dementia or confusion
Environmental incontinence	Aware of need to urinate but physically unable to reach the toilet unaided

Health History

The health history should include the patient's experiences with urinary tract disorders. Other past health problems that may be significant are a history of cancer of reproductive organs (especially if radiation therapy was used), recent surgery or trauma, labor and delivery, systemic diseases such as hypertension and diabetes mellitus, or sexually transmitted diseases. Elicit information regarding prescription and OTC drug use.

Lifespan Considerations

Perinatal. The normal physiologic changes accompanying pregnancy predispose women to postpartum urinary problems. During pregnancy and the weeks immediately following delivery, smooth muscle tone is reduced because of an increased level of progesterone. A dilated bladder with poor muscle tone is less likely to empty itself effectively. The pressure within the bladder nearly doubles during pregnancy and then rapidly returns to a prepregnancy level during the first postpartum week. This rapid change in pressure results in hypotonia of bladder muscles.

Bladder tone and sensation may be reduced as the result of operative vaginal procedures and the effects of analgesia and anesthesia. The duration of the voiding difficulty is also influenced by analgesic drugs. For example, long-acting bupivacaine can result in decreased detrusor strength for up to 8 hours after administration. Further, pain or fear of pain interferes with the woman's ability to relax. These factors in combination with postpartum diuresis frequently lead to bladder distension or to incomplete emptying of the bladder. Edema and increased blood flow to the bladder mucosa and urethra may interfere with free passage of urine.

Pediatric. Voiding experiences linked with toilet training can have long-lasting effects. A patient's positive or negative attitudes toward elimination can sometimes be traced back to this period. Reinforcement of positive behavior tends to result in continued, problem-free elimination patterns. Punishment as the primary motivating factor during toilet training may carry over into adulthood. The guilt or shame from prolonged enuresis (bed-wetting) may cause voiding dysfunction long after the enuresis has resolved.

The psychosocial impact of neurogenic atony once the patient has successfully attained bladder control can be significant. Children may feel ashamed if they can no longer control bladder function. This problem is compounded if the child's peers learn about the use of absorbent undergarments or episodes of incontinence.

Older Adults. The aging process affects the act of voiding. The bladder becomes funnel shaped as a result of alterations in connective tissue and weakening of pelvic floor muscles. Irritability of the bladder wall often increases, adding more urgency to the normal desire to void. Impairment of the detrusor muscle's ability to elongate results in decreased bladder capacity. Because of these changes, the older adult may have problems with incontinence, frequency, retention, and dysuria.

Urinary retention in the older adult is not uncommon. Causes include phimosis, meatal stenosis, urethral trauma or stricture, BPH, prostate cancer, and bladder tumor. Bleeding with clot formation, uterine prolapse, fecal impaction, and neurologic impairment (diabetes mellitus, nerve damage related to neoplasms) may also contribute to urinary retention. Box 11-2 provides a listing of drug classifications commonly associated with urinary retention and obstruction.

Cultural/Social Considerations

Cultural teachings lead most people to consider the act of voiding a private matter. Western society and child-rearing practices support this view by providing locks on bathroom doors, separate public bathrooms for men

---

BOX 11-2 **Drugs Associated with Varying Degrees of Urinary Retention and Obstruction**

Central Nervous System

baclofen
carbamazepine
clonazepam
Opioids and opioidlike drugs
phenytoin

Bladder

Anticholinergic drugs
Antihistamines
Antiparkinson drugs
Beta-adrenergic agonists
Calcium channel blockers
Diuretics
Ganglionic blockers
Muscle relaxants
Prostaglandin inhibitors
Phenothiazines
Tricyclic antidepressants

Detrusor Muscle

Alpha-adrenergic agonists
Amphetamines
Beta-adrenergic blockers
Estrogen combinations
levodopa
Tricyclic antidepressants

and women, and so forth. This attitude may inhibit the micturition reflex if the patient is in an environment where privacy is missing.

Patients with chronic urinary retention may have lifestyle adjustments to make, some of which are related to the underlying cause of the retention and some to the retention itself. Most patients with neurogenic atony have experienced overflow incontinence at some point. Fear of incontinence may keep these individuals from participating fully in school, vocational, and social activities. Some patients may choose to use external, indwelling, or intermittent catheterization rather than drugs to control the disorder. This is particularly true for patients unable to sense that they have been incontinent or who cannot perform personal hygiene tasks independently. Knowledge of the patient's current lifestyle, level of independence, and anticipated changes helps determine treatment goals and methods.

Physical Examination

The physical examination is based on information obtained from the history. Most of the necessary data comes directly from examining the urinary system. The ability to palpate the bladder above the symphysis pubis indicates urinary retention. Depending on the patient's size and weight, palpation may be difficult, even of a distended bladder. In very thin patients, it may be possible to visualize bladder distension. A dull sound is produced when a distended bladder is percussed. Patients voiding more than once per hour or in amounts smaller than 50 mL are probably experiencing urinary retention with overflow and may become diaphoretic or restless as a result of discomfort from the distended bladder. Urinary retention should always be considered when fluid intake is considerably greater than urinary output.

Assess the patient also for urinary incontinence, particularly if epidural analgesia has been administered.

Laboratory Testing

Urodynamic studies evaluate the motor and sensory function of the bladder. These tests are used primarily to diagnose voiding problems or loss of bladder control (as with incontinence) and to evaluate the effectiveness of treatment used for voiding disorders. Urine flow rates (uroflowmetry) or a cystometrography may be performed. Cystometrography measures bladder pressures during filling and voiding. It is a measure sensitive to filling compliance, capacity, and detrusor contraction. Electromyography measures striated perineal muscle activity, including the sphincters, during bladder filling and emptying.

If urinary retention is suspected despite a patient having voided, postvoiding catheterization is performed,

and the amount of voided urine is measured. This allows comparison of the amount of urine voided with the amount obtained through catheterization. Patients may think they are voiding adequately when in reality they are voiding only a small amount and most of the urine remains in the bladder. In some cases, it may be necessary to perform an ultrasound examination to estimate bladder size.

GOALS OF THERAPY

The treatment goal for the patient with urinary retention is to stimulate complete bladder emptying. Cholinergic drugs are used on a short-term basis until the effects of surgery, childbirth, or other drugs have diminished. Avoidance of urinary retention also minimizes the risk of damage to the urinary system and urinary tract infection. Establishing a routine schedule for voiding is a major factor in the patient's ability to be independent and function in the community.

Not all cases of urinary retention require treatment. Using a drug that stimulates bladder contraction is generally not advised if swelling of perineal tissues is obstructing urine flow. If the patient is unable to void because of positioning or privacy concerns, stimulating bladder contractions probably will not help. However, for patients whose bladders are not contracting adequately, use of a cholinergic drug may be appropriate. Bethanechol is the only drug in this class that is prescribed for urinary retention. Subcutaneous administration typically results in a more rapid and stronger response than that seen with oral administration. However, oral administration results in longer duration of action. Bethanechol is not suitable for use in patients who have questionable structural integrity of the urinary or gastrointestinal tract. It should be used very cautiously in patients with a previous history of bronchial asthma or cardiac disease.

When bethanechol is used in the acute care setting, both the oral and subcutaneous forms are used. Bethanechol is rarely used in the ambulatory care environment. Use of the subcutaneous formulation in the home setting requires the patient or caregiver to have adequate vision to prepare the drug correctly for administration. This may be an issue for individuals with poor vision related to diabetes, stroke, or aging. Patients who have had a stroke or a high-level spinal cord injury may not have the manual dexterity to prepare and administer the drug.

INTERVENTION
Administration

Monitor blood pressure, pulse, and respirations before administering bethanechol and for at least 1 hour following subcutaneous administration. A test dose is ordinarily given before maintenance therapy to determine the minimum effective dosage. Oral and subcutaneous dosage formulations are not interchangeable; attention to the dosage is therefore important. The parenteral formulation is designed for subcutaneous administration only; it should not be given intramuscularly or intravenously. Regardless of the formulation used, the health care provider should assure the patient that a bathroom, bedside commode, or bedpan is readily available. Intake and output should be carefully monitored to evaluate drug effectiveness.

Equipment to support respiratory function and atropine, the cholinergic antagonist, should be readily available in the event of respiratory depression.

Education

Instruct the patient to take the drug exactly as directed. Forgotten doses should be taken as soon as possible if it is within 2 hours of the scheduled administration time. If it is past the 2-hour limit, the regular administration schedule should be followed. Double dosing is not recommended. Teach the patient to take the drug during the day, when fluid intake is higher, to minimize nocturnal voiding patterns. However, advise the patient to report flushing, salivation, and abdominal cramping to the health care provider, because these symptoms suggest overdose.

Caution the patient taking bethanechol chloride to change positions slowly, particularly when first starting the drug, to minimize orthostatic blood pressure changes. This measure is especially important for patients with spinal cord injuries, who are already at risk for orthostatic hypotension.

EVALUATION

The expected outcome for patients using bethanechol chloride is regular, complete emptying of the bladder. For hospitalized patients, this would be observed as relative balance between fluid intake and urine output, no distension of the bladder, and no complaints of pelvic discomfort. The health care provider should expect urinary output to exceed 50 mL per void. For patients using bethanechol chloride on a regular basis, regular emptying of the bladder without incontinence should be expected.

Bibliography

Adams T, Page S: New pharmacological treatments for Alzheimer's disease: implications for dementia care nursing, *J Adv Nurs* 31(5):1183-1188, 2000.

Mead M: New acetylcholinesterase inhibitors improve options, *Pract Nurs* 16(9):586, 1998.

Melum MF: Emergency. Organophosphate toxicity: symptoms of insecticide poisoning may mimic those of the flu, *Am J Nurs* 101(5):57-58, 2001.

Miracle VA: What makes bradycardia tick? First of a series, *Nursing* 31(2):44-45, 2001.

Newton M, Kosier JH, Smith D: Medication minute: treatments for overactive bladder, *Urol Nurs* 20(4):267-268, 2000.

Page S: Dementia care and cholinesterase inhibitors, *Prof Nurse* 16(10):1421-1424, 2001.

Pharmacology update, *J Neurosci Nurs* 33(3):172-173, 175, 2001.

Potter DC, Wogoman HA, Nietch P: Understanding nocturnal enuresis and its treatments, *J Pract Nurs* 49(3):16-25, 1999.

Shaw F: Continence: it's never too late, *Nurs Times* 94(6):68, 70, 72, 1998.

Stewart KB: Actionstat: myasthenia gravis cholinergic crisis, *Nursing* 28(12):33, 1998.

Internet Resources

Mercer University: Anticholinergic drugs. Available online: http://www.mercer.edu/pharmacy/faculty/holbrook/paralyt.html.

Pharmacy Central: Cholinergic drugs. Available online: http://www.pharmcentral.com/cholinergics.htm.

University of Toledo: Acetylcholine. Available online: http://www.neurosci.pharm.utoledo.edu/MBC3320/acetylcholine.htm.

University of Toledo: Acetylcholinesterase inhibitors. Available online: http://www.neurosci.pharm.utoledo.edu/MBC3320/AChEase.htm.

The Upstate South Carolina Chapter of the Alzheimer's Association: Facts about FDA-approved cholinesterase inhibitors. Available online: http://www.upstatescalz.org/Cholinesterase.htm.

CHAPTER

12

Drugs Affecting Adrenergic Mechanisms

JOSEPH A. DiMICCO • KATHLEEN GUTIERREZ

 Visit **http://evolve.elsevier.com/Gutierrez/** for additional information.

KEY TERMS

Alpha$_1$-adrenergic receptors, p. 155

Alpha$_2$-adrenergic receptors, p. 155

Anaphylactic shock, p. 155

Anaphylaxis, p. 157

Baroreflex, p. 155

Beta$_1$-adrenergic receptors, p. 160

Beta$_2$-adrenergic receptors, p. 160

Beta blockers, p. 162

Cardiogenic shock, p. 155

Cardioselective, p. 162

Hemorrhagic (hypovolemic) shock, p. 155

Hypertension, p. 155

Indirect sympathomimetic, p. 156

Intrinsic sympathomimetic activity, p. 162

Orthostatic (postural) hypotension, p. 155

Pheochromocytoma, p. 158

Prejunctional (presynaptic) receptor, p. 155

Prodrug, p. 157

Septic shock, p. 155

Shock, p. 155

Sympathomimetics, p. 156

OBJECTIVES

- Discuss alpha$_1$-, alpha$_2$-, beta$_1$-, and beta$_2$-adrenergic receptors and the effect of stimulation of these receptors.

- Indicate three major uses for drugs that stimulate alpha-adrenergic receptors.

- Define direct- and indirect-acting adrenergic drugs.

- List the important effects of blocking alpha-adrenergic receptors and indicate two important uses for drugs that do so.

- Indicate and explain the major uses for beta-adrenergic receptor agonist drugs.

- List the important effects of blocking beta-adrenergic receptors and indicate two important uses for drugs that do so.

- Develop a nursing care plan for a patient receiving a drug affecting the sympathetic nervous system.

PHYSIOLOGY • Alpha-Adrenergic Receptors

The single most important function of the sympathetic nervous system is the maintenance of arterial pressure on a moment-to-moment basis, and this control is exerted primarily through activation of alpha–adrenergic receptors. Arterial pressure—or simply blood pressure—is the driving force for delivering oxygen and nutrients to all the tissues of the body through the bloodstream. Pressure in the arteries is the result of the pumping activity of the heart and the resistance to flow in the small blood vessels of the body. Norepinephrine released from sympathetic nerves stimulates cardiac activity through activation of beta-adrenergic receptors in the

heart. However, control of blood pressure by the sympathetic nervous system occurs primarily through the release of norepinephrine at alpha$_1$-receptors on small blood vessels (Figure 12-1). When these blood vessels are constricted, resistance to flow through them is increased. Total peripheral resistance, or the resistance to blood flow in all the blood vessels of the body, is the single most important determinant of blood pressure. As resistance increases, arterial blood pressure rises. This careful regulation is necessary because blood pressure must always be sufficient to drive blood through the tiny blood vessels supplying vital tissues and organs of

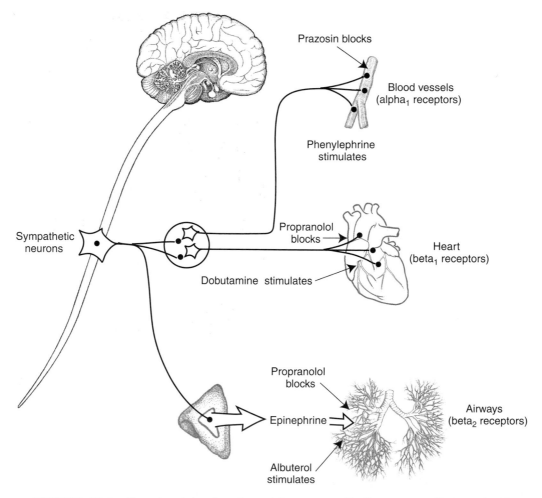

FIGURE 12-1 Norepinephrine is released from sympathetic nerve endings and epinephrine is secreted by the adrenal medulla to act at three major receptor populations. Each receptor population is characterized by an agonist and an antagonist. Phenylephrine is an agonist and prazosin is an antagonist at alpha$_1$-adrenergic receptors in blood vessels, as shown, and in certain other tissues. Dobutamine is an agonist and propranolol is an antagonist at beta$_1$-adrenergic receptors, which are found primarily on the heart. Albuterol acts as an agonist and propranolol as an antagonist at beta$_2$-adrenergic receptors in smooth muscle of the airways.

the body, particularly the brain and the heart. At the same time, excessive blood pressure must be avoided to prevent damage in certain susceptible tissues and to the heart.

The task of this close regulation of blood pressure falls to the brain, the source of sympathetic nerve activity, and is achieved primarily through the **baroreflex** (*baro-*, pressure). The brain receives a constant stream of information about the level of arterial pressure from special receptors called *baroreceptors*. These receptors are found in the carotid arteries that provide blood flow to the brain and in the aortic arch. Pressure in these blood vessels causes the baroreceptors to fire impulses to the brain. The brain uses this information to adjust the activity of sympathetic nerves so that blood pressure is always adequate to perfuse the brain and heart. For example, when a normal individual who has been lying down suddenly stands up, gravity immediately affects the circulation, causing blood to tend to pool in the legs and making it harder for the heart to pump "uphill" to deliver blood to the brain. The baroreceptors sense the resulting falling arterial pressure and the brain responds immediately to increase sympathetic nerve activity to blood vessels and the heart so that arterial pressure is maintained. If arterial pressure rises above normal levels, the opposite occurs—that is, the same baroreceptors detect the increase, and the brain responds by decreasing sympathetic activity, thereby reducing pressure to normal levels. (In the case of sudden or severe increases in arterial pressure, the brain may also increase the activity of the vagus nerve fibers innervating the heart. This parasympathetic mechanism acts as a "brake" to slow heart rate.) When arterial pressure is greatly elevated even for a short time, the heart may fail or blood vessels in the brain may rupture, causing a stroke. However, even relatively modest increases in arterial pressure above normal levels over months or years can cause permanent damage to the heart and to blood vessels, especially those in the kidney, retina, and brain. This is the situation in patients with untreated **hypertension**, or high blood pressure.

If arterial pressure is too low, so that perfusion of the brain is inadequate even for a few moments, the individual may feel faint and lose consciousness. This is commonly seen in a condition called **orthostatic (postural) hypotension**, which is defined as a decrease of 20 mm Hg in systolic or 10 mm Hg diastolic blood pressure for at least 3 minutes on rising to a standing position. Orthostatic hypotension may result when drug or disease impairs the normal activity of the sympathetic nervous system, especially when the affected person suddenly changes position from lying down to standing. Without the normal activity of the sympathetic nervous system to compensate, blood pressure and blood

flow to the brain may suddenly fall, causing dizziness and fainting. Older adults often have a sluggish baroreflex response that leads to hypotension on rising. However, the person can avoid problems by changing from a lying to a standing position slowly so that blood pressure can adjust adequately.

A more extreme situation occurs in a variety of settings that fall under the heading of **shock.** Shock is defined as a condition in which adequate tissue perfusion cannot be maintained, and is usually associated with hypotension. Note that any condition where the sympathetic nervous system is depressed or impaired may cause severe hypotension requiring circulatory support with drugs. This impairment of sympathetic function may occur as a result of general or spinal anesthesia or in spinal cord or brain injury. However, there are many other types of shock, including (1) **hemorrhagic (hypovolemic) shock,** where the cause is excessive loss of blood volume, (2) **cardiogenic shock,** reflecting acute failure of the heart as a pump, often seen after severe myocardial infarction, and (3) **septic** or **anaphylactic shock,** caused by vasodilation secondary to systemic infection or severe allergic reaction, respectively. In each case, similar physiologic mechanisms attempt to maintain adequate blood flow to the brain and heart at the expense of other organs. Under these conditions, certain other organs such as the kidney are especially sensitive to reduced blood flow and may be permanently damaged. Ultimately, shock will cause generalized failure of many organs and systems.

In addition to regulation of vascular smooth muscle tone, sympathetic nerves act through **alpha$_1$-adrenergic receptors** to play other important roles. One of these roles is in the bladder, where stimulation of alpha$_1$ receptors constricts the muscle at the neck of the bladder and inhibits outflow. This action inhibits micturition, or emptying of the bladder. Another role for alpha$_1$ receptors is in the eye, where sympathetic activity causes contraction of the radial muscles to open the pupil and allow light to enter.

Alpha$_2$-adrenergic receptors play a unique role in the peripheral sympathetic nervous system. This subtype of receptor is found on sympathetic nerve endings, and is therefore called a **prejunctional (presynaptic) receptor.** Activation of the prejunctional alpha$_2$ receptors has an inhibitory effect on the release of neurotransmitter from the terminal. When norepinephrine leaves the terminal, it binds to these receptors to inhibit further release. In this way, excessive release is prevented and neurotransmitter is conserved.

Alpha$_2$ receptors are also found in the central nervous system where they regulate sympathetic nerve activity. These central alpha$_2$ receptors are the targets for several antihypertensive agents (see Chapter 41).

DRUG CLASS • Alpha-Adrenergic Receptor Agonists

dopamine (Intropin, Revimine*)

ephedrine

epinephrine (Adrenalin)

norepinephrine (Levophed)

mephentermine (Wyamine)

metaraminol (Aramine)

midodrine (Pro-Amatine)

⚕ **phenylephrine (Neo-Synephrine)**

MECHANISM OF ACTION

All of the drugs listed above are called **sympathomimetics** because they mimic the effects of the sympathetic nervous system wherever alpha-adrenergic receptors are found. All produce primary therapeutic effects by increasing the stimulation of alpha$_1$-adrenergic receptors on vascular smooth muscle to cause vasoconstriction. For most drugs this effect is accomplished by a direct action on the receptors. Some of these drugs also produce effects by stimulating the release of norepinephrine from sympathetic nerve endings. This is called an **indirect sympathomimetic** effect (see Table 12-1).

Phenylephrine, the prototype alpha receptor agonist in this class, acts directly and selectively to stimulate alpha$_1$ receptors (see Figure 12-1). However, some sympathomimetic drugs have other actions that add to their usefulness in specific clinical settings. Epinephrine is active at all adrenergic receptors including beta receptors on the heart, blood vessels, and bronchioles. Norepinephrine, too, is an effective stimulant of beta-adrenergic receptors on the heart (beta$_1$ receptors) but is practically ineffective at beta receptors in the blood vessels and bronchioles (beta$_2$ receptors). Dopamine has the potential to act at its own receptors on blood vessels in the kidney where it produces vasodilation. At higher doses, dopamine can act both directly and indirectly to produce effects at alpha- and beta-adrenergic receptors. Effects caused by stimulation of beta-adrenergic receptors are discussed later.

Mephentermine, methoxamine, and metaraminol are relatively selective alpha-adrenergic receptor agonists but may also produce indirect effects (mephenter-

---

TABLE 12-1

Receptor Specificity of Selected Adrenergic Agonist Drugs

Generic Name	Alpha Receptor	Beta$_1$ Receptor	Beta$_2$ Receptor	Central Nervous System	Main Therapeutic Use
Catecholamines					
dobutamine	0	D	0	0	Increases cardiac contractility with little increase in heart rate or conductivity
dopamine	(I)	(I)	0	0	Dilates renal arteries at low doses by activating dopamine receptors and preventing renal failure in shock
epinephrine	D	D	D	(D)	Treats anaphylactic shock
isoproterenol	0	D	D	0	Improves bronchodilation for asthma
norepinephrine, levarterenol	D	D	0	0	Counteracts hypotension of spinal anesthesia
Noncatecholamines					
albuterol	0	0	D	0	Improves bronchodilation
ephedrine	I, D	I, D	D	(I)	Improves bronchodilation; reduces nasal congestion
metaraminol	I, D	I, D	0	0	Counteracts hypotension of spinal anesthesia
midodrine	D	0	0	0	Treats orthostatic hypotension
naphazoline	D	0	0	0	Nasal decongestant (local spray)
pseudoephedrine	I, D	I, D	D	(I)	Nasal decongestant (systemic)
ritodrine	0	0	D	0	Stops premature labor

D, Stimulates by direct action on receptors; *I*, stimulates by indirect action on receptors; *0*, no effect.

mine and metaraminol) or stimulation at beta receptors on the heart at higher doses (methoxamine).

Ephedrine, first isolated from a plant, works primarily by an indirect action, releasing stored norepinephrine from sympathetic nerve endings. Therefore ephedrine may produce stimulation of alpha$_1$ receptors on blood vessels and beta$_1$ receptors in the heart as well.

Midodrine is actually a **prodrug.** This means that it is inactive in the form that is given to the patient but is changed in the body into an active substance. Thus, the effects of midodrine are exerted after it is enzymatically transformed to desglymidodrine, which stimulates alpha$_1$ receptors.

USES

The therapeutic value of the drugs listed above is based primarily on their ability to stimulate alpha receptors in blood vessels and produce vasoconstriction. Systemic administration of these drugs is used to support the circulation in the treatment of shock or hypotensive states. Some of these drugs are also used to produce vasoconstriction restricted to a specific region.

Phenylephrine is used intravenously to treat a variety of conditions, including hypotensive emergencies and shock. The ability of phenylephrine to cause a systemic pressor effect (i.e., increase in blood pressure) is sometimes used in the treatment of certain types of tachycardia. The basis for its therapeutic effect is that the increase in blood pressure triggers the baroreflex to cause increased parasympathetic activity to the heart. One of the most versatile of the alpha receptor agonists, phenylephrine is also employed as a nasal decongestant (in oral cold remedies and as a nasal spray; Chapter 54) and topically in the eye to dilate the pupil (Chapter 65).

Epinephrine's ability to stimulate beta-adrenergic receptors as well as alpha receptors makes it a particularly useful drug in the treatment of **anaphylaxis,** or acute allergic reactions. Besides hypotension, another feature of anaphylaxis that may be life threatening is bronchospasm. Epinephrine can relieve this symptom by stimulating beta$_2$ receptors in the bronchioles, causing relaxation of the smooth muscle and relief of bronchoconstriction. In addition to its systemic administration alone, epinephrine is also commonly injected along with a local anesthetic to produce vasoconstriction in a limited region. This action reduces local blood flow and thereby slows the rate at which the local anesthetic drug is removed from the area. As a result, the duration of action is prolonged and lower doses can be injected (see Chapter 16). Epinephrine is sometimes used in resuscitation following cardiac arrest and is one of several sympathomimetic amines used in the eye (see Chapter 65).

Dopamine has special value in shock, particularly in septic shock where it is often used along with norepineph-

rine. Dopamine stimulates dopamine D$_1$ receptors in blood vessels in the kidney to cause vasodilation and also stimulates alpha receptors to cause vasoconstriction in most other places. The result is an increase in peripheral resistance, which elevates arterial pressure while improving blood flow to the kidneys, which are especially susceptible to permanent damage caused by low blood flow. Dopamine also has the ability to stimulate beta-adrenergic receptors on the heart, thus improving cardiac function.

Mephentermine, methoxamine, metaraminol, and phenylephrine are all used to maintain arterial pressure in diverse settings, especially where sympathetic function is impaired or depressed. Ephedrine is sometimes used for this purpose and has the added advantage of being effective when given orally. Ephedrine, its chemical cousin pseudoephedrine, and several other closely related drugs are used as nasal decongestants (see Chapter 54). Drugs that stimulate alpha-adrenergic receptors relieve nasal congestion by constricting swollen blood vessels in the nasal mucosa.

Midodrine is used in the management of autonomic failure and postural hypotension.

PHARMACOKINETICS

The naturally occurring catecholamines (dopamine, norepinephrine, epinephrine) are all ineffective when given orally and are rapidly cleared from the systemic circulation with plasma half-lives of 1 to 2 minutes. Therefore, a sustained effect requires constant intravenous infusion. None of these drugs enter the CNS to any significant degree, although infusion of epinephrine may cause excitation in some individuals. The mechanism for this effect is unknown.

Mephentermine, metaraminol, and methoxamine are all given only by the parenteral route. These drugs are biotransformed by the liver and cleared by the kidneys. When administered intramuscularly or intravenously, the effects last from 15 to 60 minutes. Intravenous phenylephrine has a similar duration of action. Phenylephrine is also effective when given orally and is administered by this route as a nasal decongestant (see below).

Like phenylephrine, ephedrine is effective when given orally and oral doses are useful to treat nasal congestion. Ephedrine has a half-life of 3 to 6 hours and when given intravenously can produce pressor effects for an hour or more. Most of the drug is excreted unchanged by the kidney. Unlike other drugs in this class, ephedrine enters the CNS where it produces significant stimulation, often referred to as an amphetamine-like effect.

ADVERSE EFFECTS
AND CONTRAINDICATIONS

All sympathomimetic drugs have the potential to provoke excessive increases in arterial pressure and marked vasoconstriction in the extremities. The latter may result in tissue necrosis at high doses or in the presence of pre-existing vascular disease. Any of these drugs has the potential to cause cerebral hemorrhage (stroke) as a result of excessive increase in arterial pressure. Restlessness and CNS stimulation are seen occasionally with epinephrine and more often with ephedrine. Midodrine sometimes causes supine hypertension. Certain sympathomimetics, especially those with indirect or beta receptor agonist activity, may cause cardiac rhythm disturbances by a combination of action directly on the heart and through baroreflex reactions to increased blood pressure.

When given systemically as nasal decongestants, sympathomimetics such as phenylephrine and ephedrine may cause urinary retention. This is especially true in middle-aged men with benign prostatic hyperplasia (BPH).

INTERACTIONS

Epinephrine may provoke a life-threatening hypertensive crisis in patients taking nonselective beta-adrenergic blocking drugs. This is because under normal conditions epinephrine causes both relaxation of blood vessels through stimulation of beta$_2$-adrenergic receptors and constriction of blood vessels through stimulation of alpha-adrenergic receptors. The result of these opposing actions is a moderate effect on blood pressure. However, in a patient whose beta receptors are blocked, the vasoconstricting action of epinephrine is unopposed, leading to severe hypertension. Beta blockers may also interfere with other therapeutic actions of epinephrine, such as bronchorelaxation. Concurrent treatment with alpha-adrenergic receptor antagonists or any drugs with alpha-adrenergic blocking action (such as haloperidol or phenothiazines) will interfere with the therapeutic effect of any adrenergic pressor drug.

Many gaseous anesthetics increase the possibility of arrhythmias caused by sympathomimetic pressor drugs, especially epinephrine or those with indirect action or the ability to stimulate cardiac beta receptors. Patients taking drugs that inhibit monoamine oxidase (MAO) inhibitors may have exaggerated responses to sympathomimetic drugs, especially those that work through an indirect action.

DRUG CLASS • Alpha-Adrenergic Receptor Antagonists (Alpha Blockers)

Nonselective

phenoxybenzamine (Dibenzyline)

phentolamine (Regitine, Rogitine✳)

tolazoline (Priscoline)

Alpha$_1$ Selective

doxazosin (Cardura)

 prazosin (Minipress)

tamsulosin (Flomax)

terazosin (Hytrin)

MECHANISM OF ACTION

Alpha blockers produce their effects by blocking alpha-adrenergic receptors. Except for phenoxybenzamine, all of the drugs listed above act as competitive antagonists at alpha-adrenergic receptors. Phenoxybenzamine binds irreversibly to alpha receptors and therefore causes effects that persist until new receptors are made. Phenoxybenzamine and the other nonselective drugs do not differentiate between alpha$_1$ and alpha$_2$ receptors to any significant degree and so block all alpha receptors. In contrast, alpha$_1$ selective drugs such as prazosin block only alpha$_1$ receptors at doses used clinically (see Figure 12-1).

In addition to blocking alpha receptors, tolazoline both releases endogenous histamine and directly stimulates histamine receptors.

USES

The nonselective alpha receptor antagonists have extremely limited clinical use (see Table 12-2). Tolazoline is occasionally used in the treatment of pulmonary hypertension in newborns. Phentolamine and phenoxybenzamine are sometimes used in the management of the hypertension associated with pheochromocytoma, a tumor of the adrenal medulla. Patients with these tumors are in danger of increases in blood pressure great enough to produce stroke because the tumor can secrete large amounts of epinephrine or norepinephrine into the bloodstream. Phentolamine and phenoxybenzamine are effective in controlling blood pressure until the tumor can be removed. However, adverse reactions limit their usefulness in other cases (discussed later).

Drugs acting as selective antagonists at alpha$_1$-adrenergic receptors are much more useful than nonselective drugs. These drugs are used primarily in the treatment of hypertension (see Chapter 41), but also in the treatment of BPH, a condition where an enlarged

TABLE 12-2

Selected Drugs that Block Adrenergic Receptors

Generic Name	Alpha Receptor	Beta$_1$ Receptor	Beta$_2$ Receptor	Central Nervous System	Main Therapeutic Use
Alpha-Adrenergic Receptor Antagonists					
phenoxybenzamine	X	0	0	0	Used in the management of pheochromocytoma (Raynaud's syndrome); treats hypertension related to pheochromocytoma
prazosin	X	0	0	0	Treats chronic hypertension; benign prostatic hyperplasia
Beta-Adrenergic Receptor Antagonists					
atenolol	0	X	0	0	Treats chronic hypertension; prophylactic for angina
betaxolol	0	X	0	0	Treats glaucoma (topical)
esmolol	0	X	0	0	Controls supraventricular tachycardia
labetalol	X	X	0	0	Treats chronic hypertension; prophylactic for angina
metoprolol	0	X	0	X	Cardioselective; treats chronic hypertension; prophylaxis for angina
propranolol	0	X	X	X	Treats chronic hypertension; prophylactic for angina, migraine, and arrhythmias
timolol	0	X	X	0	Treats chronic hypertension; glaucoma (topical)

X, Inhibition; *0*, no effect.

prostate gland makes urination more difficult, and in heart failure. Tamsulosin is more selective for producing effects in the bladder than in blood vessels and so is used only in the treatment of BPH.

PHARMACOKINETICS

Phenoxybenzamine is given orally. Its absorption is somewhat variable, averaging about 30%. Because the drug combines irreversibly with alpha receptors, a single dose produces effects that may last 3 or 4 days. Phentolamine is given intravenously and has a half-life of less than 30 minutes.

Alpha$_1$ selective drugs are effective orally and generally have excellent pharmacokinetics. All are highly protein bound and biotransformed in the liver, but they differ individually in their duration of action. Prazosin has the briefest action, with a plasma half-life of 2 to 3 hours and a duration of action of 6 to 8 hours, whereas doxazosin, the longest acting, has a plasma half life of almost 20 hours and a duration of action of nearly 36 hours.

ADVERSE REACTIONS AND CONTRAINDICATIONS

The nonselective alpha receptor antagonists may cause excessive reductions in blood pressure and orthostatic hypotension. Sedation and nasal congestion can also occur with these drugs, and ejaculation may be inhibited in men. However, one of the most troubling adverse effects of nonselective alpha blockers is an unusually large increase in heart rate, which can put a dangerous strain on a diseased heart. The tachycardia is thought to result from excessive release of norepinephrine from sympathetic nerve endings because of the blockade of presynaptic alpha$_2$ receptors. Phentolamine may cause GI stimulation, resulting in nausea and pain.

In contrast, the alpha$_1$ selective antagonists have a low incidence of adverse effects and do not usually provoke increases in heart rate. Alpha$_1$ selective antagonists may cause orthostatic hypotension, especially shortly after the first dose is given. This reaction is sometimes called the "first dose phenomenon." To avoid potential problems associated with this initial response, patients are often instructed to take these drugs at bedtime. Tamsulosin, which is more selective in producing effects in the bladder, is unlikely to cause hypotension.

INTERACTIONS

Alpha blockers interfere with the pressor and vasoconstrictor actions of any of the sympathomimetic amines described above.

PHYSIOLOGY • Beta-Adrenergic Receptors

Beta-adrenergic receptors are responsible for many important effects of norepinephrine released from sympathetic nerve endings or epinephrine circulating in the bloodstream. The two major subtypes, beta$_1$- and beta$_2$-adrenergic receptors, are involved in very different effects.

The most important beta$_1$ receptors are found in the heart (see Figure 12-1). Norepinephrine released from sympathetic nerves or epinephrine from the adrenal gland stimulate these receptors to increase heart rate, speed the conduction of the cardiac impulse from the atria to the ventricles, and increase the strength of the cardiac contraction. Also, stimulation of beta$_1$ receptors in the kidney increases the secretion of renin, an enzyme responsible for the generation of angiotensin II, a powerful vasoconstrictor.

Important physiologic effects caused by activation of beta$_2$ receptors are all based on relaxation of smooth muscle. The most significant of these effects is in the upper airways where simulation of beta$_2$-adrenergic receptors dilates the bronchioles, making it easier to move air into and out of the lungs (see Figure 12-1 and Table 12-1). Activation of beta$_2$ receptors in blood vessels in the skeletal muscle, brain, and heart causes vasodilation and shunts blood to these regions. Another site where stimulation of beta$_2$ receptors can provoke relaxation is in the pregnant uterus. Unlike beta$_1$ receptors, norepinephrine has little or no ability to stimulate beta$_2$ receptors. Instead, these responses are generally produced under natural conditions by epinephrine released from the adrenal medulla.

DRUG CLASS • Beta-Adrenergic Receptor Agonists

Nonselective

 isoproterenol (Isuprel)

Beta$_1$ Selective

 dobutamine (Dobutrex)

Beta$_2$ Selective

 albuterol (Ventolin, Proventil, Gen-Salbutamol,✱ Novo-Salmol✱)

bitolterol (Tornalate)

formoterol (Foradil)

isoetharine (Bronkosol)

levalbuterol (Xopenex)

metaproterenol (Alupent)

pirbuterol (Maxair)

ritodrine (Yutopar)

salmeterol (Serevent)

terbutaline (Brethaire, Brethine, Bricanyl)

MECHANISM OF ACTION

These drugs all act by binding reversibly to and stimulating beta-adrenergic receptors. Only isoproterenol has similar activity at both beta$_1$ and beta$_2$ receptors. All the others are relatively selective agonists at beta$_1$ receptors (dobutamine) or at beta$_2$ receptors (albuterol, for example; see Figure 12-1), but it is important to understand that this selectivity is not absolute.

USES

The most important use for beta agonists is in the treatment of patients with restricted airways, primarily caused by asthma or chronic obstructive pulmonary disease (COPD). Beta agonists are especially useful in the acute treatment of asthmatic attacks (except for salmeterol; see pharmacokinetics) but may also be used prophylactically, that is, to prevent attacks. Stimulation of beta$_2$ receptors relaxes bronchial smooth muscle, and this decreases airway resistance and makes it easier to breathe. Although the nonselective drug isoproterenol is effective as a bronchodilator and sometimes is used for this purpose, beta$_2$-selective drugs such as albuterol are generally preferred (see below). The uses of bronchodilators are discussed further in Chapter 52.

Drugs acting through stimulation of beta$_2$ receptors, such as ritodrine and terbutaline, are also used to stop premature labor by relaxing the uterus. This use is discussed in Chapter 60.

Stimulation of beta$_1$ receptors on the heart would seem to be a logical approach to help support a failing or damaged heart by increasing the strength of the contraction. In fact, the use of a drug such as isoproterenol for this purpose is generally not helpful for three reasons. First, isoproterenol causes marked increases in heart rate that may put an excessive strain on the heart. Second, isoproterenol stimulates beta$_2$ receptors in blood vessels to decrease arterial pressure at the same time that the heart needs more oxygen because it is working harder. The result of these two effects could be dangerous to a patient with heart problems or coronary artery disease. Finally, isoproterenol is a catecholamine and therefore is ineffective orally and would have to be given intravenously to affect the heart.

Dobutamine is a beta$_1$ agonist that is unusual because it produces a greater effect on the strength of the heart than on heart rate. Although dobutamine is sometimes useful in the management of severe heart failure, this usefulness is greatly limited by its pharmacokinetics as described below. Drugs used to manage or treat the failing heart are discussed further in Chapter 38.

PHARMACOKINETICS

Isoproterenol, isoetharine, bitolterol, and dobutamine are subject to extremely rapid enzymatic degradation in the body. Therefore, these drugs are not effective when given orally and have a half-life of only a few minutes in systemic circulation. Isoproterenol, isoetharine, and bitolterol are still useful as bronchodilators when they are taken by inhalation because this applies them directly to the target tissue in the airways. However, the usefulness of dobutamine to support a failing heart is ex-

tremely limited by its rapid biotransformation, so it must be given by continuous intravenous infusion to produce a sustained effect. The other beta$_2$ selective agonists can be given orally, although inhalation is still the preferred route of administration to treat bronchodilation. When given by this route, these drugs produce an effect within 5 to 10 minutes that lasts from 3 to 6 hours. The exception is salmeterol, which may take as long as 25 minutes to produce bronchodilation, although once this effect is seen it may persist for as long as 12 hours. Because of the long time to onset of therapeutic action, salmeterol is used to prevent attacks in asthmatic patients but not to treat them acutely.

Ritodrine is effective when given orally in the treatment of premature labor. The drug may also be infused intravenously if a rapid effect is needed.

ADVERSE REACTIONS AND CONTRAINDICATIONS

The most serious potential adverse reaction produced by beta agonists is increased heart rate and cardiac stimulation. In severe cases or in susceptible individuals, chest pain (angina), arrhythmias, or myocardial infarction may result. This is more likely to occur with isoproterenol than with beta$_2$ selective drugs, and after oral or intravenous administration of any drug rather than after inhalation. Muscle tremor is sometimes seen when treatment is started, but it usually disappears with continued administration. Hyperglycemia and even ketoacidosis may occur in patients who have diabetic tendencies or frank diabetes mellitus because of the metabolic effects produced by stimulation of beta-adrenergic receptors in the liver and adipose tissue.

INTERACTIONS

The therapeutic effects of beta receptor agonists will be greatly attenuated or blocked in patients treated with beta-adrenergic receptor antagonists (see next section). Alternatively, severe adverse cardiac effects of beta agonists can be treated very effectively with these drugs.

DRUG CLASS • Beta-Adrenergic Receptor Antagonists (Beta Blockers)

acebutolol (Sectral, Monitan✷)

atenolol (Tenormin, Apo-Atenolol,✷ Novo-Atenol✷)

betaxolol (Kerlone, Betoptic)

bisoprolol (Zebeta)

carteolol (Cartrol)

carvedilol (Coreg)

esmolol (Brevibloc)

labetalol (Normodyne)

levobunolol (Betagan)

metipranolol (OptiPranolol)

metoprolol (Lopressor, Toprol XL, Betaloc,✷ Lopressor,✷ Novo-Metoprol✷)

nadolol (Corgard)

penbutolol (Levatol)

pindolol (Visken, Novo-Pindol,✷ Syn-Pindolol✷)

△ propranolol (Inderal, Apo-Propranolol,✷ Detensol,✷ Novo-Pranol,✷ PMS-Propranolol)

sotalol (Betapace, Sotacor✷)

timolol (Blocadren, Timoptic, Apo-Timol,✷ Novo-Timol✷)

MECHANISM OF ACTION

Beta blockers are competitive antagonists at beta-adrenergic receptors. In the healthy person, blockade of the $beta_1$ receptors in the heart causes only a modest decrease in heart rate at rest but limits the cardiac stimulation normally seen under conditions where the sympathetic nervous system is activated, such as exercise and emotional stress. The action on $beta_1$ receptors in the heart is thought to be the basis for most of the clinical uses of beta blockers discussed below. Many beta blockers—including propranolol, the prototype drug in this class—are called nonselective because they also antagonize $beta_2$ receptors in smooth muscle (see Figure 12-1 and Table 12-2), and this action may lead to adverse effects. Some beta receptor antagonists are called **cardioselective** because they produce a greater effect on $beta_1$ receptors on the heart, and are therefore preferred in certain patients.

Certain beta blockers have additional actions that may contribute to their usefulness in some disease states. Propranolol has a membrane stabilizing effect (sometimes called a "quinidine-like" effect) and so has the ability to depress all excitable tissue, including the heart and nerves. However, this action may only be significant at relatively high doses of propranolol. Pindolol, and to a lesser extent, acebutolol are partial agonists that actually cause a low degree of stimulation when they occupy beta receptors. Because of this property, often referred to as **intrinsic sympathomimetic activity** or simply **ISA**, these drugs are more likely to protect the heart from the effects of nervous stimulation while avoiding excessive cardiac depression. Labetalol and carvedilol also block alpha receptor antagonists and so lower peripheral resistance. Sotalol blocks potassium channels in the heart.

USES

Propranolol, the first beta receptor antagonist approved for clinical use in the United States, as well as many other nonselective and cardioselective beta blockers are used extensively in the treatment of a number of the most important cardiovascular disease states, including angina (Chapter 39), hypertension (Chapter 41), and arrhythmias (Chapter 40). Sotalol is especially useful in the treatment of certain arrhythmias because it also affects potassium channels. It is now standard practice to administer beta blockers to patients who have had heart attacks in order to protect their hearts from the potentially harmful effects of excessive sympathetic stimulation. Low doses of carvedilol and several other beta blockers have even been found to be beneficial in patients suffering from heart failure (Chapter 38).

Beta blockers are effective in treating hypertension as monotherapy. The mechanism by which beta blockers lower blood pressure in hypertensive patients is not fully understood, but they act in an additive fashion when combined with diuretics to lower blood pressure. Also, when a beta blocker is given with a vasodilator drug, the beta blocker inhibits the reflex activation of the heart caused by the drop in blood pressure. Therefore a beta blocker combined with a diuretic and vasodilator is an especially effective combination for treating hypertension. Labetalol, one of a number of beta blockers used in the treatment of hypertension, also works to lower blood pressure by blocking alpha-adrenergic receptors.

A blockade of $beta_2$ receptors may cause bronchoconstriction in patients with asthma or asthmatic tendencies and therefore can severely compromise pulmonary function. This effect has led to the development of $beta_1$ selective antagonists (cardioselective antagonists) such as atenolol, metoprolol, and acebutolol that are thought to be less likely than nonselective drugs to cause respiratory problems. Esmolol is another cardioselective beta blocker with a special use in critically ill or surgical patients because of its rapid pharmacokinetics.

Timolol, betaxolol, levobunolol, and metipranolol are examples of beta receptor antagonists effective in treating glaucoma by reducing the production of aqueous humor in the eye. They are discussed along with other ophthalmic drugs in Chapter 65.

Beta blockers are also useful in the prevention or treatment of hyperthyroidism, migraine headache, performance anxiety, and even alcohol withdrawal. The connections between the therapeutic effects of these drugs and the physiologic roles of beta receptors in most of these conditions are often not clear.

PHARMACOKINETICS

The prototype beta blocker, propranolol, and several others that followed have low oral bioavailability because they are subject to a first-pass effect and are rapidly cleared from the bloodstream by biotransformation in the liver. These characteristics are important issues for drugs used in the treatment of chronic conditions such as hypertension because they must be taken more than once a day to maintain their effects. For this reason, a significant improvement came with drugs whose pharmacokinetics allow once-daily dosing. Such drugs include nadolol, with a half-life of up to 20 hours, acebutolol, which is biotransformed to an active metabolite, and atenolol.

On the other hand, esmolol is useful in certain settings where a very short duration of action is desired. Because enzymes in the blood rapidly destroy it, esmolol has a half-life of only 5 to 10 minutes in the circulation. Therefore, this drug is given by continuous intravenous infusion usually in critical care or surgical settings where the heart must be protected from excessive stimulation. Because of its ultra-short half-life, the degree of blockade can be quickly adjusted in either direction by increasing or decreasing the rate of infusion.

ADVERSE REACTIONS AND CONTRAINDICATIONS

Beta blockers depress the function of the heart by blocking the effects of the sympathetic nervous system. This action results in bradycardia (slowed heart rate) in a normal heart but may provoke heart failure or other significant cardiac problems in certain patients with damaged or abnormal hearts. Exercise tolerance is also impaired by beta blockers because an important physiologic adjustment to exercise involves increased sympathetic tone to the heart.

Beta blockers may cause bronchospasm or asthmatic attacks in patients with asthma or asthmatic tendencies. Cardioselective beta blockers may be less likely to cause these respiratory problems, but in general all beta blockers should be avoided in susceptible patients.

Troublesome CNS effects caused by beta blockers include fatigue, depression, and nightmares.

In patients with diabetes, beta blockers may prevent the tachycardia that typically warns the patient when blood sugar levels drop excessively.

INTERACTIONS

Beta blockers interfere with bronchodilator effects of epinephrine in the acute treatment of anaphylaxis or of any of the beta receptor agonists used in the treatment of chronic obstructive pulmonary disease (COPD) to produce bronchodilation. Allergenic challenges that would not be considered dangerous otherwise may cause anaphylaxis in a patient being treated with a beta blocker. In addition, the bronchodilator activity of epinephrine administered to such a patient would be impaired or prevented if the patient is also taking a beta blocker. As discussed above, when epinephrine is given at usual therapeutic doses to a patient being treated with a beta blocker, an excessive increase in blood pressure may result.

Insulin-dependent patients with diabetes have an increased risk for severe hypoglycemia when a beta blocker is used. Beta receptor blockade prevents the tachycardia that usually warns such a patient of excessively low blood glucose levels. Also, beta receptor blockade interferes with physiologic mechanisms that would normally respond to hypoglycemia by producing more glucose.

General anesthesia with halothane, which also causes cardiac depression, may cause an excessive reduction in cardiac output in a patient taking a beta blocker.

Other Drugs Acting on Sympathetic Mechanisms

All the drugs discussed in this chapter influence sympathetic mechanisms by acting more or less selectively on one of the types or subtypes of adrenergic receptors. However, there are also drugs that interfere with the function of sympathetic nerve endings themselves. Because these drugs act on sympathetic nerves everywhere and not only on certain receptors, they generally cause many unwanted adverse reactions. Therefore, these drugs, which are termed adrenergic neuron blockers, have a limited use in the management of hypertension and hypertensive emergencies, and are discussed in Chapter 41.

APPLICATION TO PRACTICE

ASSESSMENT
History of Present Illness

Inquire about the onset, intensity, and duration of the patient's symptoms. What has been done to relieve the symptoms? What activities or interventions make the symptoms worse? Determine whether the patient has had the symptoms previously and what treatment was rendered.

Health History

Because of the urgency with which many sympathetic nervous system drugs are used, there may be little time to obtain a thorough patient history. However, ask about a history of pheochromocytoma, tachyarrhythmias such as ventricular fibrillation, hypovolemia, general anesthesia, and occlusive vascular disease. Elicit information regarding a history of narrow-angle glaucoma, organic brain damage, cerebral arteriosclerosis, coronary insufficiency, and renal dysfunction. Information about diabetes, hyperthyroidism, prostatic hyperplasia, and seizure disorders should also be elicited. Ask about drugs the patient is currently taking, including over-the-counter and prescription drugs. Determine whether the patient has sensitivities to specific drugs or components of the drug preparation to be used.

Lifespan Considerations

Perinatal. Blood loss from vaginal delivery or cesarean section is notoriously underestimated. Compensatory mechanisms may provide a normal blood pressure until blood loss exceeds 1000 to 1500 mL. Blood loss can be concealed (e.g., abruptio placentae) and not appreciated until shock occurs. Patients at risk for obstetric hemorrhage are those of multiparity or those who have been diagnosed with placenta previa. Because of the young age of most obstetric patients and their lack of underlying disease, mortality from septic shock is distinctly uncommon. This is true despite the frequent presence of infections in the upper and lower genital tracts. As in hemorrhage, compensatory mechanisms may mask the severity of sepsis, and shock may occur suddenly when they are overcome. Acute respiratory distress syndrome (ARDS) and disseminated intravascular coagulation may accompany septic shock. Adrenergic drugs are usually avoided during lactation.

Pediatric. The circulatory system of a healthy child is able to transport oxygen and nutrients to meet essential needs of the body tissues. The cardiac output and distribution of blood flow to various body tissues can change rapidly in response to intrinsic (myocardial and intravascular) or extrinsic (neuronal) control mechanisms. In shock states, these mechanisms are altered or challenged. Septic shock is the most common form of shock seen in newborns.

Older Adults. The physiologic changes in the cardiovascular system of an older adult manifest in a variety of ways. The efficiency and contractile strength of the myocardium declines, resulting in a 1% per year reduction in cardiac output. It is thought that stroke volume decreases by 0.7% yearly. The systolic and diastolic phases of the myocardial cycle are prolonged. Ordinarily, older adults adjust to these changes without much difficulty. However, when unusual demands are placed on the heart (e.g., shoveling snow, running to catch a bus), the changes become more evident. Pulse rates may not reach the levels of younger people, and tachycardia lasts longer.

Resistance to peripheral blood flow increases by 1% each year. Decreased elasticity of the arteries is responsible for vascular changes of the heart, kidneys, and pituitary gland. The rigidity of vessel walls and narrowing of lumens require more force to move blood through the vessels. These changes lead to a higher diastolic blood pressure. There is also a decrease in the ability of the aorta to distend, in turn causing an increase in systolic pressure. Vagal tone increases and the heart becomes more sensitive to carotid sinus stimulation. Reduced sensitivity of baroreceptors contributes to orthostatic hypotension. The normal changes of aging do not usually influence venous circulation.

Cultural/Social Considerations

There are few social and cultural considerations in the use of sympathetic nervous system drugs with the exception of cost. Many of these drugs are costly even though there may only be a one-time use. However, there is evidence that significant short- and long-term emotional distress occurs in patients with chronic cardiorespiratory disorders or a history of anaphylaxis. The distress can manifest as sleep disturbances, restlessness, irritability, and a strong identification with death although long-term emotional disturbances are rare. The perceived vulnerability and powerlessness complicate the plan of care. For some patients, the sense of vulnerability is alleviated by surgery (e.g., coronary artery bypass graft) because it is perceived as curative or by their ability to attribute the arrhythmia to a specific correctable cause (i.e., potassium imbalance). The sense of powerlessness stems from real and perceived losses, including losses of employment and financial security, role status, physical or social independence, short-term memory, and control over their illness.

Physical Examination

Body weight and skin color should be noted. Temperature, pulse rate and rhythm, blood pressure, and respiratory rate and depth should evaluated. The chest should be auscultated for adventitious sounds. Urinary output should also be noted. In some patients, the prostate is palpated to note any enlargement.

Laboratory Testing

Most patients require blood tests for serum electrolytes, hemoglobin and hematocrit, prothrombin time (PT), partial thromboplastin time (PTT), thyroid function, glucose, blood urea nitrogen (BUN), and creatinine. An electrocardiographic tracing is also used to determine the heart's response. For patients with reactive airway disease, a chest x-ray, peak expiratory flow rate, or pulmonary function test may be indicated as well as measurement of arterial blood gas levels.

GOALS OF THERAPY

The treatment goals for a patient in shock are determined by the type of shock but, in general, are threefold: (1) maintain mean arterial pressure above 60 mm Hg (in a normal adult) to ensure adequate perfusion of vital organs, (2) maintain blood flow to those organs most often damaged by shock (i.e., kidneys, liver, CNS, lungs), and (3) maintain arterial blood lactate levels below 22 mmol/L. In hypovolemic shock, the goal is to restore vascular volume. In cardiogenic shock, treatment is directed at reducing the workload of the heart while improving pumping efficacy. Treatment goals for the patient with anaphylaxis are directed toward maintaining adequate respiratory gas exchange, cardiac output, and tissue perfusion. Treatment goals for the patient with septic shock include maintenance of adequate organ system perfusion and function.

INTERVENTION
Administration

Extreme caution should be used when calculating and preparing doses of sympathetic nervous system drugs. Some adrenergics are very potent; thus, small errors in dosage can cause serious adverse reactions. Double check pediatric dosages. When adrenergics are used as a pressor drug, fluid volume deficit is corrected with volume expanders before initiating dopamine, epinephrine, or norepinephrine therapy. Adrenergic inhalation may be alternated with other drug administration (e.g., steroids, other adrenergics) if necessary, but should not be administered simultaneously because of the danger of excessive tachycardia. Tachy-

phylaxis or tolerance may develop after prolonged or excessive use.

The drugs used in an emergency should be administered in large veins of the antecubital fossa in preference to veins of the hand or ankle. Phentolamine, a nonselective alpha antagonist, should be available in the event of extravasation of an alpha agonist drug.

The cardiovascular effects of sympathetic nervous system drugs should be monitored carefully, particularly in patients with a history of hypertension or other cardiovascular disorders. A rapid-acting alpha blocker such as phentolamine or a vasodilator (a nitrite) should be available in the event of an excessive hypertensive reaction. Patients diagnosed with atrial fibrillation who are to be treated with dobutamine will require digitalization (see Chapter 38) before being given dobutamine. Dobutamine facilitates atrioventricular conduction.

Education

Because sympathetic nervous system drugs are most often used in emergency situations, patient teaching depends on the patient's awareness and medical status. Advise patients using these drugs to notify the health care provider if they experience chest pain, dizziness, insomnia, weakness, tremor, or irregular heart beat.

When the drugs are used in the outpatient setting, instruct the patient to continue taking the drug, even if he or she is feeling well. Abrupt withdrawal may cause rebound hypertension. Drug therapy controls but does not cure some of the disorders for which these drugs are used. Instruct the patient and family on proper technique for monitoring blood pressure. Advise them to check the blood pressure weekly and report significant changes. Caution the patient to make position changes slowly to minimize orthostatic hypotension. Advise the patient that exercise or hot weather may enhance the hypotensive effects of adrenergic-blocking drugs. Emphasize the importance of follow-up examinations to monitor progress.

EVALUATION

The desired outcome of drug therapy with sympathetic nervous system drugs is correction of hemodynamic imbalance and increase in cardiac output, blood pressure, peripheral circulation, and urinary output.

Bibliography

Braunwald E, Hauser S, Fauci A, et al., eds.: *Harrison's principles of internal medicine*, ed 15, New York, 2001, McGraw-Hill.

Edwards S: Shock: types, classifications and explorations of their physiological effects, *Emergency Nurse* 9(2):29-39, 2001.

Hardman J, Limbird L: *Goodman and Gilman's the pharmacological basis of therapeutics,* ed 10, New York, 2001, McGraw-Hill.

Haviland MD: Making sense of the beta-agonist debate: a guide for nurse practitioners, *J Ped Health Care* 11(5):215-221, 1997.

Spolarich AE: Drugs used to manage cardiovascular disease. Part II. Adrenergic agonists and antagonists, *Access* 15(3):34-39, 2001.

Zusman RM: The role of alpha$_1$-blockers in combination therapy for hypertension, *Int J Clin Pract* 54(1):36-41, 2000.

Internet Resources

University of Kentucky: Adrenergic pharmacology. Available online: http://www.mc.uky.edu/pharmacology/instruction/pha824ar/PHA824ar.html.

Centenary Cardiology Associates: Beta blockers. Available online: http://www.centenarycardiology.com/Therapies/Medications/Beta_Blockers.htm.

Healthwise: Alpha blockers for benign prostatic hyperplasia (BPH). Available online: http://www.healthwise.org/kbase/topic/detail/drug/hw59707/detail.htm.

Health Evolution: Alpha blockers. Available online: http://www.healthevolution.com/Articles/AlphaBlockers.html.

Drug Digest: Alpha blockers. Available online: http://www.drugdigest.org/DD/HC/HCDrugClass/0,4055,5,00.html.

Pharmacology Central: Adrenergics. Available online: http://www.pharmcentral.com/adrenergics.htm.

Pharmacology 2000: Sympathomimetic agents. Available online: http://www.pharmacology2000.com/Autonomics/Adrenergics/sympclin1.htm.

International Program on Chemical Safety: Intox Project: Alpha adrenergic crisis. Available online: http://www.intox.org/pagesource/treatment/english/alphaadrenergic.htm.

CHAPTER

13

Opioid Analgesics

MICHAEL R. VASKO • KATHLEEN GUTIERREZ

 Visit http://evolve.elsevier.com/Gutierrez/ for additional information.

KEY TERMS

Acute pain, p. 170

Analgesics, p. 168

Antitussives, p. 174

Chronic pain, p. 170

Endogenous peptides, p. 168

Mixed agonist-antagonist, p. 171

Opioids, p. 168

Opioid receptors, p. 171

Phantom pain, p. 170

Physical dependence, p. 178

Placebo, p. 171

Psychologic dependence, p. 178

Referred pain, p. 170

Tolerance, p. 177

Vascular pain, p. 170

Withdrawal (abstinence) syndrome, p. 178

OBJECTIVES

- Explain the action of morphine in the central nervous system (CNS) and other parts of the body.

- Explain the differences among opioid agonists, antagonists, and mixed agonist-antagonists, and identify the clinical uses of each group of drugs.

- Explain the reasons for alternative drug delivery of opioids.

- Describe the roles of endogenous opioid peptides and the three types of opioid receptors in providing pain relief.

- Discuss tolerance and dependence with opioids.

- Describe the symptoms and treatment of acute opioid toxicity.

- Develop a nursing care plan for the patient receiving an opioid analgesic.

Analgesics are drugs that relieve pain without significantly affecting other sensory input, such as touch. The major classes of drugs that produce analgesia are the opioids, the nonsteroidal antiinflammatory drugs (NSAIDs, see Chapter 14), and for acute localized pain the local anesthetics (see Chapter 16). This chapter discusses the opioids, which are drugs formerly referred to as narcotic analgesics, and describes the nature of pain and its treatment with opioids. **Opioids** can be classified as *agonists*, drugs that activate specific opioid receptor subtypes; *mixed agonist-antagonists*, drugs that are agonists at one receptor subtype but are antagonists at others; and "pure" *antagonists*, drugs that have no activity at opioid receptors but block the effects of agonists. The pharmacology of morphine, the prototype opioid agonist, is reviewed, followed by a discussion of the specific characteristics of other clinically used opioids.

HISTORY OF OPIOIDS

Opium has been used throughout history to produce analgesia, to treat dysentery and diarrhea, and to produce euphoria. The earliest recorded use of juice from the opium poppy was in the third century BC. The word opium comes from the Greek, *opion*, meaning poppy juice, which is collected from the seedpod of *Papaver somniferum*, a variety of poppy. About 10% of the content of opium is morphine. Codeine and other alkaloids such as the nonopioid papaverine can also be extracted from the juice of the opium poppy. Morphine was isolated in 1806 by Serturner and was named after Morpheus, the Greek god of dreams. Morphine was the first pure chemical substance extracted from a natural product that mimicked the pharmacologic effects of that product. In the nineteenth century, opium and

morphine were readily available in the United States and were often ingredients of patent drugs. By the late nineteenth century, attempts were made to modify the structure of morphine to keep the analgesic property but eliminate the addictive potential. The first semisynthetic opioid was heroin, but heroin produces drug dependence more readily than morphine. Today heroin is not a legal drug in the United States or Canada, although it is in other countries. Most other opioids are listed as controlled substances in the United States and Canada. The first purely synthetic morphinelike compound was meperidine, which came into clinical use in the 1940s. Because meperidine was not a chemical modification of morphine, it was commonly thought not to cause drug dependence. Today, meperidine is considered a drug with high abuse potential (schedule II) similar to morphine. The search for drugs that could have the therapeutic actions of morphine without the adverse effects led to the discovery of nalorphine, a mixed opioid agonist and antagonist and naloxone, a pure opioid antagonist. Naloxone is important for two reasons: first, it is an antagonist for opioids and rapidly reverses the effects of the agonist in cases of acute overdose; second, the discovery of a specific antagonist for opioids suggested that the drugs acted at specific receptor sites in the brain. In the early 1970s opioid receptors were discovered, followed 2 years later by the discovery of **endogenous peptides** that had selective opioidlike actions through binding to opioid receptors. Today, we know of three clinically important opioid receptors, *mu*, *kappa*, and *delta*, and five distinct groups of endogenous opioid peptides, *enkephalins*, *endorphins*, *dynorphins*, *orphanins*, and *endomorphins*.

PHYSIOLOGY • Pain

Pain is a normal manifestation of everyday life and is an essential defense mechanism. Pain is defined by the International Association for the Study of Pain as an unpleasant sensory and emotional experience arising from actual or potential tissue damage, or is described in terms of such damage. A useful working definition, however, is put forth by Margo McCaffery, a registered nurse who is a recognized pain expert, *"pain is whatever the experiencing person says it is and exists whenever he says it does."* This definition requires that the patient be seen as the authority on his pain and the only person who can define the experience. Acute pain is useful because it signals a pathologic situation and protects us from injury caused by extreme temperatures, mechanical pres-

sure, or penetrating wounds. A person in pain usually takes action to eliminate the pain or its cause. Indeed, it is the main symptom that causes people to seek health care intervention. With chronic pain states, however, the clinical picture is much more complicated. Conventional acute pain therapies are often ineffective or need to be administered with other interventions that address the affective component of chronic pain. Unmanaged or undermanaged chronic pain dramatically diminishes the quality of life more than any other single health-related problem.

There are many pathologic origins of pain, including central or peripheral nervous system disorders, musculoskeletal damage, vascular disease, inflammation, or malignancy. Back pain is one of the most common pain complaints, second only to headache. Psychogenic pain, although not related to physiologic dysfunction, can nonetheless result in pain. Pain is a response to the trauma of surgery; over 23 million operations have been performed in the United States since 1989. In addition, pain related to malignancy occurs in 60% to 80% of patients with solid tumors.

The prevalence of pain in patients with human immunodeficiency virus (HIV) infection range from 25% to 40% in early and ambulatory patients to 60% to 100% in patients with end-stage disease. There are many sources of pain in this population, including gastrointestinal (GI) pain related to oropharyngeal candidiasis or herpes, esophagitis, gastritis, or colitis; herpes and cytomegalovirus infections; peripheral neuropathy; headache; pleuritic pain from pneumonia; and pain from lymphatic obstruction caused by Kaposi's sarcoma.

Regardless of the etiology, pain has both sensory *(perception)* and affective *(interpretation)* components. An understanding of the elements that control pain perception from damaged tissues, the spinal cord, and higher brain centers is needed to provide effective pain management. However, pain interpretation varies among patients and health care providers alike, which, in turn, strongly influences pain management strategies.

PAIN PATHWAYS

The perception of pain begins when sensory nerve endings or *nociceptors* in the periphery are stimulated by a noxious stimulus. Noxious stimuli can be mechanical (e.g., stretching of organs or pressure), thermal (i.e., extremes of heat or cold), or chemical (e.g., bradykinin, serotonin, potassium ions, acids, or acetylcholine). The sensory neurons that conduct noxious information are the small diameter A-delta or C fibers that have a slow conduction velocity and a high threshold for activation. The numerous chemicals released in response to tissue trauma change the sensitivity of these neurons and augment their activation at lower thresholds. This leads to an enhanced perception of a painful stimulus *(hyperalgesia)* or the perception of a normally nonpainful stimulus as painful *(allodynia)*. A good example of the latter is the pain of a simple touch after a burn. An important class of chemicals that sensitizes sensory neurons is the *prostaglandins*. These locally released chemicals are produced from arachidonic acid by enzymes known as *cyclooxygenases*. A major action of NSAIDs (nonsteroidal antiinflammatory drugs) is to inhibit this activity of cyclooxygenases, thereby preventing prostaglandin production (see Chapter 14).

After activation of nociceptors, nerve impulses travel through A-delta or C sensory fibers in the periphery to reach the spinal cord, unless they are blocked by local anesthetics (see Chapter 16). The cell bodies for these sensory neurons lie within the dorsal root ganglion, outside the central nervous system, and the nerve fibers terminate in laminae I, II, and V of the dorsal spinal cord. These areas receive, transmit, and process noxious sensory input and are thought to be the site of the gating of noxious input originally described by Melzack and Wall in their gate control theory of the mid-1960s. The dorsal spinal cord is also the site where the pain signal can be regulated by a number of drugs, including opioids and alpha$_2$-adrenergic agonists.

From the dorsal spinal cord, the pain signal is conducted to higher brain centers by distinct pathways, the major pathways being ascending spinothalamic tracts. The most direct pathway is along the neospinothalamic tract, which begins in the dorsal horn of the spinal cord and projects into the posterior nucleus of the thalamus to provide discriminatory functions such as the location, intensity, and duration of the painful stimulus. This pathway has few synapses and thus permits rapid impulse conduction. A more diffuse pathway is the paleospinothalamic tract, which leads to the thalamus indirectly through synapses in the brainstem. Impulse transmission through this structure is associated with autonomic nervous system responses and the unpleasant emotional aspects of pain. From the thalamus, the pain signal is communicated to various regions in the forebrain. These regions are associated with the perception of pain, the affective component of pain, and autonomic responses to pain.

An analogous pathway conducting noxious impulses from the neck and head is through the trigeminal system. The trigeminal ganglion is the site of sensory cell bodies that project from the periphery to the trigeminal nucleus. From there, the fibers conduct noxious impulses to the ventral posterior thalamus via the ventral trigeminothalamic tract.

There are wide variations among individuals in the perception and interpretation of pain. Peripheral pain perception is modulated by a number of proinflammatory substances and possibly opioids. At the level of the dorsal horn of the spinal cord, interneurons and descending pathways modify the incoming pain signal. For the most part, this modulation is inhibitory, but evidence suggests that in certain chronic pain states, there might be a descending activation. In general, the interneurons in the dorsal horn inhibit the pain signal by releasing endogenous opioids or gamma-aminobutyric acid (GABA), whereas descending pathways involve the neurotransmitters serotonin and norepinephrine. Because there are a number of sites in the body and factors that regulate the perception of pain, there can be a wide range of patient responses to injury.

TYPES OF PAIN

There are several ways to define types of pain, including the onset of occurrence, duration, severity or intensity, mode of transmission, location or source, and causation. The pain threshold, which is the lowest intensity of stimulus perceived by the patient as pain, is essentially the same for all people as long as the central and peripheral nervous systems remain intact. However, the threshold may vary within each person based on a number of physiologic and psychosocial factors (e.g., age, gender, disease or condition, fatigue, insomnia, anxiety, the meaning of the pain, past experiences with pain, depression, isolation, religious beliefs, and cultural expectations). Pain tolerance, on the other hand, is different for each person and varies based on many subjective factors. In reality, pain tolerance refers to the amount of pain the patient is willing to endure. Only the patient can relate what that tolerance level is, not the health care provider.

In general, pain is defined as either acute or chronic. **Acute pain** is short term, generally lasting only for the duration of tissue damage. It has an identifiable cause (e.g., inflammation, trauma, or surgery) and an immediate onset. Acute pain is relieved once the trauma or injury is addressed and the chemical mediators of pain are removed. In contrast, chronic pain is long lasting and can persist in the absence of pathology. There are a number of determinants of the severity of chronic pain including physiologic, psychologic, and social issues.

Acute pain can be classified further as somatic or visceral. *Somatic* pain originates in cutaneous tissues such as skin and superficial tissues. Pain in these structures is well defined and localized. Although the pain is of low to moderate intensity, it stimulates the sympathetic nervous system to increase blood pressure, pulse rate, and respirations; dilates pupils; and increases the tension of skeletal muscles. In contrast, deep pain originates in bone, nerves, muscles, blood vessels, and other supporting tissues of the abdominal or thoracic cavities. It produces a dull, aching sensation that is hard to localize. Deep pain stimulates the parasympathetic nervous system, reducing blood pressure and pulse, but often causing nausea and vomiting, weakness, syncope, and possibly loss of consciousness.

Visceral pain arises from body organs and the pain sensations are diffuse and poorly localized. Visceral nociceptors are insensitive to cuts and temperature extremes, but they are sensitive to ischemia, inflammation, and stretching. Nerve fibers in body organs follow sympathetic nerves to the spinal cord. This may explain why autonomic manifestations (i.e., diarrhea, cramps, sweating, and hypertension) frequently accompany visceral pain. Typical visceral pain includes that associated with acute appendicitis, cholecystitis, biliary and pancreatic tract inflammation, gastroduodenal disease, cardiovascular disease, pleurisy, and renal and ureteral colic. Visceral nociceptors transmit referred pain.

Referred pain occurs because visceral nerve fibers synapse at a level in the spinal cord close to fibers supplying certain subcutaneous tissues of the body. This type of pain is peculiar in that it is sometimes intense, although there is little or no pain at the point of the noxious stimulus. For example, pain associated with cholecystitis is referred to the back and the scapula. Pleural pain from the diaphragm is referred to the shoulder, and myocardial ischemia is often felt in the left arm, shoulder, or jaw.

Vascular pain is believed to originate from a pathologic condition of vascular or perivascular tissues. Distention, displacement, or pulling on cranial vessels may account for a large portion of migraine headaches and headaches associated with arterial hypertension, brain tumors, and variations in the hydrodynamics of cerebrospinal fluid. Blood vessel responses are thought to be associated with pain induced by cold.

Chronic pain is defined as pain of at least 6 months' duration. It may occur with or without evidence of tissue damage and, unlike other types of pain, it serves little if any useful purpose. When allowed to persist, chronic pain results in fatigue and irritability. Chronic pain is not characterized by physical signs but is often accompanied by depression and changes in personality, lifestyle, and reduced functional ability. Chronic pain is difficult to describe and difficult to manage because it is often unresponsive to conventional management strategies. One form of chronic pain, neuropathic pain, is caused by injury or damage to nerve fibers in the periphery or by damage to the CNS. Neuropathic pain is often present in the absence of pathologic processes known to produce pain or in the absence of otherwise painful stimuli. **Phantom pain** is associated with the traumatic or surgical amputation of a body part. Patients describe the pain as residing in the missing body part, with the sensations described as itching, tingling, stabbing, or burning.

The pain of cancer has multiple causes and can be composed of several types at any given time. Cancer pain can be caused by pressure on or displacement of nerves, interference with blood supply, or blockage within hollow organs. Metastasis to the bone is a common cause of cancer pain. Other causes are the result of cancer treatments, such as surgery, radiation therapy, and antineoplastic therapy. Immobility and inflammation contribute to cancer pain.

Other types of pain, although they are not encountered as frequently, deserve a brief discussion. Central pain is associated with lesions, tumors, trauma, or inflammation in the brain. This pain manifests as high-frequency bursts of impulses that patients describe as severe, spontaneous, and often unyielding. Central pain can occur with any disorder that produces CNS damage, including cancer, diabetes, stroke, multiple sclerosis, or trauma. Thalamic pain is extremely rare, may occur after a thalamic injury. It is described by patients as hyperesthesia (abnormally increased sensitivity to stimuli) in one half of the body. Thalamic pain can range in intensity from paresthesias (i.e., numbness, tingling, or prickling) to agonizing, boring, burning pain.

Psychogenic pain is distress primarily caused by psychologic factors rather than to physiologic dysfunction, but it is very real to that patient. The tension or stress the patient feels may lead to pronounced physiologic changes. Unfortunately, this type of pain is often thought to be "all in the head," and the diagnosis is assigned to the patient prematurely. However, careful assessment may uncover a treatable physiologic cause for the pain. Further, pain relief obtained with a **placebo,** a supposedly inert substance such as a sugar pill or injection of saline solution given under the guise of effective pain treatment, does not mean the patient does not have pain. Paradoxically, a placebo may exert either a positive or negative effect on the recipient. When the psychogenic effects of stress, anxiety, fear, and anger produce painful physiologic responses, the pain is known as psychophysiologic pain.

DRUG CLASS • Opioid Agonists

℞ morphine (Contin)

The opioids can be divided into three classes (Table 13-1): natural and semisynthetic opiate alkaloids (e.g., morphine, codeine, oxymorphone, hydromorphone, oxycodone, hydrocodone, levorphanol, and heroin), piperidines and phenylpiperidines (e.g., meperidine, diphenoxylate, fentanyl, sufentanil, alfentanil), and methadone-like drugs (e.g., methadone, levomethadyl acetate, propoxyphene). The pharmacology of morphine, the prototype opioid, provides the standard for describing and comparing the actions of all opioid agonists. Therefore the general activities of morphine are described in depth, including the biochemical basis of action and the central and peripheral physiologic effects. Differences in uses, pharmacokinetics, and toxicity of individual drugs will be discussed separately.

MECHANISM OF ACTION

In the early 1970s scientists demonstrated that specific receptors for opioids exist in the brain, spinal cord, and gut. These receptors bind opioids in a stereo-specific manner (i.e., only one of the two mirror image forms binds) and the binding was blocked by naloxone. At the present time three subtypes of clinically important opioid receptors have been characterized. The mu receptor mediates central analgesia, euphoria, respiratory depression, and physical dependence. It is activated by both exogenous opioid agonists and by various endogenous opioids. Pharmacologic studies suggest that there are a number of mu receptor subtypes.

The kappa receptors mediate spinal analgesia, miosis, sedation, and appetite regulation. The kappa$_1$ receptor is associated with spinal analgesia, whereas the kappa$_2$ receptor is associated with analgesia in regions of the brain associated with pain modulation. The kappa receptors are activated by opioids with **mixed agonist-antagonist** activity, but these drugs act as antagonists at mu receptors. Kappa receptors are also activated by the naturally occurring dynorphins. Unlike the euphoria associated with mu receptors, the kappa receptors are associated with disoriented or depersonalized feelings.

The delta receptor appears to mediate analgesia both spinally and in brain structures. It is thought to be the primary receptor for some group of endogenous opioids, and to date there are no selective drugs available for clinical use. Using various molecular biologic techniques, unique receptors with sequence homology to known opioid receptors have been identified. One such "orphan receptor" (a term that refers to a receptor without a known agonist) is the N/OFQ receptor, which has a low affinity for classic opioid peptides and a high affinity for the peptide nociceptin (orphanin FQ).

All **opioid receptors** are G protein–coupled receptors. Activation of these receptors is involved with inhibiting activity of neurons. This inhibition could result from either activation of potassium channels, which contributes to the hyperpolarization of neurons or an inhibition of calcium channels, which could diminish transmitter release. The properties and pharmacology of opioid receptor subtypes are actively being studied. Future research should clarify the nature of analgesia and the development of the opioid type of drug dependence and provide the basis for understanding the role of opioid peptides in mental disorders, seizure activity, and behavior patterns involving the reward system, eating, and drinking.

TABLE 13-1			

Opioid Agonists, Mixed Agonists-Antagonists, and Antagonists

Generic Name	Brand Name	Uses	Comments
Agonists			
codeine	Generic, Paveral✽	Mild to moderate pain	When combined with nonopioid analgesics (aspirin or acetaminophen): #2 = 15 mg codeine, #3 = 30 mg codeine, and #4 = 60 mg codeine.
Transdermal fentanyl	Duragesic	Chronic pain	Transdermal fentanyl is not recommended for control of postoperative or mild intermittent pain. Additional short-acting opioids should be available for breakthrough pain until conversion from other opiods is successful.
hydrocodone	Lorcet, Lortab, Vicodin, Hycodan, Dolagesic, Hydrocet	Moderate to severe pain	Available in combination with acetaminophen or aspirin. May be administered with food or milk to minimize GI irritation.
hydromorphone	Dilaudid, Dilaudid HP	Moderate to severe pain	An initial bolus of two times the hourly rate in milligrams may be given with subsequent breakthrough boluses of 50% to 100% of the hourly rate in milligrams.
levophanol	Levo-Dromoran, Levorphan	Moderate to severe pain	Unlabeled for use in children. Use with extreme caution in patients receiving MAO inhibitors.
meperidine	Demerol	Moderate to severe pain, obstetric analgesia, preoperative sedation, adjunct to anesthesia	Do not confuse with morphine or hydromorphone—fatalities have occurred. May be administered with food or milk to minimize GI irritation. Local irritation is possible with repeated SC administration. Oral dose is 50% less effective than parenteral formulation.
methadone	Dolophine, Methadose	Severe pain, suppression of opioid withdrawal symptoms	May be administered with food or milk to minimize GI irritation. Diskettes (dispersible tablets) are to be dissolved and used for detoxification and maintenance treatment only.
morphine	Morphine HP,✽ MS Contin, Roxanol, Statex✽	Moderate to severe pain, pulmonary edema, myocardial infarction	Larger doses may be required for chronic therapy. IV infusion rates vary greatly; up to 440 mg per hour have been used.
oxycodone	Oxycontin, Roxicodone, Percodan, Percocet Supeudol,✽ Oxycocet,✽ Oxycodan✽	Moderate to severe pain	May be administered with food or milk to minimize GI irritation. Controlled-release tablets should be taken whole, not crushed or chewed. Empty matrix tablets may appear in the stool with controlled release formulation.
oxymorphone	Numorphan	Moderate to severe pain	Suppositories should be stored in the refrigerator.
propoxyphene	Darvon, Darvocet-N, Darvon Compound, Darvon-N✽	Mild to moderate pain	Doses may be administered with food or milk to minimize GI irritation.
Opioid Agonist-Antagonists			
butorphanol	Stadol	Moderate to severe pain, obstetric analgesia, preoperative sedation, adjunct to anesthesia	Instruct patient on proper use of nasal spray. Use with extreme caution in patients taking MAO inhibitors.
buprenophrine	Buprenex	Moderate to severe pain	Doses should be given only IM in deep, well-developed muscle.

GI, Gastrointestinal; *IM,* intramuscular; *IV,* intravenous; *MAO,* monoamine oxidase; *SC,* subcutaneous.

| TABLE 13-1 | | | |

Opioid Agonists, Mixed Agonists-Antagonists, and Antagonists—cont'd

Generic Name	Brand Name	Uses	Comments
Opioid Agonist-Antagonists—cont'd			
nalbuphine	Nubain	Moderate to severe pain, obstetric analgesia, preoperative sedation, adjunct to anesthesia	Coadministration with nonopioid analgesic may have additive effects and permit lower doses. Administer deep IM into well developed muscle.
pentazocine	Talwin, Talwin NX	Severe pain, obstetric analgesia, preoperative sedation, adjunct to anesthesia	Patients requiring doses that exceed 100 mg should be switched to an opioid agonist. Patients taking concurrent MAO inhibitors should have the dosage of pentazocine reduced by 25% to 50% to minimize unpredictable adverse reactions. Pentazocine is not recommended for prolonged use or as first-line therapy for acute pain.
Opioid Antagonists			
nalmefene	Revex	Opioid-induced CNS depression of refractory circulatory shock (unlabeled use)	IV route is preferred. May also be given by IV infusion at rate adjusted to patient response.
naloxone	Narcan	Management of opioid or alcohol dependence	Analyze urine for opioids and follow with naloxone challenge before administration. Assess patient for suicidal tendencies.
naltrexone	ReVia		Patients must be opioid free for 7-10 days before starting naltrexone.

USES
Analgesia

The major use of morphine and other opioid agonists is to relieve moderate to severe pain of various causes, such as traumatic injuries, burns, biliary or renal colic, cancer-related pain, and pain related to surgery. The analgesic action of opioids is characterized by an increase in the threshold for pain perception, thus making patients less aware of pain, and by a reduction in anxiety and fear, the emotional reactions to pain. At therapeutic doses, opioids decrease pain perception without significantly altering other sensations. Morphine and related drugs do produce sedation (discussed below), and although this may be beneficial, the analgesia is not caused by sedation.

The biochemical mechanism of opioid pain relief is its ability to mimic the endogenous peptides that act through opioid receptors at many sites in the brain to modify the perception of and reaction to pain. Opioid receptors are distributed throughout the pain pathway in the forebrain, the thalamus, the brainstem, and the dorsal spinal cord. In the forebrain limbic regions, morphine alters mood and subjective response to pain. In other regions, it suppresses the perception of pain. Opioids exert a powerful analgesic action at the level of the spinal cord, which accounts for their epidural or subdural administration (discussed below). Mu, kappa, and delta opioid receptors are localized on neurons in the dorsal spinal cord and on the sensory neurons that carry the pain signal. The action of opioid agonists is to inhibit the release of excitatory neurotransmitters (e.g., glutamate and substance P) from sensory neurons and to inhibit second-order nociceptive neurons in the dorsal horn directly.

The relative potency of opioids as analgesics is the dosage ratio of two opioids that produce the same effect. Estimates of the relative potency afford a basis for determining the dose to be used when changing from one drug to another or from one administration route to another. Table 13-2 lists the equianalgesic doses of selected opioid agonists compared with the prototype morphine. Note, for example, that 30 mg of morphine given orally is equivalent in analgesia to 300 mg of meperidine given by the same route or to 10 mg of morphine given intramuscularly. Because not every patient responds the same to a given dose of opioid, the dosage and dosage frequency may need to be adjusted to gain optimum pain relief.

TABLE 13-2

Equianalgesia: Dosing Data for Opioid Analgesics

Drug	Approximate Equianalgesic Oral Dose	Approximate Equianalgesic Parenteral Dose
Opioid Agonists		
morphine	30 mg q3-4h (around-the-clock dosing) 60 mg q3-4h (single dose or intermittent dosing)	10 mg q3-4h
codeine*	130 mg q3-4h	75 mg q3-4h
hydromorphone	7.5 mg q3-4h	1.5 mg q3–4h
hydrocodone	30 mg q3-4h	Not available
levorphanol	4 mg q6-8h	2 mg q6-8h
meperidine	300 mg q3-4h	100 mg q3h
methadone	20 mg q6-8h	10 mg q6-8h
oxycodone	30 mg q3-4h	Not available
oxymorphone	Not available	1 mg q3-4h
Opioid Agonist-Antagonists and Partial Agonists		
buprenorphine	Not available	0.3-0.4 mg q6-8h
butorphanol	Not available	2 mg q3-4h
nalbuphine	Not available	10 mg q3-4h
pentazocine	150 mg q3-4h	60 mg q3-4h

NOTE: Published tables vary in the suggested doses that are equianalgesic to morphine. Clinical response is the criterion that must be applied for each patient; titration to clinical response is necessary. Because there is not complete cross-tolerance among these drugs, it is usually necessary to use a lower than equianalgesic dose when changing drugs and to retitrate to response.
CAUTION: Recommended doses do not apply to patients with renal or hepatic insufficiency or other conditions affecting drug biotransformation and kinetics.
CAUTION: Doses listed for patients with body weight less than 50 kg cannot be used as initial starting doses in babies less than 6 months of age. Consult specialty references.
*Codeine doses greater than 65 mg often are not appropriate because of diminishing incremental analgesia with increasing doses but continually increasing adverse effects.

Antitussive

Morphine and other opioid agonists inhibit the area of the medulla that controls cough. Thus these drugs are effective cough suppressants or **antitussives.** Since morphine is poorly absorbed orally and has many potential adverse effects, codeine and hydrocodone are the major opioids used to relieve serious cough. Even these drugs, however, have limited use because of their adverse effect profile and abuse potential. The most widely used opioid derivative for cough is dextromethorphan. Unlike codeine and other opioid agonists, this drug is a D-isomer and therefore has no analgesic or euphorogenic actions. Dextromethorphan acts in the central nervous system at nonopioid receptors to suppress coughs; it has a low incidence of toxicity and no abuse potential. Only in high amounts is depression of the CNS observed.

Antidiarrheal

Morphine has a profound depressant effect on the GI tract, including the ability to decrease secretions, delay gastric emptying, and reduce peristaltic contractions of the small and large intestine. This effect is due to an inhibition of nerves in the gut that cause contraction of smooth muscle. The result is a decrease in the passage of bowel contents and greater reabsorption of water. Actions in the large intestine to decrease motility and to increase anal sphincter tone can result in constipation, a major adverse effect of opioids. Although morphine is not used to treat nonspecific diarrhea, piperidines and phenylpiperidine drugs such as loperamide or diphenoxylate are used.

Sedation

Acute administration of therapeutic doses of morphine-like drugs produce sedation, whereas progressively larger doses cause drowsiness, sleep, or coma. A few individuals become excited rather than depressed by acute administration of opioid agonists. Sedation and drowsiness result in impaired mental and physical abilities, so patients receiving opioid agonists should be instructed to avoid tasks such as driving or operating machinery. The sedative effects can be compounded by concurrent use of other CNS depressants. Tolerance develops to the sedative effects of these drugs. The sedation can be seen as a therapeutic use of the drugs or as an adverse effect. This effect is beneficial when opioids are used as pre-anesthetic medication or in surgical anesthesia. As pre-anesthetic medication, opioids relieve anxiety and provide sedation so that the patient is not in a fearful state before surgery. More potent analgesics, including morphine, meperidine, fentanyl, and hydromorphone, are widely used in combination with nitrous oxide and a muscle relaxant such as tubocurarine as components of surgical anesthesia. This combination of opioid, nitrous oxide, and muscle relaxant is called balanced anesthesia (see Chapter 16). The duration of anesthesia is controlled by the duration of action of the opioid used. Note that morphine has a longer onset and duration of action than fentanyl, alfentanil, and sufentanil; thus these latter drugs are often preferred for surgical anesthesia.

Miscellaneous Uses

Morphine and meperidine are used to treat the pain of an acute myocardial infarction. At analgesic dosages, morphine not only relieves the pain but also reduces the anxiety without altering the cardiovascular system. Additionally, morphine is the drug of choice in pulmonary edema. The beneficial actions of morphine include relief of anxiety and vasodilation, which reduce the workload of the heart (preload) so that it pumps more efficiently. This increased cardiac efficiency relieves the pulmonary edema that arises when the left side of the heart cannot adequately pump the blood being supplied by the pulmonary veins.

PHARMACOKINETICS

Opioids are variably absorbed from mucosal surfaces of the nose and GI tract as well as from intramuscular and subcutaneous injection sites. Rectal absorption can be erratic. The onset of analgesia is rapid by most routes (Table 13-3). The highly lipid-soluble drugs (e.g., alfentanil and sufentanil) generally have a more rapid onset of action. There are advantages and disadvantages to administering opioids by different routes. Obviously the oral route is the most convenient and has the least potential for toxicity. Unfortunately many opioids are poorly absorbed when given orally and the onset of pain relief is slow. Parenteral administration of opioids provides more rapid onset of action. Intramuscular administration can still have variable absorption, whereas intravenous administration allows titration of dosage, but requires careful monitoring. Opioids are also administered into the subdural space (epidurally) or the

subarachnoid space (intrathecally). By delivery to the sites of nociceptive input to the dorsal horn of the spinal cord, much smaller doses of opioids can be used. As a result, there is significantly less toxicity, although there is a risk of infection and spinal cord injury. Using these routes, health care providers can titrate the dose of highly lipid-soluble opioids, but they must be cautious about late onset toxicity caused by drug redistribution.

Opioids are distributed to a variety of tissues, such as the lungs, liver, kidneys, and spleen. Methadone, sufentanil, and alfentanil are highly bound to plasma proteins, whereas other agonists are intermediately or poorly bound. Skeletal muscle and fatty tissues act as storage sites, although opioid concentration in brain tissue is less than that of other areas. Slow penetration of morphine to brain sites and biotransformation as a result of the first-pass effect influence the onset, peak, and duration of drug action. The difference in oral versus parenteral doses of opioid agonists is accounted for by the bioavailability of these drugs. For example, morphine is subject to a large first-pass effect, and thus higher doses must be given orally. Opioids are converted to metabolites by the liver and are excreted in the urine. The half-life of each opioid varies. These drugs also pass into the milk of a nursing mother and affect the infant.

ADVERSE REACTIONS AND CONTRAINDICATIONS
Respiratory Depression

Opioids depress the medulla's respiratory center, so the major adverse effect of morphinelike drugs is respiratory depression. The depression ranges from slow, shallow respirations to respiratory arrest. The medullary response to carbon dioxide becomes reduced. Respiratory depression is noted about 7 minutes after intravenous administration, 30 minutes after intramuscular injection, and 90 minutes after a subcutaneous injection of morphine. Depressant effects can last from 4 to 5 hours. Death from an opioid overdose is commonly caused by respiratory arrest; the victim stops breathing. This occurs most often in patients who have not received opioids in the past or when CNS depressants are used concurrently. For overdose to occur, doses well above the therapeutic level have to be given. Accumulated doses, especially in patients with liver or renal failure and in the older adult, can cause an overdose. As mentioned above, tolerance develops to the respiratory depression, so individuals who chronically use opioids can tolerate doses of opioids that would cause fatal respiratory depression in nontolerant individuals.

Important drug interactions with opioids are those arising from a synergistic depression of the respiratory center, such as with any of the sedative-hypnotic drugs,

TABLE 13-3

Pharmacokinetics of Selected Opioids, Agonist-Antagonists, and Antagonists

Drug	Route	Onset	Peak	Duration	Protein Binding (%)	$t_{1/2}$
Opioid Agonists						
codeine	po	30-45 min	60-120 min	4 hr	50	2.5-4 hr
	IM, SC	10-30 min	30-60 min			
fentanyl	TD	Slow	12-24 hr	24-48 hr*	79-87	13-22 hr
hydrocodone	po	10-30 min	30-60 min	4-6 hr	UA	3.8 hr
hydromorphone	po	30 min	90-120 min	4 hr	UA	2-4 hr
	IM	15 min	30-60 min	4-5 hr		
	IV	10-15 min	15-30 min	2-3 hr		
	SC	15 min	30-90 min	4 hr		
levorphanol	po	10-60 min	90-120 min	4-5 hr	50	12-16 hr
	IM	UA	60 min			
	IV	Immed-20 min				
	SC	UA	60-90 min			
meperidine	po	15 min	60-90 min	2-4 hr	60-80	3-8 hr
	IM	10-15 min	30-50 min			
	IV	1 min	5-7 min			
	SC	10-15 min	30-50 min			
methadone	po	30-60 min	90-120 min	4-6 hr	90	4-6 hr
	IM	10-20 min	60-120 min	4-5 hr		
	IV	Immediate	15-30 min	3-4 hr		22-48 hr†
morphine	po	10-30 min	60-120 min	4-5 hr	33	2-3 hr
	IM	10-30 min	30-60 min			
	IV	5-10 min	20 min			
	SC	10-30 min	50-90 min			
	EP	15-60 min	—	24 hr	—	
oxycodone	po	10-15 min	60-90 min	3-4 hr	50	2-3 hr
oxymorphone	IM	10-15 min	30-90 min	3-6 hr	33	2-3 hr
	IV	5-10 min	15-30 min	3-4 hr		
	SC	10-20 min	UA	3-6 hr		
propoxyphene	po	15-60 min	120 min	4-6 hr	50	6-12 hr
Opioid Agonist-Antagonists						
butorphanol	IM	10 min	30-60 min	3-4 hr	96	2.5-4 hr
	IV	Immediate	30 min			
buprenorphine	IM	15 min	60 min	6 hr‡	96	4-5 hr
	IV	Immediate	60 min	6 hr		
nalbuphine	IM	15 min	60 min	3-6 hr	30	5 hr
	IV	2-3 min	30 min	3-4 hr		
	SC	15 min	UA	3-6 hr		
pentazocine	po	15-30 min	60-90 min	3 hr	60	2-3 hr
	IM	15-20 min	30-60 min	2-3 hr		
	IV	2-3 min	15-30 min			
	SC	15-20 min	30-60 min			
Opioid Antagonists						
naloxone	IM	2-5 min	UK	45 min	50	60-100 min
	IV	1-2 min	Varies§			
	SC	2-5 min				
naltrexone	po	5-60 min	UK	Varies‖	UA	4-13 hr¶

TD, Transdermal; *PB*, protein binding; $t_{1/2}$, elimination half-life; *UK*, unknown; *UA*, unavailable; *EP*, epidural; *SUP*, suppository.

*Duration of action of fentanyl patch after the patch is removed.

†Duration of action and half-life of methadone's active metabolites with repeated dosing. May be even longer in elderly patients and patients with renal dysfunction. Extended half-life is not related to analgesic effects.

‡Respiratory depressant effects of buprenorphine occurs 1 to 3 hours after IM injection.

§Duration of action of naloxone varies with dose administered and route of administration.

‖Duration of action of naltrexone is dose dependent;. 25 mg can block effects of IV heroin for up to 24 hours, whereas a 100- to 150-mg dose can last 48 to 72 hours, respectively.

¶The half-life of naltrexone metabolites.

antianxiety drugs, alcohol, general anesthetics, or phenothiazines. Tolerance does not develop to the respiratory depression produced by these latter drug classes. An individual who is abusing an opioid and a drug of another class, such as alcohol or one of the other sedative-hypnotic drugs can readily succumb to drug-induced respiratory depression. It should also be noted that opioid antagonists such as naloxone reverse the respiratory depression of opioids (discussed below), but do not affect arrest caused by other CNS depressants.

Gastrointestinal Effects

A common adverse effect of opioids is constipation. Constipation is caused by diminished peristaltic contractions in the small and large intestine and delay in passage of gastric contents through the duodenum. There is also decreased lower GI smooth muscle tone and glandular secretion and increased water reabsorption from the intestines. Tolerance does not develop to constipation as it does to the other adverse effects of opioids. Morphine treats the pain associated with biliary colic, but it may exacerbate rather than relieve the pain in some patients because the biliary tract may go into painful spasms in the presence of morphine.

The chemoreceptor trigger zone is another medullary center affected by morphine. Morphine stimulates this center to produce nausea and vomiting. This effect is transient, so repeated doses do not usually cause nausea and vomiting. Individuals vary in their sensitivity to this emetic action.

Cardiovascular Effects

In a supine patient, therapeutic doses of morphine or the synthetic opioids have very little effect on blood pressure and cardiac rate or rhythm. However, some patients experience orthostatic hypotension when moving from a supine position to a head-up or standing position. This hypotension results from a direct dilating action on peripheral blood vessels caused by the opioids, which reduces the capacity of the cardiovascular system to respond to gravitational changes. Morphine also releases histamine from mast cells, which can cause vasodilation. Therefore, opioids are used with caution in patients who are volume depleted because the hypotensive effects are more pronounced. Increasing blood volume decreases the orthostatic changes. In large doses morphine slows the heart rate.

Miscellaneous Effects

Ureteral spasm, spasm of urinary sphincters, urinary retention or hesitancy oliguria, antidiuretic effects, and reduced libido have been noted with opioid use. Urinary retention is especially problematic in patients with prostatic hypertrophy. Opioids (except meperidine) also

tend to prolong labor. They pass through the placenta to the fetus and can produce respiratory depression in the neonate. In the case of an opioid-dependent mother, the newborn is also dependent on the drug.

Severe hypersensitivity reactions to opioids are rare, but when they occur, they appear as urticaria or a skin rash. Some patients experience itching or wheal formation at the site of injection, but this effect is usually a local, histamine-mediated response. Anaphylaxis is rare.

All opioids except meperidine cause pupillary constriction. Some patients experience blurred vision, dry eyes, and lens opacities. A pinpoint pupil is one characteristic of an opioid overdose. However, if the victim is near death, hypoxia causes the release of epinephrine, which dilates the pupil. Opioids also stimulate the release of antidiuretic hormone, prolactin, and human growth hormone.

Opioids are not recommended for use, or must be used very cautiously, in people with chronic lung disease, respiratory depression, liver or kidney disease, and in persons with a previous hypersensitivity reaction. They should also be used with caution in patients with head injuries, increased intracranial pressure, adrenal insufficiency, Addison's disease, alcoholism, undiagnosed abdominal pain, urethral stricture, and prostatic hypertrophy. In patients with head injury, opioids can decrease respirations, thus increasing carbon dioxide retention. Carbon dioxide, in turn, dilates intracranial blood vessels, worsening the situation. Because of the potential for neonatal respiratory depression, opioids are used with caution during labor and delivery.

Because opioids can cause hypotension, they must be used cautiously in patients with shock or blood loss, conditions worsened by a hypotensive action.

Drug Tolerance

Tolerance to opioids develops quickly, depending on the dose, dosage frequency, and frequency of use. **Tolerance is characterized by a shorter duration of pain relief, a decrease in peak analgesic effect, and an increase in the amount of opioid needed to relieve pain.** Tolerance is one of the main limitations of using opioids for treating some types of chronic pain. With tolerance, increasingly larger doses of the drug are needed to achieve the same clinical effect. Some individuals tolerate doses that are 10 to 20 times the initial dose. This leads to increased severity and incidence of adverse effects. When individuals stop using the drug, symptoms of withdrawal appear. Tolerance to the sedative and euphoric effect of opioids develops rapidly. Individuals who abuse opioids keep increasing the dosage to maintain the good feelings associated with the drug. Tapering the dosage of the drug is usually sufficient for a patient to discontinue opioid therapy.

178 PART IV *Central Nervous System Drugs*

Tolerance also develops to the respiratory depressant effects of opioids, which is why patients with cancer pain can tolerate large doses of these drugs. Little or no tolerance develops to the pupillary constriction or to the constipating effect of the opioids.

Drug Dependence

Euphoria caused by opioid administration may be experienced if the individual has been in pain or has been fearful and anxious. These drugs produce positive reinforcing effects that can result in recreational or long-term use. It is important to point out, however, that chronic use of opioids for pain rarely results in dependency. Patients are unlikely to become drug dependent because as the pain subsides, so will the need and use of the drug. However, patients who receive therapeutic doses of morphine several times a day for an extended period do develop some degree of **physical dependence**, defined as an involuntary altered physiologic state produced by repeated administration of a drug. Continued administration of the drug is required to prevent **withdrawal (abstinence) syndrome**. In drug abusers, chronic use of opioids results in **psychologic dependence** as well as a physical dependence. Withdrawal symptoms after stopping long-term morphine use include a characteristic mix of CNS and autonomic nervous system responses such as tactile hallucinations, irritability, sleeplessness, restlessness, yawning, tremors, and joint and muscle pains. Anorexia, nausea, vomiting, diarrhea, dehydration, abdominal cramps, ketosis, weight loss, distorted vision, and photophobia also plague the individual. Peak severity of withdrawal symptoms occurs 36 to 72 hours after the last dose of morphine, with symptoms gradually waning over 2 to 5 weeks. Withdrawal symptoms that lasted for months have been documented. Withdrawal is usually not life threatening in an otherwise healthy individual. Clonidine, an antihypertensive drug activates central alpha$_2$-adrenergic receptors (see Chapter 12) to reduce sympathetic overactivity. Because of the reduction in centrally mediated sympathetic activity, clonidine is useful in treating opioid withdrawal symptoms since it reduces symptoms without producing its own withdrawal syndrome.

In the United States the most widely used treatment for dependency on opioids is to substitute methadone, which can be given orally in a daily dose. Because tolerance already has developed to the euphoria level in these individuals, the methadone maintains this tolerance while protecting against withdrawal symptoms. The goal of maintenance therapy is to discourage the individual from continuing to seek drugs and to participate instead in rehabilitation programs. If detoxification (elimination of drug) is the goal, methadone is ad-

ministered first when withdrawal symptoms appear, and then the dosage of methadone is gradually reduced to zero over 1 to 3 weeks. Because methadone has a long half-life in the body, the withdrawal symptoms are not as severe as with morphine or heroin. Detoxification of dependent individuals is rarely sufficient to prevent relapse. Drugs such as methadone may help in a drug rehabilitation program, but educational and psychosocial interventions are also needed.

TOXICITY

As discussed previously, opioids produce sedation in therapeutic doses. Patients may experience dizziness or be drowsy. The overdosed individual is stuporous or in a deep sleep, and initially is warm and has flushed wet skin. The next stage is coma, in which respiration is depressed. As the individual becomes hypoxic (starved for oxygen), the skin becomes cold, clammy, and mottled, and the pupils dilate.

INTERACTIONS

Opioids interact with other CNS depressants such as alcohol, anesthetics, barbiturates, and sedative-hypnotics to enhance CNS depression (Table 13-4). Severe constipation and urinary retention may result with the concurrent use of tricyclic antidepressants, phenothiazines, and anticholinergic drugs. The paralyzing effects of neuromuscular blockers are enhanced in the presence of opioids. Smoking and nicotine use decrease the analgesic effect of opioids. Concurrent use of diuretics can result in additive orthostatic hypotension. Cimetidine inhibits the biotransformation of the opioids, leading to increased respiratory and CNS depression.

INDIVIDUAL AGONISTS
Codeine

An oral dose of 32 or 65 mg of codeine produces analgesia, but at these low dosages codeine seldom produces adverse effects. At high dosages the adverse effects of codeine are similar to those of morphine. Because codeine causes significant histamine release if given intravenously, it is given only intramuscularly or by mouth. A portion of codeine dose is metabolized to morphine in the liver. Codeine is a schedule II drug when given in analgesic dosages. When formulated with an NSAID analgesic, it is usually a schedule III drug. Codeine is an effective cough suppressant at low dosages and is available for this purpose in dilute solutions as a schedule V drug.

Fentanyl/Alfentanil/Sufentanil

Fentanyl, alfentanil, and sufentanil are highly lipid soluble compared to morphine and are useful in anesthesia because of their rapid onset and short duration of action.

TABLE 13-4

Drug-Drug Interactions of Selected Opioids, Agonist-Antagonists, and Antagonists

Drug	Interactive Drugs/Class	Interaction
Opioid Agonists		
Opioids	Alcohol	Enhanced CNS depression, respiratory depression, and hypotension
	Anesthetics	
	Antianxiety drugs	
	Antihistamines	
	Antipsychotic drugs	
	Barbiturates	
	Sedative-hypnotics	
	Tricyclic antidepressants	Severe constipation and urinary retention
	Phenothiazines	
	Anticholinergics	May inhibit opioid biotransformation, leading to increased respiratory and
	cimetidine	CNS depression
	Diuretics	Orthostatic hypotension
	MAO inhibitors	CNS excitation, severe hypotension, or hypertension
	phenorphine	May precipitate opioid withdrawal in dependent patients
	pentazocine	
	Skeletal muscle relaxants	Enhances neuromuscular blocking action of interactive drug
	Nicotine	Decreases analgesic effect
meperidine	MAO inhibitors	Additive CNS depression with hypotension and respiratory depression, or CNS stimulation with hyperexcitability and seizures
methadone	Hydantoins	Induces biotransformation of methadone
propoxyphene	carbamazepine	Decreased biotransformation and increased serum concentrations of interactive drug
	naltrexone	Withdrawal symptoms
Opioid Agonist-Antagonists		
buprenorphine	MAO inhibitors	Increased CNS and respiratory depression, hypotension
butorphanol		
dezocine	Alcohol	Additive CNS depression
nalbuphine	Antihistamines	
pentazocine	Antidepressants	
	Sedative-hypnotics	
	Opioids	Decreased effectiveness of interactive drug
Opioid Antagonists		
naloxone, naltrexone	Opioids	Withdrawal symptoms

Fentanyl is available in transdermal patches for the treatment of pain. These drugs rapidly redistribute from the CNS after epidural or intrathecal injection and thus are used extensively by this route. The ability to titrate the dosage and allow rapid recovery is beneficial.

Hydrocodone

Hydrocodone is a semisynthetic derivative of morphine. In Canada it is available as a syrup for cough suppression and in tablet form for analgesia or cough suppression. In the United States hydrocodone is commercially available only in combination with aspirin or acetaminophen.

Hydromorphone

Hydromorphone is a semisynthetic derivative of morphine. A full opioid agonist, it is more potent but shorter acting than morphine. Oral doses require more time to become effective but are longer acting than parenteral doses. The actions of hydromorphone are identical to those of morphine.

Levorphanol

Levorphanol (Levo-Dromoran) has actions identical to those of morphine, but the effective dose is about one fourth that of morphine.

Methadone

Methadone (Dolophine) can be taken orally. Although the onset of action for a single analgesic dose is similar to that for morphine, methadone is highly bound to protein and is not readily metabolized. Methadone has a half-life of 25 hours. Methadone currently is used in the treatment of opioid dependence because it is effective orally and only one dose per day is necessary. In addition, the long plasma half-life more easily allows for a gradual reduction in dosage without adverse effects. Methadone is a second-line opioid for the management of cancer pain and is very effective. It is best administered by an experienced professional because of its high potency, long half-life, and the unpredictable individual response.

Meperidine

Meperidine was the first of the synthetic opioids. It is shorter acting than morphine and does not have an antitussive effect. Meperidine is widely used for obstetric and surgical analgesia since therapeutic doses do not prolong labor. It is more likely than most opioids to cause adverse effects associated with histamine release, convulsions, and constipation. Meperidine is biotransformed to normeperidine, which is active and also neurotoxic. If meperidine is administered over several days, especially to patients with impaired renal or hepatic function, symptoms of normeperidine toxicity may be seen. These signs and symptoms include significant mood changes (paranoia and hallucinations), increased irritability, quivering, fever or convulsions, and sinus tachycardia.

Morphine

Chemically, morphine is a base that is positively charged at the pH of the GI tract and therefore is not readily absorbed when taken orally. Morphine is commonly given by intramuscular or subcutaneous routes. Because morphine is readily biotransformed within the gut and by the liver, larger dosages may be required when given orally. Older adults usually require a smaller dose because they do not biotransform morphine as readily as younger patients.

Oxymorphone

Oxymorphone is a semisynthetic derivative of morphine that has all the actions of morphine except the antitussive action. Oxymorphone is more potent than morphine, but must also be given by injection or rectally.

Oxycodone

Oxycodone is a semisynthetic derivative that is taken orally. Oxycodone has an onset of 10 to 15 minutes and a duration of action of 3 to 6 hours. In the United States and Canada oxycodone is also available as a combination product with aspirin or acetaminophen.

Propoxyphene

Propoxyphene, an opioid related to methadone, is not a very potent analgesic. A 65-mg dose of propoxyphene is the analgesic equivalent of two tablets (650 mg) of aspirin or acetaminophen. Propoxyphene is commonly formulated in combination with aspirin or acetaminophen. Alone or in combination, propoxyphene is a schedule IV drug. Adverse effects are uncommon at analgesic dosages. Propoxyphene has low abuse potential but has been implicated as a cause of death when used in combination with alcohol and other CNS depressant drugs.

 DRUG CLASS • Mixed Agonist-Antagonists and Partial Agonists

Nalbuphine (Nubain)

The mixed opioid agonist-antagonists were developed in an attempt to produce analgesics without classic opioid adverse effects. However, this effort has been less than successful. Drugs included in this group are pentazocine, butorphanol, nalbuphine, and anileridine (see Table 13-1). Although they differ in some respects from opioid agonists, they produce analgesia and respiratory depression at therapeutic doses that are similar to those of morphine (see Table 13-2 for equianalgesic doses). However, there is a ceiling effect for analgesia and respiratory depression with these drugs.

MECHANISM OF ACTION

These drugs act as agonists at kappa opioid receptors and as partial antagonists at mu receptors. In contrast to the above drugs, buprenorphine is a partial mu agonist that is more potent than morphine as an analgesic.

USES

Opioid agonists-antagonists are used to relieve moderate to severe pain. These drugs alter the perception of and response to painful stimuli while producing generalized CNS depression. Butorphanol, buprenorphine, and nalbuphine can be used for patients who have a hypersensitivity to meperidine or who are intolerant of morphine. Butorphanol, nalbuphine, and pentazocine have been used for analgesia during labor, for sedation before surgery, and as a supplement in balanced anesthesia. These drugs have little antitussive action.

PHARMACOKINETICS

Absorption of opioid agonist-antagonists readily occurs with parenteral formulations. The drugs are distributed to most body tissues, including the placenta and breasts (the drugs are excreted in breast milk). Some variation exists in the onset, peak, and duration of action of parenterally administered drugs (see Table 13-3). The agonist-antagonists vary in protein binding from less than 30% for nalbuphine to 96% for butorphanol and buprenorphine. Opioid agonist-antagonists are biotransformed in the liver and excreted in the urine. More than 10% of a butorphanol dose and a small amount of pentazocine are eliminated via the GI tract. The plasma half-life of these drugs varies from 2 to 13 hours.

ADVERSE REACTIONS AND CONTRAINDICATIONS

Common adverse effects include nausea, vomiting, light-headedness, sedation, and euphoria. Visual hallucinations, disorientation, dysphoria, and confusion can also occur. As with opioid agonists, respirations may be depressed with initial doses. Insomnia and disturbed dreams can develop, especially with nalbuphine and pentazocine. Both pentazocine and butorphanol have adverse cardiovascular effects, including increased pulmonary arterial pressure and cardiac workload, and, in the case of pentazocine, increased blood pressure. Nalbuphine has fewer cardiovascular effects. These drugs can precipitate withdrawal symptoms in patients who are physically dependent on an opioid agonist. Hypersensitivity reactions to opioid agonist-antagonists are possible. Parenteral use of pentazocine may lead to severe, potentially fatal reactions, including pulmonary emboli, vascular occlusion, ulceration, and abscess.

INTERACTIONS

Additive CNS depression may result when opioid agonists-antagonists are taken concurrently with other CNS depressants (see Table 13-4). Decreased effectiveness of an opioid agonist may occur in the presence of an opioid agonist-antagonist. Monoamine oxidase inhibitors used concurrently with opioid agonist-antagonists can result in unpredictable reactions including, but not limited to, increased CNS and respiratory depression and hypotension. Antihypertensive drugs and other drugs that lower blood pressure can exacerbate opioid-induced orthostatic hypotension.

INDIVIDUAL DRUGS
Buprenorphine

Buprenorphine is a partial mu receptor agonist that is administered intramuscularly. The onset of action is 15 minutes, and the duration of action is about 6 hours. Buprenorphine is effective for moderate to severe pain associated with surgery, cancer, neuralgias, labor, renal colic, and myocardial infarction. The respiratory depression produced by buprenorphine can be prevented by prior administration of opioid antagonists, but is not readily reversed by naloxone or nalmefene, suggesting that buprenorphine binds tightly to opioid receptors.

Butorphanol

Butorphanol has a mixed agonist-antagonist opioid. Administered intramuscularly, butorphanol has an onset of action of 10 to 30 minutes with a duration of action of about 4 hours. It is also available in a nasal spray formulation that is especially useful for patients with migraine. In general, its actions resemble those of morphine, except that butorphanol increases pulmonary arterial pressure and the cardiac workload, which makes it undesirable for treating the pain of a myocardial infarction.

Nalbuphine

Nalbuphine is a semisynthetic derivative of morphine and is a mixed agonist-antagonist opioid. It may be preferable for treating the pain of a myocardial infarction because it appears to reduce the oxygen needs of the heart without reducing blood pressure. Nalbuphine is a stronger antagonist than pentazocine, which suggests that the degree of tolerance and drug dependence should be low. However, withdrawal symptoms are seen when nalbuphine is abruptly discontinued, and it causes withdrawal symptoms when administered to an individual already dependent on one of the more common opioids.

Pentazocine

Pentazocine is a mixed agonist-antagonist opioid. Unlike morphine, pentazocine increases blood pressure and cardiac workload, making it less desirable than morphine for treating the pain of myocardial infarction or pulmonary hypertension. Pentazocine causes dysphoria rather than euphoria, producing nightmares, feelings of depersonalization, or visual hallucinations. Large doses can induce seizures. Although there are reports of indi-

viduals who have become dependent on pentazocine, its administration to a person dependent on another opioid results in withdrawal symptoms because of its antagonistic properties. It does not, however, reduce the respiratory depressant effects of morphine.

DRUG CLASS • Opioid Antagonists

 naloxone (Narcan)

MECHANISM OF ACTION

Opioid antagonists produce few effects when used by themselves under usual circumstances. They are effective, however, in reversing the therapeutic and toxic effects of opioid agonists and mixed agonist-antagonists. The clinically available drugs are naloxone, naltrexone, and nalmefene (see Table 13-1). As antagonists, these drugs have an affinity for opioid receptors but do not activate them. Instead they attach to the receptors and prevent opioids (both exogenous and endogenous) from producing effects. They competitively displace opioids already present and block further binding.

USES

Pure opioid antagonists are used when an antagonist is required to reverse opioid-induced respiratory depression or coma. Naloxone is usually the drug of choice, but both naltrexone and nalmefene are equally effective. Naltrexone also blocks the effects of opioids and is used in behavioral therapy to discourage resumption of opioid use. Naltrexone recently was approved for use in prevention of recidivism in alcohol dependence. These drugs have no effect when the overdose is not caused by an opioid.

PHARMACOKINETICS

Absorption of opioid agonist-antagonists readily occurs with parenteral formulations. The drugs are distributed to most body tissues, including the placenta, and excreted in breast milk. Some variation exists in the onset, peak, and duration of action of parenterally administered drugs (see Table 13-3). These drugs are biotransformed by the liver and excreted via the kidneys.

ADVERSE REACTIONS AND CONTRAINDICATIONS

The adverse reactions of antagonists are minimal and only occur with high doses. They include nausea, vomiting, and occasionally, elevated blood pressure and tachycardia. For opioid-dependent patients, withdrawal symptoms associated with antagonist administration develop within a few minutes to 2 hours. The severity of

symptoms depends on the opioid involved, the dose of antagonist, and the degree of physical dependence.

INDIVIDUAL ANTAGONISTS
Naloxone

Naloxone is especially useful in emergency room situations. When a comatose patient is brought to the emergency department because of a drug overdose, the first goal is to support respiration and the second is to determine which drug was used. If an opioid is suspected, naloxone is administered intravenously; if the overdose is a result of an opioid, the patient will respond in 2 to 3 minutes with improved respiration and will return to consciousness. The patient must still be monitored carefully, however, because naloxone has a short duration of action and its effect may wear off before the overdosed drug has been sufficiently eliminated. If the patient again becomes comatose, naloxone must be given a second time.

Naltrexone

Naltrexone produces withdrawal symptoms and prevents the euphoria associated with opioid use, but it does not reduce the craving for the drug. Thus prophylactic treatment of drug dependence is less successful with naltrexone than with methadone therapy. Additional adverse effects of naltrexone include anxiety, dizziness, headache, nervousness, abdominal pain, nausea, and vomiting. Naltrexone should be used with caution in patients with acute hepatitis or liver failure. It is not advisable for use in patients in acute opioid withdrawal; it should be used with caution in patients younger than 18 years of age and in pregnant or nursing women.

Nalmefene

Nalmefene is an opioid antagonist that has a longer duration of action than naloxone. Nalmefene is intended for the management of known or suspected opioid overdose. It will bring a complete or partial reversal of the effects of various opioids, including respiratory depression, and will precipitate withdrawal symptoms in persons with opioid dependence.

DRUG CLASS • Miscellaneous Drugs

There are a number of nonopioid drugs used for the treatment of pain as either first line drugs or as adjunctive therapy. Tramadol is a centrally acting analgesic with about one tenth the analgesic potency of morphine. The mechanism of action for tramadol is not well understood but may include binding to the mu opioid receptor and inhibiting norepinephrine and serotonin uptake. Tramadol and its metabolite are effective in suppressing a cough. Tramadol is recommended for pain after orthopedic and gynecologic procedures. It is being evaluated in the long-term treatment of chronic pain syndromes as cancer pain, low back pain, neuropathic pain, and orthopedic and joint conditions. Unlike NSAIDs, tramadol does not have antiinflammatory activity.

In neuropathic pain states, opioids and NSAIDs are often not effective in relieving the pain. As such, it is important to understand that the mechanism of chronic pain is not just an extension of acute pain. Thus, a number of additional drugs may be useful in chronic pain treatment and these will be discussed in detail in other chapters. These drugs include tricyclic antidepressants (Chapter 18), carbamazepine (Chapter 22), gabapentin (Chapter 22), and capsaicin cream (Chapter 14).

APPLICATION TO PRACTICE

ASSESSMENT
History of Present Illness

Patient self-report is the single most reliable indicator about the existence and intensity of pain and related psychologic distress. Because pain is a subjective phenomenon that varies in intensity and severity, it is important that the location of the pain, onset, pattern (e.g., intermittent, continuous, or cyclical), intensity, character (e.g., sharp, dull, boring, aching, burning, or viselike), duration, and frequency be elicited. Determine how the pain affects activities of daily living. Elicit factors that precipitate, aggravate, and alleviate the patient's pain. Ask if the pain extends from where it started to other areas. Elicit information about what pain relief measures the patient has used to relieve the pain and their effectiveness.

Multiple pain complaints are common in patients with advanced disease and need to be prioritized and classified. It is also important to clarify the patient's level of anxiety or depression. Because we all have our own perception of the meaning of pain, it is useful to have the patient elaborate on this meaning. Does he or she think it represents recurrent tumor, as in the case of a patient with cancer? Is the patient convinced that it is simply arthritis? The more serious the nature of the pain diagnosis, the more likely its meaning may produce psychologic distress.

Health History

Determine whether or not the patient has a personal history or a family history of acute or chronic pain. Information on how the patient has handled previous painful events provides insight into whether the patient is reluctant or afraid to take an opioid. Information about previously used strategies for pain management, helpful or not, should be elicited.

Lifespan Considerations

Perinatal. The gate-control theory has two important implications for childbirth. First, pain can be controlled by tactile stimulation; and second, pain can be modified by activities that affect the CNS such as the use of back rubs, effleurage, suggestion, distraction, and physical conditioning.

Pain during the first stage of labor is, for the most part, related to dilation of the cervix. During the second stage of labor, pain is related to distention of the vagina and perineum, and pressure on surrounding structures. Uterine contractions and cervical dilation as the placenta is expelled produces pain during the third stage of labor. The absence of crying or moaning during labor does not necessarily mean the woman has no pain. Alternatively, crying or moaning does not necessarily mean that pain relief is desired.

Pediatric. In general, pain in children younger than 5 years old is difficult to assess. Language development and comprehension; the confounding variables of anxiety, fear, or loneliness; lack of a good understanding of pain phenomena; and the relative lack of valid and reliable pain assessment instruments contribute to the difficulty. Infants may cry and display muscular rigidity and thrashing behaviors. Preschoolers can be aggressive or verbally complain of discomfort. School-age children express pain verbally or behaviorally, often displaying regressive behaviors. Adolescents are often reluctant to admit that they are uncomfortable or need help.

Observing the expression of pain in another child or a parent also influences the child's pain experiences. Such observations can result in anxiety and negative social modeling that leads children to act much like the person in pain. In contrast, if the child views another child or adult coping well with the painful situation, pain expression and acting out behaviors can be reduced.

Older Adults. Pain assessment presents unique problems for older adults. Physiologic and psychologic influences, and cultural changes associated with aging cause pain to be perceived differently in this population. Many institutionalized older adults are stoic about pain. In addition, they often have altered presentations of common illnesses such as so-called silent myocardial infarctions and painless intraabdominal emergencies.

The widespread belief that aging increases the pain threshold is a myth. Cognitive impairment, delirium (common among acutely ill, frail older adults), and dementia are serious barriers to pain assessment. Whether behavioral observations (agitation, restlessness, groaning) are sensitive and specific for pain assessment among demented older adults remains uncertain. Also, visual, hearing, and motor impairments impede the use of assessment instruments. Many older adults with moderate to severe cognitive impairment are reliably able to report acute pain when it occurs, however, pain

recall and integration of the pain experience over time may be less reliable.

Older adults, especially the frail and old-old (i.e., those older than 75), are at particular risk for both too much and too little pain management, although age-related responses are variable. Older adults experience a higher peak and longer duration of drug action than their younger counterparts. Age-related changes in drug distribution and elimination make the older adult more sensitive to sedation and respiratory distress.

Cultural/Social Considerations

Pain perception and reactions are heavily influenced by culturally derived expectations and learned responses. Psychosocial factors influencing pain perception include anxiety, feelings of powerlessness, and ineffective coping mechanisms (Figure 13-1). In addition to personality, ethnicity, and other factors that cannot be changed (e.g., age and gender), variables that influence pain experiences include insomnia, fatigue, fear, anger, sadness, depression, mental isolation, introversion, and past experiences with pain. Factors that tend to increase the pain threshold include symptom relief, sleep, rest, empathy, diversion, elevation of mood, analgesics, antianxiety drugs, and antidepressants.

A particularly important factor influencing severe, chronic pain is its significance to the patient as an actual or potential loss, with associated losses of personal con-

PSYCHOSOCIAL INFLUENCES

Family and occupational roles—Past experiences—Spiritual belief system
Meaning of pain—Cultural/societal influences—Sexual identity and stereotypes
Communication skills—Level of growth and development—Motivations
Personality—Presence of fear—Level of excitement or distraction at time of injury
Attitude toward pain—Level of anxiety—Fatigue

PAIN THRESHOLD
GENERAL STATE OF HEALTH
PAIN INTENSITY
PAIN FREQUENCY
INTEGRITY OF NERVOUS SYSTEM PATHWAYS
AGE
PHYSICAL INFLUENCES
(SLEEP, STRESS)

PAIN TOLERANCE
UNDERLYING CAUSE OF PAIN
PAIN QUALITY
PAIN LOCATION
PAIN DURATION
TYPE OF PAIN
PRIOR EXPERIENCE WITH PAIN

I'M UNIQUE!

FIGURE 13-1 Factors influencing responses to pain. (From Black JM, Matassarin-Jacobs E: *Medical-surgical nursing: clinical management for continuity of care*, ed. 6, p. 363, Philadelphia, WB Saunders. Used with permission.)

trol and autonomy. Patients may deny severe pain for a variety of reasons, including fear of inadequate pain control or a perception that stoicism is expected or rewarded (see Case Study: Postoperative Analgesia).

Physical Examination

Objective findings associated with unmanaged or undermanaged pain can be divided into three categories: sympathetic responses, parasympathetic responses, and behavioral responses. Although the responses are not diagnostic in and of themselves, they provide clues as to the cause of pain. Sympathetic responses occur with minimal to moderate pain intensity and include tachycardia, increased blood pressure and respirations, skeletal muscle tension, dilated pupils, and diaphoresis.

Parasympathetic responses occur with intense, severe pain, or with deep pain. Objective manifestations include pallor, decreased blood pressure and heart rate, nausea and vomiting, weakness, prostration, and loss of consciousness. It also delays return of bowel and gastric functioning.

Behavioral responses to pain include a guarded, rigid position. The patient is restless; facial expression is drawn; he or she may cry or appear frightened. Moaning, sighing, grimacing, clenching of the jaws or fist, and withdrawal from others may be noted.

Laboratory Testing

Although many pain assessment tools exist, three common self-report instruments are useful for adults and many children. Numeric rating scales, visual analog scales, and adjective rating scales can be used to assess pain intensity and affective distress. These tools are easy to use and provide the patient and health care provider with a means to quantify pain. The tools are valid and reliable as long as the end points and adjective descriptors are carefully identified. Visually impaired or confused patients may have difficulty using the scales.

GOALS OF THERAPY

The primary goal of pain management is to remove the cause and alleviate suffering by using the least toxic, most effective drug, and the one with the least amount of sedation. The importance of effective pain management, however, goes beyond alleviating patient suffering. Additional benefits are gained when earlier mobilization, shortened hospital stays, reduced cost, and improved quality of life are realized. Preventing anxiety, fear, and learned responses that augment pain and pain-related behaviors contribute to effective pain management.

INTERVENTION

Pain management strategies are many and varied (Figure 13-2). Cognitive-behavioral strategies include relaxation,

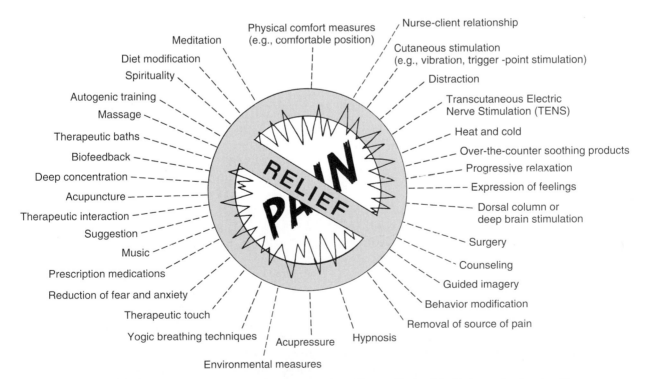

FIGURE 13-2 Pain management strategies. (From Black JM, Matassarin-Jacobs E: *Medical-surgical nursing: clinical management for positive outcomes*, ed. 6, p. 497, Philadelphia, WB Saunders. Used with permission.)

distraction, imagery, and biofeedback. Physical agents such as massage, the application of heat and cold, or transcutaneous electrical nerve stimulation (TENS) are also effective for some patients. These strategies can be used alone or in alliance with systemic analgesics and other adjunctive drug measures.

Management of mild to moderate pain begins with the use of nonsteroidal antiinflammatory drugs (NSAIDs) unless otherwise contraindicated (see Chapter 14). Moderate to severe pain should be managed initially with an opioid. The requisites for rational opioid therapy include: knowledge of drugs used for acute and chronic pain, their mechanism of action, the relationships between drug action and potentially serious adverse effects, pharmacokinetic variability, and the variability between patient and disease condition as it relates to the magnitude of effects. Drug selection, dose, route, and treatment regimen should be based also on anticipated pain. That is, drug therapy should correspond with the overall pain syndrome. Using the placebo effect (potentially present in all patients) and reducing sensory input that aggravates pain provide for the most effective and complete pain relief. Agonist-antagonists are not recommended for prolonged use or as first-line therapy for acute or cancer pain.

Placebos have little place in modern pain management as the sole treatment modality, albeit pain relief from placebos can frequently be equivalent to that produced by high doses of morphine. It should be noted that there is a placebo effect with essentially all drugs, and that illness and illness behaviors provide some degree of secondary gain. A positive response to a placebo permits no diagnostic conclusion about the patient's pain. A response to placebo cannot be taken to mean that the patient is faking, that the patient's pain is not real, or that the patient is imagining some illness or symptom. Lastly, in most cases, patients tell the truth.

Administration

Oral administration is the route of choice for opioids and is as effective as parenteral routes when used in appropriate doses. The oral route should be used if the patient tolerates oral intake. Oral formulations are also convenient and less expensive.

Intravenous administration is the parenteral route of choice for opioids. It is suitable for a titrated bolus or for continuous administration, including use of intermittent self-administration of opioids (patient-controlled analgesia [PCA]). The disadvantage of an intravenous route is that the patient requires continual monitoring and there is a significant risk for respiratory depression. The potential dependency-producing aspects of opioid infusions are negligible. When intravenous access is difficult or impossible, the subcutaneous route is preferable to the intramuscular.

PCA infusion pumps offer two modes for drug administration: demand dosing with a fixed dose taken intermittently, or constant-rate infusion plus demand dosing. PCA begins with setting infusion pump parameters. A loading dose is determined along with the background infusion rate, the dose to be administered per demand, the lockout interval (i.e., the minimum time between demand doses), and the maximum dosage to be received over a specified time interval (e.g., a demand dose of 1 mg of morphine with a lockout time of 5 to 10 minutes).

The patient should be reassessed every 1 to 2 hours, and if the pain is not well managed, the bolus dose may be increased 25% to 50%. If pain relief from the bolus is adequate but the duration of pain relief is too short, the lockout time is decreased.

Rescue doses of opioids should be available for the patient with breakthrough pain or for children with poorly controlled pain who are receiving PCA. Request drug orders that permit the patient, child, or parent to refuse or omit the drug if they are asleep or not in pain. However, keep in mind that a steady-state drug level is necessary for a drug to be continuously effective. Interruption of an around-the-clock (ATC) schedule may cause resurgence of pain as blood levels of the drug decline.

Epidural or intrathecal administration is suitable in some circumstances and can provide effective pain relief; however, respiratory depression remains a significant risk. The onset of respiratory depression is sometimes delayed, thus requiring careful monitoring, the use of infusion pumps, and a specially educated staff.

Opioid analgesia should be provided ATC or by continuous infusion rather than on an as-needed basis. It has been well established that a pro re nata (prn) regimen is not effective for pain management and should be avoided. Further, a prn order is not recommended because it requires the patient to communicate the presence of pain and the need for the drug. In addition, a prn schedule promotes delays in drug administration and subsequent periods of inadequate pain relief. The best strategy to prevent progression of acute pain to a chronic pain syndrome is the appropriate and adequate treatment of acute pain.

Blood pressure, pulse, and respiratory rate should be assessed before and periodically during administration of an opioid. If the respiratory rate falls below 10 breaths per minute, the patient's level of sedation should be assessed. Physical stimulation may be sufficient to prevent significant hypoventilation. The initial drowsiness associated with opioid use diminishes with continued use.

Treatment of Opioid Overdose. Naloxone is the drug of choice when an antagonist is required to reverse opioid-induced CNS and respiratory depression. The dosage is titrated to avoid withdrawal, seizures, and severe pain and may be given by direct intravenous push, intramuscular, or subcutaneous routes every 2 to 3 minutes. Naloxone can also be given by continuous infusion with supplemental doses given intramuscularly or subcutaneously to provide longer-lasting effects. Patients who have been receiving opioids for longer than 1 week are remarkably sensitive to the effects of naloxone; hence, the drug should be diluted and administered carefully.

For opioid-dependent patients, withdrawal symptoms associated with the use of naloxone develop within minutes to 2 hours. Symptom severity depends on the opioid involved, the dose of naloxone, and the degree of physical dependence. Lack of significant response suggests that symptoms may be caused by a disease process or to a nonopioid CNS depressant not responsive to naloxone.

Education

Patients should be taught to take the opioid analgesic as directed. Although this principle applies to all drugs, it is particularly important with analgesics because of potentially serious adverse effects and because analgesics may mask or enable the patient to tolerate pain for which medical attention would otherwise be required. Patients should be advised not to take an opioid previously used for other disorders and not to let anyone else use the prescription.

Teach patients to avoid concurrent use of alcohol or other CNS depressants with opioids without first checking with the health care provider. Teach them to store their analgesics in a secure place away from the bedside to prevent unintentional overdose. They should be told not to smoke when taking an opioid because smoking when less alert is unsafe, and it reduces the effectiveness of opioids.

Some patients report a history of gastric upset when taking an opioid analgesic. Instruct the patient to take the drug with small amounts of food to reduce the potential for nausea.

Assess bowel sounds on a regular basis. Constipation can be prevented or at least minimized by consuming high-fiber foods such as whole-grain cereals, fruits, and vegetables; drinking 2 to 3 liters of fluids daily, and remaining as active as possible. A bowel program should be instituted for patients receiving an opioid for longer than 24 hours. A stool softener such as docusate sodium may be taken daily. Bulk-forming laxatives such as psyllium hydrophilic mucilloid (Metamucil) (see Chapter 49) are effective for most patients, as long as adequate hydration is maintained. Warm prune juice may also be effective in producing a bowel movement. It is better to prevent constipation than to begin treatment after it develops.

All patients should be advised to change positions slowly to minimize the potential for orthostatic hypotension, particularly if they are also taking antihypertensive drugs or diuretics. Hospitalized patients should be taught the reasons for raising the side rails on the bed after they have received an opioid. Side rails promote safety by serving as a reminder to stay in bed or to call for assistance.

Patients who are taught the importance of turning, coughing, deep breathing, and ambulation during the preoperative period report less pain, use fewer analgesics, and have shorter lengths of stay than patients who do not receive instruction.

EVALUATION

Evaluation of opioid effectiveness depends in part on the reason for use. Patients may offer a verbal statement of pain relief, demonstrate decreased behavioral manifestations of pain or discomfort, and progressively increase the usual activities of daily living. There may be a decrease in blood pressure and pulse rate as well as slower and deeper respirations. The frequency of pain evaluation should be based on the knowledge of how quickly the drug works.

CASE STUDY

Postoperative Analgesia

ASSESSMENT

HISTORY OF PRESENT ILLNESS

AB is a 24-year-old woman admitted to the surgical unit via the operating room and the postanesthesia care unit. She was in a motor vehicle accident and was sent to surgery from the emergency room for splenectomy and internal fixation of a compound fracture of the left leg. It is now 12 hours later, and AB is reporting that she is thirsty and feeling weak and "out of it," but states that her left side and leg hurt "somethin' awful." She has had three doses of 75 mg of meperidine administered intramuscularly since surgery; the last dose was given 3 hours ago, but without much relief. She refuses to cough or breathe deeply, and is lying very still and rigidly. She is becoming more irritable and communicates in yes or no answers only. She occasionally answers questions inappropriately. She also refuses to use the overhead trapeze because of pain from her incision and does not move unless someone turns her.

HEALTH HISTORY

AB's records indicate she has a history of intravenous opioid drug abuse (crack) and hepatitis B since age 19 but has been drug free for the last 3 months. She has been in and out of drug abuse treatment programs since age 21. She admits to smoking 1 to $1\frac{1}{2}$ packs of cigarettes a day for the past 8 years.

LIFESPAN CONSIDERATIONS

AB admits her sense of responsibility appropriate for this age has been lacking. She has been unable to maintain impulse control, has lacked the ability to implement realistic goals and develop a career, and has been unable to enter into mature, intimate relationships. Since she has been in a substance abuse program, she has been working on these age-appropriate behaviors.

CULTURAL/SOCIAL CONSIDERATIONS

AB is reluctant to ask for pain medication, afraid that she will once again become "addicted" and that the nurses will think "bad" of her for asking. She admits to searching for the "meaning of life." AB recently returned to work after leaving a drug treatment program. She is not eligible for health insurance through her employer for another 3 months. A social worker has been contacted to explore financial alternatives with AB. It is anticipated that AB will be off work for approximately 3 to 4 months during rehabilitation.

PHYSICAL EXAMINATION

Temperature is 99.6° F, BP is 140/92 mm Hg, pulse 128, respirations 28, and shallow. Urinary output is over 50 mL/hr; skin is cool and clammy. Breath sounds are clear to auscultation bilaterally. Abdominal and leg dressings are dry and intact.

LABORATORY TESTING

Results of CBC with differential and electrolytes are within normal limits (WNL); wound cultures negative. Pain assessment using numeric scale (1-10) indicates pain level of 9. AB reports her pain has been at this level since she came out of surgery.

PATIENT PROBLEM(S)

Postoperative pain within the framework of past substance abuse.

GOALS OF THERAPY

Prevention and alleviation of pain and minimize anxiety, fear, and learned responses that may augment pain and pain-related behaviors.

CRITICAL THINKING QUESTIONS

1. What are the two components of pain? Which is affected by opioids?
2. The health care provider wants AB to have a morphine PCA. What information is needed by the nurse to implement the order for the PCA morphine?
3. What five common adverse reactions to morphine should be monitored?
4. What drug should be available on the nursing unit in the event AB receives too much morphine? What is the action of this drug? Why is it a good drug for treating opioid overdose?
5. After 3 days on the morphine PCA, AB begins to complain of constipation. What nursing interventions would be appropriate to help relieve the constipation?
6. The health care provider wants to move AB to oral analgesics once she is off the PCA. Which opioid analgesic(s) would be equianalgesic to 10 mg parenteral morphine given every 3 to 4 hours?
7. What properties of methadone make it useful for maintaining or withdrawing from opioid dependence?

Bibliography

Akil H, Owens C, Gutstein H, et al: Endogenous opioids: overview and current issues, *Drug Alcohol Depend* 51:127-140, 1998.

Barber D: The physiology and pharmacology of pain: a review of opioids, *J Perianesth Nurs* 12(2):95-99, 1997.

Dray A, Urban L: New pharmacological strategies for pain relief, *Ann Rev Pharmacol Toxicol* 36:253-280, 1996.

Fishman SM, Wilsey B, Yang J, et al: Adherence monitoring and drug surveillance in chronic opioid therapy, *J Pain Symptom Manage*, 20(4):293-307, 2000.

Goodwin SA: A review of preemptive analgesia, *J Perianesth Nurs* 13(2):109-114, 1998.

Gutstein HB, Akil H: Opioid analgesics. In Hardman JG, Limbird LL, Gilman A, eds: *Goodman and Gilman's The pharmacologic basis of therapeutics*, ed. 10, New York, 2000, Pergamon Press.

Harris LG: Spinal and combined spinal epidural techniques for labor analgesia: clinical application in a small hospital, *AANA J* 66(6):587-594, 1998.

MacConnachie AM: Analgesics in the management of chronic pain, Part five: Step 3 parenteral analgesic drug therapy, *Intensive Crit Care Nurs* 15(1):58-60, 1999.

Martin LA, Hagen NA: Neuropathic pain in cancer patients: mechanisms, syndromes, and clinical controversies, *J Pain Symptom Manage* 14(2):99-117, 1997.

McCaffery M: How to use the new AHCPR cancer pain guidelines, *Am J Nurs* 94(7):42-47, 1994.

McCaffrey M, Ferrell B: Nurses' assessment of pain intensity and choice of analgesic dose, *Contemporary Nurse* 3(2):68-74, 1994.

Melzack R, Wall PD: Pain mechanisms: a new theory, *Science* 150(699):971-979, 1965.

Payne R: Transdermal fentanyl: suggested recommendations for clinical use, *J Pain Symptom Manage* 7:540-544, 1992.

Pereira J, Lawlor P, Vigano A, et al: Equianalgesic dose ratios for opioids: a critical review and proposals for long-term dosing, *J Pain Symptom Manage* 22(2):672-687, 2001.

Pleuvry B, Lauretti G: Biochemical aspects of chronic pain and its relationship to treatment, *Pharmacol Ther* 71:313-324, 1996.

Resch L: Agonist narcotics, *AANA J* 6:637-639, 1998.

Rospond RM: A new transmucosal fentanyl for breakthrough cancer pain, *Cancer Pract* 7(6):317-320, 1999.

Wall PD, Melzack R: *Textbook of pain*, ed. 3, London and New York, 1994, Churchill Livingstone.

Internet Resources

American Pain Society: Opioids. Available online at http://www.ampainsoc.org/advocacy/opioids.htm.

HIV Positive.com: Opioids. Available online at http://www.hivpositive.com/f-PainHIV/Pain/PainMenu3a.html.

Hospital Practice: Chronic pain 2: the case for opioids. Available online at http://www.hosppract.com/issues/2000/09/brook.htm.

Pain and palliative care reporter: Using opioids to control pain. Available online at http://www.painlaw.org/opioids.html.

The Medical Letter: Drugs for pain (#1085). Available online at http://www.medicalletter.com.

United States Drug Enforcement Administration. Available online at http://www.usdoj.gov/dea.

CHAPTER
14

Nonsteroidal Antiinflammatory Drugs (NSAIDs) and Disease-Modifying Antirheumatic Drugs (DMARDs)

MICHAEL R. VASKO • KATHLEEN GUTIERREZ

 Visit http://evolve.elsevier.com/Gutierrez/ for additional information.

KEY TERMS

Analgesia, p. 193

Antipyresis, p. 192

COX-2 inhibitors, p. 202

Cyclooxygenases, p. 192

Encephalopathy, p. 198

Gout, p. 207

Hyperuricemia, p. 207

Prostaglandin, p. 192

Pyrogens, p. 194

Reye's syndrome, p. 198

Salicylism, p. 198

Tinnitus, p. 198

Tophus, p. 207

Uricosuric drugs, p. 208

OBJECTIVES

- Differentiate between aspirin and acetaminophen in terms of action, adverse effects, and uses.
- Discuss therapeutic uses and adverse effects of nonsteroidal antiinflammatory drugs (NSAIDs) and differentiate among individual drugs.
- Distinguish between selective COX-2 inhibitors and nonselective COX inhibitors.
- Discuss drug therapy for arthritic conditions.
- Discuss drug therapy for gout.
- Develop a nursing care plan for the patient receiving an NSAID, DMARD, or antigout drug.

Inflammation, pain, and fever are common manifestations of many conditions, including tissue trauma and infection. In chronic diseases such as rheumatoid arthritis and osteoarthritis, inflammation and pain are major debilitating symptoms. In this chapter, we discuss nonsteroidal antiinflammatory drugs (NSAIDs) and related drugs that are used to alleviate acute pain, inflammation (including hypersensitivity) and to reduce fever **(antipyresis)**. These drugs are called analgesic-antipyretics, and acetylsalicylic acid (aspirin) is the prototype. Though not an antiinflammatory drug, acetaminophen is included in this chapter because of its extensive use as an analgesic and antipyretic. Aspirin and acetaminophen are commonly found in over the counter (OTC) and combination prescription drugs marketed for relief of colds and allergies. The newer

NSAIDs are similar to aspirin in that they are also antiinflammatory, antipyretic, and analgesic. Except for ibuprofen, ketoprofen, and naproxen, most NSAIDs are prescription drugs used primarily to treat inflammation and resulting pain. These drugs relieve symptoms and contribute to a patient's comfort and quality of life; they do not cure the underlying disorder producing the symptoms. Corticosteroids, which make up the other class of antiinflammatory drugs, will be discussed in Chapter 57.

This chapter also discusses drugs used to treat gout. Gout is a metabolic disease in which crystals of uric acid form in a joint, typically the base of the big toe. Drugs are available that decrease the amount of uric acid produced or maintained in the body and reduce the pain and inflammation associated with gout.

PATHOPHYSIOLOGY • Inflammation

The body uses inflammation to limit the extent and severity of an injury, to clean the traumatized area, and to promote healing. Thus, under normal circumstances, the symptoms of acute inflammation are designed to protect. These symptoms include pain, redness, warmth, and swelling and they are immediate responses to various stressors. The redness, warming, and swelling are caused by local vasodilation and increased capillary permeability. Swelling is followed by an infiltration of leukocytes and phagocytes. The final stage is a chronic proliferative phase of tissue degeneration and fibrosis. Acute inflammation usually resolves entirely in 8 to 10 days if no complications interfere with healing. In some instances, however, the inflammation does not disappear and instead becomes chronic. Chronic inflammation involves the same signs as acute simple inflammation, but it is relentless and damaging and can last for weeks, months, or years.

Different cell types and a number of chemicals produced and released in response to trauma contribute to the signs of inflammation. Chemical mediators are synthesized and released by activated granulocytes, lymphocytes, macrophages, mast cells, and sensory nerve endings. The chemicals include histamine, prostaglandins, leukotrienes, cytokines, platelet activating factor, oxygen radicals, and enzymes. In addition, bradykinin is generated by cleavage of kininogenin by plasma and tissue kallikreins. Histamine is released early in the inflammatory response and produces venous dilation and plasma extravasation. The role and effects of histamines and antihistamines are discussed in Chapter 53. Bradykinin produces pain, increases vascular permeability, and increases the synthesis of prostaglandins.

Selective antagonists to both bradykinin receptor subtypes (B_1 and B_2) are currently under investigation as potential antiinflammatory agents.

Prostaglandin production is associated with a variety of conditions characterized by pain and inflammation, including inflammatory arthritic conditions and musculoskeletal injury. Large amounts of prostaglandin E_2 (PGE_2) have been found in the synovial fluid of affected joints in patients with rheumatoid arthritis, synthesized by cells in the mesenchymal synovial lining. Presumably this production of PGE_2 contributes to the swelling and eventual bone erosion seen in cases of rheumatoid arthritis. Inflammatory bowel disease and dysmenorrhea also are associated with high production of prostaglandins. Leukotrienes (slow-reacting substances of anaphylaxis) are proinflammatory mediators synthesized by the lipoxygenase pathway. This pathway generates LTA_4, LTB_4, LTC_4, LTD_4, and LTE_4. LTB_4 in particular is a potent chemotactic agent that causes aggregation of granulocytes. These leukotrienes produce smooth muscle contraction, greater vascular permeability, and neutrophil and eosinophil chemotaxis in addtion to altering pulmonary physiology. Leukotrienes are thought to be important in the later stages of the inflammatory response because the effects they produce are slower and more prolonged than those of histamine or prostaglandins.

Prostaglandins and leukotrienes are metabolic products of the 20-carbon fatty acid, arachidonic acid. This fatty acid is released from cell membranes in response to trauma via activation of phospholipase A_2. The fatty acid can be metabolized by a number of enzymes (Figure 14-1), including **cyclooxygenases**,

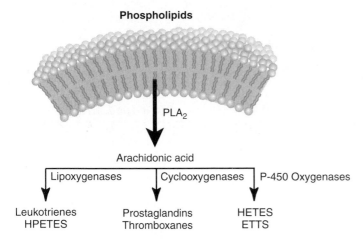

Phospholipids

PLA$_2$

Arachidonic acid

Lipoxygenases | Cyclooxygenases | P-450 Oxygenases

Leukotrienes
HPETES

Prostaglandins
Thromboxanes

HETES
ETTS

FIGURE 14-1 Metabolic pathways of arachidonic acid that result in production of eicosanoids. Arachidonic acid is liberated from membrane phospholipids by phospholipase A$_2$ (PLA$_2$) and then metabolized by one of three major classes of enzymes—cyclooxygenases, lipoxygenases, or P-450 oxidases—to a number of active substances including prostaglandins. The cyclooxygenases are inhibited by NSAIDs, preventing the synthesis of prostaglandins and thromboxanes. The lipoxygenases make leukotrienes and hydroperoxyeicosatetraenoic acids (HPETES), whereas P-450 catalyzes the synthesis of hydroxyeicosatetraenoic acids (HETES) and eposyeicosatetraenoic acids (ETTS).

which result in the synthesis of prostaglandins and thromboxanes, *lipoxygenases,* which make a number of products including leukotrienes, and the enzyme cytochrome *P-450 mixed function oxidases,* which synthesize eposyeicosatetraenoic acids (ETTS). Of all the products of arachidonic acid (called eicosanoids), the most important for inflammation, pain, and fever are the prostaglandins. Indeed, the major pharmacologic actions and adverse effects of NSAIDs can be attributed to their ability to inhibit cyclooxygenase and thus prevent the synthesis of prostaglandins and thromboxanes. Since these eicosanoids are not stored in cells but are synthesized on demand, the inhibition of their synthesis results in a loss of their actions on cells. This is advantageous if the effects of the prostanoids are deleterious, but if the effects of the prostaglandins are important in maintaining homeostasis, then inhibiting their synthesis could be detrimental to the patient.

Cyclooxygenases are now recognized to exist in at least two isoforms. Cyclooxygenase-1 (COX-1) is especially prevalent in blood vessels, the stomach, and the kidneys, although low levels are constantly present in most tissues. Cyclooxygenase-2 (COX-2) is not normally present in many cell types but it is induced by agents such as cytokines and growth factors. In some cell types, however, it also may be constitutively produced. COX-2 contributes to the production of prostaglandins associated with inflammation. Because COX-2 is inducible and appears to augment prostaglandin production during trauma or stress, the selective inhibition of this enzyme should reduce the harmful effects of prostaglandins while minimizing toxicity.

PATHOPHYSIOLOGY • Pain

One of the major pharmacologic effects of NSAIDs is **analgesia** (the relief of pain). In the previous chapter, we discussed the cause of pain and the pain pathway in detail. In this chapter we focus on the ability of prostaglandins to sensitize nociceptors (sensory nerve endings activated by noxious stimuli, such as heat or pressure) as the critical event prevented by NSAIDs. Free nerve endings of small-diameter sensory neurons are found throughout the body in cutaneous and visceral tissues. Although these endings are activated by high-threshold noxious stimuli, exposure to proinflammatory prostaglandins such as PGE$_2$ and PGI$_2$ enhances their excitability and lowers the threshold for activation. The result is that pain perception is heightened (hyperalgesia) or a harmless stimulus is perceived as noxious (allodynia). By blocking cyclooxygenase, the prostaglandins are not produced, and pain arising from stimulation of peripheral nerve endings is therefore lessened. Recent evidence also suggests that prostaglandins are produced in the spinal cord in response to peripheral injury and contribute to enhanced pain perception at this level. Thus NSAIDs may also act in the central nervous system to reduce pain.

PATHOPHYSIOLOGY • Fever

Under normal conditions, an area of the hypothalamus maintains a balance between heat production and heat dissipation. With infection, chronic inflammation, cancer, and other conditions, however, substances are introduced to or produced in the body that elevate the set point for body temperature. The substances producing fever are called **pyrogens**. The major endogenous pyrogens are the cytokines, including interleukin-1 beta (IL-1β), interleukin-6 (IL-6), and tumor necrosis factor alpha (TNFα). Cytokines are synthesized and released by almost all nucleated cells. They activate growth and function of neutrophils, lymphocytes, and macrophages as well as promote the release of additional mediators that influence the immune response. They also appear to contribute to the production of prostaglandins by inducing the COX-2 enzyme. Known exogenous pyrogens include microorganisms and their endotoxins, certain drugs (e.g., bleomycin and colchicine), and a few steroids. Bacterial endotoxins cause neutrophils to release prostaglandins and endogenous pyrogens.

Cytokines and exogenous pyrogens produce fever by augmenting the production of PGE$_2$ in the hypothalamus. The prostaglandins in turn act on neurons to elevate the body temperature. Even exogenous administration of PGE$_2$ into the hypothalamus of laboratory animals produces fever. Because PGE$_2$ is the local hormone that produces fever, blockade of its synthesis can reduce fever. Interestingly, both nonselective COX inhibitors and COX-2 selective inhibitors reduce fever, suggesting that COX-2 is the important isozyme. NSAIDs do not reduce body temperature in the absence of fever, presumably because the synthesis and release of PGE$_2$ in the hypothalamus is not involved in maintaining normal body temperature but only in fever production.

ADDITIONAL ACTIONS OF PROSTAGLANDINS

One way to remember the major pharmacologic actions and adverse effects of NSAIDs is to understand the various physiologic functions of prostaglandins and thromboxanes in the body. Because these eicosanoids are only produced on demand and the major action of NSAIDs is to block their synthesis, the actions of these drugs are generally opposite to the effects of prostaglandins and thromboxanes. As discussed above, prostaglandins are proinflammatory agents that also produce hyperalgesia and fever. Thus the NSAIDs are antiinflammatory (except acetaminophen), antipyretic, and analgesic. In addition to these actions, the prostaglandins and thromboxanes have a number of additional physiologic and pathologic actions (Table 14-1).

TABLE 14-1

Function of Eicosanoids

Eicosanoid	Physiologic or Pathologic Effects
Prostaglandins E$_1$, E$_2$ (PGE$_1$, PGE$_2$)	Hyperalgesia Fever Vasodilation of most vascular beds Bronchodilation Contraction of GI smooth muscle Contraction of pregnant uterus (low doses) Relaxation of nonpregnant uterus Inhibition of GI acid secretions Stimulation of GI mucous secretion Diuresis, naturiuresis
Prostaglandin F$_2$ (PGF$_2$)	Vasodilation/vasoconstriction based on vascular bed Bronchoconstriction Contraction of GI smooth muscle Contraction of nonpregnant or pregnant uterus
Prostaglandin I$_2$ (PGI$_2$; prostacyclin)	Hyperalgesia Vasodilation of vascular beds Inhibition of platelet aggregation Bronchodilation Relaxation of pregnant uterus (low doses) Inhibition of GI acid secretions Stimulation of GI mucous secretion Diuresis, naturiuresis
Prostaglandin D$_2$ (PGD$_2$)	Vasodilation of most vascular beds Vasoconstriction of pulmonary vascular beds Bronchoconstriction
Thromboxane A$_2$ (TXA$_2$)	Vasoconstriction Induction of platelet aggregation
Leukotriene B$_4$ (LTB$_4$)	Chemotaxis Hyperalgesia Contraction of GI smooth muscle
Leukotrienes C$_4$, D$_4$, E$_4$ (LTC$_4$, LTD$_4$, LTE$_4$) (slow-releasing substance of anaphylaxis)	Plasma extravasation Anaphylaxis Contraction of GI smooth muscle Bronchoconstriction

Thromboxane A_2 (TXA_2) and prostacyclin (PGI_2) have potent but opposite actions on platelet aggregation. TXA_2 is synthesized and released from platelets to induce aggregation. Therefore inhibition of thromboxane synthesis augments bleeding, which is one adverse effect of aspirinlike drugs. Prostacyclin and PGE_2 are vasodilators in most vascular beds, whereas $PGF_{2\alpha}$ has mixed effects, depending on the area of the body, and TXA_2 is a vasoconstrictor. Because of its ability to dilate the ductus arteriosus, PGE_1 (alprostadil) is used to maintain the vascular opening.

The prostanoids also affect smooth muscle other than that in the vasculature. Prostacyclin is a bronchodilator useful in treating pulmonary hypertension. PGE_2 and $PGF_{2\alpha}$ both contract the uterus in pregnancy and can induce labor, and PGE_2 is useful in promoting cervical dilation. Both these eicosanoids can be used as abortifacients.

Both PGE_2 and PGI_2 inhibit acid secretion in the stomach and promote the secretion of mucus, thereby producing a protective action. Blockade of prostaglandin production can lead to gastric irritation and damage, which are adverse effects of NSAIDs. Conversely, the PGE_1 analog misoprostol, is used to suppress gastric acid secretion and ulceration especially during chronic therapy with NSAIDs. Interestingly, there appears to be little COX-2 in stomach cells, which could explain why COX-2 selective inhibitors produce significantly fewer adverse effects in the gastrointestinal (GI) tract than nonselective NSAIDs. Prostaglandins also act on the kidneys to promote diuresis and naturiesis. These chemicals play a role in enhancing renal blood flow and in electrolyte balance. Thus there is concern for patients with compromised renal function who are administered NSAIDs.

DRUG CLASS • Salicylates

Aspirin (acetylsalicylic acid) is the prototype of the NSAIDs and the most widely used salicylate. It is available in OTC form and is a component of a number on preparations. Table 14-2 lists additional salicylates and brand names, including difunisal, choline salicylate, choline magnesium salicylate, olsalazine, salsalate sodium salicylate, and sulfasalazine. The first report of salicylate use was in the fifth century BC, when willow leaves were used as an analgesic. In the eighteenth century, the Reverend Edmund Stone presented a paper to the Royal Society on the use of willow bark to reduce fever. The active ingredient in the bark was salicin, which is converted to salicylic acid in the body. Aspirin was first synthesized by Hoffmann in 1879 and has been commercially available since 1899.

MECHANISM OF ACTION

Aspirin irreversibly inhibits both forms of cyclooxygenases, the key enzymes catalyzing the formation of prostaglandins. Other salicylates also inhibit COX-1 and COX-2, but the inhibition is reversible. The fact that aspirin irreversibly inhibits cyclooxygenase is what distinguishes this drug from other NSAIDs with respect to the extent of antiplatelet effects (see next section).

USES

Small doses of aspirin reduce fever and relieve mild pain. Two aspirin tablets are the analgesic equivalent of 60 mg of codeine. Aspirin is an effective analgesic for most mild to moderate common headaches and generalized mild muscular aches. Aspirin or aspirin-codeine combinations are used to treat mild to moderate pain of tooth extractions, episiotomies, cancer, and bone fractures.

Because aspirin inhibits platelet aggregation, it is also widely taken as a prophylactic drug to prevent myocardial infarction (MI), stroke, and other thromboembolic conditions. A unique property of aspirin is that it irreversibly acetylates cyclooxygenase of platelets, an effect that persists for 3 to 7 days. Because platelets do not synthesize new enzymes, production of TXA_2, a potent promoter of platelet aggregation, is blocked for the life of the platelet. Even one aspirin tablet inhibits blood clotting by inhibiting platelet aggregation.

Aspirin administered at high dosages is often the initial treatment to control the symptoms of inflammatory arthritis. These dosages are associated with considerable gastric irritation with or without bleeding, salicylism (see below), decreased platelet aggregation, and interactions with other drugs. Aspirin must be taken continuously for a long period before an improvement may be noted. Timed-release or enteric-coated formulations (see Table 14-2) may improve patient compliance by decreasing the number of times aspirin must be taken each day and by bypassing the stomach, thereby reducing gastric irritation.

Salicylates are used topically as keratolytic drugs (skin-eroding product) and as counterirritants. The keratolytic effect is useful in treating warts, corns, fungal infections, and certain types of eczematous dermatitis. Methyl salicylate (oil of wintergreen) is used as a counterirritant in the treatment of inflamed muscles caused by physical exercise or viral infections. When it is placed

TABLE 14-2

Nonsteroidal Antiinflammatory Drugs

Generic Name	Brand Name	Comments
Aspirin and Other Salicylates		
aspirin (acetylsalicylic acid)	A.S.A., Aspergum, Bayer Aspirin, Children's Aspirin, Ecotrin	Oral doses should be taken with large glass of water or milk to decrease stomach irritation; some patients may need to take aspirin after a meal to avoid GI distress; nonprescription
aspirin (acetylsalicylic acid), buffered	Alka-Seltzer, Bufferin, various others	Alka-Seltzer contains 1.9 g sodium bicarbonate and 1 g citric acid per tablet, so to avoid acid-base disturbances, limit ingestion to occasional use only; remaining products contain magnesium and aluminum antacid salts; these salts are not absorbed systemically to any great extent; nonprescription
aspirin (acetylsalicylic acid)	Bayer Timed-Release, Bufferin Arthritis Strength, various others	Dosage needed to achieve blood levels for antinflammatory activity of 20-30 mg/dl may vary from person to person; children who have viral illness and are given aspirin have increased risk of Reye's syndrome
choline salicylate	Arthropan	Mint-flavored liquid formulated for patients with arthritis
choline magnesium trisalicylate	Trilisate	Used in rheumatoid arthritis, osteoarthritis, and acute painful shoulder
diflunisal	Dolobid	Long-acting salicylic acid derivative; has lower incidence of same adverse effects as aspirin
magnesium salicylate	Doan's, Magan, Sero-Gesic✤	Contains no sodium, low incidence of GI upset; not recommended for patients with renal failure
olsalazine	Dipentum	Prophylaxis for inflammatory bowel disease for patients intolerant to sulfasalazine
salsalate	Amigesic, Disalcid	Dimer of salicylate. Absorption is from intestine only after hydrolysis to salicylic acid; delayed onset compared with free salicylic acid
sodium salicylate	Dodd's Pills,✤ generic	Less effective than equal doses of aspirin; may be tolerated in patients allergic to aspirin; does not affect platelet aggregation but is a vitamin K antagonist
sulfasalazine	Azulfidine, PMS-Sulfasalazine✤	Primary use in inflammatory bowel disease; also for treating rheumatoid arthritis
Para-Aminophenols		
acetaminophen	Tylenol, Datril, Panadol, Liquiprin, various others	Acts as analgesic and antipyretic only; has little antiinflammatory action and no ability to inhibit platelet aggregation
NSAIDs: Propionic Acid Derivatives		
fenoprofen	Nalfon	For mild to moderate pain, dysmenorrhea, and rheumatoid arthritis
floctafenine	Idarac✤	For mild to moderate pain and inflammation
flurbiprofen	Ansaid, Froben✤	For arthritis or dysmenorrhea
ibuprofen	Advil, Motrin, Nuprin, various others	Nonprescription for mild pain, fever, or dysmenorrhea; higher dosages available in prescription form for arthritis
ketoprofen	Orudis, Oruvail	For rheumatoid arthritis and dysmenorrhea
naproxen	Anaprox, Naprosyn, Naprelan, various others	For dysmenorrhea, mild to moderate pain, acute gout, and rheumatoid arthritis
oxaprozin	Daypro	For rheumatoid arthritis and osteoarthritis; patients with renal impairment should be started at half the normal dose
tiaprofenic acid	Surgam✤	For rheumatoid arthritis and osteoarthritis

✤ Available only in Canada.

TABLE 14-2

Nonsteroidal Antiinflammatory Drugs—cont'd

Generic Name	Brand Name	Comments
NSAIDs: Acetic Acid Derivatives		
diclofenac	Arthrotec, Novo-Difenac, ✷ Voltaren, various others	For rheumatoid arthritis, osteoarthritis, and ankylosing spondylitis
etodolac	Lodine	For pain and osteoarthritis
indomethacin	Apo-Indomethacin, ✷ Indocid, ✷ Indocin, Novomethacin ✷	Administer with meals or antacids to minimize gastric irritation; for acute inflammatory episodes; also given to premature infants to close ductus arteriosus
ketorolac tromethamine	Toradol	NSAID with analgesia equivalent to morphine; useful for outpatient surgery
sulindac	Apo-Sulin, ✷ Clinoril, Novo-Sundae ✷	For rheumatoid arthritis, acute gout, and bursitis
tolmetin	Tolectin	For rheumatoid arthritis, osteoarthritis, ankylosing spondylitis, juvenile arthritis, and psoriatic arthritis
NSAIDs: Enolic Acids		
meloxicam	Mobic	Approved for treatment of osteoarthritis
piroxicam	Apo-Piroxicam, ✷ Feldene, Novopirocam ✷	For rheumatoid arthritis and osteoarthritis; administer after meals to avoid gastric irritation
tenoxicam	Mobiflex ✷	For rheumatoid arthritis, acute gout, and bursitis
NSAIDs: Fenamates		
meclofenamate	Meclomen	For rheumatoid arthritis; not available in Canada
mefenamic acid	Ponstel, Ponstan ✷	For mild to moderate pain; administer after meals to avoid gastric irritation
NSAIDs: Alkanones		
nambumetone	Relafen	For rheumatoid arthritis and osteoarthritis
NSAIDs: COX-2 Inhibitors		
celecoxib	Celebrex	Minimal GI adverse effects; used for patients with rheumatoid arthritis and osteoarthritis
rofecoxib	Vioxx	Minimal GI adverse effects; used for patients with rheumatoid arthritis and osteoarthritis for short-term pain relief
valdecoxib	Bextra	For osteoarthritis, rheumatoid arthritis, and menstrual pain; not associated with increased risk of cardiovascular or renal complications

on the skin, it obscures the pain and discomfort by causing a feeling of warmth or slight burning. However, methyl salicylate is a common pediatric poison and its use is discouraged.

Sodium salicylate is marketed as an analgesic and antipyretic. Magnesium and choline salicylates are also marketed for the relief of muscle aches. Diflunisal is a prescription drug used to relieve the symptoms of rheumatoid arthritis and osteoarthritis. The major use of sulfasalazine is in the treatment of inflammatory bowel disease, but it is also used occasionally for the treatment of rheumatic diseases. The active principal for rheumatic diseases may be the sulfapyridine component, which has suppressive effects on lymphocytes. Olsalazine is a salicylate that is only recommended as prophylactic therapy for patients in remission from ulcerative colitis who do not tolerate sulfasalazine.

PHARMACOKINETICS

Aspirin is rapidly absorbed from the stomach and upper small intestine. Once aspirin is absorbed, 50% to 90% binds loosely to plasma albumin. Aspirin is rapidly hydrolyzed in the blood. The acetyl group of aspirin is readily transferred to the COX enzymes. Salicylic acid is the other product of the hydrolysis of aspirin. Salicylate is an analgesic-antipyretic and a reversible inhibitor of prostaglandin synthesis. Salicylate does not affect platelet aggregation to a significant degree, and therefore a salicylate salt is sometimes used in place of aspirin.

In acidic urine, salicylic acid is uncharged and therefore diffuses back into the blood. Vitamin C (ascorbic acid) maintains an acidic urine when taken in large doses and can therefore delay the excretion of salicylic acid. This interaction can be dangerous if large doses of aspirin are taken, such as for arthritis. In alkaline urine, salicylic acid dissociates to its charged form, cannot diffuse back into the blood, and is therefore eliminated in the urine. Salicylate is biotransformed to inactive salicyluric acid by the liver. However, a 325-mg aspirin tablet will saturate this liver inactivation system; the liver cannot readily biotransform large doses of aspirin.

Buffering agents are present in several aspirin brands to hasten dissolution of and to reduce gastric irritation from the tablet. The advantages of buffering agents are minimal, and if several doses are taken, the buffering agents may cause loose stools. Alka-Seltzer contains so much sodium and bicarbonate that it should be used only on a short-term basis.

Diflunisal is a fluoridated derivative of salicylic acid with a long duration of action. It is not converted to salicylic acid. Because it does not penetrate the central nervous system (CNS), it does not reduce fever.

ADVERSE REACTIONS AND CONTRAINDICATIONS

Approximately 2% to 10% of those taking an occasional aspirin tablet experience GI irritation, which may be felt as heartburn or nausea. When aspirin is taken regularly in large doses for arthritis, this incidence rate reaches 30% to 50% and may be the primary factor limiting the use of aspirin. Sometimes antacids are prescribed to minimize stomach irritation, but they also raise the pH of the urine and increase the rate of excretion of salicylic acid. Alternatively, enteric-coated or timed-release preparations may be tried to decrease gastric irritation. Sodium salicylate, magnesium salicylate, and choline salicylate are all salicylate salts that produce less gastric irritation than aspirin.

Aspirin is directly irritating and damaging to gastric mucosal cells because inhibition of COX-1 results in reduced synthesis of protective prostaglandins. Patients with active peptic ulcers should be advised not to use aspirin.

Because of the effects on platelet aggregation, aspirin is contraindicated for patients with bleeding disorders and those on anticoagulants. Long-term aspirin inges-

tion can cause the loss of 10 to 30 mL of blood daily from GI irritation. This loss may lead to iron deficiency anemia in women with heavy menses. Rarely, massive GI bleeding occurs in patients who take aspirin on a long-term basis. Salicylate salts do not alter platelet function, as does aspirin.

Some people develop an allergy to aspirin; the most common form of intolerance manifests as a rash. However, patients with a skin rash caused by aspirin may tolerate other salicylates. A few people develop nasal polyps and sometimes later an asthma triggered by aspirin. Patients hypersensitive to aspirin may be sensitive to a variety of other compounds. Most commonly, these individuals may show cross-sensitivity to salicylin-containing foods (e.g., apples, oranges, bananas), processed foods or drugs containing tartrazine (a food additive, FDA yellow dye #5), sodium benzoate, iodide-containing substances, or various other NSAIDs. The origin of these cross-sensitivities is not always the classic cross-reactivity caused by structural similarities of the drugs. Sulfasalazine contains sulfur in its structure; thus persons with intolerance to sulfa drugs should avoid using this compound.

Aspirin is contraindicated for treating children and teenagers who have an acute febrile illness such as influenza or chicken pox, because aspirin puts them at increased risk for developing **Reye's syndrome,** a rare but serious disorder characterized by vomiting and rapidly progressive **encephalopathy.** Acetaminophen and other NSAIDs have not been so implicated. Nonprescription aspirin products now contain a warning against administration to children and teenagers who manifest chicken pox or flu symptoms.

Although aspirin was used in the past to treat gout, low doses decrease uric acid secretion and therefore worsen symptoms. Only high levels of aspirin increase uric acid loss. Because of the potential to worsen gout and the existence of superior drugs to treat this problem (see later discussion), aspirin should not be used for this purpose.

TOXICITY

Intoxication with aspirin is called **salicylism** and is commonly experienced when the daily dosage exceeds 4 g (Box 14-1). **Tinnitus** (ringing in the ears) is the most common symptom and may be accompanied by a degree of reversible hearing loss. Because salicylate stimulates the respiratory center, hyperventilation (rapid breathing) may occur. Fever may also result because salicylate interferes with the metabolic pathways coupling oxygen consumption and heat production. Acute overdose of aspirin causes serious disturbances in the body's acid-base balance. Initial toxicity is characterized by respiratory alkalosis secondary to stimulation of respira-

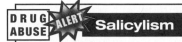 **Salicylism**

The Problem

Salicylism is a well-described syndrome resulting from intentional or accidental overdosage with aspirin (or another salicylate). The fatal dosage is variable, depending on patient size, rate of absorption, and so forth. Mild salicylate toxicity is usually due to drug accumulation following chronic administration of 150 to 250 mg/kg body weight. Severe to lethal toxicity is found with doses exceeding 250 mg/kg. Methyl salicylate is particularly toxic in low doses, with fatalities reported following ingestion of even a single teaspoon (approximately 5 g). Toxicity is classified as mild, moderate, or severe based on the following plasma salicylate levels:

- Mild toxicity: 45 to 65 mg/dL
- Moderate toxicity: 65 to 90 mg/dL
- Severe toxicity: over 90 mg/dL
- Severe to lethal toxicity: over 120 mg/dL

Early symptoms of salicylism include tinnitus, headache, nausea and vomiting, dizziness, and dimness of vision. The tinnitus is caused by vasoconstriction of auditory microvasculature or increased pressure within the cochlear labyrinth and effects on its hair cells. High-frequency hearing loss is correlated with salicylate concentration but is reversible by discontinuing the drug.

Hyperventilation, an early sign of salicylate overdose, is almost always present. It is attributable to direct CNS-stimulating effects on respiratory centers and to the CO_2 generated by uncoupling of oxidative phosphorylation. The result is an initial respiratory alkalosis compensated in about 3 days by enhanced renal elimination of sodium and potassium bicarbonate. Compensated respiratory alkalosis in combination with the aforementioned symptoms is the usual presentation of salicylism in adults. Without intervention, respiratory alkalosis will be followed by metabolic acidosis as the patient's respiratory efforts weaken and CO_2 builds up.

Salicylism in children presents a more serious picture. They display profound CNS effects, including respiratory depression, marked hyperthermia, vomiting, diarrhea, and diaphoresis. The combined signs and symptoms produce a mixed acid-base imbalance as well as respiratory and metabolic acidosis, ultimately leading to seizures, coma, and death.

The Solution: *Prevention!*

- Store NSAIDs in a childproof container out of sight in a locked cabinet.
- Never call aspirin or other drugs candy.
- Avoid concurrent use of salicylates and other NSAIDs. Teach patients to read labels carefully to avoid duplicate sources of aspirin and ibuprofen and potential overdose.
- Advise the patient to discard salicylate tablets with a vinegar-like odor, a sign of salicylate deterioration.
- Encourage the patient to report hearing changes, because bilateral hearing loss of 30 to 40 decibels occurs with prolonged salicylate use. Reassure the patient that hearing usually returns to normal within 2 weeks after treatment is stopped.

The Treatment

- Undissolved tablets are removed by inducing vomiting or by absorption with activated charcoal.
- Plasma salicylate, blood gas, glucose, sodium, and potassium levels are monitored every 4 to 5 hours.
- Hyperthermia is treated with sponge baths.
- Hypovolemia, dehydration, and acid-base and electrolyte imbalances are corrected with intravenous fluids.
- Additional interventions may include hemodialysis, peritoneal dialysis, or exchange transfusions if salicylate levels do not fall with supportive treatment.

tion. Patients with overdose rapidly develop metabolic acidosis, perhaps because of the acidic nature of aspirin and its metabolites and because salicylate inhibits biotransformation in a manner that favors the accumulation of organic acids, which would normally have been changed to carbon dioxide and water. Furthermore, respirations are depressed, leading to respiratory acidosis. The hyperthermia also produced with this metabolic block must be treated quickly.

Profuse sweating can produce dehydration. The supportive treatment of aspirin toxicity therefore consists of careful monitoring of the acid-base balance and electrolyte levels as well as appropriate fluid administration. Intravenous sodium bicarbonate can counter the tendency toward metabolic acidosis and produce an alkaline urine that hastens the excretion of salicylate. Osmotic diuretics or dialysis may be necessary in extreme cases to remove salicylate. A day or two after massive aspirin ingestion, increased bleeding tendency and signs of minor hemorrhaging may be noted. A child is more likely than an adult to die from a large overdose of aspirin. Fatalities among children have been dramatically reduced since 1970, when the Poison Prevention Packaging Act required that orange-flavored baby aspirin (in 81-mg tablets) be limited to 36 tablets per bottle and that safety caps be used. If a child ingests more than 150 mg/kg (36 baby tablets [one bottle] or 9 adult tablets [for a 45-lb child]), vomiting may be induced, or gastric lavage used to eliminate undissolved tablets. Because charcoal absorbs about half its weight in aspirin, it is given orally to reduce aspirin absorption. Diflunisal does not cause tinnitus and has a lesser incidence of GI and antiplatelet adverse effects than aspirin.

INTERACTIONS

The drug interactions associated with aspirin are especially important because of its widespread and noncritical use. Aspirin enhances the potential for GI bleeding and ulcers with corticosteroids and alcohol. Aspirin should not be taken when alcohol is in the stomach; the combination of alcohol and aspirin increases the risk of gastric bleeding. Aspirin and other salicylates can displace oral anticoagulants, oral hypoglycemic drugs, phenytoin, and methotrexate from plasma protein binding. Because the unbound drug is the active form, free drug may reach toxic levels when displaced by aspirin.

 DRUG CLASS • **Other NSAIDs**

There are a number of additional classes of NSAIDs (see Table 14-2), including the *propionic acid derivatives* fenoprofen, floctafenine, flurbiprofen, ibuprofen, ketoprofen, naproxen, oxaprozin, and tiaprofenic acid; the *acetic acid derivatives* diclofenac, etodolac, indomethacin, ketorolac, sulindac, and tolmetin; the *enolic acids*, piroxicam, tenoxicam, and meloxicam; the *fenamates*, meclofenamate and mefenamic acid; and the *alkanone* nabumetone. Oxaprozin is available in the United States but not in Canada; floctafenine and tiaprofenic acid are available in Canada but not in the United States. These drugs are discussed as a group because the pharmacologic and toxicologic actions are similar. Choice of which drug to use in a patient is largely empirical and may be related to the adverse effects profile or the duration of action.

MECHANISM OF ACTION

As with salicylates, the primary mechanism of action of the other NSAIDs is the inhibition of the enzyme cyclooxygenase so that prostaglandins are not formed. All of these drugs are reversible inhibitors and are not selective for COX-1 or COX-2 at therapeutic doses. These drugs may have other actions that contribute to their antiinflammatory actions, including reducing the motility of leukocytes and inhibition of various other enzymes.

USES

NSAIDs are widely used as first-line therapy for inflammatory diseases, including rheumatoid arthritis, ankylosing spondylitis, and juvenile arthritis. Osteoarthritis is not characterized by a high level of inflammation, but lower dosages of NSAIDs can be used to treat the pain associated with osteoarthritis. NSAIDs are also useful in treating pain and inflammation in athletic injuries, bursitis, synovitis, and other soft tissue injuries involving strains and sprains.

NSAIDs are effective analgesics for mild to moderate pain from a variety of conditions, including dental, obstetric, or orthopedic surgery. They can help to avert menstrual cramps, particularly if therapy is begun a few days before the start of menses. Ibuprofen and naproxen are used to reduce fever.

Propionic acid derivatives provide effective analgesic and antiinflammatory action and are often used to treat rheumatoid arthritis, osteoarthritis, and gout. In addition to its use as an analgesic and antipyretic, ibuprofen is effective in treating dysmenorrhea. Fenoprofen also is used to treat the pain of gout and to relieve vascular headaches and dysmenorrhea. Floctafenine is primarily used as an analgesic. Flurbiprofen, which has also been formulated as a solution for ophthalmic use, is used to treat and prevent vascular headaches as well. Ketoprofen is used as an analgesic, especially for headaches and dysmenorrhea. Etodolac may also be used to treat acute gout attacks, dysmenorrhea, vascular headaches, and musculoskeletal conditions. Ketorolac tromethamine is given by intramuscular injection for the short-term management of moderate to severe pain, particularly in postoperative patients. Mefenamic acid is prescribed for mild to moderate pain, whereas meclofenamate is prescribed for rheumatoid arthritis and osteoarthritis. Nabumetone treats rheumatoid arthritis and osteoarthritis. Piroxicam is prescribed principally for rheumatoid arthritis and osteoarthritis. Tenoxicam is available in Canada but not in the United States for treatment of rheumatoid arthritis, osteoarthritis, ankylosing spondylitis, bursitis, and tendonitis.

PHARMACOKINETICS

NSAIDs are generally well absorbed after oral administration and produce effective pain relief within 30 to 60 minutes. When used to treat arthritis, significant relief of other inflammatory symptoms may take several days. NSAIDs are well distributed to body tissues, placental membranes, and most transcellular fluids through pH-dependent passive processes. Some NSAIDs are highly bound to plasma proteins. Significant drug levels are found in the plasma in less than 30 minutes; peak levels are reached 2 to 4 hours after a single dose. The duration of drug action ranges from 3 to 48 hours depending on the NSAID. Ibuprofen, available in OTC form, is rapidly absorbed and has a plasma half-life of 2 hours. Flurbiprofen is taken orally every 6 to 12 hours. An extended-release form of flurbiprofen is available for once-daily dosage. Ketoprofen is available in OTC form in the United States and is taken every 4 to 6 hours; extended-release forms are available for once-daily dosage. Naproxen is longer-acting than aspirin or ibuprofen and can be taken twice a day. Piroxicam is well absorbed and has a long half-life of 45 hours, making once-daily dosing adequate. Sulindac has a plasma half-life of 8 hours and can be taken less often than indomethacin or tolmetin. Tolmetin is absorbed rapidly and has a plasma half-life of only 1 hour.

Biotransformation of NSAIDs occurs in the liver and many other tissues. The drugs are rapidly cleared in the urine as free drug and other metabolites. For example, piroxicam is rapidly excreted in the urine as a glucuronide. Although it is variable, the elimination of free drug in the urine depends on both the dose and urinary pH. A small portion of some NSAIDs is eliminated through the feces. Nabumetone is a prodrug that undergoes hepatic biotransformation to the active substance. It requires only once-daily administration, although larger dosages may be divided. Sulindac also is a prodrug activated after conversion by the liver. The active metabolite is excreted in the bile and reabsorbed from the intestine.

ADVERSE REACTIONS AND CONTRAINDICATIONS

The major adverse reaction to NSAIDs is gastric irritation leading to an increase in ulceration. This effect can be minimized by taking the drugs with meals. All prescription NSAIDs now carry a warning to reflect concern about the adverse gastric effects seen with their long-term use. Irritation and bleeding occurs less often with ibuprofen than with aspirin and may be further reduced by taking the drug with meals.

Inhibition of platelet aggregation is another common side effect of the NSAIDs. Although this effect is irreversible with aspirin, it is reversible with the other NSAIDs. Oxaprozin is an especially potent inhibitor of platelet aggregation and should be discontinued 1 to 2 weeks before elective surgery.

Patients who develop a rash or other allergic reactions to one of the NSAIDs may be intolerant of the others. This is especially true of patients who have experienced bronchospasm resulting from aspirin ingestion or who are sensitive to aspirin because they have asthma. Other adverse reactions include dizziness, headache, and water and sodium retention. Finally, much like the salicylates, overdose with NSAIDs causes auditory and visual disturbances accompanied by fever and changes in blood pH. Coma occasionally occurs.

Older adults are more likely to develop GI distress, liver toxicity, or renal damage while taking NSAIDs and should be carefully monitored. In addition, patients with clinical conditions such as heart failure, cirrhosis, and renal insufficiency are at risk for impaired renal function when taking NSAIDs. These patients require the local synthesis of vasodilating prostaglandins to maintain renal perfusion. NSAIDs, by inhibiting these prostaglandins, allow unopposed vasoconstriction. This renal ischemia can lead to a deterioration of renal function.

NSAID use places a fetus at risk for amniotic fluid deficiency caused by a decrease in fetal urine elimination. There is also a theoretic risk of premature closure of the ductus arteriosus in utero. Thus NSAIDs are generally contraindicated during pregnancy and lactation. In addition to the previously mentioned adverse effects, indomethacin use can cause confusion, lightheadedness, fainting, or drowsiness. Therapy with mefenamic acid is limited to 1 week because of the common occurrence of toxicity associated with the GI, renal, and blood-forming systems. Adverse reactions may include GI irritation, diarrhea, and rash.

INTERACTIONS

In general, the NSAIDs are highly bound to protein and displace other drugs, particularly hydantoins, sulfonamides, sulfonylureas, and calcium-channel blockers, leading to exacerbation of adverse effects of these drugs when elimination is compromised. NSAIDs may increase the risk of renal damage if used with acetaminophen over long periods. The risk of GI complications, especially ulceration or hemorrhage, is increased if NSAIDs are taken concurrently with alcohol, anticoagulants, thrombolytics, or glucocorticoids. NSAIDs may diminish the effectiveness of diuretics and intensify the risk of renal failure. They also potentiate drugs that inhibit platelet aggregation. NSAIDs should be discontinued when a gold compound or methotrexate is administered to treat rheumatoid arthritis because of their potential for renal damage.

DRUG CLASS • Cyclooxygenase-2 Inhibitors

celecoxib (Celebrex)

etodolac (Lodine)

meloxicam (Mobic)

rofecoxib (Vioxx)

valdecoxib (Bextra)

MECHANISM OF ACTION

Three major COX-2 inhibitors (see Table 14-2) are currently marketed in the United States—celecoxib, rofecoxib, and valdecoxib. These drugs selectively inhibit the activity of COX-2, one of two isozymes that catalyze the synthesis of prostaglandins and thromboxanes. At therapeutic doses, these drugs do not inhibit the activity of COX-1. At lower concentrations, etodolac and meloxicam also block COX-2 activity more than they inhibit COX-1, but they can have the capability of fully blocking COX-1.

USES

These drugs are indicated for the treatment of rheumatoid arthritis or osteoarthritis. Rofecoxib is also used for short-term pain relief (5 days) after minor surgery and for dysmenorrhea. The drugs are analgesics and antipyretics as well as having antiinflammatory action. Valdecoxib also is approved for the symptomatic relief of primary dysmenorrhea. The major advantage of these drugs over other NSAIDs appears to be the limited adverse effects.

PHARMACOKINETICS

As with most other NSAIDs, the COX-2 inhibitors are well absorbed orally; peak serum concentrations occur in 2 to 3 hours. These drugs are highly bound to plasma proteins and therefore have the potential to displace other drugs. They are biotransformed in the liver with a small percentage of a given dose excreted in the feces unchanged. The half-lives of celecoxib, rofecoxib, and valdecoxib are about 11, 17, and 8 to 11 hours, respectively. One of the metabolites of valdecoxib also is a COX-2 inhibitor.

ADVERSE REACTIONS AND CONTRAINDICATIONS

In general, the adverse effect profile for these drugs is less severe when compared with that of other NSAIDs. These drugs do not produce the incidence of GI distress seen with aspirin and even with other NSAIDs since they do not inhibit COX-1 in the GI tract. They also have no effect on platelet aggregation where the COX-1 isozyme predominates. These drugs can produce edema and skin rashes, coughing and congestion in the chest. Although rare, they can cause gastritis, GI pain or bleeding, or ulceration. Celecoxib and rofecoxib can also cause flulike symptoms and shortness of breath. The drugs should be used with caution in patients with hypersensitivity to other NSAIDs, because these drugs can produce bronchoconstriction or anaphylaxis in such individuals. Since celecoxib contains sulfur, patients with an allergy to sulfa drugs should avoid using it. Overdose of the COX-2 inhibitors can result in acute renal failure, drowsiness, epigastric pain, and gastrointestinal bleeding.

INTERACTIONS

These drugs are relatively new, so information on potential drug interactions is limited. Because they are highly bound to plasma proteins, they have the potential to displace other drugs from binding sites. The increased free drug can have negative consequences, especially if drug elimination is compromised. Celecoxib has the potential to interact with fluconazole, causing the latter to inhibit biotransformation and thus increase plasma concentration of celecoxib. Patients taking these drugs concurrently with lithium may develop a higher lithium blood level and thus should be monitored for this effect. These drugs may also diminish the antihypertensive effects of ACE–inhibitors, and valdecoxib may decrease responsiveness to other antihypertensives and to some diuretics. As with other NSAIDs, concurrent use with aspirin can worsen adverse effects on the GI tract.

 ACETAMINOPHEN

MECHANISM OF ACTION

Acetaminophen is a paraaminophenol derivative and a popular OTC drug with several brand names (see Table 14-2). It is also found in combination preparations with caffeine or codeine analogs.

Acetaminophen is believed to act principally by inhibiting prostaglandin synthesis in the CNS. The extent of its activity in the periphery is unclear. It has very weak antiinflammatory action.

USES

Acetaminophen is a drug of choice for mild pain and fever. It is also an effective analgesic for tension headaches; muscle, joint, postpartum, and postoperative pain;

and the chronic pain of cancer. Acetaminophen is often combined with codeine to provide analgesia for moderate to severe pain. Acetaminophen does not interfere with blood coagulation and platelet function; therefore it can be given to patients with clotting disorders or those on anticoagulants. It also does not typically cause gastric irritation. In addition, acetaminophen is not associated with Reye's syndrome when administered to children or adolescents with influenza or chicken pox. It is important to note, however, that it does not have significant antiinflammatory actions and therefore is not useful for dysmenorrhea, sunburn, rheumatic diseases, or juvenile arthritis except as a pain reliever.

PHARMACOKINETICS

Acetaminophen is rapidly and completely absorbed from the GI tract. Analgesia is usually apparent within 20 minutes, with peak plasma concentrations reached in 30 to 60 minutes. The duration of action is 3 to 4 hours. Acetaminophen is biotransformed in the liver to glucuronide and sulfate conjugates, which are eliminated in the urine.

ADVERSE REACTIONS AND CONTRAINDICATIONS

Persons with a known glucose-6-phosphate (G6P) dehydrogenase deficiency can develop hemolytic anemia if they take acetaminophen. Chronic daily ingestion of acetaminophen also has been associated with an increased risk of renal disease. Overdose of acetaminophen causes extensive liver damage. Children rarely experience permanent liver damage from the drug, but adults who take more than 2.6 g in 24 hours may show mild symptoms of liver damage such as loss of appetite, nausea, vomiting, and slight jaundice. In deliberate overdoses of 10 g or more, adults are highly susceptible to severe liver damage; death has been reported after ingestion of 15 g. This toxicity arises because the liver normally conjugates toxic metabolites of acetaminophen with a sulfhydryl compound, glutathione, to produce an inactive, readily excreted compound. The amount of glutathione available for conjugation is exceeded when large amounts of acetaminophen are ingested. The unconjugated metabolites then bind to and destroy liver cells. Damage to the kidneys in the form of renal tubular necrosis has also been associated with acetaminophen overdose, especially in conjunction with liver damage. Box 14-2 discusses acetaminophen toxicity.

INTERACTIONS

Hepatotoxic drugs and chronic alcohol use can augment the hepatotoxicity of acetaminophen. Caution should be exercised in patients on other NSAIDs because of the added risk of renal toxicity.

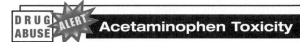

DRUG ABUSE ALERT: Acetaminophen Toxicity

The Problem

Acetaminophen overdose may be intentional or accidental. It is the most common form of poisoning in childhood. Toxicity from therapeutic use is rare but may occur with ingestion of double the recommended maximum therapeutic dosage of 90 mg/kg/day for several days. The clinical manifestations of acetaminophen toxicity occur in the following four stages:

1. Within 2 to 4 hours after ingestion: nausea, vomiting, sweating, pallor
2. After 24 to 36 hours: symptoms lessen and patient's condition improves, but levels of toxic metabolite continue to rise
3. After 2 to 7 days: hepatic damage as evidenced by right upper quadrant pain, jaundice, confusion, stupor, abnormal laboratory test results (increased levels of AST, ALT, LDH; increased prothrombin time, hypoglycemia); hepatic damage may be permanent
4. After 7 days: patients who do not die during the stage of hepatic involvement gradually recover.

The Solution

Liver damage related to acetaminophen overdose can be minimized by the timely administration of acetylcysteine (Mucomyst). This drug provides the sulfhydryl groups needed to conjugate and inactivate the toxic metabolites of acetaminophen. Acetylcysteine is most effective when administered as soon as possible after the overdose. If it is administered 12 to 24 hours after ingestion, the likelihood of severe liver damage is as high as 85%. Thus the time between ingestion and treatment is critical.

First, the stomach is emptied of its contents by inducing emesis or with gastric lavage. Since acetylcysteine has the pervasive flavor of rotten eggs, it must be disguised in a flavored iced drink such as juice, cola, or water to increase the palatability. It should be taken through a straw to minimize contact with mucous membranes of the mouth. If vomiting interferes with oral administration, the drug can be given through a nasogastric or orogastric tube. Treatment is discontinued when the acetaminophen blood level indicates a low risk of hepatotoxicity.

DRUG CLASS • **Disease-Modifying Antirheumatic Drugs**

anakinra (Kineret)

azathioprine (Imuran)

hydroxychloroquine (Plaquenil)

leflunomide (Arava)

methotrexate (Folex, Mexate, Rheumatrex)

penicillamine (Cuprimine, Depen)

In addition to NSAIDs and glucocorticoids, there are other drugs used in treating rheumatoid arthritis and osteoarthritis. Since rheumatoid arthritis appears to be an autoimmune disease, a number of immune suppressive and antineoplastic drugs are used to relieve symptoms of the disease. Additional information on azathioprine, leflunomide, and methotrexate can be found in Chapters 36 and 37. An additional group of drugs used in the treatment of rheumatoid diseases are the gold compounds (see next drug class).

MECHANISM OF ACTION

Although the mechanism of action of these drugs remains to be determined, azathioprine, leflunomide, and methotrexate have the ability to suppress the immune response. Azathioprine antagonizes purine metabolism with subsequent inhibition of DNA and RNA synthesis. The benefits are the result of suppression of cell-mediated immunity and altered antibody formation. Methotrexate is a folic acid antagonist that inhibits DNA synthesis and cell reproduction, whereas leflunomide is an immunomodulator that inhibits dehydroorotate dehydrogenase. Both leflunomide and methotrexate have antiinflammatory activity.

The mechanisms of action of hydroxychloroquine and penicillamine are not known. Hydroxychloroquine has antimalarial actions (see Chapter 34) and acts as an immunosuppressant, whereas the antirheumatic effect of penicillamine may be related to multiple mechanisms. It reduces immunoglobulin synthesis by monocytes and lymphocytes, inhibits polymorphonuclear leukocytes and T-cell function, and possibly protects tissues from oxygen radical damage. Anakinra is a unique drug in that it is a competitive inhibitor of the cytokine IL-1 at its receptor (see Chapter 36).

USES

Azathioprine is a cytotoxic immunosuppressive drug used in the treatment of severe, active, erosive rheumatoid arthritis that is unresponsive to more conventional therapy. Hydroxychloroquine is prescribed earlier in the management of severe rheumatoid arthritis. It is also used for the suppression and prophylaxis of malaria (see Chapter 34). Methotrexate and leflunomide relieve

symptoms of severe arthritis, and in some cases, methotrexate may induce prolonged remission. Penicillamine is used in the management of progressive rheumatoid arthritis that is unresponsive to conventional therapy. It is also used for prophylaxis and treatment of copper deposition in Wilson's disease and in the management of recurrent cystine calculi. Anakinra is recommended for symptoms of rheumatoid arthritis in adults who have failed treatment with at least one of the other disease-modifying antirheumatic drugs.

PHARMACOKINETICS

Azathioprine is readily absorbed following oral administration. The onset of antiinflammatory effects occurs within 6 to 8 weeks; peak action is noted in 12 weeks. Azathioprine is biotransformed to mercaptopurine, which is broken down further. Hydroxychloroquine is well absorbed when given orally, is widely distributed in body tissues, and has a delayed onset of action. It is 45% bound to plasma proteins and has a half-life of 72 to 120 hours. Full therapeutic effects take 3 to 6 months to develop. Partial biotransformation takes place in the liver, and a portion of the drug is eliminated unchanged in the urine. There is some indication that the drug enters breast milk.

Leflunomide is a prodrug converted by the liver to the active metabolite M1. M1, in turn, is highly bound to plasma proteins and inactivated by liver biotransformation. It has a half-life of 1 to 2 weeks. Small doses of methotrexate are completely absorbed from the GI tract, whereas larger doses are incompletely absorbed. It is actively transported across cell membranes to be widely distributed. The drug crosses the placenta and enters breast milk in low concentrations. Methotrexate is eliminated mostly unchanged by the kidneys.

Penicillamine is well absorbed following oral administration, although its oral bioavailability is decreased in the presence of food, antacids, and iron supplements. The onset of antirheumatic effects occurs 1 to 3 months after administration. Anakinra is given subcutaneously, is well absorbed by this route, and has a half-life of 2 to 6 hours.

ADVERSE REACTIONS AND CONTRAINDICATIONS

Because of the potential toxicity of these drugs, they are usually only given when other therapies for rheumatoid arthritis fail. The most common adverse effects of azathioprine are fever, chills, anorexia, nausea, vomiting, and hepatotoxicity. Leukopenia, anemia, pancytopenia, and thrombocytopenia have also been noted. Serum sickness can be life threatening. Azathioprine is teratogenic and should not be used during pregnancy. The drug may also be carcinogenic.

There are many adverse effects of hydroxychloroquine, but the most common include nausea, vomiting, diarrhea, corneal changes, pruritus, and bleaching of the hair. The most serious adverse effects are retinal damage, agranulocytosis, and aplastic anemia. The retinal damage may be irreversible and can produce blindness. Visual loss is directly related to drug dosage. Because retinal damage is progressive and may continue even after drug use has been discontinued, therapy should be stopped at the first sign of retinal changes. Fatalities have occurred with the ingestion of even three or four tablets of hydroxychloroquine, so the drug must be kept out of children's reach.

Common adverse effects of methotrexate include stomatitis, anorexia, nausea, vomiting, and hepatotoxicity. Anemia, leukopenia, thrombocytopenia, and neuropathy are also fairly common occurrences. Pulmonary fibrosis is life threatening. Methotrexate should be used with caution in patients with low creatinine clearance and those who are of childbearing age. Cautious use also is warranted in patients with active infections and decreased bone marrow reserve, in older adults, and in patients with chronic debilitating illnesses.

Leflunomide administration can result in bronchitis, hypertension, or hepatotoxicity as well as an increase in the incidence of respiratory or urinary tract infections. The most common adverse effects of penicillamine include anorexia, oral ulcerations, epigastric pain, nausea, vomiting, diarrhea, and altered taste perception. Bone marrow depression, proteinuria, and a generalized pruritus have also been noted.

Polymyositis and a myasthenic syndrome are life-threatening adverse effects.

Major adverse effects of anakinra are reactions at the injection site and an increased incidence of serious infections. This drug is not recommended for patients hypersensitive to products made from *Escherichia coli* and patients with serious infections.

INTERACTIONS

Drug-drug interactions include an additive myelosuppression with antineoplastics, cyclosporin, and myelosuppressants. Allopurinol inhibits the biotransformation of azathioprine, thus increasing the risk of toxicity. Azathioprine also decreases the antibody response to live virus vaccines and increases the risk of adverse effects. There is increased risk of hepatotoxicity when hydroxychloroquine is administered concurrently with other hepatotoxic drugs. When used concurrently with drugs having dermatologic toxicity, the patient's risk of dermatitis increases. Serum digoxin levels may be increased, and urinary acidifiers may increase the renal elimination of hydroxychloroquine.

Many drug-drug interactions are associated with methotrexate. Additive toxicity can occur with concurrent use of other hepatotoxic and nephrotoxic drugs including leflunomide. Methotrexate decreases antibody response to live virus vaccines and increases the risk of adverse effects. When used with antineoplastic or immunosuppressive drugs, penicillamine increases the risk of adverse hematologic effects. Iron supplements decrease drug absorption and serum digoxin levels. Daily requirements for pyridoxine (vitamin B_6) may be increased.

DRUG CLASS • Gold Salts

auranofin (Ridaura)

aurothioglucose (Solganal)

gold sodium thiomalate (sodium aurothiomalate, Myochrysine)

MECHANISM OF ACTION

The exact mechanism by which gold reduces symptoms and induces remission of arthritis has not been determined. It is thought that the gold salts are taken up by macrophages, followed by inhibition of phagocytosis and activity of lysosomal enzymes. They decrease concentrations of rheumatoid factor and immunoglobulins, although the mechanisms are not clearly known. Whether this is their mechanism in the treatment of rheumatoid arthritis is yet to be determined.

USES

Gold salts are used in the management of progressive rheumatoid arthritis that has been unresponsive to traditional therapies. They can relieve pain and stiffness and may arrest the progression of joint degeneration for some patients. These drugs do not reverse damage that has already occurred.

PHARMACOKINETICS

Orally administered auranofin is 20% to 25% absorbed from the GI tract. Aurothioglucose and gold sodium thiomalate are rapidly absorbed following intramuscular injection. The onset of antiinflammatory drug action takes from 6 to 8 weeks for intramuscular formulations and 3 to 6 months for orally administered drugs. Gold salts are widely distributed, concentrating in arthritic joints more than in uninvolved joints. They are also found in breast milk. The kidneys eliminate 60% to 90% of gold salts for up to 15 months. Up to 40% is eliminated in the feces. The half-life of gold salts in the blood is 3 to 26 days; however, in tissues the half-life ranges from 40 to 128 days.

ADVERSE REACTIONS AND CONTRAINDICATIONS

Gold salts have a number of toxicities that limit their use. Adverse reactions force 15% to 20% of patients to discontinue treatment. The most common adverse effects are a metallic taste, stomatitis, and diarrhea accompanied by abdominal pain and cramping. Some patients develop a rash, dermatitis, or dizziness. Although thrombocytopenia is a possible adverse effect, aplastic anemia and agranulocytosis are more important concerns. Interstitial pneumonitis, fibrosis, and acute tubular necrosis have been noted in patients receiving aurothioglucose. Renal toxicity, manifested as proteinuria, occurs frequently. Oral gold formulations cause less renal toxicity than intramuscular formulations.

Gold salts are not recommended for patients with hypersensitivity to gold, those with severe hepatic or renal dysfunction, or patients who have a history of heavy metal intoxication. Cautious use of gold salts is warranted in patients with a history of colitis, exfoliative dermatitis, uncontrolled diabetes mellitus, tuberculosis, heart failure, systemic lupus erythematosis (SLE), and recent radiation therapy. Gold salts should not be used in debilitated patients or in women who are pregnant or breast-feeding.

INTERACTIONS

Additive bone marrow toxicity may occur when gold salts are used in conjunction with other myelosuppressive drugs such as antineoplastics. Combined use of gold salts with radiation therapy can also contribute to myelosuppression.

 DRUG CLASS • **Miscellaneous Drugs for Osteoarthritis**

capsaicin cream (Zostrix)

hylan G-F 20 (Synvisc)

sodium hyaluronate (Hyalgan)

MECHANISM OF ACTION

There are some relatively novel therapies used to treat osteoarthritis, including hyaluronate injections into the knee. Synovial fluid surrounding a joint contains hyaluronate, a material that acts as a lubricant and shock absorber. In osteoarthritis of the knee, the synovial fluid may be deficient in hyaluronate. New drugs have been developed to replace the synovial fluid of the osteoarthritic knee. Hylan G-F 20 is an injectable elastic and viscous mixture of hylan polymers, whereas sodium hyaluronate is a solution of hyaluronate.

Another new therapy is the topical application of capsaicin-containing cream. Presumably, the effects of capsaicin cream arise from the drug's ability to deplete the neurotransmitters in small-diameter sensory nerve endings (nociceptors) and desensitize them.

USES

In some individuals, hyaluronate injections produce pain relief that persists for several months. This therapy is reserved for patients experiencing pain that cannot be relieved by analgesics. Capsaicin is a newer topical analgesic used for the temporary management of pain from rheumatoid arthritis and osteoarthritis. It has also been shown effective for pain associated with neuralgias (e.g., shingles or diabetic neuropathy). Pain relief lasts only as long as capsaicin is used regularly. The patient should be advised that any burning sensation usually disappears after the first few days of use but can continue for 2 to 4 weeks or longer.

PHARMACOKINETICS

The onset of drug action after a hyaluronate injection occurs in approximately 1 to 2 weeks; peak effects are noted in 2 to 4 weeks. For patients with head and neck neuralgias, it may take up to 6 weeks for peak effects of capsaicin to be reached. The duration of action of capsaicin and the results of its biotransformation are unknown, as are its elimination route and half-life.

ADVERSE REACTIONS AND CONTRAINDICATIONS

Hyaluronate therapy may result in mild local pain or swelling at the site of injection, but this is rare. Capsaicin's adverse effects are few, but include cough and transient burning sensation at the site of administration. Hypersensitivity to capsaicin, hot peppers, or other components used in the preparation makes its use inadvisable. It should not be used near the eyes or on broken skin. Safe use during pregnancy, lactation, or in children has not been established. Patients should also be advised that the burning sensation is increased by heat, sweating, bathing in warm water, humidity, and clothing. Patients with herpes zoster should be advised not to apply capsaicin cream until the lesions have completely healed. Patients should also be advised to discontinue use of capsaicin and to notify the health care provider if pain persists longer than 1 month, worsens, or if signs of infection are present.

PATHOPHYSIOLOGY • Gout

Gout is a metabolic disease in which total body pools of uric acid (the end product of purine metabolism) are elevated. Acute gout occurs as a result of an inflammatory reaction to deposits of sodium urate crystals in joints or, less commonly, in tendons or bursae. These deposits occur because of **hyperuricemia** (high levels of uric acid in the body). There is a local infiltration of tissues by granulocytes, which phagocytize urate crystals. With an acute attack, the patient experiences excruciating pain and inflammation in one or more small joints, usually the metatarsophalangeal joint of the great toe. Inflammation of the great toe joint as an initial manifestation occurs in 75% of all patients with gout. Middle-aged and older men as well as postmenopausal woman make up 85% to 90% of patients with gout. Persons of Polynesian heritage are often affected. The peak onset of gout is between the ages of 30 and 40.

Chronic gout appears after repeated bouts of the acute form. Deposits of urate crystals develop within major organ systems, particularly in the kidneys and under the skin. Some patients develop a **tophus** in a joint (crystals of uric acid surrounded by fibrous tissue). Patients with tophi or recurrent attacks of gouty arthritis must receive long-term treatment, often for the rest of their lives, with drugs that will reduce uric acid levels in the body. If present, tophi often regress with long-term drug therapy, restoring the joint to a normal range of function. About 25% of such patients overproduce uric acid.

If gout is diagnosed early and therapy begun promptly, the disease can be arrested and complications prevented.

DRUG CLASS • Antigout Drugs

allopurinol (Zyloprim)
colchicine (generic only)

MECHANISM OF ACTION

Acute attacks of gout are treated with colchicine, indomethacin, or other NSAIDs (see previous section) to relieve the pain and inflammation or with intraarticular injections of corticosteroids (Chapter 57). Colchicine is particularly effective in acute gout, probably because of its effect on the mobility of granulocytes. It binds to microtubular proteins to interfere with function of the mitotic spindles and inhibits the migration of granulocytes to the inflamed area. The inhibition reduces the release of lactic acid and proinflammatory enzymes during phagocytosis. In other words, it breaks the cycle leading to inflammation. Colchicine also inhibits the release of histamine from mast cells and the secretion of insulin from beta cells of the pancreas. Allopurinol, used for chronic gout, inhibits the formation of uric acid from xanthine or hypoxanthine (the purine metabolites of DNA and RNA metabolism), so xanthine or hypoxanthine is excreted instead.

USES

Colchicine is a unique antiinflammatory drug in that it is largely effective against gouty arthritis. It provides dramatic relief of acute gout and is effective for prophylaxis, especially when there is frequent recurrence of attacks. Prophylaxis is recommended on initiation of long-term use of allopurinol or uricosuric drugs because acute attacks often increase in frequency during the early months of therapy. Colchicine is also of benefit for patients with primary biliary cirrhosis, although the underlying disease may not be altered. It has also been used to treat a variety of skin disorders, including psoriasis and Behçet's syndrome (a multisystem illness characterized by lesions of the oral mucosa, genitalia, eyes, and skin). It has been approved as an orphan drug to arrest the progressive neurologic disability caused by multiple sclerosis.

Allopurinol is effective for the treatment of hyperuricemia. A patient whose morning urine has a ratio of uric acid to creatinine greater than 0.75 or whose 24-hour urine contains more than 600 mg of uric acid is classified as an overproducer of uric acid. These overproducers and patients with renal uric acid crystals or impaired renal function are those for whom allopurinol will be most effective. It is also effective for patients with gout resulting from drug therapy that increases uric acid production, particularly cancer drug therapy. Allopurinol is generally used to treat patients with severe chronic forms of gout characterized by one or more of the following conditions: hyperuricemia not readily controlled by uricosuric drugs, tophaceous deposits, gouty nephropathy, renal urate stones, and impaired renal function.

PHARMACOKINETICS

Colchicine is absorbed from the GI tract and then undergoes enterohepatic recirculation, where more absorption may occur. It also concentrates in white blood cells. When the drug is given orally, its onset of action occurs in 12 hours; peak effects are noted in 24 to 72 hours. Its duration of action is unknown. The plasma half-life is about 20 minutes, but the half-life in white blood cells is 60 hours. It is 30% to 50% bound to protein. Biotransformation of colchicine takes place in the liver before elimination in the feces.

Allopurinol is rapidly absorbed following oral administration. Peak plasma concentrations are reached in 30 to 60 minutes. It is rapidly cleared from plasma, and approximately 20% of the drug is eliminated in the feces in 48 to 72 hours. The half-life of allopurinol is 2 to 3 hours, after which the drug is primarily converted to alloxanthine. The plasma half-life of alloxanthine is 18 to 30 hours in patients with normal renal function.

ADVERSE EFFECTS
AND CONTRAINDICATIONS

Colchicine commonly causes nausea, vomiting, and diarrhea, effects that limit the dosage tolerated. Older adults and those with hepatic or renal disease need a lower dosage to avoid toxic reactions. The onset of acute toxicity is seen in 24 to 72 hours, with the first sign commonly a fever. A burning feeling may be noted in the throat or GI tract. Hair loss may be experienced 10 days after an overdose. The adverse effects in the GI tract may be almost completely avoided if colchicine is given intravenously, but in doing so, there is a greater risk for bone marrow suppression, kidney and renal damage, and injury to the CNS. Colchicine also produces a temporary leukopenia that is soon replaced by leukocytosis. Long-term administration of colchicine entails some risk of agranulocytosis, aplastic anemia, myopathy, and alopecia.

Allopurinol's most common adverse effect is hypersensitivity. The reaction can occur even after months or years of drug use. The reaction is characterized predominantly by pruritus or an erythematous or maculopapular eruption. Occasionally, the lesions are exfoliative, urticarial, or purpuric. Fever, malaise, and muscle aches also are present. Transient leukopenia or leukocytosis and eosinophilia are rare reactions but may require stopping the drug. Other undesirable adverse effects include headache, drowsiness, nausea and vomiting, vertigo, diarrhea, and GI irritation but usually do not require stopping treatment. Allopurinol is not recommended for patients who have had serious adverse reactions, nursing mothers, and children except those who have a malignancy or certain inborn errors of purine metabolism.

INTERACTIONS

Colchicine has few drug-drug interactions. It may, however, cause a reversible malabsorption of vitamin B_{12}. Phenylbutazone, radiation therapy, and drugs causing bone marrow depression all increase the likelihood of bone marrow depression of colchicine and should not be administered concurrently. Allopurinol interferes with hepatic inactivation of other drugs, including oral anticoagulants. It is thought that there is an increased incidence of skin rash with concurrent administration of ampicillin. Hypersensitivity reactions have been reported in patients with compromised renal function who receive allopurinol and thiazide diuretics. Concurrent use of allopurinol and theophylline preparations leads to an increased concentration of theophylline's active metabolites.

DRUG CLASS • Uricosuric Drugs

probenecid (Benemid, Probalan)

sulfinpyrazone (Anturane)

MECHANISM OF ACTION

In contrast to antigout drugs, uricosuric drugs increase the rate of uric acid secretion, thus reducing plasma concentration. Probenecid and sulfinpyrazone inhibit the renal tubular reabsorption of urate, which increases the urinary elimination of uric acid, decreases serum uric acid level, retards urate deposition, and promotes reabsorption of urate deposits. Probenecid also inhibits renal tubular secretion of most penicillins and cephalosporins.

USES

The use of probenecid and sulfinpyrazone for the mobilization of uric acid in chronic gout is well established. These drugs inhibit the reabsorption of uric acid by the kidney tubules and thereby promote the excretion of uric acid in the urine.

PHARMACOKINETICS

Probenecid is a highly soluble benzoic acid derivative that is completely absorbed after oral administration. Peak concentrations are reached in 2 to 4 hours. The plasma half-life is dose dependent and varies from less than 5 hours to more than 8 hours over the therapeutic range. The drug is 85% to 95% bound to plasma albumin. Biotransformation takes place in the liver, and less than 10% of the drug is eliminated unchanged in the urine. The half-life of probenecid is 4 to 17 hours.

Sulfinpyrazone is similar to probenecid in that it is well absorbed when given orally. It is highly bound to plasma albumin (98% to 99%) and tends to displace other drugs that have a high affinity for the same binding sites. After oral administration, its uricosuric effect may persist for as long as 10 hours. Approximately 50% of an oral dose appears in the urine within 24 hours 90% unchanged.

ADVERSE EFFECTS
AND CONTRAINDICATIONS

Probenecid is well tolerated by most patients. Some degree of GI irritation is noted by about 2% of patients. The incidence of hypersensitivity, usually consisting of mild skin rashes, is between 2% and 4%. Serious hypersensitivity reactions are rare. Nephrotic syndrome has been reported as a toxic reaction. A large overdose results in CNS stimulation, seizures, and death from respiratory failure.

GI irritation occurs in about 10% to 15% of patients receiving sulfinpyrazone. Hypersensitivity reactions do occur, usually consisting of a rash with fever, but they occur less frequently than with probenecid. Depression of hematopoiesis has been demonstrated. Sulfinpyrazone is not recommended for patients with allergies to phenylbutazone or other pyrazoles and patients who have blood dyscrasias or a history of peptic ulcer disease. It should be used with caution in patients with renal failure or in those who are pregnant or lactating. Probenecid and sulfinpyrazone are not recommended for patients with renal failure or a history of renal stones, because they flood the kidney tubules with uric acid.

INTERACTIONS

Probenecid increases the concentration of sulfonamide in the blood to some degree. The uricosuric action of sulfinpyrazone is additive to that of probenecid but is mutually antagonistic to that of salicylates. The effectiveness of uricosuric drugs is diminished by several other drugs. Heavy alcohol consumption produces enough lactic acid to inhibit uric acid secretion. Because aspirin at low dosages inhibits uric acid secretion, acetaminophen should be substituted for simple pain relief in patients taking uricosuric drugs.

In addition, the uricosuric drugs inhibit the secretion or degradation of several other drugs. Probenecid inhibits the renal secretion of organic acids, including drugs such as penicillin, indomethacin, methotrexate, sulfonylureas (oral hypoglycemics), sulfinpyrazone, salicylates, and rifampin, keeping their plasma levels high. Sulfinpyrazone inhibits the degradation of sulfonamides, particularly sulfadiazine and sulfisoxazole, sulfonylureas, and coumarins.

◣ APPLICATION TO PRACTICE

ASSESSMENT
History of Present Illness

The course of most disorders that require nonopioid, antipyretic, antiinflammatory drugs are variable. Thus a detailed description of symptoms must be elicited from the patient. Determine the location, severity, and length of time the disorder has been present and what the patient has done to treat the problem. Since the inflammatory response produces pain, evaluate the patient's pain level and tolerance. Ask the patient to describe tolerable pain and what he or she desires for relief. Be sure to inquire about prescription drugs and OTC preparations used. Determine whether or not the patient has been using alternative or complementary pain relief

strategies. Ask whether the symptoms the patient is experiencing have been accompanied by a fever. In many cases, the patient will note that he or she has had chills even though a temperature reading was never taken. For the patient with complaints of dysmenorrhea, elicit the timing of the discomfort and what the patient has tried for relief.

Assess the activity level of patients with rheumatoid disorders and identify which activities are most impaired by the problem. Also ask what assistance has been needed with activities of daily living. The patient should understand that fatigue or malaise is not a sign of laziness but a symptom of an underlying problem.

Health History

Determine whether or not the patient has a history of renal, hepatic, or peptic ulcer disease or bleeding disorders (e.g., hemophilia, vitamin K deficiency, hypoprothrombinemia). Ask specifically about the use of OTC analgesic, antipyretic, or antiinflammatory drugs and herbal remedies as well as prescription drugs such as anticoagulants or corticosteroids. If the patient has previously taken an NSAID, determine his or her reaction to the drug. Did the patient obtain therapeutic effects or undesirable adverse effects? Ask specifically about response to aspirin because a person allergic to aspirin is at risk for cross-allergenicity to other NSAIDs.

Determine if the patient or the family has a history of gout and goutlike symptoms. Ask also about comorbid disorders associated with gout such as obesity, hypertension, and hyperlipidemia, to name a few. Risk factors for gout include dietary excess of purines, lead poisoning, kidney disease, hemoproliferative disorders, chronic alcohol ingestion, and patients taking salicylates, aminophylline, caffeine, corticosteroids, cytotoxic drugs (e.g., cyclosporine), diazepam, diphenhydramine, L-dopa, dopamine, epinephrine, ethambutol, pyrazinamide, methaqualone, nicotinic acid, probenecid, and vitamins B_{12} and C. Diuretics may be responsible for 20% of secondary gout (see Chapter 46).

Lifespan Considerations

Perinatal. If the patient is of childbearing age, determine whether she is pregnant or nursing before giving an NSAID. DMARDs and some NSAIDs are teratogenic, and still others have not been studied during pregnancy. It is clear that any drug or chemical administered to the mother is capable of crossing the placenta to some extent to reach the fetus. Of great concern is whether the rate and extent of drug transfer are sufficient to result in significant concentrations in the fetus. Use of aspirin and other NSAIDs during labor and delivery can suppress spontaneous uterine contractions, induce premature closure of the ductus arteriosus, and intensify uterine bleeding.

Not only must maternal pharmacologic mechanisms be taken into account, but the fetus must always be kept in mind as a potential recipient of the drug. The FDA classification system for risk factors associated with systemic drug use in pregnancy should be consulted when assessing potential use of an NSAID. The upswing in breastfeeding and markedly increased parental concerns about health needs of the fetus have contributed to increased questioning of health care providers about the safety and potential toxicity of drugs. It has also increased interest in drugs and chemicals excreted in breast milk.

Pediatric. Acetaminophen is preferred over aspirin to treat chicken pox and viral illnesses. NSAIDs (particularly aspirin) are not recommended for children under the age of 18 with chicken pox or viral illnesses because of the risk of Reye's syndrome. This syndrome is characterized by sudden, persistent vomiting, signs of encephalopathy (disturbances of consciousness), listlessness, and lethargy. As intracranial pressure rises, the child becomes more agitated, irritable, and delirious. In its severest form the disorder causes seizures and coma. The mortality rate is between 20% and 30%.

Older Adults. Many older adults are prone to GI bleeding and ulceration, renal damage, decreased hepatic function, and CNS changes. These persons also easily develop sodium and fluid retention, which exacerbates other medical problems such as heart failure. Because the older adult commonly has reduced serum protein levels, drugs that are normally highly protein bound circulate freely and can reach toxic levels.

Older adults with a history of GI bleeding can develop peptic ulcerations and hemorrhage asymptomatically. Evidence suggests that histamine-1 antagonists (e.g., cimetidine, ranitidine, famotidine), antacids, and sucralfate do not prevent NSAID-induced ulcers. Misoprostol, a PGE_1 analog, acts on PGE_2 receptors to increase mucus formation and decrease gastric acid secretion (see Chapter 48). As a cytoprotective drug, misoprostol is helpful in reducing GI irritation from NSAIDs but it is expensive, and there is no firm evidence that it prevents ulcer complications and death.

NSAIDs can compromise existing renal function in the older adult, especially when the creatinine clearance is less than 30 mL per minute. Tinnitis may be a difficult and unreliable indication of toxicity because of age-related hearing loss or damage to the eighth cranial nerve. CNS adverse effects such as confusion, agitation, and hallucinations are generally seen with overdose or high-dose situations, but older adults may demonstrate these adverse effects at lower dosages than younger adults.

Cultural/Social Considerations

A psychologic assessment is important because acute or chronic inflammation, pain, and fever can cause great anxiety in both the patient and the family. Determine the meaning of symptoms to the patient. Some perceptions and reactions are heavily based on expectations and learned responses; therefore ask about actual or potential losses the patient may be experiencing, which may be contributing to discomfort.

There is a connection between nutritional status and rheumatoid conditions; hence dietary assessment is equally important. Ask specifically about consumption of milk, cheese, and yogurt because these foods have been known to reduce joint stiffness, pain, and swelling in some patients. Foods that contain eicosopentanoic acid, a fatty acid found in fish (e.g., salmon, mackerel, tuna, rainbow trout, and sardines), may also alleviate symptoms. Cereal grains (e.g., wheat, oat, rye), shrimp and foods containing sodium nitrate (a food preservative) can trigger joint problems in some patients.

Physical Examination

Objective signs of pain help verify what a patient says about pain, but such data are not used to prove or to disprove whether pain is present. Physiologic signs of moderate and superficial pain are responses to sympathetic nervous system stimulation. The signs include rapid, shallow, or guarded respirations; pallor; diaphoresis; increased pulse rate; elevated blood pressure; and skeletal muscle tension. Behavioral signs of pain may include crying, moaning, tossing about in bed, pacing the floor, lying quietly but tensely in one position, drawing the knees upward toward the abdomen, rubbing the painful part, and a pinched facial expression or grimacing. The person in pain may also have difficulty concentrating and remembering because he or she may be preoccupied with the pain. Because objective measurement of pain and inflammation is not always possible, patients usually express an opinion about the level of discomfort. Determine the patient's pain level using a measurement scale such as those discussed in Chapter 13.

Inspect all joints and body surfaces for redness, warmth, and edema even if the patient's complaint is isolated to a single joint. There may be other sources of the inflammation. Carefully examine the joints for crepitation, deformity, subluxation, and contraction. Note muscle atrophy or decreased subcutaneous tissue. Check vital signs, paying particular attention to temperature. Patients with a fever often have hot, dry skin and a flushed face. A low-grade fever is marked by oral temperature readings between 99.5° and 101° F (37.5° and 38.2° C). A high fever is present when the temperature is above 101° F (38.2° C). A prolonged fever eventually brings about tissue destruction because of the catabolism of body proteins.

Examination of the patient with gout or a goutlike condition often reflects severe pain, swelling, redness, or warmth in one or two joints (75% are monoarticular), soft tissue redness, swelling, warmth, and exquisite tenderness. Look for the presence of tophi. Gout symptoms are often accompanied by fever and chills. An attack may be isolated or recurrent. Left untreated, an attack can last 2 to 21 days. Recurrent attacks last longer and occur more frequently with each recurrence.

Laboratory Testing

A patient with pain or fever related to inflammation may have an elevated white blood cell count. Patients with arthritis and arthritis-like symptoms may have an elevated antinuclear antibody test result, elevated sedimentation rate, and a positive rheumatoid factor.

In patients with an acute gout attack, the eosinophil rate and white blood cell count will usually be elevated with a shift to the left (a predominance of young neutrophils). Hyperuricemia may be present.

GOALS OF THERAPY

The overall treatment goals for the patient receiving nonopioid analgesic, antipyretic, antiinflammatory drugs depend on the reason for their use but are directed at reducing or eliminating pain, fever, and inflammation as much and as quickly as possible using the least toxic, most effective drug. For patients with joint disorders, the treatment goals include preserving joint function, quality of life, and the patient's ability to carry out activities of daily living (see Case Study: Rheumatoid Arthritis). The treatment goal for fever is to return body temperature to a normal range and increase the patient's comfort. For the patient with gout, the goal is to reduce plasma uric acid concentrations to below 6 mg/dL and to relieve discomfort.

INTERVENTION

Interventions for a patient with inflammatory and inflammation-related disorders include conservative, nondrug measures such as alleviating anxiety, combating anticipatory fears related to pain, and providing physical and emotional care. Balancing rest and exercise regimens, physical therapy, and appropriate use of complementary, alternative therapies (e.g., acupressure, acupuncture, hypnosis) are included in the plan of care.

NSAIDs do not retard the progression of disease, but they do relieve symptoms rather quickly, are generally safer than DMARDs and corticosteroids (see Chapter 57), and require less vigorous monitoring. DMARDs may retard the progression of arthritis but are more toxic than NSAIDs and require more vigorous monitoring. Corticosteroids rapidly relieve symptoms, but because of their toxicity, they are usually reserved for short-term therapy. Figure 14-2 illustrates the stepwise progression of drug therapy for the patient with rheumatic disorders.

For reasons not understood, patients often respond better to one NSAID than another. Furthermore, some patients tolerate one NSAID better than another. Thus, to optimize therapy, treatment trials with more than one NSAID may be necessary. Since aspirin is such a familiar drug, many patients are suspicious of its efficacy. Consequently, to achieve compliance, patients may need to be persuaded that aspirin is in fact an effective drug.

Concurrent use of opioids (see Chapter 13) with NSAIDs often provides more effective analgesia than

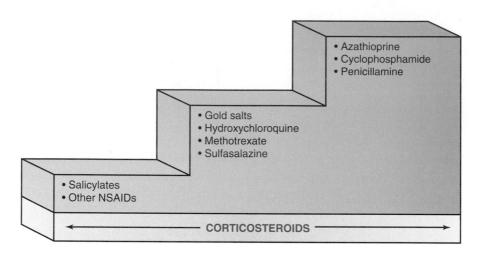

FIGURE 14-2　Stepwise progression for disease-modifying antirheumatic drugs. Treatment for rheumatic disorders is begun at the base of the steps. As the disease progresses and changes in treatment plans are warranted, drugs are chosen in an upward, stepwise fashion. Corticosteroids may be used on a short-term basis at any point in the treatment regimen. Drugs at the highest steps are considerably more toxic than those nearer the base.

either drug class alone. NSAIDs should be titrated to maximum dosage and taken on a regular schedule before the patient is placed on opioids. If regularly scheduled NSAIDs are not effective, a combination of an NSAID with an opioid (e.g., aspirin with oxycodone) may be effective.

If noninflammatory mechanisms (e.g., headache or muscle ache) are thought to be causing mild pain symptoms, acetaminophen is effective, inexpensive, and produces little, if any, GI irritation. Acetaminophen is the drug of choice for children with chicken pox or other viral illnesses.

Administration

To reduce the risk of esophageal irritation caused by NSAIDs, DMARDs, or anti-gout drugs lodging against the lining of the esophagus, such drugs should be taken with food or a full glass of fluid. Antigout and uricosuric drugs should be administered after meals to minimize GI irritation. Even though food delays drug absorption and decreases peak plasma levels of some drugs, it is probably safer to take them with food. The patient should be advised to remain upright for 15 to 30 minutes after taking the drug.

Enteric-coated formulations should be swallowed whole without chewing or crushing. Chewable NSAIDs may be crushed, chewed, or swallowed whole. If necessary, capsules may be opened and the contents mixed with food. Mix choline and magnesium salicylate oral solutions with fruit juice just before taking, and follow the dose with a full glass (8 ounces) of water. Patients

on long-term therapy may find extended-release formulations helpful, particularly at night, because the morning blood level of the drug may not be as low with this formulation. When necessary to break extended-release formulations, do so along the scored lines.

Pain relief provided by NSAIDs is subject to a ceiling effect. In other words, higher than recommended dosages may not necessarily provide additional therapeutic benefit in the treatment of pain unrelated to inflammation. Thus the patient who omits a scheduled dose should not double the next dose but should instead resume the usual dosing schedule. Once pain is controlled, the average daily dosage is usually decreased by 25% every 1 to 2 weeks until the minimum effective dose is reached. Once-daily or even as-needed dosing may be all that is required.

Plasma salicylate levels should be measured periodically when large doses of salicylates are given for antiinflammatory effects. Chronic administration of large doses saturates a major metabolic pathway, thereby slowing drug elimination, prolonging serum half-life, and causing drug accumulation. A number of OTC and prescription preparations containing aspirin can be easy sources of salicylate in overdose. The health care provider should be aware of the symptoms and signs and the treatment of salicylism (see Box 14-1).

Check the patient's stools for the presence of blood. If diarrhea or vomiting is severe or persistent, monitor intake and output. In patients with cardiovascular, renal, or hypertensive disease, assess for possible fluid retention related to the use of NSAIDs. Auscultate breath sounds and assess for jugular venous distention. Report weight gain in excess of 2 pounds per day or 5 pounds per week to the health care provider.

Education

To fully participate in treatment, the patient must know the nature and time course of expected beneficial drug effects. With this information, the patient can help evaluate the success or failure of the treatment. Although analgesic and antipyretic effects may become evident in a short time, weeks or months may be required in some cases before beneficial antiinflammatory effects are felt. As discussed in Chapter 13, teaching nondrug measures for pain relief enhances the chance of success with drug therapy.

Just as patients must know when and how to take the drug, they must also be taught when to stop. The time to stop is typically when symptoms subside. However, in some patients, lifelong treatment may be required, and still other patients may need to return for further evaluation. Patients who self-manage long-term NSAID or DMARD therapy should be advised of the importance of periodic laboratory evaluation of white blood cells, hemoglobin and hematocrit levels, blood urea nitrogen (BUN), serum creatinine levels, weight, and blood pressure. For patients taking choline or magnesium salicylates, the serum magnesium level should be monitored as well.

Teach patients to notify their health care provider when they are taking OTC aspirin, ibuprofen, or other NSAIDs on a regular basis. Patients on chronic aspirin therapy should be advised to terminate use 1 week before elective surgery.

A woman of childbearing age should be told to consult with the health care provider should she become pregnant while taking an NSAID or DMARD. If breastfeeding, the woman should be advised to contact the health care provider because many of these drugs are detected in breast milk and are cleared slowly from the body of an infant.

Patients with comorbid disorders (e.g., gastritis, ulcers, bleeding disorders, diabetes, or gout) or who are on anticoagulant therapy should discuss the use of NSAIDs with the health care provider. Teach them also that acetaminophen is an effective aspirin substitute for pain or fever but not for inflammation or to prevent heart attack or stroke. Advise the patient with hypertension not to use effervescent aspirin products because of the high sodium content.

Since fever is one way the body fights infection, drug therapy may not be necessary unless the fever is high or is accompanied by other uncomfortable signs and symptoms. Furthermore, pain is not usually associated with the common cold, so analgesic-antipyretic drugs

are used only for their fever-relieving characteristics. If acetaminophen use is required for more than 2 to 3 days, the health care provider should be contacted for further evaluation of the fever.

Patients should be advised to avoid alcohol while they are taking NSAIDs. Alcohol produces synergistic effects with NSAIDs, thus increasing the risk of GI irritation and bleeding. Some patients experience drowsiness and dizziness while taking NSAIDs. They should be cautioned about performing tasks that require alertness. Furthermore, aspirin should not be taken concurrently with vitamin C products (e.g., orange juice) because it contributes to gastric acidity.

Advise the patient with nasal polyps to avoid using acetylated salicylates for self-treatment of minor aches, pains, and fever because these drugs may induce an acute asthma attack. Nonacetylated salicylates may be used cautiously.

 Dietary Considerations for GOUT

Uric acid is produced when purines are catabolized. Gout is a problem of elevated uric acid. Dietary restriction of purine was formerly the mainstay of gout therapy. With improved drug therapy, however, purine restriction is now a less significant component of therapy. Patients may still be asked to limit excessive purine intake, unless more severe restriction is indicated on an individual basis. High purine foods to avoid or limit include the following:

- Organ meats (e.g., tongue, brain, liver, kidneys)
- Roe
- Sardines
- Scallops
- Anchovies
- Broth and consommé
- Mincement
- Herring
- Shrimp
- Mackerel
- Gravy
- Yeast

Uric acid is less likely to crystallize in alkaline urine. For this reason the patient should be advised to increase his or her intake of alkaline ash foods such as the following:

- Citrus juices
- Fresh fruits (except cranberries, plums, and prunes)
- All vegetables (except lentils and corn)
- Milk, buttermilk
- Cream
- Almonds, chestnuts, coconuts

CASE STUDY  *Rheumatoid Arthritis*

ASSESSMENT

HISTORY OF PRESENT ILLNESS

MJ is a 74-year-old woman who complains of right hip pain. She is accompanied by her daughter, who said MJ was unable to get out of bed this morning because of the pain in her hip. MJ reports she has been getting along fine by balancing rest and exercise, as well as by using aspirin several times a day for inflammation and pain. Her daughter believes that the arthritis has progressed to the point where her current drug regimen is no longer effective. Patient and daughter are now requesting additional assistance in managing the disease.

HEALTH HISTORY

MJ has a 12-year history of rheumatoid arthritis and type 2 diabetes mellitus, for which she takes 10 mg of glipizide (Glucatrol XL) daily. Her daughter indicates that the arthritis started in her left hand and gradually affected both hands as well as her feet and knees. She had her left knee replaced at age 60 and her right knee replaced at age 65. MJ has had several regimens of physical therapy since she was originally diagnosed. She has used salicylates and other NSAIDs in the past with varying degrees of success. She indicates she is careful to take her drugs with food or milk. MJ denies drug or food allergies, history of renal or hepatic disease, or GI bleeding. The health care provider, however, had prescribed indomethacin because he was worried about MJ's risk of GI bleeding.

LIFESPAN CONSIDERATIONS

When MJ's husband died last year, she moved to an assisted living facility. She interacts independently with the other adults at the facility but needs assistance with eating because of the arthritic deformities in her hands. This dependency causes her a great deal of distress. She wants to remain as independent as possible in spite of her need for assistance with eating.

CULTURAL/SOCIAL CONSIDERATIONS

MJ and her husband lived in a mobile home; he cared for her until his death. She has two married daughters who have families of their own. They visit and help with her care when possible. MJ has a limited income and would prefer to "spend money on good food rather than on expensive medicine for my [her] joints." She has Medicare coverage for hospitalization but lacks coverage for office visits and pharmacy needs. Her family is unable to assist her with health care costs.

PHYSICAL EXAMINATION

MJ has little to no effective use of her fingers, wrists, and elbows. There is lateral deviation of metacarpal joints bilaterally and a generalized discomfort of the right hip when palpated. Passive and active range of motion is painful and limited. Crepitation is noted on movement of right hip. Temperature is 98.4° F, pulse is 80 bpm.

LABORATORY TESTING

Radiograph of right hip reveals severe arthritic changes. Results of CBC, urinalysis (UA), renal function, and liver function tests are within normal limits. Erythrocyte sedimentation rate (ESR) is elevated; rheumatoid factor (RF) is positive; antinuclear antibody (ANA) is positive.

PATIENT PROBLEM(S)

Rheumatoid arthritis.

GOALS OF THERAPY

To reduce pain and inflammation while maintaining existing joint function; to preserve quality of life and ability to carry out activities of daily living.

CRITICAL THINKING QUESTIONS

1. MJ has been using aspirin to treat her rheumatoid arthritis. What are the three pharmacologic effects characteristic of aspirin? Which factors determine the biotransformation and elimination of aspirin?
2. MJ's health care provider advises her to stop taking the aspirin and prescribes methotrexate. What is the mechanism of action of this drug?
3. Which level is MJ at, considering the stepwise progression for DMARD therapy? How long will it be before MJ is likely to notice improvement in her symptoms?
4. Which other treatment options might MJ's health care provider suggest to help relieve her discomfort?
5. MJ's health care provider wants her to take ibuprofen 600 mg po qid until the desired response from the methotrexate is reached. Of which drug-drug interactions should the nurse be aware?
6. MJ tells the nurse that she heard blood tests will be required while she takes the methotrexate. What laboratory testing will be required for MJ while she is taking the methotrexate and how often?

Increasing fluid intake is one of the best measures to prevent urate stone formation. It also helps dilute the urine and prevent formation of sediment. Instruct patients taking uricosuric drugs to maintain oral intake sufficient to ensure a daily urinary output of at least 2 L. This may require 3000 mL of fluid intake per day. Patients should also be instructed to limit their intake of alcohol. Dietary restriction of purines for the patient with gout is controversial. See the Dietary Considerations box for patients with gout.

EVALUATION

Treatment effectiveness can be evaluated through patient reports of increased comfort and range of motion, increased mobility, and ability to perform the activities of daily living. Redness, warmth, edema, and pain should be reduced or absent. If the drug is used for its antipyretic effects, the patient's temperature should return to the normal range. The patient is not expected to experience untoward effects of therapy.

Treatment effectiveness for gout can be demonstrated by a decrease in the pain and swelling of affected joints, a decrease in the level of serum uric acid, resolution of tophi, and a subsequent decrease in the frequency of attacks. Several months of continuous therapy may be required before maximum benefits become apparent. Since the health care provider has information about which activities were most impaired by the problem, this information can also be used as an indicator of improvement.

Bibliography

Beehrle DM, Evans D: A review of NSAID complications: gastrointestinal and more, *Lippincott's Prim Care Pract* 3(3):305-315, 1999.

Halverson PB: Nonsteroidal antiinflammatory drugs: benefits, risks, and COX-2 selectivity, *Orthop Nurs* 18(6):21-26, 1999.

Klippel JH, Crofford L, eds: Primer on the rheumatic diseases, ed 12, Atlanta, 2001, Arthritis Foundation.

Paster RZ, McCarberg B: The spectrum of pain: the primary care physician's role in managing pain, *Intern Med World Rep* 15(suppl):8, 2000.

Pepper GA: Nonsteroidal antiinflammatory drugs: new perspectives on a familiar drug class, *Nurs Clin North Am* 35(1):223-244, 2000.

Ramsburg KL: Rheumatoid Arthritis, *Am J Nurs* 100(11):40-43, 2000.

Internet Resources

Arthritis Insight.com: Arthritis. Available online at http://arthritisinsight.com/.

Arthritis Foundation: Types of drugs. Available online at http://www.arthritis.org/conditions/drugguide/drugtypes.asp.

National Institute of Arthritis and Musculoskeletal and Skin Disorders. Available online at http://www.niams.nih.gov/.

National Institute of Diabetes and Digestive and Kidney Diseases: NSAIDs. Available online at http://www.niddk.nih.gov/health/digest/summary/nsaids.

Medicine Plus Health Information: Gout and pseudogout. Available online at http://www.nlm.nih.gov/medlineplus/goutandpseudogout.html.

Scleroderma Foundation. Available online at http://www.scleroderma.org/pdf/medicat.PDF.

Drugs to Treat Headaches

MICHAEL R. VASKO • KATHLEEN GUTIERREZ

 Visit http://evolve.elsevier.com/Gutierrez/ for additional information.

KEY TERMS

Chronic tension headaches, p. 218

Classic migraine, p. 218

Cluster headache, p. 220

Common migraine, p. 218

Ergotism, p. 223

Triptans, p. 220

OBJECTIVES

- Describe chronic tension, migraine, and cluster headaches.
- Identify lifestyle factors that may contribute to the development of headaches.
- Explain the rationales for using analgesic combinations, ergot-containing drugs, and triptans in treating headaches.
- Develop a nursing care plan for a patient taking a triptan for a headache.

PATHOPHYSIOLOGY • Headaches

The International Headache Society has classified 129 different types of headaches. It is estimated that 40% of individuals experience a severe headache at least annually. Most headaches for which patients seek medical help are one of three types: chronic tension headache, migraine, or cluster headache (Table 15-1). Many of the patients use drugs identified in Table 15-2 to relieve their headaches. People with tension headaches seek medical help if the headaches last for many days and/or recur frequently (**chronic tension headaches**). These headaches are often associated with fatigue, stress, or excessive use of tobacco or alcohol. The treatment should emphasize lifestyle changes. Biofeedback training may be helpful for those needing help with stress management.

Headaches that are severe or disabling require medical assessment. In about 10% of cases, a severe or chronic headache is a symptom of a serious illness such as a brain tumor, glaucoma, or giant cell arteritis. These headaches are secondary headaches, symptoms of a primary disorder. More commonly, headaches are the primary problem. The two principal varieties of primary headaches that are severe and recurring are migraine and cluster headaches.

Migraine is a clinical classification for a periodic headache that lasts from 4 to 24 hours. The pain is on one side of the head and can be nondescript and throbbing or severe and stabbing. Nausea and vomiting are common, as is sensitivity to light, scalp tenderness, and light-headedness. Dark surroundings and sleep can bring some relief. About 8 million Americans experience recurrent migraines. Common triggering factors include stress, menstrual period, odors, and foods. In addition, the overuse of acute drugs to treat migraine, especially the combination of analgesics and ergotamine, can trigger migraines. The **classic migraine** is associated with an aura that may precede the headache by several minutes to an hour. Usually the aura is visual, but it may be any sensory or motor symptom.

Migraine without an aura is called **common migraine** and accounts for about 80% of migraine cases. Migraines occur at all ages but commonly begin before the age of 40 years, with the highest incidence in children and young adults. Seventy-five percent of migraine sufferers are women.

Each patient with a migraine tends to have a characteristic pattern for the onset and duration of the headache. The question remains as to whether most forms of migraine are inherited. A clear genetic basis for migraine is known for only one type, familial hemiplegic migraine. For other types, genetic predisposition along with environmental factors may contribute to the headache. Although the etiology of migraine remains unknown, it likely involves both neurological and vascular events. Current theories suggest that a migraine results in part from vasodilation caused by release of neu-

---

TABLE 15-1

Comparison of Common Types of Headaches

Pattern	Tension Headache	Migraine Headache	Cluster Headache
Character	Bilateral; constant, squeezing, tight, bandlike pressure at base of skull, face, or both	Unilateral; may switch sides, commonly anterior; throbbing, synchronous with pulse	Unilateral; radiating up or down from one eye; severe, bone crushing
Frequency	Cyclical; several years	Periodic; cycles of months to years	Clusters; one to three times daily over a 4- to 8-week period, with months or years between attacks
Duration	Intermittent for months or years	Continuous for hours or days	30 to 90 minutes
Timing	Unrelated	Often preceded by aura; onset after awakening; gets better with sleep	Nocturnal; commonly awakens patient from sleep
Associated symptoms	Tender, stiff neck and shoulders; palpable tension	Nausea or vomiting; irritability, diaphoresis, photophobia; sensory, motor, or psychic aura	Facial flushing or pallor; unilateral lacrimation, ptosis, rhinitis

ropeptides from sensory nerve endings innervating the blood vessels surrounding (but not in) the brain. Blood flow studies indicate that the initial change is a modest decrease in blood flow. Activation of the trigeminal nerve by an unknown trigger causes the release of substance P, calcitonin gene-related peptide, and other substances causing vasodilation and extravasation of proteins and platelets into the perivascular areas (i.e.,

neurogenic inflammation). Neuropeptides released at central terminals of sensory neurons within the trigeminal system conduct the pain signals.

Drug development for the treatment of severe migraine headaches focuses on the key role of the neurotransmitter serotonin (5-hydroxytryptamine [5-HT]). There are at least four main families of serotonin receptors, and each receptor family has several subtypes.

TABLE 15-2

Analgesic Combinations Used to Treat Headaches

Constituents/Dosage	Trade Name	Comments
acetaminophen 500 mg + caffeine 65 mg	Aspirin Free Excedrin, Bayer Select Maximum Strength Headache Pain Relief	Chronic use can lead to caffeine dependence. Caution patients not to drink alcohol with acetaminophen (increased risk of liver damage).
acetaminophen 250 mg + aspirin 250 mg + caffeine 65 mg	Excedrin Migraine	Chronic use can lead to caffeine dependence. Caution patients not to drink alcohol with acetaminophen (increased risk of liver damage) or aspirin (gastric damage).
acetaminophen 650 mg + butalbital 50 mg	Phrenilin, Sedapap	Frequent use can lead to abuse and to rebound headaches when the drug is discontinued.
acetaminophen 325 mg + butalbital 50 mg + caffeine 40 mg	Esgic, Fioricet	Frequent use can lead to abuse and to rebound headaches when the drug is discontinued.
acetaminophen 325 mg + butalbital 50 mg + caffeine 40 mg + codeine phosphate 30 mg	Fioricet with Codeine	Frequent use can lead to abuse and to rebound headaches when the drug is discontinued. Codeine can cause nausea and vomiting.
acetaminophen 325 mg + dichloralphenazone 100 mg + isometheptene mucate 65 mg	Midrin, Migrex	Isometheptene is an indirect-acting sympathomimetic vasoconstrictor. Dichloralphenazone is a mild sedative and relaxant.
aspirin 385 mg + caffeine 30 mg + orphenadrine citrate 25 mg	Norgesic	Orphenadrine is a skeletal muscle relaxant. Caution patients to avoid alcohol and other central nervous system depressants.
acetaminophen 325, 650 mg + propoxyphene napsylate 50, 100 mg	Darvocet N50, Darvocet N100	Propoxyphene is an opioid (schedule IV).
aspirin 389 mg + caffeine 32.4 mg + propoxyphene hydrochloride 65 mg	Darvon Compound 65	Propoxyphene is an opioid (schedule IV).
acetaminophen 325 mg + hydrocodone bitartrate 5 mg	Vicodin	Hydrocodone is an opioid; overdose can be life threatening. Chronic use can lead to opioid dependence.
acetaminophen 325 mg + oxycodone hydrochloride 5 mg	Endocet, Oxycocet,✻ Percocet, Roxicet	Oxycodone is an opioid; overdose can be life threatening. Chronic use can lead to opioid dependence.
aspirin 325 mg + oxycodone hydrochloride 4.5 mg *or* oxycodone terephthalate 0.38 mg	Endodan, Oxycodan,✻ Percodan	Oxycodone is an opioid; overdose can be life threatening. Chronic use can lead to opioid dependence.

✻Available only in Canada.

Serotonin receptor types 1B and 1D appear to be acted on by ergotamine and the triptans in stopping a migraine. These drugs are also effective for cluster headaches. The serotonin 1B receptor is associated with altered vascular effects, whereas activation of the 1D receptor is thought to decrease the release of peptides for sensory neurons, thereby reducing neurogenic inflammation.

A **cluster headache** begins suddenly, reaching a peak in a few minutes and persisting for 30 minutes to 2 hours. The pain is described as sharp, boring, and excruciatingly severe. Pain is clustered on one side of the head around the eye, with lacrimation, eyelid droop, runny nose, congestion, and facial sweating. A common pattern is for one to three attacks to occur per day for 4- to 8-weeks, followed by a year of remission. However, the pattern may be chronic. Attacks tend to come at the same time each day, and the time may be during the day or at night while sleeping.

Cluster headaches most commonly occur in men between the ages of 20 and 50 years. Alcohol is a common precipitating factor in a bout of cluster headaches.

DRUG CLASS • Triptans

almotriptan (Axert)

frovatriptan (Frova)

naratriptan (Amerge)

rizatriptan (Maxalt, Maxalt-MLT)

sumatriptan (Imitrex)

zolmitriptan (Zomig)

MECHANISM OF ACTION

The **triptans** are agonists at serotonin 1B and 1D receptors (5-HT1B, 5-HT1D) receptors. Stimulation of 5-HT1B receptors produces vasoconstriction through direct activation of vascular smooth muscle. Activation of the 5-HT1D receptor is thought to reduce the release of neuropeptides (especially calcitonin gene-related peptide) from the terminals of small-diameter sensory neurons. This decreased release of neuropeptides reduces inflammation in the area of the blood vessels surrounding the brain and reduces pain signals in the trigeminal system.

USES

The triptans have rapidly become drugs of choice for relief of acute migraine headaches. They are not useful for prophylaxis or chronic treatment. They are to be administered after the start of an attack and are effective for classic and common migraine. However, because many patients know when a migraine is starting, an injection of sumatriptan or an oral dose of any triptan can abort the acute attack. Sumatriptan is also recommended for the treatment of cluster headaches. These drugs are not useful for the treatment of basilar artery migraine or hemiplegic migraine.

PHARMACOKINETICS

The triptans are rapidly absorbed after oral administration but have variable bioavailability. Only about 15% of sumatriptan is absorbed after oral administration because of incomplete absorption and the first-pass effect. Absorption through nasal passages is also low, but most of a given dose is absorbed after subcutaneous injection. Bioavailability of frovatriptan, rizatriptan, and zolmitriptan is 20% to 40%, whereas approximately 70% of an oral dose of almotriptan or naratriptan enter the circulation. Onset of action of these drugs after oral administration is approximately 30 minutes, with peak plasma levels at 1 to 4 hours depending on the drug. The onset of action for migraine relief is 10 minutes after subcutaneous administration of sumatriptan and 30 minutes after oral administration. The duration of action is 24 to 48 hours. Sumatriptan is extensively biotransformed by the liver and excreted in the urine.

For most of the triptans, half-lives are 2 to 6 hours, except for frovatriptan, which has a half-life of 26 hours. Although sumatriptan is widely distributed in the body, passage through the blood-brain barrier is low. These drugs are extensively biotransformed by the liver, with a portion excreted unchanged by the kidney. Triptans can also be deaminated by monoamine oxidase A; consequently, the use of a monoamine oxidase inhibitor (MAOI) in patients taking triptans could increase levels of the drugs and may increase the risk of adverse reactions.

ADVERSE REACTIONS AND CONTRAINDICATIONS

Triptans commonly produce mild and transient adverse effects, namely nausea, malaise, dizziness, weakness, and dry mouth. However, these are also symptoms of the migraine itself. These drugs also may cause numbness and a tingling sensation. Triptans can cause a feeling of tightness in the chest and overt chest pain. In rare instances arrhythmias may be observed. Sumatriptan and frovatriptan may cause hypersensitivity reactions.

The major concern is the vasoconstriction caused by triptans. Patients are screened for active or potential underlying cardiovascular disease, including angina, hypertension, diabetes, obesity, and smoking. These drugs are contraindicated in patients with myocardial ischemia or vasospastic coronary artery disease. These drugs should also be avoided in patients with stroke, transient ischemic attacks, and uncontrolled hypertension. The risk of triptans during pregnancy is unknown.

INTERACTIONS

Triptans should not be administered within 24 hours of dihydroergotamine or ergotamine administration (see below) because of the risk of severe vasoconstriction. In addition, potential toxic interactions can occur with the concurrent use of any of the antidepressant 5-HT uptake blockers, such as fluoxetine, fluvoxamine, paroxetine, and sertraline, or the MAOIs.

DRUG CLASS • Ergot Derivatives

dihydroergotamine (Migranal, D.H.E. 45)

ergotamine (Ergostat, Ergomar✶)

methysergide (Sansert)

MECHANISM OF ACTION

Although ergot derivatives have both agonist and antagonist activity for alpha adrenergic, serotonergic, and dopaminergic receptors, their mechanism of action for treating migraine is attributed to their agonist activity at serotonin receptors. Presumably, activation of these receptors produces vasoconstriction and decreases transmitter release from small-diameter sensory neurons. The prophylactic mechanism of methysergide is believed to be antagonist activity at the serotonin type 2 receptors.

USES

There are a number of ergot derivatives, but only two are currently used for treating migraine after onset: dihydroergotamine and ergotamine (Table 15-3). Dihydroergotamine is used to treat acute or chronic severe migraine in patients who do not get relief from analgesics. Ergotamine is administered orally for the treatment of acute migraine or for prophylactic treatment of cluster headaches. Ergotamine also is prescribed in combination with caffeine to improve absorption of the ergot (see Table 15-3). A third compound, methysergide, is used to prevent migraines but it is ineffective after the headache begins.

In addition to being formulated with caffeine to speed absorption, Canadian formulations of ergotamine include the anticholinergic drug belladonna, the sedative pentobarbital, or an antihistamine such as cyclizine, dimenhydrinate, or diphenhydramine. Methysergide is indicated for the prophylaxis of migraine and cluster headaches. If a response has not occurred after 3 weeks, treatment is discontinued. The drug can produce a number of adverse effects (discussed later), some of which can be serious. Consequently, prophylaxis is preferred in most cases.

PHARMACOKINETICS

Dihydroergotamine is administered parenterally and is well absorbed by this route, with a duration of action of about 8 hours. A nasal spray is also available. Ergotamine is administered orally, but it is poorly absorbed and has an extensive first-pass effect, which severely limits oral bioavailability. There is considerable patient variation, in part because migraines are often accompanied by a sluggish gastric motility. Caffeine increases the rate and extent of absorption. Without caffeine, the onset of action is about 2 hours, but with caffeine the onset of headache relief is reduced to about 1 hour. Another additive to ergotamine can be metoclopramide, which stimulates gastrointestinal motility, thereby increasing ergotamine absorption. Metoclopramide also has an antiemetic action.

Ergotamine and caffeine may also be administered rectally, a route that provides more extensive absorption and produces less nausea. The onset of action is about 1 hour. Sublingual ergotamine is absorbed slowly. Methysergide is well absorbed when given orally; the duration of action is 1 to 2 days.

Dihydroergotamine and ergotamine are highly bound to plasma proteins. Both drugs also are extensively biotransformed in the liver with metabolites excreted primarily in the bile. Approximately 50% of methysergide is eliminated unchanged in the urine.

ADVERSE REACTIONS AND CONTRAINDICATIONS

The major adverse effects of ergot derivatives are nausea and vasoconstriction. The antiemetic metoclopramide is commonly given 20 to 30 minutes before administration of dihydroergotamine to minimize nausea.

The vasoconstrictive action of ergot derivatives can lead to transiently cold fingers and toes, often accompanied

---

TABLE 15-3

Drugs to Treat Severe Headaches

Generic Name	Trade Name	Comments
Ergot-Containing Drugs		
dihydroergotamine mesylate	D.H.E. 45, Migranal	Has less arterial vasoconstrictive action than ergotamine. New spray form must be prepared as needed and discarded after use.
ergotamine tartrate	Ergostat, Ergomar, ✽ Gynergen, ✽ Medihaler, Ergotamine ✽	Oral preparation without caffeine has slower onset of action. Variability of oral absorption with low bioavailability.
ergotamine tartrate + caffeine	Cafergot	To reduce the risk of dependence on ergotamine, use no more than two times/week, preferably 5 days apart. Caffeine used to increase oral absorption.
ergotamine tartrate + caffeine + belladonna ✽	Wigraine ✽	To reduce the risk of dependence on ergotamine, use not more than two times/week, preferably 5 days apart. Caffeine used to increase oral absorption.
methysergide	Sansert	Prophylactic treatment for migraine and cluster headaches only.
Triptans		
almotriptan	Axert	Administered by the oral route with higher bioavailability.
frovatriptan	Frova	Has a longer half-life. Patients can show hypersensitivity.
naratriptan	Amerge	Note approximately 50% of dose excreted unchanged, so may have altered kinetics in patients with compromised renal function.
rizatriptan	Maxalt, Maxalt-MLT	MLT formulation is mint flavored and dissolves rapidly in the mouth.
sumatriptan	Imitrex	Available in both oral and parenteral forms. Should not be administered within 24 hr after ergotamine because of the risk of severe vasoconstriction. Should be administered only after headache pain begins. If the first dose is not effective, do not administer additional doses.
zolmitriptan	Zomig, Zomig ZMT	Antimigraine drug with moderate oral biovailability.

✽ Available in Canada only.

---

by tingling or numbness. Dihydroergotamine produces less vasoconstriction than ergotamine.

Ergot derivatives are contraindicated during pregnancy because these drugs stimulate the uterus. Also, the reduced uterine blood flow may be harmful to the fetus. Ergot derivatives are excreted in breast milk and can produce adverse effects in the infant, including vomiting, diarrhea, unstable blood pressure, and seizures. Other contraindications include coronary artery disease, hypertension, peripheral vascular disease, and impaired renal function since these conditions may be aggravated by ergot derivatives. Patients with angina are at risk, and nitroglycerin is less effective as a vasodilator. Patients with

impaired liver function may not biotransform the drug readily, leading to toxicity.

Adverse effects of methysergide include nausea, vomiting, diarrhea, cramps, and peripheral ischemia, which can produce abdominal pain; chest pain; itching of the skin; numbness and tingling of the toes, fingers, and face; and pale, cold hands and feet. Occasionally there are changes in vision, peripheral edema, and rashes. Orthostatic hypotension may be noted as dizziness or light-headedness. A rare adverse effect after a longer duration of therapy is fibrosis, which may occur in cardiac, penile, pleuropulmonary, or retroperitoneal tissues. Because of this risk, methysergide should be administered for no longer than 6 months, with a drug-free interval of 3 to 4 weeks. Patients with any comorbid cardiovascular, pulmonary, hepatic, or renal condition are at greater risk for adverse effects. Methysergide is not recommended for mothers who breast-feed, for children, or for older adults.

TOXICITY

The classic toxicity associated with ergot alkaloids is **ergotism,** which was called St. Anthony's fire in the Middle Ages. Ergot alkaloids are produced by a fungus, *Claviceps purpurea,* that flourishes in damp grains, especially rye. Epidemics of ergotism from contaminated grain are part of recorded history. Symptoms included hallucinations, fiery pain, prolonged vasoconstriction leading to gangrene, miscarriages, and seizures. Ergotamine poisoning from medicinal use can also occur. Severe vasoconstriction can be treated with nitroprusside infusion until the body eliminates the ergotamine.

Methysergide is chemically related to the hallucinogen LSD. Signs of an overdose include changes in vision and symptoms of central nervous system (CNS) stimulation such as excitement, difficulty in thinking, a feeling of being outside the body, or hallucinations and nightmares. The patient may show clumsiness or unsteadiness. The drug should be discontinued and the patient carefully monitored, especially for impaired respiration and convulsions. If the patient has ingested an overdose, gastric lavage may be needed. Severe peripheral vasospasm may require treatment with nitroprusside.

INTERACTIONS

Drugs that have a vasoconstrictor action are contraindicated with ergot derivatives. These drugs include cocaine, epinephrine, metaraminol, methoxamine, norepinephrine, and phenylephrine. Smoking increases the risk of vasoconstrictive adverse effects.

 APPLICATION TO PRACTICE

ASSESSMENT
History of Present Illness

The subjective and objective data that should be obtained from a patient with a headache are presented in Table 15-4. Be sure to include the specific details of the headache itself. If the patient has a history of tension-type headaches, migraines, or cluster head-aches, it is important to note if the character, intensity, or location of the headache has changed. Cluster headaches may occur at high altitudes with low oxygen levels.

Health History

Ask about previous illnesses (hypertension, cancer, stroke), head injuries or seizures, surgery (craniotomy, sinus, facial), asthma or allergies, family history, and response to drugs taken. Inquire about a history of mental illness, travel, and exposure to noxious stimuli. Ask also about the use of herbal remedies; over the counter (OTC) and prescription drugs, particularly hydralazine, bromides, nitroglycerin, ergotamine (withdrawal), nonsteroidal antiinflammatory drugs (NSAIDs) (in high daily doses), and estrogen preparations; and the use of oral contraceptives.

Lifespan Considerations

Headaches can occur at any age, from the very young to the very old. Young children are often unable to describe how they feel, and older adults may not be able to communicate their symptoms.

Cultural/Social Considerations

Headaches are a cultural/social phenomenon. Cultural factors influencing the development or persistence of headaches include taboos and myths held by the patient and the family. Treating all patients alike regardless of culture is unsafe. For example, some patients express pain openly whereas others are stoic in pain. If the nurse makes conclusions about the degree of pain based on behavior, one patient could be undertreated and another overtreated.

Social factors affecting the development or persistence of headaches include family structure and functions, roles of individuals within the family and among generations, communication patterns, educational and support systems, and socialization functions. Western and non-Western belief systems also influence how headaches are perceived and treated. Be sure to elicit cultural/social information that may influence patient care.

Physical Examination

The physical examination should include observation for signs of malaise, anxiety, apprehension, irritability, restlessness, or withdrawal. Watch for forehead diaphoresis, pallor, unilateral facial flushing with cheek edema, red eyes, lacrimation, and photophobia. Check for resistance to head movement, nuchal rigidity, and palpable neck and shoulder tension. Note any signs of vertigo or hemiparesis.

TABLE 15-4

Headache History

Subjective Data
On what part of the head do the headaches start?
After the headache starts, does it stay in one place or move around?
How would you describe the pain?
Describe the degree of pain on a scale of 1 to 10.
How long ago did the current headaches start?
How old were you when any headache started?
How long does the headache usually last?
How often does the headache occur?
Does the headache awaken you from sleep?
Is the headache getting worse, getting better, fluctuating, no change?
Previous professional treatment for headache?
Previous drugs used for headache? Name/dosage/frequency
Do any blood relatives have severe headaches? Who?
Alcohol, smoking, coffee history?
Is there a history of a head injury? When?
Was a headache diary kept?

Are Any of the Following Symptoms Associated with the Headache?

Vision Changes	*Face/Scalp Symptoms*	*GI Tract Symptoms*
Spots before eyes	Scalp/face/tooth pain	Nausea or vomiting
Blindness, blurring	Nasal congestion/discharge	Diarrhea
Red, tender eyes	Odor sensitivity	Anorexia
Eyelids droop	Noise sensitivity	Hunger
Eyes red or puffy	Circumoral numbness	Painful chewing
Eyes sensitive to light	Sweating	Difficulty opening mouth
Double vision		
Seeing only half of an object		

Mental Status Changes

Difficulty concentrating	Difficulty following instructions	Difficulty finding words
Slurred speech	Depression	Anxiety
Irritability	Dizziness	Fainting

Which of the Following Factors Trigger or Worsen the Headache?

Sexual activity	Too much or too little sleep	Missed meal
Stress, during or after	Weather changes	Depression/anxiety
Changing seasons	Physical activity	Alcohol/MSG
Erect position	Pregnancy	Straining/coughing
Cheeses	Menstrual periods	Contraceptives
Chocolate	Citrus fruits	Drugs

Which of the Following Makes/Made the Headache Better?

Rest	Activity	Darkness
Quiet	Compresses	Pregnancy
Menopause	Direct pressure	Massage
Other (specify)		

Laboratory Testing

Most laboratory testing is done for patients with secondary headaches and those who may be recalcitrant to conservative treatment. Testing may include brain imaging (CT or MRI), cerebral arteriogram, lumbar puncture, electroencephalogram, and electromyography.

GOALS OF THERAPY

The primary goal for the treatment of headaches is to prevent their occurrence. When this is not possible, the overall goal is that the patient have reduced or no pain, experience increased comfort and decreased anxiety, demonstrate an understanding of triggering events and treatment strategies, and use positive coping strategies to deal with chronic headache pain.

INTERVENTION

The most effective treatment for tension headaches is stress reduction. Help the patient to examine his or her lifestyle, recognize stressful situations, and learn to cope with them more appropriately. Precipitating factors can be identified and strategies for avoiding them developed. Daily exercise, relaxation periods, and socialization can be encouraged, since each can help decrease the recurrence of the headache. Suggest alternative ways of pain management, such as relaxation, meditation, yoga, and self-hypnosis. Massage and application of moist hot packs to the neck and head can help a patient with tension headaches.

Treatment of migraines is divided into two phases: acute treatment and prophylactic treatment. Treatment of the acute attack aims to stop or at least ameliorate the attack. Analgesics including nonsteroidal antiinflammatory drugs and codeine are used in the treatment of mild to moderate migraines and tension headaches (Table 15-2). Severe migraine may be treated with ergotamine or one of the new triptans. An antiemetic may be administered to counteract the nausea of the headache as well as the nausea caused by ergotamine; these are discussed in Chapter 50. Patients with severe migraines often benefit from prophylaxis with one of a number of drugs, including beta-adrenergic receptor blockers (e.g., propranolol, atenolol; see Chapter 12); sedative hypnotics, especially butalbital (see Chapter 17); calcium channel blockers (e.g., verapamil; see Chapter 41); and antidepressants (e.g., fluoxetine; see Chapter 18). Prophylactic treatment of chronic tension headaches also may involve use of these drugs.

Treatment of cluster headaches is also divided into acute treatment and prophylactic treatment. Because a cluster headache has a sudden and explosive onset, acute treatment is difficult. Sublingual ergotamine or parenteral dihydroergotamine may be useful. Triptans may also be effective. Inhalation of 100% oxygen (7 to 9 L/min) for 15- to 20-minute periods with a 5-minute rest between periods may be helpful. The patient should be seated and leaning forward. Prophylactic treatment of cluster headaches begins with avoidance of alcohol and smoking. A number of drugs, including lithium, ergotamine, beta blockers, thiazide diuretics (e.g., hydrochlorothiazide), nonsteroidal antiinflammatory drugs, calcium channel blockers (e.g., verapamil), and MAOIs (see Chapter 18) can be tried as prophylactic drugs.

Administration

Teach the patient appropriate drug administration techniques: intramuscular, subcutaneous, sublingual, in-halation, or rectal, depending on the drug. Take oral doses with a full glass (8 ounces) of water, swallowing the drug whole without breaking or chewing. A drug such as the immediate-release formulation of rizatriptan should be given by the sublingual route. Oral doses of methysergide should be taken with milk or a snack to reduce gastric irritation. If rectal suppositories must be divided to obtain the correct dose, instruct patient to cut lengthwise. Refrigerate suppositories to make cutting and insertion easier. Review patient instruction leaflets provided by manufacturer.

Many of these drugs will be more effective if the patient can lie down in a darkened room immediately after taking the drug. Limiting noise in the environment, turning off the lights, and applying a cold washcloth to the forehead may help relieve some of the discomfort. Monitor the patient's blood pressure. Examine the extremities and monitor peripheral pulses. Instruct the patient to report the development of chest pain. Ergot formulations may cause nausea and vomiting in some patients. This may subside with use, but antiemetics may be prescribed concurrently.

Education

Teaching objectives for the patient with headaches include avoiding the factors that can trigger the headache, where possible. The Dietary Considerations box identifies factors that trigger a headache and some that may prevent the headache.

Teach the patient about the prescribed drugs. Recognize that many products contain multiple ingredients (see Table 15-2) and that the patient needs to know about all of the component ingredients. Review the dosing schedule with the patient. Emphasize the importance of taking the drug as ordered for best effect, but not increasing the dose or frequency of administration unless approved by the health care provider. Many of these drugs are habit-forming. Remind the patient to keep these and all drugs out of the reach of children and not to share the drugs with others. Instruct the patient to seek medical help immediately if overdose with any of these drugs is suspected.

Many of the drugs used for headaches cause drowsiness or dizziness. Caution the patient to avoid driving or engaging in potentially dangerous activities until the effects of the drug are known. Remind the patient to avoid drugs that depress the CNS (sedative-hypnotics and antihistamines) and to avoid self-treating with OTC preparations unless approved by the health care provider. Tell the patient to keep all health care providers informed of all drugs taken. Instruct the patient to avoid alcohol, which may aggravate headaches, and to avoid smoking and cold temperatures, which may intensify vasoconstriction.

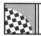

Dietary Considerations
HEADACHES

How foods may influence headaches depends on the type of headache and many specific characteristics of the individual, so it is impossible to create hard and fast rules. However, it is possible to suggest some strategies that have worked for others and might offer a basis for assuming a degree of personal control over headaches.

It is clear that several components of foods and drugs can contribute to the development of specific types of headaches. Examples include the following:

1. Phenylethylamine, which is found in dark chocolate; white chocolate is usually not a problem
2. Nitrates/nitrites, which are found in cured meats such as hot dogs, bacon, salami, and ham
3. Monosodium glutamate (MSG), which is found in prepared oriental foods as well as hydrolyzed vegetable oil (HVP), hydrolyzed plant protein (HPP), and Kombu extract
4. Tyramine, which is found in a variety of foods including:
   a. Fruit, particularly oranges, grapes, lemons, limes, pineapple, and their fruit juices; figs, dates, red plums, dates, raisins, and avocados
   b. Fermented alcoholic beverages, including all tap beer, domestic nonalcoholic beer, ales, vermouth, sherry, and wines such as Riesling or Chianti
   c. Yeast and yeast products, such as homemade breads, yeast extracts such as soup cubes, canned meats, marmite, and sour cream
   d. Cheeses, especially American (processed), blue, Boursault, brick, Brie, Camembert, cheddars, Emmentaler, Gouda, Gruyere, mozzarella, Parmesan, Romano, Roquefort, and Stilton

Other foods or components of foods that may contribute to headaches in some patients include alcohol, the artificial sweetener aspartame, caffeine (see Chapter 20), and vinegar. Legumes of many varieties have also been implicated by some patients; the products include broad beans, lima beans, fava beans, navy beans, and pea pods.

A few foods have been noted by some patients to help prevent headache. Fish and fish oils, particularly salmon, tuna, sardines, and mackerel, have been shown to be more effective in men than women but must be a regular part of the diet to have an effect. Ginger, made into a tea, may also relieve or prevent migraines.

For the patient whose headaches are triggered by food, dietary counseling should be provided. The patient should be encouraged to eliminate foods that provoke headaches (Box 15-1). Active challenge and provocative testing with specific foods may be necessary to determine the triggers. Advise the patient to also avoid exposure to triggers such as strong perfumes, volatile solvents, and gasoline fumes.

EVALUATION

Effective drug treatment should help relieve the headache within a reasonable time. Advise the patient to contact the health care provider if symptoms become more severe, last longer than usual, or are resistant to drug therapy. Report nausea, vomiting, change in vision, or fever occurring with a headache.

CASE STUDY  *Headache*

ASSESSMENT

HISTORY OF PRESENT ILLNESS

SB, a 28-year-old woman, complains of a recurring head-ache, one that is particularly severe today. She brings with her the headache diary supplied by her previous health care provider. She has not used the diary and does not re-member what type of headaches she has. She knew the headache was coming on today when she awoke to flashes of light in her field of vision. The headache developed on one side of her head, is throbbing, and appears to be syn-chronous with her pulse. The headache has now lasted for almost 36 hours. Her eyes hurt and she is nauseated. There has been no vomiting. She self-treated with ibupro-fen, Excedrin Migraine, aspirin, and naproxen, without re-lief. The headaches appear unrelated to her menses. SB is unable to identify triggers for the headache.

HEALTH HISTORY

SB has no history of hospitalization, surgeries, or major trauma. She denies history of cardiovascular disease, in-cluding angina, hypertension, diabetes, and obesity, and she takes no other drugs.

LIFESPAN CONSIDERATIONS

SB is newly married (3 weeks ago) and is trying to estab-lish a personal lifestyle with her husband and a 10-year-old child from her husband's previous marriage. She is hoping to return to school to finish her degree in journal-ism and thus would like to delay pregnancy for another 2 years.

CULTURAL/SOCIAL CONSIDERATIONS

SB's cultural/social background is Jewish; her husband and stepson are Irish Catholic. These differences have created dis-sention in the family. SB is a nonsmoker and nondrinker. She frequently stops by the family-owned delicatessen, where she has her favorite salami and Swiss cheese sandwich on home-made rye bread.

PHYSICAL EXAMINATION

BP is 120/70 mm Hg, pulse 72, respirations 20. Skin is warm and dry. SB is obviously photophobic, preferring to have the room darkened during the examination. She is withdrawn and sensitive to noise. CN II to XII are intact. Deep tendon re-flexes (DTRs) are intact bilaterally in upper and lower extrem-ities. SB has now had an emesis of undigested food.

LABORATORY TESTING

Pregnancy test was negative. No other tests were performed.

PATIENT PROBLEM(S)

Common migraine.

GOALS OF THERAPY

Relieve today's headache and prevent recurrence.

CRITICAL THINKING QUESTIONS

1. SB's health care provider orders intramuscular sumatrip-tan, 6 mg now. What is the mechanism of action of sumatriptan?
2. What assessments should be done by the nurse before administration of sumatriptan? Why are these assess-ments necessary?
3. What kinds of nondrug therapies might help SB prevent or alleviate her headaches in the future?
4. SB is prescribed rizatriptan for use at home. What patient teaching is needed for SB to safely use this drug?
5. What factor(s) in SB's history may be implicated in trig-gering her headaches?

Bibliography

Green CA: Nursing rounds: is this headache serious? *Am J Nurs* 97(2):45-46, 55, 1997.

Headache Classification Committee of the International Headache Society: Classification and diagnostic criteria for headache disorders, cranial neuralgias, and facial pain, *Cephalgia* 8(Suppl 7):1, 1988.

Lin JN: Overview of migraine, *J Neurosci Nurs* 33(1):6-13, 2001.

Marin PA: Pharmacological management of migraine, *J Am Acad Nurse Pract* 10(9):407-412, 1998.

Moloney MF, Matthews KB, Scharbo-Dehaan M, et al: Caring for the woman with migraine headaches, *Nurse Pract* 25(2):17-18, 21-24, 27-28, 2000.

Pfeiffer GM: Easing the pain of the tension headaches: a systematic approach, *Adv Nurse Pract* 5(5):24-25, 29-31, 1997.

Rosenblum RK, Fisher PG: A guide to children with acute and chronic headaches, *J Pediatr Health Care* 15(5):229-235, 2001.

Weiss J: Assessing and managing the patient with migraines. *Nurse Pract* 24(7):18-20, 23-25, 28-29, 1999.

Internet Resources

JAMA Migraine Information Center. Available online at http://www.ama-assn.org/special/migrane/migrane.htm.

MEDLINEplus Health Information. Available online at http://www.nlm.nih.gov/medlineplus/headacheandmigrane.html.

National Women's Health Information Center. Available online at www.4woman.gov.

16

Anesthetics and Related Drugs

JOSEPH A. DiMICCO • KATHLEEN GUTIERREZ

 Visit http://evolve.elsevier.com/Gutierrez/ for additional information.

KEY TERMS

OBJECTIVES

- Describe the mechanism of action of local anesthetics.

- Identify and describe the adverse effects of local anesthetics.

- Explain the differences between drugs used for surface anesthesia and those injected to produce local anesthesia.

- Differentiate among infiltration, nerve block, epidural, caudal, and spinal anesthesia.

- Describe the distinguishing characteristics of inhalation anesthetics, intravenous anesthetics, balanced anesthesia, and neurolept anesthesia.

- Explain minimum alveolar concentration.

- Discuss the action of neuromuscular-blocking drugs.

- Differentiate between nondepolarizing and depolarizing neuromuscular-blocking drugs.

- Develop a nursing care plan for a patient who has received local or general anesthesia or neuromuscular-blocking drugs.

ANESTHESIA DEFINED

Anesthesia is a state in which the perception of and response to painful stimulation is blocked. In fact, anesthesia literally means "without sensation," and anesthetic drugs have the capacity to block all sensory transmission. Note that anesthesia is different from *analgesia*, a term which refers specifically to the reduction or blockade of pain and painful stimuli. In this chapter, the use of drugs to induce two very different types of anesthesia will be discussed.

PHYSIOLOGY • Local Anesthesia and the Transmission of Painful Stimuli

Painful sensations and other sensory information are transmitted over long distances in the body by the rapid spread of action potentials down nerve processes. Action potentials are responsible for the spread of excitation and triggering events in all excitable tissues, including neurons in the central and peripheral nervous systems, cardiac muscle, and skeletal muscle. Although this process can be visualized as similar to an electrical impulse traveling down a wire, it is in fact much more complex and involves a specific protein embedded in the membrane of the nerve fiber. This protein can change shape suddenly and become a pore or channel in the membrane through which sodium ions can move. These channels open briefly when the adjacent membrane depolarizes and then close quickly. The channels are called **voltage-gated sodium channels** because they are opened by membrane depolarization, or *fast sodium channels* because they open only briefly and then close rapidly. The movement of sodium through these channels also depolarizes the membrane in which they sit, resulting in the opening of sodium channels in adjacent membrane areas. Thus an *action potential* is a wave of brief openings (and closings) of sodium channels that spreads rapidly down the nerve fiber. The speed at which action potentials spread down nerve fibers is breathtaking, approaching 400 feet per second in some cases. Painful stimuli, though transmitted somewhat more slowly, nevertheless reach the central nervous system (CNS) very quickly through such a process.

Local anesthesia is a condition in which sensory stimulation transmitted through peripheral nerves is blocked only in a restricted region of the body. Usually, the drugs are applied to the immediate vicinity of the painful stimulus or the region through which nerves travel that would carry the pain signal to the central nervous system. Local anesthesia is often relatively uncomplicated, involving a patient who is otherwise awake and alert throughout the experience.

DRUG CLASS • Local Anesthetics

Surface (Topical or Mucosal) Anesthetics

benzocaine (Americaine, Anbesol, Chloraseptic, Num-Zit, Orajel)

butamben (Butesin)

cocaine

dibucaine (Nupercainal)

dyclonine (Dyclone, Sucrets)

pramoxine (Anusol, Prame-gel, ProctoFoam, Tronolane, Tronothane)

proparacaine (Alcaine, Ocu-Caine, Ophthaine)

Parenteral Anesthetics

articaine (Astracaine, ✳ Ultracaine✳)

bupivacaine (Marcaine, Sensorcaine)

chloroprocaine (Nesacaine)

etidocaine (Duranest)

levobupivacaine (Chirocaine)

lidocaine* (Xylocaine, Dalcaine, Dilocaine, L-Caine, Octocaine)

mepivacaine (Carbocaine, Polocaine)

prilocaine (Citanest)

procaine (Novocain)

proparacaine (Ophthaine, Alcaine)

ropivacaine (Naropin)

tetracaine* (Pontocaine)

MECHANISM OF ACTION

Local anesthetics all work by blocking fast sodium channels in peripheral sensory nerve fibers and thereby preventing the pain-producing signals—or any sensory information from the affected area—from reaching the brain. This effect results when a molecule of the drug binds to a specific site near the intracellular end of the sodium channel and blocks it. Since the

---

*Also available for topical administration.

action potential is generated by the rush of sodium ions into the cell through these channels, the local anesthetic can therefore depress the action potential such that it fails to spread down the nerve fiber. The interaction of the drug with the ion channel is reversible. Sensation returns as the drug diffuses away and local concentration falls. Local anesthetics can also block voltage-gated sodium channels responsible for excitability of neurons in the brain, cardiac muscle, and skeletal muscle.

Different nerve fibers have various sensitivities to local anesthetics. The two most important factors are (1) diameter or size of the nerve fiber and (2) firing rate of the neuron. With regard to size, smaller-diameter fibers are more susceptible to blockade, whereas large-diameter fibers tend to be resistant. Since fibers that transmit pain tend to be among the smallest in diameter and those innervating skeletal muscle are the largest, local anesthetic can cause complete blockade of pain without causing motor paralysis in the affected region. Unfortunately, sympathetic postganglionic nerves have relatively small diameters and therefore can be blocked by therapeutic concentrations of local anesthetic. The firing rate of the neuron is important because the drug molecules can bind to their receptor in the channel only when the channel is open. Therefore the faster a nerve fiber is firing, the more likely that drug molecules will be able to reach their binding sites in open channels and the greater the drug's effect will be. This phenomenon, whereby firing nerves are affected more by local anesthetic than silent nerves, is called **use dependence.**

Cocaine is unique among local anesthetics in its ability to inhibit the reuptake of norepinephrine released by sympathetic nerves back into the nerve endings (see Chapter 10). In this way, cocaine can increase the local concentration of norepinephrine at innervated adrenergic receptors and thus intensify sympathetic responses.

USES

In general, local anesthetics can be divided into those applied topically to provide surface anesthesia and those injected into an area to produce local anesthesia. Only lidocaine, dibucaine, and tetracaine are used both topically and by injection.

Surface Anesthesia

Local anesthetics applied as drops, sprays, lotions, creams, or ointments, called surface anesthetics, are listed separately at the beginning of this section. A distinction must be made among those drugs as to which can be safely applied to the eyes, to skin, and to mucosal areas.

Most drugs used for surface anesthesia are very safe and effective when applied to the skin. These drugs are poorly soluble, so little systemic absorption occurs when they are applied to relieve itching or the pain of mild burns. Mucous membranes of the nose, mouth, and throat (bronchotracheal mucosa) and of the urethra, rectum, and vagina are highly vascular and allow ready absorption of the local anesthetic into systemic circulation. A local anesthetic is often used to eliminate the gag reflex when inserting an endotracheal tube or to limit the discomfort of endoscopic procedures.

Only tetracaine and proparacaine are suitable for application to the eye.

Local Anesthetics Administered by Injection

The potency and the duration of action of an injected local anesthetic increases together with its lipid solubility. The onset of anesthesia is determined by the drug concentration and the size of the nerve.

The area affected by injection of a local anesthetic depends on how and where it is injected. The anesthesia produced is described by the technique of injection: infiltration, nerve block, epidural, and spinal. These techniques are described below, along with their potential for producing toxic adverse effects.

Infiltration anesthesia refers to the superficial application of a local anesthetic. To suture a cut or to perform dental procedures, local anesthetic is injected superficially in small amounts to block the small nerves and to numb the area. To work on the scalp or to make an incision in the skin, the anesthetic is infused around the area. Small incisions require a small volume and a low drug concentration, so toxicity is seldom associated with these uses. However, systemic toxicity from local anesthetics is commonly seen in the emergency room when large cuts are infiltrated with local anesthetic.

Intravenous regional anesthesia (Bier's block) is an anesthetic technique used in surgery of the forearm and hand or foot and distal leg. The limb is cannulated and then drained of blood by applying an elastic bandage. A tourniquet is applied and inflated to 100 to 150 mm Hg above the systolic blood pressure. The local anesthetic, usually lidocaine, is then administered through the cannula. Anesthesia occurs in about 5 to 10 minutes. The duration of compression must be limited to 2 hours to avoid ischemic nerve injury. The advantage of the technique is that it can be terminated by deflation of the tourniquet with rapid return of sensation. However, a toxic level of local anesthetic may be released if the tourniquet is not left in place for a minimum of 15 to 30 minutes.

Nerve block anesthesia refers to the injection of a local anesthetic along a nerve before it reaches the surgical site. The volume and concentration of a local anesthetic for a nerve block must be larger than in infiltration anesthesia to penetrate the larger nerve. The most extensive field of local anesthesia is achieved by applying the anesthetic around the nerve roots near the spinal cord to produce epidural or spinal anesthesia. As shown in Figure 16-1, the spinal cord proper ends at the lumbar region. The spinal cord is surrounded by three membranes: (1) the *pia mater*, (2) the *arachnoid*, and (3) the outer membrane, the *dura mater*. These membranes extend below the spinal cord proper to form a sac in the lumbar and sacral region. The dura mater and arachnoid membranes are close together, and the subarachnoid space is between the arachnoid and pia mater. Cerebrospinal fluid fills the subarachnoid space throughout the spinal cord.

For **epidural anesthesia**, the local anesthetic is administered outside the dura mater (see Figure 16-1) so that the nerve roots are blocked at the point where they emerge from the dura mater. The extent of anesthesia depends on the volume and concentration of local anesthetic used. **Caudal anesthesia** is a form of epidural anesthesia achieved by administering the local anesthetic epidurally at the base of the spine. The anesthesia affects only the pelvic region and legs. Caudal anesthesia is used for obstetrics and for surgery on the rectum, anus, and prostate gland.

Spinal anesthesia is achieved by injecting local anesthetic into the subarachnoid space between the arachnoid and pia mater membranes in the lumbar area, usually between the second lumbar and first sacral vertebrae and well below the spinal cord proper (see Figure 16-1). This method blocks the nerve roots for the entire lower body. If the solution containing local anesthetic has the same density (isobaric) as cerebrospinal fluid and is administered slowly, it will stay where it is injected and will slowly diffuse into the rest of the cerebrospinal fluid. The solution of local anesthetic can be made more dense (hyperbaric) by diluting it with 5% dextrose. The solution will then gravitate downward. If

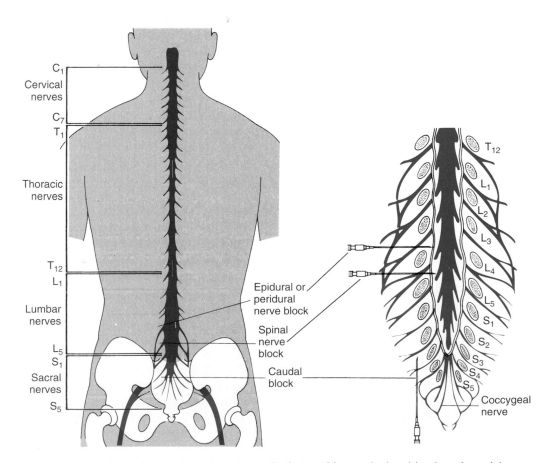

FIGURE 16-1   Sites for injection of local anesthetic to achieve spinal, epidural, and caudal anesthesia.

the patient is on a tilt bed with feet high and head low, the hyperbaric solution will travel up the spinal cord toward the head and anesthetize more of the body. The solution of local anesthetic also can be diluted with distilled water to be less dense (hypobaric). In the patient positioned on the tilt bed, this solution would move to the end of the dura mater and anesthetize only the lower part of the body. Procedures using hypobaric and hyperbaric solutions of local anesthetic require skill in positioning patients. If the level of anesthesia is adjusted to block more of the spinal cord than just the lumbar and sacral regions, there is danger of blocking the intercostal and phrenic nerves, which would paralyze spontaneous respiration.

If the patient is seated when the local anesthetic is administered as a low spinal anesthetic, only those nerves affecting the parts of the body that would be in contact with a saddle are affected—hence the name **saddle block.** This procedure is used principally in obstetrics for vaginal delivery.

With spinal anesthesia the patient is awake, breathing and cardiovascular function are not immediately affected, and muscles are relaxed, all of which are advantageous for patients with heart and lung disease or for older adults. However, the sympathetic fibers to the blood vessels are blocked, so vasodilation with hypotension is a common adverse effect of spinal anesthesia. Spinal anesthesia is widely used in obstetrics, particularly for cesarean births.

PHARMACOKINETICS

Local anesthetics eventually enter systemic circulation and can affect other organs, especially excitable tissues such as the brain and the heart. Fortunately, all these drugs are quickly inactivated by enzymatic degradation in the blood or the liver. When used in infiltration anesthesia, ester drugs (e.g., procaine and chloroprocaine) are considered relatively safe because of their especially rapid hydrolysis in the plasma by cholinesterases. They may be inactivated almost as fast they are absorbed into the systemic circulation. Other local anesthetics, which are usually amides (e.g., lidocaine or bupivacaine), are more likely to accumulate in the systemic circulation and cause toxicity because they are degraded more slowly by the liver and have a longer plasma half-life. Therefore the key to the usefulness of most local anesthetics is restricting their distribution and slowing their systemic absorption.

The rate at which local anesthetic is removed from the infiltrated area depends largely on the degree of vascularization and local blood flow. The duration of the anesthetic effect can be increased by 50% to 100% when the injection includes an adrenergic agonist such as epinephrine, which causes vasoconstriction.

ADVERSE REACTIONS AND CONTRAINDICATIONS

Although cocaine is unique in causing euphoria, all local anesthetics can act as CNS stimulants if sufficient amounts are absorbed systemically. This stimulation can be seen as anxiety, tingling (paresthesia), tremors, and ringing in the ears (tinnitus). At very high plasma concentrations, local anesthetics can cause CNS depression. Depression of CNS function is serious because vasomotor control is lost, resulting in profound hypotension; respiration may fail and finally coma may result.

In addition to the CNS effects, the direct cardiovascular effects of local anesthetics are important. The electrical properties of the heart reflect in part the activity of voltage-gated sodium channels in cardiac tissue. In fact, the local anesthetics lidocaine and procainamide are also used as antiarrhythmic drugs to block some of these sodium channels (see Chapter 40). However, local anesthetics may also cause life-threatening cardiac arrhythmia under certain circumstances. High systemic levels of local anesthetics decrease electrical excitability in the heart and may depress cardiac performance.

Local anesthetics cause direct vasodilation, thus increasing blood flow and favoring removal of the drug, because transmission in sympathetic fibers innervating vascular smooth muscle is blocked. The potent vasoconstrictor actions of cocaine lead to a unique adverse reaction: prolonged abuse of cocaine by insufflation (sniffing) can produce loss of nasal septa caused by tissue death after ischemia (insufficient blood flow).

Spinal anesthesia can also cause variable hypotension by blocking the sympathetic nerves that maintain blood pressure by constricting blood vessels. The patient may experience a severe headache after spinal anesthesia, and it may last for hours or days after the anesthetic has worn off. This postspinal headache is believed to reflect a drop in the pressure of the cerebrospinal fluid caused by a leak where the dura mater was penetrated. The chance of a spinal headache is reduced when patients are kept flat on their backs and instructed not to raise their heads for 12 hours. This maximizes the hydrostatic pressure of the cerebrospinal fluid in the head.

Local anesthetics applied to the skin, especially esters, can cause skin rash (contact dermatitis).

Epinephrine is contraindicated for infiltration of areas with end arteries (fingers, toes, ears, nose, and penis) because intense local vasoconstriction may result in ischemia leading to tissue death. Similarly, the addition of a vasoconstrictor is not recommended for epidural anesthesia during labor because of the potential vasoconstriction of the uterine blood vessels with a resultant decrease in placental circulation. Epinephrine is also contraindicated in patients with severe cardiovascular disease or thyrotoxicosis, in whom cardiac function would be compromised by added vasoconstrictors.

TOXICITY

Local anesthetics have the potential to produce life-threatening toxicity by affecting the CNS or the heart, and some may trigger anaphylaxis in susceptible patients. As discussed earlier, the principal site of acute toxicity is the CNS; signs of stimulation culminate in convulsions. Intravenous diazepam or small doses of an ultrashort-acting barbiturate such as thiopental (Pentothal) or methohexital are given to stop these convulsions.

Effects on the heart generally appear only after CNS effects are evident. Bupivacaine seems especially likely to cause cardiotoxic effects, including ventricular fibrillation in rare cases. However, through a mechanism that is unclear, accidental intravascular infusion of other local anesthetics along with epinephrine has caused sudden cardiac death.

Certain local anesthetics, especially esters such as chloroprocaine, procaine, and tetracaine, can cause acute hypersensitivity reactions (anaphylaxis) in those rare individuals who are allergic to them. Patients who are allergic to one ester-type local anesthetic usually exhibit cross-sensitivity to other esters. In addition to the three drugs named above, other esters include benzocaine and proparacaine.

INTERACTIONS

The ability of local anesthetics to produce CNS depression is greatly increased in the presence of other drugs that depress the CNS, including many that are given before general anesthesia (i.e., so-called preanesthetics). Procaine should be avoided in patients taking sulfonamides because one of the metabolites of procaine inhibits their action. The potential for systemic toxicity of ester-type local anesthetics (e.g., procaine, chloroprocaine, and tetracaine) is greatly increased in patients being treated with a cholinesterase inhibitor.

Many of the significant drug interactions seen with injected local anesthetics occur when they are administered with adrenergic vasoconstrictors to slow the systemic absorption of the anesthetic, thus prolonging their action. Because vasoconstrictors all act by stimulating alpha-adrenergic receptors, alpha blockers or drugs with alpha-adrenergic receptor antagonist properties may reduce the effectiveness and duration of action of the local anesthetic. In the presence of anesthetic gases (particularly halothane), the heart may become sensitized to the effects of these drugs, resulting in arrhythmia. Adrenergic drugs may also provoke arrhythmia and hypertension in patients treated with digoxin or tricyclic antidepressants.

PHYSIOLOGY • General Anesthesia

General anesthesia is a condition in which the subject is usually unconscious; this is the desired condition for patients undergoing most major surgical procedures. Whereas local anesthesia often involves a small area of an extremity and is relatively uncomplicated, general anesthesia is a major intervention that targets the brain. Drugs that produce general anesthesia usually cause significant depression of most brain functions. Therefore general anesthetics are almost always administered in a setting where vital functions such as respiration and cardiovascular status are constantly monitored and can be controlled or supported. The degree to which various brain functions are depressed is often related to the dosage of the drug administered. At deeper levels of anesthesia, motor and cardiovascular reflexes are depressed or absent. Preservation of cardiovascular and respiratory function is desirable during surgery, but movement and muscle tone are not. Therefore neuromuscular blockers are commonly administered in conjunction with general anesthesia to relax skeletal muscle and eliminate motor reflexes during the operation. These neuromuscular blocking drugs are considered in this chapter as well.

A combination of drugs is commonly employed simultaneously in the induction, maintenance, and management of the surgical patient, including opioid analgesics, benzodiazepines, anticholinergics, neuromuscular blockers, and inhaled anesthetics.

DRUG CLASS • Inhaled Anesthetics

desflurane (Suprane)

enflurane (Ethrane)

halothane (Fluothane)

isoflurane (Forane)

nitrous oxide

sevoflurane (Ultane)

MECHANISM OF ACTION

Although inhaled anesthetics are all known to act in the CNS to produce anesthesia, the precise mechanism by which these drugs work is still unknown. The best evidence suggests that they have an effect on receptors of the inhibitory neurotransmitter **gamma-aminobutyric acid (GABA).** GABA acts primarily at receptors that conduct chloride ions into neurons, making them less likely to fire action potentials. Most of the inhaled anesthetics somehow amplify this inhibitory action.

Acting on GABA receptors and perhaps others, inhaled anesthetics produce the classic anesthetic state, which includes *analgesia* (loss of painful sensation), hypnosis (loss of consciousness), *amnesia* (loss of memory), and *depression of reflexes*. The different aspects of the anesthetic state may be caused by drug actions at various sites. For example, depression of reflexes may result from action of these drugs on the spinal cord and brainstem, whereas loss of consciousness and amnesia are caused by actions at higher levels in the brain.

Gaseous anesthetics also produce some muscular relaxation, probably through a combination of direct action on skeletal muscle and an effect on the nervous system. However, since inhaled anesthetics alone will not completely block the potential for movement, a neuromuscular blocker is often given as well to ensure total paralysis when required.

USES

Gaseous anesthetics are used to produce and maintain general anesthesia in surgical patients. However, they are rarely used alone. The inhaled anesthetics most often used in the United States are isoflurane, sevoflurane, and desflurane. Because most are not well tolerated by fully conscious patients, an inhaled anesthetic to be used for maintenance of anesthesia is often given only after heavy sedation or induction with one or more intravenous drugs. An exception is halothane, which is well tolerated and therefore often used for induction in children in whom insertion of an intravenous catheter may be difficult.

Nitrous oxide is too weak to produce general anesthesia when used alone, but it is sometimes used for analgesia in certain dental and obstetric procedures that do not require loss of consciousness. This gas is also often used in combination with other anesthetics to produce surgical anesthesia because its effect is additive with other gaseous drugs. In addition, it is often a component of **balanced anesthesia,** in which an opioid, a skeletal muscle relaxant, and nitrous oxide are used together to produce surgical anesthesia.

Historically, the depth of anesthesia was defined by four stages: I, analgesia; II, excitement; III, surgical anesthesia; and IV, depression of brainstem functions. Today so many other drugs are administered that these stages are not useful for observational purposes. The most reliable indication of stage III surgical anesthesia is the loss of the eyelash reflex (in which the eye blinks when the eyelash is stroked) and the establishment of a respiratory pattern that is regular in depth and rate.

PHARMACOKINETICS

Inhaled anesthesia is a mixture of volatile liquids or gas and oxygen. These drugs exist as liquids that evaporate at room temperature. When inhaled drugs are administered by mask, the gases flow into the mask through a finely calibrated vaporizer. The amount of vapor the patient receives determines the depth of anesthesia. When an endotracheal tube is used, the gases flow directly into the patient's tracheobronchial tree.

Since they are administered as gases and act as gases, inhaled anesthetics have unique pharmacokinetic properties. The effective concentration of such an anesthetic in the brain does not depend on its solubility in blood or tissue. Rather, effective concentration depends on its partial or effective pressure in the atmosphere. If a constant partial pressure of an anesthetic is inhaled, the partial pressure in the alveoli rises toward the inhaled level. If the gas is not soluble in blood, little will be removed by the blood circulating around the alveoli, and the partial pressure of the gas in the blood—and therefore in the brain—quickly reaches the inhaled partial pressure. Such an anesthetic has a rapid onset of action. However, if the gas is soluble in blood, partial pressure in the alveoli quickly drops because the gas is being removed more rapidly by the blood than can be replenished by breathing. Under these conditions, time to induction is prolonged by the time required to equilibrate the blood with the gas so that the partial pressure matches that coming into the alveoli. To shorten the time to reach this steady state, anesthesia is induced using a high partial pressure of the gas and then lowering the partial pressure to maintain anesthesia.

The potency of an inhaled anesthetic is determined by the **minimum alveolar concentration (MAC),** which is defined as the alveolar concentration that produces insensitivity to a skin incision (anesthesia) in 50% of patients at equilibrium. For instance, a MAC of 10% is equivalent to a partial pressure of 0.1 atmosphere at sea level. Surgery is usually conducted at about 1.4 times the MAC value of the anesthetic chosen. In general, pediatric patients require higher concentrations of inhaled anesthetics, whereas older adult patients require lower concentrations. With the exception of nitrous oxide, all gaseous anesthetics in current use have MACs of less than 10%.

The distribution of the anesthetic is determined by the blood flow; thus the brain, liver, and kidneys reach equilibrium first. Excretion is largely through the lungs. Anesthetics in solution are biotransformed by the liver to a variable degree. Certain halogenated hydrocarbons (e.g., enflurane, halothane) have metabolites that may damage the liver and kidneys.

Emergence is the time during which the patient regains consciousness after the anesthetic has been discontinued. The duration of emergence from the inhaled anesthetics depends on the same factors as induction.

ADVERSE REACTIONS AND CONTRAINDICATIONS

Inhaled anesthetics all produce varying degrees of cardiovascular depression. Halothane and enflurane have the more pronounced effects, which include reduction in blood pressure as well as cardiac output. Desflurane and isoflurane have a greater effect in lowering blood pressure but little effect on cardiac output. Older adults are more likely than others to react with hypotension and circulatory depression to an inhaled anesthetic.

Renal function is also affected by inhaled anesthetics. Reduced blood flow to the kidney results in reduced glomerular filtration rate and renal plasma flow. Blood flow to the liver is also decreased. Consequently, inhaled anesthetics should be used with caution in patients with renal or hepatic disease or impairment. Patients with head injuries or intracranial tumors may also pose special problems because inhaled anesthetics tend to increase intracranial pressure.

All inhaled anesthetics except nitrous oxide are respiratory depressants. They decrease the ventilatory response to hypoxia. During both surgery and recovery ventilatory assistance and increased oxygen are required. With the exception of nitrous oxide, all inhaled anesthetics are also uterine muscle relaxants. This effect can assist fetal manipulation during delivery but increases bleeding during a dilation and curettage (D & C) procedure.

Nitrous oxide poses a special problem with regard to air-filled spaces in the body. Since the gas is 34 times more soluble than nitrogen in the blood, it enters these spaces faster than the blood can transport nitrogen out. As a result, these pockets of trapped gas expand. Trapped gas is common in a blocked middle ear, pneumothorax, loops of twisted intestine, renal cysts, and the skull after a pneumoencephalogram. These conditions or procedures are contraindications to nitrous oxide use because the large increases in pressure or volume that may result after administration may cause serious damage. Nitrous oxide has also been linked to an increased incidence of spontaneous abortions in women—and decreased spermatogenesis in men—who work in operating rooms. Scavenging equipment must now be used in the operating room to remove nitrous oxide.

Although inhaled anesthetics are all considered CNS depressants, enflurane is unusual in its potential to produce seizure activity at high doses.

Desflurane is highly irritating to the respiratory tract in awake patients. Therefore an intravenous drug is almost always used for induction when desflurane is to be employed for anesthesia maintenance.

Shivering is a common reaction during recovery. It is the body's response to heat loss and to the recovery of neurologic functions.

TOXICITY

In a small percentage of susceptible patients, halothane may cause hepatotoxicity, which may progress to fatal hepatic failure in about half of these. **Malignant hyperthermia** is a rare toxic reaction to inhaled anesthetics, often in combination with the neuromuscular blocker succinylcholine (see below), and occurs in genetically susceptible patients (Box 16-1).

INTERACTIONS

Many drugs increase the effect of inhaled anesthetics and thus lower the dose (or concentration) necessary to achieve the desired level of anesthesia. Such drugs include opiate analgesics and CNS depressants. Although inhaled anesthetics alone tend to produce only slight depression of neuromuscular transmission, the halogenated gases isoflurane and enflurane may significantly enhance the neuromuscular blockade produced by nondepolarizing neuromuscular blockers (see later below).

Halothane sensitizes the myocardium to exogenously administered catecholamines, which may result in arrhythmias. This effect is also seen to a lesser extent with enflurane and isoflurane. Sensitization means that a sympathomimetic drug must be used cautiously during surgery to maintain blood pressure. Catecholamines may be used topically, such as on the brain or in irrigation of the bladder to stop local bleeding.

| BOX 16-1 | Patient Problem: Malignant Hyperthermia |

The Problem

Malignant hyperthermia (MH) is a rare but potentially fatal autosomal dominant syndrome often initiated by a pharmacologic trigger, usually succinylcholine, although it may be brought on by suxamethonium and halothane as well. The incidence rate is estimated to be 1 in every 15,000 pediatric surgical cases and 1 in every 50,000 adult surgical cases. It occurs more often in male patients and in patients with muscular disorders such as Duchenne's muscular dystrophy. At one time, the mortality rate from MH was 70%, but this has now decreased to 10% with early recognition and treatment. This syndrome is believed to result from decreased calcium reuptake by the sarcoplasmic reticulum with an increased resting intracellular calcium level.

Signs and Symptoms

MH usually develops within 30 minutes after induction of anesthesia. Tachycardia is one of the first signs; other early symptoms include increased expired carbon dioxide concentration, hypoxemia, acidosis, tachypnea, cyanosis, hyperkalemia, unstable blood pressure, and myoglobinuria. Muscle rigidity is usually seen in the masseter muscles of the jaw but may occur in the chest or extremities. Elevation of body temperature is usually a late sign and results from a hypermetabolic state of the skeletal muscle. Body temperature elevation results in an oxygen consumption of two to three times the normal rate. If MH is not treated, the temperature may rise as high as 109° to 111° F (42.8° to 44° C). The patient develops a rosy, flushed appearance because of the increased metabolism. The heat produced by the increased metabolism causes vasodilation, such that the skin may become mottled or cyanotic. Blood pressure may fall, and the serum potassium level may rise. Premature ventricular contractions and ventricular tachycardia are reflected on the ECG.

The Solution

Malignant hyperthermia can be prevented in many patients and should be treated aggressively if it develops.

Prophylaxis

Patients known to be susceptible to MH should receive dantrolene intravenously 15 to 30 minutes before induction of anesthesia. A vapor-free anesthesia machine should be used and the patient should be fully monitored, including temperature and carbon dioxide level. Nontriggering anesthetics should be used. Safe drugs that may be used include nitrous oxide, barbiturates, opioids, benzodiazepines, amide and ester local anesthetics, and nondepolarizing muscle relaxants.

Teach patients who develop MH to wear a medical alert bracelet or necklace and to inform all health care providers that this syndrome has occurred.

Treatment

Treatment of MH includes immediately discontinuing anesthesia and changing the anesthetic gas circuit. The patient is then hyperventilated with 100% oxygen and given dantrolene intravenously (see Chapter 21). Cooling measures (surface, nasogastric, rectal) are instituted and correction of acid-base imbalances (e.g., sodium bicarbonate) is begun.

DRUG CLASS • Intravenous Anesthetics

Barbiturates

methohexital (Brevital)

thiopental (Pentothal)

Benzodiazepines

diazepam (Valium)

midazolam (Versed)

Opioids

alfentanil (Alfenta)

fentanyl (Sublimaze)

remifentanil (Ultiva)

sufentanil (Sufenta)

Others

droperidol (Inapsine)

etomidate (Amidate)

ketamine (Ketalar)

propofol (Diprivan)

MECHANISM OF ACTION

All of these drugs except for ketamine and the opioids are thought to produce an anesthetic-like state primarily by increasing the effect of GABA. Since GABA is important in so many brain mechanisms, these drugs have the potential to depress vital functions controlled by the brain, such as maintenance of respiration and blood pressure. Ketamine works by interfering with the action of glutamate, which acts as an excitatory neurotransmitter, at one of its receptors called the NMDA receptor. Ketamine is probably the only one of these drugs that can be considered a true anesthetic, although the specific state it induces, called **dissociative anesthesia,** differs from that produced by other anesthetic drugs. Muscle tone remains high and spontaneous movement is possible. The patient's eyes may be open, and he or she may actually appear to be conscious. Respiration is rarely depressed and arterial pressure may even be elevated. Although mechanisms involving GABA and glutamate seem to be the primary targets for these drugs, other actions may contribute to their effects as well.

Opioids (discussed in Chapter 13) act by stimulating receptors for opiates and opioid peptides in the CNS. They can provoke profound analgesia but are not actually anesthetic drugs. Droperidol is a dopamine receptor antagonist with neither anesthetic nor analgesic properties (see Chapter 19). These drugs are therefore used only in combination with other drugs when anesthesia is desired (see below).

USES

The primary use for these drugs is in the induction of the anesthetic state, usually in short surgical procedures or where inhaled anesthetics will be employed for maintenance. Most cause loss of consciousness within seconds of intravenous administration, but the duration of this action after this route of administration is relatively brief, typically lasting no more than 15 to 30 minutes. Even during this period of unconsciousness, most of these drugs do not abolish reflex reaction to pain and so are not true anesthetics. Therefore they can only be used as the principal anesthetic drug for brief surgical procedures that do not involve very painful stimulation.

Diazepam and midazolam are benzodiazepines, an important class of CNS drugs used as antianxiety and sedative-hypnotic drugs (i.e., drugs that have a calming effect and produce sleep—see Chapter 17), and in the treatment of epilepsy (see Chapter 22). In a surgical setting, these drugs are normally given intravenously to produce conscious sedation for induction but may be given intramuscularly for this purpose as well. More commonly, diazepam and midazolam are used to produce strong sedation in patients undergoing cardioversion or endoscopic, diagnostic, or dental procedures, often along with opioid analgesics. Sedation, sleep, and amnesia are achieved with little depression of cardiovascular or respiratory functions.

Deeper sedation is achieved with thiopental and the other barbiturates, ketamine, etomidate, propofol, and intravenous opioids. The patient is in a controlled state of decreased consciousness and is not easily aroused.

There is a loss of protective reflexes, an inability to maintain an open airway, and lack of response to surgical stimuli. Because etomidate does not produce analgesia, the short-acting narcotic-analgesic fentanyl citrate also may be infused for total intravenous anesthesia. Other barbiturates are used as sedative-hypnotics (see Chapter 17) and in the treatment of convulsions (see Chapter 22).

Ketamine, unlike the other drugs described above, is a true anesthetic and produces a cataleptic state in which the patient appears to be awake but neither responds to pain nor remembers the procedure. Ketamine, which can be given intravenously or intramuscularly, is sometimes used as the primary anesthetic drug for short procedures where skeletal muscle relaxation is not indicated or desired.

Droperidol and the opiates are often used in combinations with the drugs discussed above to produce general anesthesia or states that are particularly suitable for specific types of procedures. For example, balanced anesthesia refers to the combination of an opioid, nitrous oxide, and a skeletal muscle relaxant for surgical anesthesia. **Neurolept anesthesia** refers to the combination of droperidol (an antipsychotic drug of the butyrophenone class), an opioid (usually fentanyl), and nitrous oxide sufficient to cause unconsciousness and suppression of the reaction to what would otherwise be painful stimuli. A skeletal muscle relaxant may also be used if needed. Neurolept anesthesia is useful for older and high-risk patients and for bronchoscopy and carotid arteriography. A fixed combination of the opioid fentanyl and droperidol is available as Innovar. **Neurolept analgesia** refers to the combination of fentanyl and droperidol without nitrous oxide to produce a quiet state with reduced motor activity, reduced anxiety, and indifference to the surroundings. Procedures such as endoscopy, radiologic studies, and changing burn dressings can be carried out with the patient in this state.

PHARMACOKINETICS

When given intravenously, most of these drugs produce effects within seconds because (1) the brain has a very high blood flow, so a drug placed directly in the bloodstream will go first to the brain in high concentration, and (2) these drugs are very lipophilic, so they easily cross the blood-brain barrier and enter the CNS. The effect lasts only 5 to 15 minutes for most drugs under these circumstances. However, this brief duration of action is not because the drug is eliminated from the body; rather, the drug has redistributed out of the brain as it equilibrates with less highly perfused tissues, such as muscle, fat, and bone. This redistribution lowers the circulating concentration and so the concentration in the brain drops to a level that no longer maintains anesthesia.

Eventually, most of these drugs are biotransformed and thus inactivated as they pass through the liver. In contrast, diazepam produces active metabolites and has a long duration of action in systemic circulation (see Chapter 17).

ADVERSE REACTIONS AND CONTRAINDICATIONS

Barbiturates provide no analgesia per se and can cause excitement or delirium in the presence of pain in an awake patient. Changes in blood pressure or cardiac output are uncommon after intravenous administration of anesthetic doses of barbiturates unless the injection is made rapidly. However, barbiturates can markedly depress respiration, and yawning, coughing, or laryngospasm may also occur. Methohexital may cause hiccups. Solutions of barbiturates should be injected only into veins. Arterial injections can cause inflammation and clotting. The barbiturate solution damages tissue if it leaks around the injection site, a situation which can lead to gangrene.

Compared with barbiturates, benzodiazepines are less likely to cause cardiovascular or respiratory depression, but midazolam in particular should still be administered intravenously only where these functions can be monitored. Propofol is as likely as barbiturates to cause cardiovascular or respiratory depression. Etomidate produces minimum cardiovascular or respiratory changes but may provoke transient, myoclonic skeletal muscle movements.

Ketamine enhances muscle tone and increases blood pressure, heart rate, and respiratory secretions. A major adverse effect is seen in the recovery period. Here ketamine, which is chemically related to the illicit hallucinogen phencyclidine (PCP), may provoke vivid, unpleasant dreams or hallucinations. Adults are more prone than children to these experiences. Ketamine may also cause vomiting and shivering. This drug should be used cautiously in patients with seizure disorders, psychosis, or mild hypertension or in those who are undergoing eye surgery. It is generally contraindicated for patients in whom an increase in blood pressure or sympathetic activity could be dangerous, such as those with a history of coronary artery disease, severe hypertension, cerebrovascular accident (stroke), or hyperthyroidism.

Adverse effects of neurolept analgesia or anesthesia are hypotension, bradycardia, and respiratory depression. The action of droperidol persists for 3 to 6 hours, whereas the analgesic effect of fentanyl lasts for only 30 minutes. About 1% of patients who receive droperidol may have extrapyramidal muscle movements (see Chapter 19) for as long as 12 hours after administration. These movements may be controlled by administration of atropine or benztropine.

Effects of opioids are discussed at length in Chapter 13; recall that they are potent respiratory depressants.

INTERACTIONS

The CNS depression produced by any of these drugs is greatly enhanced by other CNS depressants and may result in excessive respiratory and cardiovascular depression. Severe hypotension may also result from anesthetic doses of barbiturates in patients taking antihypertensive drugs, including clonidine, guanabenz, methyldopa, and reserpine (see Chapter 41).

PHYSIOLOGY • Neuromuscular Transmission

Acetylcholine released from motor nerve endings stimulates nicotinic receptors (see Chapter 11) on the muscle cell to briefly depolarize the muscle membrane. This depolarization triggers the opening of voltage-gated (or fast) sodium channels in the membrane to cause an action potential that spreads through the muscle and produces contraction. The released acetylcholine that initiated this event is rapidly destroyed by acetylcholinesterase, allowing the muscle membrane to repolarize between nerve impulses. This repolarization is necessary so that the fast sodium channels can reset and be ready to open again before the next pulse of acetylcholine is released from the nerve. In this way, the process can be repeated again and again, many times in a second, resulting in sustained muscular contraction and movement.

DRUG CLASS • Neuromuscular Blockers

Nondepolarizing

atracurium (Tracrium)

cisatracurium (Nimbex)

doxacurium (Nuromax)

mivacurium (Mivacron)

pancuronium (Pavulon)

pipecuronium (Arduan)

rocuronium (Zemuron)

⚠ **D-tubocurarine (Turbarine✲)**

vecuronium (Norcuron)

Depolarizing

succinylcholine (Anectine, Quelicin, Sucostrin)

MECHANISM OF ACTION

Neuromuscular-blocking drugs occupy the nicotinic receptors for acetylcholine on muscles. All these drugs except succinylcholine act principally as competitive antagonists at these receptors, thus preventing muscle contraction in response to motor nerve activity. These are called **nondepolarizing neuromuscular blockers.**

Succinylcholine actually stimulates these receptors much as acetylcholine does. However, unlike acetylcholine, succinylcholine is not instantly destroyed by acetylcholinesterase. As a result, it remains bound to the receptor, which it continues to stimulate. The membrane does not repolarize between nerve impulses, and fast sodium channels cannot reset to open again, meaning that no further action potentials are possible. Therefore the typical response to an injection of succinylcholine is a transient wave of initial muscle twitching followed by relaxation and neuromuscular paralysis. This kind of blockade of the neuromuscular junction is called a depolarizing blockade and succinylcholine is a **depolarizing neuromuscular blocker.**

The muscles of the body are affected in a characteristic order after administration of neuromuscular blockers. The first muscles affected are those of fine movement—eyes and face, fingers, and larynx—followed by muscles of the limbs and then the trunk. The last muscles to relax are the muscles of respiration—the diaphragm and the intercostals. Recovery occurs in the reverse order, so that spontaneous respiration recovers first.

USES

Neuromuscular-blocking drugs provide muscle relaxation, particularly of the abdominal muscles, during surgery. By preventing movement that would normally result from sensory stimulation associated with surgical procedures, neuromuscular blockers also permit the use of a lower concentration of inhaled anesthetic, thereby reducing cardiovascular depression. Neuromuscular blockers are also used with light anesthesia to allow a tube to be passed down easily to the trachea (endotracheal intubation), to relieve spasm of the larynx, to prevent convulsive muscle spasms during electroconvulsive therapy for depression, and to allow breathing to be controlled totally by a respirator (i.e., controlled ventilation) during surgery. Skeletal muscle relaxants do not inhibit pain or provide amnesia and so are never used alone in surgery.

Because these drugs paralyze the muscles responsible for ventilation (i.e., the diaphragm and intercostal muscles), assisted ventilation is mandatory when administering nondepolarizing neuromuscular blockers. Assisted ventilation should always be available when succinylcholine is used but may not always be necessary because of its short duration of action (see below).

PHARMACOKINETICS

A paralyzed patient must remain on artificial ventilation as long as a neuromuscular blocker is effective. By comparison with many other drugs, neuromuscular blockers all have relatively short durations of action (3 hours or less). However, newer drugs with shorter times to onset and durations of action have proven to be more useful and convenient in many settings.

D-tubocurarine (the prototype nondepolarizing neuromuscular blocker), doxacurium, pancuronium, pipecuronium, and vecuronium are considered to have long durations of action (up to 2 hours) and are eliminated mostly by renal clearance (D-tubocurarine, doxacurium, and pancuronium) or by a combination of renal clearance and hepatic biotransformation (pipecuronium and vecuronium).

Other nondepolarizing neuromuscular blockers are eliminated by more efficient means and therefore have shorter durations of action. Atracurium, cisatracurium, and rocuronium have intermediate durations of action (up to about an hour). Atracurium and cisatracurium break down spontaneously in the body but are also eliminated in part by the kidney and destroyed enzymatically by cholinesterases in the plasma. Rocuronium is biotransformed primarily in the liver. Mivacurium, the shortest-acting nondepolarizing blocker, is rapidly degraded by cholinesterases in the blood and therefore produces paralysis that lasts only about 15 minutes.

Succinylcholine, the only depolarizing blocker in current use, has the shortest duration of action, producing effects within 1 minute of infusion and typically lasting 5 to 7 minutes. This drug owes its short half-life to its rapid degradation by plasma cholinesterases.

ADVERSE REACTIONS AND CONTRAINDICATIONS

Many nondepolarizing neuromuscular blockers can produce significant cardiovascular effects. These effects result from two different mechanisms. First, some drugs can trigger the release of histamine from mast cells. The released histamine can lower blood pressure markedly and may also cause troublesome bronchoconstriction in some patients. D-tubocurarine is the most likely to cause histamine release, followed by atracurium and mivacurium; other nondepolarizing blockers rarely provoke this effect.

The second way nondepolarizing blockers may alter cardiovascular function is by acting at other cholinergic receptors found in the parasympathetic nervous system. D-tubocurarine and high doses of atracurium may cause a partial block at nicotinic receptors, resulting in a fall in blood pressure. Atracurium and pancuronium may also increase heart rate by blocking muscarinic cholinergic receptors. This blockade removes the vagal tone that normally serves as a brake on heart rate.

The depolarizing drug succinylcholine may cause different adverse reactions. Its ability to stimulate cholinergic receptors provokes a brief period of muscular contraction and twitching before relaxation, and patients often complain of muscle soreness after treatment. When a nicotinic receptor is stimulated it becomes an open ion channel through which sodium and potassium can move, and potassium is always at high concentration inside cells and at low levels in the extracellular space. Because succinylcholine causes a sustained opening of these channels, large shifts of potassium occur from inside any cells where nicotinic receptors are located to the exterior. In certain patients (e.g., burn patients, patients with extensive soft tissue damage, or quadriplegics) this shift may be sufficient to produce **hyperkalemia**, resulting in life-threatening effects on the heart.

Succinylcholine may cause stimulation of nicotinic receptors at autonomic ganglia, resulting in bradycardia, tachycardia, or hypertension in some patients. A few patients are genetically deficient in plasma cholinesterase activity. In these patients, the usual dose of succinylcholine may produce extremely prolonged neuromuscular paralysis and apnea. Succinylcholine also transiently raises intraocular pressure. Succinylcholine is no longer used in children younger than 8 years.

TOXICITY

In patients with a rare genetic susceptibility, succinylcholine may trigger a life-threatening condition called malignant hyperthermia (see Box 16-1).

INTERACTIONS

A wide variety of drugs can influence the intensity and duration of the neuromuscular blockers. Many drugs that possess neuromuscular blocking activity too weak to be of clinical significance on their own may potentiate or prolong the neuromuscular blockade produced by nondepolarizing drugs. Such drugs include certain anesthetics (especially halothane and enflurane), antibiotics (e.g., aminoglycosides and clindamycin), antiarrhythmic drugs (e.g., quinidine), ganglionic blockers, and magnesium sulfate.

Cholinesterase inhibitors are used to help reverse the blockade caused by nondepolarizing drugs. Because cholinesterase inhibitors inhibit the enzyme responsible for the rapid destruction of acetylcholine, the concentration of acetylcholine increases in the vicinity of the nicotinic receptors at the neuromuscular junction. This higher concentration can better compete with the blockers for receptor sites and thus accelerate the recovery of effective neuromuscular transmission.

In contrast to their antagonism of the effect of nondepolarizing drugs, cholinesterase inhibitors may actually intensify the paralysis caused by succinylcholine, because in this instance the receptors are already being overstimulated.

APPLICATION TO PRACTICE

ASSESSMENT
History of Present Illness

Many variables influence the patient's physiologic and psychologic response to anesthetics and subsequent outcomes. Elicit from the patient information about his or her physical and mental state, the extent of disease and comorbid disorders, the magnitude of the specific procedure, and any preoperative psychologic and physiologic preparations. Identify the patient's behavioral responses to the upcoming surgery or procedure and the use of anesthesia. Recognize that anger, depression, and grief are protective mechanisms and are not signs of maladaptive coping. When these variables are considered collectively, they reveal the degree of surgical risk and can help predict how the patient will cope during the postoperative period.

Information regarding the patient's last food and fluid intake should be noted. This information is needed to assess the risk of aspiration of gastric contents during surgery and subsequent pneumonitis.

Health History

Specific information about comorbid conditions, past surgical and anesthetic history, and particularly information about family history of malignant hyperthermia should be elicited. Note whether the patient has any history of asthma, cardiovascular, hepatic, or liver disease, as well as any previous anesthesia problems in the patient or in family members. Serious neurologic conditions, such as uncontrolled epilepsy or severe Parkinson's disease, increase surgical risk and should be identified. In some cases, a menstrual and obstetric history should be included with the general review of systems. Question the patient carefully about smoking habits and alcohol use.

Information about current drug use is important because of the concern for drug interactions. For example, certain antibiotics used in combination with some muscle relaxants increase the risk of postoperative respiratory depression. Antianxiety drugs lower blood pressure, increasing the risk of shock. They also potentiate the effects of opioids and barbiturates. Thiazide diuretics contribute to potassium depletion and increase the risk for arrhythmia. Chronic corticosteroid use may impair adrenal cortex function, thus impairing physiologic response to the stress of anesthesia and surgery. Antidepressants such as monoamine oxidase inhibitors can cause hypertensive crisis when combined with anesthetics. Anti-parkinson drugs may cause hypotension or hypertension when combined with anesthetics. Remember that when patients refer to any local anesthetic, regardless of the specific drug, they often call it Novocaine.

Lifespan Considerations

Perinatal. Modern obstetrics employs both analgesics and anesthetics for pain relief. Explore various strategies for diminishing or managing the pain of labor and birth, so that informed choices can be made regarding the pain relief measures desired. There are three strategies for pain management for a woman in labor: (1) systemic drugs (e.g., barbiturates, antianxiety drugs, opioids, opioid agonist-antagonists) primarily for use during the first stage of labor; (2) regional anesthesia for use during first-stage labor (e.g., paracervical block, epidural, intrathecal injections) and second-stage labor (e.g., local infiltration, pudendal or spinal block); and (3) general anesthesia for use during second-stage labor. General anesthesia is rarely used for a normal vaginal delivery; it is reserved for emergency vaginal or cesarean birth. There are advantages and disadvantages to each type of anesthesia. Adequate assessment of previous experience with the various types helps the anesthesia provider determine the most effective method and drug to use.

Pediatric. Determine preoperatively if the family is intact. Children who have lost one or both parents may not have accepted the loss. Problems could arise on emergence from anesthesia for the child who is greeted with, for example, "Do you want to see your mom now?"

Children between 12 months and 3 years of age fear separation from parents. Children 3 to 7 years old often act out their fears through anxiety, hostility, or aggression. Children 7 to 11 years old are in their so-called quiet years; they often think good behavior will get them back to their parents sooner (i.e., they do not cry, even when in pain). After 3 years of age, children understand separation is temporary. Adolescents may exaggerate pain when pain is not always the problem. Fear and lack of control of the situation is usually the root of the problem. Keep questions and explanations to the point and at a simple level. Children and adolescents who ask questions usually need simple, honest, direct answers.

Children are not small adults. Physiologic differences between an adult and a child require special considerations. The larynx is at the C_3-C_4 level in an infant but at the C_4-C_5 level in an adult. The cross-sectional diameter of a child's larynx is 4 mm, whereas an adult's larynx is 8 mm. The epiglottis is short, narrow, stiff, and U-shaped in an infant; it is flexible and flat in an adult. The trachea is 22 to 29 cm long in a child but 74 to 76 cm long in adults. An infant's neck is very short, almost nonexistent, and intercostal muscles are poorly developed. The differences to be considered when evaluating the child include attention to respiratory effort and functional reserve, facial size and structure for use of an appropriately sized mask, and hepatic capacity for biotransformation.

Older Adults. There are minimal physiologic alterations with the use of regional anesthetics in the older adult. This method of delivery permits rapid recovery and postoperative analgesia. It also reduces the risk of cardiovascular complications and postoperative confusion. Be sure to evaluate the mental status of the patient so that a baseline is identified on the chart. The effects of spinal anesthesia are prolonged in the older adult, and hypotension may be pronounced. In contrast, epidural anesthesia has less impact on blood pressure and cardiovascular status. However, musculoskeletal changes associated with aging may make administration of spinal or epidural anesthesia difficult.

General anesthesia permits smooth induction and rapid recovery in the older adult. However, drug biotransformation and clearance are delayed, requiring lower doses of barbiturates, benzodiazepines, and opioids. Moreover, the older adult is at risk for hypothermia from age-related decrease in body fat. It can be difficult to ventilate an edentulous patient, and arthritis may restrict the cervical spine region and inhibit intubation.

Cultural/Social Considerations

Surgery and anesthesia are psychologic as well as physical stressors. Psychologic responses to stress include anticipation of actual or perceived harm. The intensity of the perception is related to the amount, imminence, and probability of the threat. Anxiety is a response to a nonspecific threat, such as the outcome of surgery or the diagnosis, whereas fear is related to an identifiable and definable threat, such as the operation itself, loss of control, or not waking from anesthesia. Physical threats to self-image include the loss of a body part, change in functional ability or appearance, the visibility of the change to self and significant others, physiologic effects of surgery, and pain. Threats to psychosocial image include changes in roles (e.g., breadwinner, care provider), dependence versus independence, perception of powerlessness, loss of control or insecurity, fear of death (especially with cardiac, major, or emergency surgery), perception of loss, and aging.

With the increased national attention on health care and health care costs, anesthesia providers are becoming more conscious of their choice of anesthetic techniques and drugs. Even so, adequate evaluation of the patient's physical, psychologic, cultural, and social state is important. Compared with general anesthesia, the use of regional or local anesthesia generally results in significant savings in hospital costs, partly because of shorter hospital stays and reduced need for intensive care.

Physical Examination

A physical examination is performed before the scheduled procedure. Upon arrival for the procedure, the nurse should obtain the patient's height and weight, auscultate the heart and breath sounds, measure the blood pressure, peripheral pulses, and evaluate venous access sites. Also included is an assessment for neurologic dysfunction, movement limitations, dentition, temporomandibular joint movement, airway patency, and range of motion of the neck.

Laboratory Testing

Laboratory tests are ordered based on the proposed surgical procedure as well as on the findings of the history and physical examination. Although fewer laboratory tests are performed today than in the past, the tests performed are for specific indications. For example, a prothrombin time (PT) and partial thromboplastin time (PTT) are often performed to check the patient's coagulation status. Baseline blood gases, pulmonary function studies, and a chest x-ray examination may be obtained to evaluate cardiopulmonary function. Urinalysis and renal function tests help determine the ability of the kidneys to eliminate urea, protein wastes, and drugs. Thyroid studies may be performed to evaluate the presence of hyperthyroidism or hypothyroidism. Hyperthyroidism can lead to thyroid crisis with hypertension, tachycardia, and hyperthermia; therefore the condition should be treated medically before surgery. Similarly, hypothyroidism increases the risk of hypotension and cardiac arrest during anesthesia.

GOALS OF THERAPY

The goals of anesthesia center around anxiety relief, sedation, amnesia, analgesia, little or no emesis, aspiration prophylaxis, reduction of oral secretions, facilitation of induction, and reduction of anesthesia requirements. To achieve these goals, the decision of which anesthetic to use is made largely by the anesthesia provider in consultation with the patient and surgeon and includes consideration of the following variables:

- Age of the patient, level of anxiety, and general physical condition
- Drug allergies and the presence of comorbid disease
- Patient preference (e.g., spinal versus general anesthesia)

- Patient history of previous adverse responses to anesthesia
- Magnitude of specific surgical procedure and its duration
- Technical intricacies of the procedure
- Outpatient or inpatient status
- Anesthesia provider preference

INTERVENTION
Administration

General Anesthesia. Techniques of general anesthesia administration are beyond the scope of this book. However, the preoperative use of antianxiety, analgesic, and other drugs is an integral part of planned anesthesia. Administer them as ordered and on time.

After surgery, monitor blood pressure, temperature, pulse, respiration, and oxygen saturation (pulse oximetry) frequently. With the exception of temperature, this monitoring may have to be every 5 minutes initially, progressing to every 15 minutes, then every 30 minutes or more. Auscultate breath sounds and check neurologic status. Do not leave the patient unattended unless the patient can call for assistance and can handle oral and respiratory secretions safely. Position the patient on the side initially, if possible, to prevent aspiration if vomiting should occur. Keep a suction machine at the bedside and keep the siderails up.

Evaluate the patient's pain during the immediate postoperative period (the first 2 to 4 hours after surgery). Factors to consider include the surgical site, vital signs, age, weight, level of consciousness, anesthetic(s) used, and whether analgesics were administered during surgery. The initial dose of analgesics may be one-half to one-fourth the ordered dose, but make reductions in dose only after consultation with the health care provider. Begin nursing measures to prevent atelectasis and pneumonia as soon as the patient is able. This may include turning and deep breathing, coughing, and early ambulation.

Ketamine is associated with unpleasant dreams, emergence delirium, irrational behavior, disorientation, and hallucinations. These adverse effects may be lessened by providing the patient with a quiet wake-up period, perhaps in the quietest corner of the postanesthesia recovery room. Avoid excessive stimulation, although vital signs must be monitored. If psychologic effects occur, provide calm reassurance and reorientation. Do not leave the patient unattended. Once the patient is returned to his or her room, keep it dimly lit and keep noise and stimulation to a minimum. Inform family members of the probable cause of the behavior and enlist their aid in patient reorientation and reassurance. Vivid dreams and hallucinations usually disappear upon waking, but some patients may experience flashbacks for up to several weeks after surgery.

The effects of anesthesia persist even after the patient appears alert and awake. When teaching about postoperative activity, diet, or drugs, as in the outpatient or day-surgery setting, do so verbally and in writing to the patient and have at least one family member present. Do not permit patients in the outpatient setting to drive themselves home if they have received general anesthesia, intravenous barbiturates or benzodiazepines, or any drug that may alter response time or level of consciousness.

Local or Regional Anesthesia. A patient receiving local anesthesia may be drowsy from preoperative drugs but will usually be alert and able to understand conversation in the room. Keep conversation and noise to a minimum. Avoid discussing other patients, complications, pathology reports, or other topics that might alarm the patient.

Monitor blood pressure, pulse, and respiration. If anesthesia is used during labor and delivery, assess fetal heart tones. Assess for the ability to void or for a distended bladder. Assist these patients when ambulating for the first time. Monitor intake and output. If the patient has not voided in 8 hours after surgery or delivery, notify the health care provider.

Position the patient carefully in bed because the patient who has received anesthesia of the lower extremities has no sensation to warn of wrinkles, tight sheets, or other skin irritants. If applying heat or cold is necessary, shield the skin well from the heat or cold source, and check the patient and skin surfaces every 5 to 15 minutes. This applies after oral and dental anesthesia as well.

Keep the patient who has received spinal anesthesia flat for 12 hours to prevent headache. Transfer the patient flat from the stretcher to the bed. Use a thin pillow.

After injection of anesthetics into tongue, lips, and gums, or after topical application of liquid, lozenges, or other drugs causing numbness to the throat or mouth, caution the patient to avoid eating or chewing until sensation returns to avoid biting the tongue or cheek and to avoid choking.

After bronchoscopy or other procedures in which surface anesthesia may have been applied to the back of the throat, assess the gag reflex and ability to swallow. Do not leave the patient unattended until the patient can safely handle oral and respiratory secretions.

Application of excessive amounts of local anesthetics to mucosal surfaces is the most common cause of systemic toxicity with these drugs. Therefore the lowest concentration possible of the local anesthetic should be used on mucosal surfaces to avoid systemic toxicity, and the total amount of drug should be recorded and matched against recommended total doses.

Although serious systemic reactions are rare with local anesthetics, have drugs, equipment, and personnel available to treat acute allergic reactions in settings where these drugs are used. Tell the patient to report any rash or skin irritation occurring as a result of application of a local anesthetic.

Education

To prepare for surgery, inform the patient and family about the surgical procedure and what to expect afterward. Have the patient give a return demonstration of any exercises or activities required, such as coughing and deep breathing. Provide the patient with an opportunity to ask questions of the anesthesia provider. Schedule a visit to the intensive care unit, if appropriate. Provide emotional support.

The patient scheduled for any procedure requiring local, regional, or general anesthesia must give informed consent before the procedure can be performed. The patient or legal guardian must be informed about potential risks, complications, and anesthesia alternatives. The expected outcome and the likelihood that the chosen anesthetic will be effective should also be addressed.

The procedure for obtaining signed consent varies from state to state and according to the policy of the health care agency. Emancipated minors (children who are younger than 18 but because of marriage or other circumstances are independent of the family) may give consent. Children under the legal age (18 in most states) who are not emancipated must have consent from their parents or legal guardian. In some cases, a court order may be needed to permit anesthesia and surgery to take place.

Reassure patients receiving anesthesia that they will be continually monitored until the effects of the drugs have dissipated. They will be kept warm and have their blood pressure, heart rate, oxygenation status, and comfort level monitored.

Advise patients who receive regional or local anesthesia that the sensation and movement in the area will return once the effects of the drug have worn off. Before discharge, review any limitations the patient may have until the effects of the anesthetic wear off. For example, a patient who has had local anesthesia to a joint should be instructed to avoid use of the joint for a certain number of hours. Instruct the patient to use surface anesthetics as instructed and not to increase the frequency of application or to use the preparation on skin surfaces for which it was not designed.

Instruct the patient using anesthetic dental paste to follow the manufacturer's instructions. Use an applicator to apply small amounts to the tender areas, and do not rub with fingers while applying, because the drug will crumble.

Instruct the patient to allow an anesthetic lozenge to dissolve in the mouth and not to bite, chew, or swallow them whole. Warn the family to make certain the child understands how to use a lozenge correctly before giving it to him or her.

Advise the patient using a benzocaine film-forming gel to dry the area with a swab where the drug is to be applied, apply the gel to a second swab, then roll the gel over the specified area. Instruct the patient to try to keep the mouth open and dry for 30 to 60 seconds after applying the gel. It will form a film that should not be removed and will slowly disappear over several hours.

For anesthetic creams or ointments that are to be inserted into the rectum, instruct the patient to use applicators provided by the manufacturer and to be careful not to insert the cap into the rectum. For rectal aerosol form, instruct the patient not to insert the container itself into the rectum but to use the applicator provided by the manufacturer. For topical forms applied to the anal area, clean the area with soap and water or a cleansing wipe, and then dry the area. Use a tissue, gauze, glove, or finger cot to apply a small amount of drug to the area.

EVALUATION

All anesthetics require time to wear off, and specific evaluation depends on the anesthesia used. For example, if the throat has been anesthetized for bronchoscopy, the ability to swallow without coughing or choking indicates resolution of the anesthesia. If the patient has had regional anesthesia, the return of movement and sensation indicates a return to normal function. If the patient has had general anesthesia, anxiety was reduced; sedation, amnesia, and analgesia were successful; there was little or no emesis or aspiration; and the requirement for anesthesia was reduced as much as possible.

Bibliography

Arbour R: Mastering neuromuscular blockade, *Dimens Crit Care Nurs* 19(5):4-16, 2000.

Arsenault C: Nurse's guide to general anesthesia, part I, *Nursing* 28(Suppl 3):32cc1-2, 32cc4, 32cc6, 1998.

Cox F: Clinical care of patients with epidural infusions, *Prof Nurse* 16(10):1429-1432, 2001.

Earl G, McMahon MB, Bartley M, et al: Development of a policy for patients receiving neuromuscular blocking agents, *J Trauma Nurs* 4(3):76-81, 1997.

Foster JGW, Kish SK, Keenan CH: A national survey of critical care nurses' practices related to administration of neuromuscular blocking agents, *Am J Crit Care* 10(3):139-145, 2001.

Golinski MA: Understanding conscious sedation in the operating room, *Plast Nurs* 18(2):90-95, 1998.

Goodwin SA: Pharmacology: a review of preemptive analgesia, *J Perianesth Nurs* 13(2):109-114, 1998.

Griffiths R: Back to basics: Anaesthetic drugs, *Br J Perioper Nurs* 10(5):276-279, 2000.

Hall J: Epidural analgesia management, *Nurs Times* 96(28):38-40, 2000.

Johnson CN: Intravenous regional anesthesia: new approaches to an old technique, *CRNA* 11(2):57-61, 2000.

Klein SM: Ambulatory anesthesia for the twenty-first century, *Surg Serv Manag* 6(9):45-47, 2000.

Kreger C: Getting to the root of pain: spinal anesthesia and analgesia, *Nursing* 31(6):36-42, 2001.

Maikler VE: Pharmacologic pain management in children: a review of intervention research, *J Pediatr Nurs* 13(1):3-14, 1998.

Malignant hyperthermia: an OR emergency! *Plast Surg Nurs* 20(4):222-226, 2000.

Malviya S, Voepel-Lewis T, Tait AR, et al: Sedation/analgesia for diagnostic and therapeutic procedures in children, *J Perianesth Nurs* 15(6):415-422, 2000.

McAuliffe MS, Hartshorn EA: Anesthetic drug interactions: quarterly update, *CRNA* 11(3):144-149, 2000.

Pasero C: Pain control: continuous local anesthetics, *Am J Nurs* 100(8):22, 2000.

Internet Resources

Anesthesia, Nursing and Medicine. Available online at http://www.anesthesia-nursing.com/.

Global Anesthesia Server Network. Available online at http://gasnet.med.yale.edu/.

The Virtual Anesthesia Textbook. Available online at http://www.virtual-anaesthesia-textbook.com/.

Anesthesia, Critical Care, Emergency. Available online at http://www.invivo.net/bg/index2.html.

CHAPTER

17

Anxiolytic and Sedative-Hypnotic Drugs

JOSEPH A. DiMICCO • KATHLEEN GUTIERREZ

 Visit http://evolve.elsevier.com/Gutierrez/ for additional information.

KEY TERMS

Agoraphobia, p. 248

Anxiety, p. 248

Anxiolytic, p. 249

Enzyme induction, p. 253

GABA-A receptor, p. 250

Generalized anxiety disorder, p. 248

Hypnosis/hypnotics, p. 249

Insomnia, p. 249

Limbic system, p. 250

Metabolic tolerance, p. 253

Non-REM sleep, p. 249

Obsessive-compulsive disorder (OCD), p. 248

Panic disorder, p. 248

Phobia, p. 248

Posttraumatic stress disorder, p. 248

Rapid eye movement (REM) sleep, p. 249

Sedation/sedative, p. 249

Serotonin, p. 249

Status epilepticus, p. 253

OBJECTIVES

- Differentiate among sedatives, hypnotics, and anxiolytic drugs.
- Describe the mechanism of action of benzodiazepines.
- Explain the role of pharmacokinetics in determining the specific uses of benzodiazepines.
- Identify the key differences between the benzodiazepines zaleplon and zolpidem.
- Identify the key differences between benzodiazepines and barbiturates.
- Develop a nursing care plan for patients receiving benzodiazepines, barbiturates, or miscellaneous anxiolytic and sedative-hypnotic drugs.

PATHOPHYSIOLOGY • Anxiety, Sleep, and Their Disorders

The universal human emotion called **anxiety** can arise from many sources. It can be a normal reaction to stress, the adverse effect of a drug or a disease process, or a distinct psychologic condition. Anxiety is experienced along a spectrum of intensity. At one end of the spectrum is mild apprehension, which produces increased awareness and anticipation, such as a runner might experience before a race. At the other extreme, however, anxiety blocks awareness of surroundings, clouds judgment, and can lead to panic with complete disintegration of coping abilities. An anxiety disorder is defined as an illness that prevents an individual from coping and that can disrupt daily life. Although the anxiety arising from the stresses of everyday life usually does not require treatment with drugs, anxiety disorders often merit intervention. Five types of anxiety disorders are recognized.

About 7 million Americans are estimated to have **generalized anxiety disorder.** This disorder persists for 6 months or longer and involves exaggerated worry and tension without a recognized cause. People with this disorder are unable to relax and have trouble falling or staying asleep. They may have physical symptoms such as trembling, twitching, muscle tension, headaches, irritability, sweating, or hot flashes. They are easily startled. They may have to go to the bathroom often or feel nauseated. The overall impairment associated with generalized anxiety disorder is usually mild. People with this disorder do not feel restricted in social situations or in their jobs. The disorder commonly begins in childhood or adolescence. It is more common in women than in men and tends to run in families. The symptoms tend to diminish with age.

An extreme variant of anxiety is seen in **panic disorder,** a sudden episode of terror that happens repeatedly. The panic attack is characterized by chest pain, heart palpitations, shortness of breath, dizziness, feelings of unreality, and fear of dying. These attacks commonly last from 2 to 10 minutes. The person may develop a phobia (see below) based on where the attacks have occurred, for instance in an elevator. Depression and alcoholism are other conditions that may accompany panic disorder. Women are more commonly affected than men, and the condition usually begins in young adults, although it can appear at any age. Many people experience only a single panic attack. It is estimated that between 3 and 6 million Americans have panic disorder. Treatment is recommended for panic disorder when attacks become frequent or disabling.

A **phobia** is any fear magnified to an intense and irrational degree. **Agoraphobia** is an extreme type of panic disorder that occurs in about one third of cases. In agoraphobia the individual fears being in any situation that might provoke a panic attack and may be housebound as a result. Phobias can be very specific so that a certain object or situation is feared, such as flying, confining spaces, specific animals, and water. Specific phobias affect about 1 in 10 persons. Childhood phobias are common and are usually outgrown. Phobias that persist usually begin in adolescence or adulthood and only about 20% disappear with time. Social phobia is a fear of being painfully embarrassed in a social setting. People with a social phobia see themselves as incompetent in public. Fear of public speaking is a common social phobia. Some social phobias involve fear of specific public areas, such as restrooms, restaurants, or public phones. Shyness is not the same as social phobia.

Obsessive-compulsive disorder (OCD) affects about 1 in 50 people and occurs equally in men and women. This disorder is characterized by anxious thoughts and rituals that cannot be controlled. The anxious thoughts include persistent and unwelcome images, and the rituals are driven by an urgent need to perform repetitive acts over and over. Most people have some behavior patterns that are necessary for comfort. However, when rituals become distressing, take 1 hour or more a day, and interfere with daily life, they are viewed as being obsessive-compulsive. OCD usually begins in adolescence or early adulthood, but about one third of cases begin in childhood. The progression of OCD is highly variable. It may increase or decrease over time and can be accompanied by depression or other anxiety disorders.

Posttraumatic stress disorder is a disabling condition that can follow a terrifying event. Memories of the ordeal come flooding back, with persistent frightening thoughts and nightmares, leaving the individual emotionally numb even to loved ones. Events that lead to posttraumatic stress disorder include war, kidnapping, rape or other violent personal attacks, and serious accidents or natural disasters. Any traumatized person will have flashbacks. Individuals who develop posttraumatic stress syndrome experience the symptoms for more than 1 month beginning within 3 months of the trauma. Posttraumatic stress disorder can occur at any age, including in childhood. Between 5 and 6 million Americans are believed to have posttraumatic stress disorder. Persons with this disorder may also abuse alcohol or other substances and be depressed or anxious. Severe symptoms include easy irritability and violent outbursts such that the individual cannot lead a normal social life or hold a job.

If fear, anxiety, and panic are at one end of the scale of physiologic states of arousal for humans, then sleep is at the other end of this scale. Sleep is defined as a period of rest in which physiologic activities and consciousness are diminished and voluntary physical activity is absent. Sleep is a normal physiologic process that is a necessary part of the usual cycle of daily living. Sleep is thought to be the result of decreased activity in the reticular-activating system, a group of neuronal pathways in the brainstem and midbrain where incoming signals from the senses (light, sound, smell, touch, taste, and balance) and viscera are collected, processed, and passed on to higher brain centers. Typically, sleep occupies about 8 hours of a 24-hour day, although persons may differ widely in the normal amount of sleep required. Sunlight is a major factor that sets the biologic clock for sleep.

Normal sleep has two major components: **rapid eye movement (REM) sleep** and **non-REM sleep.** REM sleep is characterized by fast brain waves, eye movements, and metabolic and temperature changes. The body is physiologically active during REM sleep—the heart rate is increased, breathing is irregular, stomach acid is secreted, and the clitoris or penis may become erect. Muscles lose their tone during REM sleep, so only the mind and autonomic nervous system are active during this stage. Because dreaming occurs exclusively during REM sleep, this time is also called *dreaming sleep*. Some believe that during the REM sleep period we integrate emotionally meaningful experiences. Non-REM sleep is subdivided into four stages based on brain wave patterns, with stage 1 being the lightest and stage 4 the deepest sleep. Individuals cycle between REM and non-REM sleep over a 90- to 100-minute period. During the night an individual has about four or five non-REM periods of sleep. Although REM sleep is associated with dreams, night terrors and sleepwalking occur during non-REM sleep. Older persons tend to spend less time in stages 3 and 4 of non-REM sleep, and they are more easily aroused by sounds. Children spend more total time in stages 3 and 4 of non-REM sleep.

Insomnia, the inability to get to sleep or to stay asleep, is the most common sleep complaint. Insomnia is not a disease but rather a symptom of physical or mental distress. Treatment of insomnia involves assessment of physical problems, drugs, and sleep habits. Emotionalism and anxiety are common enemies of sleep and are the most common cause of impaired sleep patterns. People who are depressed often wake early and cannot go back to sleep. Chronic alcoholism, hyperthyroidism, heart or kidney failure, and pregnancy are commonly accompanied by insomnia. Pain of arthritis or muscle aches can make sleep difficult, as can respiratory problems and urinary tract problems. More than half of people over 65 years old have difficulty falling asleep or are excessively sleepy during the day. Many drugs disrupt sleep, including decongestants, beta-blockers, and antihypertensive drugs.

Among the many neural signals involved in regulation of arousal levels, including anxiety and sleep, are the neurotransmitters gamma aminobutyric acid (GABA) (also discussed in Chapter 16 and below) and **serotonin** (5-hydroxytryptamine [5-HT]). Receptors for these substances are found in cell membranes of neurons in regions of the central nervous system (CNS) associated with these functions. Therefore drugs acting at receptors for GABA or serotonin have important effects on anxiety and sleep. **Sedation** refers to a state of calm and reduced activity, and drugs that cause it are called **sedatives.** Sedation is generally accompanied by a relief of anxiety, termed an **anxiolytic** effect. The medical term for sleep is **hypnosis** (not to be confused with the stage-show phenomenon), and drugs that induce or facilitate sleep are called **hypnotics.** Drugs that produce any of these effects are called *sedative-hypnotics*, and those that are used in the treatment of anxiety are called *anxiolytics*.

DRUG CLASS • Benzodiazepines and Related Drugs

alprazolam (Xanax, Apo-Alpraz,✸ Novo-Aprazol,✸ Nu-Alpraz✸)

chlordiazepoxide (Librium, Libritabs, Mitran, Apo-Chlordiazepoxide,✸)

clonazepam (Klonopin, Rivotril✸)

clorazepate (Tranxene, Apo-Clorazepate,✸ GenXENE,✸ Novo-Clopate✸)

⚠diazepam (Valium, Apo-Diazepam,✸ Diazemuls, Vivol✸)

estazolam (Prosom)

halazepam (Paxipam)

lorazepam (Ativan, Apo-Lorazepam,✸ Novo-Lorazem✸)

midazolam (Versed)

oxazepam (Serax, Apo-Oxazepam,✸ Novoxapam,✸ Oxpam,✸ Zapex✸)

quazepam (Doral)

temazepam (Restoril)

triazolam (Halcion, Apo-Triazo,✸ Gen-Triazolam,✸ Novo-Triolam,✸ Nu-Triazol✸)

zaleplon (Sonata)

zolpidem (Ambien)

MECHANISM OF ACTION

The most important receptor for the neurotransmitter GABA is the GABA-A receptor. This receptor is actually a large chemical complex found on all neurons. When GABA binds to its specific binding site on this receptor, the channel opens, allowing chloride ions to rush into the cell. This rush of chloride ions makes the cell membrane more negative (hyperpolarized) and therefore less excitable.

Benzodiazepines have a characteristic chemical structure that increases the inhibitory action of GABA. They do so by binding at their own specific site, the benzodiazepine receptor, on the GABA-A receptor complex. In this way, benzodiazepines strengthen the inhibitory effects of GABA on neurons in the region of the brain that plays a role in fear, anxiety, and arousal. This action results in a calming or sedative effect, and at higher doses, hypnosis or sleep. Benzodiazepines help the patient go to sleep more quickly and stay asleep for a longer time. However, the pattern of sleep they cause is not entirely normal, because more time is spent in non-REM sleep at the expense of REM sleep. The sedation and amnesia produced by benzodiazepines makes two of these drugs (diazepam and midazolam) useful in anesthesia (see Chapter 16).

Areas especially rich in benzodiazepine receptors are the limbic system and related regions of the cerebral cortex. The limbic system is the major integrating system governing emotional behavior associated with self-preservation. The presence of high numbers of receptors for benzodiazepines in this system probably accounts for their anxiolytic action.

Benzodiazepines also act on specific receptors located at other sites in the brain where GABA serves as a neurotransmitter. Because of their effects at these other sites, benzodiazepines are also useful as skeletal muscle relaxants (see Chapter 21) and in the treatment of seizures (see Chapter 22).

Zaleplon and zolpidem, though chemically unlike the benzodiazepines, are thought to act in a similar manner but at different subtypes of benzodiazepine receptors. Zaleplon produces effects very similar to those of the benzodiazepines. Zolpidem, however, appears to act through a different subset of receptors to cause benzodiazepine-like sedation but only weak antiseizure and muscle relaxant effects. In addition, the pattern of sleep induced by zolpidem is more normal than that caused by benzodiazepines because more time is spent in REM sleep.

USES

Benzodiazepines are widely used for both their sedative effects in the treatment of diverse anxiety disorders and for their hypnotic effect in the treatment of insomnia. Whether a particular benzodiazepine is more useful in the treatment of anxiety disorders or insomnia is determined largely by its pharmacokinetics (see below). In either case, however, the drugs do not cure the patient and should be used only for short-term management of either condition. Other uses of benzodiazepines are discussed in Chapter 16 (in anesthesia), Chapter 21 (as skeletal muscle relaxants), and Chapter 22 (in the treatment of seizures).

Zaleplon and zolpidem are used only in the treatment of insomnia and may be superior to benzodiazepines for this purpose. Not only does zolpidem produce a more normal sleep pattern than benzodiazepines, but both drugs are also less likely to produce next-day drowsiness because their durations of action are shorter than even the short-acting benzodiazepines.

PHARMACOKINETICS

As discussed earlier, the pharmacokinetic profile of a given benzodiazepine is the major determinant of its suitability as either an anxiolytic or a hypnotic. For the treatment of insomnia, the ideal drug should produce a rapid hypnotic effect when taken at bedtime without morning drowsiness the next day. Therefore the shorter-acting benzodiazepines (estazolam, flurazepam, quazepam, temazepam, and triazolam) are commonly used as hypnotics.

In contrast to the relatively brief action desirable for the treatment of insomnia, a sustained effect is usually necessary for a drug used to treat anxiety disorders. Many benzodiazepines used as anxiolytics have longer durations of action because they are biotransformed in the liver to active metabolites. In fact, these active metabolites sometimes have longer durations of action than the parent compounds. Benzodiazepines with prolonged action based on active metabolites include chlordiazepoxide, clorazepate, diazepam, halazepam, and prazepam. Lorazepam and oxazepam do not have active metabolites to prolong their duration of action and therefore are preferred for older adults and for patients with liver disease. Alprazolam and the anticonvulsant clonazepam are biotransformed to weakly active compounds.

Benzodiazepines are administered by a variety of routes for different purposes and indications. All are readily absorbed after oral administration, but some can also be given parenterally. Only lorazepam is rapidly and completely absorbed after intramuscular injection. Chlordiazepoxide and diazepam may be administered by intravenous or intramuscular routes, but chlordiazepoxide is not reliably absorbed after intramuscular administration. Benzodiazepines are highly lipid soluble and therefore are widely distributed in body tissues. They are also highly bound to plasma protein, usually greater than 80%. Protein binding is reduced in patients with cirrhosis and renal insufficiency as well as in newborns, and these patients often have impaired biotransformation of benzodiazepines as well, making a reduction in dosage important.

Zaleplon and zolpidem are also readily absorbed, but bioavailability is only about 30% and 70%, respectively, because of first-pass biotransformation by the liver. Both drugs are rapidly cleared from the circulation by a combination of hepatic biotransformation and renal elimination with plasma half-lives less than 3 hours.

ADVERSE REACTIONS AND CONTRAINDICATIONS

Adverse reactions common with benzodiazepines include daytime sedation, ataxia, dizziness, and headaches. Tolerance usually develops to these adverse effects. (Unfortunately, tolerance also develops to the anticonvulsant effect of benzodiazepines as well, limiting their usefulness in the chronic treatment of seizure disorders.) As discussed above, shorter-acting benzodiazepines are preferred in the treatment of insomnia to minimize or avoid drowsiness the next morning. However, the half-life of triazolam (3 hours) may actually be too short; a problem sometimes seen is rebound early-morning insomnia.

Less common adverse effects of benzodiazepines include blurred or double vision, hypotension, tremor, amnesia, slurred speech, urinary incontinence, and constipation.

Older adults are more likely to experience the typical adverse effects of benzodiazepines to a disabling degree. Moreover, older adults do not readily biotransform benzodiazepines, so the drug persists two to three times longer. Therefore the drug dosage should be reduced for older adults and for patients who have impaired liver function. Older adults taking these drugs for sleep or anxiety are at risk for falling and injuring themselves.

A key feature making benzodiazepines particularly advantageous over other sedative-hypnotic drugs is their wide therapeutic index. In contrast to other drugs, benzodiazepines are unlikely to produce notable respiratory depression in patients with normal pulmonary function, even at relatively high doses, unless taken with other CNS depressants. Nevertheless, the respiratory depressant effects of benzodiazepines may become significant in patients with pulmonary disease, making use of these drugs inadvisable for these patients.

Benzodiazepines may produce paradoxical excitement or aggression, especially in patients over 50 who have a history of psychosis. These drugs may worsen glaucoma. Benzodiazepines are associated with an increased incidence of congenital abnormalities in children whose mothers used the drugs during pregnancy. These drugs are excreted in breast milk. Infants do not readily biotransform them and can become lethargic, so benzodiazepines are not recommended for nursing mothers. They are also contraindicated during labor, to avoid excessive CNS depression of the infant.

As with many other drugs that depress the CNS, chronic use of benzodiazepines at therapeutic doses may induce dependence. However, this dependence is relatively mild compared with that seen with other CNS depressants. Thus withdrawal in such cases often provokes a rebound phenomenon that includes insomnia and anxiety as well as tremor and confusion, but does not involve the life-threatening consequences typically seen with barbiturates (see below).

Zaleplon and zolpidem may produce next-day sedation and drowsiness when taken for insomnia. However, because of their shorter half-lives, the incidence of these unwanted effects appears to be less frequent with zaleplon and zolpidem than with benzodiazepines. These drugs appear to have the same mild potential for dependence and abuse seen with benzodiazepines.

INTERACTIONS

By far the most significant drug interactions associated with benzodiazepines and benzodiazepine-like drugs is the potential for excessive and life-threatening respiratory depression when combined with other CNS depressants. The interaction with alcohol is particularly marked and important because of its widespread social use. The combination of benzodiazepines and alcohol may produce marked incoordination and motor impairment that make driving dangerous.

A number of drugs and other substances are known to interfere with the hepatic biotransformation of many benzodiazepines, thus prolonging their half-lives and leading to increased plasma levels. These substances include fluvoxamine, ketoconazole, and grapefruit juice.

 DRUG CLASS • Benzodiazepine Antagonists

flumazenil (Anexate,✱ Romazicon)

MECHANISM OF ACTION

Flumazenil is an antagonist at the benzodiazepine receptor. It has no effect itself but will block the effects of any drug that acts through benzodiazepine receptors.

USES

Flumazenil is used intravenously in the treatment of acute benzodiazepine overdose or intoxication.

PHARMACOKINETICS

Flumazenil is given intravenously to treat benzodiazepine overdose. It has a fast onset but a relatively short duration of action (1 to 3 hours) because of rapid hepatic bio-

transformation. Therefore flumazenil is sometimes administered by constant intravenous infusion to achieve a sustained blockade of benzodiazepine-induced sedation.

ADVERSE REACTIONS

Flumazenil produces few adverse reactions on its own but can precipitate emotional lability, headache, or more serious reactions in patients dependent on benzodiazepines.

INTERACTIONS

Flumazenil blocks both the sedative and the anticonvulsant actions of benzodiazepines. The risk of seizures is increased in patients who are predisposed to seizures or who have received drugs that promote seizure activity.

 DRUG CLASS • Barbiturates

amobarbital (Amytal)
aprobarbital (Alurate)
butabarbital (Butisol Sodium, Sarisol)
butalbital + acetaminophen (Axocet)
mephobarbital (Mebaral)
methohexital (Brevital Sodium)
pentobarbital (Nembutal, Novo-Pentobarb✱)
⚠ phenobarbital (Luminal, Barbital, Solfoton)
secobarbital (Seconal Sodium, Novo-Secobarb✱)
thiopental (Pentothal)

MECHANISM OF ACTION

Like benzodiazepines, barbiturates also act at the GABA-A receptor to enhance the effects of GABA. Thus they have sedative-hypnotic effects and antiseizure ac-

tivity. However, unlike benzodiazepines, barbiturates may produce effects even in the absence of GABA to allow the movement of chloride through the channel. Because of this difference, barbiturates have the potential to cause greater and more widespread CNS depression than benzodiazepines.

USES

Barbiturates that were once widely used for the treatment of insomnia and anxiety disorders include amobarbital, aprobarbital, butabarbital, and secobarbital. However, these drugs have now been largely replaced by benzodiazepines and others that are just as effective but not as dangerous. Similarly, barbiturates are no longer the drugs most commonly used in the treatment of seizures (see Chapter 22), although mephobarbital and phenobarbital were once very popular for this purpose. As discussed in Chapter 16, methohexital and thiopental are used to produce brief general anesthesia.

PHARMACOKINETICS

Most barbiturates can be administered orally for use as sedative-hypnotics and are well absorbed. (For the use of certain barbiturates as anticonvulsants or in general anesthesia, preparations are also available for intravenous or intramuscular injection and for rectal administration.) Barbiturates are subject to extensive hepatic biotransformation. Administration of barbiturates for a few days causes the liver to synthesize more of the drug-biotransforming enzymes. This increase is called **enzyme induction** (see Chapter 1). After induction of these enzymes, the barbiturates are more rapidly biotransformed, decreasing average blood levels after a given dose. Therefore, with chronic treatment, higher doses may be required to achieve and maintain the same plasma levels seen early in therapy, a phenomenon known as **metabolic tolerance**. Because many other drugs are also biotransformed by the same liver enzymes, barbiturates can induce tolerance of other drugs (see below).

ADVERSE REACTIONS AND CONTRAINDICATIONS

Barbiturates present several important problems that severely limit their usefulness as sedative-hypnotics. Most importantly, these drugs may produce excessive CNS depression, including coma and potentially lethal respiratory depression. This danger is compounded by their low therapeutic index and the fact that the depression is greatly enhanced by other CNS depressants. When used as hypnotics, next-day drowsiness and significant motor impairment are often seen.

Tolerance and dependence occur more readily with barbiturates than with benzodiazepines, and barbiturates are more likely to be abused. Secobarbital, pentobarbital, and amobarbital are schedule II drugs (those having a high potential for abuse). Butabarbital is a schedule III drug (lesser abuse potential), whereas phenobarbital and mephobarbital are considered schedule IV drugs (low abuse potential; see Chapter 7 for a discussion of schedules). Unlike with benzodiazepines, withdrawal from barbiturates in a dependent individual may be life threatening. Severe withdrawal symptoms begin within 24 hours after the drug is discontinued in an individual with severe drug dependence. Tonic-clonic seizures and delirium are common symptoms; seizures may become continuous, a potentially fatal condition known as **status epilepticus**. Because of the danger associated with barbiturate withdrawal, detoxification of a dependent person is usually performed gradually. Withdrawal is achieved by slowly reducing the dosage of the barbiturate over 10 to 20 days. Sometimes the long-acting barbiturate phenobarbital is substituted for a short-acting barbiturate for once-daily administration.

Because barbiturates induce the enzymes responsible for porphyrin synthesis, they are not recommended for patients with a history of porphyria. These drugs should be used with caution in patients known to be susceptible to drug abuse, in patients with hepatic disease or impairment, or in pregnant women (because of the potential for CNS depression and dependence in the fetus). Infrequently, barbiturates may cause paradoxical excitation, especially in children and older adult patients.

TOXICITY

Rarely, patients may develop one of several hypersensitivity reactions to barbiturates. In some cases, these may be severe and even fatal.

INTERACTIONS

A wide variety of significant drug interactions involving barbiturates are known to occur. These may be divided into pharmacokinetic and pharmacodynamic interactions.

Pharmacokinetic interactions arise primarily from the ability of barbiturates to induce the biotransforming enzymes. These include the enzymes responsible for the biotransformation of corticosteroids, the anticoagulant warfarin, oral contraceptives, and the anticonvulsants valproate and carbamazepine. In patients treated with these drugs, steady-state plasma levels are likely to fall during treatment with barbiturates, and their therapeutic effect may be diminished or lost unless the dosage is increased.

The depressant effect of barbiturates not only is additive with alcohol and other general CNS depressants but also is potentiated by antipsychotics and opioid analgesics. These interactions are important to remember for the patient scheduled to undergo surgery. If secobarbital or pentobarbital is prescribed for sleep the night before, it should be given at least 8 hours before any antipsychotics, opioid analgesics, or general anesthetics are administered to avoid undue depression of the medullary control of respiration and the cardiovascular system.

DRUG CLASS • Atypical Anxiolytic

buspirone (Buspar)

MECHANISM OF ACTION

Unlike other sedative-hypnotic drugs in common use today, buspirone has no effect on GABA-A receptors. Instead, it appears to act at certain receptors for serotonin, the 5-HT1A receptors, and may also produce actions at dopamine D_2 receptors. Nevertheless, the exact mechanism for buspirone's anxiolytic activity is presently unclear.

USES

Although buspirone has antianxiety activity comparable with that of benzodiazepines, it has no significant anticonvulsant or muscle relaxant effect and may produce less sedation as well. However, an anxiolytic effect may not be evident for up to a week after therapy with buspirone is begun, and this effect may not be maximal for a month.

PHARMACOKINETICS

Buspirone is well absorbed but because of extensive first-pass biotransformation has a bioavailability of only 4%. The drug is rapidly biotransformed by the liver and thus has a relatively short plasma half-life (less than 3 hours).

ADVERSE REACTIONS AND CONTRAINDICATIONS

Adverse reactions to buspirone are relatively rare. The drug produces little sedation or impairment and appears to lack the potential for abuse and dependence. Since bioavailability is greatly reduced and plasma half-life is normally very short because of rapid inactivation in the liver, caution should be exercised when using buspirone in patients with significant hepatic disease or impairment.

INTERACTIONS

Drugs that compete for the hepatic enzymes responsible for inactivation of buspirone may greatly enhance its bioavailability, resulting in much higher plasma levels after a typical oral dose and therefore an increase in the incidence of adverse effects. Erythromycin and itraconazole may increase peak plasma levels of buspirone about fivefold through this mechanism. Administration of buspirone to patients taking monoamine oxidase (MAO) inhibitors has been reported to provoke significant increase in blood pressure.

 DRUG CLASS • Older Sedative-Hypnotics

chloral hydrate (Noctec, Novo-Chlorhydrate,✶ PMS-Chloral Hydrate✶)
ethchlorvynol (Placidyl)
hydroxyzine (Atarax, Vistaril)
meprobamate (Equanil, Miltown, Meprospan, Trancot, Apo-Meprobamate✶)
paraldehyde

MECHANISM OF ACTION

The precise mechanism underlying the sedative-hypnotic effect of all of these drugs is unknown. However, the best evidence points to action through GABA-A receptors for all except hydroxyzine. Hydroxyzine is actually an antihistamine (see Chapter 53), but the basis for its antianxiety effect is unknown. With the exception of meprobamate, the remaining drugs seem to produce effects similar to those of the barbiturates. Meprobamate may resemble the benzodiazepines with some important differences (see below).

USES

Although all of these drugs were employed in the past as sedative-hypnotics, they are now used rarely, if at all, for this purpose. Chloral hydrate is occasionally used for preoperative sedation but is no longer used for hypnosis or to treat anxiety. Meprobamate and hydroxyzine are rarely used in the treatment of mild anxiety disorder, and ethchlorvynol is effective but infrequently employed in the short-term treatment of insomnia. Paraldehyde is only used infrequently, in the management of abstinence syndromes or other mental conditions characterized by excitement.

PHARMACOKINETICS

All of these drugs are orally bioavailable and subject to extensive hepatic biotransformation with plasma half-lives ranging from 8 to 20 hours. Chloral hydrate is biotransformed to trichloroethanol, which is thought to be responsible for its CNS effects.

ADVERSE REACTIONS AND CONTRAINDICATIONS

These drugs cause or have the potential to cause a variety of unpleasant effects, which led to their being all but abandoned as sedative-hypnotics in favor of the benzodiazepines. All of these drugs may cause excessive sedation and CNS depression, and large doses of meprobamate or ethchlorvynol alone may cause fatal cardiovascular and respiratory depression. Paraldehyde and chloral hydrate are highly irritating, unpleasant to take, and may cause hepatic or renal damage.

TOXICITY

Rarely, patients may manifest hypersensitivity reactions to ethchlorvynol.

INTERACTIONS

As with the other benzodiazepines and barbiturates, the CNS depression caused by these drugs is greatly enhanced by other CNS depressants.

 APPLICATION TO PRACTICE

ASSESSMENT
History of Present Illness

How a person with anxiety or an impaired sleep pattern presents to the health care system is important. The assessment of a patient who visits a health care professional voluntarily and complains of an inability to sleep or to cope with life is very different from that of a patient in a locked psychiatric unit showing signs of panic. Much can be learned by careful observation of the patient and the symptoms. Table 17-1 reviews the levels of anxiety and their associated characteristics.

Because high anxiety levels and panic states are associated with feelings of intense fear and doom, providing a safe environment with decreased stimulation is an essential step in the assessment process. The health care provider may find it helpful to group symptoms into one of four categories: physiologic, behavioral, cognitive, or affective.

TABLE 17-1

Levels of Anxiety

Level of Anxiety	Characteristics
Mild anxiety	Appears calm Perceptual field broadens; perceptual abilities intensified Learning and critical thinking abilities enhanced Able to connect feelings, thoughts, and actions Focuses on present problems; identifies cause-and-effect relationships
Moderate anxiety	Appears tense and restless Perceptual field narrows; perceptual abilities restricted to immediate situation Able to attend to stimuli if they are pointed out Alertness at its highest, most efficient level Uses ego-defense mechanisms
Severe anxiety	Appears tense with increased respiration, blood pressure, and pulse Perceptual field significantly reduced Learning and critical thinking abilities reduced Unable to connect feelings, thoughts, and actions Able to focus on small aspect of problem of environment Behaviors directed at immediate relief of anxiety
Panic level	Demonstrates symptoms of helplessness, hopelessness, rage Behaviors directed at gaining or maintaining control Learning and critical thinking abilities lost Perceptual field distorted; details scattered, spinning Physiologic response includes hypertension and possibly hyperventilation

Ask about factors that may have resulted in anxiety or an impaired sleep pattern (Box 17-1). Additionally, the patient's previous coping strategies and their effectiveness, as well as the total effect that anxiety or impaired sleep is having on a patient's life, should be addressed. When appropriate, significant others should be included in the assessment process. It is beneficial to explore with the patient which symptoms are the most distressing.

Health History

A health history is by far the most important tool in any assessment of the patient with anxiety or sleep cycle disorders. First, it is important to ask about medical conditions. Chronic pulmonary disease, cardiac disorders, hyperthyroidism, and hypoglycemia tend to produce relatively high levels of anxiety.

Elicit from the patient information about the drugs—prescribed, over the counter (OTC), or illicit—he or she is taking at present. Obtaining information about use of these substances is important because abrupt withdrawal itself of some drugs can precipitate anxiety, particularly if the patient is physiologically dependent.

An accurate health history is more complete if the family and significant others are involved. However, inclusion of the family may at times be inadvisable because the patient's anxiety can be compounded by overly concerned family members. In cases of anxiety in children or older adults, it may be more important to involve the family, because these patients are sometimes less willing or able to reflect on their circumstances. In all instances, the examination must always make the patient feel secure in his or her environment.

Lifespan Considerations

Perinatal. Pregnancy brings enormous changes to a woman's body. She must deal with alterations in hormone fluctuations and body image, the role change of becoming a mother, and concern for the health of her child. The possibility that anxiety can be manifested either as a normal response or as a pathologic adjustment is apparent.

Pediatric. Developmental stereotypes often lead to underestimating the prevalence of anxiety disorders in children and adolescents. In fact, such disorders are more prevalent than attention deficit disorders in this age group. Children can have so-called adult anxiety disorders as well as disorders specific to their age group, such as separation anxiety, overanxious behavior, and stranger anxiety. Children rarely have a pure anxiety disorder but instead display multiple symptoms, making diagnosis more challenging. The possibility of substance or sexual abuse should be explored. A full psychiatric review of the family is important because children with overanxious parents often learn similar behaviors.

Older Adults. The adjustments needed to cope with the multiple losses of independence, health, and family, which are so often encountered in older adults, contribute to anxiety. Many emotional dilemmas of the older adult can mimic or have the appearance of anxiety. Dysfunctional grieving, Alzheimer's disease, and confusion can all bear a striking resemblance to anxiety. The older adult may have somatic or behavioral symptoms similar to those noted in a younger patient but more frequently he or she may appear withdrawn, a behavior used commonly as a coping mechanism. A careful geropsychiatric evaluation will help define actual pathology and allow a definitive diagnosis of anxiety or sleep disorder to be made.

Cultural/Social Considerations

Since anxiety is a normal human response, a basic task for the health care provider is determining whether a patient is suffering from an abnormal anxiety response or reacting to the normal stress of life. The patient can help by identifying how severely his or her lifestyle is affected by the anxiety level. Some areas to pursue include recent work history, family disruptions, sleeping habits, and overall satisfaction with life. Patients with phobias or posttraumatic stress disorder may have episodic interruptions in their lives. Patients with agoraphobia or generalized anxiety disorder may report severely disrupted lives and minimal functioning. How patients view their current and past interactions with the health care system is important in understanding the level of trust they need. This is crucial information because the basis of all therapeutic relationships is trust (see Case Study: Panic Disorder).

Physical Examination

Anxiety and impaired sleep are frequently associated with medical problems. A thorough physical examination should be made with an eye toward discovering the underlying causes of the anxiety. The presence and severity of somatic symptoms provide important information clues about the level of anxiety of the patient. Attention should be paid to the patient's pulse and respiratory rates as well as blood pressure. The health care provider should also observe for diaphoresis, restlessness, or trembling, because these manifestations are often hallmarks of anxiety. In addition, assess for visible signs of fatigue and lack of sleep, such as reddened eyes, lack of coordination, drowsiness, and irritability. The health care provider will be able to monitor the effectiveness of anxiolytic or sedative-hypnotic therapy more accurately by referring to these baseline physical examination findings.

BOX 17-1	Patient Problem: Insomnia

The Problem

Insomnia is a difficulty in the initiation or maintenance of sleep or nonrestorative sleep associated with clinically significant distress or functional impairment. No single physiologic basis for insomnia exists; however, perceptual and psychologic factors often play an important role.

Transient insomnia strikes most people at some time, it is usually related to stress or worry, travel across several time zones, pain, or injury. Patients who are anxious, angry, frustrated, depressed, or under situational stress often experience this condition. People who overestimate the time it takes to fall asleep or the time spent awake after the initial onset of sleep are prone to complaints of insomnia, especially during times of emotional stress. In addition, insomnia can be caused by a number of different drugs or illnesses.

Patients with insomnia typically complain of malaise and fatigue, not getting enough sleep, irritability, and may doze off briefly at unanticipated or dangerous times (e.g., while driving). There may also be mild to moderate impairment in concentration and psychomotor dysfunction. In some cases, the patient's bed partner may report snoring, apparent pauses in breathing (apnea), and kicking movements.

Assessment

- Note the usual hour of sleep and rising times, as well as bedtime rituals or preferences that enhance sleep quality. For example, a patient with chronic airway limitation or gastroesophageal reflux disease may be accustomed to sleeping with several pillows or with the head of the bed elevated.
- Ask about usual bedtime activities. Inquire about how long it takes to get to sleep, the number and perceived cause of awakenings, the regularity and consistency of sleep patterns, and the frequency and duration of naps should be elicited.
- Elicit information about when the patient is likely to doze off: Sitting and reading? Watching television? Sitting inactive in a public place? Riding as a passenger in a car for an hour or more without a break? Lying down for a nap, if able? Sitting and talking? Sitting quietly after lunch without alcohol? Stopped for a few minutes in traffic?
- Elicit information about prescription, OTC, and illicit drugs used and the time of day taken. Note the patient's diet and amount of alcohol or caffeine intake.
- Obtain information about comorbid conditions and how these are treated.
- Note any history of unexplained motor vehicle or work-related accidents and changes in personality or cognitive functioning due to fatigue.
- Perform a physical examination with attention to body mass index (over 30 indicates obesity), nuchal obesity (i.e., neck size over 17 inches in males, 15 inches in females), and size of the pharynx.

The Solution

- Have the patient review and modify daily high-stress obligations. Delegate responsibilities when able or elicit help.
- Establish a daily bedtime routine; that is, the same sequence of bedtime activities and same time for bed.
- Have patient try drinking warm milk, taking a bath, getting a backrub, or performing other quiet activities before bedtime. Avoid strenuous exercise within 2 hours of bedtime. Incorporate regular exercise into an earlier daily routine.
- Avoid heavy meals, alcohol, and caffeine-containing food and drinks after 5 PM. Limit liquids after 7 PM to decrease nocturia.
- Avoid watching scary or anxiety-producing movies or television shows before bedtime. If fact, if there is a television set in the bedroom, move it to another room. Beds are for sleeping and sexual activities.
- Avoid engaging in non–sleep-related activities such as paying bills, doing homework, and so forth while in bed.
- Keep noise to a minimum. Try soft music or "white noise" (e.g., a fan or an audiotape of rain).
- Keep the temperature in the bedroom cool, but use sufficient blankets and pillows to keep warm and comfortable. Wear comfortable clothing.
- Turn off the lights. Use a night-light if necessary.
- Limit afternoon naps and try to avoid going to bed at times other than the scheduled time.
- Use sedative-hypnotics as a last resort. Ask the health care provider for further evaluation, cognitive-behavioral therapy, and if appropriate, referral to a sleep disorder center.
- Refer the patient to a specialist in sleep disorders or nose and throat disorders if abnormalities are identified.

Laboratory Testing

Baseline laboratory values alert the health care provider to electrolyte imbalances suggestive of underlying diseases that may lead to anxiety or impaired sleep. Toxicology screening is called for if drug ingestion or withdrawal is suspected. There are also a number of anxiety assessment tools available to help determine the extent of the patient's anxiety.

The primary diagnostic test for sleep disorders is polysomnography. Patients may be referred to a sleep center for an overnight recording of electroencephalogram, electrooculogram, and submental electromyogram using surface electrodes. Depending on the cause of the sleep disorder, a variety of other studies may be performed.

GOALS OF THERAPY

Treatment goals for the patient with an anxiety disorder include a decrease in or resolution of symptoms that significantly interfere with the patient's ability to perform life's tasks. Helping the patient to develop effective coping skills to deal with some aspects of the anxiety and to prevent secondary disorders such as depression or substance abuse is also an important goal. Finally, treatment goals also include preventing relapse or recurrence of the anxiety. Situational anxiety should have been previously differentiated from generalized anxiety disorders.

Treatment goals for the patient with impaired sleep are directed at promoting sleep in the short term (i.e., 1 to 4 days). Thus daytime disruptions such as fatigue, impaired work performance, and transient mood disturbances may be lessened. Sleep can also be promoted for up to 3 weeks while the patient learns alternative behavioral techniques (e.g., eliminating daytime napping, instituting relaxation exercise).

INTERVENTION

There are no specific guidelines as to when drug therapy for anxiety or impaired sleep should be initiated. Such therapy is ordinarily considered when nondrug modalities have been unsuccessful, if the patient is suicidal, or if symptoms of anxiety are severe, persistent, and recurrent enough to disrupt the patient's activities of daily living. Greater response rates occur when behavioral and drug therapies are combined.

Refer the patient with continuing anxiety or insomnia problems to appropriate resources for evaluation and counseling. Note that excessive or prolonged use of an anxiolytic or sedative-hypnotic drug may result in physical or psychologic dependence (see Drug Abuse Alert Box: Barbiturates).

Note that anxiolytic and sedative-hypnotic drugs should not be used in place of analgesics for the patient in pain. Pain alters the patient's response to hypnotic drugs, causing an increased risk of disorientation and

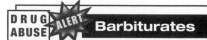

Background

Barbiturates are sedative-hypnotics. They are abused to bring about a sense of euphoria and a lessening of anxiety. They can be taken orally or injected.

Health Hazard

Pharmacodynamic tolerance develops with repeated administration of the barbiturates. This is the tolerance typically seen with CNS depressants, in which the nervous system adapts to the presence of the depressant. However, the medullary centers controlling respiration and the cardiovascular system do not adapt to general CNS depressants because they are not affected at the usual doses taken. The lethal dose of barbiturates therefore does not increase with drug dependence; this accounts for the accidental death of persons dependent on high doses of barbiturates. The lethal dose of barbiturates in nontolerant individuals is about 15 times the hypnotic dose. These margins are decreased by the ingestion of alcohol or another CNS depressant.

A barbiturate overdose causes shallow respirations; cold, clammy skin; dilated pupils; and a weak, rapid pulse and may progress to coma and respiratory arrest. Withdrawal symptoms include anxiety, insomnia, tremors, delirium, and seizures.

Interventions

Supportive care is required of the patient with a barbiturate overdose. There are no antagonists to barbiturates.

From the American Psychiatric Association: *Diagnostic and statistical manual of mental disorders (DSM-IV)*, ed. 4, Washington, D.C, 1994, The Association.

paradoxical excitement. Analgesics are discussed in Chapters 13, 14, and 15.

Administration

Vital to successful anxiolytic therapy is understanding the degree of insight a patient has into his or her anxiety or sleep disorder. Patients with anxiety levels bordering on panic ordinarily have little understanding of the reasons for their distress. Lower anxiety levels translate into heightened awareness of the reasons for distress. Anxiolytic drug dosages can be proportionately adjusted to modulate higher or lower anxiety levels. Use sleeping pills judiciously. Do not deprive patients of a needed drug, but use these drugs as an adjunct to nursing measures such as a backrub, repositioning, a small snack, or a glass of warm milk. In the institutional setting, keep siderails up and a night-light on after administering an anxiolytic or sedative-hypnotic drug. Supervise the patient's ambulation and smoking.

Patients may take a benzodiazepine with food, fruit juice, or ginger ale if gastric irritation occurs when the drug is taken on an empty stomach. Oral solutions can be diluted with liquid or semisolid food such as applesauce or pudding to help improve taste and reduce gastric irritation. Sustained-release formulations should be administered intact, without crushing or chewing. Teach patients taking a sublingual formulation to let the drug slowly dissolve under the tongue and then to swallow. If a dose is missed, it should not be doubled at the next administration time. Instead, the missed dose should be skipped unless its omission is realized within an hour of its usual time.

Read labels carefully and follow the manufacturer's instructions when preparing intravenous formulations of anxiolytic and sedative-hypnotic drugs. These formulations should be administered slowly because apnea, hypotension, bradycardia, and cardiac arrest have been reported with rapid administration. Be sure to check the location and patency of the intravenous site. Arteriospasm with resultant gangrene can result from accidental intraarterial administration.

The patient receiving a benzodiazepine or barbiturate intravenously should have his or her blood pressure and respiratory rate closely monitored for 2 to 8 hours. Keep the siderails up and do not leave the patient unattended unless he or she is sufficiently alert to handle oral and respiratory secretions and to call for assistance. Have a suction machine and intubation equipment available as well as resuscitative drugs, including flumazenil.

Intramuscular formulations should be avoided because they are highly alkaline and irritating to the tissues. Absorption by this route is also erratic.

In the outpatient setting, be alert to patients who request prescription refills on an increasingly frequent basis; this behavior may suggest improper use, abuse, or a knowledge deficit about the hazards of continued use of the drug. Some cases of chronic overdose arise because the patient receives prescriptions from more than one health care provider, each of whom is unaware of the others' prescription. Evaluate patients carefully for possible depression and suicidal ideations. Suicide is always a potential with psychoactive drugs.

For the patient on long-term anxiolytic or sedative-hypnotic therapy, monitor liver function as well as BUN and serum creatinine levels.

Education

Successful anxiolytic and sedative-hypnotic therapy depends on a close alliance between patient and health care provider. Patients must be taught that anxiolytic and sedative-hypnotic drugs are useful for short-term tension relief and to promote sleep. They are not a solution for stress. Drug therapy is most effective as an adjunct that is combined with other intervention modalities (see Box 17-1).

Any critical decisions or judgments required of the patient should be made before sedative-hypnotic drugs are administered. The validity of legal documents will be in question if they are signed while the patient is under the influence of any CNS depressant.

The patient should be advised that activities requiring mental alertness (e.g., driving or using power tools) should be avoided, particularly in the early stages of therapy. Advise parents to supervise the play of children taking these drugs. The patient should be instructed to avoid alcohol, sleep-inducing OTC drugs, and other CNS depressants while taking anxiolytic or sedative-hypnotic drugs unless specifically prescribed by the health care provider. Examples of such drugs include antiemetics, opioid analgesics, and antihistamines. Dangerous combinations are more likely to be identified if the patient purchases all drugs from the same pharmacy. Most pharmacists maintain drug profiles on their clients, monitoring records for inappropriate or potentially dangerous drug interactions.

Patients for whom sedative-hypnotics are prescribed should be cautioned about the risks inherent in their use. Advise the patient that 1 to 2 weeks of therapy may be required to see the full effects. They should be told not to increase the dosage or to abruptly stop the drug without first contacting the health care provider. Further, patients can become forgetful about their use. Supplies of the drug should be kept in a place other than on the bedside table. The place chosen should be far enough away from the bedroom so that the patient is fully alert before repeating a dose. It is thought that many cases of overdose arise from repeated doses taken by the patient during waking periods. In some cases, it may be necessary to place the drug supply under the supervision of a second person. Keep these and all drugs out of the reach of children, use childproof caps in settings where small children are present, and keep the drugs in their original, clearly labeled containers.

Caution patients taking these drugs about their anticonvulsant effects, specifically that drowsiness may continue for several days to weeks but should gradually diminish. Emphasize the importance of taking drugs as ordered and not discontinuing their use without consulting the health care provider. Encourage the patient with a history of seizures to wear a medical alert necklace or bracelet.

Since anxiolytic and sedative-hypnotic drugs are used for adjunctive therapy, it is important that patients stay in close contact with their health care provider. Dosages and administration times may need to be adjusted in the early stages of treatment. Additionally, patients should be advised to inform their health care provider of any increase in sedation, lethargy, or difficulty staying awake after initial therapy has been established. In many cases, education in sleep hygiene (e.g., reducing caffeine intake, changing sleep habits, or pain relief) might be more appropriate than a sedative-hypnotic. Early-morning waking is one of the biologic features of depression; thus an antidepressant may be appropriate (see Chapter 18).

Some drugs cause changes in libido or sexual activity. Tactfully assess for these adverse effects. Provide emotional support as appropriate and advise the patient to consult with the health care provider for possible changes in type of drug or dosage.

EVALUATION

Evaluating the efficacy of anxiolytics and sedative-hypnotics can be problematic because the essential characteristics of anxiety and insomnia cannot be adequately reproduced. Cognition, communication, and social relationships are difficult to assess objectively. However, clinical improvement should be evaluated, and patients should report a decrease of physical symptoms. They should note better concentration and less tendency toward distraction. Their sense of dread and negative anticipation should be lessened, and they could begin to gain an insight into the reasons for their anxiety. Furthermore, there should be no symptoms of dependency.

When impaired sleep has been the problem, the patient should report a decrease in symptoms of insomnia and fatigue.

CASE STUDY   *Panic Disorder*

ASSESSMENT

HISTORY OF PRESENT ILLNESS

RD is a 45-year-old white man who visits the primary care clinic complaining of not being able to concentrate or sleep at night. Additionally, he says that he feels he is suffocating or blacking out. He relates that these episodes have been occurring for at least 5 years but that their frequency and intensity have increased. Occasionally, he is unwilling to leave his home for fear that something terrible will happen.

HEALTH HISTORY

RD reports overall good health with no cardiovascular or pulmonary problems. He has smoked 1 pack of cigarettes per day for 20 years. He has abstained from alcohol for the past 4 months but has used it heavily in the past. He notes feeling the need for a drink now and then to help him concentrate and to be able to sleep. RD uses marijuana about twice a week but reports using no other illicit drugs. While in the Navy, RD injured his left knee and has had several arthroscopic procedures. RD has sought psychotherapy but reports that it was of little value: "All they did was give me drugs that put me to sleep."

LIFESPAN CONSIDERATIONS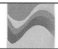

RD has been married for 10 years and is employed as a real estate agent. He reports recent sales have been slow, and he is worried about his ability to compete in the real estate market with his difficulty concentrating.

CULTURAL/SOCIAL CONSIDERATIONS

His childhood was described as normal, without episodes of abuse or neglect. His parents divorced when he was 10 years old, and he remembers this as a "very sad time." RD was in the Navy for 6 years and reports no episodes of imminent death or extreme danger. RD's knee injury is considered related to his military service, and he is therefore eligible for treatment at a local veterans hospital.

PHYSICAL EXAMINATION

Blood pressure 146/85 mm Hg, pulse 90, respirations 26, temperature is 98.6° F; lungs are clear to auscultation. RD is well groomed and articulate but rarely makes eye contact. He fidgets in the chair, attempting to position himself so that the door to the examination room is in sight at all times.

LABORATORY TESTING

ECG shows normal sinus rhythm (NSR); fasting blood glucose level is 98 mg/dL; thyroid panel within normal limits.

PATIENT PROBLEM(S)

Panic attacks with depression.

GOALS OF THERAPY

Minimize frequency and intensity of panic attacks so as to permit RD to assume his normal daily regimen with minimal sedation.

CRITICAL THINKING QUESTIONS

1. The health care provider orders paroxetine 20 mg qd, alprazolam 0.5 mg po tid prn, and cognitive-behavioral therapy. What is the purpose of each of these treatment strategies?
2. How long will it take for the alprazolam to reach a therapeutic steady-state serum level?
3. What is the mechanism of action for alprazolam?
4. To what adverse effects of alprazolam should RD be made aware?
5. Alprazolam has the potential to produce dependency; thus the dosage should be tapered gradually. Over what period of time would tapering be appropriate?
6. What information is important for RD in regard to the use of alprazolam given his history of substance abuse?

Bibliography

American Psychiatric Association: *Diagnostic and statistical manual of mental disorders*, ed 4, Washington, D.C., 2000, American Psychiatric Press.

Antai-Otong D: The neurobiology of anxiety disorders: implications for psychiatric nursing practice, *Issues Ment Health Nurs* 21(1):71-89, 2000.

Durback-Morris LF, Scharman EJ: Charcoal for overdoses, *Am J Nurs* 99(4):14, 1999.

Fishel AH: Nursing management of anxiety and panic, *Nurs Clin North Am* 33(1):135-151, 1998.

Folks DG: Management of insomnia in the long-term care setting, *Ann Long-Term Care* 7(1):7-13, 1999.

Gutierrez MA, Roper JM, Hahn P: Paradoxical reactions to benzodiazepines: when to expect the unexpected, *Am J Nurs* 101(7):34-40, 2001.

Haack MR: Treating acute withdrawal from alcohol and other drugs, *Nurs Clin North Am* 33(1):75-92, 1998.

Ring D: Management of chronic insomnia in the elderly, *Clin Excell Nurse Pract* 5(1):13-16, 2001.

Seivewright N: Theory and practice in managing benzodiazepine dependence and misuse, *J Subst Misuse Nurs Health Soc Care* 3(3):170-177, 1998.

Internet Resources

California State University: Sedative-hypnotics. Available online at http://www.csusm.edu/DandB/Sedatives.html.

California State University: Sedative-hypnotics quiz. Available online at http://www.csusm.edu/DandB/sedatives_quiz.html.

Division of Alcohol and Drug Abuse: Sedative-hypnotics. Available online at http://www.well.com/user/woa/fsseda.htm.

Emergency Medicine.com: Toxicity, sedative-hypnotics. Available online at http://www.emedicine.com/emerg/topic 525.htm.

University of Utah: Pharmacology of the sedative-hypnotic drugs. Available online at http://medlib.med.utah.edu/calendar/block4/ppt_sedatives2001/.

Antidepressant and Antimania Drugs

MICHAEL R. VASKO • KATHLEEN GUTIERREZ

 Visit http://evolve.elsevier.com/Gutierrez/ for additional information.

KEY TERMS

OBJECTIVES

- Briefly describe the symptoms of depression and of mania.
- Know the adverse effect profiles of each class of antidepressants.
- Describe the toxic symptoms of lithium and the corresponding blood level.
- Develop a teaching plan for a patient on a tyramine-restricted diet.
- Develop a nursing care plan for patients receiving a selective serotonin reuptake inhibitor, a tricyclic antidepressant, an atypical antidepressant, a monoamine oxidase inhibitor, or lithium.

PATHOPHYSIOLOGY • Depression

Depression is defined as an affective disorder characterized by disturbances in emotional, cognitive, behavioral, and somatic regulation. It is not to be confused with normal sadness or disappointment that occur in the course of living and needs to be diagnosed by a qualified health care provider. Major depressive disorder (depression) is characterized by one or more episodes of mild, moderate, or severe clinical depression that lasts for more than 2 weeks without episodes of mania or hypomania. As a primary mood disorder, depression includes both unipolar (depressive) and bipolar (manic-depressive) conditions. With unipolar depression, people of routinely normal moods suffer recurrent episodes of depression. With bipolar depression, the episodes of depression alternate with periods of mania.

At any time, 15 million Americans suffer from major depression. The prevalence of major depressive disorder in the Western industrialized nations is approximately 3% for men and 4% to 9% for women. The lifetime risk for a major depressive disorder is higher in women than in men. Depression often is not properly diagnosed or treated. Many patients with major depressive disorders have a history of one or more other psychiatric disorders.

Patients with major depressive disorder also have a higher incidence of physical and psychologic disabilities, as well as occupational difficulties, including loss of work time. In the primary care setting, depressed patients also have more physical illnesses than nondepressed patients and their use of health care resources is greater compared with that of other patients. Major depression is associated with an increased mortality rate, which is generally attributed to suicide and accidents. A large proportion of those who commit suicide (70%) have visited their primary care provider with mood or somatic complaints within 4 or 6 weeks before their suicide. The number of deaths associated with depression is estimated to be 30,000 to 35,000 suicides per year. Patients with untreated recurrent major depression have a 15% suicide rate.

Types of Depression

Depression is a syndrome that can include various symptoms, as detailed in Box 18-1. Although there are genetic components predisposing an individual to depression, stressful situations and environments may play a strong triggering role. Changes in life patterns, especially serious losses, a difficult relationship, and financial problems may underlie a depressive episode. Depression becomes a medical problem when normal functioning is significantly hampered. The three most prevalent forms of depression are major depression, dysthymia, and bipolar disorder.

Major depression is characterized by a depressed mood most of the day and a greatly diminished interest or pleasure in most daily activities. In addition, there may be weight changes, sleep problems, anxiety or lethargy, fatigue, feelings of worthlessness or guilt, inability to concentrate or make decisions, decreased libido, and thoughts of death or suicide. Although major

---

BOX 18-1 | **Signs and Symptoms of Depression and Mania**

Not everyone who is depressed or manic experiences every symptom. Some people experience a few symptoms, some many. The severity of symptoms varies with individuals.

Depression

- Persistent sad, anxious, or "empty" mood
- Feelings of hopelessness, pessimism
- Feelings of guilt, worthlessness, helplessness
- Loss of interest or pleasure in hobbies and activities that were once enjoyed, including sex
- Insomnia, early-morning awakening, or oversleeping
- Appetite and/or weight loss or overeating and weight gain
- Decreased energy, fatigue, being "slowed down"
- Thoughts of death or suicide; suicide attempts
- Restlessness, irritability

- Difficulty concentrating, remembering, making decisions
- Persistent physical symptoms that do not respond to treatment, such as headaches, digestive disorders, and chronic pain

Mania

- Inappropriate elation
- Inappropriate irritability
- Severe insomnia
- Grandiose notions
- Increased talking
- Disconnected and racing thoughts
- Increased sexual desire
- Dramatically increased energy
- Poor judgment
- Inappropriate social behavior

Reprinted with permission from the Diagnostic and statistical manual of mental disorders, ed 4, text revision. Copyright © 2000 American Psychiatric Association.

depression can occur at any age, the midtwenties are the most common time of development. Episodes typically last about 1 year, and 80% of patients will experience more than one episode in their lifetimes. Most experience two or three episodes.

Dysthymia is a depression lasting more than 2 years that is not disabling but keeps the patient from functioning fully. Common symptoms include self-criticism, low self-esteem, difficulty in making decisions, and feelings of hopelessness. Primary dysthymia (formerly called endogenous depression) has no identifiable cause. Secondary dysthymia (formerly called exogenous or reactive depression) may be precipitated by a number of factors such as environmental stress, adverse life events, drugs, or concurrent disease states.

Bipolar disorder, which is discussed in detail on p. 274, involves cycles of depression and elation or mania (see Box 18-1). In type I bipolar disorder, hypomania is more common than depressive episodes. In type II bipolar disorder, depressive episodes are more significant than mania.

Depression as an Adverse Effect

Depression can be the adverse effect of some drugs, especially antihypertensive drugs such as reserpine, methyldopa, guanethidine, and propranolol. Alcohol and antianxiety drugs often mask depression by alleviating the anxiety that commonly accompanies depression. Steroids, particularly glucocorticoids and oral contraceptives, can cause depression. Drug-induced depression mimics primary dysthymia but is treated by removing the drug or lowering the dosage.

Neurochemical Basis of Mood Disorders

Depression is a neurochemical disorder that can be treated with appropriate drug therapy. This concept arose from the observation in the 1950s that reserpine caused depression in patients treated for hypertension. Reserpine depleted the neurotransmitter norepinephrine. About the same time, iproniazid, a drug then used to treat tuberculosis, was found to elevate mood in these patients. Iproniazid inhibits the degradation of norepinephrine and serotonin (5-hydroxytryptamine [5-HT]) by inhibiting the enzyme monoamine oxidase (MAO). Later that decade it was discovered that imipramine, a drug developed in an attempt to find new antihistamines, sedatives, and analgesics, was quite effective in helping depressed patients. Imipramine belongs to the class of drugs called tricyclic antidepressants, which prevent the reuptake of serotonin and norepinephrine into nerve terminals (Figure 18-1). Since reuptake into the nerve terminal is the major way in which these transmitters are removed from the synaptic cleft for subsequent breakdown, the antidepressants restore levels of norepinephrine and serotonin at active sites (see Figure 18-1).

These observations suggested that a deficiency in the brain neurotransmitters norepinephrine and serotonin is

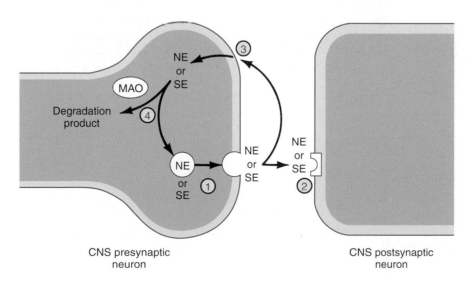

CNS presynaptic
neuron

CNS postsynaptic
neuron

FIGURE 18-1 The biogenic theory suggests that depression results from amine concentration too low to activate sufficient receptors; mania results from overabundance of amine acting at receptor. (1) Lithium inhibits release of norepinephrine (NE). (2) Tricyclic antidepressants and MAOIs increase receptor sensitivity to norepinephrine and serotonin (SE). (3) Tricyclic antidepressants and atypical antidepressants block reuptake of norepinephrine and/or serotonin. Selective serotonin reuptake inhibitors block reuptake of serotonin. (4) MAO inhibitors prevent degradation of norepinephrine and serotonin. (CNS is the central nervous system.)

associated with depression. It is important to note, however, that although the levels of the neurotransmitters increase rapidly, the onset of relief of symptoms of depression takes 1 to 4 weeks after the start of drug therapy. This delay suggests that the increased levels of norepinephrine and serotonin produce additional long-term changes in the nervous system in depressed patients that resolve the symptoms. Although the nature of these changes remains unknown, several possibilities exist, including alterations in neurotransmitter receptor function, enzyme activity or gene expression in neurons, and neuropeptide transmitters (especially corticotropin-releasing hormones). There are four major categories of antidepressants: selective serotonin reuptake inhibitors, tricyclic antidepressants, atypical antidepressants, and monoamine oxidase inhibitors. These antidepressants are presented in Table 18-1.

TABLE 18-1

Antidepressant Drugs

Generic Name	Brand Name	Comments
Selective Serotonin Reuptake Inhibitors		
citalopram	Celexa	For major depression
escitalopram	Lexapro	For depression, panic disorders
fluoxetine	Prozac	For mild to moderate depression, obsessive-compulsive disorders, and eating disorders (obesity, bulimia)
fluvoxamine	Luvox	For obsessive-compulsive disorder and mild to moderate depression
aroxetine	Paxil	For obsessive-compulsive disorder, panic attacks, and mild to moderate depression
sertraline	Zoloft	For mild to moderate depression
Tricyclic Antidepressants		
amitriptyline	Apo-Amitriptyline ✱ Elavil Endep Levate ✱ Novotriptyn ✱	Bedtime administration is preferred to lessen discomfort of sedation and anticholinergic effects prominent with this drug
amoxapine	Asendin	Related to tricyclic antidepressants; low incidence of anticholinergic, sedative, and cardiovascular adverse effects May be taken at bedtime to lessen daytime sedation or to treat insomnia
clomipramine	Anafranil	Used for obsessive-compulsive disorders, for blocking panic attacks, and to treat cataplexy associated with narcolepsy
desipramine	Norpramin Pertofrane ✱	Sedation and anticholinergic effects are not prominent; metabolite of imipramine
doxepin	Novo-Doxepin ✱ Sinequan Triadapin ✱	Bedtime administration is preferred to lessen discomfort of sedation and anticholinergic effects prominent with this drug; doxepin may have much less effect on heart than other tricyclic antidepressants

✱ Available only in Canada.

TABLE 18-1

Antidepressant Drugs—cont'd

Generic Name	Brand Name	Comments
Tricyclic Antidepressants—cont'd		
imipramine	Apo-Imipramine ✽ Novopramine ✽ Tipramine Tofranil Tofranil-PM	Prototype tricyclic antidepressant Sedative and anticholinergic effects are moderate; can be taken at bedtime
maprotiline	Ludiomil	Low incidence of anticholinergic, sedative, and cardiovascular adverse effects May be taken at bedtime to lessen daytime sedation or to treat insomnia
nortriptyline	Aventyl Pamelor	Metabolite of amitriptyline Sedative effect is moderate and anticholinergic effect is mild; can be taken at bedtime
protriptyline	Triptil ✽ Vivactil	Tricyclic antidepressant that has little sedative action and can cause insomnia if given at bedtime; preferred for patients who have been immobile and sleepy
trimipramine	Apo-Trimip ✽ Novo-Tripramine ✽ Rhotrimine ✽ Surmontil	Sedation effect is high, but anticholinergic effect is moderate
Atypical Antidepressants		
bupropion	Wellbutrin Zyban	Seizures may occur at high dosages Used to assist with withdrawal from nicotine dependence
mirtazapine	Remeron	Sedating; minimal anticholinergic effects
nefazodone	Serzone	Confusion, dizziness, dry mouth, hypotension, and nausea Elevates prolactin and growth hormone levels
reboxetine	Edronax Vestra	For depression, as initial or maintenance therapy
trazodone	Desyrel Trazon Trialodine	Sedation may be noted Low incidence of anticholinergic and cardiovascular adverse effects; may be taken at bedtime to lessen daytime sedation or to treat insomnia
venlafaxine	Effexor	For mild to moderate depression; inhibits both serotonin and norepinephrine reuptake
Monoamine Oxidase Inhibitors (MAOIs)		
isocarboxazid	Marplan	Instruct patient in food and drug interactions with MAOIs
moclobemide	Manerix	Instruct patient in food and drug interactions with MAOIs
phenelzine	Nardil	Instruct patient in food and drug interactions with MAOIs
tranylcypromine	Parnate	Instruct patient in food and drug interactions with MAOIs Has some psychomotor stimulant activity characteristic of amphetamine

DRUG CLASS • Selective Serotonin Reuptake Inhibitors (SSRIs)

citalopram (Celexa)

escitalopram (Lexapro)

⚠ fluoxetine (Prozac)

fluvoxamine (Luvox)

paroxetine (Paxil)

sertraline (Zoloft)

MECHANISM OF ACTION

Selective serotonin reuptake inhibitors (SSRIs) are chemically unrelated to any other class of antidepressants. Their mechanism of action for treating depression remains unknown, but appears to be linked to their ability to block the neuronal reuptake of serotonin. These drugs have little or no effect on the uptake of norepinephrine or dopamine (see Figure 18-1). The blockade of the uptake of serotonin allows more of this transmitter to remain in the synaptic cleft, where it exerts actions on a number of serotonin receptor subtypes. SSRIs have limited affinity for alpha$_1$-, alpha$_2$-, and beta-adrenergic receptors, as well as gamma-aminobutyric acid (GABA), histamine, and cholinergic receptors.

SSRIs (see Table 18-1) have greater pharmacologic specificity, fewer adverse effects, and lower potential for fatal overdose than tricyclic antidepressants (see Tables 18-1 and 18-2).

USES

The major use of SSRIs is the treatment of depressive disorders. The onset of antidepressant effect is faster with SSRIs than with tricyclic antidepressants but it still may take up to 4 weeks. In recent years, these drugs as well as other antidepressants have been used for other conditions. Several SSRIs (fluoxetine, fluvoxamine, paroxetine, and sertraline) are indicated for the treatment of obsessive-compulsive disorder. Both paroxetine and sertraline are used to treat panic disorder, whereas paroxetine also is indicated for social anxiety disorder. Fluoxetine is accepted as therapy for bulimia nervosa and for premenstrual dysphoric disorder (PMDD). SSRIs also are used in the treatment of anorexia nervosa, obesity, chronic pain, fibromyalgia, migraine, attention-deficit hyperactivity disorder, aggression, and posttraumatic stress disorder (PTSD).

PHARMACOKINETICS

SSRIs are well absorbed when taken orally. Their onset, peak, and duration of action range from 1 to 4 weeks and may require up to 12 weeks for complete effec-

tiveness. SSRIs are distributed throughout the body and across placental membranes. They have been found in breast milk. Most SSRIs are highly protein-bound with half-lives that vary from 5 to 72 hours. These drugs are extensively biotransformed in the liver by the P-450 oxidases. Major metabolites such as norfluoxetine and norsertraline have long half-lives (10 days and 60 to 70 hours, respectively). Norfluoxetine also is an inhibitor of serotonin reuptake. The half-lives of SSRIs are prolonged in patients with hepatic impairment. The metabolites of these drugs are largely eliminated in the urine, along with a small percentage of unchanged drug.

ADVERSE REACTIONS AND CONTRAINDICATIONS

The adverse effects of SSRIs are less pronounced than those seen with tricyclic antidepressants because of the lack of anticholinergic activity or cardiac conduction disturbances characteristic of tricyclic antidepressants (see Table 18-2). They are not without adverse effects, however, and a significant number of patients experience nausea and vomiting, headache, and sexual dysfunction (see Table 18-2). Sexual dysfunction may include lack of orgasm in women and ejaculatory delay in men. Less commonly reported adverse effects include tremor, anxiety, drowsiness, dry mouth, sweating, and diarrhea. A number of these drugs, including fluoxetine, citalopram, sertraline, and fluvoxamine can cause restlessness and agitation, whereas paroxetine has mild sedating effects.

SSRIs are contraindicated in cases of hypersensitivity and should not be used by patients with narrow-angle glaucoma or immediately after a myocardial infarction. Caution should be used in prescribing SSRIs during pregnancy or lactation, and an obstetric specialist should closely manage these drugs. They should be used cautiously in older adults and those with preexisting cardiovascular disease. Individuals with severe liver disease may have impaired ability to biotransform SSRIs, so dosages may need to be reduced and should be monitored. SSRIs should be used with caution for patients with seizure disorders.

INTERACTIONS

SSRIs bind to plasma protein and may displace other drugs, especially oral anticoagulants and phenytoin. The central nervous system (CNS) depression of other drugs can be potentiated by SSRIs. Tryptophan should not be taken concurrently with SSRIs because it also affects serotonin levels. SSRIs are potent inhibitors of

25

5

TABLE 18-2

Incidence of Adverse Effects of Antidepressant Drugs

| | Autonomic Nervous System | Central Nervous System | | Cardiovascular | | Others | | |
Drug	Anticholinergic	Drowsiness	Insomnia/ Agitation	Orthostatic Hypotension	Cardiac Arrhythmias	GI Distress	Weight Gain (0.6 kg)	Sexual Adverse Effects
Tricylic Antidepressants								
amitriptyline	++++	++++	0	++++	++++	0	++	++++
amoxapine	++	+	0/+	++	+++	0	+	+++
clomipramine	++++	+++	0	++	++++	+	++	++++
desipramine	+	+	+	+	++	0/+	+	+++
doxepin	+++	++++	0	++	++++	0/+	++	+++
imipramine	+++	+++	0/+	+++	++++	+	+++	+++
maprotiline	+++	+++	0	+++	+++	0	+	+++
nortriptyline	+	+	0	+	++	0	+	+++
protriptyline	+++	0/+	++	++	++++	0	+	+++
trimipramine	++++	++++	0	++	++++	0	++	+++
Atypical Antidepressants								
bupropion	0	0	++	0	0	+	0	0
mirtazapine	0	++++	0	0/+	0	0/+	++	0
nefazone	0	++++	0	0	0/+	+++	0/+	0/+
trazodone	0	++++	0	0	0/+	+++	+	+
venlafaxine	0	0	+	0	+	++	0	+++
SSRIs*	0	0/+	+	0	0	++++	0	++++
MAOIs†	0	0	++	++	0	+	++	+++

Modified from Clinical practice guideline: depression in primary care, *AHCPR Pub. No. 93-0552*, Rockville, MD, April 1993, U.S. Department of Health and Human Services, Agency for Health Care Policy and Research. Also modified from Bladessarini RJ, Tarazi FI: Drugs in the treatment of psychiatric disorders, psychosis and mania. In Hardman HG, Limbird LE, Gilman AF (eds): *The pharmacological basis of therapeutics*, ed 10, New York, 2001, McGraw-Hill.

KEY: *0*: effect not typically noted; *0/+*: effect may rarely occur; +, ++, +++, ++++: effect occurs, with + designating the lowest incidence and ++++ designating the highest incidence or severity.

*SSRIs, Selective serotonin reuptake inhibitors (citalopram, escitalopram, fluoxetine, fluvoxamine, paroxetine, sertraline and venlafaxine).

†MAOIs, Monoamine oxidase inhibitors (isocarboxid, moclobemide, phenelzine, and tranylcypromine).

liver enzymes and may potentiate the effect of other drugs biotransformed by the liver. These include, but are not limited to, tricyclic antidepressants, phenytoin, carbamazepine, and several antipsychotic drugs. All SSRIs are contraindicated for concomitant use with monoamine oxidase inhibitors (MAOIs) because of the dangerous and potentially lethal consequences. The combination of an SSRI and an MAOI may result in a severe **serotonergic syndrome**, which is characterized by autonomic instability, rigidity, hyperpyrexia, widely fluctuating vital signs, stuporous rigidity, and possibly death. People taking MAOIs or SSRIs should wait a minimum of 14 days after ending treatment with one type of drug to begin treatment with the other type.

DRUG CLASS • Tricyclic Antidepressants (TCAs)

amitriptyline (Elavil, Endep, Levate,✳ Meravil,✳ Novo-Triptyn✳)

amoxapine (Asendin)

clomipramine (Anafranil)

desipramine (Norpramin, Pertofrane)

doxepin (Adapin, Sinequan, Novo-Dosepin,✳ Triadapin✳)

imipramine (Tofranil, Tipramine, Janimine, Apo-Imipramine,✳ Impril,✳ Novo-Pramine✳)

maprotiline (Ludiomil)

nortriptyline (Aventyl, Pamelor)

protriptyline (Vivactil, Triptil✳)

trimipramine (Surmontil)

MECHANISM OF ACTION

Tricyclic antidepressants (TCAs) block the reuptake of norepinephrine and serotonin into the presynaptic neurons (see Figure 18-1). Blockade of reuptake by itself, however, cannot fully explain the therapeutic effectiveness of TCAs because clinical responses (antidepressant) and the biochemical effects (blockade) do not occur in the same time frame. Therefore it appears that an intermediary response must be occurring between the onset of the blockade and the onset of the therapeutic response. Recent research suggests that TCAs alter the sensitivity of receptors to the action of norepinephrine and serotonin. Although altered receptor sensitivity more closely correlates with the onset of the clinical antidepressant action, whether or not it accounts for the antidepressant actions of TCAs remains unknown. Amoxapine is a chemical metabolite of the antipsychotic drug loxapine and, as with the antipsychotic drugs, blocks dopamine receptors.

USES

TCAs are indicated for the treatment of depressive episodes of major depression, bipolar disorder, dysthymia, and atypical depression. They elevate mood, increase activity and alertness, decrease morbid preoccupation, improve appetite, and normalize sleep patterns. Relieving the depression can take a number of weeks. TCAs also are used for the treatment of chronic pain syndromes (amitriptyline, doxepin, imipramine, nortriptyline), neuropathy, migraine headache, attention-deficit hyperactivity disorder, and enuresis (imipramine only). They also are effective in severe anxiety disorders such as panic attacks, panicagoraphobia, and obsessive-compulsive disorder.

PHARMACOKINETICS

TCAs are usually given orally, although amitriptyline and imipramine are available in injectable forms for cases of severe depression. All TCAs are widely distributed throughout the body, and effective relief of depression is achieved within 2 to 6 weeks. They are over 90% bound to plasma proteins, with half-lives ranging from 8 to more than 67 hours. They also are strongly bound to tissues, especially the heart, which adds to the potential for cardiotoxicity (see below). Most TCAs are extensively biotransformed in the liver and secreted into gastric juices. Some metabolites of TCAs are active, so an active form of the drug will persist in the body for a long time. Amitriptyline is biotransformed to nortriptyline, an active TCA, whereas desipramine is a metabolite of imipramine. The rate of TCA biotransformation is rapid in children and decreases with age. People more than 55 years old generally are started at half of the regular adult dosage.

ADVERSE REACTIONS AND CONTRAINDICATIONS

The relative incidence of adverse effects among the TCAs is given in Table 18-2, with the major adverse effects being antimuscarinic or atropinelike effects and sedation. Because of these adverse effects, TCAs are usually given before bedtime so that the patient is asleep when the adverse effects are at their peak. The more sedating TCAs, amitriptyline and doxepin, are particularly effective in relieving the insomnia of depression when given at bedtime. These drugs do not interfere with normal sleep patterns.

The anticholinergic adverse effects include dry mouth, blurred vision, and constipation. Some patients may experience temporary confusion or speech blockage. Patients with glaucoma or those at risk for glaucoma must have this condition evaluated, because the anticholinergic effect may increase intraocular pressure. The anticholinergic action also may adversely affect patients, particularly older adults with urinary retention or obstruction.

Cardiac effects have been a major limitation of TCAs, including actions such as anticholinergic effects, blockade of alpha-adrenergic receptors, blockade of reuptake of norepinephrine from sympathetic nerves, and a quinidinelike action. Therefore the final cardiac effect is complex and depends on the dosage. The anticholinergic action increases heart rate. The quinidinelike adverse effects (i.e., decreased heart rate, myocardial contractility, and coronary blood flow) are seen with high concentrations of TCAs. Both mechanisms increase the risk of arrhythmias (premature atrial and ventricular contractions, ST segment depression, flattened or inverted T waves, and a prolonged QRS segment). Heart failure can be worsened. Therefore TCAs are contraindicated for patients with a recent myocardial infarction and they present special concern for the patient with cardiac disease. Patients who have hyperthyroidism and who are at risk for developing arrhythmias have this risk potentiated by TCAs.

Orthostatic hypotension is also a common adverse effect of TCAs. It is caused, in part, by the blockade of alpha$_1$-adrenergic receptors on blood vessels. The action to prevent the reuptake of norepinephrine into neurons tends to deplete norepinephrine stores in peripheral neurons. This decrease in blood pressure affects the heart by reducing the workload.

Sedation, muscle tremors or twitches, numbness, fatigue, weakness, and seizures may occur with overdose or in patients with known seizure disorders. Maprotiline may cause a higher incidence of seizures, even in patients with no known seizure disorder. Concurrent administration of other drugs known to lower the seizure threshold is to be avoided. The chemical structure of amoxapine is similar to some antipsychotic drugs; thus there is a remote possibility of neuroleptic malignant syndrome and extrapyramidal symptoms. In addition, hallucinations, delusions, and activation of schizophrenic or manic states may also occur.

Adverse gastrointestinal (GI) effects include nausea, vomiting, and heartburn, as well as weight loss and weight gain. TCAs can also cause sexual dysfunction, which is manifested as decreased libido, reduced arousal, and impaired orgasm. A comparison of the relative severity of the adverse effects of TCAs is found in Table 18-2.

TOXICITY

TCAs are not addictive, and their abuse potential appears limited. A major problem is their acute toxicity when depressed patients overdose on TCAs in a suicide attempt. Indeed, TCAs do not decrease the suicide potential among depressed patients during the early weeks of therapy. The toxic effects of overdose are analogous to anticholinergic poisoning. The early symptoms are confusion, inability to concentrate, and, sometimes, visual hallucinations. More severe signs include delirium, seizures, and coma. Respirations may be depressed. The patient may have a low body temperature early but an elevated body temperature later. The pupils are dilated, the eyeballs are restless, the reflexes are hyperactive, and motor coordination is compromised. Depending on the patient's cardiac status and the degree of overdose, the overall cardiac effects may range from increased heart rate (tachycardia) to a slow heart rate (bradycardia) to various arrhythmias related to an atrioventricular (A-V) block. Especially serious is the slowing of conduction in the A-V node by the quinidinelike action, which can result in heart block. Sudden death from arrhythmias may occur several days after an overdose. Physostigmine, a peripherally and centrally active anticholinesterase drug, reverses the anticholinergic toxic effects of a TCA overdose. This drug must be administered often because it is short acting, whereas TCAs are long acting.

INTERACTIONS

TCAs can potentiate CNS depression, anticholinergic actions, and sympathomimetic effects for a number of drug classes, including antihistamines, phenothiazines, thioxanthenes, and sympathomimetics. Because they are highly bound to plasma proteins, TCAs can interact with other drugs that are extensively bound. Cimetidine and methylphenidate inhibit the metabolism of TCAs, potentially leading to an overdose. Metrizamide may increase the risk of seizures, whereas antithyroid drugs increase the risk of agranulocytosis. The interaction of guanethidine and a TCA is classic; the TCA inhibits the uptake of guanethidine by the neurons so that guanethidine cannot reach its site of action and is therefore ineffective in lowering blood pressure. Clonidine also is blocked by TCAs and may be rendered ineffective. Monoamine oxidase inhibitors and antiarrhythmics have potentially fatal drug interactions with TCAs and should not be administered concurrently.

DRUG CLASS • Atypical Antidepressants

bupropion (Wellbutrin, Zyban)

mirtazapine (Remeron)

nefazodone (Serzone)

reboxetine (Edronax, Vestra)

trazodone (Desyrel, Trazon, Trialodine)

venlafaxine (Effexor)

MECHANISM OF ACTION

Various antidepressant drugs have been introduced that are neither TCAs, SSRIs, nor MAOIs (see Table 18-1). As with other antidepressants, the mechanism of action of the atypical antidepressants remains unknown, but they block the reuptake of norepinephrine, serotonin, or both. Bupropion differs from TCAs in having a stimulant rather than a sedative effect. It weakly blocks the uptake of norepinephrine, dopamine, and serotonin. Mirtazapine blocks noradrenergic and serotonergic reuptake, is an antagonist at presynaptic alpha$_2$-adrenergic receptors, and blocks 5-HT$_2$ and 5-HT$_3$ receptors. Nefazodone is structurally related to trazodone; it blocks presynaptic serotonin and norepinephrine reuptake and antagonizes alpha$_1$-adrenergic receptors. Reboxetine is a selective inhibitor of norepinephrine reuptake and antagonizes presynaptic alpha$_2$-adrenergic receptors. Trazodone inhibits serotonin uptake but also inhibits alpha-adrenergic receptors. Venlafaxine is a potent inhibitor of serotonin reuptake, is slightly less potent at preventing norepinephrine reuptake, and is a weak inhibitor of dopamine reuptake. It does not appear to have significant actions on adrenergic or serotonergic receptors.

USES

The atypical antidepressants are primarily used to treat depression. As with other drugs, the onset of effectiveness is 1 to 4 weeks. An extended-release form of bupropion is used in nicotine dependence to aid smoking cessation efforts. In addition to treating depression, trazodone is used for chronic pain in diabetic neuropathy and other neuropathic pain conditions. Venlafaxine is also used to treat anxiety.

PHARMACOKINETICS

The atypical antidepressants are rapidly absorbed after oral administration and peak plasma concentrations occur within 1 to 2 hours, depending on the drug. Mirtazapine, nefazodone, and venlafaxine have a significant first-pass effect in which approximately 50%, 20%, and 45%, respectively, of an oral dose enters systemic circulation. In contrast, reboxetine is well absorbed and has a high bioavailability. An extended-release preparation of venlafaxine is available. The atypical antidepressants are widely distributed throughout the body and all except venlafaxine are highly bound to plasma proteins. They are biotransformed in the liver, with a large portion of the elimination of metabolites occurring in the kidney and a small portion in the feces. Fifty-six percent of venlafaxine is converted to its active metabolite O-desmethylvenlafaxine (ODV).

ADVERSE REACTIONS AND CONTRAINDICATIONS

The atypical antidepressant drugs have, to a varying degree, a lower incidence of anticholinergic adverse effects, and less cardiotoxicity than TCAs. Adverse effects of bupropion include agitation, anxiety, restlessness, insomnia, anorexia, and weight loss. It carries a significant risk of seizures and is specifically of concern in patients who have a history of seizures, head injury, anorexia or bulimia (i.e., electrolyte imbalance), and those who are taking other drugs that lower the seizure threshold. Cardiac effects are uncommon. Mirtazapine causes shortness of breath, edema, flulike symptoms, sexual dysfunction, mood changes, and, rarely, agranulocytosis and seizures. Its adverse effect profile includes weight gain and sedation. Nefazodone can cause sedation, gait disturbances, abnormal vision, skin rash, and itching. Rare allergic reactions and photosensitivity have been noted. GI effects may include anorexia, altered taste, nausea, vomiting, dry mouth, dyspepsia, and constipation. Reboxetine can significantly increase resting heart rate and slightly increase blood pressure. Other adverse effects include blurred vision, dry mouth, insomnia, sweating, and constipation. Trazodone can produce sedation, confusion, muscle tremors, and GI distress. Rarely, men may experience priapism (prolonged painful erection). Venlafaxine has an adverse effect profile that includes headache, sexual dysfunction, decreased libido, nausea (especially in high or rapidly increased dosages), vision disturbances, nervousness, constipation, dizziness, sweating, and fatigue. Venlafaxine is also associated with sustained increase in blood pressure in some patients. A comparison of the adverse effect profile of these drugs is found in Table 18-2.

INTERACTIONS

The atypical antidepressants are contraindicated in patients taking MAOIs, since serious or fatal interactions can occur. Bupropion should not be combined with alcohol, levodopa, or drugs that lower the seizure threshold. Mirtazapine also interacts with alcohol and its effects are additive with those of CNS depressants. Because nefazodone, reboxetine, and trazodone are extensively bound to plasma proteins, concurrent administration of another highly protein-bound drug may cause increased free concentrations of the drug, possibly resulting in adverse events. This risk is especially great when the drug or drugs interacting with the antidepressants compete for biotransformation in the liver. Hepatic impairment by other drugs for disease has the potential of significantly increasing levels of the atypical antidepressants in the plasma. Concurrent administration of trazodone with antihypertensive drugs can increase the incidence of hypotension.

DRUG CLASS • Monoamine Oxidase Inhibitors (MAOIs)

isocarboxazid (Marplan)

moclobemide (Manerix✱)

phenelzine (Nardil)

tranylcypromine (Parnate)

Monoamine oxidase inhibitors (MAOIs) were synthesized in the early 1950s as a byproduct of research into newer, more effective antituberculosis drugs. It was soon found that iproniazid had mood-elevating effects in tuberculosis patients. The patients became energized, hyperactive, and, in some cases, manic. As investigators assessed patient responses they concluded that iproniazid was capable of inhibiting the enzyme monoamine oxidase (MAO). Thus, MAOIs had an important impact on the development of modern biologic psychiatry. (These drugs also are listed in Table 18-1.)

MECHANISM OF ACTION

MAOIs exert their effects primarily on organ systems influenced by monoamine oxidases, the enzymes that biotransform norepinephrine and serotonin. MAOIs cause the amount of these transmitters to increase (see Fig. 18-1). The increased transmission that results is thought to be key to relief of depression. There are two major isozymes of MAO: monoamine oxidase A (MAOA) and monoamine oxidase B (MAOB). MAOA preferentially has serotonin as a substrate, whereas MAOB prefers phenethylamine. These drugs (except moclobemide) produce irreversible inhibition of intraneuronal MAO, which is largely MAOA, but also block MAOB.

USES

MAOIs are less commonly used because of their potential for drug interactions and poor safety profile that requires strict adherence to dietary limitations. Because their use can be hazardous, they are reserved for patients who have not responded to TCAs, SSRIs, newer drugs, or electroconvulsive therapy (ECT). However, for patients with atypical depression, MAOIs may be the drugs of first choice. They also have been used with some success in the treatment of panic disorder, bulimia, obsessive-compulsive disorders, and agoraphobia.

PHARMACOKINETICS

MAOIs are well absorbed when taken orally. They are biotransformed in the liver to inactive forms and excreted in urine. The onset of action requires 2 to 3 weeks. Because MAOIs act by irreversible inhibition, their effect persists for 2 to 3 weeks after discontinuation, reflecting the time needed to synthesize new enzymes.

ADVERSE REACTIONS AND CONTRAINDICATIONS

Sedation and orthostatic hypotension are adverse effects associated with MAOIs. Restlessness, insomnia, anorexia, constipation, nausea, vomiting, dry mouth, urinary retention, impotence, drowsiness, headache, rash, dizziness, and weakness have also been noted. Tranylcypromine can have a stimulatory action similar to amphetamine.

Adverse effects of MAOIs are dose dependent for the most part; however, they cause severe hypertension when taken with foods containing large amounts of tyramine (Box 18-2). Following ingestion of tyramine, there is a rapid displacement and release of norepinephrine from noradrenergic neurons. Under normal conditions, the ingested tyramine is metabolized by MAOA in the gut and liver so a limited amount circu-

 Dietary Considerations: Monoamine Oxidase Inhibitors and Tyramine

Patients taking monoamine oxidase inhibitors may experience a hypertensive crisis (characterized by severe chest pain, hypertension, severe headache, photophobia, clammy skin, nausea, and palpitations) if they ingest foods containing a large amount of tyramine. Foods high in tyramine include the following:

- Avocados
- Bananas
- Beer
- Bologna
- Canned figs
- Chocolate
- Cheese (except cottage cheese)
- Cheese-containing food (e.g., pizza, macaroni and cheese)
- Liver
- Meat extracts (e.g., Marmite, Bovril)
- Papaya products, including meat tenderizers
- Paté
- Pickled and kippered herring
- Pepperoni
- Pods or broad beans (fava beans)
- Preserved meat products (e.g., potted ham)
- Raisins
- Raw yeast or yeast extracts
- Salami
- Sausage
- Sour cream
- Soy sauce
- Wine and Chianti
- Yogurt

lates. In addition, the released norepinephrine is taken back up by the nerve terminals and broken down by MAO. In the presence of MAOIs, the tryamine and norepinephrine are not biotransformed and the norepinephrine accumulates, resulting in severe hypertension. This hypertensive crisis is the most serious and potentially fatal adverse effect of MAOI therapy. Severe headache, nausea, vomiting, sweating, neck stiffness and soreness, and mydriasis also occur. Intracranial hemorrhage also can result, which may lead to death.

TOXICITY

Symptoms of toxicity appear within 12 hours of an overdose of an MAOI and reflect increased adrenergic activity such as restlessness, anxiety, and insomnia, progressing to include tachycardia and sometimes seizures. Dizziness and hypotension may occur, whereas some patients have severe headaches and develop high blood pressure. Some patients develop a high fever. Treatment is supportive to maintain respiration and circulation. Because the effect of MAOIs is persistent, patients must be monitored for at least 1 week.

INTERACTIONS

Several clinically significant problems arise from the interaction of MAOIs with other drugs and certain foods containing tyramine. A hypertensive crisis may be precipitated when a food containing tyramine (see Box 18-2) or

---

CASE STUDY  *Major Depression*

ASSESSMENT

HISTORY OF PRESENT ILLNESS

MG is a 76-year-old white woman who complains of sad mood, intermittent crying, hypersomnia, weight loss, and lack of appetite. She has decreased energy, focus, and concentration. She notes feelings of hopelessness and helplessness, anhedonia, and vague suicidal ideation. Her symptoms have been present now for more than 2 months. Her daughter suspects she is depressed because her husband of 55 years died 4 months ago.

HEALTH HISTORY

MG has a history of mild depression, as well as hyperlipidemia and coronary artery disease confirmed by a cardiac catheterization 2 months ago. She is a nonsmoker with no history of alcohol abuse. She has a family history of depression, Alzheimer's disease, and alcoholism. She had a head injury 4 years ago as a result of a fall, but she takes no drugs and has had no seizures since the original injury. Her current drug regimen includes nifedipine 10 mg tid, Transderm-Nitro patch once daily, 1 baby aspirin qd, atorvastatin 20 mg, and phenytoin sodium 300 mg at hs.

LIFESPAN CONSIDERATIONS

MG considers herself "old" and is having a difficult time adapting to a decline in her speed of movement, reaction time, sensory abilities, and problem-solving capabilities. She is unhappy with her increasing dependence on her daughter for transportation.

CULTURAL/SOCIAL CONSIDERATIONS

MG is a retired accountant. Her health has kept her from working part-time with her former partners. Her degree of compliance is judged to be adequate. MG has health insurance that covers prescriptions.

PHYSICAL EXAMINATION

The examination results are unremarkable; vital signs are stable (VSS); MG appears withdrawn.

LABORATORY TESTING

CBC, thyroid function tests, B_{12}, and folate levels are within normal limits.

PATIENT PROBLEM(S)

MG meets DSM-IV criteria for major depression.

GOALS OF THERAPY

Relieve major depression. Reestablish sleeping, eating, and normal ADL patterns.

CRITICAL THINKING QUESTIONS

1. What factors in MG's life may be contributing to her depression?
2. The health care provider orders sertraline daily for MG. What other classes of drugs could be effectively used to treat her major depression?
3. Why do you think the health care provider ordered an SSRI for MG rather than a TCA?
4. What potential drug interactions may occur with MG's sertraline therapy? What activity is required to monitor for this drug interaction?
5. After 1 week on sertraline, MG's daughter calls you aside and seems very upset. "She's just not any better! I expected my mother to be more cheerful by now! What is going on here?" What is the best response to her concerns?
6. Of which adverse effects of sertraline should MG and her daughter be aware?

indirect-acting sympathomimetic drugs (e.g., cough and cold drugs, asthma drugs, phenylephrine, ephedrine, and amphetamine) are ingested. The necessity of avoiding these substances to avert a life-threatening hypertensive crisis is the major limitation of MAOIs. Meperidine can cause hyperpyrexia. Thus, if an analgesic is needed, a drug other than meperidine should be chosen. The use of antihypertensive drugs with MAOIs may cause excessive lowering of blood pressure.

When MAOIs are taken in combination with TCAs, they can produce hypertensive episodes or crises. They should also not be administered with SSRIs or tryptophan since this can produce a serotonergic syndrome consisting of altered mental status with confusion, agitation, disorientation, poor concentration, and restlessness along with muscle spasms and exaggerated reflexes, shivering, and sweating.

PATHOPHYSIOLOGY • Bipolar Disorders

Bipolar disorder (previously known as manic-depressive disorder) is a mood disorder characterized by expansive emotional states, flight of ideas, hyperactivity, destructive behaviors, and psychotic processes. It consists of periods of depression alternating with mania, usually separated by periods of near-normal function. It is estimated that approximately 40% of all patients with mania present with a mixture of depressed mood and hyperactivity. They report feeling dysphoric, depressed, and unhappy yet exhibit the characteristic energy associated with mania. This state is often complicated by concomitant substance abuse because it is common to find bipolar patients attempting to self-treat with drugs and alcohol. Patients with bipolar disorder may cycle only a few times within a lifetime, or they may cycle once or twice a year. Patients with rapid-cycling bipolar disorder may have four or more distinct, complete cycles within a year. Some patients with ultrarapid cycling describe almost constant, quick up-and-down cycling. Bipolar disorders appear to have a strong genetic component, and at least 2 million Americans have bipolar disorder.

Mania is thought to be caused by increased levels of some of the same neurotransmitters that cause depression (i.e., serotonin, norepinephrine, and others). In theory, if a relative lack of neurotransmitters contributes to depression, then a relative excess may contribute to what appears to be an opposite mood state, mania.

Hypomania

Hypomania is an expansive, energized portion of the mood cycle, characterized by disturbances in speech, cognition, judgment, self-concept, and behavior. Hypomania is a mood state that must last at least 4 days. Accompanying this mood are other disturbances, such as inflated self-esteem, flight of ideas, distractibility, increased involvement in goal-directed activity, or psychomotor agitation. Another symptom of hypomania is excessive involvement in pleasurable activities that have a high potential for painful consequences. Hypomania may progress in some individuals to full mania, which is characterized by a more amplified and sustained version of hypomania, as well as delusions or hallucinations.

Mania

A full manic mood state lasts at least a week and is accompanied by the other characteristics noted previously. The disturbance is severe enough to cause significant impairment in social or occupational functioning. Hallucinations or delusions must be present since they are the defining characteristics that delineate hypomania from full mania; in some cases, hospitalization is required. The mood is often euphoric, characterized by unceasing, indiscriminate enthusiasm, and may be intrusive. The mood, however, may be consistently irritable or labile, alternating between euphoria and irritability.

It is common for an individual in a manic state to give advice to anyone encountered and write letters to or communicate with important officials, offering direction. Manics may believe that they have a special relationship with famous people or religious figures, including God. Manic individuals may dress in loud clothing or wear excessive makeup, jewelry, or extreme hairstyles. There is almost invariably a decreased need for sleep, and the person may not sleep at all for days at a time. Manic speech is typically loud, pressured, tangential, nonstop, rapid, and difficult to interrupt. Irritable manics are critical and make cutting remarks. Manic individuals complain of racing thoughts that cannot be stopped or slowed down. While acutely manic, they frequently engage in reckless and dangerous activities, such as excessive, inappropriate, or unprotected sexual relations, poor business investments and decisions, and buying sprees, and they may exercise poor judgment in other areas of life. These activities are all pursued despite the painful consequences the acts may cause. The person does not recognize illness and resists treatment, often adamantly.

DRUG CLASS • Antimania or Mood-Altering Drugs

carbamazepine (Atretol, Tegretol, Apo-Carbamazepine✽)

divalproex sodium (Depakote, Epival✽)

⚕ lithium (Eskalith, Lithane, Lithizine✽)

valproic acid (Depakene)

MECHANISM OF ACTION

The mechanism by which lithium and anticonvulsants are effective in mania remains unknown. Lithium decreases the release of norepinephrine and dopamine in the CNS, an action that supports the theory that an excess of these transmitters contributes to manic episodes. Lithium also affects transduction cascades in neurons, especially interfering with phosphatidylinositol metabolism and blocking the actions of protein kinase C. This latter action is shared by valproic acid. Lithium and valproic acid also alter gene expression in neurons, but whether this is related to their mood stabilizing actions remains to be determined.

USES

Although lithium is the drug of choice for treating the manic phase of bipolar disorders, its slow onset of action limits its effectiveness in acute manic episodes. Rather, it is the drug of choice to prevent manic episodes. If a patient is having an acute manic attack, an antipsychotic drug such as haloperidol (see Chapter 19) or a benzodiazepine with sedative properties (see Chapter 17) is used to control the agitation. Continuous lithium therapy is indicated for patients in whom lithium reduces the frequency and intensity of their manic-depressive disorder. Evidence shows that lithium may be effective in treating the depression component of bipolar disorder and even endogenous depression. Carbamazepine and valproic acid are used for patients who fail to respond to lithium or who cannot tolerate lithium's adverse effects. These mood-stabilizing drugs are most often used for the treatment of rapid-cycling bipolar disorder (Table 18-3).

PHARMACOKINETICS

Lithium is administered orally as the carbonate or citrate salt and is rapidly and completely absorbed in the GI tract in 1 to 2 hours. It is widely distributed to many tissues and body fluids, crossing placental membranes and entering breast milk in low concentrations. Because lithium is an element related in the atomic table to sodium and potassium, it is not biotransformed but is eliminated by mechanisms similar to those for sodium and potassium. Of the lithium filtered in the kidney, 80% is reabsorbed in the proximal tubule, and 20% is eliminated in the urine. The plasma half-life of lithium is 24 hours but is increased to 36 hours in older adult

---

TABLE 18-3

Antimanic Drugs

Generic Name	Brand Name	Comments
Lithium		
lithium carbonate	Eskalith Lithane Lithizine ✽ Lithonate Lithotabs	Blood should not be drawn for determination of lithium levels earlier than 8 hr after last dose; levels above 2 mEq/L are toxic Patients should be instructed not to make up missed dose of lithium
lithium citrate	Cibalith-Si	
Other Drugs		
carbamazepine	Apo-Carbamazepine ✽ Atretol Tegretol Others	Used alone or in combination with lithium and/or antidepressants to treat bipolar illness in patients unresponsive to lithium alone
valproic acid	Depakene Depakote Epival ✽ Others	For treating acute manic symptoms Delayed-release tablets lessen GI side effects

✽ Available only in Canada.

patients, so the relative dosage of lithium must be decreased to avoid the accumulation to toxic levels. When lithium therapy is stopped, there is a rapid and slow phase of elimination. Factors that decrease lithium elimination include sodium deficiency, extreme exercise, diarrhea, and postpartum status, whereas those that increase lithium elimination include high sodium intake and pregnancy.

The absorption of carbamazepine is slow, but it is almost completely absorbed from the GI tract. It is moderately protein bound at 55% to 75% and is biotransformed in the liver. Carbamazepine can induce its own biotransformation as well as that of many other drugs. With repeated dosing, the half-life is 8 to 29 hours, with an average of 12 to 17 hours.

Valproic acid is rapidly and efficiently absorbed from the GI tract. The divalproex sodium formulation is enteric coated, so absorption is delayed by 1 to 4 hours. Food may significantly slow the rate but not the extent of absorption. Peak serum concentrations are reached 1 to 4 hours after administration of the capsule or syrup. Delayed-release capsules reach peak serum concentrations in 3 to 4 hours. Valproic acid is rapidly distributed throughout the body and 90% to 95% plasma protein bound. It is primarily biotransformed in the liver, with minimal amounts eliminated unchanged in the urine.

ADVERSE REACTIONS AND CONTRAINDICATIONS

The adverse effects of lithium can be categorized as those that occur at therapeutic levels and those most likely to occur at toxic levels (Table 18-4). In the therapeutic range, these responses may include GI effects (e.g., anorexia, nausea, bloating, and diarrhea), transient headache, fatigue, confusion, memory impairment, and muscle weakness. Early in treatment 30% to 50% of patients experience thirst and polyuria, which can continue with chronic lithium use. Drug-induced fine hand tremors that interfere with writing and other motor skills may be noted.

Secretion of the thyroid hormone thyroxine is inhibited by lithium, and a few patients develop an enlarged thyroid gland and may become hypothyroid. A few patients who receive lithium therapy develop nephrogenic diabetes insipidus, which is reversed when the lithium dosage is lowered or discontinued. A more serious consequence is permanent renal damage (initially without symptoms), which may develop with long-term lithium therapy. Renal function should be evaluated periodically for patients on long-term therapy. Lithium is contraindicated in early pregnancy because an increased incidence of congenital malformations in infants of treated mothers has been noted.

Carbamazepine's adverse effects include nausea, blurred vision, and ataxia. There are also cases of leukopenia, thrombocytopenia, and aplastic anemia. Patients must be monitored for renal, liver, and bone marrow functions. Valproic acid has most commonly been associated with indigestion, nausea, and vomiting. Hepatotoxicity is the most serious adverse effect. Other adverse effects include drowsiness, sedation, headache, dizziness, ataxia, and confusion.

TOXICITY

The therapeutic index for lithium is relatively small, and at the start of treatment, patients are tested at least weekly to ensure that the plasma level is in the therapeutic range. The therapeutic range is 0.6 to 1.2 mEq/L but can be as low as 0.2 mEq/L in older adults. Toxic symptoms begin to appear at 1.5 to 2 mEq/L and by 4 mEq/L may be fatal. The symptoms of toxicity are listed in Table 18-4 and include myoclonic jerks, seizures, impaired consciousness, coma, and, ultimately, death. Renal failure and nephrogenic diabetes insipidus are common consequences of toxicity. Although toxicity usually resolves without complications once dosages are lowered or stopped, some patients die and others develop persistent neurologic disabilities. The most common cause of lithium accumulation in compliant patients is sodium depletion and dehydration, which reduces the volume of distribution of lithium and increases lithium levels.

Hastening lithium excretion while maintaining fluid and electrolyte balance treats acute lithium toxicity. Lithium excretion is increased by administration of an osmotic diuretic such as urea or mannitol. The drugs

TABLE 18-4
Toxic Symptoms of Lithium at Various Blood Levels

Blood Level (mEq/L)	Signs and Symptoms
1.5	Fine tremor of hands, dry mouth, increased thirst, increased urination, nausea
1.5-2	Vomiting, diarrhea, muscle weakness, uncoordination (ataxia), dizziness, confusion, slurred speech
2-2.5	Persisitent nausea and vomiting, blurred vision, muscle twitching (fasciculations), hyperactive deep tendon reflexes
2.5-3	Myoclonic twitches or movements of an entire limb, choreoathetoid movements, urinary and fecal incontinence
>3	Seizures, arrhythmias, hypotension, peripheral vascular collapse; death

aminophylline and acetazolamide increase lithium excretion, and one may be given concurrently with the osmotic diuresis. Peritoneal dialysis, or preferably hemodialysis, may be used for severe toxicity or when renal failure occurs.

INTERACTIONS

A large number of drug interactions occur with lithium. Thiazide and loop diuretics, potassium-sparing diuretics, amiloride, and nonsteroidal antiinflammatory drugs (except aspirin) create a definite reduction in renal elimination of lithium. An especially problematic combination may be lithium, carbamazepine, and diuretics because these drugs may dramatically alter normal renal function and fluid and electrolyte balance. Lithium potentiates the effects of haloperidol, TCAs, phenothiazines, benzodiazepines, and neuromuscular-blocking drugs.

 APPLICATION TO PRACTICE

ASSESSMENT
History of Present Illness

The assessment of the depressed patient should include a determination of physical and psychologic symptoms that occurred during the month before the visit to the health care provider. Information about the onset, duration, and course of these symptoms should be obtained. How severe and frequent are the symptoms? How long have they been present? Are these symptoms new or have they occurred before? Does the patient have difficulty functioning in the workplace or at home? Are interpersonal relationships affected by these symptoms?

The first objective in obtaining a history of present illness for the patient with mania is to establish the current mood state (e.g., depression, mania, hypomania, or mixed). This is often difficult when the patient is acutely ill. During episodes patients rarely complain of the symptoms that comprise hypomania or mania but are more likely to acknowledge symptoms when asked a direct question (e.g., "This week, how many hours have you actually been sleeping?"). Even with direct questions, denial of symptoms should be expected, not because patients are necessarily attempting to deceive the health care provider, but because the patient with mood elevation is, in general, insensitive to problems. Many patients with mania do, however, report their mood as depressed and are very aware when they are feeling irritable or annoyed. Accuracy of diagnosis is improved by a brief systematic inquiry into mood and symptoms associated with acute episodes. Useful questions include: How many days in the past 10 days has your mood been depressed or abnormally elevated, even briefly? How many of those days has your mood been depressed, abnormally elevated, or excessively irritable most of the day? Did you do anything this month that you or people who know you would regard as unusual behavior for you? If any of present history responses are positive, inquire about recent changes in diet and hydration, history of infection, head trauma or loss of consciousness,

sleep patterns, menstrual regularity, plans for conception, delivery, and lactation.

Health History

Elicit information about the patient's current and past psychiatric history, particularly regarding anxiety disorders and substance abuse. These conditions are quite common in patients with depressive disorders, particularly unipolar disorder. Ask about medical disorders that may be associated with the emergence of depressive symptoms such as hypothyroidism, folate deficiency, hypoadrenalism, rheumatoid arthritis, and Parkinson's disease. The patient may also note other problems along the illness continuum, such as attention-deficit hyperactivity disorder, panic attacks, eating disorders, anxiety, and obsessive-compulsive disorder. There may also be a family history of these disorders, especially bipolar disorder. There may be a personal or family history of drug and alcohol abuse or dependence, or unrestrained sexual behaviors.

Assess the patient's use of psychotropic drugs, alcohol, and dietary habits (in particular carbohydrate intake). Ask about the use of OTC drugs, including dietary supplements and herbal remedies (Box 18-3). Psychoactive substances can cause symptoms that mimic some of those of depressive or bipolar disorders. In addition, the use of these substances may increase when symptoms of depressive disorders worsen, perhaps as an attempt to obtain relief from the psychologic stress. Ask about recent bereavement (i.e., the loss of a loved one in the past month).

Lifespan Considerations

Perinatal. Although earlier reports suggested that pregnancy is a time of decreased risk for the onset of mood disorders, a growing body of literature supports the clinical observation that the prevalence of major and minor depression during pregnancy is approximately 10%. It may be difficult to distinguish the symptoms of depression during pregnancy from the normal symptoms as-

EVIDENCE-BASED PRACTICE
St. John's Wort as an Antidepressant

Setting

Depression, a primary mood disorder characterized by a despondent mood or anhedonia, is estimated to affect 5% to 20% of the American population in a lifetime. Extracts of the plant *Hypericum perforatum* (popularly known as St. John's wort) has long been used in folk medicine for a range of indications, including depressive disorders.

Objective of Literature Review

To determine whether extracts of *Hypericum* are more efficacious than placebo and at least as effective as standard antidepressants in the treatment of depression in adults; and to determine if *Hypericum* has fewer adverse effects than standard antidepressant drugs.

The search was carried out using Medline, Embase, Psychlit, Psychindex, Cochrane Complementary Medicine Field, Cochrane Depression and Neurosis Collaborative Review Group, and Phytodok. In addition, reference lists from the articles were reviewed and the retrieved studies searched for further potentially relevant citations.

Criteria for Inclusion of Studies in Review of Literature

Investigators included randomized studies that compared formulations of *Hypericum* (alone or in combination with other botanicals) with placebo and standard antidepressants. Studies were included if they also included tools to measure depressive symptoms.

Data Extraction and Analysis

Two reviewers independently performed the extraction and analysis of the data and the quality of the studies. Outcome measures for comparing the effectiveness of *Hypericum* to placebo and standard antidepressants used descriptive statistics.

Results of Review

In the 27 studies (*N* = 2291 patients) reviewed, *Hypericum* formulations were significantly superior to placebo and at least as effective as standard antidepressants. Most of the studies were 4 to 6 weeks long and included patients with mild to moderately severe depressive disorders or neurotic depression. Seventeen of the 27 studies were placebo-controlled (16 studies addressed single formulations and one with four other botanicals). Ten of the studies compared *Hypericum* with standard antidepressants or sedative drugs (eight studies addressed single formulations and two with combinations of *Hypericum* and valerian).

The percentage of patients reporting adverse effects to single-ingredient formulations of *Hypericum* were approximately half that of standard antidepressants.

Investigators' Conclusions

Extracts of *Hypericum* are more effective than placebo and at least as effective as standard antidepressants for the short-term treatment of depression. Further research is needed that compares different extracts and dosages of *Hypericum* in defined patients over time to confirm safety and efficacy of the botanical.

Mulrow L: St. John's wort for depression (Cochrane Review). In *The Cochrane Library*, Issue 2, Oxford, 2002: Update Software.

sociated with pregnancy, including impaired sleep, fluctuating appetite, lower energy, and changes in libido. However, these symptoms should not be dismissed, since depression that develops during pregnancy may place both the mother and the fetus at risk. New-onset depression during pregnancy in particular should not be dismissed. It demands the same assessment as that of any other patient with an emerging affective illness. Depression during pregnancy is clinically important since there is no stronger predictor of postpartum depression than affective disturbance during pregnancy. However,

given the concerns about the known and unknown risks of prenatal drug exposure, as well as the risk of untreated psychiatric disorders during pregnancy, health care providers frequently are caught between a "teratogenic rock and a clinical hard place."

Pediatric. Children who have major difficulties in one area of functioning often demonstrate symptoms and difficulties in other areas of their lives. Studies have shown that fewer than 30% of children with substantial dysfunction are recognized, and of these less than half are referred to mental health providers. Often recognition depends on parental complaint or school report of overt behavioral problems. Early recognition, prevention, and less overt dysfunction (e.g., adolescent depression or family factors such as divorce) are much less likely to be addressed. Approaches that may be helpful during the interview include focusing on key, high-risk issues, building a relationship with the child and family, and communicating an interest in psychosocial issues. Ask parents for a family history of psychiatric disorders and about any parental discord or divorce. For a newborn, assess parental coping skills, family supports, and possible maternal depression. Review the infant's temperament and the parents' ability to cope with these traits. Ask about a toddler's autonomy and ability to separate. For an early school-age child, ask about social functioning in first grade. For a child in elementary school, ask about academic ability and extracurricular activities. For the adolescent patient, ask about autonomy, mood, sexual relations and behaviors, and substance abuse.

Confirm screening findings or further define the nature of the parent's or school's complaint, and elaborate on the child's symptoms. Add the context of the family history of psychiatric disorders and current family functioning (e.g., discord or divorce, relationship with child, key losses) to the database. Confirm the safety of the child in his or her current environment.

Older Adults. Older adults are at risk for depression and mood disorders much like other population groups. However, taking a history from an older adult may require patience, close observation, and a systematic approach. Older adults and their families tend to underreport symptoms or to blame the altered physical responses of illness on advancing age. For example, malaise, a decline in mental status, or impaired cognition may be a symptom of an infection, myocardial infarction, or stroke. Visual and auditory impairments, cognitive decline, slowed responses to questions, and vague complaints are other obstacles that can make an interview arduous and less informative.

Many older adults are unable to formulate a single complaint or problem; the problem is often wrapped in a complex array of vague complaints and family issues. A complaint related to mental status may be buried among complaints related to multiple organ systems and chronic conditions. Confusion, personality change, lack of interest, and fatigue may be the only complaints relating to an acute medical illness. However, medical symptoms such as malaise, constipation, chronic pain, and a decline in physical function may be somatic manifestations of psychiatric illness in the older adult. Direct questioning of family members rather than the patient usu-

ally does not aid in history taking and may distance the health care provider from the patient because the family is often baffled by the behavior of their older adult.

Be sure to ask about the older adult's social history. Determine whether the patient lives independently in his or her own home or apartment and whether the patient or family want to continue with the current arrangements. Ask, tactfully, if the patient lives on a fixed income. Expensive drugs, food, housing, and transportation issues lead to poor compliance. Proper nutrition depends on multiple factors so ask about medical and psychiatric health, dentition, and financial status. Asking a patient what he or she does in a typical day provides insight into the patient's dependent or independent ability to carry out the activities of daily living. The issues of advanced directives, durable medical power of attorney, and health care proxy should be addressed.

The misuse of psychoactive drugs may obscure an undiagnosed medical disorder, increase the risk of falls and hypotensive reactions, or allow use of drugs as a quick solution when environmental or interpersonal interventions would be far more appropriate. Because of these concerns, a set of federal guidelines has been constructed for the rational use of psychoactive drugs in nursing home patients (see Chapter 19). Further, the physical changes of aging in older adults must be considered, because elimination of these drugs is primarily through the kidneys.

Cultural/Social Considerations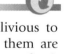

Patients with bipolar disorder are often oblivious to their mood cycling, although those around them are acutely aware of the situation. Manic patients are frank about missing their highs, and this factor contributes to their discontinuation of drug therapy. Therefore they may actively resist treatment and may be particularly reluctant to have the euphoric, energized periods of mania controlled.

Bipolar patients may also be actively self-treating their painful mood states with alcohol, street drugs, or prescription drugs such as benzodiazepines, opioids, or sedative-hypnotics. The patient and health care provider may be unaware of the underlying disorder until after the other substances are removed.

Because bipolar disorder is a life-long, unremitting, chronic medical and psychiatric disease characterized by multiple relapses, it is common for patients to become reluctant to comply with complex or demanding drug regimens. Treatment regimens may be complicated further by annoying or dangerous adverse effects and the need for frequent laboratory monitoring.

It may be particularly difficult for bipolar patients who lack family or social support, easily accessible community caregivers, structured housing or day programs, or financial resources to consistently comply with therapeutic regimens. Drug, dietary, or sleep hygiene practices that assist with management of the disorder and its treatment protocols are warranted.

Many bipolar patients respond favorably to treatment and continue to live extremely productive lives. They may be successful in their careers and personal lives, particularly if their energy and creativity can be constructively harnessed (see Case Study: Rapid-Cycle Bipolar Disorder).

Physical Examination

In addition to obtaining the psychiatric and medical history, a mental status examination of the patient should be included, possibly along with physical examination, and laboratory tests, when indicated. The mental status examination of the patient with unipolar depressive disorder is often unremarkable. The patient's symptoms typically include a depressed mood accompanied by irritability and diminished interest or motivation. Decreased concentration and attention may affect the patient's performance on the Mini-Mental State Examination (MMSE), geriatric depression scale, or other evaluation tool. The physical examination is either unremarkable or nonspecific.

For the patient with mania, emphasis is placed on evaluation of neurologic and endocrine systems. In the absence of psychotic features (e.g., hallucinations) primary mood disorders do not involve alteration in cranial nerves, reflexes, or sensation. Note the patient's speech patterns, cognition, and affect.

Laboratory Testing

Laboratory tests should be performed when there is a specific concern about a medical condition that underlies the depression. Many studies have failed to document significantly higher rates of medical conditions (e.g., hypothyroidism) among outpatients with depressive disorders. For this reason, there is usually no need to obtain standard and specific tests in the evaluation of the patient who is depressed. However, laboratory testing can be helpful when assessing patients who do not respond to standard treatments for depression. In particular, thyroid function tests and B_{12} and folate levels should be checked in these patients since these abnormalities are known to be associated with depression and can be easily corrected.

For the patient with mania, routine laboratory tests focus on ruling out other medical causes of mood disturbance. There are no laboratory tests to diagnose bipolar disorder. Complete blood cell (CBC) count, serum chemistries, thyroid function tests, and screening for toxic substances are usually indicated at the time of evaluation. Additional testing may be necessary, based on the patient's clinical presentation. Any patient who has psychotic symptoms should have at least one electroencephalogram (EEG) or brain imaging study (CT or MRI).

GOALS OF THERAPY

Treatment objectives for the patient with depression, bipolar disorder, or mania are to correct the neurotransmitter imbalance through the appropriate use of drugs and to return the patient to an optimal level of functioning. Mood disorders are not cured, however they are dealt with by treatment, management, and prevention of relapse. Thus rapid stabilization of mood, reestablishment of normalized sleep patterns, prevention of self-injurious acts, and long-term stabilization are necessary. Untreated or inadequately treated bipolar disorder tends to become more serious over time and more difficult to arrest.

INTERVENTION
Administration

The use of antidepressants and antimania drugs requires careful planning, administration, and monitoring. These drugs are usually administered two to three times daily, which requires the patient to take doses while at work, school, away from home, and on vacation.

Before initiating antidepressant or antimania therapy, baseline renal and thyroid function, white blood cell (WBC) count with differential, serum electrolytes, and glucose levels should be obtained. It is also important to establish that the female patient is not pregnant. If there is any possibility of pregnancy, a human chorionic gonadotropin pregnancy test should be done. In addition, tests of liver function, bilirubin, urinalysis, and blood urea nitrogen should be routinely performed for patients taking carbamazepine and valproic acid.

Antidepressants are usually taken with food to minimize gastric distress. Carefully ascertain that the drug is swallowed and not hidden in the mouth to be discarded or saved for later use. Enteric-coated or sustained-release formulations should be taken whole. They should not be broken or chewed because this causes throat irritation and alters drug absorption. Liquid formulations should be shaken well before pouring, and a calibrated measuring device used to ensure accurate dosage. Once-a-day drugs should be taken in the morning. If daytime drowsiness becomes a problem, the patient may take daily doses at bedtime. For doses usually taken at bedtime but forgotten, instruct the patient not to take the dose the next morning and to check with the health care provider. For missed doses taken more than once daily, tell the patient to take the missed dose as soon as remembered, unless it is almost time for the next dose, then omit the missed dose and resume regular dosage schedule. Do not double up for missed doses.

To prevent premature dissolution, valproic acid should not be taken with milk. Doxepin concentrate should be diluted in 4 ounces of recommended liquid (water, milk, or fruit juice, but not grape juice or carbonated beverages) before taking. Imipramine may be used in the treatment of enuresis in children over 6 years of age. The drug should be taken about 1 hour before bedtime, although early nighttime bedwetters may have a better response if part of the dose is given in the afternoon and the rest at bedtime. The treatment of enuresis can be complex; provide emotional support as needed.

Assess the patient for suicidal ideations. The risk of suicide may persist for several weeks after antidepressant drug therapy has begun. Some patients who were not suicidal may become so during initial therapy.

Monitor the patient's weight periodically throughout therapy because as mood improves, appetite may also improve. In addition, some antidepressants contribute to weight gain. If weight gain is significant, the patient should be counseled about weight-reduction strategies and exercise regimens. Provide emotional support for these changes and consult the health care provider about possible changes in drug or dosage.

Many antidepressants alter the seizure threshold. In the hospitalized patient with a history of seizures, the use of padded siderails and watchful supervision is warranted until the effects of the drugs can be evaluated.

Therapeutic drug levels of certain antidepressant and antimania drugs should be monitored closely throughout therapy. For example, lithium levels should be monitored once or twice weekly during the acute manic phase until serum concentrations have stabilized and the patient's condition has improved. Serum drug levels are measured approximately 10 to 12 hours after the previous dose (Table 18-4). Lithium drug concentrations in children, adolescents, older adults, those with chronic illnesses, and especially those with any renal involvement should be maintained at lower levels. Lithium level evaluations should be repeated every 2 to 3 months during long-term therapy and more frequently in older adults, who are more prone to dehydration, hypothyroidism, and CNS toxicity. If urinary output is excessive, assess the patient taking lithium for diabetes insipidus (dilute, high-volume urine with a specific gravity of 1.000 to 1.003).

Education

The patient and family require education concerning the course of the illness, its symptoms, and its management. Inform the patient and family that several weeks of therapy may be necessary before full effects of a specific drug regimen may be known. One point that should be reinforced is the importance of compliance with the drug regimen. Inform the patient that antidepressants must be taken regularly as ordered, even if he or she begins to feel better. Instruct the patient to consult the health care provider before changing or discontinuing the drug regimen.

The patient should notify all health care providers of all drugs being taken. Advise the patient to use caution when driving or operating machinery if drowsiness or dizziness occurs and to avoid alcohol unless approved in moderation by the health care provider. Remind the patient to keep these and all drugs out of the reach of children. Advise patients with diabetes mellitus to monitor blood glucose levels regularly since antidepressants may alter them. A change in diet or insulin dosage may be necessary in some patients.

The patient should be instructed about the necessity of maintaining adequate hydration and salt in the diet (particularly for the patient taking lithium), especially during periods of illness, fever, vomiting, diarrhea, or profuse sweating. Caffeinated beverages such as coffee, tea, and colas should be limited. Fluid consumption should be increased during periods of hot weather to avoid dehydration.

Encourage the patient to stay in touch with the health care provider and to seek assistance from other health care personnel as appropriate, including psychologists, psychiatrists, and therapists. Sleep hygiene, regular daily routine, cognitive-behavioral therapy, group therapy, and family support are all factors that optimize functioning. The patient should be warned to report promptly any deterioration of sleep patterns because often it is the first warning sign of an impending episode of hypomania or mania.

Patients should be encouraged to obtain information from advocacy groups, the Alliance for the Mentally Ill, employee assistance programs, and drug manufacturers. For example, Abbott Laboratories has a sample program and an indigent patient program available for those who are uninsured or who cannot afford divalproex (Depakote). Solvay Pharmaceuticals has a program available to supply patients with lithium (Lithobid).

Families require information and support because the depression or bipolar disorder has an impact on the entire family system: roles, relationships, responsibilities, finances, and parenting. The patient should be assisted to understand that although the illness needs to be an important focus, it should not be the only focus of life, and it is important to resume life and make it as normal, productive, and stable a life as possible.

EVALUATION

Indications that drug therapy and any other measures employed have been effective include the resolution of mania or hypomania, the establishment of euthymia (normal mood), the resolution of dysphoric symptoms

CASE STUDY

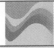

Rapid-Cycle Bipolar Disorder

ASSESSMENT

HISTORY OF PRESENT ILLNESS

SN is a 26-year-old Hispanic woman who complains of frequent, rapid mood fluctuations for the past several years. She reports at least four complete mood cycles per year. When depressed, her symptoms include feeling irritable, crying, hopelessness, helplessness, insomnia, decreased appetite, and weight loss. She loses interest in usually pleasurable activities and is unable to care for her 2-year-old son. She made a suicide attempt by ingesting large amounts of alcohol, benzodiazepines, and aspirin. When her mood is elevated, she feels alternatively euphoric and irritable; she may not sleep for several days at a time; has engaged in reckless activities; and exercises poor judgment in relationships, sexual encounters, and care of her child. She tends to wear excessive makeup and jewelry when manic, and spends large amounts of money and charges her credit cards beyond their limit.

HEALTH HISTORY

SN's health history is unremarkable. She has a 10 pack-year smoking history and drinks alcohol primarily when manic but occasionally while depressed. She has one child born by vaginal delivery. She has no known allergies and no renal, hepatic, or coagulation problems. She is taking oral contraceptives.

LIFESPAN CONSIDERATIONS

Although she is a single parent, SN expresses interest in having another child before age 30.

CULTURAL/SOCIAL CONSIDERATIONS

SN lives on emergency assistance from the state. She has been unable to maintain employment because of her mood lability, poor judgment, and need to care for her child. She has a 10th grade education. Her potential for compliance is judged to be fair to good. She reports that she is highly mo-

tivated to control her mood cycling so she can be a better parent, complete her education, and start a career. SN has access to any required drugs through her emergency assistance entitlement program.

PHYSICAL EXAMINATION

Vital signs are stable (VSS). SN is an underweight woman with no physical stigmata; otherwise the examination was unremarkable.

LABORATORY TESTING

CBC, thyroid function tests, B_{12}, and folate levels are within normal limits.

PATIENT PROBLEM(S)

SN meets DSM-IV criteria for rapid-cycle bipolar disorder.

GOALS OF THERAPY

Correct the neurotransmitter imbalance contributing to rapid-cycle bipolar disorder. Return SN to optimal level of functioning.

CRITICAL THINKING QUESTIONS

1. Why did the health care provider order divalproex for SN?
2. What is the mechanism of action of divalproex?
3. Considering the adverse reactions and potential for toxicity, why do you think divalproex was ordered for SN rather than lithium?
4. What concerns might you have regarding the laboratory tests required to monitor SN's divalproex therapy?
5. Considering the acute nature of SN's bipolar disorder, which pharmacokinetic factors were important in the decision to use divalproex rather than carbamazepine or lithium?

(if they were present), and a therapeutic, nonproblematic physiologic response to the drug. If adverse effects develop, they are tolerable, non–life threatening, noncompromising, and do not compel the patient to discontinue the drug.

The patient and family should express knowledge and some degree of acceptance of the disorder and demonstrate an awareness of the nature, course, and treatment of the illness. Evidence should also include documentation that the patient actually has a means for ongoing care, obtaining the prescribed drugs, and is actually using the resources. The patient should be aware of psychosocial supports and rights as a disabled person

under the Americans with Disabilities Act. When applicable, the patient should express a desire to stop or actually stops the use of alcohol or street drugs.

Bibliography

American Psychiatric Association: Diagnostic and statistical manual of mental disorders, ed 4 (text revision), Washington, DC, 2000, American Psychiatric Press.

Bladessarini RJ, Tarazi FI: Drugs in the treatment of psychiatric disorders, depression and anxiety disorders. In Hardman JG, Limbird LE, Gilman AF, eds: *The pharmacological basis of therapeutics*, ed 10, New York, 2001, McGraw-Hill.

Bladessarini RJ, Tarazi FI: Drugs in the treatment of psychiatric disorders, psychosis and mania. In Hardman JG, Limbird

LE, Gilman AF, eds: *The pharmacological basis of therapeutics*, ed 10, New York, 2001, McGraw-Hill.

Blows WT: The neurobiology of antidepressants, *J Neurosci Nurs* 32(3):177-180, 2000.

Britton GR: Selective serotonin reuptake inhibitors: implications for advanced nursing practice, *J Am Acad Nurse Pract* 11(9):389-395, 1999.

Davis KM, Mathew E: Pharmacologic management of depression in the elderly, *Nurse Pract* 23(6):16-18, 26, 28, 1998.

Depression Guideline Panel: Depression in primary care. Vol. 1. Detection and diagnosis. In *Clinical practice guideline*, No. 5, AHCPR Pub. No. 93-0550, Rockville, MD, April 1993, U.S. Department of Health and Human Services, Public Health Service, Agency for Health Care Policy and Research.

Heffern WA: Psychopharmacological and electroconvulsive treatment of anxiety and depression in the elderly, *J Psychiatr Ment Health Nurs* 7(3):199-204, 2000.

Lynch A, Glod CA, Fitzgerald F: Psychopharmacologic treatment of adolescent depression, *Arch Psychiatr Nurs* 15(1): 41-47, 2001.

Martin AC: Major depressive illness in women: assessment and treatment in the primary care setting, *Nurse Pract Forum* 11(3): 79-86, 2000.

Nichols MR: The use of bupropion hydrochloride for smoking cessation therapy, *Clin Excell Nurse Pract* 3(6):317-322, 1999.

St Dennis C, Synoground G: Medications for early onset bipolar illness: new drug update, *J Sch Nurs* 14(5):29-41, 1998.

Stern TA, Herman JB, Slavin PL: *The MGH guide to psychiatry in primary care*, New York, 1998, McGraw-Hill.

Thobaben M: Successful treatment for major depressive episodes, *Home Care Provid* 3(3):131-134, 1998.

Williams JW, Mulrow C, Chiquette E, et al: A systematic review of newer pharmacotherapies for depression in adults: evidence support summary: clinical guideline, Part 2, *Ann Intern Med* 132(9):743-756, 2000.

Internet Resources

A site with links to clinical descriptions from the Mayo Clinic and to various print resources. Available online at http://www.psycom.net/depression.central.bipolar.html.

Internet Mental Health. Available online at http://mental heath.com.

National Depressive and Manic-Depressive Association web site, with links to various resources. Available online at http://www.ndmda.org.

National Institute of Mental Health site on bipolar disorder, with links to publications. Available online at http://www. nimh.nih.gov/publicat/bipolar.cfm.

National Institute of Mental Health site on depression, with links to publications. Available online at http://www.nimh. nih.gov/publicat/depressionmenu.cfm.

Pharmacology Central. Available online at http://www. pharmcentral.com.

CHAPTER
19

Antipsychotic Drugs

MICHAEL R. VASKO • KATHLEEN GUTIERREZ

 Visit http://evolve.elsevier.com/Gutierrez/ for additional information.

KEY TERMS

OBJECTIVES

- Outline the kinds of psychoses discussed.
- Discuss the role of neurotransmitters, dopamine, norepinephrine, and acetylcholine in the actions and adverse effects of antipsychotic drugs.
- Describe the signs and symptoms of extrapyramidal reactions to antipsychotic drugs.
- Develop a nursing care plan for a patient receiving one of the antipsychotic drugs discussed.

PATHOPHYSIOLOGY

PSYCHOSES

Psychosis is a major emotional disorder with an impairment of mental function great enough to prevent the individual from participating in everyday life. The hallmark of a psychosis is the loss of contact with reality. A functional psychosis may be an isolated breakdown caused by a major traumatic event and is usually amenable to treatment with an antipsychotic drug.

An organic psychosis results from damage to the brain by an infectious disease, a deficiency disease, lead poisoning, a tumor, and injury through trauma or interrupted blood supply, such as in a cerebrovascular accident (stroke) and Alzheimer's disease. Organic psychoses do not respond to treatment with antipsychotic drugs as successfully as functional psychoses.

A toxic psychosis can arise during withdrawal from alcohol or other drugs. Some toxic psychoses are treated with diazepam, an antianxiety drug, rather than with antipsychotic drugs. However, a toxic psychosis can be caused by amphetamines because they release dopamine in the CNS. In this case, the specific therapy is the blockade of dopamine receptors provided by antipsychotic drugs.

SCHIZOPHRENIA

The term schizophrenia is used to describe a group of psychotic disorders characterized by fragmented perception, thought, and emotion; gross distortions of reality; disorganization; and withdrawal from social interactions. A diagnosis of schizophrenia is made on the basis of characteristic symptoms, one or more areas of social or occupational dysfunction, and the duration of the symptoms (see DSM-IV, Criteria for Schizophrenia and Related Disorders). About 1% of Americans develop schizophrenia during their lifetime. Men and women are affected equally. Men typically experience their first psychotic episode in their teens or twenties, and women in their twenties or early thirties. Symptoms may develop gradually or may appear abruptly.

About 14% to 30% of patients with a single psychotic episode have total recovery. For others, treatment is maintained throughout their lifetime, although patients may not require medication for several weeks or months during a disease remission. About 75% of patients will relapse within 18 months after discontinuation of antipsychotic drug therapy. Many individuals with schizophrenia can live in the community with strong family or group support and vocational training. However, about 5% to 15% of patients have relatively severe continuous psychosis. About 40% of patients in long-term institutions have schizophrenia. Studies indicate that 30% to 40% of America's homeless population have severe mental illness, including schizophrenia. The appropriate societal oversight of individuals with severe schizophrenia has not been resolved.

Psychotic symptoms are a hallmark of schizophrenia. This disease influences perception, thought content, thought process, affect, and daily functioning. The behavioral manifestations can be grouped as positive, negative, and cognitive symptoms. *Positive symptoms* are those behaviors existing in addition to or outside of the range of usual human responses (e.g., hallucinations and delusions). *Negative symptoms* are behaviors that are lessened or diminished and that are not typical of a healthy individual (e.g., flat affect, poverty of speech, attention impairment). The distinction between positive and negative symptoms is important because different psychotropic drugs tend to affect each group of symptoms differently. The *cognitive symptoms*, which may also be listed among the positive and negative symptoms, seem to be the least responsive to drug therapy. Examples of cognitive disturbances include looseness of association, a tangential or circular thought process, and neologisms (words that have a meaning known only to the patient). The older antipsychotic drugs specifically reduce the positive symptoms, such as delusions, hallucinations, bizarre behavior, catatonia, and thought disorder, so that patients can think and function more coherently. The newer antipsychotics are also effective in treating the negative symptoms, such as low levels of emotional arousal, mental activity, and social drive. These negative symptoms tend to be debilitating for persons with chronic schizophrenia.

Persons suffering from schizophrenia also demonstrate psychomotor and affective disturbances, including an overall reduction in emotional responsiveness, flat affect, anhedonia (loss of interest in normally pleasurable activities), abnormal emotions, and inappropriate responses. Psychomotor disturbances may include impulsivity, overexcitement, aggression, automatic obedience, echopraxia (stereotyped imitation of the movements of another person), stupor, or catalepsy.

Defects Underlying Schizophrenia

The exact cause of schizophrenia is unknown; however, it appears to have a genetic link with a high concordance rate among blood relatives. The neurotransmitter dopamine has long been associated with theories regarding schizophrenia. It is hypothesized that excess dopamine in the limbic system structures (i.e., the hippocampus, anterior cingulate, and amygdala) causes psychotic symptoms. In an effort to modulate the overactivity caused by the excess dopamine, the frontal areas of the brain may become hyporesponsive to this neurotransmitter, resulting in defective information processing.

Five subtypes of dopamine receptors have been identified in the brain. The clinical potency of antipsychotic drugs such as chlorpromazine and haloperidol is correlated with their ability to inhibit the dopamine-2 (D_2) receptor. They also block other subtypes of dopamine receptors. Inhibition of the D_2 receptor also correlates with appearance of extrapyramidal adverse effects (see below). The antipsychotic drugs clozapine and olanzapine are weak blockers of dopamine D_2 receptors. However, they do block D_4 receptors and the serotonin 5-HT_{2A} receptor effectively.

DRUG CLASS • Antipsychotics

Antipsychotic or antischizophrenic drugs are also called **neuroleptic drugs**. Neuroleptic refers to the ability of these drugs to cause a general quiescence and a state of psychic indifference to the surroundings, thus quieting a severely agitated patient. The phenothiazines are the largest class of antipsychotic drugs and are subdivided into three subgroups based on chemical differences in side groups on the three-ringed main structure. These subgroups are the aliphatic, the piperidine, and the piperazine phenothiazines, and the prototype of each drug class is listed below. Other phenothiazines are listed in Table 19-1. The three subgroups differ in potency and in the incidence of key adverse effects (see below and Table 19-4).

TABLE 19-1

Antipsychotic Drugs

Generic Name	Brand Name	Comments
Phenothiazines		
chlorpromazine hydrochloride	Largactil, ✽ Novo-Chlorpromazine, ✽ Sonazine, Thorazine	Control of initial acute psychotic episodes is achieved with high dosages, which are then tapered to lowest maintenance dosage when patient's condition stabilizes. Best tolerated by patients less than 40 years of age and those hospitalized less than 10 years. Sedation is pronounced at start of therapy, which may be desired for highly agitated patients. Incidence of hypotension, ophthalmic changes, and dyskinesia is high in older adult patients. Antiadrenergic and anticholinergic side effects usually diminish after first week.
fluphenazine decanoate	Mediten, ✽ Prolixin Decanoate	Long-acting depot forms last at least 2 weeks. Dosage should be stabilized in hospital because severe episodes of parkinsonism can appear. Not recommended for older adult patients or those who have had difficulty with extrapyramidal reactions.
fluphenazine enanthate	Moditen Enanthate, ✽ Prolixin	Most potent of phenothiazines used for management of psychotic disorders.
fluphenazine hydrochloride	Moditen, ✽ Permitil, Prolixin	See above.
mesoridazine besylate	Serentil	Management of psychotic disorders. Metabolite of thioridazine with antiemetic activity and no reported retinopathy.
methotrimeprazine	Nozinan ✽	Used as antipsychotic, analgesic, antianxiety agent as well as sedative. For moderate to severe pain of bedridden patients, obstetric pain, anxiety before surgery, and adjunctive therapy in general anesthesia to increase effects of anesthetics.

✽ Available only in Canada.

Continued

TABLE 19-1

Antipsychotic Drugs—cont'd

Generic Name	Brand Name	Comments
Phenothiazines—cont'd		
pericyazine	Neuleptil ❋	To treat psychotic disorders.
perphenazine	Apo-Perphenazine, Trilafon	For acute psychotic disorders. Lower dosages needed when used as an antiemetic.
perphenazine/amitriptyline	Etrafon, PMS-Levazine, ❋ Proavil, ❋ Triavil ❋	Combination of antipsychotic and antidepressant. Available in United States as generic.
pipotiazine palmitate	Piportil ❋	To treat psychotic disorders.
prochlorperazine	Compazine, Compro, Nu-Prochlor ❋	More widely used to control severe nausea and vomiting than for psychiatric treatment. Hypotension is seen when given intravenously for surgical procedures.
prochlorperazine edisylate	Compazine Edisylate	More widely used to control severe nausea and vomiting than for psychiatric treatment. Hypotension is seen when given intravenously for surgical procedures.
prochlorperazine maleate	Compazine Maleate, PMS-Prochlorperazine, ❋ Stemetil ❋	More widely used to control severe nausea and vomiting than for psychiatric treatment. Hypotension is seen when given intravenously for surgical procedures.
promazine hydrochloride	Sparine	Total daily dose for adults should not exceed 1000 mg.
thioproperazine mesylate	Majeptil ❋	To treat psychotic disorders.
thioridazine hydrochloride	Apo-Thioridazine, ❋ Mellaril, Novo-Ridazine, ❋ Thioridazine Intensol	Little antiemetic activity. Safe for patients with epilepsy. Possibly effective in alcohol withdrawal syndrome, intractable pain, and senility. One of the least likely of antipsychotic drugs to cause extrapyramidal reactions. Dosages higher than 800 mg daily have produced serious pigmentary retinopathy.
trifluoperazine	Apo-Trifluoperazine, Stelazine, Terfluzine ❋	Management of psychotic disorders.
triflupromazine hydrochloride	Vesprin	Management of psychotic disorders. Control of nausea and vomiting.
Thioxanthenes		
chlorprothixene	Taractan	Incidence of side effects is same as for aliphatic phenothiazines, including high sedation, autonomic effects, and few extrapyramidal effects.
flupenthixol decanoate	Fluanxol Depot ❋	Management of psychotic disorders.
flupenthixol hydrochloride	Fluanxol ❋	
thiothixene	Navane	Incidence of side effects same as for piperazine phenothiazines, including low incidence of sedation and autonomic effects and high incidence of extrapyramidal effects.
Butyrophenones		
droperidol	generic	Rapid onset and short duration; rarely used as an antipsychotic.
droperidol/fentanyl	Innovar	Used for dissociative anesthesia (see Chapter 16).

TABLE 19-1		

Antipsychotic Drugs—cont'd

Generic Name	Brand Name	Comments
Butyrophenones—cont'd		
haloperidol	Apo-Haloperidol,✱ Haldol, Novo-Peridol,✱ Peridol✱	Management of psychotic disorders. Likely to produce extrapyramidal reactions in patients. In severely hyperkinetic retarded patients, large doses may bring improvement in social behavior and concentration. Drug of choice for treatment of Tourette's syndrome. Also used for acute manic episodes. Spectrum of side effects is similar to that of piperazine phenothiazines: low incidence of sedation and autonomic effects but high incidence of extrapyramidal reactions.
haloperidol decanoate	Haldol Decanoate, Haldol LA✱	Depot form of haloperidol for severe chronic schizophrenics not compliant with oral medication.
Other Heterocyclic Antipsychotics		
clozapine	Clozaril	Indicated only in management of severely ill schizophrenic patients failing to respond to other drugs. Monitor for agranulocytosis and seizures.
loxapine succinate	Loxitane, Loxapac✱	Effective for schizophrenia and acute psychoses.
molindone hydrochloride	Moban	Effective for schizophrenia and acute psychoses.
olanzapine	Zyprexa	Risk of orthostatic hypotension minimized by starting with 5 mg daily.
pimozide	Orap	Indicated for control of Tourette's syndrome.
quetiapine fumarate	Seroquel	
risperidone	Risperdal	Skin may be more sensitive to sunlight.
ziprasidone	Geodon	

Another major class of antipsychotic drugs, the thioxanthenes, has a three-ringed main structure that differs by only one atom from that of the phenothiazines. The remaining drug classes are chemically different from the phenothiazines and from each other. These include butyrophenones and the newer heterocyclic compounds (see Table 19-1). All of these drugs are similar in many ways and thus are discussed in this chapter.

Phenothiazines

chlorpromazine (Largactil, Sonazine, Thorazine)

fluphenazine (Prolixin, Modecate, Moditen)

thioridazine (Mellaril, Novo-Ridazine,✱ Apo-Thioridazine✱)

Thiozanthenes

chlorprothixene (Taractan)

thiothixene (Navane)

Butyrophenones

droperidol (Inapsine)

haloperidol (Haldol, Apo-Haloperidol,✱ Novo-Peridol,✱ Peridol✱)

Other Heterocyclic Compounds

clozapine (Clozaril)

loxapine (Loxitane, Loxapac✱)

molindone (Moban)

olanzapine (Zyprexa)

pimozide (Orap)

quetiapine (Seroquel)

risperidone (Risperdal)

ziprasidone (Geodon)

MECHANISM OF ACTION

Most antipsychotic drugs block D_2 receptors in the postsynaptic areas. Symptoms of schizophrenia are affected by blocking D_2 receptors in the mesolimbic area of the brain. Blocking D_2 receptors in the chemoreceptor trigger zone of the medulla is thought to produce antiemetic effects. Blocking D_2 receptors in the tuberoinfundibular region of the hypothalamus accounts for the increase in prolactin that occurs with antipsychotic therapy, whereas D_2 receptor antagonism in the nigrostriatal pathways produces extrapyramidal adverse effects. Clozapine and olanzapine selectively act at dopamine sites in the cortical and limbic regions of the brain but have much less effect in the nigrostriatal region. They have less affinity for D_1, D_2, and D_3 receptors, and bind more frequently with D_4 receptors. These drugs and quetiapine, risperidone, and ziprasidone also are antagonists at 5-HT_{2A} receptors. This dual action is believed to account for their effectiveness in blocking the positive symptoms of psychosis with minimal extrapyramidal adverse effects and in relieving the negative symptoms of schizophrenia.

Antipsychotic drugs also block a number of other neurotransmitter receptors to varying degrees, including alpha$_1$-adrenergic, cholinergic muscarinic, and histamine receptors. The sedative effect of the phenothiazines and the thioxanthenes may result from their blockade of alpha$_1$-adrenergic receptors. The blockade of norepinephrine receptors in the vasomotor center also inhibits peripheral sympathetic tone and causes orthostatic hypotension. Drowsiness and weight gain may result from the partial antagonism of histamine.

USES

The primary use of antipsychotic drugs remains in the management of schizophrenia. They do not cure psychotic disorders but do ease many of the most distressing symptoms, including thought disorders, hallucinations, bizarre behaviors, agitation, and hyperactivity. They are also useful in the treatment of other disorders such as schizoaffective disorder, severe mania or the acute manic phase of bipolar disorder, drug-induced psychosis, and delusional disorders. Haloperidol and pimozide are indicated for the control of the tics and vocalizations of Tourette's syndrome.

Several antipsychotic drugs are prescribed to control vomiting (see Chapter 50). Chlorpromazine, triflupro-

---

TABLE 19-2

Pharmacokinetics of Selected Antipsychotic Drugs

Drugs	Route	Bioavailability (%)	Time to Peak	Half-Life	Plasma Protein Binding (%)
Phenothiazines					
chlorpromazine	po	32 ± 19	2-4 hours	8-35 hours	~95
fluphenazine	po	Low	2-4 hours	14-24 hours	>95
mesoridazine	po	NA*	4-7 days	24-48 hours	>95
perphenazine	po	NA	1-3 hours	8-24 hours	NA
trifluoperazine	po	NA	2-4 hours	14-24 hours	> 90
Butyrophenone					
haloperidol	po	60 ± 18	2-6 hours	12-36 hours	90-95
Other Heterocyclic Antipsychotics					
clozapine	po	55 ± 12	1-3 hours	8-16 hours	>95
loxapine	po	NA	1-3 hours	3-4 hours	NA
molindone	po	NA	30-90 minutes	6-24 hours	NA
olanzapine	po	~60	4-8 hours	20-54 hours	~93
pimozide	po	~50	8-12 hours	29-111 hours*	~99
quetiapine	po	~9	1-2 hours	6 hours	~83
risperidone	po	66 ± 28	~1 hour	20-24 hours	~89
ziprasidone	po	~60	6-8 hours	12-36 hours	>99

NA, not available.

*Multiphasic elimination.

mazine, perphenazine, and prochlorperazine in particular are widely used as antiemetics. Chlorpromazine is also prescribed for intractable hiccups. Because of the numerous adverse effects of these drugs, their use as antiemetics is restricted to management of postoperative nausea and vomiting, radiation and chemotherapy sickness, nausea and vomiting caused by toxins, and intractable vomiting. The antiemetic dosage is much smaller than the antipsychotic dosage.

PHARMACOKINETICS

Oral absorption of antipsychotic drugs can be variable, and in a number of instances bioavailability is poor (Table 19-2). Although parenteral administration of these drugs diminishes the variable absorption, these drugs are routinely administered orally. Haloperidol, fluphenazine, and flupenthixol (in Canada), are available as the decanoate ester in depot forms for intramuscular injection, which requires administration only every 3 to 6 weeks.

The antipsychotic drugs are lipophilic, readily entering the brain and most other body tissues. In addition, many of the antipsychotic drugs are highly bound to plasma proteins. Peak plasma levels of most drugs are reached in 2 to 8 hours when given orally, although they can range up to 7 days. The half-life of these drugs ranges from 3 hours to days (see Table 19-2).

The drugs are biotransformed in the liver, with metabolites eliminated by the kidneys. Excretion is slow, however, and active metabolites may be found in urine as long as 6 months after the drug is discontinued.

ADVERSE REACTIONS AND CONTRAINDICATIONS

The major adverse effects of the antipsychotic drugs are summarized in Table 19-3. In general, these drugs share common adverse effects, but the incidence can vary as shown in Table 19-4. One of the major adverse effects is the onset of movement disorders, called extrapyramidal symptoms, which can manifest as acute dystonia,

TABLE 19-3

Adverse Effects of Antipsychotic Drugs

Type of Effect	Signs and Symptoms	Comments
Central nervous system	Sedation, lower seizure threshold (except molindone), relief of nausea or vomiting (except thioridazine), neuroleptic malignant syndrome	Usually transient
Adrenergic blockade	Postural (orthostatic) hypotension	Occurs when patient stands quickly
Cholinergic blockade	Atropinelike effects: dry mouth, blurred vision, constipation, delayed micturition, confusion (especially in older adult)	Usually transient
Endocrine	Weight gain, thyroid disturbances Men: erection problems, breast engorgement Women: menstrual irregularities, galactorrhea	Usually transient
Extrapyramidal (dopamine blockade)	Acute dystonia: neck twisting, facial grimacing, abnormal eye movements, involuntary muscle movements	Most common during first few days of therapy; usually disappears after brief treatment with antiparkinson drugs
	Akathisia: restlessness, difficulty in sitting still, strong urge to move about	Most common after first week of therapy; control with antiparkinson drugs or diazepam
	Parkinsonism: motor retardation, masklike face, tremor, rigidity, salivation, shuffling gait	Most common after first weeks of therapy; control with antiparkinson drugs
	Tardive dyskinesia: protrusion of tongue, puffing of cheeks, chewing movements, involuntary movements of extremities, involuntary movements of trunk	Most common when dosage is lowered after prolonged therapy; older adult women at greatest risk; may not be reversible; no drug treatment available
Allergic reactions	Photosensivity Cholestatic hepatitis, agranulocytosis	Common Rare

akathisia, parkinsonism, neuroleptic malignant syndrome, perioral tremor, or tardive dyskinesia. It is important to recognize these bizarre reactions as adverse effects of drug therapy that require palliative drugs or reduction or discontinuance of therapy. These reactions should not be treated as manifestations of the psychotic disease being treated, and the drug dosage should not be increased. Extrapyramidal symptoms wax and wane over time and disappear during sleep. They can be aggravated by emotional stress.

The highest incidence of extrapyramidal reactions are observed with piperazine phenothiazines and haloperidol, whereas aliphatic phenothiazines and many of the newer drugs have a relatively low incidence (see Table 19-4). Clozapine and quetiapine do not appear to produce significant extrapyramidal symptoms.

Acute dystonia is a spasm of muscles of the tongue, face, neck, or back and may mimic seizures. Dystonia is usually seen in the first 5 days of antipsychotic therapy. It may be treated with an antihistamine or anticholiner-

---

TABLE 19-4

Classic Antipsychotic Drugs: Drug Class and Major Adverse Effects

Drug	Relative Incidence of Adverse Reactions			
	Sedative Effect	Orthostatic Hypotension	Anticholinergic Effects	Extrapyramidal Symptoms
Phenothiazines				
Aliphatic				
chlorpromazine	High	Moderate	Moderate/high	Moderate
methotrimeprazine	High	High	Moderate	Low/moderate
promazine	Moderate	Moderate	High	Moderate
triflupromazine	High	Moderate	Moderate/high	Moderate/high
Piperidine				
mesoridazine	High	Moderate	Moderate	Low
pericyazine	High	Moderate	High	Moderate
pipotiazine	Low	Low	Low	Low
thioridazine	High	Moderate	Moderate/high	Low
Piperazine				
fluphenazine	Low/moderate	Low	Low	High
perphenazine	Low/moderate	Low	Low	Moderate/high
prochlorperazine	Moderate	Low	Low	High
thioproperazine	Low	Low	Low	High
trifluoperazine	Low	Low	Low	High
Thioxanthenes				
chlorprothixene	High	Moderate	Moderate/high	Moderate
thiothixene	Low/moderate	Moderate	Low	Moderate
Other Heterocyclic Antipsychotics				
clozapine	Moderate/high	Moderate/high	Moderate/high	None
haloperidol	Low	Low	Low	High
loxapine	Moderate	Low	Low/moderate	Moderate
molindone	Moderate	Low/moderate	Moderate	Moderate
olanzapine	Low	Moderate	High	Low
pimozide	Low	Low	Moderate	Moderate/high
quetiapine	Moderate/high	Moderate	Low	None
risperidone	Moderate	Moderate/high	Low	Moderate
ziprasidone	Moderate/high	Moderate	Moderate/high	Low/moderate

gic antiparkinson drug (see Chapter 23). Dystonia can occur at any age, but it is more common in patients less than 35 years old and rarely persists during treatment. Some of the classic movements observed in dystonia include neck twisting (torticollis), upward gaze paralysis **(oculogyric crisis),** stereotyped motions of the jaw, and a spasm in which the head and feet create a horseshoe configuration (opisthotonos). Dystonia may be seen in some patients after a short course of phenothiazines used to treat nausea and vomiting.

Akathisia is a motor restlessness and may be mistaken for psychotic restlessness or agitation. Akathisia commonly appears after the first few days of therapy, and if not recognized, the antipsychotic drug dosage may be mistakenly increased to relieve the agitation, thus resulting in a worsening of the adverse effect. Patients experiencing akathisia have difficulty sitting still and may pace about, fidget, or constantly move their legs. Anticholinergic drugs or a muscle relaxant such as diazepam can alleviate these symptoms. If these treatments are not effective, a different antipsychotic drug may have to be tried. Akathisia disappears when the drug is discontinued.

Parkinsonism is marked by motor retardation **(bradykinesis)** and rigidity, symptoms virtually the same as those seen with idiopathic Parkinson's disease. Patients find it difficult to initiate movements or to carry them out. The face resembles a mask because emotions do not register on it. The patient has a shuffling gait and hypersalivates. Tremor is seen in the hands and legs. These parkinsonian symptoms commonly appear 5 to 30 days after initiation of therapy and are treated with antiparkinson drugs (see Chapter 23). The parkinsonian symptoms do not diminish with continued therapy and if antiparkinson drugs cannot control them, the antipsychotic drug must be changed.

Neuroleptic malignant syndrome (NMS) is a rare adverse effect but has a mortality of 10% (Box 19-1). Perioral tremor also is rare and develops months to years after therapy begins. It is characterized by excessive tremor of the lower face and is sometimes called the rabbit syndrome because the movement is similar to the twitching of a rabbit's face. Antiparkinson drugs are often helpful in reducing the excessive movement.

Tardive dyskinesia is associated with long-term, high-dose antipsychotic drug therapy. Tardive dyskinesia is the worst of the extrapyramidal reactions because it cannot be readily treated, is persistent, and may not altogether disappear when the drug therapy is discontinued. It usually appears months to years after therapy is started. The exact mechanism for the disorder is unknown but it may result from the development of receptors that are supersensitive to dopamine after prolonged blockade by the antipsychotic drugs. At present,

there is no specific treatment other than to stop the drug. Interestingly, the symptoms may become more severe for several weeks after the drug is withdrawn. The flare-up is then followed by a slow, gradual improvement over many months or years, although in some instances the dyskinesia is irreversible. Antiparkinson drugs also worsen the condition. Some common symptoms of tardive dyskinesia are protrusion of the tongue, puffing of the cheeks or the tongue in a cheek, chewing movements, and involuntary movements of the extremities and trunk.

Additional CNS effects of antipsychotic drugs include the reduction in seizure threshold and sedation. Most of these drugs lower seizure threshold, which is particularly problematic in patients with a preexisting seizure disorder, abnormal electroencephalogram, or other CNS pathology. This is especially true for the aliphatic phenothiazines, the thioxanthenes, clozapine,

BOX 19-1 **Patient Problem: Neuroleptic Malignant Syndrome**

The Problem

Neuroleptic malignant syndrome (NMS), a potentially fatal syndrome, may occur at any time during therapy with neuroleptics. Although rare, NMS is more commonly seen at the start of therapy, after patients are switched from one drug to another, after a dosage increase, or when a combination of drugs is used.

Signs and Symptoms

The patient may have convulsions, difficult or fast breathing, tachycardia or irregular pulse rate, fever, high or low blood pressure, increased sweating, loss of bladder control, skeletal muscle rigidity, pale skin, excessive weakness or fatigue, or an altered level of consciousness. There may be severe extrapyramidal side effects such as difficulty swallowing, excessive salivation, oculogyric crisis, and dyskinesia. The white blood cell count may be elevated in the range of 9500 to 26,000 cells/mm³, and liver function test results and creatine phosphokinase (CPK) level may be elevated as well.

The Solution

The patient with NMS requires intensive care. Monitor vital signs, notify the physician, and discontinue neuroleptic therapy. Monitor electrocardiographic changes. Administer antipyretics and use a cooling blanket to lower temperature. Monitor electrolytes and administer intravenous fluids. Drug treatment for NMS includes dantrolene and bromocriptine (experimental).

and olanzapine. Molindone has the lowest incidence of lowering the seizure threshold. Because antipsychotic drugs lower the convulsive threshold, they are unsuitable for treating drug withdrawal that is likely to produce seizures, such as withdrawal from alcohol, barbiturates, and other sedative-hypnotic drugs. Sedation is an adverse effect of all antipsychotics, but the degree of sedation is related to the specific drug, dosage, and individual patient. Sedation usually occurs with initial administration of the drug and is experienced for the first few days of therapy. After several weeks of treatment, the patient develops a tolerance to the sedative effects.

There are two primary cardiovascular adverse effects. Orthostatic hypotension is related to alpha-adrenergic receptor blockade, which inhibits reflex vasoconstriction and has a CNS component. This form of hypotension is common during the first hours or days of treatment, but tolerance develops over time. Aliphatic phenothiazines (see Table 19-4) are the most likely to produce nonspecific changes in the T wave of the electrocardiogram (ECG). Although this change is not clinically significant it is undesirable in a patient with concomitant heart disease who is being monitored for ECG changes.

The antipsychotic drugs, especially the aliphatic phenothiazines, chlorprothixene, and olanzapine have anticholinergic actions. The atropinelike effects include dry mouth and eyes, blurred vision (from ciliary muscle paresis), constipation, and urinary hesitancy and retention (related to increased sphincter tone). Urinary retention can lead to incontinence and enuresis. However, a central anticholinergic action may be beneficial in controlling some extrapyramidal reactions. In general, there appears to be an inverse relationship between the incidence of anticholinergic actions and extrapyramidal actions of many of these drugs. Indeed, anticholinergic drugs are often the initial therapy for the treatment of Parkinson's disease (see Chapter 23).

Antipsychotic drugs can produce a number of endocrine-related adverse effects. One is weight gain, which occurs with chronic drug administration, especially clozapine and quetiapine. Dopamine inhibits the release of the hormone prolactin by the pituitary gland through an action at D_2 receptors in the hypothalamus. As a result, blockade of dopamine leads to hypersecretion of prolactin and secondarily to endocrine disturbances of the reproductive system by mechanisms not yet understood. Women may experience delayed ovulation and menstruation, lack of menstruation (amenorrhea), milk production (galactorrhea), or weight gain. Men may experience impotence, decreased libido, retrograde ejaculation, or moderate breast growth (gynecomastia). Risperidone has a high incidence of increasing prolactin, whereas clozapine, olanzapine, and quetiapine have a low incidence.

Sexual dysfunctions also occur as a result of antipsychotic drug therapy. These include disturbances in ejaculation (delayed or blocked), prolonged erection, impotence, decreased libido, and changes in the quality of orgasm or the ability to experience orgasm. The exact mechanism for these effects is unknown.

Photosensitivity occasionally develops during therapy. This condition is fairly common and represents an allergic reaction to a metabolite produced not by the body but by a reaction to sunlight (Box 19-2). The long half-life of antipsychotic drugs allows them to accumulate in the skin, where sun exposure causes chemical changes that can cause skin allergies. Patients taking antipsychotic drugs should not sunbathe because they risk a painful

---

BOX 19-2 Patient Problem: Photosensitivity

The Problem

Some drugs can cause the skin to become especially sensitive to the effects of ultraviolet rays, so patients become sunburned with minimal exposure to the sun.

Signs and Symptoms

Sunburn develops after relatively brief exposure to the sun or other sources of ultraviolet light. Blisters, red skin, pain, or discomfort over skin surfaces may also occur.

The Solution

Patients should be advised of the following suggestions:

- Avoid sunbathing or tanning at tanning salons.
- Limit outdoor activities during the middle part of the day (10 AM to 2 PM) as much as possible.
- When outside, wear a wide-brimmed hat, long-sleeved shirt or jacket, long pants, and socks or other foot covering.
- Use a sunblock lipstick of at least SPF 15 and reapply regularly.
- Use a maximum-strength sunblock on exposed skin surfaces (SPF 15 or higher). Read product labels carefully and choose one that blocks both ultraviolet rays A and B. Apply liberally to exposed skin surfaces and repeat application every 1 to 2 hours. If you suspect that the sunblocking agent is causing skin irritation or rashes, try another agent or a product labeled hypoallergenic, which may be less irritating.
- If you experience moderate to severe sunburn, notify the health care provider.

skin rash. Some patients develop slate-blue patches on their skin. This is an accumulation of drug metabolites, not an allergy, and is not dangerous. Additional allergic reactions include a maculopapular rash of the face, neck, upper chest, and extremities, erythema multiforme, and localized or generalized urticaria (hives).

Cholestatic hepatitis can also develop with antipsychotic therapy. Jaundice develops when the bile duct becomes blocked by an allergic inflammation caused by metabolites excreted in the bile. It is commonly seen in the first month of therapy with an aliphatic phenothiazine. It is normally mild and self-limiting, but if jaundice is detected, the drug taken should be replaced with an antipsychotic drug from a different chemical class.

Blood dyscrasias occur with a number of the antipsychotic drugs. Depression of leukocytes is common but is usually transient and not serious. However, agranulocytosis, in which leukocytes are no longer produced, is serious and often fatal. This condition is most commonly seen within 3 months of the start of therapy. Any sign of fever or sore throat indicates the possible onset of agranulocytosis and should be checked immediately. Clozapine carries a risk of agranulocytosis at the rate of 1% to 2% per year, and patients on this drug should have weekly monitoring of their white blood cell (WBC) count. Risperidone and olanzapine do not carry this risk.

Given the potential adverse effects of antipsychotic drugs, caution should be used in administering these drugs to patients with dyskinesias, orthostatic hypotension, or hyperprolactinemia. Patients with cardiovascular disease and breast cancer may be at increased risk for worsening of these conditions. Care is also warranted for patients with seizure disorders, those taking anticonvulsants, and persons who have hepatic, renal, or cardiovascular disorders.

INTERACTIONS

Antipsychotic drugs potentiate the action of CNS depressants, including alcohol and other sedative-hypnotic drugs, opioids, and anesthetics. The effects of an alcoholic beverage or a sleeping pill are greatly exaggerated in patients taking an antipsychotic drug. A toxic overdose of alcohol or other sedative-hypnotic drug therefore becomes possible at a lower dosage. Clinical use is made of the potentiation of opioids by antipsychotic drugs. Droperidol is widely used with a narcotic to produce a state of quiescence and indifference to stimuli, which allows bronchoscopy, radiographic examinations, burn dressing, and cytoscopy to be performed. Nitrous oxide can be added to this neuroleptic-opioid combination to produce general anesthesia for surgery, called neurolept-anesthesia (see Chapter 16).

Antacids, activated charcoal, and aluminum salts limit gastrointestinal absorption of the drugs, thereby diminishing antipsychotic drug effectiveness. Anticholinergics and certain tricyclic antidepressants add to the anticholinergic adverse effects (e.g., blurred vision, constipation, dry mouth, and urinary retention). Levodopa therapy or dopamine agonists (see Chapter 23) can reduce the antipsychotic effects of these drugs and worsen psychosis.

Because some antipsychotics are highly bound to plasma proteins, other drugs with a high degree of affinity for plasma proteins can displace them. This displacement produces a transient increase in free drug levels that can be sustained if metabolism is compromised. Drugs that increase or decrease the activity of the cytochrome P-450 oxidases (see Chapter 1) can alter the biotransformation of the antipsychotics, resulting in higher or lower drug concentrations in the body.

APPLICATION TO PRACTICE

ASSESSMENT
History of Present Illness

Initial assessment of baseline functioning and mental status are imperative because antipsychotic drug therapy is aimed at treating symptoms and behaviors. Make the patient as comfortable as possible to facilitate description of abnormal experiences. Allow the patient to talk freely and do not take a dismissive stance.

Inquire and take note of the patient's thoughts. Are they tangential, grossly disorganized, or loose and difficult to follow (as seen in mania), or is there a decreased thought production (as seen in depression and some forms of schizophrenia)? Paranoid ideation occurs in many psychoses, whereas ideas of reference (e.g., the be-

lief that one is receiving special messages from the television or radio) and beliefs in thought manipulation or broadcasting are typically seen in schizophrenia.

Determine whether the patient is experiencing hallucinations through any sensory modality (i.e., visual, auditory, olfactory, gustatory, or tactile) and ascertain the level of insight into the experience. If auditory hallucinations are suspected, ask about command hallucinations. If patients are hearing commanding voices, they will generally acknowledge this if asked directly but rarely volunteer this information. Directed questions (e.g., "Do you feel safe here?" "Are there voices that are bothering you?") may elicit an acknowledgment of the psychosis.

The presence of command hallucinations may increase the risk of suicide. As many as 10% of patients with schizophrenia eventually carry through on suicidal ideations, mostly during periods of improvement from a relapse or during episodes of depression.

Ask the patient about specific behaviors. When did the unusual behaviors begin? Was there an identifiable precipitating situation, event, or element linked to the onset of behaviors? Have the symptoms ever occurred before? If so, what treatment was received? Family members and others may need to be interviewed if the patient cannot provide the necessary information.

Health History

Previous psychiatric disorders should be identified and documented. Pay attention to any preexisting psychotic or mood disorder as well as evidence of posttraumatic stress or personality disorder (e.g., borderline or schizotypal). Ask the patient about a history of neurologic disorders such as seizures, degenerative disorders, neoplasms, traumatic brain injury, and stroke. These disorders often cause hallucinations and delusions. Infections and demyelinating diseases also should be noted.

Multiple medical conditions such as metabolic disturbances, poisonings, myelin diseases, nutritional deficiency states, and the use of mind-altering substances can lead to abnormalities of perception and thought. Pay attention to endocrine and autoimmune disorders as well as conditions resulting in acute confusional states.

Because of the genetic predisposition for many primary psychiatric disorders, a family history of similar symptoms or other psychiatric history can provide valuable information. Effective management strategies used to treat a family member will often be successful in the patient who has a similar psychotic presentation. This is particularly important in a family with a history of schizophrenia, major depression, or bipolar disorder (see Chapters 17 and 18).

Determine whether the patient has taken psychoactive drugs in the past. Information about the drug, dosage, route, responses, and if applicable, reason for stopping therapy should be gathered. An in-depth assessment of all drugs that the patient is taking is necessary.

Substance abuse is known to predispose a person to develop psychosis, especially with substantial ingestion of substances such as alcohol, lysergic acid diethylamide (LSD), phencyclidine (PCP), and cocaine or with acute alcohol withdrawal. Substance-induced psychotic symptoms may persist long after the cessation of the offending drug (e.g., posthallucinogen perceptive disorder months or years after LSD use).

Lifespan Considerations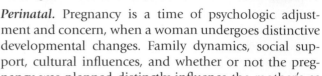

Perinatal. Pregnancy is a time of psychologic adjustment and concern, when a woman undergoes distinctive developmental changes. Family dynamics, social support, cultural influences, and whether or not the pregnancy was planned distinctly influence the mother's as well as the family's adjustment to the pregnancy.

Determine whether or not the woman has a previous history of psychosis that may be now complicated by the pregnancy. During the first trimester, the woman normally feels some ambivalence about the pregnancy, even if it was planned. Discuss these feelings with the woman, because she may feel the need to hide negative feelings, thinking they are abnormal. The ambivalence usually ends by the beginning of the second trimester. Treatment of psychosis during pregnancy is complicated because many of the antipsychotic drugs are pregnancy category C drugs. This means that they are given only after taking into account the risks to the fetus; animal studies have shown adverse reactions, but no studies in humans are available.

Pediatrics. The term childhood schizophrenia is no longer used when discussing mental disorders of childhood. Children adapting to life experiences exhibit symptoms that in an adult would be characteristic of mental illness. Psychotic behaviors generally appear after 5 years of age. Speech disorganization, behavior disorganization, and catatonia are most often found in children.

Psychotic behavior in an adolescent may be obvious from childhood or it can be triggered by a developmental crisis. Some health care providers believe that an individual must at least reach the developmental stage of adolescence before the diagnosis of schizophrenia can be made. The disease process during adolescence is noted by a gradual disintegration in several areas of mental functioning. The youth's lack of integration of thought processes is manifested most often by disturbed behavior, emotions, and speech patterns. In children it is necessary to exclude pervasive developmental disorders.

An adolescent is not a miniature adult but rather a developing person within a family system. The adolescent's needs are not those of an adult but rather those of an individual in an emotional and often confusing world. Therefore information should be collected from the parents and adolescent about the history and progress of the illness. Observations of parent-adolescent interactions and the effectiveness of those interactions with the environment are documented. Additionally, the extent to which an adolescent can distinguish self from the environment and whether there is evidence of self-mutilation or aggressive behavior can help determine if the individual can distinguish between reality and fantasy. The adolescent may be unaware of anything but a growing sense of unhappiness. To an adolescent, asking for help is developmentally inconsistent with the internal drive for mastery and control. Until recently, seeking professional help also carried a social stigma. Since adolescents are particularly prone to emotional disturbances, the health care provider needs to incorporate assessment of mental health as part of the database.

Older Adults. An older adult's sense of self and security is threatened when it becomes necessary to adapt to various personal changes. Changes in physical status, loss of significant other, hospitalization, or movement to a long-term care facility have a profound effect on the older adult's sense of independence. Uncharacteristic behaviors may emerge or existing personality traits may be exaggerated when a person is confined to an acute-care setting, or is in a crisis state, or is receiving treatment and drugs.

The greatest risk factor for late-life psychosis appears to be progressive dementia. Psychosis related to dementia often presents itself as aggressive behavior accompanied by paranoia and delusions. Current estimates project that 33% to 73% of individuals with Alzheimer's disease (see Chapter 23) experience psychotic symptoms.

An accurate assessment of the older adult should include recent changes or new stressors, a drug history, and the use of stimulants such as caffeine, nicotine, or OTC drugs, including cold remedy preparations. A formal examination of the patient's cognitive status (e.g., mini-Mental State Examination [MMSE]) is particularly useful in an older adult patient to help rule out dementia.

Cultural/Social Considerations

Stressful life events tend to occur before an episode of psychosis but do not cause the psychosis. Rather, these events can be viewed as destabilizing factors that exacerbate a preexisting tendency to develop psychosis. People with prolonged psychosis tend to experience a phenomenon known as *social drift*; that is, their impairment causes a downward shift in social class. Whether this change in social class is a cause or an effect of a prolonged psychotic state is not always clear. Most current data suggests that lower social class is a consequence of the psychosis.

Physical Examination

Although it may be difficult to perform a full physical examination on a psychotic individual, it is vital to establish baseline parameters. The baseline information is used to identify underlying medical problems and to monitor both progression of the disorder and responsiveness to the antipsychotic drug or potential adverse effects.

The patient's appearance (attention to personal hygiene and clothing, posture, and general nutritional state) may indicate an underlying psychotic thought process.

Laboratory Testing

Most routine laboratory tests ordered are appropriate for the patient with acute-onset or chronic psychosis. The purpose in ordering these evaluations is to uncover secondary causes for the psychosis (e.g., hyperthyroidism, Huntington's chorea, dementia, substance abuse). A urine drug screening should be considered for patients with acute-onset psychosis or the reemergence of a previously controlled psychosis when visual hallucinations are prominent.

Although no specific testing is required, it is prudent to gather information about liver, heart, and neurologic functioning whenever possible. CBC count, liver function tests, and ECG results should be recorded. A CT scan may be used to determine the presence of structural abnormalities in patients experiencing first-time or acute-onset psychosis. Magnetic resonance imaging (MRI), positron emission tomography (PET), and single proton emission computed tomography (SPECT) scans may indicate abnormalities consistent with schizophrenia.

GOALS OF THERAPY

The primary goal for the patient with a psychotic disorder is to diminish the psychotic behaviors, thus preventing harm to the patient or others, improving thought disorders, reducing the duration of inpatient hospitalization, and preventing or decreasing the severity of future exacerbations. Reduction of psychotic symptoms also facilitates a higher level of functioning. Accomplishing these goals permits the patient to participate more fully in psychotherapy. However, in so doing, the safety and functioning of the patient are key factors.

INTERVENTION

Antipsychotic drugs are the primary treatment option for patients with psychosis. Whether the patient is hospitalized, is in a community-based outpatient program, or is residing at home or in a long-term care facility, little improvement can be made without the drugs. Electroconvulsive therapy may be used to control psychotic behaviors in some patients.

Despite the wide variety of available antipsychotic drugs, there are no convincing data that one antipsychotic drug is necessarily more effective than another.

Furthermore, there is no evidence to suggest that higher doses of antipsychotic drugs are likely to improve psychosis faster than lower doses, although higher doses increase the risk of adverse effects and should be avoided. Additionally, caution must be exercised when antipsychotic drugs are used for persons residing in long-term care facilities. Antipsychotic drugs used as chemical restraints must be justified in the patient's records (Box 19-3).

Administration

Typically, antipsychotic drugs are first given orally for at least 1 to 2 weeks before the patient is switched to a depot formulation. After the depot form is administered the oral dosage is tapered. At this time, no specific guidelines for tapering the oral dose have been developed. Tapering is handled on an individual basis, and the health care provider must remain cognizant that the steady state of the parenteral formulations is not achieved for several weeks.

The first oral dose of an antipsychotic drug should be given 12 to 24 hours after administration of the last parenteral dose. An intramuscular injection is the preferred route (for the most rapid effect) when prompt control of an acutely agitated patient is desired. The injection should be given in a large muscle mass. The patient should be warned that the drug may cause a burning sensation while being injected. The administration sites should be recorded and rotated. The patient should be kept recumbent for at least 30 minutes after administration to minimize the drug's hypotensive effects.

If the patient refuses the injection, a liquid formulation may be used. Liquid formulations provide a more rapid response than tablets. Oral formulations are to be taken with food, milk, or a full glass of water to minimize gastric irritation. Concentrated oral formulations of many antipsychotic drugs are available for institutional use. Most concentrates can be diluted in 120 mL of water or fruit juice just before administration. The solution should be handled with caution because it can cause contact dermatitis.

For missed doses, if the drug is ordered once daily, advise the patient to take the missed dose as soon as remembered on the day it was due; otherwise omit the missed dose and resume the regular dosing schedule the next day. If the drug is ordered more than once daily, advise the patient to take the missed dose as soon as re-

---

BOX 19-3   Patient Problem: Chemical Restraints in Nursing Homes

The Problem

A chemical restraint is the use of a drug to control an individual's behavior. Such use is legally appropriate only if used to ensure the physical safety of residents or other individuals. The usage rates of inappropriate chemical restraints in nursing homes has been increasing since 1995. As a result, the Senate Committee on Aging has requested that the Office of the Inspector General look into the matter. They found that psychoactive drug use in nursing homes is appropriate in 85% of cases. However, legislative guidelines were imposed to reduce inappropriate use.

The Solution

Chemical restraints may be used only upon the written order of a health care provider. The order must specify the duration and circumstances under which the restraints are to be used. The following situations require written assessment and documentation for continued use of psychoactive drugs:
- Continuous use of hypnotic drugs for more than 30 days
- Concurrent use of two or more antipsychotic or hypnotic drugs at the same time
- Anxiolytic, hypnotic, or antipsychotic drugs administered in excess of listed maximum dosages
- Use of psychoactive drugs in dementia unless the condition is associated with psychotic or agitated features subjectively disturbing to the patient or leading to agitated or dangerous behavior that interferes with patient safety or care
- Use of antipsychotic drugs for the sole purpose of controlling anxiety, wandering, restlessness, or insomnia
- Use of antipsychotic drugs for less than 3 days unless to control acute episodes of agitation
- Use of anticholinergic drugs in combination with antipsychotic drugs in the absence of extrapyramidal symptoms

Federal guidelines require monitoring for tardive dyskinesia (using the Abnormal Involuntary Movement Scale [AIMS] assessment tool) every 6 months in recognition of the older adult's vulnerability to this disorder. Patients must be provided with drug holidays, gradual dosage reductions, and behavioral management in an effort to discontinue the drugs.

membered, if within 1 hour of when it was scheduled; otherwise omit the dose and resume regular dosing schedule with the next dose. Missed doses should not be doubled up.

Supervise the patient carefully to determine that the drug is swallowed and not hidden in the mouth to be discarded or stored for later use. Some antipsychotic drugs are available in syrup, injection, or depot formulations to ensure that the patient receives the prescribed dose. In an outpatient situation, it may be necessary for a responsible family member to supervise drug administration.

The patient's blood pressure should be monitored every 4 hours until the patient is stable; this may require several days to 2 weeks. Some health care providers prefer that blood pressure be monitored with the patient in lying, sitting, and standing positions. Monitor fluid intake and output until the patient is stabilized. The patient should be weighed weekly on the same scale and in the same type of clothing, and the blood glucose level should be checked periodically.

Adverse effects may make the patient unsteady when ambulating. Supervise ambulation and assist when appropriate. The patient should be watched closely and seizure precautions should be instituted for the patient with a history of seizures, because antipsychotic drugs may alter the seizure threshold.

The patient should be monitored closely for evidence of extrapyramidal effects, and the health care provider notified right away if any of these adverse effects are observed.

Education

The patient and support individuals who assist the patient (e.g., family or assisted living supervisor) must be taught about the psychotic disorder, its possible causes, associated behaviors, and the importance of drug therapy in managing symptoms. Because some symptoms subside before others, it is helpful to educate the patient and his or her support group about which behaviors are likely to change first, how long after initiation of treatment the change will take place, and how to recognize extrapyramidal symptoms. Because there is no effective treatment for tardive dyskinesia, its appearance should be reported immediately. Fine vermicular (worm-like) movements of the tongue may be the first sign of this adverse effect. Instruct the patient and family to report any new signs and symptoms and not to discontinue therapy abruptly without consulting with the health care provider. Warn the patient to avoid driving or operating hazardous equipment until the effects of the drug are known.

Assess tactfully for changes in libido, gynecomastia, galactorrhea, and other endocrine problems that may develop in some patients. If priapism (prolonged, painful, inappropriate erection of the penis) develops, notify the health care provider. Instruct female patients to keep a record of the menstrual cycle. Some of these drugs may cause amenorrhea or other changes in the cycle. If pregnancy is suspected, instruct the patient to notify the health care provider immediately.

Advise the patient taking chlorpromazine, mesoridazine, thiothixene, or trifluoperazine that it may color the urine pink or reddish brown. Yellowing of the skin and eyes is common with molindone. Patients taking trifluoperazine should be cautioned to avoid prolonged exposure to the sun to minimize photosensitivity reactions.

Antipsychotic drugs interfere with the body's ability to regulate temperature. Instruct patients about how to care for the transient fevers that may occur during the first 3 weeks of therapy. Warn the patient to avoid prolonged exposure to extremes of temperature, to allow for frequent cooling-off periods when exercising or in hot environments, and to dress warmly for exposure to the cold.

The patient and family should be informed about any additional drugs that may be prescribed to manage the adverse effects of antipsychotic drugs. For example, benztropine (Cogentin) may be administered to diminish the anticholinergic effects of haloperidol. The patient should be taught that chewing sugarless gum might assist in relieving the dry mouth associated with the drug, and that frequent rinsing with cool water refreshes a dry mouth. If hypotensive effects are experienced, the patient should be shown how to change positions and rise slowly from lying or seated positions.

The patient should be advised to carry medical alert identification containing information about the antipsychotic drugs taken. He or she should be instructed to inform all health care providers (e.g., nurses, physicians, practitioners, dentists, and physical therapists) of their regimen. In so doing, therapeutic effects as well as adverse drug effects and interactions can be monitored.

EVALUATION

The effectiveness of antipsychotic therapy is demonstrated by a decrease in the symptoms and the severity of the psychosis. Agitation should be diminished within hours of initiating therapy, and significant improvement should be seen within 24 to 48 hours. Sleep disturbances should improve within days, hallucinations within weeks, and thought disorders within 1 to 2 months. Negative symptoms such as anhedonia and restricted or blunted affect take weeks to months to improve. In some cases, negative symptoms may not improve at all. Some patients require 8 to 12 weeks of therapy at typical doses before full response.

The dosage of the antipsychotic drug is maintained for at least 4 to 6 weeks and the patient's response is evaluated before a different drug or dosage is considered. Because first-generation antipsychotic drugs tend to have a slow onset of action, the direct correlation between dosage and therapeutic effectiveness is difficult to judge. If improvement is observed at 4 weeks, therapy is continued for an additional 2 weeks, at which point the patient is reevaluated. The duration of therapy depends on the patient's specific diagnosis. However, in schizophrenia, maintenance therapy is usually necessary to maintain patient functioning.

Over time, patients who have responded positively to treatment may be permitted a gradual reduction in dosage to allow for a drug holiday and to determine the need for ongoing therapy.

Patients should be monitored weekly for signs of decompensation. There is a 50% relapse rate at 6 months.

Delusions, paranoia, disorganized thinking, and command hallucinations can interfere with compliance. Compliance is particularly problematic if the illness, its treatment, or the health care provider is incorporated into the psychosis. One year after therapy is discontinued, the relapse rate is approximately 70%, but if therapy is continued, only 40% of patients relapse. As a rule, after the first episode of decompensation, the patient should be treated continuously for 1 year. After a second episode, he or she should be treated continuously for at least 3 years. With a third episode of decompensation, treatment should extend for at least 5 years before attempting a drug holiday. However, the risk of developing tardive dyskinesia increases with the length of therapy and the patient's age.

CASE STUDY   *Schizophrenia*

ASSESSMENT

HISTORY OF PRESENT ILLNESS

NC is a 55-year-old man with a long history of psychoses resulting from damage to the brain from lead poisoning as a child. He is brought to the psychiatrist's office today by his brother, who is his legal guardian. The brother notes that NC's condition has deteriorated in recent weeks despite adherence to antipsychotic drug therapy. He has been hostile, combative, and more paranoid than usual. He appears to hallucinate at times.

HEALTH HISTORY

NC has no significant health care problems except for gingivitis, for which he sees a periodontist every 3 months. His current medications include chlorpromazine 300 mg daily in divided doses.

LIFESPAN CONSIDERATIONS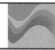

NC has been unable to relate to his spouse, who is thinking about filing for divorce. His two college-age children have all but disowned him. His younger brother remains in close contact.

CULTURAL/SOCIAL CONSIDERATIONS

NC's disease has prevented him from seeking and holding onto gainful employment. He has had 6 different positions in the last 6 months and thus has no health or pharmacy insurance. The brother would like assistance in filing for Social Security disability.

PHYSICAL EXAMINATION

NC glances around the room as if responding to internal stimuli. There is little to no direct eye contact with the health care provider, and he delays answering questions.

LABORATORY TESTING

None.

PATIENT PROBLEM(S)

Organic psychosis.

GOALS OF THERAPY

Reduce positive symptoms and improve negative symptoms associated with schizophrenia.

CRITICAL THINKING QUESTIONS

1. The health care provider considers the use of clozapine and risperidone. The decision is made to use risperidone for NC's psychosis. What are the advantages and disadvantages of this drug over clozapine?
2. What is the mechanism of action of risperidone?
3. Of which adverse effects should NC and his family be made aware? How are these adverse effects monitored?
4. Which four actions of antipsychotic drugs can be attributed to blockade of dopaminergic receptors?
5. For which types of psychoses are antipsychotic drugs generally effective?

Bibliography

American Psychiatric Association: *Diagnostic and statistical manual of mental disorders: DSM-IV,* ed 4, Washington, DC, 1994, American Psychiatric Press.

Antai-Otong D: Schizophrenia in the elderly, *Adv Nurse Pract* 8(3):38-40, 46, 2000.

Barron M: Tardive dyskinesia, *Nurse Pract* 24(4):144-147, 1999.

Bennett J: Antipsychotic drug treatment, *Nurs Stand* 13(24):49-53, 55-56, 1999.

Coffey M: Psychosis and medication: strategies for improving adherence, *Br J Nurs* 8(4):225-230, 1999.

Coffey M: Schizophrenia: a review of current research and thinking, *J Clin Nurs* 7(6):489-498, 1998.

Ecdeu GW: Assessment Manual for Psychopharmacology, revised ed, Washington, DC, 1976, U.S. Department of Health, Education, and Welfare.

Gray R, Gournay K: What can we do about acute extrapyramidal symptoms? *J Psychiatr Ment Health Nurs* 7(3):205-211, 2000.

Kalinyak CM: Schizophrenia treatment: the use of atypical drugs—risperdal, zyperexa, and clozaril, *Int J Psychiatr Nurs Res* 4(2):445-451, 1998.

Marland GR, Sharkey V: Depot neuroleptics, schizophrenia and the role of the nurse: is practice evidence based? A review of the literature, *J Adv Nurs* 30(6):1255-1262, 1999.

Pickford M: Antipsychotic drug overdose, *Emerg Nurse* 7(9):17-22, 2000.

Psychotropic drug use in nursing homes, Doc. OEI-02-00-00490, Rockville, MD, 2001, U.S. Department of Health and Human Services, Office of Inspector General.

Internet Resource

Clinical Evidence, London, BMJ Publishing Group. Available online: www.clinicalevidence.org.

Central Nervous System Stimulants

MICHAEL R. VASKO • KATHLEEN GUTIERREZ

 Visit **http://evolve.elsevier.com/Gutierrez/** for additional information.

KEY TERMS

Analeptic, p. 311

Anorexiants, p. 309

Attention-deficit hyperactivity disorder (ADHD), p. 304

Cataplexy, p. 303

Narcolepsy, p. 303

Obese, p. 308

OBJECTIVES

- Identify the appropriate clinical uses of CNS stimulants.
- Discuss the adverse effects of these drugs.
- Differentiate among drugs used to treat narcolepsy, attention-deficit hyperactivity disorder, or obesity.
- Develop a nursing care plan for a patient who is receiving a CNS stimulant.

 PATHOPHYSIOLOGY • Narcolepsy

Narcolepsy is a sleep disorder characterized by unexpected and unwanted falling asleep during times of normal activity such as while typing, driving a car, or talking. In addition to the sleepiness, patients with narcolepsy can also exhibit periodic episodes of cataplexy (sudden brief episodes of muscle weakness and paralysis), sleep paralysis, hypnagogic hallucinations, and automatic behavior. Hypnagogic hallucinations are brief, fragmented, and vivid dreamlike experiences that occur while the patient is not fully asleep (usually when falling asleep). Cataplexy affects 70% to 80% of patients with narcolepsy, and can range from slight weakness of muscles to abrupt collapse. Patients may exhibit cataplexy at any time but are particularly prone to attacks during emotional disturbances, such as excitement, crying, or even laughter. Sleep paralysis manifests as a loss of muscle tone, paralysis, and the inability to speak for a brief time when falling asleep or waking up. During the episodic attacks, an observer may notice the patient performing automatic behaviors, mindless and simple repetitive tasks that cannot be remembered by the patient after the attack is over.

Less observable symptoms are by far the most frequent in patients with narcolepsy. Patients may note a slight buckling of the knees, but the buckling is imperceptible to an observer. The observer may notice only that the patient used a wall for support. A weakening of the jaw, similar to that accompanying REM sleep, may occur. Jaw weakness affects speech or causes wide masticatory (chewing) movements or brief stutter. Patients also may complain of clumsiness, especially when they are startled or laughing.

Narcolepsy occurs in 5 of 1000 adults. Although the first episode can occur at any time up to the age of 60 years, it usually begins when patients are in their twenties. There appears to be a genetic component to some

narcolepsy, but unknown environmental factors may also be responsible for the disease. The patient who experiences narcolepsy may also have one or more natural sleep activities disturbed.

There are a number of theories as to the causes of narcolepsy; however, the mechanisms for the disease remain unknown. Recent studies suggest that a defect in the neuropeptides hypocretin I or II may play a role. One of the important features of narcolepsy is the possibility of REM sleep cycles occurring during wakefulness, which produce the major symptoms of narcolepsy. REM sleep is initiated by acetylcholine neurons in the brainstem and is inhibited by norepinephrine-containing neurons. Hypocretin neurons projecting from the hypothalamus to the brainstem excite noradrenergic neurons, thereby inhibiting REM sleep. The theory is that when the hypocretin level is low or its receptors are not functioning, the ability of monoamine neurons to suppress REM sleep is reduced. Animal studies support this theory because dogs with a genetic defect in hypocretin receptors have a narcoleptic syndrome, and specific mice that do not make hypocretin have narcoleptic-like behavior.

PATHOPHYSIOLOGY • Attention-Deficit Hyperactivity Disorder

Attention-deficit hyperactivity disorder (ADHD) manifests itself in one of three major behavioral types: hyperactivity and impulsivity, inattentiveness, or both inattentiveness and hyperactivity. Patients with ADHD display a variety of symptoms that impair their ability to learn or to maintain appropriate social interactions. To be diagnosed with ADHD, the individual's behavior must match six of nine defined criteria for both inattentiveness and hyperactivity-impulsivity (Box 20-1). Because other disorders (especially anxiety and depression) may cause similar symptoms, a diagnosis of ADHD must be made with care. The disorder may persist into adolescence and adulthood for many patients. The diagnosis in adults is the same as in children, with emphasis on impaired function in daily activities.

Controversy has surrounded the diagnosis and treatment of children with ADHD. Some authorities have claimed the disorder is diagnosed more often than it exists and suggest that thousands of children may be receiving CNS stimulants unnecessarily, pointing to the lower rate of drug use for this condition in Europe and England. The adoption of more rigorous criteria for diagnosis has reduced the risk of inappropriate drug treatment. At the same time, numerous clinical trials have shown the efficacy of CNS stimu-

lants in reducing hyperactivity, impulsivity, and inattentiveness in patients with ADHD. Dietary manipulation for ADHD has failed to control symptoms, whereas counseling assists in achieving favorable long-term outcomes.

Theories about the causes of ADHD include a genetic relationship, trauma or infection in utero, nutritional deficits or allergies, and an imbalance in dopamine or norepinephrine in the brain. However, a single cause of the disorder has yet to be identified, possibly because ADHD represents several different conditions. There is evidence of a genetic link in a number of families with individuals diagnosed with the disorder.

ADHD may occur as a result of a reduction in functional dopamine or norepinephrine, especially in the prefrontal cortex and the basal ganglia. Studies suggest that patients with this disorder have decreased blood flow and decreased dopamine activity in brain regions associated with it. The drugs commonly used to treat ADHD augment dopamine activity in the brain. Norepinephrine may act to inhibit the processing of irrelevant information in the prefrontal cortex, thereby enhancing focus on tasks. Thus a decrease in the function of this transmitter might contribute to attention deficits.

BOX 20-1 | **Diagnostic Criteria of Attention-Deficit Hyperactivity Disorder**

Symptoms from Either 1 or 2 Below

1. Six or more of the following symptoms of *inattention* persisting for at least 6 months and to a degree that is maladaptive and inconsistent with developmental level
   - Fails to give close attention to details in schoolwork, work, or other activities
   - Has difficulty sustaining attention in tasks or play activities
   - Does not seem to listen when spoken to directly
   - Does not follow through on instructions and fails to finish schoolwork, chores, or duties in the workplace (not because of oppositional behavior or failure to understand instructions)
   - Has difficulty organizing tasks and activities
   - Avoids, dislikes, or is reluctant to engage in tasks requiring sustained mental effort
   - Loses things necessary for task or activities (e.g., toys, school assignments, pencils, books, or tools)
   - Is easily distracted by extraneous stimuli
   - Is forgetful in daily activities
2. Six (or more) of the following symptoms of *hyperactivity-impulsivity* persisting for at least 6 months and to a degree that is maladaptive and inconsistent with developmental level

Hyperactivity
- Fidgets with hands or feet or squirms in seat
- Leaves seat in classroom or other situations in which remaining seated is expected
- Runs about or climbs excessively in situations in which it is inappropriate (in adolescents or adults, may be limited to subjective feelings of restlessness)
- Has difficulty playing or engaging in leisurely activities quietly
- Is constantly "on the go" or often acts as if driven by a motor
- Talks excessively

Impulsivity
- Blurts out answers before questions have been completed
- Has difficulty awaiting turn
- Interrupts or intrudes on others (e.g., butts into conversations or games)

3. Clear evidence of clinically significant impairment in social, academic, or occupational functioning
4. Some hyperactive, impulsive, or inattentive symptoms that caused impairment present before age 7
5. Some impairment from the symptoms present in two or more settings (e.g., school, workplace, home)
6. Symptoms not occurring exclusively during the course of (or are not accounted for by) another mental disorder

From the American Psychiatric Association: *Diagnostic and statistical manual of mental disorders (DSM-IV)*, ed 4, Washington, DC, 1994, American Psychiatric Press.

DRUG CLASS • CNS Stimulants

amphetamine

dextroamphetamine (Dexedrine, Dextrostat)

methamphetamine (Desoxyn)

methylphenidate (Ritalin, Ritalin SR, Concerta, Methylin ER, Metadate CD)

modafinil (Provigil)

oxybate (Xyrem)

pemoline (Cylert)

The drugs used to treat narcolepsy and ADHD will be discussed together because a number of these drugs overlap (Table 20-1). It is important to note, however, that modafinil and oxybate are only indicated for narcolepsy, whereas pemoline is used only for ADHD. Additional drugs used in the management of ADHD are the antidepressants imipramine, desipramine, protripty-line, bupropion, and venlafaxine, which are discussed in detail in Chapter 18, and the alpha-adrenergic receptor agonists guanfacine and clonidine (see Chapter 41). Selective antidepressants are also employed for the treatment of cataplexy in patients with narcolepsy.

MECHANISM OF ACTION

The actions of amphetamines, such as dextroamphetamine and methamphetamine, result from their ability to increase the release of norepinephrine and dopamine from nerve terminals in the central and peripheral nervous systems. Amphetamines may affect many sites in the brain, but the clinically observed actions may be related to stimulation of the reticular activating system, increasing alertness and sensitivity to stimuli. Another area of the brain stimulated by amphetamines is the reward center. Actions affecting dopamine at this site are

---

TABLE 20-1

CNS Stimulants for Narcolepsy and Attention-Deficit Hyperactivity Disorder

Generic Name	Brand Name	Comments
amphetamine (also called racemic or D-amphetamine sulfate)	Adderall, Adderall-XR	Schedule II drug (U.S.). Dosage is adjusted according to patient's needs and tolerance to adverse effects. Dosage should be minimum required for control of symptoms. New, longer-acting formulation available to extend duration.
dextroamphetamine	Dexedrine, Dextrostat, Dexedrine-SR	Schedule II drug (U.S.); Class C drug (Canada). Dosage should be minimum required for control of symptoms. New, longer-acting formulation available to extend duration.
methamphetamine	Desoxyn	Schedule II drug. Dosage should be minimum required for control of symptoms.
methylphenidate	Ritalin, Concerta, Ritalin-SR, Methylin ER, Metadate ER, Metadate CD	Schedule II drug (U.S.); Class C drug (Canada). Drug of choice for most children with ADHD. New, longer-acting formulations available to extend duration.
modafinil	Provigil	Schedule IV drug (U.S.). Less overall activation of the CNS. Used only for narcolepsy.
oxybate (gamma-hydroxybutyrate, GHB)	Xyrem	Schedule III drug (U.S.). Orphan drug for treating narcolepsy. GHB has potential for substance abuse and is known as the date-rape drug.
pemoline	Cylert	Schedule IV drug (U.S.). Clinical effects develop over 3 to 4 weeks.

thought to be the source of the dependency potential of amphetamines.

Methylphenidate is a mild CNS stimulant. Its exact biochemical mechanism of action is unknown but it may involve blockade of dopamine uptake in specific regions of the brain. Although pemoline apparently stimulates the CNS by acting on dopaminergic systems, the exact biochemical mechanism of action for this drug remains unknown. Modafinil's action differs from that of amphetamines and methylphenidate in that it appears to activate discrete brain regions, but its mechanism and that of oxybate remain unknown. The orphan drug oxybate is actually gamma hydroxybutyrate (GHB), which is a CNS depressant yet it somehow decreases daytime sleep.

USES

Psychomotor stimulants such as amphetamines promote arousal, alleviate symptoms of narcolepsy, and are particularly helpful in the management of patients with moderate to severe ADHD. In addition to managing ADHD behavior, these stimulants may also increase cognition. Amphetamines, however, have a high incidence of adverse effects, and their potential for abuse limits their usefulness. As a result, methylphenidate is currently the preferred drug for the management of ADHD. It is also useful in the management of narcolepsy because of its mild CNS stimulatory effects on the cortex and other portions of the brain. Pemoline is recommended only for the management of ADHD, but it is not used routinely as initial therapy because of its potential for liver toxicity (see below). Modafinil and oxybate are only used to treat narcolepsy.

PHARMACOKINETICS

Amphetamines for medical uses are given orally. These drugs are well absorbed from the gastrointestinal (GI) tract and produce peak serum concentrations within 2 to 3 hours after ingestion. Recently, several slow-release amphetamine preparations have been marketed (see Table 20-1) to lengthen the duration of action. The half-lives of the various amphetamines in the blood range from 4 to 30 hours. These drugs easily penetrate the blood-brain barrier to produce their CNS effects. Amphetamines are biotransformed in the liver and are eliminated primarily through the kidneys. The elimination rate varies with urinary pH and therefore can be enhanced by acidifying the urine.

Methylphenidate is adequately absorbed orally when taken with meals. Orally administered methylphenidate is extensively biotransformed during the first pass through the liver. Peak plasma concentration is achieved within 2 hours for the regular tablets, 1 to 8 hours for extended-release formulations, and 6 to 8 hours for methylphenidate delivered by oral administration of a mini-osmotic pump (Concerta). Most of the drug is biotransformed into inactive compounds, then eliminated through the kidney, with less than 1% of the parent compound excreted unchanged. Pemoline is well absorbed orally, and produces its peak serum level within 2 to 4 hours. The serum half-life for the drug is about 12 hours and thus can be given once daily. The kidneys eliminate 50% of the pemoline as unchanged drug and the rest as metabolites after liver biotransformation. Although the blood level reaches a plateau within a few days after therapy is begun, the therapeutic effects of pemoline are not immediately evident in hyperkinetic children. Dosage is gradually increased over 2 to 4 weeks after therapy is started. Significant clinical response may not be seen until the third or fourth week of therapy.

Oral absorption of modafinil is rapid and the peak plasma level occurs in 2 to 4 hours. The drug is extensively biotransformed in the liver, with less then 10% eliminated unchanged. The half-life is approximately 15 hours.

ADVERSE REACTIONS AND CONTRAINDICATIONS

Amphetamines stimulate the CNS, causing excitation, irritability, nocturnal sleep disturbances, tremor, restlessness, amphetamine psychosis, seizures, and euphoria. Because they enhance feelings of well-being and control, they have a high potential for abuse (see Chapter 9). They are not recommended for patients with psychosis, because they can exacerbate the illness.

Amphetamines also produce cardiac stimulation and can increase blood pressure. Thus they are contraindicated in patients with cardiovascular disease (e.g., hypertension, angina, arrhythmia) or hyperthyroidism. Patients with glaucoma should not be given psychomotor stimulants. Amphetamines in general have teratogenic effects, and their use during pregnancy should be avoided. Uterine response varies, but there is usually an increase in uterine muscle tone. Children receiving amphetamines may experience growth retardation as a result of loss of appetite. Instituting drug holidays can minimize this effect. These drugs may also cause difficulty in falling asleep.

Methylphenidate often causes nervousness and insomnia as well as anorexia, nausea, and abdominal pain, which can reduce the appetite. Cardiovascular ef-

DRUG ABUSE ALERT Methylphenidate

The Problem

Methylphenidate rarely causes toxic psychosis but may cause psychologic drug dependence. Both effects are observed after long-term use with dosages exceeding therapeutic levels. The patient is most at risk for developing dependency, but health care providers must also be alert to the problem among caregivers. For example, adult guardians of children receiving methylphenidate may divert the drug from the child and use it themselves. Adolescents treated with methylphenidate may also share the drug with friends and acquaintances.

The Solution

- Confirm that dosages are not being extemporaneously increased by the patient or the health care provider.
- Be alert for signs that the drug is being diverted from the patient to inappropriate recipients.
- Advise the patient to seek medical advice if the drug seems to become less effective after several weeks.
- See that dosage is reduced gradually so that withdrawal symptoms are minimized.

fects similar to those produced by amphetamines are also seen and include hypertension and tachycardia. Methylphenidate causes a temporary slowing of growth in prepubertal children, probably resulting from appetite suppression. Most children overcome the deficit and ultimately gain normal stature. There is a risk of psychologic dependency on the drug (see the box above). Methylphenidate should be avoided by patients with severe anxiety, depression, motor tics (e.g., Tourette's syndrome), or glaucoma because the drug may worsen these conditions.

Pemoline often causes insomnia, anorexia, and weight loss. Irritability, mild depression, dizziness, headache, and hallucinations are rare. Children do not seem to experience permanent growth retardation, but careful records of the child's growth should be maintained to allow assessment during therapy. Pemoline should be avoided by patients with impaired hepatic function because the drug may cause liver failure. Pemoline has been associated with cases of liver failure that required transplantation or caused the death of the child, many of whom seemed to have normal liver function before therapy.

Modafinil may cause anxiety, headache, nausea, insomnia, and nervousness, whereas the adverse effects of oxybate include dizziness, nausea, headache, and enuresis.

TOXICITY

The CNS toxicity of amphetamines is an extension of effects observed at therapeutic dosages. At high dosages, amphetamines cause restless behavior, tremor, irritability, talkativeness, insomnia, and mood changes. Excessive aggression, confusion, panic, and increased libido also may occur. With long-term use, patients sometimes experience toxic psychosis, which resembles schizophrenia in that hallucinations or delirium may occur. The ability of amphetamines to stimulate adrenergic receptors also can cause various cardiovascular reactions. Patients report headache, chills, and palpitations. Pallor or facial flushing may be present. Angina and arrhythmia may arise. Hypertension or hypotension may be observed at various stages during intoxication. Severely intoxicated patients may die in circulatory collapse.

Very high dosages of methylphenidate and pemoline can cause dangerous CNS effects (agitation, confusion, delirium, seizures, and coma) and cardiovascular effects (arrhythmia and hypertension). Though rare, there is a risk of thrombocytopenia, anemia, leukopenia, and neuroleptic malignant syndrome with methylphenidate (see Box 19-1). Symptoms of withdrawal seen after prolonged use at high dosages include bizarre behavior, depression, and unusual tiredness or weakness.

INTERACTIONS

Most of the dangerous interactions with amphetamines involve cardiovascular symptoms. For example, amphetamines administered with tricyclic antidepressants increase the risk of arrhythmia and hypertension. Use of amphetamines with beta-adrenergic blockers may cause hypertension and slow heart rate as a result of unopposed alpha-adrenergic activity. Use of amphetamines with meperidine may lead to hypotension, respiratory depression, and vascular collapse. Cardiac glycosides or thyroid hormones may increase the risk of arrhythmia or coronary insufficiency when used in combination with amphetamines. Amphetamines also should not be used in combination with monoamine oxidase inhibitors. Death may occur from hypertensive crisis or cerebral hemorrhage.

Methylphenidate, like the amphetamines, interacts with many other medications. Interactions that result in toxicity can occur with monoamine oxidase inhibitors, sympathomimetic drugs, or vasopressors. Pimozide should be avoided by patients receiving methylphenidate because the risk of tics is increased. Pemoline may cause additive stimulation if used with other CNS stimulants. Significant drug interactions with modafinil and oxybate have yet to be determined.

PATHOPHYSIOLOGY • Obesity

More than half the adult population in the United States is overweight and a significant portion of these are **obese** (defined as a body mass index (BMI) of 30 kg/m^2 or more). The normal BMI range for both men and women is between 20 and 25 kg/m^2. Obesity is associated with several different problems, including hypertension, hyperlipidemia, carbohydrate intolerance, cardiac problems, back problems, and stroke.

Maintaining a certain body weight depends on keeping the balance between caloric intake and caloric needs. Consequently, the shift during the twentieth century from a diet high in carbohydrates to one that is high in fat is a major cause of obesity. Another contributing factor is the decrease in the amount of energy expended in daily activities (e.g., a shift from manual labor to sedentary jobs). Although a certain level of energy is expended when at rest, varying with the individual, the overall decrease in exercise and activity in our society contributes to the caloric imbalance and thus to weight gain.

Evidence clearly points to a genetic component in the tendency toward obesity, although the mechanisms for this disorder remain unknown. Energy expenditure

and fat distribution appear to be particularly influenced by heredity. In recent years, a number of unique proteins have been identified that regulate body weight, providing insight into potential mechanisms for obesity. Of major importance is the hormone leptin, which is released from fat cells and communicates to the brain to maintain body weight. Animals with a leptin deficiency or inactive leptin receptors are obese. In addition, mutations of leptin and leptin receptors have been found in a minority of obese humans. Studies are in progress to determine if leptin treatment is effective in treating obesity.

Other work focuses on the role of neurons containing neuropeptide Y (NPY) neurons and melanocyte-stimulating hormone (MSH) in regulating weight. Neurons containing leptin receptors also contain NPY and agouti-related peptide. Release of NPY activates NPY receptors, which in turn affect the autonomic nervous system to regulate energy balance. Agouti-related peptide is expressed in obesity and may inhibit the action of MSH on melanocortin-4 receptors. Activation of this receptor by MSH is believed to suppress appetite, so that when agouti-related peptide is present, appetite becomes excessive. Finally, there is ongoing work to determine if obesity could involve mutations in adipocytes that affect their production and ability to store fat. One such protein under investigation is peroxisome proliferator-activated receptor–gamma (PPARgamma), which may regulate differentiation of fat cells.

DRUG CLASS • Antiobesity Drugs

Anorexiants

benzphetamine (Didrex)

diethylpropion (Depletite, Dospan, Tenuate, Tepanil)

mazindol (Sanorex, Mazanor)

phendimetrazine (Bontril, X-trozine)

phentermine (Adipex-P)

sibutramine (Meridia)

Lipase Inhibitor

orlistat (Xenical)

Prescription medications used in weight control (exception for orlistat) are listed as Schedule II or IV drugs in the United States because they have the potential to produce drug dependency as a result of CNS stimulation. The antidepressant fluoxetine also is prescribed for the treatment of obesity by many health care providers, although this is not an FDA-approved use at the present time. Fluoxetine is discussed in detail in Chapter 18. There are also a number of OTC weight-loss products that contain chromium, ephedra, and numerous other so-called "natural" products. Some of these products are discussed in Chapter 8.

MECHANISM OF ACTION

Anorexiants suppress appetite, but the mechanism is unclear. CNS stimulants may work by acting on the hypothalamus (Table 20-2). D-Amphetamine and methamphetamine were the original CNS stimulants used to control obesity, but because of the risk of dependency and the tolerance that rapidly develops to the anorexic effects, they are no longer used for this purpose. These drugs increase the release of catecholamines from nerve terminals. Other CNS stimulants, including benzphetamine, diethylpropion, phendimetrazine, and phentermine, also increase catecholamine release. Mazindol and sibutramine appear to act by preventing the reuptake of norepinephrine as well as norepinephrine and serotonin, respectively. Only orlistat does not act by a central mechanism. Rather, this drug is a reversible lipase inhibitor that acts in the GI tract to prevent breakdown of triglycerides to fatty acids, thereby reducing absorption.

TABLE 20-2

Appetite Suppressants

Generic Name	Brand Name	Comments
benzphetamine	Didrex	Schedule III drug (U.S.).
diethylpropion	Depletite, Dospan, Tenuate, Tepanil	Schedule IV drug (U.S.); Class C drug (Canada). Safest anorexiant for use in patients with mild cardiovascular disease.
fluoxetine	Prozac	SSRI antidepressant approved for treatment of bulimia. Prescribed for weight loss by some physicians.
mazindol	Mazanor, Sanorex	Schedule IV drug (U.S.). May be used in patients with arteriosclerosis or hyperthyroidism.
orlistat	Xenical	Inhibitor of intestinal lipases preventing triglyceride breakdown and absorption of fatty acids.
phendimetrazine	Bontril, X-tropine	Schedule III drug (U.S.).
phentermine	Adipex-P	Schedule IV drug (U.S.); Class C drug (Canada).
sibutramine	Meridia	Inhibitor of norepinephrine and serotonin uptake.

USES

These drugs are used for the short-term management of obesity. When prescribed, they are intended to act as adjuncts to other therapies such as behavior modification, exercise, and calorie restrictions. Tolerance develops to all appetite-suppressing drugs in clinical use except orlistat. Drugs to suppress appetite may help a patient during the initial stages of a weight-reduction program, but these drugs are not the key to long-term success.

PHARMACOKINETICS

Anorexiants are well absorbed after oral administration, and sibutramine in particular has an extensive first-pass effect. Orlistat is not absorbed to any significant degree; thus systemic actions are unlikely. Half-lives of the various stimulants range from 4 to 24 hours. Diethylpropion and phentermine are available in extended-release forms that have a duration of action of 12 to 14 hours. Sibutramine is the only drug of this class that is highly bound to plasma proteins (97% to 99%). These drugs are biotransformed in the liver, in some cases to active drugs. Benzphetamine is biotransformed to amphetamine and methamphetamine, whereas sibutramine is biotransformed to forms that have anorexic activity. Elimination of unchanged drugs and metabolites takes place largely through the kidney. Acidifying the urine increases the excretion of benzphetamine, diethylpropion, mazindol, phendimetrazine, and phentermine. Orlistat is eliminated in the feces.

ADVERSE REACTIONS AND CONTRAINDICATIONS

Stimulant anorexiants can elevate mood and increase motor activity. They can also produce nervousness, irritability, restlessness, dizziness, insomnia, and weakness (Table 20-3), as well as nausea, constipation, and dry mouth. They have the potential to worsen psychosis or agitated states. Heart rate and blood pressure may also become elevated with these drugs, and they should be avoided by patients with hypertension, hyperthyroidism, or glaucoma and, except for diethylpropion, by patients with cardiovascular disease. Mazindol is contraindicated in patients with hepatic insufficiency. Orlistat has few adverse effects except fecal urgency, gas, and oily rectal seepage. This drug is not recommended for patients with cholestasis or chronic malabsorption syndrome. It and other anorexiants can also cause hypersensitivity reactions in some patients.

Many effective appetite suppressants have a high potential for abuse, and patients often experience some level of dependence on these drugs. Therefore most appetite suppressants should be avoided by patients with a history of drug or alcohol abuse. Children less than 12 years old should not be given anorexiant drugs.

TOXICITY

Overdosage with stimulant anorexiants produces dangerous cardiovascular and CNS effects, including aggressiveness, convulsions, coma, hallucinations, hostility, panic, restlessness, tremors, arrhythmia, fluctuating blood pressure, and cardiovascular collapse. Symptoms of overdose also include GI distress (e.g., abdominal cramping, diarrhea, nausea, vomiting). Symptoms of withdrawal seen after prolonged use at high dosages include GI distress, insomnia, depression, trembling, and unusual fatigue or weakness.

INTERACTIONS

Anorexiants interact with many other drugs. For example, adrenergic agonists may have a much greater effect in patients receiving appetite suppressants, because the appetite-suppressing drugs tend to increase the effectiveness of catecholamines. This precaution should be mentioned to patients, and they should be warned to avoid cold remedies, allergy medications, and nasal decongestants that include adrenergic drugs. For the same reasons, monoamine oxidase inhibitors should not be used within 14 days of taking an anorexiant. Anorexiants may also block the effects of antihypertensive drugs.

TABLE 20-3

Systemic Effects of Stimulant Appetite Suppressants

Drug	Mood	Motor Activity	Heart Rate	Blood Pressure	Abuse Potential
benzphetamine	Elevated	May increase	May increase	May increase	High
diethylpropion	May be elevated	May increase	Unchanged	Unchanged	Relatively low
mazindol	May be elevated	May increase	Increased	Usually no change	Relatively low
phendimetrazine	Highly elevated	Increased	Usually no change	Usually no change	High
phentermine	Usually no change	May increase	Increased	Increased	Relatively low
sibutramine	May be depressed	Usually no change	Increased	Increased	Relatively low

DRUG CLASS • Analeptics

aminophylline

caffeine

cocaine

doxapram (Dopram)

nicotine

theophylline

The discussion below focuses on caffeine and doxapram as **analeptic** drugs, that is, drugs that increase responsiveness to external stimuli and stimulate respiration. Aminophylline and theophylline are also respiratory stimulants but are discussed in Chapter 52. Nicotine and cocaine are discussed as drugs capable of producing dependence in Chapter 9, whereas cocaine as a local anesthetic is covered in Chapter 16.

MECHANISM OF ACTION

Caffeine can stimulate any level of the CNS, depending on the dosage, but it stimulates the medullary centers controlling respiration, vasomotor tone, and vagal tone only at relatively high dosages. It also stimulates cardiac activity, secretion of gastric acid, and diuresis. On the cellular level, caffeine increases the calcium permeability in the sarcoplasmic or endoplasmic reticulum, thereby increasing free intracellular calcium. It also promotes the accumulation of cyclic adenosine monophosphate (cAMP) and blocks adenosine receptors.

Doxapram stimulates respiration in two ways. At low dosages the drug stimulates carotid chemoreceptors, which increases sensitivity to carbon dioxide and thereby increases the impulse to breathe. At slightly higher dosages, doxapram stimulates CNS medullary centers controlling respiration. The result is that patients breathe more deeply and may breathe slightly more rapidly.

USES

Analeptics are used to stimulate respiration, but their use has become less common because modern techniques of respiratory therapy allow a patient to be adequately ventilated even when the natural reflex is absent. Caffeine is used as a treatment adjunct for apnea in neonates and prophylactically in children for apnea after surgery. This drug is also commonly used as an aid to stay awake. Caffeine is an adjunct in analgesic formulations, largely to aid in drug absorption. Doxapram is indicated only for postanesthesia respiratory depression or acute respiratory insufficiency in chronic obstructive pulmonary disease.

PHARMACOKINETICS

The effects of caffeine begin within 15 minutes of oral administration and peak in 15 to 45 minutes. The duration of action is 3 to 4 hours. The drug is biotransformed in the liver and eliminated in the urine. It crosses placental membranes and passes into breast milk.

Doxapram is administered intravenously. The drug acts very rapidly and effects are observed within 1 minute after injection. The duration of respiratory stimulation is usually 5 to 12 minutes. Doxapram may be given repeatedly or by continuous infusion to sustain a patient throughout a period of respiratory depression, but the maximum dosage should not be exceeded. Doxapram is biotransformed in the liver and eliminated in the urine.

ADVERSE REACTIONS AND CONTRAINDICATIONS

CNS adverse effects of caffeine most often include insomnia, restlessness, excitement, tachycardia, and diuresis. Headaches, light-headedness, nausea, vomiting, diarrhea, and abdominal pain also have been reported. Caffeine withdrawal manifests as anxiety, increased muscle tension, and headache. Doxapram can produce increased reflexes and blood pressure. Laryngospasm, bronchospasm, and seizures have been reported and can be life threatening. Other, less common adverse reactions include headache, dizziness, disorientation, hyperactivity, diaphoresis, and flushing. Nausea, vomiting, and diarrhea can be troublesome reactions as well with this drug.

Caffeine is generally not recommended for patients with a history of depression, duodenal ulcers, and diabetes mellitus, as well as in lactating women. Doxapram is contraindicated in patients with epilepsy, head injury, cerebrovascular accident, severe hypertension, flail chest, pneumothorax, acute asthma, and pulmonary fibrosis. It is to be used cautiously during pregnancy and lactation.

TOXICITY

If doxapram is injected too rapidly, hemolysis may occur. Extreme agitation, hallucinations, or convulsions usually occur only with overdose, but certain patients may be more susceptible to these reactions.

INTERACTIONS

There are increased CNS effects of caffeine when it is taken with cimetidine, oral contraceptives, disulfiram, or ciprofloxacin. Since doxapram increases blood pressure, this drug should not be used in combination with other drugs tending to elevate blood pressure, such as adrenergic agonists and MAO inhibitors. Adverse interactions can also occur between doxapram and inhalation anesthetics that sensitize the heart to catecholamines (e.g., halothane, enflurane). A delay of 10 minutes or more between the end of inhaled anesthesia with these drugs and the administration of doxapram is suggested to lessen the possibility of excessive cardiac toxicity.

APPLICATION TO PRACTICE

ASSESSMENT
History of Present Illness

Narcolepsy is identified primarily by its symptoms. When obtaining the patient history, ask about daytime somnolence, sleep paralysis, and hypnagogic hallucinations. Elicit information from the patient about impaired daytime performance due to sleepiness or disturbances in nighttime sleeping.

When obtaining the history of present illness for a patient with ADHD, the chief complaints usually arise from parents and teachers. Ask about the signs and symptoms of inattention, hyperactivity, and impulsivity identified in Box 20-2.

The general history for the patient who is obese should aim to identify complications of obesity and conditions that may contribute to it. Clarify the patient's chief complaint to determine the agenda and motivation for the patient; this clarification may suggest a cause for the obesity. A chief complaint focused on dissatisfaction with appearance should lead to an assessment of body image distortion and overvaluation or preoccupation with body weight or shape. Inquire about an exercise history. Determine the age of onset of obesity (i.e., childhood, adolescence, or adulthood) and potential precipitating factors, such as pregnancy, injury, concomitant illness, personal or family crisis, depression, or changes in activity level. Establish whether there is a history of weight cycling and weight fluctuation. Ask about maximum and minimum weights the patient has had during adulthood and what he or she feels the desired weight should be. Unrealistic or inappropriate expectations on the patient's part may be revealed. Previous attempts to lose weight should be chronicled with attention to successes, failures, and complications. The patient should be asked about professional guidance (e.g., a weight loss clinic), self-help groups (e.g., Overeaters Anonymous), and other treatment strategies (e.g., dieting, exercise, fasting, purging, diet pills, diuretics, or laxative use) that have been tried to lose weight.

Determine the general nutritional adequacy of the diet, caloric intake, the amount of dietary fat, and note patterns of food consumption (e.g., grazing versus sitting down for a scheduled meal, eating alone or when bored). Ask the patient about early learning patterns and familial interactions around food and eating that may perpetuate the obesity. Also elicit information about the amount, type, and patterns of exercise, which can provide clues to motivation and suggest specific treatment strategies.

Tobacco, alcohol, and substance abuse should be carefully assessed, both to establish whether alcohol consumption contributes to excess caloric intake and to determine whether other drugs (e.g., cocaine, nicotine) are used as a means of weight control. Substance abuse is a relative contraindication to treatment with anorexiant drugs.

Health History

A history of periodic amnesia or accidents may be the presenting symptoms for the patient with narcolepsy because of the patient's so-called "sleep attacks" and cataplexy. A history of psychiatric disorders and medical diseases should be elicited.

The behaviors exhibited by the child with ADHD are not unusual aspects of child behavior. The difference lies in the quality of the motor activity and the developmentally inappropriate inattention, hyperactivity, and impulsivity that the child displays. To have a diagnosis of ADHD, the signs and symptoms must have been present before the age of 7 and in at least two different environments. In addition, the persistence of developmentally inappropriate behaviors and marked inattention must not be a symptom of another disorder. Ask about the child's past learning abilities or disabilities and classroom activities. About half the children with ADHD also have learning disorders. Most of these children have average or above-average intelligence and are often very creative (see the Case Study: Attention-Deficit Hyperactivity Disorder).

The obese patient's psychiatric history may have some bearing on or pose special considerations for weight management. The patient often has a history of multiple and varied attempts at dieting. Many may overeat in response to stress, depression, or boredom. Approximately 30% of patients seeking treatment suffer from binge-eating disorder.

Also ask about physical illnesses that may contribute to obesity, including hypothyroidism, Cushing's disease, or polycystic ovary syndrome. Identifiable obesity-related conditions include coronary artery disease, cerebrovascular accident, gout, diabetes mellitus, hypertension, hyperlipidemia, degenerative arthritis, menstrual irregularities, infertility, gallbladder disease, and sleep apnea. The family history may reveal risk factors contributing to or associated with obesity and should include obesity or eating disorders in first-degree relatives.

Drugs that may contribute to obesity should also be identified. Ask about the patient's past use of marijuana or other illicit drugs, antidepressants such as monoamine oxidase inhibitors, lithium, valproic acid, selective serotonin reuptake inhibitors, and neuroleptics, because many of these drugs may contribute to weight gain.

Lifespan Considerations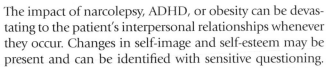

The impact of narcolepsy, ADHD, or obesity can be devastating to the patient's interpersonal relationships whenever they occur. Changes in self-image and self-esteem may be present and can be identified with sensitive questioning.

Birth weight offers no clue to detection and prediction of childhood obesity. However, there is a high degree of correlation of childhood adiposity with both parental adiposity and the child's daytime activity level.

Cultural/Social Considerations

The psychosocial implications of ADHD, narcolepsy, and obesity are far reaching. For example, the patient with narcolepsy may have been detained by law enforcement officers who initially thought that the individual was under the influence of illicit drugs or alcohol. Daytime somnolence and falling asleep or displaying excessive weakness at unexpected times can lead to personal safety issues and interfere with relationships with others.

In an attempt to cope with attention deficit, many children with ADHD develop maladaptive behavior patterns that become a deterrent to psychosocial adjustment. Their behavior evokes negative responses from others, and repeated exposure to such feedback adversely affects the child's self-concept, especially in boys.

Cultural and social values related to ethnicity, gender, and educational background concerning dietary, weight, or body image issues may motivate or complicate weight management and should be explored. Obesity is more prevalent among women, certain ethnic groups (e.g., African Americans, Mexican Americans, and Pacific Islanders), and within socioeconomically disadvantaged groups. The higher rates are likely based not only on a genetic predisposition but also on lifestyles that support weight gain and on cultures that tolerate or encourage heavier weights.

Physical Examination

Objective data related to narcolepsy may reflect visible signs of fatigue and lack of sleep, such as puffiness around the eyes, lack of coordination, drowsiness, and irritability. The frequency of cataplexy episodes and their duration should be noted.

The child with ADHD may display nonlocalized, so-called "soft" neurologic signs, motor-perceptual dysfunction (e.g., poor hand-eye coordination), and electroencephalographic abnormalities. The child may have difficulty distinguishing between the left and right hands or standing on one foot without falling. The child is often described as clumsy by the parents.

Obese patients will weigh more than normal in relation to their height and body build. The patient's height and weight are measured and compared with a standardized measure for BMI (see Appendix A). This method is inexpensive and accurate. The major disadvantage is that the percentage and distribution of body fat are not measured (possibly causing, for example, the muscular athlete to appear obese).

Laboratory Testing

Several different tests can be used to diagnose and manage narcolepsy, among them the human leukocyte antigen (HLA). Nearly 100% of patients with narcolepsy have the HLA subtypes DR_2 and DQw1. Therefore if the patient lacks these antigens, the diagnosis of narcolepsy may well be wrong. Pupillography is a research tool that may be used as an objective test for narcolepsy based on the fact that the pupil is large when the patient is alert, small when asleep, and intermediate when drowsy. It is an accurate method of evaluating a patient's ability to stay awake and has been used in evaluating sleepy drivers. Other evaluative tests include the Stanford Sleepiness Scale, the Multiple Sleep Latency Test (MSLT), and the nocturnal polysomnogram. The MSLT measures the severity of the problem. Sleep studies using 24- to 36-hour formats have been useful in measuring the sleep-wake cycle. The abrupt transition into REM sleep is a necessary criterion for a diagnosis of narcolepsy. The polysomnogram is used to find the underlying cause of the sleepiness, especially if it is disease related.

There are no definitive tests to identify or manage ADHD. The child is primarily assessed and monitored based on clinical signs and symptoms.

Few tests are routinely indicated for the obese patient. Because of the concomitant increased rates of non–insulin-dependent diabetes, hypercholesterolemia, and hypertriglyceridemia in obese individuals, however, blood glucose level and a fasting lipid panel are usually obtained.

GOALS OF THERAPY

The major treatment goal for the patient with narcolepsy is to combat somnolence and restore normal function. None of the CNS stimulants are appropriate to treat general fatigue. Some patients with narcolepsy respond well to nondrug therapies if their symptoms are not too severe. Others require therapy to remain alert throughout the day. Although psychomotor stimulants are effective for many patients, they do not work for all.

For ADHD, treatment goals are directed toward correction of cognitive and behavioral problems. However, not all children who exhibit signs of ADHD should be treated with CNS stimulants. The decision for drug therapy depends in part on societal expectations and demands. Because drug therapy is intended as an adjunct to other modalities, an evaluation of the interest and ability to comply with therapy should be determined; however, drug therapy is not indicated if symptoms are mild.

The health care provider has many options in the management of ADHD. The drug of choice is the one best expected to target the symptoms. Whatever the drug chosen, the dosage should be titrated for 1 month and the results evaluated. If the first drug is not effective, a second may be tried. It is not unusual to try three different types of stimulants before finding one that is effective. Drug holidays should be initiated periodically to assess the need for continuance. In no case should treatment continue for more than one school year without interruption.

Drug therapy for overweight or obese individuals is reasonable for those who are 40% or more above the desired body weight. The goal is to reduce and stabilize the patient's weight at a more desirable level. The desirable level may not necessarily be within normal limits but rather reduced sufficiently to lower the risk of major health problems. For patients who are less than 40% overweight, self-help and behavioral programs are usually preferable to drug therapy.

INTERVENTION
Administration

Blood pressure, pulse, respiration, mental status, and behavior are monitored before administering a psychomotor stimulant, anorexiant, or analeptic drug, and periodically during therapy. Assess also for restlessness, irritability, confusion, insomnia, mood changes, and GI distress.

Psychomotor stimulants are usually taken on an empty stomach. Mazindol, however, may be taken with meals or a snack to reduce gastric irritation. The last dose of an amphetamine or anorexiant is usually given several hours (e.g., 6 hours for regular dosage forms and 14 hours for extended-release formulations) before bedtime to avoid insomnia. Insomnia caused by methyl-phenidate use may lessen with continued use, but may be better treated by eliminating the final dose during the day. Additionally, intake of a large amount of caffeine should be avoided. Rinsing the mouth frequently with water as well as chewing sugarless gum or sucking on sugarless hard candy can minimize the dry mouth associated with psychomotor stimulants.

Weigh the patient taking a drug to treat narcolepsy, ADHD, or obesity two or three times weekly until the effects of the drug can be evaluated. Most CNS stimulants suppress appetite. Review periodic CBC counts with differential and platelet counts to monitor for methylphenidate-induced anemia and leukopenia. Check urine catecholamines before and during methyl-phenidate therapy to determine any increase in the level of dopamine.

For the patient taking respiratory stimulants, monitor pulse, blood pressure, respiration, temperature, and ECG tracing. Note, however, that analeptic drugs are seldom used outside of the intensive care setting. Anticipate that seizures may occur; have a suction machine at the bedside. Keep the siderails up and use padding. Do not leave the patient receiving an analeptic drug unattended.

Anorexiant drugs quickly become ineffective as tolerance develops. Once tolerance occurs, the drug should be discontinued and doses should not be increased to suppress appetite.

Education

Patients taking a psychomotor stimulant, anorexiant, or analeptic drug require thorough patient teaching about the disorder, the purpose and the expected outcome of drug therapy, possible adverse effects, and the importance of following up. The patient should be instructed not to increase the dosage of the prescribed drug or to abruptly stop therapy without first consulting with the health care provider. Abrupt cessation of high doses may cause extreme fatigue and mental depression.

Instruct the patient taking a CNS stimulant once daily to take a missed dose as soon as remembered but not too close to bedtime; otherwise omit the missed dose and resume the usual dosing schedule the next day. If two or more doses per day are prescribed, instruct the patient to take the missed dose if remembered within 1 hour of when scheduled, otherwise omit the missed dose and resume the usual dosing schedule. The patient should not double up for missed doses. Remind patients taking long-acting formulations to swallow tablets whole, that is, without chewing or crushing them.

The patient should take these drugs only as directed and not change the dosage or frequency without consulting with the health care provider. Review the dosage schedule with the patient and family. Some patients require daily dosage, whereas others may require drugs during school or work but can be drug-free on the weekends or during the summer months for children.

Make sure the patient understands that several weeks of therapy may be necessary until the full effects of the drug therapy can be evaluated. Advise him or her to inform the health care provider of adverse effects such as tachycardia, loss of appetite, insomnia, abdominal pain, or weight loss.

The patient should be informed that CNS stimulants impair judgment. Caution the patient to avoid driving or operating hazardous machinery if dizziness, nervousness, agitation, or other CNS effects occur and to consult the health care provider if these symptoms become severe. Advise the patient to avoid alcohol and OTC drugs unless first approved by the health care provider. Point out that these drugs are habit forming.

CNS stimulants should not be used during pregnancy unless specifically prescribed by the obstetrician. Counsel the patient regarding contraceptives as needed.

Warn patients who have diabetes mellitus to monitor their blood glucose level because these drugs may alter it. A sustained elevation in blood glucose may require a change in diet or the use of an antidiabetic drug.

The patient with narcolepsy should be instructed to document the frequency and character of attacks. They may be able to counteract the effects of daytime sleepiness by engaging in frequent short walks or other forms of exercise as well as avoiding large meals, caffeinated beverages, and eating lunch before important meetings, and by taking short naps throughout the day.

Parents of a child with ADHD should periodically monitor the child's height and inform the health care provider if growth is inhibited. Drug-free periods may be used periodically to assess whether the drug is still needed and to allow growth if the prescribed drug has caused growth retardation. For example, a 6-week course of therapy might be followed by a 3-week discontinuation.

Refer the obese patient for appropriate counseling and instruction as well as for weight and exercise programs. Many commercial programs (e.g., Weight Watchers) and support groups (e.g., Overeaters Anonymous) are available. In addition, the patient should be encouraged to follow through with behavior modification therapies.

EVALUATION

Treatment success for the patient with narcolepsy is measured by the patient's ability to stay alert and functional throughout the day. Some patients with severe narcolepsy may not overcome fatigue and sleepiness even with stimulants. In this case, success can be measured by relative improvement in functioning.

ADHD treatment success is determined by the child's marked improvement in behavior and cognition and in the child's ability to focus and pay attention. It is estimated that drug-related improvements occur in 60% to 90% of children. Teacher ratings of the child should note improvement in behavior and attention span as well as improved performance on visual-motor tasks. Although a child with ADHD may become quieter with an increase in dosage, the academic performance declines. Thus the child should be monitored closely so that the smallest effective dosage can be used.

The effectiveness of anorexiant therapy can be demonstrated by a decrease in appetite and subsequent decrease in weight. The use of prescription appetite suppressants has been shown to significantly increase weight loss relative to placebo. However, the differences are usually modest, averaging 0.25 to 0.5 pounds per week, with a total weight loss of 5%. The long-term safety of appetite suppressants has not been demonstrated, and patients tend to regain their weight when the drugs are discontinued. These drugs also may interfere with the effectiveness of behavioral modification.

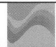

CASE STUDY — *Attention-Deficit Hyperactivity Disorder (ADHD)*

ASSESSMENT

HISTORY OF PRESENT ILLNESS

TC is a 10-year-old boy who has difficulty concentrating, a short attention span, irritability, hyperactivity, is unable to follow parent and teacher directives, is easily distracted, and has poor social skills, poor academic performance, and low frustration tolerance. His parents say that he was "born antsy" and seems to be driven by a motor that he cannot turn off. His sixth-grade teacher recommended that TC be evaluated by a health care provider for the possibility of ADHD.

HEALTH HISTORY

TC has no known allergies. He had the usual childhood illnesses but no major health problems. He has a history of risky behaviors that have resulted in injuries. At age 5, he climbed a 30-foot tree in the yard and had to be rescued by the local firefighters. At 7, he dislocated his shoulder when he fell from the same tree. Last year he had stitches after he injured himself while chasing the family cat into the street. His risky behaviors and activities have increased over the last 3 years.

LIFESPAN CONSIDERATIONS

TC is an only child. His parents have tried to compensate for his lack of friends, but when he hangs around his parents he is quickly labeled a loser by other children. TC's social skills with peers have been adversely affected by his lack of self-control. Despite his poor academic performance, his teachers agree with his parents that he is a bright child.

CULTURAL/SOCIAL CONSIDERATIONS

TC's inability to control his behavior makes him unpredictable and often the brunt of teasing by other children. As a result, he has learned to amuse himself and to find playmates in the family pets. TC's parents are tenured faculty at the local university, and philosophically they are not strong supporters of drug therapy for children. They waited to

Continued

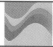

bring him to treatment after exhausting many other treatment avenues. The parents have both the means and desire to provide TC with the care they think is needed for him.

PHYSICAL EXAMINATION

TC falls within the average height and weight category for his age, sex, and developmental level. The results of his physical examination were within normal limits. TC weighs 75 pounds and is 4'6" tall.

LABORATORY TESTING

Diagnosis of ADHD was confirmed by history and observation. Psychologic tests sensitive for the ability to focus attention and to perform motor tasks suggest deficits. TC's behavior and history ruled out other possibilities to explain his symptoms, such as thyroid problems, toxins, other CNS disturbances, or metabolic problems.

PATIENT PROBLEM(S)

Attention-deficit hyperactivity disorder.

GOALS OF THERAPY

Control impulsive behavior, increase ability to attend and focus, improve academic and social skills.

CRITICAL THINKING QUESTIONS

1. The health care provider prescribes methylphenidate 5 mg po bid, to be titrated to a maximum of 60 mg daily. What is the mechanism of action for methylphenidate?
2. TC's parents should be informed of which adverse effects that may occur with methylphenidate use?
3. Which signs of toxicity are associated with the use of methylphenidate?
4. Which drug would be used to treat neuroleptic malignant syndrome?
5. Which laboratory tests would be appropriate to monitor TC's methylphenidate therapy?
6. Which information does the nurse need to evaluate the effectiveness of methylphenidate for TC?

Bibliography

American Psychiatric Association: *Diagnostic and statistical manual of mental disorders (DSM-IV)*, ed 4, Washington, DC, 1994, American Psychiatric Press.

Aronne LJ: Treating obesity: a new target for prevention of coronary heart disease, *Prog Cardiovasc Nurs* 16(3):98-106, 115, 2001.

Brooks SN, Guilleminault C: New insights into the pathogenesis and treatment of narcolepsy, *Curr Opin Pulm Med* 7(6):407-410, 2001.

Crombie N: Obesity management, *Nurs Stand* 13(47):43-46, 1999.

Edwards A: Attention deficit-hyperactivity disorder not just for children anymore, *Adv Nurse Pract* 7(5):47-50, 1999.

Hechtman L: Assessment and diagnosis of attention-deficit/hyperactivity disorder, *Child Adolesc Psychiatr Clin N Am* 9(3):481-498, 2000.

Holm, K, Li S, Spector N, et al: Obesity in adults and children: a call for action, *J Adv Nurs* 36(2):266-269, 2001.

Jensen PS: ADHD: Current concepts on etiology, pathophysiology, and neurobiology, *Child Adolesc Psychiatr Clin N Am* 9(3):557-569, 2000.

Leslie M: Weighing in on clinical guidelines for obesity. Tools to assist your patients, *Adv Nurse Pract* 8(3):78-81, 2000.

MacLeod V, Shneerson J: Narcolepsy: nursing the sleeping sickness, *Nurs Times* 94(22):48-50, 1998.

Meaux JB: Stop, look, and listen: the challenge for children with ADHD, *Issues Compr Pediatr Nurs* 23(1):1-13, 2000.

Murray-Tait M: Preventing and managing the problem of obesity, *Community Nurse* 5(10):13-14, 1999.

O'Brien C: Dieting fads: the facts, *Nurs Times* 96(1):46-47, 2000.

Valente SM: Treating attention deficit hyperactivity disorder, *Nurse Pract* 26(9):14-15, 19-20, 23-29, 2001.

Internet Resources

Internet Mental Health on methylphenidate. Available online at http://www.mentalhealth.com/drug/p30-403.html.

National Institute of Mental Health site on attention-deficit hyperactivity disorder. Available online at http://www.nimh.nih.gov/publicat/adhd.cfm.

National Heart, Lung, and Blood Institute site on obesity. Available online at http://www.nhlbi.nih.gov/guidelines/obesity/ob_home.htm.

CHAPTER

21

Skeletal Muscle Relaxants

MICHAEL R. VASKO • SUSAN SCIACCA

 Visit **http://evolve.elsevier.com/Gutierrez/** for additional information.

KEY TERMS

Clasp-knife phenomenon, p. 320

Clonic, p. 318

Deep tendon reflexes (DTRs), p. 317

Hypertonus, p. 319

Spasms, p. 318

Spasticity, p. 319

Tonic, p. 318

OBJECTIVES

- Discuss the differences between spasticity and muscle spasm.
- Differentiate between centrally acting and peripherally acting skeletal muscle relaxant drugs.
- Describe the most common adverse effects of skeletal muscle relaxant drugs.
- Identify patient outcomes that indicate successful drug therapy in the treatment of muscle spasms and spasticity.
- Develop a nursing care plan, including a teaching plan, for a patient receiving drug therapy to treat muscle spasms and spasticity.

The neuromuscular system is controlled by a complex interrelationship between the central nervous system (CNS) and the skeletal muscles. Many disorders of the neuromuscular system result in muscle tone imbalances. Although the exact mechanisms of neuromuscular disorders are not fully understood, physical and drug therapy provide clues to the pathways and medical management.

Deep tendon reflexes (DTRs) are used to assess the integrity of the neuromuscular system. These muscle contractions or "jerks" are elicited with a quick tap of a reflex hammer to the muscle's tendon insertion.

317

The strength of the reaction gives the health care provider a wealth of information. A normal reaction demonstrates that neuromuscular synapses are operative and muscle fibers can contract. It also indicates that the spinal cord, dorsal root ganglion, and extrapyramidal and pyramidal systems are functional. Abnormal reactions may indicate a neuromuscular disorder.

PATHOPHYSIOLOGY • Spasms and Spasticity

SPASMS

Spasms are sudden, violent, painful, involuntary contractions of a muscle or group of muscles. Most muscle spasms are related to local injury of muscles, joints, tendons, or ligaments. Specific trauma-related causes of spasms include sprains, whiplash injuries, herniated discs, and lower back syndrome (Table 21-1). In addition, bursitis, myositis, neuritis, dislocations, fractures, muscle strains from excessive stretching or overuse, and sprains from joints with stretched or torn ligaments can also cause spasms. Although hypocalcemia and epileptic myoclonic seizure activity also produce spasms, the discussion in this chapter is limited to spasm resulting from musculoskeletal injury.

The delicate balance between musculoskeletal movement and body posture allows the execution of fine and gross motor skills. The physical hierarchy controlling this balance includes the motor cortex, extrapyramidal and pyramidal systems, basal ganglia, cerebellum, descending brainstem circuitry, spinal cord, and motor neurons in the ventral spinal cord. Feedback from muscle and tendon joint afferent nerves to the spinal cord via projections to the thalamus and higher brain centers helps to complete the information loop that regulates movement and posture.

Motor neurons in the ventral regions of the brainstem and spinal cord are directly responsible for motor function. Action potentials from motor neurons are conducted directly to nerve terminals in muscle fibers that form synapses called *neuromuscular junctions* (NMJ). Acetylcholine is released from the nerve terminal and stimulates nicotinic receptors on the muscle, producing contraction. A deficiency in synaptic activity at the NMJ causes myasthenia gravis (see Chapter 23). A number of drugs block nicotinic receptor activation and serve as neuromuscular blockers; they are discussed in Chapter 16.

The stretch reflex maintains muscle tone (Figure 21-1), which can be described as *hypotonic* (less than normal), *flaccid* (absent), or *hypertonic* (excessive, rigid, spastic, tetany). Motor neurons in the ventral horn link spinal cord reflexes to muscles. When the motor neuron axon or cell body is damaged, a pattern of hyperexcitability develops that can produce multiple contractions of the nerve. These muscle spasms can be mild or severe, and acute or chronic. Muscle spasms may also be **clonic**, characterized by alternate contraction and relaxation, or **tonic**, sustained contractions of striated muscle. Depending on their location, spasms can be aggravated by movement, sneezing, coughing, or straining. Muscle atrophy may develop as a consequence of motor neuron lesions.

Patterns of movement organized in the frontal cortex of the brain are carried out by the motor cortex.

TABLE 21-1

Comparison of Spasm and Spasticity

	Spasm	*Spasticity*
Definition	Sudden, violent, painful involuntary contractions of a muscle or group of muscles	Increased muscle tone or contractions that cause stiff, awkward movement
Mediator	Motor neurons	Premotor neurons/descending motor systems
Etiology	Cervical root syndrome; bursitis, overuse syndrome; dislocation or fracture; epilepsy; herniated disc; hypocalcemia; myositis, neuritis; sprains, strains; whiplash injuries	Cerebrovascular accident; closed head injury; hemiplegia, paraplegia, quadriplegia; multiple sclerosis; poliomyelitis; spinal cord trauma or tumor; tetanus

The basal ganglia and cerebellum provide ongoing support functions that contribute to the gracefulness and the temporal smoothness of movement. If the motor system is diseased or injured, skilled movement is lost, but the extrapyramidal system can elicit crude movement.

SPASTICITY

In contrast to spasm, **spasticity** is an increase in the passive stretch resistance of a muscle or muscle group. The increased muscle tone or contractions cause movements to be stiff and awkward. Spasticity is considered a permanent condition and unless physical and drug therapy are instituted, it can progress to disabling contractures. Disorders of the CNS such as closed head injuries, cerebral palsy, multiple sclerosis, and cerebrovascular accident (stroke) are common causes of spasticity. Two

thirds of patients with multiple sclerosis have moderate to severe spasticity. Patients with spinal cord trauma, spinal tumors, poliomyelitis, hemiplegia, paraplegia, quadriplegia, and tetanus also may experience spasticity (see Table 21-1).

Although the mechanisms that cause spasticity remain unknown, it is likely that it involves abnormalities in the descending motor system, since various areas of the brain control muscle tone and reflexes. Clonus, flexor spasms, mass reflexes, and a positive Babinski's sign are identifiable signs of spasticity. **Hypertonus** (excessive level of skeletal muscle tension or activity) likely results from either an increase in excitatory influences or decrease in inhibitory influences in descending pathways. As a result, the stretch reflex is augmented and muscle fibers may lengthen in an exaggerated way (see Figure 21-1). With spasticity there is little or no muscle

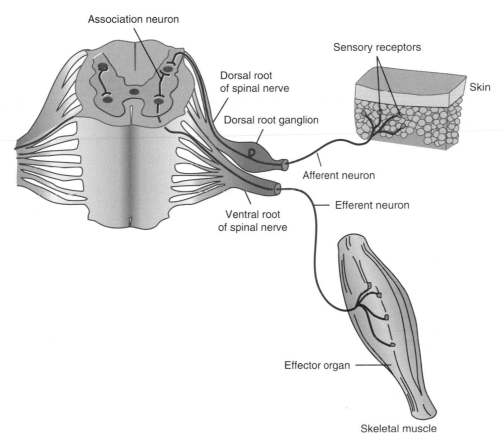

FIGURE 21-1 Reflex arc. The stretch reflex maintains muscle tone. When communication between sensory receptors and muscles is broken, a pattern of hyperexcitability develops that produces multiple contractions or spasms. Hyperactive reflexes can also result in spasticity. (From Black JM, Matassarin-Jacobs E: *Medical-surgical nursing: clinical management for continuity of care*, ed 5, Philadelphia, 1997, WB Saunders. Used with permission.)

atrophy such as that seen with diseases of motor neurons, and the effects are generally more diffuse, affecting a number of muscle groups.

Spasticity does not develop immediately after a neural injury occurs. Therefore, severity may vary throughout the progression of the disorder. A gradual increase in muscle tone triggers increases in resistance until tone is suddenly reduced resulting in a very painful **clasp-knife phenomenon** (a motion similar to the sudden closing of a jackknife). Urinary tract infections, decubitus ulcers, and other painful stimuli can exacerbate spasticity.

Two types of spasticity have been identified. *Spinal spasticity* is characterized by a discernible loss of inhibitory influences. Hyperactive deep tendon reflexes, clonus, primitive withdrawal reflexes, and a flexed posture are present. In contrast, *cerebral spasticity* produces hypoactive deep tendon reflexes, increased muscle tone, or inappropriate posture. Ordinarily, there are no primitive withdrawal reflexes or flexed postures with cerebral spasticity. Dystonia or disordered muscle tone may be present in persons with cerebral spasticity.

DRUG CLASS • Drugs Used to Treat Spasticity

baclofen (Lioresal; Alpha-Baclofen✱)

botulinum toxin type A (Botox)

dantrolene (Dantrium)

diazepam (Valium)

tizanidine (Zanaflex)

MECHANISM OF ACTION

The exact mechanisms of action for drugs used to treat spasticity (Table 21-2) are unknown. Baclofen, diazepam, and tizanidine are believed to act at the level of the spinal cord to restore inhibitory tone, whereas botulinum toxin type A and dantrolene have peripheral actions. Baclofen is an agonist at the B receptor subtype for the inhibitory neurotransmitter gamma-aminobutyric acid (GABA). Presumably it inhibits synaptic reflexes by inhibiting primary afferent neurons, thus decreasing transmitter release from them. Diazepam is a benzodiazepine commonly prescribed as an antianxiety drug, and the details of its actions and adverse effects are discussed in Chapter 17. Diazepam enhances inhibitory descending pathways in the spinal cord that govern muscular activity, apparently by enhancing the activity of GABA. Tizanidine is a centrally acting agonist for alpha$_2$-adrenergic receptors. It increases presynaptic inhibition of motor neurons thereby reducing spasticity caused by motor neuron activity.

Botulinum toxin type A blocks neurotransmission at the NMJ by entering the motor nerve terminals and inhibiting the release of acetylcholine. Dantrolene is unique in that it acts directly on muscle cells by interfering with the intracellular release of calcium necessary to initiate contraction. At therapeutic dosages, this effect is limited to skeletal muscle and is not seen in the heart or smooth muscle.

USES

Baclofen is most effective in relieving spasticity caused by spinal cord injury and is less effective in relieving spasticity from brain damage. It can be administered directly into the thecal space so it has direct access to the spinal cord. Botulinum toxin type A is used to treat spasticity caused by multiple sclerosis, stroke, brain injury, or spinal cord injury and as an adjunctive therapy in cerebral palsy. It has recently been approved for the reduction of the appearance of facial wrinkles. Diazepam is effective in relieving spasticity associated with spinal cord injury, multiple sclerosis, and cerebral injury and in treating muscle spasms. Relatively high dosages are required to relieve muscle hyperactivity. Dantrolene is most useful for the patient whose spasticity causes pain, discomfort, or limits functional rehabilitation. In addition to the spasticity caused by spinal cord injury, dantrolene relieves spasticity of stroke, cerebral palsy, and multiple sclerosis, for which the other drugs have limited effectiveness. Dantrolene is also used in the preoperative and intraoperative management of malignant hyperthermia. Tizanidine is used for the intermittent management of increased muscle tone associated with spasticity, especially that associated with spinal cord injury or multiple sclerosis.

PHARMACOKINETICS

The pharmacokinetics of drugs used to treat spasticity is summarized in Table 21-3. Most drugs are readily absorbed from the gastrointestinal (GI) tract following oral administration. Baclofen is sometimes given intrathecally either in individual doses or by infusion. The absorption of dantrolene from the GI tract is slow and incomplete, but it is thought to be sufficient to provide dose-related plasma concentrations. Although tizanidine is well absorbed orally, it has an extensive

TABLE 21-2

Centrally Acting Skeletal Muscle Relaxants

Generic Name	Brand Name	Comments
Drugs for Spasticity		
baclofen	Apo-Baclofen,✤ Lioresal, PMS-Baclofen✤	Diminishes reflex responses by decreasing transmission in spinal cord
botulinum toxin type A	Botox	Neuromuscular blocking drug
dantrolene	Dantrium	Acts peripherally to inhibit calcium release within muscle
diazepam	Valium	Benzodiazepine used to treat spasticity or muscle spasm
tizanidine	Zanaflex	For intermittent management of spasticity
Drugs for Muscle Spasms		
carisoprodol	Soma, Vanadom	Related to meprobamate; may cause drowsiness
chlorphenesin	Maolate	May cause drowsiness and dizziness
chlorzoxazone	Paraflex, Parafon Forte DSC, Relaxone	May cause drowsiness; watch for signs of liver damage (rare)
cyclobenzaprine	Cycloflex, Flexeril	Related to tricyclic antidepressants; does not cause drug dependence but may cause changes in liver
diazepam	Valium	Benzodiazepine used to treat spasticity or muscle spasm
metaxalone	Skelaxin	Monitor patient for development of liver toxicity
methocarbamol	Carbacot, Robaxin, Skelex	Not recommended for patients with epilepsy; do not administer parenterally to patients with impaired renal function because drug vehicle may worsen kidney function
orphenadrine	Disipal,✤ Flexoject, Norflex✤	Anticholinergic effects are common adverse effects; not for patients with glaucoma, myasthenia gravis, tachycardia, or urinary retention
vigabatrin	Sabril✤	Adjunct treatment for epilepsy used in treating infantile spasms

✤ Available only in Canada.

first-pass effect with a bioavailability of approximately 40%. Dantrolene is highly bound to plasma proteins, whereas the other drugs are not highly bound. Dantrolene and tizanidine are almost entirely biotransformed by the liver, and metabolites are eliminated in the urine. In contrast, 70% to 85% of a dose of baclofen is excreted unchanged.

ADVERSE REACTIONS AND CONTRAINDICATIONS

Most drugs used to treat spasticity are associated with some degree of sedation, drowsiness, light-headedness, ataxia, and dizziness. Caution should be used when the patient has preexisting conditions that produce weakness, ataxia, or light-headedness. Other adverse effects and contraindications are drug specific. Adverse effects

of baclofen include drowsiness, weakness, confusion, insomnia, and occasional GI upset. Symptoms of baclofen overdose include visual disturbances (blurred vision, diplopia), vomiting, seizures, respiratory difficulties, and severe muscle weakness. Sudden withdrawal of drug in patients who have been receiving intrathecal baclofen may cause high fever, progressing muscle rigidity or destruction and has caused death. Patients receiving botulinum toxin type A can develop antibodies to the toxin and are at some risk for cardiovascular collapse. Dantrolene causes muscular weakness and can worsen the overall condition if the patient already has only marginal strength. It can produce transient depression of GI smooth muscle. Tizanidine's most common adverse effects are sleepiness, dizziness, and loss of vitality. Dry mouth, hypotension, bradycar-

TABLE 21-3

Pharmacokinetics of Selected Skeletal Muscle Relaxants

Drug	Route	Onset	Peak	Duration	PB (%)	$t_{1/2}$
baclofen	po	Hrs to wks	<2	8 hr	30	2-4 hr
	Intrathecal	6-8 hr	1-2 days	4-8 hr	30	1.5 hr
carisoprodol	po	30 min	4 hr*	4-6 hr	30	8 hr
chlorphenesin	po	UA	1-3 hr	UA	UA	2.5-5 hr
chlorzoxazone	po	60 min	1-2 hr	3-4 hr	UA	1-2 hr
cyclobenzaprine	po	60 min	3-8 hr	12-24 hr	93	1-3 days
dantrolene	po	1 hr§	5 hr	6-12 hr	>90	6-9 hr
metaxalone	po	60 min	2 hr†	4-6 hr	30	2-3 hr
methocarbamol	po	30 min	2 hr	3-6 hr	UA	1-2 hr
orphenadrine	po	60 min	3 hr‡	8 hr	UA	14 hr
tizanidine	po	30 min	1-2 hr	3-6 hr	30	2.5 hr
vigabatrin	po	UA	2 hr	UA	Minimal	5-8 hr

PB, Protein binding; $t_{1/2}$, half-life; *UA*, unavailable.
*Peak drug activity for 350 mg dose of carisoprodol.
†Peak drug activity for 800 mg of metaxalone.
‡Peak drug activity for 50 mg of orphenadrine.
§Time for dantrolene to reach blood levels; therapeutic effect may take 1 to 2 weeks.

dia, and fever have also been observed. There are no absolute contraindications to baclofen or tizanidine therapy other than hypersensitivity.

INTERACTIONS

Alcohol is the most commonly used drug that interacts with skeletal muscle relaxants. Other interacting drugs include CNS depressants (e.g., opioids), monoamine oxidase inhibitors, antihistamines, anticonvulsants, cimetidine, levodopa, barbiturates, phenothiazines, propoxyphene, tricyclic antidepressants, and contraceptives. Concurrent use of dantrolene in women more than 35 years old who are receiving estrogen replacement therapy increases the potential for hepatotoxicity. Verapamil and other calcium-channel blockers increase the risk of ventricular fibrillation and cardiovascular collapse when administered in conjunction with intravenous dantrolene.

DRUG CLASS • Skeletal Muscle Relaxants

carisoprodol (Soma, Rela)

chlorphenesin (Maolate)

chlorzoxazone (Paraflex, Parafon Forte✳)

cyclobenzaprine (Flexeril)

diazepam (Valium)

metaxalone (Skelaxin)

methocarbamol (Robaxin, Marbaxin)

orphenadrine (Norflex, Banflex)

vigabatrin (Sabril✳)

MECHANISM OF ACTION

The mechanism of action of the muscle relaxants remains unknown but is related to their ability to inhibit activity in the CNS. Carisoprodol, chlorphenesin, and chlorzoxazone presumably block transmission between neurons in the descending pathways and the spinal cord. Cyclobenzaprine acts in the brainstem to reduce muscle tone and hyperactivity. Both metaxalone and methocarbamol produce a generalized CNS depression and methocarbamol can also produce sedation. Orphenadrine produces mild analgesia and has some anticholinergic properties. Vigabatrin appears to produce muscle relaxation by preventing the breakdown of GABA in the CNS, thereby increasing the levels of this inhibitory transmitter.

USES

Muscle spasms occur with sprains, bursitis, arthritis, and lower back pain. The primary treatment includes analgesics, antiinflammatory drugs, immobilization of the affected part (if possible), and physical therapy. If relief is not achieved through these means, skeletal muscle relaxants may be added. Thus, these drugs are used for the relief of muscle spasm associated with acute musculoskeletal injury. Vigabatrin is an adjunct treatment for epilepsy and is also used to treat spasms in infants.

In addition to the individual drugs listed above, some of these drugs are found in combination with analgesics. These preparations include orphenadrine and aspirin (Norgesic, Norphadine), carisoprodol and aspirin (Soma Compound), carisoprodol, aspirin, and codeine (Soma Compound W), and chlorzoxazone with acetaminophen (Parafon Forte✳). Quinine has been used for the relief of nocturnal leg cramps although more effective, less toxic drugs have largely replaced it.

PHARMACOKINETICS

The pharmacokinetics of selected skeletal muscle relaxants are summarized in Table 21-2. These drugs are readily absorbed from the GI tract following oral administration. Methocarbamol and orphenadrine are available for intravenous or intramuscular administration. The only drug that is highly bound to plasma proteins is cyclobenzaprine. These drugs (except vigabatrin) are biotransformed in the liver and eliminated via the kidneys. Carisoprodol is chemically related to meprobamate, which is its principal metabolite. Approximately 70% of a dose of vigabatrin is excreted unchanged by the kidney.

ADVERSE REACTIONS AND CONTRAINDICATIONS

Drowsiness and dizziness are common adverse effects of all skeletal muscle relaxants. Headaches, sleepiness, and visual disturbances are common. Nausea, vomiting, constipation, and diarrhea have been associated with carisoprodol, chlorzoxazone, cyclobenzaprine, methocarbamol, and orphenadrine. Most of these drugs can produce hypersensitivity reactions and are contraindicated in patients who exhibit allergic reactions. Carisoprodol may cause ataxia, tremor, tachycardia, and hypotension. It is contraindicated in patients with acute intermittent porphyria. Carisoprodol, dantrolene, and tizanidine may be excreted in breast milk.

Chlorphenesin is contraindicated during pregnancy or for nursing mothers and should be given with caution to patients with impaired liver function. Cyclobenzaprine is chemically related to the tricyclic antidepressants and can produce hypothermia, tachycardia, and arrhythmias. Overdosage can produce confusion, hallucinations, agitation, fever, seizures, and coma. Cyclobenzaprine is contraindicated for patients with hyperthyroidism, arrhythmias, heart block, conduction disturbances, heart failure, or recent myocardial infarction. Metaxalone is associated with hemolytic anemia or hepatotoxicity and contraindicated for patients with a history of these conditions. When administered intravenously, methocarbamol may cause convulsions, fainting, slow heartbeat, muscle weakness, nystagmus, and facial flushing, especially if administered rapidly. Orphenadrine has anticholinergic properties, so adverse effects include dry mouth, blurred vision, tachycardia, urinary retention, and mental confusion in older adults. Orphenadrine is contraindicated in patients who have closed-angle glaucoma, pyloric or duodenal obstruction, prostate hypertrophy, or myasthenia gravis. Vigabatrin is associated with amnesia, increased seizure frequency, and ophthalmic abnormalities.

INTERACTIONS

Alcohol and other CNS depressants (e.g., opioids) can exacerbate the depressive effects of muscle relaxants. Monoamine oxidase inhibitors should not be used concurrently with many muscle relaxants, especially cyclobenzaprine.

APPLICATION TO PRACTICE

ASSESSMENT
History of Present Illness

When obtaining the patient's history of present illness, it is important to elicit information about the cause of the spasm or spastic state. Questions that may be asked include the following: Is the injury or illness related to employment or to recreational activities? When did the symptoms occur in relation to activities? What actions or situations aggravate or alleviate the discomfort? What has been used for self-treatment and how effective was the treatment?

Pain is the prominent symptom of muscle spasm and is usually aggravated by movement. Therefore, assessment should include a subjective description of the discomfort or pain. The location of the spasm or spasticity should be identified as precisely as possible, as well as the intensity, duration, and any precipitating factors. The potential for secondary gain related to spasms also should be considered, given Workman's Compensation and insurance issues.

With spasticity, the patient should be assessed for pain and impaired function (e.g., eating, dressing, bathing). Determine whether the spasticity interferes with joint and muscle mobility as well as the ability for self-care. Factors contributing to the development of spasticity also should be elicited.

Health History

The health history helps to determine the progress of the disease or condition and in developing treatment objectives. The health history should include information regarding previous or concurrent GI disorders (e.g., peptic ulcer disease); neuromuscular, musculoskeletal, and renal disorders; hepatic impairment; seizure disorder; and a drug history. Of significance is the patient's report of symptoms that may have been noticed several years earlier, but because they disappeared medical attention was not sought. When possible, the month and year when the patient first noticed the symptoms should be noted.

Lifespan Considerations

Perinatal. Skeletal muscle relaxants are not used during pregnancy unless the anticipated benefits outweigh the risks. Most skeletal muscle relaxants cross placental membranes and some cross into breast milk.

Pediatric. Skeletal muscle relaxants are not usually needed in children, with the exception of children who have spinal cord injuries or cerebral palsy. Most drugs are not recommended for children less than 5 years old, and others are not recommended until the child is 12 years old. When skeletal muscle relaxants are required, the dosage should be calculated on a milligram per kilogram (mg/kg) basis.

Older Adults. Spasms and spasticity are not uncommon in older adults. All skeletal muscle relaxants have adverse effects that can alter the functional abilities of an older adult. To prevent falls or injuries, precautions should be taken if dizziness or weakness is exacerbated.

Cultural/Social Considerations

The psychologic response to spasms or spasticity is determined by the cause of the disorder, the severity of symptoms, and the impact of those symptoms on the patient's lifestyle. Chronic or recurrent spasm and spasticity cause the patient to fear incapacitation if the symptoms cannot be managed effectively. Considerations should be given to the potential for secondary gain associated with the patient's illness or condition. The illness or condition affects, and is affected by, the patient's emotional response.

Emotional distress associated with spasm and spasticity can manifest as sleep disturbances, restlessness, irritability, decreased appetite, and loss of interest in daily activities. The perceived vulnerability and associated powerlessness complicate the plan of care for some patients. The sense of powerlessness stems from real and perceived losses, including employment and financial security, role status, physical or social independence, and control of home environment (see Case Study: Multiple Sclerosis and Case Study: Low Back Pain with Spasm).

The potential impact of spasticity on a patient's physical condition, functional status, and adaptation to disability is significant. Perceived susceptibility to disease and its seriousness influences the plan of care. Also, many of the skeletal muscle relaxants have unpleasant or undesirable adverse effects; therefore, the likelihood of noncompliance is a concern.

Physical Examination

The clinical presentation of spasm and spasticity depends on the location of the injury in the neuromuscular system. For this reason, the physical examination should include an assessment of DTRs, Babinski's sign, muscle strength, range of motion, gait, balance, coordination, and dexterity. Muscle size, tone, symmetry, and the presence of tremor, spasms, or spasticity should be noted. Clonus, flexor spasms, mass reflexes, and a positive Babinski's sign are identifiable signs of spasticity. In patients with spasms, muscle firmness and tenderness may be noted over the affected area and are accompanied by limited movement and guarding. DTRs may be hyperactive. Adduction contractions can cause difficulties with personal hygiene, particularly of the perineal and axillary regions.

Assessment of other body systems should include neurologic symptoms such as weakness, skin color and temperature, the presence of edema, erythema, ecchymosis, or crepitus. The effect of the spasm or spasticity on urinary and bowel function also should be determined.

Laboratory Testing

There are no definitive testing methods for spasms. An electromyogram is helpful to confirm nerve damage associated with spasticity. Magnetic resonance imaging is useful in detecting abnormalities of the spine or lesions in the gray or white matter of the brain. Radiography assists in determining the presence of fractures, dislocations, bony spurs, soft tissue swelling, and the presence of foreign objects that may be causing the spasm.

GOALS OF THERAPY

The goals of therapy in treating spasms and spasticity is based on the cause and issues of pain and mobility. Skeletal muscle relaxants are used to minimize or stop unwanted spasm and spasticity, with the ultimate goal of establishing normal muscle tone and function. Additionally, effective treatment regimens improve activity tolerance, range of motion, strength, and mobility.

INTERVENTION

Most spasms are self-limiting, responding rapidly to rest and physical measures, such as application of cold or warm compresses, whirlpool baths, and physical therapy. No completely satisfactory form of therapy is available to alleviate spasticity. The cornerstone of any treatment is the management of the underlying disease and physiotherapy. Measures that can be used include physical therapy for stretching, strengthening, range-of-motion exercises, assistive-adaptive devices, and hydrotherapy. A combination of treatments, when augmented with drug therapy, provides the greatest functional benefit. Because no studies indicate that any one skeletal muscle relaxant has superiority over another, drug selection is largely based on the preference of the health care provider and the patient's response.

Administration

In general, the dosage of skeletal muscle relaxants is increased gradually to reduce the likelihood of adverse effects. Administer the skeletal muscle relaxant with food or beverages to minimize GI distress. For ease of administration, tablet formulations can be crushed and mixed with applesauce, jelly, or other food. Relief from dry mouth caused by cyclobenzaprine and tizanidine can be obtained with sips of water, ice chips, or sugarless chewing gum. Frequent mouth rinses and sugarless hard candy may also help. Warn the patient that intramuscular injections may cause a burning sensation at the injection site.

Consult the manufacturer's recommendations for information about intravenous administration of skeletal muscle relaxants. For intravenous administration, keep the patient supine and the siderails up. Monitor vital signs. Keep the patient recumbent until the blood pressure is stable.

In some cases of severe spasticity, baclofen is administered intrathecally via an implantable infusion pump. A test dose determines responsiveness and maintenance therapy is determined based on the screening dose that elicited an adequate response. Intrathecal formulations must never be given by intravenous, intramuscular, or subcutaneous routes.

Assess the patient for adverse effects and sensitivity reactions during drug therapy. Monitor the patient's blood pressure every 4 hours until it is stable. Be alert to signs of hypotension when assisting patients to ambulate, especially if they have been immobilized or mostly sedentary before starting drug therapy.

Assess the patient's mental status. Watch for signs of depression, including withdrawal, lack of interest in personal appearance, insomnia, anorexia, and weight loss. In addition, monitor the stools and urine for occult blood and keep track of the patient's intake and output. The use of skeletal muscle relaxants such as dantrolene, tizanidine, and chlorzoxazone require monitoring of liver function to identify adverse hepatic effects. Warn the patient to avoid alcoholic beverages when taking skeletal muscle relaxants.

Watch for hepatitis (fever and jaundice), severe diarrhea, and severe weakness. Check the respiratory rate, breath sounds, and assess for dyspnea. Inspect for skin changes and edema. Monitor the CBC count and urinalysis. Tactfully question the patient regarding impotence and provide emotional support as needed. Remind the patient not to discontinue the drug without first consulting with the health care provider.

Be alert for idiosyncratic reactions when administering the first four doses of carisoprodol, including weakness, ataxia, visual and speech difficulties, fever, skin eruptions, and mental changes. Additionally, monitor the patient for severe reactions, including bronchospasm, hypotension, and anaphylactic shock. Should the patient exhibit these symptoms, hold the dose and notify the prescriber immediately.

Botulinum toxin type A is injected directly into one or more muscles of the affected limb. Monitor cardiovascular status and assess for visual disturbances during therapy.

Document the amount of relief obtained from the administration of the ordered skeletal muscle relaxant and assist the prescriber in determining the lowest effective dosage.

A gradual reduction in dosage over 2 weeks is recommended when the patient is being withdrawn from therapy. Abrupt withdrawal (from baclofen in particular) may cause hallucinations, paranoia, nightmares, confusion, and rebound spasticity. Dosages of carisoprodol should also be tapered to avoid insomnia, headaches, nausea, and abdominal cramps.

Despite their different chemical structures, all skeletal muscle relaxants are sedating and are abused primarily for this effect. At high doses, they have been described as producing a buzz (baclofen), euphoria (carisoprodol), and mood enhancement and pleasant perceptual alterations (orphenadrine). Carisoprodol has been abused more often than other drugs in this class, presumably because of its close similarity to meprobamate. Abusers of any of these drugs demonstrate signs of tolerance to the drugs and also experience withdrawal symptoms.

Potential for Abuse. The extent to which these drugs are abused is unclear since they are often used in conjunction with other CNS depressants (e.g., alcohol, benzodiazepines, opioids). When abused, skeletal muscle relaxants potentiate and prolong the effects of CNS depressants. In addition, prescriptions for skeletal muscle relaxants are often easier to obtain and are less costly. Substance abusers occasionally substitute a skeletal muscle relaxant when an opioid is not available.

Health care providers today are conscious of patient requests for opioids or benzodiazepines and are rightly concerned about the dependency potential of these drugs. However, few health care providers are aware of the potential for dependency that skeletal muscle relaxants hold. Because skeletal muscle relaxants are not controlled substances, health care providers may become complacent about their use. Some of the drugs, such as carisoprodol, can even be ordered by mail through veterinary supply houses. Watch for frequent refills or requests for refills before the expected completion of a prescription.

Education

The patient should be encouraged to comply with additional therapies prescribed for muscle spasms (e.g., rest, heat/cold, physical therapy). Correct posture and lifting techniques should be taught. Stooping rather than bending to lift objects, carrying heavy objects close to the body, and not lifting excessive amounts of weight should be stressed. Regular exercise and the use of warm-up and cool-down exercises minimize the potential for injury. Strenuous exercise performed infrequently is more likely to cause acute muscle spasms.

The patient and family should be educated about the drug prescribed, including the name, purpose, dosage, administration times and frequency, and potential adverse effects. Missed doses should be taken within 1 hour of their scheduled time or omitted. Double doses should not be taken. If the drug is to be discontinued, the patient should be advised not to suddenly stop the drug, but to taper the dosage as instructed. Suggest that the patient take the final dose of the day at bedtime.

If drowsiness occurs, the patient should avoid activities that require mental alertness, judgment, and physical coordination, such as operating a motor vehicle. Alcohol and other CNS depressants increase CNS depression and place the patient at risk for injury. Further, because postural hypotension is common when taking these drugs, the patient should be instructed to change positions slowly.

The patient should also be told not to take other drugs without the health care provider's knowledge, including nonprescription drugs. The major risks occur with concurrent use of alcohol, antihistamines, sleeping aids, or other drugs that cause drowsiness.

The patient taking baclofen should be advised that maximum benefit may not be reached for 4 to 8 weeks. The sedative effects are generally transient and usually disappear with continued therapy. Baclofen and metaxalone have been shown to elevate the blood sugar level. Patients with diabetes mellitus should be instructed to monitor their blood glucose level more frequently.

Inform the patient taking chlorzoxazone that the drug may discolor his or her urine orange or purple-red. Further, instruct the patient to immediately notify the prescriber about any fever, rash, anorexia, nausea, vomiting, fatigue, right upper quadrant pain, dark urine, or jaundice because these may indicate hepatocellular toxicity.

Inform the patient taking methocarbamol that his or her urine may turn green, black, or brown, and the patient may develop a metallic taste in his or her mouth. Advise the patient taking vigabatrin to report visual changes.

Teach the patient receiving botulinum toxin type A injections and the patient taking dantrolene how to avoid photosensitivity reactions (e.g., use sunscreen and wear protective clothing). Further, advise the patient to report any fever, yellowed skin or eyes, itching, or abdominal discomfort. The patient receiving botulinum type A therapy should be advised that a decrease in spasticity typically does not occur until 2 weeks after treatment and wanes after 3 to 6 months, thus requiring repeat dosing.

EVALUATION

Criteria for evaluating the therapeutic outcome of therapy for spasms include decreased pain and tenderness, increased mobility, and the ability to participate in the activities of daily living. When a skeletal muscle relaxant is used for the spasticity of chronic neurologic disorders, therapeutic effects include increased ability to maintain posture, balance, and self-care, improvement in strength and muscle tone, improved coordination, and ease of movement. Reduction in spasticity does not necessarily correlate with overall functional improvement.

CASE STUDY | *Multiple Sclerosis*

ASSESSMENT

HISTORY OF PRESENT ILLNESS

DJ is a 40-year-old woman with a 10-year history of multiple sclerosis (MS). She now complains of reduced strength and mobility, increased cutaneous, flexor and extensor spasms, and pain that started 1 month ago. The spasms disturb her sleep. DJ states that she is unable to carry out routine activities of daily living and daily range of motion exercises as before. She used a cane until recently but now must use a walker. She denies having any recent illness, infection, unusual stress, or trauma.

HEALTH HISTORY

DJ has been taking alternate-day low dose prednisone for the past year with general improvement in symptoms. She was actively employed until the recent change in her health status. She usually follows her prescribed exercise regimen and, according to her record, she is a motivated patient. DJ is postmenopausal; she takes estrogen/progesterone daily. She has no known food or drug allergies.

LIFESPAN CONSIDERATIONS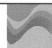

DJ is single and lives alone. She works as a secretary-receptionist and is age-appropriate for chronologic and developmental stage.

CULTURAL/SOCIAL CONSIDERATIONS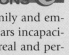

DJ copes well with her disease overall. Her family and employer are emotionally supportive. She most fears incapacitation and has a sense of powerlessness from real and perceived losses. She has changed jobs several times in the past 3 years due to her MS and now perceives her financial, physical, and social independence as threatened. DJ is interested in the theater and arts and attends shows on a regular basis with a theater group.

PHYSICAL EXAMINATION

DJ is 5'4" tall and weighs 125 lbs. Her vital signs are BP 122/72, apical pulse 72 and regular, respirations 20, temperature 98.6° F. Extensor and flexor spasms and clonus are observed; DTRs are exaggerated. DJ has an unsteady gait and borderline muscle strength.

LABORATORY TESTING

Results of CBC count and electrolyte, BUN, creatinine levels are within normal limits. Cerebrospinal fluid reflects slightly elevated WBC, cell, and protein counts. Electromyelogram (EMG) reflects slow-wave activity compared to examination 2 years ago. Repeat computed tomography (CT) scan shows increased density in the white matter with MS plaques.

PATIENT PROBLEM(S)

Spasticity related to MS; decreased activity tolerance, range of motion (ROM), strength, and mobility related to MS; postmenopausal receiving hormone replacement therapy.

GOALS OF THERAPY

Minimize severity of spasticity and improve activity tolerance, ROM, strength, and mobility.

CRITICAL THINKING QUESTIONS

1. Baclofen 5 mg po bid-tid has been ordered initially to treat DJ. The health care provider orders an increase of 5 mg/dose every 3 to 7 days until the desired response is achieved. What is the mechanism of action of this drug?
2. What other drug can be used to treat DJ's MS?
3. What adverse effects should the nurse look for during therapy with baclofen?
4. DJ takes estrogen/progesterone therapy daily. Why would consideration of this information in DJ's health history be an important factor in the choice of the skeletal muscle relaxant ordered?

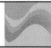

CASE STUDY   *Low Back Pain with Spasm*

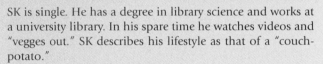

ASSESSMENT

HISTORY OF PRESENT ILLNESS

SK is a 37-year-old man with complaints of low back pain described as "knife-like burning." The pain radiates from the lumbar region to the right midbuttock and hip. He is unable to sit or stand comfortably and complains, "Any movement hurts." SK was helping to unpack and transfer oversize library books to a high shelf when the pain occurred.

HEALTH HISTORY

SK denies having a history of neuromuscular, musculoskeletal, renal, or peptic ulcer disease. He has a history of acute intermittent porphyria. SK has not gained or lost weight in the past year; his routine exercise regimen is limited to walking to and from his car and the library. He denies taking any other medications or consuming alcohol.

LIFESPAN CONSIDERATIONS

Accomplishing age-appropriate developmental tasks.

CULTURAL/SOCIAL CONSIDERATIONS

SK is single. He has a degree in library science and works at a university library. In his spare time he watches videos and "vegges out." SK describes his lifestyle as that of a "couch-potato."

PHYSICAL EXAMINATION

SK is 5'9" tall and weighs 255 lbs. Vital signs: BP 132/88, apical pulse 120, respirations 24, temperature 98.6° F. SK is pacing in the examination room, holding his right lower back and hip. Muscle firmness and tenderness noted from L_4-S_3 on palpation and tautness of the sacrospinalis and gluteal muscles. Straight leg raises aggravate the low back pain. Severe discomfort when toe walking. Unable to twist or bend at the waist without obvious discomfort. Muscle tone increased on affected side. Abdomen soft, flat, nontender. No costovertebral (CVA) tenderness.

LABORATORY TESTING

Radiograph of kidneys and upper bladder (KUB), flat plate films of lower back, CT scan, and MRI are all within normal limits. CBC count, electrolytes, BUN, creatinine, urinalysis are within normal limits as well.

PATIENT PROBLEM(S)

Low back syndrome with spasm; acute intermittent porphyria.

GOALS OF THERAPY

Establish normal muscle tone and function; improve functional state and minimize discomfort.

CRITICAL THINKING QUESTIONS

1. Cyclobenzaprine 10 mg tid has been ordered for 2 weeks. What is the mechanism of action of this drug?
2. Why is cyclobenzaprine ordered for a 2-week period?
3. Why is carisoprodol contraindicated in SK's case?
4. What adverse effects should the nurse look for during therapy with cyclobenzaprine?

Bibliography

Bhakta B: Management of spasticity in stroke, *Br Med Bull* 56(2):476-485, 2000.

Brown M: Stroke management: beginnings, *Outcomes Manag Nurs Pract* 4(1):34-39, 2000.

Gormley Jr M., Glenn M: Management of spasticity in children. Part 2. Oral medications and intrathecal baclofen, *J Head Trauma Rehabil* 14(2):207-214, 1999.

Gouzd B: Emergency: whiplash injury, *Am J Nurs* 100(3):41-43, 2000.

Lagalla G, Danni M, Reiter F, et al: Post-stroke spasticity management with repeated botulinum toxin injections in the upper limb, *Am J Phys Med Rehabil* 79(4):377-384, 2000.

Murphy M: Traumatic spinal cord injury: an acute care rehabilitation perspective. *Crit Care Nurs Q* 22(2):51-59, 1999.

Panizza M, Castagna M, di Summa A, et al: Functional and clinical changes in upper limb spastic patients treated with botulinum toxin, *Funct Neurol* 15(3):147-155, 2000.

Reeves R, Liberto V: Abuse of combinations of carisoprodol and tramadol, *South Med J* 94(5):512-514, 2001.

Schretzman D: Acute ischemic stroke, *Dimens Crit Care Nurs* 20(20):14-20, 2001.

Smith HS, Barton AE: Tizanidine in the management of spasticity and musculoskeletal complaints in the palliative care population, *Am J Hosp Palliat Care* 17(1):50-58, 2000.

Vitztum C, Olney B: Intrathecal baclofen therapy and the child with cerebral palsy. *Orthop Nurs* 19(1):43-48, 2000.

Yanko J, Mitcho K: Acute care management of severe traumatic brain injuries, *Crit Care Nurs Q* 23(4):1-23, 2001.

Internet Resources

National Institute of Neurological Disorders and Stroke web resource site. Available online at http://www.ninds.nih.gov/health_and_medical/disorders/cerebral_palsy.htm.

National Library of Medicine: Medline site for health information. Available online at http://www.nlm.nih.gov/medlineplus/druginfo/skeletalmusclerelaxantssystemi202523.html.

CHAPTER
22

Anticonvulsants

MICHAEL R. VASKO • SUSAN SCIACCA

 Visit **http://evolve.elsevier.com/Gutierrez/** for additional information.

KEY TERMS

Aura, p. 330

Epilepsy, p. 330

Fetal hydantoin syndrome, p. 333

Generalized seizures, p. 330

Gingival hyperplasia, p. 333

Partial seizures, p. 330

Postictal depression, p. 330

Seizures, p. 330

Status epilepticus, p. 330

Tonic-clonic seizures, p. 330

OBJECTIVES

- Define epilepsy.
- Characterize the major syndromes of tonic-clonic seizures, absence seizures, myoclonus epilepsy, psychomotor epilepsy, focal motor seizures, and status epilepticus.
- Discuss the principles of drug therapy for epilepsy.
- Explain the use of diazepam or lorazepam for controlling status epilepticus.
- Describe the most common adverse effects of anticonvulsants.
- Develop a nursing care plan, including a teaching plan, for a patient receiving anticonvulsant drug therapy.
- Identify patient outcomes that indicate successful drug therapy in the treatment of epilepsy or seizures.

PATHOPHYSIOLOGY • Epilepsy

Seizures are a pattern of abnormal neuronal discharges within the brain, resulting in changes in the level of consciousness, motor activity, sensory phenomena, and behavior. **Epilepsy** is a neurologic disorder characterized by recurrent seizures. The seizures may be preceded by an **aura**, a sensation peculiar for that patient that warns of an impending seizure. Between 1% and 2% of the population is estimated to have epilepsy.

The cause of epilepsy may be unknown (idiopathic) or may be traced to an identifiable brain lesion. In general, epilepsy appearing in childhood or adolescence is likely to be idiopathic, whereas epilepsy appearing in adulthood is likely to relate to a definable cause, such as a head injury, cerebrovascular accident (stroke), or brain tumor. A single-episode seizure can be caused by events such as fever, hypoglycemia, or hyponatremia, and drug withdrawal and does not mean that the patient has epilepsy.

An appropriate choice of drugs, taken on a long-term basis, can control epileptic seizures in about 80% of patients. The choice of drugs depends on a careful diagnosis of the seizure pattern, which ideally is made after observing a seizure and recording the brain wave pattern with an electroencephalogram (EEG) during the seizure. The diagnosis is critical to the drug selection because some drugs are better suited than others at controlling different types of seizures. Other causes of the seizures must be ruled out because seizures may be a result of an organic disorder such as a brain tumor, poisoning, fever, hypoglycemia, and hypocalcemia. Abrupt withdrawal of some drugs such as barbiturates and most other sedative-hypnotic drugs, including alcohol, can precipitate seizures.

CLASSIFICATION OF EPILEPSY

The Commission of Classification and Terminology of the International League Against Epilepsy classified epilepsy into two broad groups: partial seizures and generalized seizures (Table 22-1). **Partial seizures** arise from a focal area in the cerebral cortex and the location of the focal discharge determines the type of seizure observed: motor, cognitive, behavioral, or sensory. **Generalized seizures** involve both hemispheres of the brain and involve reciprocal firing of neurons from the cortex to the thalamus. Tonic-clonic seizures, absence seizures, and myoclonic seizures are examples of generalized seizures.

Partial seizures can be simple or complex and can potentially become generalized (see Table 22-1). The major characteristic that distinguishes a simple seizure from a complex one is that the patient does not lose consciousness during a simple seizure. Depending on the particular part of the brain in which the seizure originates, simple partial seizures may be visual, such as flashes of light, or tactile, such as a feeling of numbness or tingling. Focal motor seizures can involve just a finite motion, such as turning of the head. Other motor seizures begin with clonic jerking of a few muscles on half of the face or in one extremity; the seizure then progresses to include more body musculature (e.g., finger, hand, arm). Complex partial seizures often arise in the temporal lobe and include symptoms such as aura, automatism, and motor seizures, either independently or in combination. Automatism may consist of chewing or swallowing motions, temperamental changes, confusion, feelings of unreality, or unexplained bizarre behavior. A detailed neurologic examination may be required to differentiate complex partial epilepsy from psychotic mental illness.

Generalized seizure types include tonic-clonic (formerly called grand mal), absence (formerly petit mal), and myoclonus. **Tonic-clonic seizures** involve the contraction of all skeletal muscles, and before the seizure begins, the patient may experience an aura. The patient then suddenly loses consciousness and may utter a cry as the diaphragm contracts and expels air from the lungs. The seizure consists of sustained (tonic) contractions or intermittent (clonic) contractions of the muscles. The patient may become incontinent. When the contractions cease, the patient regains consciousness. Usually, the patient is confused and drowsy and lapses into prolonged sleep **(postictal depression)**.

Absence seizures occur mainly in children 4 to 12 years old, and loss of consciousness occurs for only a few seconds. Body tone is seldom lost and consciousness is regained with no confusion. The appearance is one of inattention or daydreaming and may be accompanied by slight blinking or hand movements. Attacks usually occur several times a day. Myoclonic seizures consist of sudden involuntary contractions of skeletal muscles, which are aggravated by purposeful activity and by visual, auditory, tactile, and emotional activity.

Status epilepticus occurs when a patient has seizures in rapid succession or continuous seizures lasting 30 minutes or more. There are several types of status epilepticus, including absence status epilepticus, myoclonic status epilepticus, and tonic-clonic status epilepticus. Status epilepticus has many causes, and patients who develop it may have no previous history of epilepsy. In these cases, the cause is often related to acute brain infections, head trauma, cerebrovascular disease, and toxic or metabolic disorders.

The most severe form of status epilepticus is the tonic-clonic form. The patient experiences an unrelenting series

TABLE 22-1

Types of Seizures with Associated Characteristics and Manifestations

Seizure Type	Characteristics and Manifestations
Partial Seizures	
Simple partial seizures	Consciousness is not impaired. Duration: 1 to 2 minutes. Functional disturbance in motor, sensory, and/or autonomic nerves and regions of the brain. Sensory symptoms (i.e., odor, taste) most common. Psychic symptoms (fearful feeling, sense of déjà vu).
Complex partial seizures	Consciousness impaired at onset. Start as simple partial seizures and progress to impairment of consciousness (i.e., amnesia, unresponsiveness). Duration: 1 to 2 minutes. Characterized by automatisms (e.g., staring; chewing; lip smacking; bizarre, purposeless motor or psychic activity; mumbled speech; unintelligible sounds).
Partial seizures evolving to secondarily generalized seizures	Duration: minutes. Simple partial seizures evolving to generalized seizures. Complex partial seizures evolving to generalized seizures. Simple partial seizures evolving to complex partial seizures evolving to generalized seizures.
Generalized Seizures	
Absence seizures	Brief loss of consciousness, amnesia, lack of awareness. Duration: 10 to 30 seconds. Onset in childhood with approximately 40% ending in adolescence. Typical absence seizures (petit mal seizures) or atypical absence seizures.
Myoclonic seizures	Characterized by single or multiple, short, abrupt muscular contractions of arms, legs, and/or torso and brief loss of consciousness. Duration: 1 to 5 seconds. May be confined to face and trunk or to one or more extremities.
Clonic seizures	Repetitive clonic jerks that lack tonic component. Duration: seconds. Movements may be symmetric or asymmetric; synchronous or asynchronous.
Tonic seizures	Altered consciousness, tonic contraction of muscle groups with no progression to clonic movement. Duration: 30 seconds to several minutes. Ocular phenomena common (e.g., fixed gaze, eyelid retraction, superior ocular deviation, nystagmus, mydriasis). Autonomia (e.g., tachycardia, hypertension, respiratory distress).
Tonic-clonic seizures (grand mal)	Vague aura, loss of consciousness, sudden tonic contraction. Duration: 10 to 30 seconds after falling to ground. Tonic phase gives way to clonic phase, which lasts 30 to 50 seconds. Muscle relaxation interrupts tonic contraction with tone returning as rhythmic flexor spasms that become less frequent as seizure subsides. Urinary and fecal incontinence may occur during clonic phase. Amnesia after seizure with postictal period.
Atonic seizures	Characterized by abrupt, selective loss of muscle tone or of all muscle tone. Duration: 10 to 30 seconds. Referred to as drop attacks if attacks are brief and patient slumps to ground; injury possible. May be followed by postictal confusion.
Unclassified epileptic seizures	Seizures cannot be classified because of inadequate or incomplete data. Duration: 10 to 30 seconds.

From Santilli N: *Managing seizure disorders: a handbook for health care professionals*, Philadelphia, 1996, Lippincott-Raven.

of tonic-clonic attacks. Loss of consciousness extends throughout the entire attack. The sudden withdrawal of a drug or noncompliance with anticonvulsant therapy can precipitate status epilepticus. Because of the sudden withdrawal of a drug, the blood level of the drug abruptly drops and the seizure activity is no longer suppressed. Status epilepticus requires immediate intervention and aggressive treatment to prevent damage to the CNS.

MECHANISMS UNDERLYING SEIZURES

The basis of seizures is a regional imbalance of inhibitory and excitatory neuronal inputs and alterations of membrane stability. Gamma-aminobutyric acid (GABA) is the major inhibitory transmitter in the brain, whereas glutamate is the major excitatory transmitter. The GABA-A receptor mediates much of the inhibitory activity of GABA by increasing the chloride conduction in neurons, usually resulting in hyperpolarization. Drugs that enhance this activity of GABA have an anticonvulsant effect. Such drugs include benzodiazepines, barbiturates, valproate, tiagabine, and vigabatrin. Activation of glutamate receptors results in depolarization and enhanced excitation of neurons. Consequently, drugs that inhibit the release of glutamate or inhibit activation of glutamate receptors can be anticonvulsants. One possible action of lamotrigine may be to decrease glutamate release, whereas felbamate reduces activation of glutamate receptors.

As neurons begin to depolarize, voltage-gated sodium channels are activated. After activation, these channels have a period of inactivation. Under normal conditions, prolonging this inactivation period has no clinical significance since neurons do not fire too rapidly and thus have time for the channels to return to a state where they can be activated. With bursts of action potentials, which can occur at a seizure focus, prolonging the time that the channel is in the inactive state can reduce high-frequency firing, thus reducing seizure activity. Carbamazepine, lamotrigine, phenytoin, topiramate, valproic acid, and zonisamide are capable of prolonging the inactivation period of sodium channels.

Through activation of a certain voltage-gated calcium channel, called the T channel, thalamic neurons can exhibit action-potential bursting. These bursts can produce the abnormal electrical activity associated with absence seizures. A number of anticonvulsants used in treating absence seizures—including ethosuximide, lamotrigine, trimethadione, and valproic acid—reduce the T-type calcium current in thalamic neurons.

Some types of epilepsy are inherited or result from genetic mutation. Both juvenile myoclonic epilepsy and childhood absence epilepsy may have genetic causes. Severely mutated genes are associated with idiopathic epilepsies, including mutations of a subunit of sodium channels, of two potassium channels, and of the nicotinic cholinergic receptors. However, these mutations are rare and account for a very small percentage of epilepsy cases.

DRUG CLASS • Hydantoins

ethotoin (Peganone)

fosphenytoin (Cerebyx)

mephenytoin (Mesantoin)

⚠ phenytoin (diphenylhydantoin, Dilantin, Diphenylan)

MECHANISM OF ACTION

Phenytoin and other hydantoins reduce the rate of recovery of sodium channels from the inactivated state in areas of a seizure focus and thus reduce sustained high-frequency firing of neurons. There is little if any reduction in normal neuronal activity at concentrations that affect sodium channels, but at higher concentrations there is a decrease in neuronal activity.

USES

Hydantoins are used to treat generalized tonic-clonic seizures, status epilepticus, and refractory cases of simple and complex partial seizures. Phenytoin is the most commonly used drug in this group, followed by ethotoin and mephenytoin. Sodium phenytoin is given intravenously to control status epilepticus alone or after intravenous diazepam has initially controlled the seizures. Phenytoin has largely been replaced by fosphenytoin for this indication. Phenytoin is also used as an antiarrhythmic drug (see Chapter 40).

PHARMACOKINETICS

Ethotoin and mephenytoin are fairly rapidly absorbed from the gastrointestinal (GI) tract, but phenytoin, depending on the formulation, is slow, variable, and often incomplete in its absorption. Hydantoins, particularly phenytoin, are rapidly distributed to all tissues, with the highest concentrations occurring in the brain, liver, and salivary glands. Hydantoins cross the placenta and are found in breast milk. Phenytoin is highly bound to plasma proteins.

Hydantoins are biotransformed by the microsomal enzyme system in the liver. Phenytoin follows zero-order kinetics, that is, the rate of elimination is independent of concentration; thus the half-life of the drug depends on the total amount of drug in the body. At therapeutic concentrations, the half-life is approximately 18 to 24 hours but is much longer with high amounts. Phenytoin is primarily eliminated in the bile, then reabsorbed from the GI tract, and eliminated in urine. Approximately 5% of phenytoin is eliminated unchanged. Mephenytoin is eliminated in urine. Ethotoin is eliminated in urine, feces, and in small amounts in the saliva.

ADVERSE REACTIONS AND CONTRAINDICATIONS

Common adverse effects of hydantoins include dizziness, ataxia, sensory neuropathies, nausea, vomiting, diarrhea, nystagmus, and diplopia. About 20% of patients taking phenytoin experience **gingival hyperplasia** (overgrowth of the gums), which can be particularly severe in children. Hypertrichosis (excessive body hair), exfoliative dermatitis (excessive shedding of skin), coarsened facial features, impaired cognition, dyskinesia (impaired voluntary movement), urinary incontinence, and thyroid disorders occur in some patients. Occasionally, folic acid or vitamin D deficiency can occur because phenytoin interferes with the normal metabolism of these vitamins. Phenytoin can also cause an allergic rash that can be mistaken for measles or infectious mononucleosis. The most serious adverse effects include agranulocytosis, encephalopathy, and coma. Phenytoin is contraindicated in patients who are hypersensitive to hydantoins. This hypersensitivity (fever, skin rash) usually occurs within the first 3 to 8 weeks of therapy but may occur up to 12 weeks later. It can lead to renal failure, rhabdomyolysis, or hepatic necrosis. Phenytoin hypersensitivity can be fatal. Cautious use of phenytoin is warranted in patients with hypotension, porphyria, severe myocardial insufficiency, renal or hepatic disease, and hypoalbuminemia.

A high fosphenytoin blood level may produce ataxia, nystagmus, double vision, lethargy, slurred speech, nausea, vomiting, and hypotension. As the level increases, extreme lethargy and coma develops. The most serious adverse effects of ethotoin include agranulocytosis, thrombocytopenia, leukopenia, aplastic anemia, and megaloblastic anemia. It should be used with caution in patients who have diabetes mellitus and in patients who slowly biotransform hydantoins. Ethotoin is contraindicated for patients who are hypersensitive to hydantoins or who have blood dyscrasias, hematologic disease, hepatic disorders, or porphyria.

Mephenytoin has many of the same adverse effects as ethotoin as well as lethargy, exfoliative dermatitis, palpitations, tachycardia, and hypertension. Mephenytoin should be used with caution in patients with cardiac disorders, hyperthyroidism, diabetes mellitus, or prostatic hypertrophy, as well as those with alcoholism, hepatic or renal disease, and blood dyscrasias.

Teratogenic effects can occur with the use of hydantoins. **Fetal hydantoin syndrome** includes numerous craniofacial abnormalities (e.g., cleft lip, cleft palate), hypoplasia of the digits, dislocated hips, congenital heart defects, microcephaly, and prenatal growth deficiencies. These infants are also at risk for hemorrhage and coagulation deficiencies at birth, which can be corrected with vitamin K.

Effective serum concentrations of phenytoin are 10 to 20 mcg/mL, and adverse effects are seen at higher serum concentrations. At greater than 20 mcg/mL, involuntary movement of the eyeballs (nystagmus) appears; at greater than 30 mcg/mL, ataxia and slurred speech develop. Tremors and nervousness, or drowsiness and fatigue may be seen at higher serum concentrations.

INTERACTIONS

Serious drug interactions can occur with phenytoin. Phenobarbital increases the biotransformation of phenytoin in some individuals by inducing liver microsomal enzymes, but in others, phenobarbital decreases the rate of drug biotransformation of phenytoin by competing with the enzymes for degradation. The oral anticoagulant dicumarol and the anticonvulsant carbamazepine decrease the biotransformation of phenytoin by competing with the enzymes for degradation. The anticonvulsant valproic acid displaces bound phenytoin from plasma protein, thereby increasing the free concentration of phenytoin while decreasing its total concentration since more phenytoin is available for biotransformation. Phenytoin enhances the rate of estrogen biotransformation, which can decrease the effectiveness of some oral contraceptives. Hydantoins interact with a variety of other drugs, including but not limited to rifampin, beta-blockers, calcium channel blockers, tricyclic antidepressants, estrogens, and oral antidiabetic drugs.

DRUG CLASS • **Iminostilbenes**

carbamazepine (Epitol, Tegretol, Apo-Carbamazepine, ✳)

oxcarbazepine (Trileptal)

MECHANISM OF ACTION

Carbamazepine is chemically related to the tricyclic antidepressants. As with phenytoin, it limits seizure propagation presumably by increasing the amount of time that sodium channels are inactivated, thereby reducing their ability to depolarize neurons. Oxcarbazepine is a prodrug with a similar mechanism of action.

USES

Carbamazepine is one of the drugs of choice in the management of tonic-clonic seizures. It is also used to manage complex partial, simple partial, and mixed seizures, but it is ineffective for absence and myoclonic seizures in adults. Carbamazepine can be used for the relief of pain caused by trigeminal neuralgia or glossopharyngeal neuralgia, although it is not an analgesic. It is also somewhat useful in treating bipolar depression. Oxcarbazepine is used largely as an adjunct therapy for partial seizures.

PHARMACOKINETICS

Carbamazepine is absorbed slowly and erratically after oral administration; thus it has been formulated in a sustained release capsule for twice-daily dosage. This formulation decreases fluctuations in serum concentrations by 50%, thereby reducing adverse effects. Distribution to tissues is wide and the drug is rapidly found in the brain, cerebrospinal fluid, bile, and saliva. Approximately 75% of the drug in the blood is bound to plasma proteins. Carbamazepine crosses placental membranes and can be found in fetal tissues and in breast milk. The plasma half-life is 12 hours, so the drug must be given in divided doses. Biotransformation occurs in the liver via the microsomal enzyme system, and 72% of the metabolites are excreted in the urine and 28% in the feces. Carbamazepine induces its own biotransformation

and that of other drugs biotransformed by P-450 mixed-function oxidases. Oxcarbazepine is a prodrug that is rapidly converted in the liver to an active drug, which in turn is further biotransformed in the liver by the P-450 oxidases. Oxcarbazepine does not induce drug biotransformation as much as carbamazepine.

ADVERSE REACTIONS AND CONTRAINDICATIONS

The most common adverse effects of carbamazepine are drowsiness, dizziness, ataxia, visual disturbances (particularly double vision), and GI irritation. Restlessness, aggression, irritability, and agitation may also occur. Although serious adverse effects are rare, carbamazepine occasionally causes rashes, liver damage, leukopenia, and aplastic anemia, which require its discontinuance. Blood counts should be done often in the early course of treatment and occasionally thereafter.

Carbamazepine is contraindicated in patients with hypersensitivity, bone marrow depression, or blood dyscrasias. It should be used cautiously with patients who are recovering from alcoholism and in those with behavioral problems, heart disease, metabolic disorders, renal and hepatic impairments, diabetes mellitus, or increased intraocular pressure.

INTERACTIONS

Drugs that tend to lower the plasma concentration of carbamazepine by increasing its biotransformation include many other anticonvulsants, tricyclic antidepressants, and antipsychotics. Some drugs increase the plasma concentration of carbamazepine by inhibiting its . Other drugs that potentiate its action by increasing its plasma concentration include cimetidine, propoxyphene, diltiazem, verapamil, erythromycin, and isoniazid. Carbamazepine can lower the effectiveness of several drugs by increasing their biotransformation. Drugs that are affected include estrogen, quinidine, glucocorticoids, monoamine oxidase inhibitors, and oral anticoagulants. Prolonged use of carbamazepine with acetaminophen can lead to liver damage.

DRUG CLASS • Barbiturates

mephobarbital (Mebaral)

⚠ phenobarbital (Solfoton)

primidone (Mysoline, Apo-Primidone,✱
Sertan,✱ PMS-Primidone✱)

MECHANISM OF ACTION

The anticonvulsant effects of barbiturates occur by enhancing the activity of the inhibitory neurotransmitter GABA at GABA-A receptors. Phenobarbital also decreases the repetitive firing of neurons. Primidone has a similar mechanism.

USES

Although all barbiturates possess anticonvulsant effects, the long-acting barbiturates (phenobarbital and mephobarbital) and the deoxybarbiturate primidone are the only ones used to provide oral anticonvulsant action in subhypnotic doses. The use of barbiturates as sedative-hypnotics is discussed in Chapter 17. Phenobarbital is used in the prevention and treatment of tonic-clonic, simple partial, and complex partial seizures, but it is ineffective for absence seizures. Mephobarbital is used to treat partial and generalized tonic-clonic seizures, and as a replacement drug for phenobarbital when there is paradoxic excitement in children or behavior changes in adults. It can be used alone or with other anticonvulsant drugs. Primidone can be substituted for phenobarbital to treat partial and generalized seizures, but it is not used for the treatment of absence seizures. Phenobarbital may be used to stop seizures of status epilepticus that are unresponsive to benzodiazepines and phenytoin, but respiratory and blood pressure support must be available.

PHARMACOKINETICS

Barbiturates are absorbed from the GI tract in varying degrees (approximately 50% for mephobarbital to 90% for phenobarbital). Distribution of barbiturates occurs throughout all tissues and fluids, particularly the brain, cerebrospinal fluid, liver, and kidneys. Barbiturates readily cross the placenta and can be found in breast milk. Phenobarbital has a long half-life and can be administered once a day. Biotransformation occurs in the liver by the microsomal enzyme system. Primidone is biotransformed to phenobarbital and the active metabolite phenylethylmalonamide. However, 15% to 40% of primidone is eliminated unchanged in the urine. Phenobarbital is a classic inducer of liver microsomal enzymes and thus can increase its own biotransformation and that of other drugs. Mephobarbital is eliminated almost entirely as metabolites in the urine, and phenobarbital is eliminated 25% to 50% unchanged in the urine.

ADVERSE REACTIONS AND CONTRAINDICATIONS

The main adverse effects of the barbiturates are sedation, drowsiness, dizziness, lethargy, and behavioral changes, which occur at the beginning of treatment. Tolerance usually develops to these effects. Phenobarbital tends to impair thinking, mood, and behavior. Sudden withdrawal of the drug can precipitate convulsions. In older adults and in children, a paradoxic excitement may be seen that impairs learning ability. Phenobarbital increases the incidence of congenital malformations in the fetus but not to the degree associated with phenytoin and trimethadione.

Barbiturates are contraindicated for patients with the metabolic disorder porphyria and for patients who are depressed and might consider suicide. Patients with respiratory depression or obstruction, asthma, heart failure, severe anemia, hepatic dysfunction, hypoadrenalism, hypothyroidism, or depression, or those experiencing acute or chronic pain should only use phenobarbital with caution.

The most common adverse effects of primidone are drowsiness, ataxia, vertigo, lethargy, and anorexia. Systemic lupus erythematosus, blood dyscrasias, megaloblastic anemia, and hypersensitivity reactions are possible. Phenobarbital toxicity may increase when it is used with primidone, causing additive sedation. Primidone must be used with caution in patients with renal impairment, hepatic dysfunction, and pulmonary insufficiency. It is not recommended for patients with porphyria.

INTERACTIONS

There are numerous drug interactions with barbiturates. Barbiturates interact in a synergistic manner with other CNS depressants, including alcohol. The effects of certain drugs, such as acetaminophen, oral anticoagulants, some antibiotics, tricyclic antidepressants, and oral contraceptives are reduced. Orthostatic hypotension can occur with concurrent use of furosemide. Barbiturates induce liver enzymes and can thereby decrease the levels of other drugs that are biotransformed by this system.

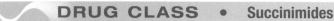

DRUG CLASS • Succinimides

⚠ **ethosuximide (Zarontin)**

methsuximide (Celontin)

phensuximide (Milontin)

MECHANISM OF ACTION

At therapeutic concentrations ethosuximide suppresses the activity of T calcium currents in thalamic neurons, thereby reducing bursts of action potentials.

USES

Ethosuximide is the drug of choice for absence seizures but it is not effective in treating tonic-clonic seizures. It has replaced trimethadione in the treatment of absence seizures because of the high incidence of adverse effects. Phensuximide is not as effective as ethosuximide for childhood absence epilepsy. Methsuximide is used as an adjunct therapy for refractory partial complex seizures.

PHARMACOKINETICS

The succinimides are readily and rapidly absorbed from the GI tract. They are distributed to the tissues and body water, cross placental membranes, and are excreted into breast milk. The plasma half-life of ethosuximide is about 30 hours in children and 60 hours in adults, with steady-state plasma concentrations reached in about 4 to 6 days in children and over a longer period in adults. Biotransformation occurs in the liver. Ethosuximide is eliminated slowly in the urine with 25% to 50% of the drug unchanged. Small amounts are eliminated via the bile and feces. Methsuximide is eliminated in the urine with less than 1% of the drug unchanged. Phensuximide is mainly eliminated in the urine as the parent compound and hydroxylated metabolites.

ADVERSE REACTIONS AND CONTRAINDICATIONS

The adverse reactions to succinimides influence the CNS, GI tract, skin, and hematologic systems. Drowsiness, ataxia, and dizziness are common adverse effects as well as nausea, vomiting, diarrhea, and anorexia. Eosinophilia, thrombocytopenia, aplastic anemia, bone marrow depression, leukopenia, agranulocytosis, monocytosis, and pancytopenia can be life threatening. The tendency of these drugs to cause blood dyscrasias may show up as periodontal problems such as increased mouth infection and gingival bleeding. Stevens-Johnson syndrome, systemic lupus erythematosus, and renal damage are also possible.

Peripheral neuropathies are associated with phensuximide. Nephropathies have occurred with the succinimides, and phensuximide causes the urine to be discolored. Contraindications for ethosuximide include blood dyscrasias, intermittent porphyria, and hepatic or renal disease.

INTERACTIONS

Ethosuximide enhances the CNS depressive effects of other drugs. When used with haloperidol, it can cause changes in the pattern or frequency of seizures, and the dosage of either drug may need to be changed. Carbamazepine and phenytoin increase the biotransformation of ethosuximide, whereas valproate decreases the biotransformation. Succinimides also increase serum hydantoin concentrations. Reduced primidone and phenobarbital levels have been noted with concurrent use of succinimides.

DRUG CLASS • Valproates

divalproex sodium (Depakote)

⚠ **valproic acid (Depakene)**

MECHANISM OF ACTION

Valproic acid increases the time sodium currents are inactive in a manner similar to phenytoin and carbamazepine. Thus, valproate can decrease the bursts of high-frequency action potentials. Valproate also increases the concentration of GABA by augmenting the activity of the synthetic enzyme glutamic acid decarboxylase and by inhibiting the enzymes that biotransform GABA (GABA transaminase and succinic semialdehyde dehydrogenase). Divalproex is a combination of the acid and salt forms of valproic acid.

USES

Valproic acid is used in the treatment of tonic-clonic seizures, absence seizures, myoclonic seizures, and partial seizures. Clinical studies suggest that valproate is effective in treating bipolar disorders and for prophylaxis in patients with migraine headaches.

PHARMACOKINETICS

Valproic acid is rapidly and efficiently absorbed after oral administration. Divalproex sodium is a combination of valproic acid and sodium valproate with an enteric covering to delay absorption for 1 to 4 hours after ingestion. In the GI tract the complex dissolves into valproate. Valproic acid is rapidly distributed to plasma and extracellular fluids; it crosses the blood-brain barrier and placental membranes and is found in breast milk. Peak serum concentrations are reached 1 to 4 hours after taking the capsule or syrup. Delayed-release capsules reach peak serum concentrations in 3 to 4 hours. Valproic acid is highly protein bound at 90% to 95% at serum concentrations of 50 mcg/mL. At serum concentrations above 50 mcg/mL, binding sites become saturated and the fraction of free drug increases, which can dramatically increase the incidence of adverse effects and toxicity. The liver biotransforms valproate and some metabolites are active. Children biotransform the drug more rapidly than adults. Infants and older adults biotransform the drug more slowly than other age groups. The drug and its metabolites are excreted in the urine as glucuronides.

ADVERSE REACTIONS AND CONTRAINDICATIONS

The most common adverse effects seen with valproic acid are anorexia, nausea, and vomiting. Sedation is marked at the beginning of treatment unless the dosage is increased gradually. A hand tremor is occasionally seen with higher dosages. Overdosage has produced coma but patients usually recover fully with no subsequent impairment. Hepatotoxicity and pancreatitis are rare but potentially serious adverse effects. These effects usually appear in the first 6 months of treatment. Chil-

dren less than 2 years old or children receiving other anticonvulsant drugs with valproate are at the greatest risk for liver failure. Nonspecific symptoms include loss of seizure control, malaise, weakness, lethargy, loss of appetite, vomiting, and edema, as well as symptoms similar to those of Reye's syndrome. Valproate also may raise ammonia concentrations in the blood, but this is not associated with any clinical manifestations.

Valproate is contraindicated for patients with liver disease because of the potential for liver failure. Valproate also interferes with platelet aggregation; prolonged bleeding, anemia, and thrombocytopenia can occur. Valproate should be used with caution in patients with bleeding disorders.

INTERACTIONS

Valproate potentiates the CNS depressant effect of other drugs, especially that of alcohol and barbiturates. Other anticonvulsants that induce liver microsomal enzymes, including phenobarbital, primidone, phenytoin, and carbamazepine, can reduce valproate blood concentrations. Phenytoin can also raise the concentration of free-plasma valproic acid by displacing the fraction bound to plasma proteins. Drugs that alter coagulation—including oral anticoagulants, heparin, platelet aggregation inhibitors, and thrombolytic drugs—also increase the risk for bleeding when taking valproate.

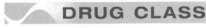

DRUG CLASS • Benzodiazepines

clonazepam (Klonopin, Rivotril)

clorazepate (Gen-Xene, Tranxene, Apo-Clorazepate, ✱ Novo-Clopate ✱)

⚠ **diazepam (Diastat, Valium)**

lorazepam (Ativan)

MECHANISM OF ACTION

Benzodiazepines act at specific receptors in the brain that are part of the GABA-A receptor complex to augment the openings of the chloride channel. The result is an enhanced hyperpolarization and suppression of the spread of seizures.

USES

Benzodiazepines are discussed in detail in Chapter 17 for their use as antianxiety sedative-hypnotic drugs. The discussion here is limited to their use as anticonvulsants.

Clonazepam is effective in controlling generalized absence seizures and myoclonic seizures, whereas clo-

razepate is used concurrently with other anticonvulsant drugs to treat partial seizures. Tolerance often develops to clonazepam and seizures recur in about a third of patients. Therefore clonazepam is not a first-line drug for epilepsy. Lorazepam is the drug of choice for the initial treatment of status epilepticus. Lorazepam usually stops seizures within 3 minutes and has a duration of action of 12 to 24 hours. Diazepam administered intravenously also terminates the tonic-clonic seizures of status epilepticus and seizures of eclampsia. In contrast to lorazepam, however, diazepam has a short duration of action for blocking seizures (15 to 30 minutes). Thus, additional treatment may be required to control the seizures.

PHARMACOKINETICS

Benzodiazepines are rapidly and efficiently absorbed after oral administration. Peak plasma concentrations of clonazepam occur 1 to 4 hours after administration. Clorazepate is inactive until it is biotransformed to desmethyldiazepam. Diazepam is slowly and erratically absorbed when administered intramuscularly, but it has a rapid onset when given intravenously because distribution to the brain occurs seconds after injection and immediate anticonvulsant effects are obtained. Redistribution to tissues occurs fairly rapidly, causing the central effects of intravenous benzodiazepines to quickly diminish. A rectal formulation of diazepam allows patients with status epilepticus to be treated before arrival at the emergency room. This form is also used for the patient with intractable epilepsy who has frequent clusters of seizures. Benzodiazepines are biotransformed in the liver and eliminated via the kidneys, with less than 1% as unchanged drug.

ADVERSE REACTIONS AND CONTRAINDICATIONS

Adverse reactions to benzodiazepines include drowsiness, ataxia, and sedation. Respiratory depression is possible with intravenous administration. Neurologic adverse effects are commonly seen during therapy with clonazepam and include drowsiness, ataxia, and personality changes. Children may become hyperactive, irritable, aggressive, violent, or disobedient. Slurred speech, tremors, abnormal eye movements, dizziness, and confusion also may be noticed. Children taking clorazepate also may exhibit hyperactivity. These effects are dose related and may subside with time or after the dosage is lowered. Increased salivation and bronchial secretions sometimes occur and create respiratory problems in children.

Benzodiazepines should be used cautiously in patients with chronic respiratory conditions and in children, older adults, and those patients who are in a debilitated state. They should also be used with caution in anyone who has a tendency toward physical or psychologic dependency. Benzodiazepines are contraindicated in patients who are hypersensitive to clonazepam and other benzodiazepines and in those with severe liver disease or with optic nerve or retinal disease.

INTERACTIONS

Benzodiazepines enhance the CNS depression produced by other drugs, especially barbiturates and alcohol. Clonazepam does not alter the activity of other anticonvulsant drugs. This allows clonazepam to be added to anticonvulsant therapy as a second drug more readily than other drugs. When clonazepam is given with primidone, behavioral disorders may be seen. Cimetidine, oral contraceptives, and disulfiram can increase the plasma concentration of clonazepam and slow the biotransformation of desmethyldiazepam, resulting in higher plasma concentrations of the active drug and increasing adverse actions. For additional discussion of drug interactions with benzodiazepines see Chapter 17.

DRUG CLASS • Oxazolidinediones

paramethadione (Paradione)
 trimethadione (Tridione)

MECHANISM OF ACTION

The anticonvulsant action of the oxazolidinediones appears to be caused by their ability to inhibit the T calcium current in thalamic neurons.

USES

Trimethadione was the first drug effective in controlling absence epilepsy. Today it is a third-choice drug for absence seizures because of the high incidence of serious adverse effects, and oxazolidinediones are used only for absence seizures refractory to other drugs.

PHARMACOKINETICS

Paramethadione and trimethadione are rapidly absorbed from the GI tract. They are freely and uniformly distributed throughout the tissues and body water, and cross the placenta. Paramethadione and trimethadione are biotransformed by demethylation in the liver and are slowly eliminated by the kidneys, almost entirely as the metabolite dimethadione.

ADVERSE REACTIONS AND CONTRAINDICATIONS

The mild adverse effects of trimethadione include drowsiness, nausea, and vomiting. The most severe CNS adverse effects include encephalopathy and coma. Trimethadione can produce serious allergic dermatitis, kidney and liver damage, agranulocytosis, and aplastic anemia. Blood counts and urinalyses are done routinely with trimethadione therapy. In adults the drug often produces an intolerance to light (photophobia). The incidence of spontaneous abortions or congenital anomalies in infants of mothers taking trimethadione is high. Oxazolidinediones are contraindicated in patients with hypersensitivity, hematologic disturbances, and hepatic or renal disease. They should be used with caution in patients with optic nerve or retinal disease, intermittent porphyria, and myasthenia gravis.

DRUG CLASS • Miscellaneous Anticonvulsants

acetazolamide (Diamox, Cetazolam✽)

felbamate (Felbatol)

gabapentin (Neurontin)

lamotrigine (Lamictal)

levetiracetam (Keppra)

tiagabine (Gabitril)

topiramate (Topamax)

vigabatrin (Sabril)

zonisamide (Zonegran)

MECHANISMS OF ACTION

Although not new, acetazolamide is a carbonic anhydrase inhibitor that lowers serum pH and is thought to reduce excessive neuronal discharge and seizure activity. The pharmacology of acetazolamide is discussed in detail in Chapter 46. A number of the newer anticonvulsants seem to have more than one potential mechanism to reduce seizures. In addition to being a weak carbonic anhydrase inhibitor, topiramate prolongs the inactive state of sodium channels thereby inhibiting their activity. Lamotrigine and zonisamide also prolong sodium channel inactivation and lamotrigine inhibits the release of the excitatory neurotransmitter glutamate. Zonisamide also inhibits the T-type calcium current. Felbamate has dual actions to inhibit the *N*-methyl-D-aspartate (NMDA) glutamate receptor and potentiate the actions of GABA at its receptor. Tiagabine and vigabatrin both increase the amount of GABA available in the brain, the former by inhibiting the reuptake of GABA into neurons (by blocking the GABA transporter) and the latter by blocking GABA transaminase, the enzyme that biotransforms GABA. The mechanisms of action of gabapentin and levetiracetam are unknown.

USES

The uses of the various additional anticonvulsants are summarized in Table 22-2. Acetazolamide is used as an adjunct in managing tonic-clonic and refractory absence seizures. Its usefulness is limited, however, because of the rapid development of tolerance to its action.

TABLE 22-2

Anticonvulsant Drugs

Generic Name	Brand Name	Comments
Hydantoins		
ethotoin	Peganone	Alternative therapy for tonic-clonic and simple or complex partial seizures.
fosphenytoin	Cerebyx	A soluble prodrug of phenytoin, packaged as phenytoin equivalents. Rapidly converted by blood and liver enzymes to phenytoin.
mephenytoin	Mesantoin	Alternative therapy for simple partial seizures in patients not responsive to other drugs.
phenytoin (diphenylhydantoin)	Dilantin, Phenytek	First-line drug for tonic-clonic seizures and simple or complex partial seizures. Used for prophylaxis and treatment of seizures during and after neurosurgery. May be used for sustained control of status epilepticus. Used for correction of atrial and ventricular arrhythmias induced by digoxin.
Iminostilbenes		
carbamazepine	Apo-Carbamazepine, ✽ Epitol, Tegretol, others	First-line drug because of relative lack of serious adverse effects and low behavioral and psychologic toxicity. Controls partial seizures with simple or complex symptoms; generalized tonic-clonic seizures; mixed seizure patterns; other partial or generalized seizures. Also indicated for treatment of trigeminal neuralgia and glossopharyngeal neuralgia.
Oxcarbazepine	Trileptal	Prodrug with effects analogous to carbamazepine.

✽ Available only in Canada.

Continued

TABLE 22-2

Anticonvulsant Drugs—cont'd

Generic Name	Brand Name	Comments
Barbiturates		
mephobarbital	Mebaral	*N*-Methylphenobarbital converted to phenobarbital in the body.
phenobarbital	Generic, Solfoton	Alternative drug for treatment of tonic-clonic seizures and simple partial seizures.
primidone	Apo-Primidone, ✱ Mysoline, PMS Primidone ✱	Adjunct or alternate therapy for generalized tonic-clonic, nocturnal myoclonic, complex partial, and simple partial seizures. One metabolite of primidone is phenobarbital.
Succinimides		
ethosuximide	Zarontin	First-line drug for absence seizures.
methsuximide	Celontin	Alternative therapy for absence seizures refractory to other drugs.
phensuximide	Milontin	Alternative therapy for absence seizures refractory to other drugs.
valproic acid	Depakene, Depakote, Epival, ✱ others	First-line drug for simple and complex absence seizures. Also effective for partial seizures, tonic-clonic seizures, and myoclonic seizures. Monotherapy is preferred because there are complex drug interactions affecting plasma levels of valproate and many other anticonvulsants.
Benzodiazepines		
clobazam	Novo-Clobazam, ✱ Frisium ✱	For status epilepticus and severe recurrent convulsive seizures. Only available in Canada.
clonazepam	Klonopin, Rivotril ✱	Treatment for Lennox-Gastaut syndrome; akinetic seizures, myoclonic seizures, absence seizure pattern; adjunctive therapy for simple partial seizure pattern, complex partial seizure patterns.
clorazepate	Apo-Clorazepate, ✱ Gen-Xene, Novo-clopate, ✱ Tranxene	Adjunctive therapy for refractory partial or generalized seizures.
diazepam	Diastat, Epam, ✱ Novo diapam, ✱ Valium, Vivol ✱	For status epilepticus and severe recurrent convulsive seizures. Rectal formulation is absorbed completely. Instruct caregiver in proper use.
lorazepam	Ativan	For status epilepticus and severe recurrent convulsive seizures.
Oxazolidinediones		
paramethadione	Paradione	Alternative therapy for absence seizures refractory to other drugs.
trimethadione	Tridione	Alternative therapy for absence seizures refractory to other drugs.
Additional Anticonvulsants		
acetazolamide	Diamox, Cetazolam, ✱ others	Carbonic anhydrase inhibitor used as adjunct therapy in partial and generalized seizures including absence and myoclonus.
felbamate	Felbatol	Adjunctive therapy for children with Lennox-Gastaut syndrome not responsive to other treatment; monotherapy for partial seizures refractory to other drugs. Reports of aplastic anemia severely limit its use.

TABLE 22-2

Anticonvulsant Drugs—cont'd

Generic Name	Brand Name	Comments
Additional Anticonvulsants—cont'd		
gabapentin	Neurontin	Adjunct therapy for partial seizures with or without generalization. Effective for treatment of some chronic pain syndromes.
lamotrigine	Lamictal	Monotherapy or adjunct therapy for partial seizures with or without secondary generalization, for myoclonus and for absence.
levetiracetam	Keppra	Adjunct therapy for partial seizures.
tiagabine	Gabitril	Adjunct therapy for partial seizures with or without generalization.
topiramate	Topamax	Adjunctive therapy for children with Lennox-Gastaut syndrome. Adjunct therapy for partial seizures with or without generalization.
vigabatrin	Sabril	Adjunct therapy for partial seizures.
zonisamide	Zonegran	Adjunctive therapy for partial seizures, absence seizures, infantile spasms, and Lennox-Gastaut syndrome.

Felbamate and lamotrigine are effective when given alone or as an adjunctive therapy for partial seizures with or without secondary generalization of seizures. They are also effective as adjunctive therapy in the treatment of partial and generalized seizures associated with the Lennox-Gastaut syndrome. This rare and severe seizure syndrome in children is characterized by frequent absence-like seizures and mental retardation.

Lamotrigine is also useful in absence and myoclonic epilepsy. It should be noted that felbamate is recommended only for the most severe and refractory patients because it is associated with a high incidence of aplastic anemia.

Gabapentin, levetiracetam, tiagabine, topiramate, vigabatrin, and zonisamide are effective as adjunctive therapies for partial seizures. Gabapentin is also used for various chronic pain syndromes and may be useful to treat bipolar depression. Topiramate and zonisamide are also effective in treating seizures in patients with Lennox-Gastaut syndrome. Zonisamide is also used for absence seizures and infantile spasm as is vigabatrin (see Chapter 21).

PHARMACOKINETICS

These anticonvulsants are rapidly absorbed after oral administration and the onset of action occurs in hours.

Felbamate has a half-life of 16 to 19 hours. The drug is excreted in urine unchanged (50%) or as metabolites. Gabapentin has a plasma half-life of 5 to 9 hours. Gabapentin is not biotransformed so a vast majority of the drug is excreted unchanged in urine. Consequently, dosages must be adjusted proportionally in patients with impaired renal function as determined if the creatinine clearance is less than 60 mL/min. Lamotrigine has a plasma half-life in adults of about 25 to 35 hours. Lamotrigine is extensively biotransformed by the liver and metabolites are excreted in urine. In contrast, approximately 65% to 70% of levetiracetam, topiramate, and vigabatrin are excreted unchanged. Zonisamide has the longest half-life of the newer agents at approximately 60 hours.

ADVERSE REACTIONS AND CONTRAINDICATIONS

Most of these drugs are well tolerated and have mild adverse effects including somnolence, dizziness, fatigue, ataxia, nausea, and, with some drugs, anorexia. Toxic adverse effects, however, have emerged to limit the use of felbamate. Aplastic anemia appears in an estimated 1 of 2000 patients who take felbamate for more than a few weeks. In addition, a few cases of acute liver failure have been reported for patients taking felbamate; therefore its use is contraindicated in patients with liver function abnormalities. Markers of liver function (ALT, AST, and bilirubin) should be monitored weekly for patients on felbamate.

Adverse reactions with lamotrigine also include headache, diplopia, blurred vision, rash, and, rarely, the emergence of Stevens-Johnson syndrome. Vigabatrin use is also associated with amnesia and ophthalmic abnormalities. Gabapentin, levetiracetam, topiramate, and vigabatrin should be used with caution in patients with renal insufficiency, and dosages should be adjusted as needed.

INTERACTIONS

Felbamate decreases the plasma level of carbamazepine, but it also increases phenytoin and valproic acid levels.

Carbamazepine and valproic acid both decrease plasma levels of felbamate. No significant drug interactions have been described with the use of gabapentin. Valproic acid significantly retards the biotransformation of lamotrigine raising the lamotrigine level and decreasing the valproic acid level. Lamotrigine used concurrently with carbamazepine may result in decreased levels of lamotrigine and increased levels of an active metabolite of carbamazepine. Valproate and topiramate mutually lower serum concentrations by 10% when given concurrently. The patient taking anticonvulsants that induce the liver biotransformation enzymes (e.g., barbiturates, carbamazepine, and phenytoin) may require a higher dosage of tiagabine, lamotrigine, or topiramate to offset their increased biotransformation.

APPLICATION TO PRACTICE

ASSESSMENT
History of Present Illness

Obtain information regarding events before, during, and after a seizure. This data should be obtained from the patient when possible, however, because alterations in consciousness often accompany seizures. Information about patient activities may be obtained from family or friends. Establish a trend in the patient's behavior before the seizure as well as during and after. Ask about the course and duration of the seizure activity. Where in the body did the seizures begin? Do the seizures travel throughout the body? Does the muscle tone seem tense or limp? Were color changes noted in the face or lips? Was there a loss of consciousness? Did the patient experience an aura before the seizure? Were there precipitating events? After the seizure, does the patient sleep or have any confusion, weakness, headache, or muscle aches? How have the seizures affected the patient's life and ability to perform activities of daily living?

Health History

The patient's health history provides information about previous seizure activity, prior anticonvulsant drug therapy, allergies, injuries, previous illnesses, and hospitalizations. Details about prenatal, birth, and developmental history, family history, and history of previous trauma are necessary. Conditions to be noted in adults include syncope (e.g., cardiac, vasovagal, or reflex) as well as narcolepsy, sleep apnea, and pseudoseizures. In children, note vertigo and periodic syndromes (including childhood migraine headaches), hyperventilation or breath holding, staring spells, and daydreaming. A

drug history is important to obtain because many drugs interact with anticonvulsants.

Lifespan Considerations

Perinatal. Many factors must be considered in the treatment of epilepsy in women. This is particularly true for women of childbearing age, when hormones, contraception, fertility, pregnancy, and sexuality may influence epilepsy. Hormones can affect the seizure threshold and seizure frequency, intensity, and duration by altering the excitability of the neurons. Fertility may be adversely affected, as well as the effectiveness of oral contraceptives.

Although most women receiving anticonvulsants bear normal children, approximately two to three times the average number of birth defects occur in children born to mothers (and sometimes fathers) who take anticonvulsant drugs. Because of the risk to women, particularly during pregnancy, anticonvulsant therapy requires careful planning, monitoring, and special interventions to safeguard both the mother and the infant. Breast-feeding is not recommended during drug therapy because anticonvulsants are excreted in breast milk.

Pediatric. The diagnosis and treatment of epilepsy in infancy, childhood, and adolescence is complicated because of the cause of the condition, the age of the child, and the need for family involvement. Most children with epilepsy can lead normal, active lives. However, for some, their seizure disorder can be disabling and can lead to social, emotional, and academic problems. When this occurs, children need additional resources from their family, school, and community.

Older Adults. The treatment of seizure disorders in older adults is complex. Older adults may have diseases and conditions that increase their vulnerability to seizures. They are susceptible to organ failure, metabolic disturbance, infection, CNS lesions, falls, trauma, alcohol withdrawal, and the adverse effects of polypharmacy. Management with anticonvulsant drugs takes special assessment, intervention, and evaluation skills, as well as an understanding of the health needs of the older adult.

Cultural/Social Considerations

There are numerous cultural and social considerations related to epilepsy. Of major concern are the negative attitudes and stigma associated with the disorder. The fear of having a seizure affects the patient's lifestyle and may affect the social, academic, or vocational aspects as well. For parents, family, or friends, seeing their loved one have a seizure is a frightening experience. The patient may have feelings of guilt, anger, isolation, and frustration. Of greatest consequence is the patient's sense of loss and grief associated with the vulnerability of having a potentially life-long disability. Epilepsy can influence the patient's self-esteem and self-confidence and therefore have an impact on decisions regarding education, driving a car, participating in sports, and childrearing. To obtain a driver's license, most states require that the patient be seizure free for a defined period.

Physical Examination

Seizures are classified by clinical symptoms and electrophysiologic data. The clinical symptoms observed during the seizure and functional deficits found at physical examination, such as weakness, sensory and thought process disturbances, and reflex alteration are essential to the classification of seizures. The examination should include evaluation of cranial nerves, muscle strength, cerebellar function, sensory system, deep tendon reflexes (DTRs), and level of consciousness.

Laboratory Testing

The diagnosis of a seizure disorder is based on data collected from careful patient observation, comprehensive health history, and clinical examination. EEG, routine skull radiographs, magnetic resonance imaging (MRI), and computed tomography (CT) scans may reveal neurologic abnormalities or structural lesions and are of value in localizing the pathologic processes associated with epilepsy.

Serum drug levels of hydantoins, valproates, iminostilbenes, and succinimides should be measured routinely throughout therapy to monitor therapeutic blood level, to verify compliance with therapy, and to manage combinations of anticonvulsant drugs that may inter-

act. Complete blood cell (CBC) counts, serum calcium levels, and liver function tests should be done periodically throughout the course of hydantoin therapy. All patients taking succinimides should have a CBC count with differential and liver enzyme test on a regular basis throughout therapy. Liver function should be monitored weekly during felbamate therapy. Patients receiving valproate therapy require baseline and periodic monitoring of liver function, prothrombin time (PT) and INR values, and platelet counts. A baseline urinalysis, BUN, liver function test, CBC, platelet and reticulocyte counts, and serum iron levels are typically ordered for patients taking carbamazepine. Oxcarbazepine therapy may require monitoring of serum sodium level.

GOALS OF THERAPY

The treatment objectives for epilepsy are to prevent seizures (or at least reduce the number of seizures and their severity as much as possible), to assist the individual in maintaining the highest level of independent functioning achievable, and to minimize the occurrence of adverse effects.

Although anticonvulsant drugs may control seizures, they do not cure the underlying disorder. In cases where epilepsy is ruled out as the cause of seizures, the condition that lowers the seizure threshold or precipitates a seizure (e.g., hypoglycemia, electrolyte imbalances, fever, exposure to toxins, and drug overdoses or withdrawal) must be controlled in addition to treating the seizures themselves. It is important to identify the cause of the seizures as early as possible because this may influence the choice of drug and the duration of therapy.

Drug treatment typically begins with one anticonvulsant drug; the dosage is increased gradually until seizures are controlled, clinical manifestations of toxicity are experienced, or serum drug levels reach the high end of the therapeutic range without controlling the seizures. In most cases, a single drug can control seizures. In cases where this is not true, other anticonvulsant drugs may be tried—each alone—before attempting multidrug therapy. Combining drugs does not appear to be as effective as monotherapy because drug interactions decrease effectiveness and increase the risk for adverse effects (Table 22-3).

Arriving at an appropriate dosage of the anticonvulsant drug involves trial and error, because drug absorption and elimination vary widely from one patient to another. In determining what dosage is appropriate, therapy is started at low levels (often one fourth to one third of the recommended therapeutic dosage) of a single drug and then slowly increased or decreased to achieve the desired effect (see the Case Study: Epilepsy).

TABLE 22-3

Primary Drugs of Choice for Different Types of Seizures

Seizure Type	Conventional Drugs of Choice	Newer Effective Drugs	Adjunct Drugs
Partial (simple and complex)	carbamazepine, phenytoin, valproate	lamotrigine, topiramate	felbamate, gabapentin, levetiracetam, tiagabine, vigabatrin, zonisamide
Partial with secondary generalized tonic-clonic	carbamazepine, phenobarbital, phenytoin, primidone, valproate	lamotrigine, topiramate	gabapentin, levetiracetam, tiagabine, zonisamide
Absence (generalized)	ethosuximide, valproate	clonazepam, lamotrigine	zonisamide
Generalized tonic-clonic	carbamazepine, phenobarbital, phenytoin, primidone, valproate	lamotrigine, topiramate	gabapentin
Myoclonic, atonic	valproate	clonazepam, lamotrigine	topiramate
Status epilepticus	diazepam, lorazepam, phenytoin	fosphenytoin	phenobarbital

INTERVENTION
Administration

Orally administered anticonvulsant drugs should be taken regularly as prescribed, at the same time of the day, and with meals to decrease the risk of GI upset. Oral suspensions should be shaken before measuring the dose. If this is not done, a subtherapeutic dose will be obtained from the top of the bottle and a supertherapeutic dose from the bottom of the bottle. Extended-release formulations of some anticonvulsants are available for once-daily dosing.

Anticonvulsant drugs administered parenterally should be given with caution. ECG and vital sign monitoring (including blood pressure and respirations) are required to reduce the risk of cardiorespiratory complications of treatment.

Chewable phenytoin tablets and phenytoin sodium capsules are not bioequivalent and thus are not interchangeable. Extended-release preparations may be used for once-daily dosing. Capsules labeled "prompt-release" may result in toxic serum concentrations if they are used for once-daily dosing. Abrupt discontinuation of hydantoins after long-term use may precipitate seizure activity.

Phenytoin may be administered intravenously as a bolus or a continuous infusion, but should not be given intramuscularly or subcutaneously because it causes irritation and precipitates in the tissues. An intravenous bolus should be administered at a slow rate.

Intravenous clonazepam solution should be mixed in a glass bottle because the drug binds to plastic. It may be administered slowly by direct injection or by slow in-travenous infusion. Divalproex is administered intravenously only when the patient is unable to take the drug orally.

Intravenous phenobarbital is reserved for emergency treatment. Administer slowly while closely monitoring the respiratory status and with resuscitation equipment available. Do not exceed the manufacturer's recommended administration rate.

For patients on enteral feedings, 2 hours should elapse between the feeding and drug administration. If phenytoin or carbamazepine is given via a nasogastric tube, the dose should be mixed with an equal volume of water and the tube flushed with 100 ml of water after administering the dose.

Monitor the patient for adverse reactions and signs of toxicity during drug therapy. Monitor appropriate laboratory values and inform the health care provider of the results. Monitor serum glucose levels closely in diabetic patients receiving hydantoin therapy. As with many anticonvulsants, the serum concentration of phenytoin correlates well with therapy and toxicity. Consequently, therapeutic drug monitoring is a useful tool to control the seizure disorder.

Seizure Precautions. The risk of injury for the seizure-prone patient is minimized by keeping all four siderails up and by accompanying the patient during ambulation. A bed alarm may be necessary to alert hospital personnel if the patient attempts to ambulate without calling for assistance.

Should the patient have a seizure, agency protocol should be followed and the patient should be protected from further injury by placing him or her in a left-sided lying position, loosening or removing restrictive clothing, and protecting the head. The patient should not be left alone during a seizure. A call for assistance, emergency anticonvulsant drug therapy, oral suctioning, and CPR may be necessary. Documentation after a seizure should include the type and duration of the seizure, the patient's level of consciousness, and the patient's actions and behaviors before, during, and after the seizure.

Education

Development of a treatment plan that prevents or arrests the seizures requires weeks of drug trial, error, and adjustment. Anticonvulsant drugs require time to take effect and to attain an acceptable level in the blood. During this time the patient must be compliant. The patient and family should be counseled regarding the importance of continuing drug therapy even when there has been an extended seizure-free period. Observation of the effects of the drug and documentation of any seizure activity are essential. Once the seizure disorder is controlled with anticonvulsant drugs, major risk factors are noncompliance, lack of medical supervision, and discontinuation of the drug.

The patient should be taught to take the anticonvulsant drug with food to minimize gastric distress. A missed dose of anticonvulsant should be taken as soon as remembered, unless it is close to the time for the next dose. In this case, the missed dose should be omitted. Teach the patient that enteric-coated tablets should be swallowed whole. Oral suspensions should be shaken well before pouring. Sprinkle capsules may be swallowed whole or opened and the contents sprinkled on a teaspoonful of soft food that should then be swallowed immediately without chewing. The patient should be advised to consult the health care provider before taking any OTC drugs.

No drug used to treat epilepsy is without adverse effects; thus a high rate of noncompliance is often seen. Teach the patient taking these drugs about their adverse effects, including neurologic symptoms, GI disturbances, visual disturbances, blood dyscrasias, and hepatic and renal impairment. Reinforcement of the risk/benefit ratio is essential to ensure that the patient understands and accepts the importance of compliance with the treatment plan.

Teach the family how to care for the member who is at risk for a seizure. It is important that the family understand precautions needed before a seizure to prevent serious injury and appropriate measures to take during a seizure.

Driving and other hazardous activities that require mental alertness should be avoided until the drug's CNS effects are known. Alcoholic beverages should be avoided. The patient should be advised not to abruptly discontinue drug therapy because this may precipitate seizures.

It is essential that the patient report adverse reactions to the health care provider. Anorexia may be suggestive of excessive blood levels, and malaise, fever, or lethargy may precede hepatotoxicity. In some cases, a rash may be a sign of a life-threatening allergic reaction warranting immediate cessation of drug therapy. Further, the patient should immediately report fever, sore throat, mouth ulcers, easy bruising, bleeding, back or abdominal pain, facial edema, or vomiting. The appearance of these reactions may necessitate a change in therapy or discontinuation of the drug.

Teach the patient with diabetes mellitus who is receiving hydantoin therapy to monitor blood glucose levels closely because these drugs may cause hyperglycemia. Caution the patient taking phenytoin that his or her urine may turn pink, red, or reddish brown. Also inform the patient about the need for good oral hygiene and the need for regular dental examinations because gingival hyperplasia may occur as an adverse reaction to phenytoin.

Advise women of childbearing age that contraceptives are recommended during anticonvulsant drug therapy. It is important for the woman who becomes pregnant or who is considering pregnancy to discuss anticonvulsant drug therapy with her health care provider. Additionally, women taking oral contraceptives should be advised to use a second form of birth control as well, because the effectiveness of the contraceptive is decreased.

The patient also needs to understand the following factors and precautions necessary to drug therapy.

- The nature of epilepsy
- How epilepsy affects the patient's life and the lives of family members and friends
- The care required during a seizure
- The importance of keeping a journal of all seizure activity
- What constitutes an adequate diet, fluid intake, sleep, and moderate recreation and exercise
- The importance of avoiding alcoholic beverages and illicit substances
- The significance of wearing a medical alert bracelet and identification with pertinent information
- Where to obtain legal information regarding protection of employment
- The availability of resources such as the Epilepsy Foundation of America

The duration of treatment with anticonvulsants is influenced by several considerations, including the probability of the patient remaining seizure free without drugs, the adverse consequences of recurrent seizures, and the adverse effects of long-term anticonvulsant drug therapy. In some cases the patient with epilepsy may have therapy discontinued. There are a number of factors to consider in this regard. It is recommended that the patient be seizure free for at least 4 years. The decision to discontinue drug therapy is made with careful consideration of the patient's desire and motivation, along with the likelihood of success and the risks associated with the recurrence of a seizure (including the possible loss of driver's license). Patients should be advised not to drive during the withdrawal period and for 3 to 4 months thereafter. This restriction makes it difficult for some patients to try withdrawal.

Before withdrawal from anticonvulsant therapy, patients should be informed that about 33% of those at low risk (for seizures) experience relapse. The longer the patient remains seizure free, the less likely seizures are to recur. Recurrence of seizures usually happens within the first 6 months after the drug is discontinued. Patients at low risk for recurrence include those with primary epilepsy, seizure onset between the ages of 2 and 35 years, and those with a normal EEG.

Patients at high risk have a 50% chance of recurrence. High-risk patients include those who have partial complex seizures and seizures with an identifiable lesion. Patients with a history of frequent seizures or status epilepticus, multiple seizure types, persistently abnormal EEG, and the development of altered cognition are poor candidates for drug withdrawal.

When the decision to withdraw therapy is made, the patient should be taught that the drugs will be withdrawn one at a time, withdrawing the least effective or most toxic drug first. The dosage will be decreased slowly over 3 to 6 months until the drug is completely withdrawn. Sufficient time is required so that a new steady state is reached before continuing with dosage reductions. If the patient remains seizure free for 1 month, the second drug can be discontinued in the same manner, and so on. If seizures recur, therapy will be restarted using the last drug withdrawn.

EVALUATION

The goal of successful anticonvulsant therapy is to prevent seizures or at least to reduce their frequency and severity

---

CASE STUDY    *Epilepsy*

ASSESSMENT

HISTORY OF PRESENT ILLNESS

PS is a 29-year-old woman who underwent emergency surgery, during which she showed marked and sudden changes in neurologic function and experienced seizures. She was found to have a basal ganglion hematoma with an infarction.

HEALTH HISTORY

PS has no significant health history and no history of seizures. She has a 2-month-old infant. Her pregnancy and delivery were uncomplicated. PS found the past 2 months physically and emotionally stressful.

LIFESPAN CONSIDERATIONS

PS has special concerns that are associated with childbearing and childrearing.

CULTURAL/SOCIAL CONSIDERATIONS

The fear of seizures may affect PS's confidence and self-image. This could raise questions about intimacy, sexual activity, and parenting. A plan for child care may necessitate additional support and safety measures. Breast-feeding is not appropriate while she is taking anticonvulsant drugs because the drugs enter the breast milk.

PHYSICAL EXAMINATION

PS experienced generalized seizures of the tonic-clonic type. During the physical examination, signs of localized brain abnormalities were detected. A comprehensive neurologic examination was conducted.

LABORATORY TESTING

EEG revealed altered electrophysiologic activity of the brain and abnormal waveforms.

PATIENT PROBLEM(S)

The patient has tonic-clonic seizures and is a new mother caring for a 2-month-old infant.

GOALS OF THERAPY

Provide maximum control of seizures with minimal adverse effects.

CRITICAL THINKING QUESTIONS

1. The health care provider orders a 20 mg/kg loading dose of phenytoin to be followed by 300 mg daily. What is the mechanism of action of this drug?
2. What adverse effects should the nurse look for during phenytoin therapy?
3. Why has PS been advised not to breast-feed during phenytoin therapy?
4. What purpose will be served by monitoring PS's serum blood level of phenytoin during therapy?

as much as possible. Accurate diagnosis of the seizure type, drug administration and compliance, and helping the patient deal with any adverse effects of the drug are essential to achieving this goal. The influence of epilepsy on the patient's lifestyle and well-being is an important component in the care and support of the patient and his or her family and is essential for treatment success.

Bibliography

Anderson G, Miller J: The newer antiepileptic drugs: their collective role and defining characteristics, *Formulary* 36(2):114-135, 2001.

Calli J, Farrington E: Vigabatrin, *Pediatr Nurs* 24(4):357-361, 1998.

Crawford P, Nicholson C: Epilepsy management, *Prof Nurse* 14(8):565-569, 1999.

Crowder K: An algorithm for monitoring phenytoin therapy, *J Am Acad Nurse Pract* 12(8):317-321, 2000.

Faught E: Epidemiology and drug treatment of epilepsy in elderly people, *Drugs Aging* 15(4):255-269, 1999.

Garrard J, Cloyd J, Gross C, et al: Factors associated with antiepileptic drug use among elderly nursing home residents, *J Gerontol* 55(7):384-392, 2000.

Gilbert K: An algorithm for diagnosis and treatment of status epilepticus in adults, *J Neurosci Nurs* 31(1):27-29, 34-36, 1999.

Hutt N: Fosphenytoin for seizure control, *Am J Nurs* 99(3):52-53, 1999.

Kopec K: New anticonvulsants for use in pediatric patients (part I), *J Pediatr Health Care* (?):81-86; quiz 87-88, 2001.

Kwan I, Ridsdale L, Robins D: An epilepsy care package: the nurse specialist's role, *J Neurosci Nurs* 32(3):145-152, 2000.

New Drugs of 2000. *J Am Pharm Assoc* 41(2):229-272, 2001.

Rumbach L, Sablot D, Berger E, et al: Status epilepticus in stroke: report on a hospital-based stroke cohort, *Neurol* 54(2)350-354, 2000.

Sagraves R: Febrile seizures—treatment and prevention or not? *J Pediatr Health Care* 13(2):79-83; quiz 84-85, 1999.

Schlicher ML: Dilantin jeopardy: avoiding the dangers of phenytoin, *Med Surg Nurs* 7(6):343-347, 356, 1998.

Shafer PO: Epilepsy and seizures: advances in seizure assessment, treatment, and self-management, *Nurs Clin North Am* 34(3):743-759, 1999.

Shafer PO: New therapies in the management of acute or cluster seizures and seizure emergencies, *J Neurosci Nurs* 31(4): 224-230, 1999.

Stephen L, Brodie M: Epilepsy in elderly people, *Lancet* 355(9213):1441-1446, 2000.

Valente MB, Valente SM: Pediatric epilepsy: primary care treatment and health care management, *Nurse Pract* 23(11):38, 43-44, 47, 1998.

Winkelman C: A review of pharmacodynamics and pharmacokinetics in seizure management, *J Neurosci Nurs* 31(1):50-53, 1999.

Internet Resources

Epilepsy Foundation website with links to other resources. Available online at http://www.efa.org/index.cfm.

National Institute for Neurologic Disease and Stroke website with information sheets. Available online at http://www.ninds.nih.gov/health_and_medical/disorders/epilepsy.htm.

National Library of Medicine: Medline site for health information on epilepsy. Available online at http://www.nlm.nih.gov/medlineplus/epilepsy.html.

Pharmacology 2000: Epileptic drugs. Available online at http://www.pharmacology2000.com/learning2.htm#specialtopics.

Drugs to Treat Movement Disorders, Myasthenia Gravis, and Alzheimer's Disease

MICHAEL R. VASKO • SUSAN SCIACCA

 Visit http://evolve.elsevier.com/Gutierrez/ for additional information.

KEY TERMS

Akinesias, p. 350

Alzheimer's disease, p. 369

Bradykinesia, p. 350

Dyskinesias, p. 350

Huntington's disease, p. 350

Micrographia, p. 350

Myasthenia gravis, p. 362

Parkinson's disease, p. 350

Rigidity, p. 350

Tremor, p. 350

OBJECTIVES

- List three classic symptoms of Parkinson's disease, and explain the role of acetylcholine and dopamine in this disease.

- Explain the use of edrophonium in the diagnosis of myasthenia gravis.

- Describe the rationale for administering drugs to patients with Alzheimer's disease.

- Describe the most common adverse effects of the drugs used to treat Parkinson's disease, myasthenia gravis, and Alzheimer's disease.

- Identify patient outcomes that indicate successful drug therapy in the treatment of Parkinson's disease, myasthenia gravis, and Alzheimer's disease.

- Develop a nursing care plan for patients receiving anticholinergic drugs, drugs that replace dopamine, or drugs that mimic dopamine actions to treat Parkinson's disease.

- Develop a nursing care plan, including a teaching plan, for a patient receiving drug therapy to treat myasthenia gravis and Alzheimer's disease.

Movement disorders are caused by functional disturbances in one of a number of nuclei in the basal ganglia, which includes the striatum, globus pallidus, subthalamic nuclei, and the substantia nigra. These nuclei and their afferent and efferent pathways make up the extrapyramidal motor system, which controls fine and coordinated movement. In these regions of the brain, lesions or an imbalance of neurotransmitters can result in disorders of excessive movement called **dyskinesias** or disorders of diminished movement termed **akinesias**. The major dyskinetic disorders include Huntington's disease, dystonia, ballismus, and Tourette's syndrome; the major disorder characterized by lack of movement is Parkinson's disease. **Huntington's disease** is a progressive disorder that is inherited in an autosomal dominant manner. Symptoms of the disease

begin to manifest when subjects carrying the Huntington's gene are 30 to 50 years old. There are three major symptoms: excessive choreoathetotic movement, progressive dementia, and behavioral changes including depression, apathy, and irritability. To date there are no effective therapies to treat the disease except for potent antipsychotic drugs, especially haloperidol, which attempts to diminish movement (see Chapter 19).

Tourette's syndrome is characterized by uncontrolled and intermittent motor or vocal tics, including touching, hitting, jumping, swearing, sputtering, grunting, or screaming. Again, the only effective therapy to reduce these tics is the use of the potent antipsychotics. Ballism is an uncontrolled jerking of extremities, and these patients may benefit from antipsychotic drugs to reduce the incidence of movement.

PATHOPHYSIOLOGY • Parkinson's Disease

Parkinson's disease is a progressive neurologic disease that results from the degeneration of neurons involved in motor control and is characterized by tremor, rigidity, and bradykinesia (slowness of movement). This disorder most commonly appears in people more than 50 years old and it progresses over decades. Approximately 500,000 Americans have Parkinson's disease. The lifetime risk of developing Parkinson's disease is estimated to be 1% to 2%. The rate of progression of the disease is variable.

Tremor is usually the first symptom to appear in this disease, and it is an asymmetric, purposeless, regular, and rhythmic movement. The resting tremor of eight to ten cycles per second disappears with voluntary movement and reappears when the limb is at rest. A movement of the thumb against the fingers is also seen. This pill-rolling tremor occurs at four to six cycles per second and may begin asymmetrically. It becomes bilateral as the disease progresses.

Rigidity is a state of involuntary contraction of all skeletal muscles. It is observed as the disease worsens, impeding active and passive movement. It is present during the entire arc of movement of a joint. Cogwheel rigidity is a jerky, ratcheting movement demonstrated during passive motion, usually at the wrist or elbow.

Bradykinesia is a general slowness characterized by difficulty initiating movement and an inability to perform rapid repetitive movements. It is one of the cardinal symptoms of Parkinson's disease and probably the most crippling of all symptoms. The severity of bradykinesia may fluctuate markedly throughout the day. *Hypokinesia* is an abnormally diminished motor response to a stimulus. It is seen in patients with Parkinson's disease when

they sit or lie down for long periods without an accompanying shift in weight. There is a decreased tendency to cross the legs when sitting, to gesture with the hands when talking, or to swing the arms when walking.

The combination of rigidity and bradykinesia results in a number of characteristic signs. Masked facies (loss of facial expression), decreased frequency of blinking, fixed flexion of the trunk, neck, and extremities, a slow and hesitant gait, and postural instability are seen. **Micrographia** (handwriting that gets progressively smaller), dysarthria, dysphagia, and general poverty of movement are also noted.

Parkinson's disease is currently understood to be caused by a loss of dopamine neurons that project from the pars compacta of the substantia nigra to the striatum (Figure 23-1). This degeneration results in a deficiency in the neurotransmitter dopamine. Under normal conditions, dopamine is believed to exert an inhibitory influence on cholinergic neurons in the striatum. When dopamine is lacking, muscle tone increases because of the unopposed action of acetylcholine, resulting in muscular rigidity, inhibition of spontaneous movements, and tremor. Why the dopamine neurons degenerate remains unknown, but it may result from genetic predisposition, environmental toxins, oxidative stress, infection, or other as yet unknown processes. It should be noted that a number of other neurotransmitters are involved in regulating movement, including GABA and glutamate. Thus it is likely that Parkinson's disease involves an imbalance of a number of neuronal systems. Because the therapies for Parkinson's disease involve manipulations of either cholinergic or dopaminergic transmission (Table 23-1),

TABLE 23-1

Drugs to Treat Parkinsonism

Generic Name	Brand Name	Comments
Anticholinergic Drugs		
benztropine	Apo-Benztropine, ✽ Cogentin	To treat Parkinson's disease and drug-induced extrapyramidal reactions. Particularly effective in reversing acute dystonic reaction to antipsychotic drugs.
biperiden	Akineton	To treat Parkinson's disease and drug-induced extrapyramidal reactions.
diphenhydramine	Benadryl	To treat Parkinson's disease and drug-induced extrapyramidal reactions. Antihistamine with anticholinergic actions. Marked sedative effects.
ethopropazine	Parsidol, Parsitan ✽	To treat Parkinson's disease. Phenothiazine with only anticholinergic effects and devoid of antidopaminergic effects.
procyclidine	Kemadrin, PMS-Procyclidin, Procyclid ✽	To treat Parkinson's disease and drug-induced extrapyramidal reactions.
trihexyphenidyl	Apo-Trihex, ✽ Artane PMS, Trihexyphenidyl ✽	To treat Parkinson's disease and drug-induced extrapyramidal reactions.
Drugs Affecting Dopaminergic Transmission		
amantadine	Symadine, Symmetrel	Antiviral drug that augments release of dopamine and blocks reuptake.
bromocriptine	Alti-Bromocriptine, ✽ Apo-Bromocriptine, ✽ Parlodel	Ergot dopamine D_2 receptor agonist. May be added to levodopa or levodopa-carbidopa therapy. Can be used alone to replace levodopa therapy.
levodopa-carbidopa	Sinemet	Carbidopa inhibits degradation of dopamine outside the CNS. Levodopa-carbidopa ratio is 10:1.
entacapone	Comtan	Adjunct therapy that inhibits degradation of dopamine by inhibiting catechol-O-methyltransferase.
levodopa	Dopar, Larodopa	Levodopa is chemical precursor of dopamine.
pergolide	Permax	Ergot dopamine D_2 receptor agonist. May be added to levodopa or levodopa-carbidopa therapy. Can be used alone to replace levodopa therapy.
pramipexole	Mirapex	Dopamine receptor agonist to treat early Parkinson's disease or to add to therapy in advanced stages.
ropinirole	Requip	Dopamine receptor agonist to treat early Parkinson's disease or to add to therapy in advanced stages.
selegiline	Carbex, Eldepryl, Novo-Selegiline ✽	Adjunct therapy that inhibits degradation of dopamine by inhibiting monoamine oxidase B. No significant interaction with foods containing tyramine.
tolcapone	Tasmar	Adjunct therapy that inhibits degradation of dopamine by inhibiting catechol-O-methyltransferase. Can produce hepatotoxicity; not often used.

✽ Available only in Canada.

NORMAL PARKINSON'S DISEASE

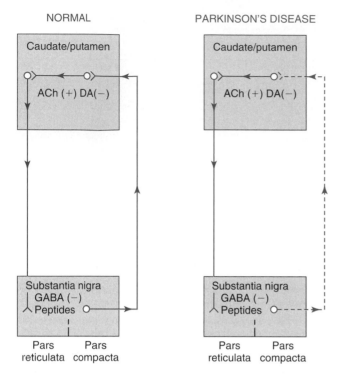

FIGURE 23-1 Schematic representation of a simple neurochemical model of Parkinson's disease (see text for details): *ACh,* acetylcholine; *DA,* dopamine; *GABA,* gamma aminobutyric acid. The dotted line indicates a loss of the projecting neurons. (From Clark WG, Brater DC, Johnson AR: *Goth's medical pharmacology,* ed 13, St Louis, 1988, Mosby.)

TABLE 23-2	
Drugs Known to Cause Parkinsonism	
Generic Name	*Brand Name*
Antiemetics	
metoclopramide	Reglan
prochlorperazine	Compazine
trimethobenzamide	Tigan
Antihypertensives	
diazoxide	Hyperstat
methyldopa	Aldomet
reserpine	Novo-Reserpine
Antipsychotics	
chlorpromazine	Thorazine
chlorprothixene	Taractan
fluphenazine	Prolixin
haloperidol	Haldol
loxapine	Loxitane
molindone	Moban
perphenazine	Trilafon
pimozide	Orap
prochlorperazine	Compazine
promazine	Sparine
risperidone	Risperdal
thiothixene	Navane
trifluoperazine	Stelazine
triflupromazine	Vesprin
ziprasidone	Geodon

we focus on these two neurotransmitters as critical for the symptoms of the disease.

In addition to Parkinson's disease (which is an idiopathic condition), infection, tumor, trauma, and a variety of drugs can produce parkinsonian symptoms (Table 23-2). Acute parkinsonism is observed in drug abusers exposed to *N*-methyl-4-phenyl-1,2,3,6-tetrahydropyridine (MPTP). Poisoning with manganese, carbon monoxide, mercury, methanol, or cyanide also produces clinical abnormalities similar to those of Parkinson's disease. Reserpine, which depletes neuronal stores of dopamine and norepinephrine, and antipsychotic drugs, which block dopamine receptors, are the usual causes of drug-induced parkinsonism. These symptoms depend on the presence of the drug, so lowering the dosage or discontinuing the drug eliminates the symptoms. Parkinsonian symptoms have been seen in patients who attempted suicide by drug overdose, during which there was a presumed hypoxic/ischemic injury from respiratory depression and hypotension. In addition, repeated head trauma may result in parkinsonian symptoms.

Other movement disorders include dystonia, essential tremor, and tardive dyskinesia. The anticholinergic drugs described below are useful for treating dystonia, whereas beta blockers (see Chapter 12) and benzodiazepines (see Chapter 17) are used to diminish essential tremor. There is no effective drug therapy for tardive dyskinesia. It is important to note that the treatment of any movement disorder involves providing symptomatic relief of the diminished or excessive movement, but does not cure the disease nor slow its progression.

DRUG CLASS • Anticholinergic Drugs

benztropine (Cogentin, Apo-Benztropine,✲
    PMS-Benztropine✲)

biperiden (Akineton)

diphenhydramine (Benadryl)

ethopropazine (Parsidol)

procyclidine (Kemadrin, Procyclid,✲ PMS-
    Procyclidine✲)

trihexyphenidyl (Artane, Apo-Trihex✲)

MECHANISM OF ACTION

Anticholinergic drugs act by competitively inhibiting the action of acetylcholine at muscarinic receptors (see Chapter 11). These receptors are found in smooth muscle, cardiac muscle, and parasympathetically innervated glands, as well as in the brain. This mechanism presumably restores the cholinergic-dopaminergic balance in the striatum.

USES

Anticholinergics are useful early in the course of Parkinson's disease more to control tremor than to treat the other manifestations of the disease. They are a reasonable treatment choice in middle-aged patients who have tremor but little rigidity or bradykinesia. Anticholinergic drugs also are useful in controlling salivation and drooling. For many years, atropine and scopolamine were used to treat symptoms of Parkinson's disease, but they have been replaced with newer, synthetic drugs that produce fewer peripheral adverse effects. The antihistamine diphenhydramine, is also used in the treatment of Parkinson's disease presumably because of its anticholinergic properties. These drugs also are used as an adjunct to levodopa-carbidopa therapy (see below).

Anticholinergics also are the drugs of choice for treatment of extrapyramidal reactions (akathisia, acute dystonia, and parkinsonism) caused by antipsychotic drugs. Anticholinergic drugs do not reverse tardive dyskinesia. These extrapyramidal reactions are described in Chapter 19. The adverse effects of anticholinergics have limited their usefulness and are particularly problematic in older adults. Additional uses of anticholinergic drugs as well as adverse effects are discussed in detail in Chapter 11.

PHARMACOKINETICS

Anticholinergic drugs are well absorbed when taken orally. The dosage is started low and increased gradually until the symptoms decrease or the adverse effects become prominent. When the drug is discontinued, the dosage should be tapered off to lessen a rebound appearance of the parkinsonian symptoms. Benztropin, biperiden, and diphenhydramine may be administered orally, intravenously, or intramuscularly. These drugs are active within a few minutes of injection. When administered orally, benztropine has an onset of action of 1 to 2 hours. The duration of action is about 24 hours.

Ethopropazine and procyclidine given orally have an onset of action within about 30 minutes and a duration of action of about 4 hours, whereas trihexyphenidyl has an onset of action of 1 hour and a duration of action of 6 to 12 hours. For patients stabilized with the drug, an extended-release capsule formulation (Artane Sequels) is available for twice-daily administration.

ADVERSE REACTIONS AND CONTRAINDICATIONS

Common adverse effects of anticholinergic drugs are dry mouth, constipation, urinary retention, and blurred vision. Common mental effects include impairment of recent memory, confusion, insomnia, and restlessness. Mental effects can become serious with the development of agitation, disorientation, delirium, paranoid reactions, or hallucinations. Such problems are more common with the older adult who has a preexisting mental disturbance. Cardiovascular effects include tachycardia and palpitations. Patients who have glaucoma, particularly narrow-angle glaucoma, men with prostatic hypertrophy, patients with another type of urinary or intestinal obstruction, or those with tachycardia are not good candidates for anticholinergic drug therapy.

INTERACTIONS

The anticholinergic drugs increase the sedative effect of alcohol and other CNS depressants. Additive anticholinergic effects may be noted with drugs that share anticholinergic properties, such as antihistamines, quinidine, disopyramide, and tricyclic antidepressants. Antacids and antidiarrheals decrease the absorption of anticholinergic drugs. The concurrent use of an anticholinergic drug and amantadine increases the incidence of the anticholinergic adverse effects. The effects disappear when the dosage of the anticholinergic drug is reduced.

When anticholinergic drugs are combined with levodopa, gastric motility may decrease, increasing the deactivation of levodopa and reducing intestinal absorption. A reduction in the efficacy of levodopa may thus be noted. Therapeutic effects of phenothiazines also may be diminished with concurrent use of anticholinergic drugs.

![banner] **DRUG CLASS** • Dopaminergic Drugs

levodopa (L-dopa) (Dopar, Larodopa)
levodopa-carbidopa (Sinemet)

MECHANISM OF ACTION

Levodopa is the chemical precursor of dopamine. Dopamine is unable to cross the blood-brain barrier, but levodopa crosses into the CNS and is converted to dopamine by the enzyme dopa decarboxylase (L-amino acid decarboxylase). Consequently, the administration of levodopa is a direct way of augmenting the amount of dopamine available in the brain (Figure 23-2). A majority (90% to 95%) of levodopa is converted to dopamine in the periphery. Carbidopa is a dopa decarboxylase inhibitor that does not enter the CNS. When administered with levodopa, it prevents the amino acid from being converted to dopamine in the periphery but does not prevent its conversion in the brain. Thus carbidopa reduces the required dose of levodopa by 75%. Because the gastrointestinal (GI) effects of levodopa reflect peripheral dopamine concentrations, the incidence of nausea and vomiting is reduced greatly with a levodopa-carbidopa combination.

USES

The combination of carbidopa and levodopa is the treatment of choice for moderate to severe cases of Parkinson's disease. Levodopa is rarely administered without the decarboxylase inhibitor carbidopa for reasons noted in the previous paragraph. Levodopa reduces tremors, rigidity, and bradykinesis. Although the patient's mood is often elevated, it is not an effect of levodopa; rather, it usually results from improvement of mobility. Levodopa therapy does not stop the progression of Parkinson's disease, but it relieves the symptoms and dramatically improves the ability to function. This relief, however, is limited in that levodopa loses its effectiveness after years of use, likely because of the progression of the disease. Levodopa-carbidopa is also recommended for the management of idiopathic, postencephalitic, and symptomatic parkinsonism associated with cerebral arteriosclerosis. It is not indicated for parkinsonism resulting from antipsychotic drug therapy because it can worsen the underlying psychosis.

PHARMACOKINETICS

Levodopa is well absorbed when taken orally, but its bioavailability is only 15% to 30% because a major portion of the drug is decarboxylated in the GI tract. The peak plasma concentration occurs 1 to 2 hours after administration. About 95% of a dose of levodopa is converted to dopamine in the periphery rather than in the brain, and the high plasma concentration of dopamine is responsible for the nausea and cardiac effects that occur with this therapy. For these reasons, levodopa is almost always given in combination with carbidopa (see Mechanism of Action). The plasma half-life ranges from 1 to 4 hours, requiring the patient to take multiple doses daily to maintain an even intermittently effective plasma level. Indeed, there is a phenomenon observed in patients where the effects of levodopa wear off at the end of a dosing period. There is also a so-called on-off effect, where the relief of symptoms is intermittent. These effects might be averted with smaller doses of drug given more often, with sustained-release preparations, or with adjunct therapy (see below). The drug is eliminated primarily in the urine.

ADVERSE REACTIONS AND CONTRAINDICATIONS

Nausea and vomiting are common adverse effects of levodopa therapy. These effects are minimized by the combination of carbidopa and levodopa. Euphoria, restlessness, anxiety, irritability, hyperactivity, insomnia, and vivid dreams often occur with levodopa. Patients occasionally become paranoid and experience psychotic episodes. Respiratory effects such as cough, hoarseness, and disturbed breathing may also appear. Because of these adverse effects, levodopa therapy is used cau-

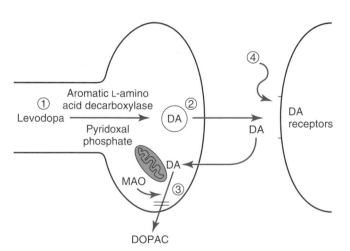

FIGURE 23-2 Model of therapeutic strategies to treat Parkinson's disease by augmenting dopamine (DA) function. These include administration of *(1)* levodopa to increase the synthesis of DA, *(2)* drugs that enhance DA release, *(3)* drugs that prevent DA breakdown by monoamine oxidase (MAO), and *(4)* drugs that function as agonists at postsynaptic DA receptors. (From Clark WG, Brater DC, Johnson AR: *Goth's medical pharmacology*, ed 13, St Louis, 1988, Mosby.)

tiously in patients with a history of heart disease, asthma, emphysema, or peptic ulcer disease. Blurred vision or dilated pupils may be caused by levodopa, so therapy with this drug is not considered for patients with narrow-angle glaucoma and should only be used with careful monitoring for patients with chronic (wide-angle) glaucoma.

Another adverse effect sometimes seen at the start of levodopa therapy is orthostatic hypotension. The mechanism is unknown but is believed to be a CNS effect rather than a peripheral effect. This hypotension tends to decrease with time. An increase in heart rate and force of contraction may also be apparent at the start of therapy. These cardiac actions are caused by the direct action of dopamine on the heart. Cardiac arrhythmia may develop and must be controlled with appropriate medication.

After prolonged therapy with levodopa, abnormal involuntary movements (dyskinesias) may appear. Dyskinesias usually comprise abnormal involuntary movements of the mouth, tongue, face, or neck. They appear 1 to 2 hours after the latest dose of levodopa and represent mild levodopa toxicity. When carbidopa is combined with levodopa, the dyskinesias and other CNS adverse effects occur more rapidly than when levodopa is used alone. Dyskinesias may require dosage reduction. End-of-dose akinesia also may occur just before a new dose is to be taken and usually can be avoided by increasing frequency of administration.

As mentioned earlier, patients taking levodopa often exhibit an on-off phenomenon. Improvement of symptoms suddenly wanes and the loss of therapeutic effect manifests as an abrupt onset of akinesia. The phenomenon is most often associated with long-term treatment, usually occurring after 2 to 3 years and increasing in frequency after 5 years. This phenomenon affects 90% of patients who have been treated for 10 or more years.

Contraindications to the use of the dopaminergic drugs include hypersensitivity, narrow-angle glaucoma, hypertension, coronary sclerosis, and concurrent use of monoamine oxidase inhibitors. Cautious use is warranted in patients with a history of heart disease (e.g., myocardial infarctions, arrhythmia), psychiatric disorders (e.g., psychosis, neurosis, convulsions), or ulcer disease.

INTERACTIONS

Drugs that reduce the effectiveness of levodopa include the antipsychotic drugs, the rauwolfia alkaloids, phenytoin, papaverine, methyldopa, and metoclopramide. A hypertensive crisis may be precipitated when levodopa and monoamine oxidase inhibitors are given concurrently. Because pyridoxine (vitamin B_6) is a cofactor in the conversion of levodopa to dopamine, this vitamin may increase the peripheral biotransformation of levodopa.

DRUG CLASS • Dopamine Receptor Agonists

bromocriptine (Apo-bromocriptine,✲ Alti-bromocriptine,✲ Parlodel)

pergolide (Permax)

pramipexole (Mirapex)

ropinirole (Requip)

MECHANISM OF ACTION

Dopamine receptor agonists serve as substitutes for dopamine by directly stimulating dopamine receptors in the corpus striatum (see Figure 23-2). Bromocriptine and pergolide are ergot derivatives and share many common adverse effects. They are both agonists at D_2 dopamine receptors. Pergolide is also an agonist at D_1 receptors, whereas bromocriptine is a partial antagonist. Pramipexole and ropinirole are agonists at D_2 and D_3 dopamine receptors.

USES

These drugs are useful in treating the symptoms of Parkinson's disease, whether used as adjunct therapies or alone. As natural or synthetic compounds that directly activate dopamine receptors, dopamine agonists can produce an acute antiparkinsonian effect equal to that of levodopa as well as minimize the on-off phenomenon observed with levodopa. Furthermore, the concurrent administration of these drugs with levodopa reduces its required dosage. Pramipexole and ropinirole were initially used as adjunct therapy for patients receiving levodopa-carbidopa but are used more as initial therapies for patients early in the disease. Bromocriptine has also been used to prevent lactation following childbirth and to correct infertility and amenorrhea in women with high prolactin levels (see Chapter 61).

PHARMACOKINETICS

Bromocriptine is poorly absorbed from the GI tract. It has an onset time of 30 to 90 minutes, peaking in 1 to 3 hours. It is 90% protein bound, with a duration of action of 6 to 24 hours. Bromocriptine is completely biotransformed in the liver and eliminated in the feces. Its half-life is 3 to 7 hours in the initial phase and up to 50 hours in the terminal phase. Pergolide is well absorbed when taken orally, peaks in 1 to 2 hours, and has a duration of action of 5 to 9 hours. It has a half-life of approximately

24 to 72 hours. Biotransformation occurs in the liver, and metabolites are eliminated primarily in the urine.

Pramipexole and ropinirole therapy can be titrated more quickly than the ergot derivatives because they are better tolerated. Bioavailability is high, and the peak plasma concentration is achieved in approximately 2 hours. They are widely distributed and not highly bound to plasma proteins. Half-lives for pramipexole and ropinirole are 8 to 12 hours and 6 hours, respectively. Ropinirole is metabolized in the liver and less than 10% of the drug excreted is unchanged. In contrast, pramipexole is eliminated unchanged by excretion through the kidneys by both glomerular filtration and secretion in the renal tubules.

ADVERSE REACTIONS AND CONTRAINDICATIONS

Common adverse effects of bromocriptine and pergolide include nausea, vomiting, dyspepsia, hypotension, hallucinations, psychosis, and dyskinesias. Because these drugs are ergots, vasoconstriction in the fingers and toes also occurs occasionally in response to cold. Orthostatic hypotension and GI disturbances result from the peripheral and central dopaminergic effects of dopamine agonists. Central dopaminergic effects include confusion, hallucinations, and dyskinesias, which tend to worsen if the dose of the agonist or the levodopa (in the combination) is not reduced.

Pramipexole and ropinirole can also produce GI distress, but it is less common than that observed with the ergot derivative. Common complaints include fatigue and nausea, and these drugs can also cause confusion, orthostatic hypotension, and dyskinesias.

Bromocriptine should be used cautiously in patients with liver disease because of its biotransformation in the liver and elimination via the biliary tract. These drugs should also be used cautiously in patients with a history of heart disease, Raynaud's syndrome (for bromocriptine and pergolide), and seizure disorders. Dosage adjustment of pramipexole may be required in patients with renal disease.

INTERACTIONS

Dopamine agonists taken concurrently with antihypertensive drugs can cause an excessive drop in blood pressure. When dopamine agonists are taken with phenothiazines or other antipsychotic drugs, the effects of the dopamine agonists are reduced; thus concurrent administration of dopamine agonists with dopamine antagonists should be avoided. Antihistamines, alcohol, opioids, and sedative-hypnotics have been known to cause additional CNS depression when taken with bromocriptine. Levodopa and dopamine agonists taken together can produce additional neurologic effects in patients with Parkinson's disease.

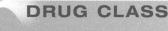

DRUG CLASS • Miscellaneous Drugs Used to Treat Parkinson's Disease

amantadine (Endantadine, Gen-Amantadine, ✽ Symmetrel)

entacapone (Comtan)

selegiline (Eldepryl)

tolcapone (Tasmar)

MECHANISM OF ACTION

Amantadine's mechanism of action is unknown. It appears capable of enhancing the release of dopamine from nerve terminals and can block reuptake at the synapse (see Figure 23-2). It also has agonist activity at NMDA glutamate receptors.

Selegiline irreversibly inhibits the enzyme monoamine oxidase B (MAOB), which contributes to the catabolism of dopamine in the brain (see Figure 23-2). Because dopamine is not rapidly degraded in the presence of selegiline, the duration of action of levodopa is enhanced and its dosage is reduced.

Entacapone and tolcapone are inhibitors of the enzyme catecholamine-O-methyltransferase (COMT), an enzyme that inactivates catecholamines, including dopamine. When administered, these drugs prevent the conversion of levodopa to 3-O-methyldopa, thereby allowing more levodopa to enter the CNS. This is especially important in the presence of inhibition of decarboxylase by carbidopa, because levodopa biotransformation by COMT is increased.

USES

Amantadine is an antiviral drug used to treat respiratory tract infections caused by influenza A viruses (see Chapter 31 for detailed discussion). It also reduces the severity of symptoms of idiopathic Parkinson's disease and postencephalitic parkinsonism. Amantadine is often used in the early stages of the disease to control symptoms, but it may also be used with anticholinergic drugs or with levodopa because it enhances their effectiveness and allows a reduction of their dosage. Selegiline is indicated as an adjunct to levodopa-carbidopa in all stages of Parkinson's disease. It is more effective when used early in the progression of the disease, but even in advanced stages, it lessens the wearing-off effects of levodopa or levodopa-carbidopa therapy. Entacapone and tolcapone are used as adjunct therapies in patients receiving levodopa-carbidopa therapy as well. These drugs improve the therapy by diminishing the wearing-off effect.

PHARMACOKINETICS

Amantadine is well absorbed from the GI tract. Its effects are not seen until about 48 hours after administration. The half-life is 11 to 15 hours, and the drug is distributed to various body fluids and tissues, including the brain. Amantadine is not biotransformed but rather eliminated unchanged in the urine.

Selegiline is well absorbed when given orally; peak plasma concentration is reached in 0.5 to 2 hours. It is rapidly biotransformed into three active metabolites: *N*-desmethyldeprenyl, amphetamine, and methamphetamine. The half-lives of the metabolites differ, ranging from 2 to 20.5 hours. Since new MAOB enzyme synthesis must occur for a patient to regain activity, it takes several weeks for the clinical effects of selegiline to disappear fully.

Entacapone and tolcapone have bioavailabilities of 35% and 65%, respectively, and are widely distributed. Peak plasma concentrations are achieved in approximately 2 hours. Both drugs are highly bound to plasma proteins; tolcapone is 99% bound and entacapone 95%. The liver biotransforms these drugs. The half-life of entacapone is biphasic (2.5 and 4 to 7 hours), and the half-life of tolcapone is 2 to 3 hours. A majority of tolcapone metabolites are excreted in the urine, whereas most entacapone metabolites are eliminated in the bile.

ADVERSE REACTIONS AND CONTRAINDICATIONS

Adverse reactions to amantadine include dizziness, nervousness, inability to concentrate, ataxia, slurred speech, insomnia, lethargy, blurred vision, dry mouth, GI irritation, and rash.

Selegiline has no life-threatening or irreversible adverse effects, although it may produce anxiety, insomnia, and cardiovascular abnormalities. As with dopamine agonists, the drug can cause dyskinesias, hallucinations, orthostatic hypotension, and mental changes. Once the drug dosage is lowered or discontinued, the adverse effects cease. Selegiline is contraindicated in patients with hypersensitivity.

The COMT inhibitors also can cause orthostatic hypotension, dyskinesias, hallucinations, and nausea. Tolcapone can cause severe hepatotoxicity and therefore is not the COMT inhibitor of choice for patients with hepatic disease. Entacapone use is associated with occurrence of pulmonary fibrosis and rhabdomyolysis.

INTERACTIONS

Amphetamine and amphetamine-like stimulant drugs amplify the effects of amantadine by causing adverse behavioral effects. Concurrent use of selegiline and meperidine may result in agitation, rigidity, fever, hypertension or hypotension, and coma. Selegiline should not be administered with other monoamine oxidase inhibitors or serotonin uptake inhibitors. Because it is selective for MAOB, there is no significant interaction with foods that contain tyramine, as occurs with other monoamine oxidase inhibitors (see Chapter 18).

Entacapone and tolcapone should be used with caution when patients are on drugs biotransformed by COMT (such as some sympathomimetics) and on nonselective monoamine oxidase inhibitors. Because entacapone is eliminated in the bile, drugs that interfere with biliary secretion such as ampicillin or erythromycin might alter the elimination. Tolcapone is highly bound to plasma proteins, so caution is warranted when giving warfarin and other highly bound drugs.

APPLICATION TO PRACTICE

ASSESSMENT
History of Present Illness

There are several important questions that help screen for Parkinson's disease: Why did the patient come to the hospital or clinic? When did the symptoms start? What does the patient think caused the symptoms? Has the patient experienced these symptoms in the past? If so, when? Complaints of interference with the activities of daily living precede the recognition of Parkinson's disease by months or years.

Health History

Health history questions should elicit information about any drug, toxin, or food allergies and the reaction the patient exhibited. Past or present alcohol or drug use, current drugs taken, recent infection or trauma, and any exposure to environmental toxins should be noted. Information related to a history of renal, hepatic, cardiovascular, or GI disorders should also be elicited.

Lifespan Considerations

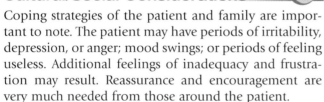

Perinatal. Antiparkinsonian drugs should not be used during pregnancy unless the anticipated benefits outweigh the risks arising from failure to treat Parkinson's disease. It is not known whether antiparkinsonian drugs cause fetal harm or affect reproductive capacity. Rodent studies have shown that these drugs produced alterations in fetal and postnatal growth and viability.

Pediatric. Antiparkinsonian drugs are usually not needed in children. Furthermore, the safety and efficacy of antiparkinsonian drugs have not been established for this age group. Juvenile parkinsonism may occur but is usually associated with Wilson's disease, progressive lenticular degeneration, or Huntington's chorea.

Older Adults. Frail older adults receiving multiple drugs for nonneurologic purposes should be monitored for drugs that could influence response to antiparkinsonian therapy. Existing dementia as well as occasional confusion should be noted before the start of any drug therapy. Normal changes of aging alter the biotransformation and elimination of antiparkinsonian drugs, increasing the risk for adverse effects.

Cultural/Social Considerations

Coping strategies of the patient and family are important to note. The patient may have periods of irritability, depression, or anger; mood swings; or periods of feeling useless. Additional feelings of inadequacy and frustration may result. Reassurance and encouragement are very much needed from those around the patient.

Physical Examination

Parkinson's disease is defined solely by clinical signs and symptoms. A characteristic tremor, rigidity, and bradykinesia are found during physical examination. However, the examination may not reveal a patient's inability to perform outside the office or to carry out activities of daily living. Nonetheless, a thorough assessment is required so that proper intervention can be undertaken.

Observation of the patient during the interview may reveal changes in speech and facial expression, arm swing, and gait. The examination can reveal valuable clues as to the extent of interference with activities of daily living. Assessment of the neurologic system may

be the greatest diagnostic aid. Other areas of importance are the musculoskeletal system, head, neck, and skin.

Assess the patient's mental status. Commonly, the patient with Parkinson's disease is emotionally labile, demonstrates a depressed affect, is easily upset, and shows signs of paranoia. When questioned, the patient may respond slowly because of cognitive impairments. The same impairments may be evident as delayed reactions in the completion of a requested task. Evidence of dementia and acute confusion are common in the older adult with this disease.

Observation of posture and gait is helpful. Because postural reflexes are lost, abnormalities may occur as early signs. The patient may experience involuntary flexion of the head and neck. When walking or standing, the patient exhibits a flexed, stooped posture. Truncal rigidity is noted when the patient attempts to change position from sitting to standing. The patient tends to move the body as a unit and may be unable to correct position when changing from one position to another or merely when rolling over. A characteristic propulsive gait is noted in patients with Parkinson's disease. The patient may be slow to initiate walking but may spontaneously break into a run. When pushed forward or backward, the patient may have difficulty recovering balance.

Typically, the arms are flexed at the elbows, with the wrists slightly dorsiflexed and the fingers adducted and flexed at the metacarpophalangeal joint. During walking, the arm swing is decreased or absent. There may be difficulties with handwriting (micrographia), using kitchen utensils, grooming, and fastening buttons. Rapid repetitive movements, such as tapping of the fingers or pronation and supination of the hand, are common.

The patient may have a masklike facial expression resulting from limited ability to perform facial muscle movements. A blank expression, decreased blinking, and characteristic stare are all common. These effects have other associated head and neck symptoms, such as difficulties in swallowing and chewing. Drooling may be noted as the disease progresses. In addition, the patient's speech may become softer and less distinct.

Other red flags in the physical examination center on hypothalamic function, including both autonomic and neuroendocrine systems. Autonomic symptoms include diaphoresis, orthostatic hypotension, and constipation. Neuroendocrine dysfunction accounts for the excessively oily skin, especially on the face.

Severity Scales. Many scales have been developed to rate the severity of Parkinson's disease. These weighted numerical scales are based on an evaluation of signs and symptoms. Each scale differs according to which symptoms are evaluated and the value assigned to each. A relatively common scale divides the progression of the disease into the following stages:

Mild Disease
Stage 0: No visible disease
Stage I: Disease involves only one side of the body
Stage II: Disease involves both sides of the body but does not impair balance
Moderate Disease
Stage III: Disease impairs balance or walking
Advanced Disease
Stage IV: Disease markedly impairs balance or walking
Stage V: Disease results in complete immobility

Laboratory Testing

There are no laboratory tests to confirm or refute the clinical diagnosis of Parkinson's disease. Blood chemistry tests are most commonly used to seek treatable causes of dementia with parkinsonism, especially hypothyroidism. Imaging or laboratory techniques are useful to rule out other disorders.

Although unreliable in diagnosing idiopathic parkinsonism, magnetic resonance imaging (MRI) has proven to be the single most useful means of looking for other causes of symptoms. Computed tomography (CT) is also useful. If a CT scan shows calcification of the basal ganglia, the possibilities of hyperparathyroidism and hypoparathyroidism should be investigated by measuring blood calcium, phosphorus, and parathormone levels.

GOALS OF THERAPY

Management of the patient with Parkinson's disease is aimed at maintaining function and independence while reducing the symptoms and disabilities caused by the disease as much as and for as long as possible. This is best accomplished by maintaining a balance between dopaminergic and cholinergic activity in the basal ganglia. In general, 85% of patients with early, mild Parkinson's disease can achieve at least 50% improvement in level of function with appropriate drug therapy. Treatment for Parkinson's disease is lifelong (see the Case Study: Parkinson's disease.)

INTERVENTION
Administration

Blood pressure and pulse should be monitored throughout the treatment regimen. This intervention is necessary because some antiparkinsonian drugs have a tendency to cause orthostatic hypotension and hypertension.

Check the patient's pulse before administering an anticholinergic drug. Withhold the dose if the resting pulse exceeds 90 to 100 beats per minute (bpm) in an adult. Administer anticholinergic drugs with caution to patients with a history of heart disease characterized by tachycardia. Auscultate bowel sounds. Keep a record of bowel movements.

Anticholinergic drugs are taken by mouth with food or meals to minimize gastric irritation. The tablets may be crushed and administered with food if the patient has difficulty swallowing. The sustained-release capsules should not be broken, crushed, or chewed (see Chapter 11). If antacids are used concurrently, give the anticholinergic 30 minutes before or 2 hours after the doses of antacid.

Excessive dosage of anticholinergics may cause dry mouth, a burning sensation of the mouth, difficulty swallowing, restlessness, tachycardia, increased respiration, muscle incoordination, dilated pupils, paralysis, tremors, seizures, hallucinations, and death. If overdosage is suspected, gastric lavage or induction of emesis followed by administration of activated charcoal is the treatment of choice. Anticholinergic effects can be reversed by administering one of the anticholinesterase drugs physostigmine or neostigmine methylsulfate (see Chapter 11). Artificial respiration should be instituted if respiratory muscles are paralyzed.

Assess for urinary retention, especially in older men with preexisting prostatic hyperplasia. Monitor fluid intake and output. Instruct the patient to report an inability to void, increasing difficulty in initiating urination, or a sensation of incomplete bladder emptying. Instruct the patient to void before taking each dose of anticholinergic.

The patient taking benztropine can develop paralytic ileus. Auscultate bowel sounds and monitor for intermittent constipation, abdominal distention, and pain. Keep a record of bowel movements. In addition to the oral route, benztropine may be given by intramuscular or intravenous routes. The intravenous route is seldom used because of the small difference in onset when compared with the intramuscular route.

Anticholinergic drugs should be used cautiously in hot weather, particularly in outpatients, because drug-induced anhidrosis may cause hyperthermia. Therapy with trihexyphenidyl requires gonioscopic evaluation and monitoring of intraocular pressure, especially in patients more than 40 years old.

Excessive gastric acidity can cause erratic gastric emptying and decrease the absorption of levodopa. Gastric emptying, and consequently the absorption of levodopa, can be accelerated by taking the drug with antacids or warm liquids and by chewing the tablets before swallowing. Food has less effect on the absorption of the controlled-release preparations than on that of the regular levodopa formulations. When levodopa-carbidopa capsules are opened or the tablets crushed, the drug should be used immediately because levodopa oxidizes in the presence of moisture. Levodopa-carbidopa should be taken with food to minimize GI irritation.

To alleviate the on-off phenomenon, the dose of the dopaminergic drug should be kept low or saved entirely for severe cases. The notion of starting low and going slow definitely applies to antiparkinsonian drugs; however, the use of drug holidays from levodopa may be dangerous and is generally not recommended.

Monitor for evidence of overdose with levodopa. The symptoms include muscle twitching, facial grimacing, eye twitching, exaggerated protrusion of the tongue, behavioral changes, and blepharospasm. These adverse effects may require a dose reduction or withdrawal of the drug. Overdosage of levodopa is treated immediately with gastric lavage. The airway should be maintained and intravenous fluids given.

Check also for the presence of occult blood in the stools. Inspect the skin daily for changes. Monitor the CBC count and differential, platelet count, blood urea nitrogen (BUN) and serum creatinine levels, and liver function tests at the start of therapy and periodically thereafter.

It is thought that protein-restricted diets minimize the fluctuations (decreased response to levodopa at the end of each day or at various times of the day) that occur in some patients. Total dietary protein should be reduced from the average daily intake of 1.6 g/kg body weight to the recommended daily allowance of 0.8 g/kg. Dietary protein may be divided into portions eaten throughout the day or may be consumed in the evening meal.

The dopamine receptor agonist amantadine produces insomnia in some patients, so it is best not to administer it near bedtime. Divided doses of this drug will help reduce CNS adverse effects. Amantadine, bromocriptine, and pergolide may be taken with or following meals. Capsules may be opened for administration, if necessary.

A small initial dose of pergolide is used for patients more than 60 years old. Close observation is needed because these patients are more susceptible to adverse effects, including confusion, agitation, hallucinations, and postural hypotension. Monitoring of cardiovascular status during pergolide therapy is necessary for the patient prone to arrhythmia.

Monitor the patient taking a dopamine receptor agonist for common adverse effects including nausea, vomiting, dyspepsia, hypotension, hallucinations, psychosis, dyskinesias, somnolence, and dry mouth. Approximately 68% of patients experience adverse reactions, although these are usually mild to moderate; nausea is the most common. Most adverse reactions can be minimized by gradually adjusting dosages as ordered.

Overdosage with dopamine receptor agonists manifests as increased severity of adverse effects. The serum blood levels should be checked and the drug withheld or the dosage lowered to maintain optimal effects. Acute overdosage is treated by induction of emesis or gastric lavage followed by administration of activated charcoal.

COMT inhibitors should be taken at the same time as levodopa-carbidopa. They may be administered with either standard or sustained-release preparations of levodopa-carbidopa and can be taken without regard to food. Levodopa-carbidopa dosage requirements are usually lower during therapy with COMT inhibitors. The levodopa-carbidopa dosage will typically be decreased or the dosing interval increased to avoid adverse effects. The patient should be monitored for adverse reactions. Diarrhea is common and typically begins within 4 to 12 weeks of starting therapy. Hallucinations may occur or worsen over time.

Selegiline is given as an adjunctive treatment with levodopa-carbidopa. The usual dose should be taken with breakfast and lunch. An attempt to reduce the dosage of levodopa-carbidopa by 10% to 30% may be made after 2 to 3 days of selegiline therapy. At low doses, there are no dietary restrictions with this drug. At higher doses, the patient should avoid foods high in tyramine (see Dietary Considerations: Monoamine Oxidase Inhibitors and Tyramine in Chapter 18). In addition, instruct the patient to avoid alcoholic beverages, large quantities of caffeine, and OTC cold and cough drugs.

Antiparkinsonian drugs must be discontinued slowly while monitoring the patient closely. Rapid withdrawal or an abrupt reduction in the dose could lead to an exacerbation of parkinsonian symptoms or hyperpyrexia and confusion, a symptom complex resembling neuroleptic malignant syndrome.

Education

Antiparkinsonian drugs should be taken as prescribed to achieve maximum therapeutic effects while minimizing adverse effects. The patient and family should be taught what the drug is, why it is being taken, the anticipated benefits, correct dosage, and the warning signs of adverse effects. In some cases, several weeks or months may be required to obtain the full benefit of drug therapy. Provide emotional support during that time.

The patient should be instructed to inform the health care provider of adverse reactions and not to abruptly discontinue the drug. A sudden withdrawal of the drug can cause a drastic increase in parkinsonian symptoms and deterioration of control. Inform the family that confusion in an older adult is often an adverse effect of a drug and should not be attributed to Parkinson's disease until fully evaluated. If a dose is missed, the patient must never take a double dose. It is better to wait 2 to 4 hours (depending on the drug) before taking the second dose. Patients should avoid OTC drugs and alcoholic beverages (in small amounts) unless approved by the health care provider.

The patient and the family should be taught that antiparkinsonian drugs may cause drowsiness or dizziness. The patient should avoid driving or other activities that require alertness until the response to the drug is known. The patient should be cautioned to make position changes slowly to minimize orthostatic hypotension. The patient should also be warned that perspiration may decrease, so that overheating could occur during hot weather. Patients should remain indoors in an air-conditioned environment during hot weather. Some antiparkinsonian drugs cause photosensitivity reactions; patients should therefore use sunblock.

Check with the health care provider regarding any dietary restrictions, but in general the patient should be advised to increase bulk and fluid in the diet as well as physical activity as much as possible to minimize the constipating effects of the drugs. Most antiparkinsonian drugs are recommended to be taken with or shortly after food or milk to lessen GI irritation. Instruct the patient to void before taking scheduled doses of anticholinergics to minimize the adverse effects of urinary retention. Furthermore, the importance of maintaining a low-protein diet when taking levodopa-carbidopa should be addressed. The daily protein intake can be divided among all meals, but the majority should be consumed in the evening.

Instruct the patient that frequent rinsing of the mouth, good oral hygiene, and use of sugarless gum or candy may decrease the dry mouth associated with antiparkinsonian drugs. The patient should notify the health care provider if dryness persists. Saliva substitutes may be required. A dentist should be notified if mouth dryness interferes with denture use. The patient should also inform the dentist of the drug regimen before undergoing oral surgery or dental work.

Alcohol should be avoided by a patient taking antiparkinsonian drugs. The combined effects of the drug and alcohol may exaggerate the sedative and blood pressure–reducing effects of the drug. Patients taking levodopa should avoid foods containing large quantities of pyridoxine (vitamin B_6) and multivitamins, because pyridoxine interferes with the action of levodopa.

Patients should be informed that harmless darkening of urine and sweat may occur with some antiparkinsonian drugs. They should also be taught to monitor themselves for skin lesions that might be new or changed, which could indicate malignant melanoma.

Patients with diabetes mellitus who are taking levodopa-carbidopa should be taught to perform fingerstick glucose monitoring rather than testing of urine, because false results are possible with Clinitest and Ketostix. Advise men receiving levodopa-carbidopa therapy to inform the health care provider if priapism (an often painful condition of prolonged penile erection) develops.

Advise the patient taking bromocriptine to use contraceptive methods other than oral contraceptives or subdermal implants. Estrogens and progestins interfere with the therapeutic effects of bromocriptine.

Additionally, bromocriptine therapy may lead to an early postpartum return of fertility. Inform the patient that frequent pregnancy testing will be necessary.

Patients receiving long-term levodopa-carbidopa therapy should be tested for diabetes mellitus and acromegaly. Liver, renal, and hematopoietic function should be periodically monitored as ordered. Amantadine increases concentrations of liver enzymes and may increase BUN. Periodic evaluations of the white blood cell count, liver function, and renal function tests are necessary. Baseline and periodic evaluations of cardiac, hepatic, renal, and hematopoietic function are recommended during prolonged dopamine agonist therapy.

Support groups and psychotherapy for patients with Parkinson's disease and their families have proved beneficial. Patients should be encouraged to pursue as many of their predisease activities as possible.

EVALUATION

The management of Parkinson's disease is guided by the impact of the patient's symptoms on activities of daily living. The patient should be seen at regular intervals—every 2 to 6 months—to monitor response to therapy and to assess for adverse effects. Therapeutic effectiveness of antiparkinsonian therapy is noted as a decrease in symptoms. Therapeutic effects usually become evident after 2 to 3 weeks of therapy but may require up to 6 months in some patients.

PATHOPHYSIOLOGY • Myasthenia Gravis

Myasthenia gravis is a disease in which the skeletal muscles quickly show weakness and become fatigued. Muscles controlling facial movements are most commonly involved, and one early sign of myasthenia gravis is a drooping eyelid (ptosis). As the disease progresses, chewing and swallowing become increasingly difficult, and the voice becomes less distinct. Death can result if the intercostal muscles and the diaphragm (muscles essential for breathing) become affected. Myasthenia gravis affects about 25,000 people in the United States. The incidence among women is most frequent between the ages of 20 and 30; in men between the ages 50 and 70.

Myasthenia gravis is an autoimmune disease with a basic defect in synaptic transmission at the neuromuscular junction caused by a reduction in the available nicotinic receptors for acetylcholine (Figure 23-3). This reduction is caused by autoantibodies against the nicotinic receptors that block the active site for acetylcholine on the receptors and increase the rate at which the cell degrades the receptors.

Although at one time fatal or disabling, myasthenia gravis is now effectively treated in most patients. Anti-

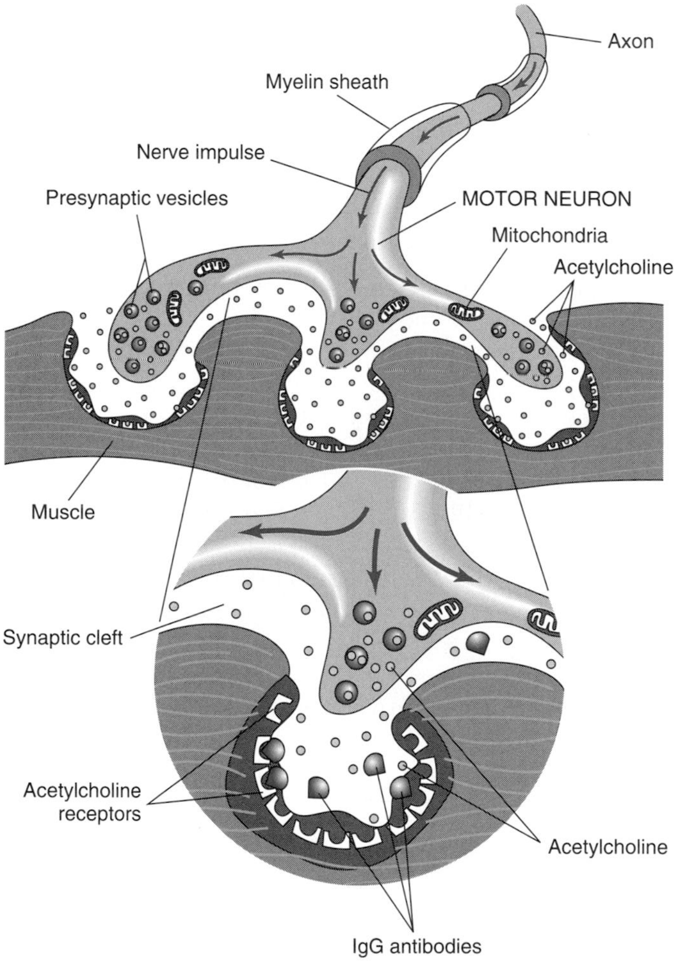

FIGURE 23-3 Myasthenia gravis. Synaptic vesicles normally contain large amounts of acetylcholine (ACh). ACh is released, accumulates within the synaptic cleft, and stimulates postsynaptic neurons. The result is a large depolarization and the production of an action potential. In myasthenia gravis, the same amount of ACh is present but it is not available to the membrane receiving the impulse. Immunoglobulin G (IgG) antibodies fix to receptor sites in postsynaptic membranes and block the binding of acetylcholine. More ACh is exposed to acetylcholinesterase breakdown. The electrical impulse from the nerve to the muscle is diminished, and the muscle contraction is weak.

BOX 23-1 Drugs that Weaken a Patient with Myasthenia Gravis

Adrenocorticotropic Hormones and Glucocorticoids

Anesthetics
halothane
lidocaine
Antiarrhythmics
procainamide
propranolol
quinidine
Antibiotics
gentamicin
kanamycin
paromomycin
streptomycin
Anticonvulsants
Antimalarials
quinine
Diuretics
Muscle Relaxants
gallamine
metocurine
pancuronium
succinylcholine
tubocurarine
Opioids
Thyroid Hormones

cholinesterases are the first choice for treatment, and most patients achieve significant improvement with these drugs (Table 23-3; see also Chapter 11). Thymectomy (removal of the thymus gland) is a common procedure performed to treat patients with myasthenia gravis. About 75% of patients with myasthenia gravis have an abnormal thymus, commonly in the form of hyperplasia or thymomas. Cells in the thymus are thought to be a major source of the autoantigen-stimulating antibody production. Removal of the thymus brings overall improvement with essentially no complications for about 85% of patients.

When anticholinesterase drugs are not adequate to treat myasthenia gravis, immunosuppressive therapy is indicated. Corticosteroids and azathioprine are used for long-term immunosuppressive therapy (see Chapters 14 and 57). Plasmapheresis to remove antibodies from circulation is another form of therapy, but it produces only short-term improvement and is used for patients in myasthenic crisis or those undergoing thymectomy.

A number of drugs have weak anticholinergic effects of their own and are contraindicated for the patient with myasthenia gravis. These drugs, listed in Box 23-1, can dangerously weaken the patient with myasthenia gravis but do not noticeably block the neuromuscular receptors of a healthy person.

TABLE 23-3

Drugs Used for the Treatment of Myasthenia Gravis

Generic Name	Brand Name	Comments
Acetylcholinesterase Inhibitors		
ambenonium chloride	Mytelase	Acetylcholinesterase inhibitor that is rapidly absorbed.
edrophonium chloride	Enlon, Tensilon	Very short-acting acetylcholinesterase inhibitor used to diagnose myasthenia gravis. Diagnosis is positive if muscle strength increases within 3 min (duration 5-10 min).
neostigmine bromide	Prostigmin bromide	An acetylcholinesterase inhibitor with a high incidence rate of adverse effects.
neostigmine methylsulfate	Prostigmin methylsulfate	An injectable form of neostigmine for diagnosis of myasthenia gravis.
pyridostigmine bromide	Mestinon, Regonol✶	The drug of choice for controlling muscular weakness caused by myasthenia gravis.
Immunosuppressants		
azathioprine	Imuran	Complete blood count should be performed weekly for first month; twice monthly for second and third month; monthly thereafter. Liver function tests should be performed every 1 to 3 months.
Corticosteroids		
betamethasone	Celestone	Provides clinical improvement, but long-term use limited by adverse effects (see Chapter 57).
cortisone	Cortone	Provides clinical improvement, but long-term use limited by adverse effects (see Chapter 57).
dexamethasone	Decadron	Provides clinical improvement, but long-term use limited by adverse effects (see Chapter 57).
hydrocortisone	Cortef	Provides clinical improvement, but long-term use limited by adverse effects (see Chapter 57).
prednisone	Deltasone	Provides clinical improvement, but long-term use limited by adverse effects (see Chapter 57).

✶ Available only in Canada.

DRUG CLASS • Acetylcholinesterase Inhibitors

ambenonium chloride (Mytelase)

edrophonium chloride (Enlon, Reversol, Tensilon)

neostigmine (Prostigmin)

pyridostigmine (Mestinon, Regonol)

MECHANISM OF ACTION

These drugs inhibit the enzyme acetylcholinesterase, thereby reducing the degradation of acetylcholine. Because acetylcholinesterase is present throughout the neuromuscular junction, inhibition of the enzyme allows acetylcholine to accumulate at the neuromuscular junction, ensuring that available receptors are activated. The pharmacology of these drugs is discussed in detail in Chapter 11.

USES

Acetylcholinesterase inhibitors are used in the diagnosis and treatment of myasthenia gravis. They effectively and rapidly restore muscle strength in the majority of patients. Because the drugs do not increase the production of acetylcholine, they are effective only as long as the transmitter is released at motor nerve endings and acetylcholine receptors are available. Acetylcholinesterase inhibitors used to treat myasthenia gravis are also used to reverse the effects of nondepolarizing neuromuscular blockers used in surgery.

Edrophonium is useful primarily as a diagnostic aid in myasthenia gravis. A test dose is given and muscle strength assessed. If there is no improvement, a second dose is given. Improvement in muscle strength suggests the diagnosis of myasthenia gravis. Furthermore, edrophonium and neostigmine are useful in determining whether a patient with confirmed myasthenia gravis is in cholinergic or myasthenic crisis. Neostigmine is also prescribed to relieve the symptoms of myasthenia gravis, but pyridostigmine is the preferred drug for treatment. Compared with neostigmine, pyridostigmine is better absorbed from the GI tract and is longer-acting. Ambenonium is slightly longer-acting than pyridostigmine or neostigmine. Ambenonium is not a bromide salt, as pyridostigmine and neostigmine are, so it is the preferred drug for patients allergic to bromides.

PHARMACOKINETICS

Anticholinesterase drugs are positively charged compounds that are not lipid soluble. These drugs are therefore not readily absorbed orally; the oral dose is 30 times the parenteral dose. The most widely used anticholinesterase drugs are pyridostigmine and neostigmine. The anticholinesterases are biotransformed by plasma esterases and hepatic enzymes to inactive compounds. The drugs and their metabolites are excreted in the urine (see Chapter 11).

The effective dose must be individualized for each patient. Stress and infection can increase the requirement. Women in the premenstrual part of their cycle may also require higher dosages. Very ill patients may become unresponsive to their drug, but temporary reduction or withdrawal of the dose over a 3-day period may restore their responsiveness.

ADVERSE REACTIONS AND CONTRAINDICATIONS

Adverse effects arising from overstimulation of neuromuscular (nicotinic) receptors include muscle cramps, rapid small contractions (fasciculation), and weakness. Acetylcholinesterase inhibitors also can result in actions at sites other than neuromuscular sites. By preventing acetylcholine breakdown, they augment cholinergic actions at muscarinic receptors, producing excessive salivation, perspiration, abdominal distress, and nausea and vomiting.

Anticholinesterase drugs are contraindicated for patients with intestinal or urinary tract obstruction. These drugs should be used cautiously in patients with bronchial asthma. Persons sensitive to bromide should be given neostigmine methylsulfate or ambenonium chloride instead of the more commonly used bromide-containing anticholinesterases.

INTERACTIONS

When used concurrently, atropine, guanethidine, procainamide, quinidine, or quinine decreases the effect of the acetylcholinesterase inhibitors. The actions of these drugs may be antagonized by any drug with anticholinergic properties (e.g., antihistamines, antidepressants). With concomitant alcohol use, weakness and unsteadiness are exacerbated.

DRUG CLASS • Immunosuppressive Drugs

azathioprine (Imuran)
Corticosteroids (see Table 23-3)

Although other immunosupressants also can be used to treat advanced cases of myasthenia gravis, this discussion will focus on azathioprine, because it is the usual drug of choice. For detailed discussion of other immunosuppressant drugs see Chapters 14 and 37. For additional discussion of corticosteroids see Chapter 57.

MECHANISM OF ACTION

Corticosteroids are thought to somehow protect acetylcholine receptor sites from immunologic attack by immunoglobulin G (IgG), thus increasing the amount of acetylcholine available at the site. Another hypothesis is that the drugs reduce the total number of circulating antibodies and the degradation of the receptor sites, thereby increasing the effectiveness of acetylcholine. Overall, corticosteroids suppress the patient's immune response. Azathioprine is an analog of the antineoplastic drug mercaptopurine. In patients with myasthenia gravis, it appears to affect T cell proliferation and the synthesis of antibodies.

USES

Corticosteroids are useful in the patient with myasthenia gravis whose thymus gland has been removed, who has a pure ocular form of the disease, or who is more than 50 years old and cannot be managed with cholinesterase inhibitors. These drugs also benefit the patient with severe generalized myasthenia gravis. In many cases, the disease goes into remission and the possibility of relapse is minimized in response to corticosteroids. Therapy with azathioprine is directed toward reducing receptor antibody production. Azathioprine is useful for myasthenia gravis that is not responsive to corticosteroids.

PHARMACOKINETICS

Corticosteroids are well absorbed when taken orally. The onset of action for oral prednisone is approximately 1 hour, and the peak drug level occurs within 1 to 2 hours. The duration of the drug's action may be as long as 1 to 2 days. Prednisone is biotransformed in the liver to prednisolone and has a half-life of more than 3 hours. Prednisone is about three to five times more potent than cortisone or hydrocortisone.

Azathioprine is readily absorbed from the GI tract, with a bioavailability of 80% to 90%. The drug is 30% bound to plasma proteins. The onset of action of oral azathioprine occurs at 6 to 8 weeks, with a peak at 12 weeks. It is biotransformed to mercaptopurine and metabolites. Azathioprine is eliminated through the kidneys, with minimal elimination of unchanged drug.

ADVERSE EFFECTS AND CONTRAINDICATIONS

The adverse effects of adrenal corticosteroids are many and varied, and some may be life threatening (see Chapter 57). Azathioprine therapy is limited by its adverse effects, the most serious and limiting of which is bone marrow suppression. Symptoms common to bone marrow suppression include macrocytic anemia, thrombocytopenia, pancytopenia, and leukocytopenia. Bruising and bleeding may also occur as a result.

Corticosteroids are contraindicated in cases of active, untreated infections, because these drugs mask infection. They are also contraindicated in patients who are lactating or who have psychoses, Cushing's syndrome, active tuberculosis, heart failure, varicella, or peptic ulcer disease. These drugs should be used cautiously during pregnancy and in children, because their safety for these groups has not been established.

INTERACTIONS

The dose of prednisone may have to be increased for a patient who is also taking an antacid, a barbiturate, phenytoin, or rifampin. Prednisone taken concurrently with an oral anticoagulant increases the effect of the anticoagulant, thus increasing the risk of hemorrhage. Women taking oral contraceptives should be warned that corticosteroids can cause a loss of contraceptive effectiveness. In addition, estrogen increases the antiinflammatory effect of corticosteroids by reducing its breakdown in the liver.

Azathioprine is partially biotransformed by xanthine oxidase. Allopurinol, an inhibitor of this enzyme, increases the potential for toxicity by decreasing the biotransformation of azathioprine in the liver. Captopril, when given concurrently with azathioprine, worsens the patient's leukopenia. Erythromycin increases the absorption of azathioprine.

APPLICATION TO PRACTICE

ASSESSMENT
History of Present Illness

When taking the history of the present illness, it is important to get the patient's and family's descriptions of symptoms, including their duration. The disease is often exacerbated by factors such as stress, infection, menstruation, and pregnancy. .

The patient may complain of symptoms that interfere with daily activities and of the need for frequent rest periods. Ask the patient to identify the specific areas or body parts that are weak. When the weakness started (slowly or suddenly), its progress, whether it affects one or both sides of the body, if breathing is affected, and whether it interferes with activities such as combing hair, eating, swallowing, or walking should also be investigated. The patient should be questioned about bladder and bowel incontinence as well.

Health History

The health history is important in identifying factors contributing to the current state of the patient's health. Elicit information regarding past operations, anesthetics received, allergies, history of exposure to toxins or food, and the reaction noted. Past drug and alcohol use, history of rheumatoid arthritis, and any vision changes within the past few years are important to note.

Lifespan Considerations

Perinatal. The pregnant patient with myasthenia gravis should be in the care of a neurologist who specializes in neuromuscular disease. No specific effects of pregnancy on myasthenia gravis have been documented; however, either significant improvement in symptoms or drastic worsening may occur. Labor proceeds as in the nonmyasthenic patient. Sedatives and opioid analgesics should be used sparingly and with attention to changes in vital signs. The obstetrician should have injectable cholinesterase inhibitors available in case of myasthenic crisis and for use during labor, when nausea may preclude oral administration.

The second stage of labor is associated with muscle fatigue and increased risk of myasthenic crisis. The vaginal route is the preferred method of delivery. Cesarean section is thought to be too stressful, possibly precipitating myasthenic crisis. An epidural anesthetic is best to decrease fatigue and provide adequate anesthesia.

Pediatric. Neonatal myasthenia gravis develops in approximately 10% to 12% of infants born of myasthenic mothers. No prenatal prognostic factors or tests have yet identified infants at risk for this problem. The pediatri-

cian should be equipped with full resuscitation equipment at birth, and the neonate should be closely monitored for 12 to 72 hours. The infant may have a weak cry and may be unable to take a bottle because of decreased muscle tone. Breast-feeding, however, is not advised, because the antibodies of myasthenia gravis cross into the breast milk. Breast-feeding prolongs the myasthenic state for the neonate. In children with seizure disorders, bronchial asthma, urinary tract infections, or severely impaired kidney function, myasthenia gravis drugs should be used with caution.

Older Adults. The older adult is not immune to myasthenia gravis, although the disease is more likely to have been diagnosed earlier in life. However, older adults are more prone to complications and more frequent crisis situations than younger populations. Stress factors tending to precipitate crisis in the older adult include complications of immobility, fractures secondary to falls, sepsis, pneumonia, and a generalized poor state of health.

Cultural/Social Considerations

A patient's adjustment to myasthenia gravis depends on the extent of loss of independence, the resultant body changes, and the nature of the disease. Factors such as age, gender, available support systems, and occupation all play important roles in the patient's ability to cope with the disease. Social adjustment may change dramatically over the course of the disease from minimal to overall maximal adjustment.

The generalized weakness and fatigue associated with myasthenia gravis contributes to social isolation and changes in body image. Neck and shoulder muscle weakness and loss of fine motor control add to the problem. The patient may become frustrated with the changes. Rest is critical after periods of activity.

Physical Examination

Patients with myasthenia gravis exhibit a characteristic picture. Note the presence of a nasal voice or aphonia, changes in facial expressions, ptosis, or a snarl instead of a smile. A sagging jaw and an inability to hold up the head suggest the presence of neck muscle involvement.

Check the temperature, pulse, respiration, and blood pressure. A patient's inability to hold the thermometer in the mouth without help is relevant. The ability to chew and swallow should be evaluated. An important clue to dietary problems may be any weight loss experienced over the past few months. An eye examination also contributes valuable information as to whether the patient has ocular palsy.

Any muscle weakness during the physical examination should be noted. Distinguish between proximal and distal weakness. Does the patient tire easily after performing a simple act such as combing hair? If leg muscles are involved, the health care provider should evaluate the risk of falling by noting the gait.

Note any weakness of cough, attacks of dyspnea following exertion, difficulty clearing the respiratory tract, and skin color changes. In severe disease, respiratory muscle weakness may lead to ventilatory failure.

Laboratory Testing

Pulmonary function tests, nerve conduction tests, and nerve stimulation tests are helpful in determining the baseline status. Laboratory testing should include a lupus screen (to rule out lupus erythematosus); tests for antinuclear antibodies, rheumatoid factor, and antithyroglobulin antibodies; a tuberculin test; and a measurement of fasting blood sugar. Approximately 5% of patients with myasthenia gravis have thyrotoxicosis. The serum antiacetylcholine (ACh) receptor antibody titer may be elevated.

In most cases, the diagnosis of myasthenia gravis is obvious from the history and physical examination findings. However, edrophonium testing can confirm the diagnosis of myasthenia gravis and help monitor for worsening of symptoms. The procedure for edrophonium testing is as follows:

- A 2-mg dose of edrophonium is given intravenously.
- The patient is observed for an increase in muscle strength within 1 to 3 minutes.
- If no response occurs, an additional 8 to 10 mg of edrophonium is given over the next 2 minutes.
- Muscle strength is again assessed. If an increase in the muscle strength occurs within 10 to 30 seconds, myasthenia gravis is diagnosed.

Immediately following the administration of the edrophonium, the patient may complain of feeling dizzy, flushed, or faint and may experience a drop in blood pressure. However, because the drug action is short-lived, these effects rarely last longer than 5 minutes.

Electromyography is helpful in demonstrating the fatigability of affected muscles. A 10% or greater decrease in amplitude during progressive stimulation generally indicates defective neuromuscular transmission.

Approximately 10% to 15% of persons with myasthenia gravis have a tumor of the thymus gland. Routine anteroposterior and lateral chest x-ray studies, chest CT scans, and possibly MRIs have been useful in identifying a thymoma.

GOALS OF THERAPY

The primary treatment goal for the patient with myasthenia gravis is to achieve the maximum muscle strength and endurance possible with the fewest adverse effects (excessive salivation, sweating, nausea, diarrhea, abdominal cramps, or tachycardia). The myasthenic stage and the extent of disability determine the treatment regimen. The regimen for each patient is individualized and is developed on a trial-and-error basis for the most part. The optimal dose and administration schedule will fluctuate during periods of stress (see the Case Study: Myasthenia Gravis).

INTERVENTION
Administration

The importance of taking an antimyasthenic drug as prescribed cannot be overstated. The risk of a myasthenic or cholinergic crisis increases with improper dosing or administration. All drugs used in the management of myasthenia gravis should be taken with food or milk. Doses should be evenly spaced to minimize gastric distress and adverse effects. In older adults, it is often helpful to have a family member oversee the treatment regimen.

The patient's vital signs, especially respirations, should be monitored frequently during drug therapy with an anticholinesterase drug. Atropine injection should be available, if needed, to reverse the drug effects. Additionally, respiratory support may be needed.

The patient's response should be monitored and documented after each dose because optimum dosage is difficult to judge. Observe for improvement in strength, vision, and ptosis 45 to 60 minutes after drug administration.

Myasthenic crisis is the sudden onset of muscular weakness. It can be caused by a late dose or inadequate dosing with an anticholinesterase drug. Symptoms are noted approximately 3 hours after the dose was due (Table 23-4). Symptoms of cholinergic crisis arise within 1 hour of an excessive dose of a cholinesterase inhibitor. Testing with edrophonium may determine whether the patient is in myasthenic or cholinergic crisis.

Antimyasthenic drugs for intravenous administration should be readily available to treat myasthenic or cholinergic crisis. Administer intravenous injection no faster than 1 mg per minute. Rapid intravenous infusion may cause bradycardia and seizures. Antimyasthenic drugs given intravenously are fast-acting and peak very quickly compared with those given orally. Before drug administration, it is important that the patency of the intravenous line be double-checked. The concentration of the solution, the administration time, possible drug-drug interactions, and the desired patient response are also important.

Corticosteroid therapy requires monitoring of patient's blood pressure, weight, and blood glucose level.

TABLE 23-4

Comparison of Cholinergic and Myasthenic Crises

	Cholinergic Crisis	*Myasthenic Crisis*
Cause	Excessive cholinergic drug	Insufficient anticholinesterase drug
Timing	Within 1 hour of when dose was due	Within 3 hours of late or inadequate dose
Signs and symptoms	Nausea, vomiting, diarrhea, abdominal cramping, blurry vision, pallor, facial muscle twitching, pupillary miosis, hypotension, fasciculations, increased sweating and salivation, extreme danger of respiratory arrest	Tachycardia, tachypnea, elevated blood pressure, anoxia, cyanosis, bladder and bowel incontinence, decreased urinary output, absence of cough or swallow reflexes, extreme danger of respiratory arrest, extreme quadriplegia, and quadriparesis

Report hypertension, weight gain, and an elevated blood glucose level to the health care provider. Watch for depression, psychotic episodes, and cushingoid effects, including moonface, buffalo hump, central obesity, and thinning hair.

Immunosuppressant drug therapy may lead to hepatotoxicity. Early signs include clay-colored stools, dark urine, pruritus, and yellow skin and sclera. Azathioprine specifically affects renal, hepatic, and hematologic functions. Monitor CBC and platelet counts, renal function, and liver enzymes as ordered. Levels of serum and urine uric acid and plasma albumin all may fall. Increases in serum alkaline phosphatase, bilirubin, aspartate aminotransferase (AST), alanine aminotransferase (ALT), and amylase all signal hepatotoxicity. Bone marrow depression may be suspected when there is a decrease in hemoglobin. A leukocyte count less than 3000/mm^3 or a platelet count less than 100,000/mm^3 may indicate the need to decrease dosage.

Education

Teach the patient and family strategies to facilitate chewing and swallowing to help prevent weight loss and aspiration. Remaining upright while eating, using thick liquids, and eating a soft diet all reduce the risk of aspiration. Small, frequent meals with high-calorie snacks may help minimize weight loss. Patients should be encouraged to take small bites and eat slowly. As the disease worsens, patients may require tube feedings.

Impaired verbal communication is often an area of frustration. It may be necessary to identify effective communication strategies before impairment becomes severe. The patient may be taught to read lips or to use sign language or an erasable board.

Visual difficulties compound the other problems. Ptosis and ocular palsy lead to the patient's inability to close the eyes, increasing the risk of corneal abrasions. If necessary, the patient should be taught to use a patch and shield to protect the eyes. The eyes also have a tendency for excessive dryness. Artificial tears can be used to keep the eyes moist. Alternating eye patches may help to relieve diplopia.

Conserving energy through rest, planning, and priority setting helps prevent or alleviate fatigue. Alternate activity periods with periods of rest. Activities that can be completed in short periods of time or divided into several segments are desirable; for example, read one chapter of a book at a time or avoid scheduling two energy-draining activities for the same day.

Explain to the patient and family that therapy for myasthenia gravis is lifelong. The patient and family should be informed of the names of the drugs prescribed along with the dosage, the benefits, and the possible adverse effects. Advise the patient to report adverse effects to the health care provider. Proper administration technique for the dosage form should be stressed to both patient and family. Teach them also how to recognize symptoms of cholinergic and myasthenic crises. The importance of taking drugs on time—not too late or too early—and how to intervene in a crisis situation should also be explained. If extended-release formulations are prescribed, the patient should be instructed not to crush the tablets or to take them less often than every 6 hours. The patient should also be advised not to take other drugs without first contacting the health care provider to avoid or minimize potential drug interactions. Breast-feeding is not advised for patients with myasthenic exacerbation, for those receiving high doses of cholinesterase inhibitors, or for those with high circulating antibody titers.

The patient and family should be aware that it may take weeks or months before the full benefits of a particular drug are seen. The drug should not be stopped abruptly or without the health care provider's consent.

Patients should be advised to avoid immunizations while taking immunosuppressants, which decrease the effectiveness of any therapy that enhances immunity. Women of childbearing age and their partners should be instructed that immunosuppressant drugs may interfere with the effectiveness of contraceptives. Safe use of immunosuppressant drugs during pregnancy has not been established. Furthermore, women should be advised to avoid conception for at least 4 months after drug therapy with immunosuppressants. Additionally, advise the patient receiving immunosuppressant therapy to report even mild infections (colds, fever, sore throat, malaise) and unusual bleeding or bruising.

Warn the patient on long-term corticosteroid therapy about cushingoid effects (e.g., moonface, buffalo hump, central obesity, thinning hair, hypertension, and increased susceptibility to infection). The patient should be instructed to report sudden weight gain, swelling, slow healing of wounds, and signs of infection (fever, sore throat, or dysuria) to the health care provider.

Furthermore, the patient should be advised to wear a form of medical alert identification and to carry written information regarding prescribed drugs and dosages. It is also important for the patient to carry a list of drugs contraindicated for persons with myasthenia gravis (see Box 23-1). Patients and families can be referred to local, state, or national myasthenia gravis support groups for additional information.

EVALUATION

Drug therapy for myasthenia gravis is considered successful if the patient experiences improved muscle strength and endurance with few troublesome adverse effects. The highest possible level of functioning should be achieved. The patient and family should be able to identify community resources that will help them maintain an effective level of functioning. The patient should also be able to identify measures that will help prevent or lessen fatigue.

PATHOPHYSIOLOGY • Alzheimer's Disease

Alzheimer's disease is a disorder of progressive mental degeneration. There is a gradual decline in cognitive abilities over 7 to 10 years. Disturbances in judgment, memory, and language are the earliest manifestations. Dementia, the decline in intellectual functioning and memory severe enough to interfere with normal daily activities, occurs as the disease progresses. Alzheimer's disease is the most common cause of dementia, accounting for about 50% of cases. The next level of loss is control of the bladder and bowel. Eventually patients are unable to walk, and finally unable to swallow. Alzheimer's disease appears primarily in persons more than 65 years old, although some genetic forms have been identified with early onset. The number of persons with Alzheimer's disease is increasing because the general population is aging.

At death, brains of persons with Alzheimer's disease show atrophy of cortical regions and abnormal plaques and neurofibrillary tangles in the affected areas. The cerebral cortex has a significant loss of neurons and a reduction in neurotransmitters, especially acetylcholine.

Research has been directed at understanding what causes the abnormal plaques and tangles associated with Alzheimer's disease. These plaques are composed of a protein fragment called beta amyloid that folds abnormally into strands that accumulate. Through a process not understood, this induces another protein, tau, to form into abnormal strands in the neuron. Because tau is important to maintaining structures for a normal neuron, this abnormality is believed to contribute to neuronal death.

The genetics of certain proteins associated with Alzheimer's plaques is being studied. An increased prevalence of the gene for apolipoprotein E4 has been found in patients with Alzheimer's disease. How this variant of the cholesterol-carrying protein is involved in the pathology of Alzheimer's disease is unclear. Genetic studies of families with early-onset Alzheimer's disease have identified a gene for amyloid precursor protein and two presenilin genes (which may affect amyloid production) as associated with this early-onset form of Alzheimer's disease.

EVIDENCE-BASED PRACTICE
Donepezil as a Treatment for Alzheimer's Disease

Setting

Alzheimer's disease is a degenerative organic mental disease characterized by progressive intellectual deterioration and dementia. Approximately 40% of persons over age 85 are affected. The goal of therapy is to improve the patient's well being, but some cholinesterase inhibitors such as tacrine are also associated with hepatotoxicity. Donepezil is thought to be more specific in action and therefore safer.

Objective of Literature Review

The objective of this review was to determine the clinical effectiveness of donepezil in treating the cognitive function and global clinical state of patients with mild to moderate Alzheimer's disease. The search was carried out using the Cochrane Dementia and Cognitive Improvement Group specialized register, the Donepezil Study Group, and Eisai, Inc.

Criteria for Inclusion of Studies in Review of Literature

Investigators included randomized controlled, quality studies that examined the use of donepezil versus placebo in patients with Alzheimer's disease.

Data Extraction and Analysis

One reviewer performed extraction of data that were then pooled when possible. Available outcome data covering the cognitive function and global clinical state were analyzed. Data included intention-to-treat as well as inferential statistics.

Results of Review

Eight studies (*N* = 2663 patients) lasting 12, 24, and 52 weeks were reviewed. At 24 weeks there was statistically significant improvement for patients given either 5-mg or 10-mg daily doses of donepezil as compared to placebo, as well as at 52 weeks for patients treated with 10-mg daily doses compared to placebo. The Alzheimer's Disease Assessment Scale for Cognition (ADAS-Cog) and the Mini-Mental Status Examination (MMSE) scales were used to evaluate the drug's effectiveness.

Three studies showed some improvement in the patients' global clinical state at 12 and 24 weeks in those treated with either 5-mg or 10-mg daily doses of donepezil as compared to placebo. Noticeably more patients on the 10-mg daily regimen stopped the drug before the end of the treatment period compared to placebo, which may have resulted in overestimation of benefits.

Investigators' Conclusions

Donepezil produced modest improvement in the cognitive function and global clinical state in patients with mild to moderate Alzheimer's disease. Patients' self-report of their quality of life showed no benefit of donepezil over placebo. The day-to-day implications of these findings are unclear.

Birks JS, Melzer D, Beppu H: Donepezil for mild and moderate Alzheimer's disease. In *The Cochrane Library,* Issue 2, Update Software, 2002, Oxford.

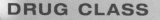

DRUG CLASS   •   Acetylcholinesterase Inhibitors Used to Treat Alzheimer's Disease

donepezil (Aricept)

galantamine (Reminyl)

rivastigmine (Exelon)

tacrine (Cognex)

MECHANISM OF ACTION

These drugs reversibly inhibit the activity of acetylcholinesterase, thereby increasing acetylcholine concentrations in the brain and enhancing the activity at cholinergic synapses. Tacrine is a centrally acting acetylcholinesterase inhibitor that also blocks potassium channels and may have some direct cholinergic activity.

USES

These acetylcholinesterase inhibitors have been specifically approved by the FDA for use to improve cognitive functions in the early stages of Alzheimer's disease. They are indicated for symptomatic treatment of mild to moderate dementia in Alzheimer's disease. Efficacy of these drugs is limited, and they do not slow the progression of the disease.

PHARMACOKINETICS

These drugs are well absorbed when given orally, but tacrine has a low bioavailability because of a significant first-pass effect. The time to peak plasma concentrations of these drugs ranges from 1 to 4 hours. Donepezil is highly bound to plasma proteins (96%), whereas the other drugs are not. These drugs are extensively biotransformed by cytochrome P-450 enzymes in the liver. Donepezil and tacrine have active metabolites, the latter being transformed into 1-hydroxytacrine, which has central cholinergic activity. Elimination of donepezil is slow; its half-life is about 70 hours. In contrast, the half-lives of galantamine, rivastigmine, and tacrine are 7 hours, 1.5 hours, and 1.5 to 4 hours, respectively. The metabolites of the drugs are eliminated largely by the kidney.

ADVERSE REACTIONS AND CONTRAINDICATIONS

The most common adverse effects of these drugs are nausea, diarrhea, anorexia, and vomiting. About 20% of patients are unable to tolerate tacrine because of the cholinergic effects, largely consisting of GI distress.

TOXICITY

Hepatotoxicity limits the use of tacrine. Up to 50% of patients develop elevated levels of liver enzymes. When the dosage is reduced or the drug discontinued, results of liver function studies commonly return to normal limits within 6 weeks. Unlike tacrine, however, donepezil, galantamine, and rivastigmine do not cause hepatotoxicity or elevated transaminase levels.

INTERACTIONS

Drugs that inhibit liver enzymes, such as ketoconazole and quinidine, inhibit the biotransformation of these acetylcholinesterase inhibitors, and drugs that induce the P-450 enzymes such as phenobarbital or phenytoin augment their biotransformation. Because the acetylcholinesterase inhibitors increase gastric acid secretion, they can increase the gastric irritation and potential for bleeding of nonsteroidal antiinflammatory drugs (NSAIDs). They also have the potential to attenuate the actions of muscarinic receptor antagonists and exacerbate the actions of succinylcholine and similar neuromuscular blockers.

APPLICATION TO PRACTICE

ASSESSMENT
History of Present Illness

Many older adults have or have had relatives with Alzheimer's disease. These individuals may be reluctant to consider the possibility that they are developing symptoms of the same disease. Forgetfulness and difficulty learning new information may be attributed to aging. Contact with the health care system may be initiated by the patient or by significant others. If the memory deficits and judgment impairments are significant, it will probably be the significant others who schedule an evaluation. Interview the patient and the informant to determine the timing of symptom onset and the rate of deterioration. Ask specifically about difficulties with activities of daily living, judgment, increasing forgetfulness, and changes in personality. Family members or significant others may relate episodes of leaving a stove on, not shutting the front door, or blaming others when objects have been misplaced. They may note that the patient does not initiate activities that were previously enjoyable and does not socialize with friends.

Inquire about the patient's reactions to changes in routine or in the environment. It is not uncommon for a patient with Alzheimer's disease to become extremely agitated over small changes. Similarly, apathy, social isolation, and irritability may be noted. As the brain atrophies, the patient often exhibits paranoia, uses abusive language, and becomes suspicious of others.

Health History

The patient, family, or significant other should be questioned closely about the patient's use of prescription and OTC drugs. Particular attention should be paid to any recently added drugs. Older adults are particularly prone to drug interactions, partly because of slower biotransformation of drugs and partly because of multidrug therapies for comorbid conditions. If patients are receiving care and prescriptions from several health care providers, the possibility of drug interactions increases.

Ask about a history of head injury, recent falls, headache, transient ischemic attacks (TIAs), or stroke. Has the patient ever felt numbness or clumsiness in one arm or leg? Has he or she ever been unable to speak for a brief period of time? Patients may have had episodes of ischemia to the brain without realizing what was happening. Multiple infarctions, whether symptomatic or not, may result in dementia. Also ask about use of alcohol and illicit drugs. Do not assume that an individual is not a substance abuser based simply on age.

Ask if anyone else in the family has had similar symptoms. Although Alzheimer's disease is not directly inherited, there is evidence to suggest a familial tendency. If the patient is unable to remember, it may be necessary to contact members of the extended family. This line of questioning should be approached with sensitivity. The possible diagnosis of Alzheimer's disease is frightening in itself. The possibility that it could affect several members of the family may be new information.

Lifespan Considerations

Perinatal. Alzheimer's disease is a disorder of late middle to old age. The gene associated with this disease is found on chromosome 21, the same chromosome responsible for Down's syndrome. Most individuals with Down's syndrome begin exhibiting changes in brain structure associated with Alzheimer's disease by 20 years of age. By the time these individuals reach 40 years of age, they may begin showing symptoms of Alzheimer's disease. Individuals with Down's syndrome may be the only population group to use drugs for the treatment of Alzheimer's disease during childbearing years, although the likelihood of such use is very small. No studies of the use of drugs in the treatment of Alzheimer's disease specifically targeting this group have been conducted.

Generally, drugs used in the treatment of Alzheimer's disease should be taken during pregnancy only if the benefit justifies the risk to the fetus. Although data is inconclusive, breast-feeding should be avoided.

Pediatric. Alzheimer's disease does not affect children. Drugs used in the treatment of the disease have not been widely studied as a treatment for childhood dementia.

Older Adults. Drugs approved for use in the treatment of Alzheimer's disease are used primarily by the older adult population. Alterations in body system functioning need to be taken into account.

Cultural/Social Considerations

Alzheimer's disease is a devastating disorder. Be sure to assess for its effect on family members. Determine their strengths and weaknesses, their ability to provide care for the patient, and their financial concerns. The caregiver burden is commonly found in families of Alzheimer's patients.

Physical Examination

Alzheimer's disease does not typically manifest as changes in physical examination findings. In the early stages, the patient has relatively normal physiologic function. As the disease progresses, however, the ability to walk, talk, and care for oneself deteriorates. Most patients are diagnosed in the first stage of the disease. A Mini-Mental State Examination may provide objective data for ongoing evaluation of the patient. Screening to determine the presence of depression assists in formulating an appropriate treatment plan.

Laboratory Testing

The definitive diagnosis of Alzheimer's disease can be made only by examining the brain for pathologic changes following the patient's death. However, most health care providers will rule out other causes of symptoms based on clinical examination and the findings of cognitive tests as well as by ruling out other causes of symptoms. Laboratory testing used to rule out other disorders includes blood chemistries, a complete blood cell count, determination of serum levels of vitamin B_{12}, and tests for syphilis and thyroid function. Neurofibrillary tangles and neuritic plaques can be identified on CT and MRI scans. A positron emission tomography (PET) scan may detect areas of the brain that have reduced metabolism.

A recently developed test shows promise in confirming the diagnosis of Alzheimer's disease. This test examines the amount of a protein called AD7C in the cerebrospinal fluid of the patient. This neural thread protein is believed to function in the regeneration of brain tissue and repair of neurons. Because patients with Alzheimer's disease have a pathologic degeneration of neurons, one would expect to find a higher level of neural thread protein in the cerebrospinal fluid. The AD7C test has detected elevations of the protein level in 80% to 90% of patients. The presence of Alzheimer's disease in these patients was confirmed at autopsy. AD7C has a low incidence rate of false positive results.

GOALS OF THERAPY

The goal of drug therapy is to slow the cognitive deterioration that inevitably occurs in patients with Alzheimer's disease. No treatment yet exists to reverse the progressive decline of the disease. Drug therapy may allow the patient to maintain a more independent lifestyle and lessen the burden on family and significant others. A longer duration of independence can promote family functioning, prevent caregiver burnout, and reduce the financial strain of placement in a skilled health care facility. The cost of cholinesterase inhibitors to treat Alzheimer's disease ultimately results in savings by significantly delaying institutionalization.

INTERVENTION
Administration

Drugs used in the treatment of Alzheimer's disease are initially administered in low doses; the dosage is then gradually increased as tolerated for optimal benefit.

Monitor the patient for adverse reactions and document the therapeutic response.

Tacrine should be taken between meals, although it is rarely used in current therapy, because it is more likely than the newer drugs to cause adverse reactions and drug interactions. Additionally, liver function tests must be monitored during tacrine therapy due to the significant risk of hepatotoxicity. Concurrent use of tacrine with cimetidine or theophylline should be avoided without careful monitoring of serum concentrations and dosage. The dosage of tacrine should not be decreased abruptly or therapy discontinued suddenly to avoid a relapse in patient symptoms.

Approximately 50% of patients taking tacrine will have at least one episode of an elevated ALT level. Of these patients, 25% will have elevations that are three times the upper limits of normal. Approximately 7% of patients taking tacrine have ALT levels ten times the upper limits of normal. The extreme elevation usually occurs 6 weeks from the time of the first elevation. Patients should be monitored biweekly for at least 6 weeks after any dosage increase. The ALT level ordinarily returns to normal 4 to 6 weeks after therapy is discontinued.

Donepezil should be taken just before bedtime. Administer rivastigmine with food in the morning and evening. Treatment with donepezil and rivastigmine requires monitoring for evidence of active or occult GI bleeding. Monitor the patient taking rivastigmine for severe nausea, vomiting, and diarrhea, which may lead to dehydration and weight loss.

CASE STUDY *Parkinson's Disease*

ASSESSMENT

HISTORY OF PRESENT ILLNESS

DP is a 75-year-old woman who complains of a general feeling of stiffness, mild to moderate tremors in both arms, and increasing difficulty dressing and eating. Her family noticed that her handwriting has changed and her speech is slower than normal. She does not exercise but has started to lose weight.

HEALTH HISTORY

DP denies allergies to food or drugs. Her last physical examination 6 years ago was unremarkable. She has mild arthritis and takes aspirin for discomfort. She denies a history of hospitalizations, illnesses, smoking, consumption of alcohol, or use of illicit drugs. Current drugs taken include 3 grains of aspirin prn for shoulder and knee discomfort (requires about four tablets per week).

LIFESPAN CONSIDERATIONS

Age-related physiologic changes to body systems.

CULTURAL/SOCIAL CONSIDERATIONS

DP retired from working in a grocery store at the age of 55. She is currently living in a retirement community with her husband, who is in good health. She has an attentive daughter and two grandchildren who live within 5 miles. They visit often. Her sister lives out of town.

PHYSICAL EXAMINATION

DP is 5'1" tall and weighs 93 lbs (5 lbs less than usual). Her vital signs are stable; she is afebrile. DP displays slight pill-rolling movements of the thumb against the fingers in the left hand with mild to moderate resting tremors and rigidity noted bilaterally. Her voice is low-pitched, and her speech is poorly articulated and lacks modulation.

LABORATORY TESTING

Chest x-ray study, ECG, MRI, CBC count, and electrolytes level are all within normal limits.

PATIENT PROBLEM(S)

Parkinson's disease; mild arthritis.

GOALS OF THERAPY

Reduce disease symptoms and enhance the quality of life. Maintain function and independence for as long as possible. Provide patient with lowest possible dosage effective in controlling symptoms.

CRITICAL THINKING QUESTIONS

1. The health care provider initially orders low-dose levodopa-carbidopa: half of scored 100-mg levodopa/25-mg carbidopa tablet daily. The dosage will be increased by half a tablet at weekly intervals until improvement or toxicities are noted. What is the mechanism of action of this drug combination?
2. What adverse effects should the nurse look for during levodopa-carbidopa therapy?
3. What rationale would you give the patient when providing education regarding abrupt cessation of levodopa-carbidopa therapy?
4. What is the on-off phenomenon often experienced by patients after long-term levodopa-carbidopa therapy?

Patients with clinical jaundice and a total bilirubin level over 3 mg/dL should have therapy discontinued, and a new trial period should not be attempted.

Education

The patient, family, and significant others need to understand that acetylcholinesterase inhibitors do not cure Alzheimer's disease. Explain to the patient and family that these drugs do not alter the underlying degenerative disease but rather slow the progression of the disease and alleviate symptoms. As the disease worsens, the effectiveness of cholinesterase inhibitors eventually declines. This fact should also be clearly explained. Mental stimulation and exercise can be effective in delaying functional decline.

The anticholinesterase drug should not be stored in a location accessible to the patient because of the possibility of overdose. Advise the patient and caregivers

---

CASE STUDY  *Myasthenia Gravis*

ASSESSMENT

HISTORY OF PRESENT ILLNESS

DD is a 56-year-old white man in moderate distress with complaints of blurred vision and an inability to open his left eye. These symptoms were first noticed when he returned home from sailing 2 days ago. He reports that bright sunlight worsens the droopy eyelid. He has noticed more fatigue recently than in the past. He states, "I'm just getting older." He jogs 2 miles a day, down from 5 miles a day 3 months ago. He follows a low-cholesterol diet.

HEALTH HISTORY

DD is allergic to aspirin and penicillin. He has no food allergies. His last physical examination was 1 year ago. He denies hospitalizations but has been told he has borderline high cholesterol. He denies history of alcohol, smoking, or illicit drug use. He takes no routine drugs.

LIFESPAN CONSIDERATIONS

DD is 56 years old with age-related physiologic changes to body systems. He has had no disabilities until recently.

CULTURAL/SOCIAL CONSIDERATIONS

DD is currently working as the manager of a local discount store. He is married and his wife is in excellent health. He is very health conscious and visits his physician twice a year for a complete physical.

PHYSICAL EXAMINATION

DD is 5'11" tall, and weighs 165 lbs. with no recent weight loss or gain. His vital signs are stable. Results of large Snellen are 20/200 corrected in both eyes (OU); ptosis of left eye is noted. Weakness noted in lifting and movement of the left shoulder only. Remainder of examination unremarkable.

LABORATORY TESTING

Result of edrophonium test is positive; DD's shoulder felt much better with improved strength, and ptosis and diplopia were lessened. CT scan and chest x-ray study show no presence of thymoma. ECG shows sinus bradycardia at a rate of 56 bpm. Antiacetylcholine receptor antibody titer is elevated.

PATIENT PROBLEM(S)

Stage 1 myasthenia gravis.

GOALS OF THERAPY

Alleviate current ocular problems, muscular weakness, and worsening fatigue. Achieve maximal benefit (muscle strength and endurance) with fewest adverse effects.

CRITICAL THINKING QUESTIONS

1. DD responds positively to a test dose of edrophonium. What is the rationale for diagnosing myasthenia gravis based on this test?
2. Pyridostigmine 600 mg po is ordered in divided doses to provide maximum relief. What is the mechanism of action of this drug?
3. What adverse effects should the nurse look for during pyridostigmine therapy?
4. The addition of low-dose prednisone will be considered based on patient response to pyridostigmine. What is the mechanism of action of prednisone?
5. What adverse effects should the nurse look for during prednisone therapy?

to report adverse effects or changes in overall health status immediately and to consult the health care provider before the patient takes any new prescribed or OTC drug. They should also be instructed to tell all health care providers, including dentists, about the patient's use of drugs to treat Alzheimer's disease because of special considerations in administering anesthesia.

Instruct the patient taking rivastigmine to report nausea, vomiting, or diarrhea. Instruct the patient and caregiver that tacrine should not be abruptly stopped because of possible behavioral disturbances and a decline in cognitive function.

EVALUATION

The effectiveness of therapy is evaluated by the patient's ability to perform activities of daily living, improvement in cognition, and a reduction in behavioral symptoms. The degree of supervision needed and the relative safety in performing tasks are evaluated. Many health care providers use the Mini-Mental State Examination as an objective measure of cognitive functioning. Although the family and significant others provide the most comprehensive information, the Mini-Mental State Examination is subjective in nature. Functional assessment may be colored by the strong desire for drug therapy to be effective.

CASE STUDY 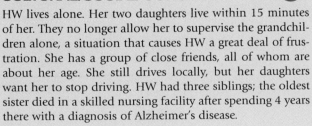 *Alzheimer's Disease*

ASSESSMENT

HISTORY OF PRESENT ILLNESS

HW is a 74-year-old Hispanic woman who states that she has developed some memory difficulty over the past 6 months. She also reports pain in her hips and knees. She is accompanied by two of her daughters. Her daughters state that their mother is experiencing significant memory and judgment impairment in addition to not maintaining her personal hygiene and diet as well as she did in the past.

HEALTH HISTORY

HW gives no significant medical history. She currently takes ibuprofen prn for joint pain. She denies use of alcohol or tobacco, which her daughters confirm.

LIFESPAN CONSIDERATIONS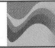

HW may have diminished effective hepatic function because of the changes of aging.

CULTURAL/SOCIAL CONSIDERATIONS

HW lives alone. Her two daughters live within 15 minutes of her. They no longer allow her to supervise the grandchildren alone, a situation that causes HW a great deal of frustration. She has a group of close friends, all of whom are about her age. She still drives locally, but her daughters want her to stop driving. HW had three siblings; the oldest sister died in a skilled nursing facility after spending 4 years there with a diagnosis of Alzheimer's disease.

PHYSICAL EXAMINATION

HW's vital signs are stable. Her daughters state that she has lost 5 lbs in the last 6 months. HW ambulates independently but slowly. She is essentially expressionless.

LABORATORY TESTING

MRI of the brain reveals neurofibrillary tangles and neuritic plaques. HW's Mini-Mental State Examination score is 26.

PATIENT PROBLEM(S)

Alzheimer's disease; osteoarthritis.

GOALS OF THERAPY

Slow the rate of cognitive deterioration as much as possible and allow patient to function as independently as possible.

CRITICAL THINKING QUESTIONS

1. Donepezil 5 mg po daily at bedtime has been ordered initially. The dosage will be increased to 10 mg after the first 4 to 6 weeks of therapy. What is the mechanism of action of this drug?
2. What adverse effects should the nurse look for during therapy with donepezil?
3. What education would you provide the patient and family regarding expectations from therapy with donepezil?
4. Why is it necessary to include family and significant others when obtaining a patient health history and during education regarding drug therapy?

Bibliography

Davitt BV, Fenton GA, Cruz OA: Childhood myasthenia, *J Ophthalmic Nurs Technol* (2):74-83, 2000.

Derbyshire M, Marsden V: Parkinson's disease: drug treatment in old age, *Elder Care* 11(2):31-34, 1999.

DiBartolo MC: Caregiver burden: instruments, challenges, and nursing implications for individuals with Alzheimer's disease and their caregivers, *J Gerontol Nurs* 26(6):46-53, 2000.

Dick A: Nursing care of Parkinson's disease, *Elder Care* 10(6):39-42, 1999.

Galvin T: Dysphagia: going down and staying down, *Am J Nurs* 99(6):44-47, 2001.

Goldsmith C: Clinical snapshot: Parkinson's disease, *Am J Nurs* 99(2):46-48, 1999.

Hagell P: Restorative neurology in movement disorders, *J Neurosci Nurs* 32(5):256-262, 2000.

Herndon CM, Young K, Herndon AD, et al: Parkinson's disease revisited, *J Neurosci Nurs* 32(4):216-221, 2000.

Hussar D: New drugs 2000: part II, *Nurs 2000* 30(6):20-28, 2000.

Jacobs LA, Deatrick JA: The individual, the family, and genetic testing, *J Prof Nurs* 15(5):313-324, 1999.

Kennedy-Malone LM, Loftus SL: Parkinson's disease, *Lippincott Prim Care Pract* 3(2):169-173, 1999.

Kernich CA, Kaminski HJ: Myasthenia gravis: pathophysiology, diagnosis and collaborative care, *J Neurosci Nurs* 27(4):207-218, 1995.

Korczyn A, Brunt E, Larsen J, et al: A 3-year randomized trial of ropinirole and bromocriptine in early Parkinson's disease, *Neurology* 53(2):364-370, 1999.

Lieberman A, Olanow C, Sethi K, et al: A multicenter trial of ropinirole as adjunct treatment for Parkinson's disease, *Neurology* 51(4):1057-1062, 1998.

Maier-Lorentz MM: Effective nursing interventions for the management of Alzheimer's disease, *J Neurosci Nurs* 32(3):153-157, 2000.

Maier-Lorentz MM: Neurobiological bases for Alzheimer's disease, *J Neurosci Nurs* 32(2):117-125, 2000.

Matheson A, Spencer C: Ropinirole: a review of its use in the management of Parkinson's disease, *Drugs* 60(1):115-137, 2000.

Mignor D: Effectiveness of use of home health nurses to decrease burden and depression of elderly caregivers, *J Psychosoc Nurs Ment Health Serv* 38(7):34-41, 2000.

New drugs of 2000, *J Am Pharm Assoc* 41(2):229-272, 2001.

O'Hanlon-Nichols T: Neurologic assessment, *Am J Nurs* 99(6):44-47, 1999.

Rascol O, Brooks D, Korczyn A, et al: A five-year study of the incidence of dyskinesia in patients with early Parkinson's disease who were treated with ropinirole or levodopa, *N Engl J Med* 342(20):1484-1491, 2000.

Ross AP: Neurologic degenerative disorders, *Nurs Clin North Am* 34(3):725-742, 1999.

Schrag A, Brooks D, Brunt E, et al: The safety of ropinirole, a selective nonergoline dopamine agonist, in patients with Parkinson's disease, *Clin Neuropharmacol* 21(3):169-175, 1998.

Schweiger J, Huey R: Alzheimer's disease: your role in the caregiving equation, *Nursing* 29(6):34-41, 1999.

Scott L, Goa K: Galantamine: a review of its use in Alzheimer's disease, *Drugs* 60(5):1065-1122, 2000.

Stahl S: The new cholinesterase inhibitors for Alzheimer's disease, part 1: their similarities are different, *J Clin Psychol* 61(10):710-711, 2000.

Steele CD: The genetics of Alzheimer disease, *Nurs Clin North Am* 35(3):687-694, 2000.

Tappen R, Roach K, Applegate E, et al: Walking and talking may slow the decline of Alzheimer's disease, *Alzheimer Dis Assoc Disord* 14:196-201, 2000.

Weuve J, Boult C, Morishita L: The effects of outpatient geriatric evaluation and management on caregiver burden, *Gerontologist* 40(4):429-436, 2000.

Zurad E: New treatments of Alzheimer disease: a review, *Drug Benefit Trends* 13(7):27-40, 2001.

Internet Resources

Birks J, Flicker L: Selegiline for Alzheimer's disease. In *The Cochrane Library*, Issue 2, Oxford, 2001, Update Software.

Birks J, Grimly E, Iakovidou V, et al: Rivastigmine for Alzheimer's disease. In *The Cochrane Library*, Issue 2, Oxford, 2001, Update Software.

Filho C, Birks J: Physostigmine for Alzheimer's disease. In *The Cochrane Library*, Issue 2, Oxford, 2001, Update Software.

The Medical Letter: Galantamine (Reminyl) for Alzheimer's disease (#1107). Available online at http://www.medical letter.com.

The Medical Letter: Rivastigmine (Exelon) for Alzheimer's disease. Available online at http://www.medicalletter.com.

The National Institute of Neurological Disorders and Stroke website on Huntington's disease. Available online at http://www.ninds.nih.gov/health_and_medical/disorders/huntington.htm.

The National Institute of Neurological Disorders and Stroke website on Alzheimer's disease. Available online at http://www.Ninds.nih.gov/health_and_medical/disorders/alzheimersdisease_doc.htm.

The National Library of Medicine Medline website for health information. Available online at http://www.nlm.nih.gov/medlineplus/parkinsondisease.html.

CHAPTER

24

Introduction to the Use of Antimicrobial Drugs

SHERRY F. QUEENER • KATHLEEN GUTIERREZ

 Visit http://evolve.elsevier.com/Gutierrez/ for additional information.

KEY TERMS

Acquired resistance, p. 381

Antibiotic-associated colitis, p. 385

Antimicrobial spectrum, p. 381

Bactericidal, p. 379

Bacteriostatic, p. 379

Minimum bactericidal concentration (MBC), p. 381

Minimum inhibitory concentration (MIC), p. 381

Plasmids, p. 381

Pyrogens, p. 379

Selective toxicity, p. 379

Septicemia, p. 379

Superinfections, p. 385

Therapeutic index (TI), p. 380

OBJECTIVES

- Discuss the principle of selective toxicity.
- Describe the difference between bactericidal and bacteriostatic drugs.
- Explain why antibiotic resistance can be passed between bacteria.
- Describe the factors that influence the outcome of antibiotic therapy.
- Outline important patient teaching points related to general use of antimicrobial drugs.

PATHOPHYSIOLOGY • Infectious Disease

Although the world of microbes was discovered by Anton Van Leeuwenhoek in 1676, the impact of these tiny organisms on human lives was not appreciated until the late 1800s. At this time Louis Pasteur and Robert Koch, working in separate laboratories and on different microorganisms, showed that bacteria could cause disease in humans. After these discoveries, microbiologists and physicians began to classify human diseases in terms of the organism that produced the disease. By the early 20th century, microorganisms that cause cholera, typhus, bubonic plague, gonorrhea, leprosy, malaria, syphilis, and other diseases had been identified. Today, ever increasing numbers of organisms are known to cause human diseases (Table 24-1). Infectious diseases that have emerged or been linked to a causative agent within the last 25 years include AIDS (caused by HIV), gastric ulcer (e.g., *Helicobacter pylori*), hemorrhagic fevers (e.g., Ebola virus and others), encephalitis (e.g., West Nile virus), and an acute fulminating pneumonia (e.g., Hanta virus).

Not all microbes are harmful; in fact, most microorganisms that live on or in the human body do not cause disease. Our normal microbial flora even have some beneficial effects, such as competing with and preventing more harmful organisms from becoming established. Bacteria in the bowel contribute to the body's energy production by digesting plant material that resists human digestive processes. These bacteria may also produce vitamin K, which can be absorbed by the host.

To cause disease, microbial pathogens must adhere to cell surfaces, colonize or invade the host, and proliferate. Humans have evolved a complex set of defense mechanisms to prevent these processes from occur-

---

TABLE 24-1

Microbial Pathogens of Humans

Organisms	Common Diseases Produced
Viruses	
Influenza	Flu and upper respiratory tract infection
Herpes simplex	Skin, eye, and brain infections
HIV	Immunodeficiency, AIDS
West Nile	Encephalitis
Chlamydia	Psittacosis, eye and genital infections
Rickettsia	Typhus, Q fever, Rocky Mountain spotted fever
Spirochetes	
Treponema pallidum	Syphilis
Borrelia burgdorferi	Lyme disease
Eubacteria, Gram-Negative	
Escherichia	Peritonitis, urinary tract infections
Haemophilus	Bronchitis, ear infections, meningitis, pneumonia, sinusitis
Klebsiella	Urinary tract infections
Neisseria	Gonorrhea, meningitis
Proteus	Urinary tract infections
Pseudomonas	Pneumonia (hospital-acquired), urinary tract infections, wound infections
Salmonella	Gastroenteritis, typhoid
Shigella	Dysentery
Eubacteria, Gram-Positive	
Enterococcus	Endocarditis, skin or wound infections
Staphylococcus	Empyema, soft tissue infections
Streptococcus	Pharyngitis, pneumonia
Mycobacteria	Leprosy, tuberculosis
Actinomycetes	Organ lesions and abscesses
Fungi	
Candida	Skin, mouth, or vaginal infections
Cryptococcus	Meningitis
Histoplasma	Pulmonary infection
Pneumocystis carinii	Pneumonia in immunosuppressed patients

ring, thus preventing disease. Nonspecific defenses include intact skin and mucous membranes as well as the ciliated epithelium of the respiratory tract that sweeps away most microorganisms attempting to attach to the surface. Chemical defenses include the strong acid of the stomach, which destroys many microorganisms before they can colonize the bowel, and enzymes found in tears or saliva that can damage or destroy bacteria. Microorganisms to which a person has been previously exposed may trigger a specific immune response. Specific antibodies or specific immune cells may target the microorganism and inactivate or destroy it.

These responses may occur without a person knowing he or she is under attack. In other situations, the attack may be painfully obvious because the pathogen evokes an inflammatory response (see Chapter 14). An inflammatory response can vary from a localized lesion surrounding an infected site in skin, with redness, tenderness, and swelling, to a systemic inflammatory response such as that seen in Lyme disease, which is caused by the spirochete *Borrelia burgdorferi*. Viruses may also cause symptoms by destroying specific cells in the human host. For example, HIV causes immunodeficiency by destroying T cells, and influenza causes upper respiratory disease by infecting respiratory tract epithelial cells.

A few important pathogens produce strong toxins that cause symptoms of disease. Exotoxins released by bacteria may cause severe local or systemic tissue damage. Examples include *Streptococcus pyogenes*, which releases a toxin that evokes shock; *Clostridium tetani*, which releases a toxin that targets nerves and causes paralysis; and *Escherichia coli* strain O157:H7, which releases a toxin that damages the kidneys. Other strains of *E. coli* release toxins with local actions on cells in the bowel, producing severe diarrhea. Endotoxins are components of the cell walls of gram-negative bacteria. These complex cell walls release endotoxins such as lipopolysaccharide (LPS) mostly when the bacteria die and the cell wall breaks down; these toxins are potent **pyrogens** (fever inducers) and may cause profound changes in the immune system of the host. **Septicemia** is a severe condition in which infection has spread into the blood. Endotoxins and exotoxins released during septicemia can contribute to the severe generalized symptoms of sepsis, which include impaired blood flow and shock; thus, sepsis is a severe, life-threatening condition.

STRATEGIES FOR CONTROLLING INFECTIOUS DISEASE

The realization that microbes cause disease allowed strategies for controlling infectious diseases to be developed. The first strategy was prevention. Thus when it was understood that bacteria in the feces of infected persons could contaminate water supplies and spread diseases such as cholera and typhoid fever, there was a strong impetus to protect public water supplies. These public health measures have prevented disease in millions of people and have saved innumerable lives.

The second strategy to control infectious disease was immunization (see Chapter 35). This approach prevented certain diseases, but immunization is not effective for all diseases, nor is it effective once the disease is established. Moreover, separate immunizations are needed for each disease.

The third strategy was to discover drugs that could destroy invading pathogens in a living patient. The validity of drug therapy for infectious diseases was established by Paul Ehrlich, who in 1912 introduced salvarsan, a drug for syphilis. In 1935 a synthetic drug that could cure streptococcal infections was discovered, and in 1939 research was begun on an extract of culture fluid from the mold Penicillium. These discoveries marked the beginnings of sulfonamides and penicillins, respectively. The search for more effective antimicrobial drugs has not ceased. As later chapters show, that search has been very fruitful.

Drug therapy of infectious disease is based on the principle of **selective toxicity**, that is, the selective poisoning of an invading disease-causing organism by a drug that has little or no effect on the person in whom the disease exists. Selective toxicity is possible because microbial pathogens differ in specific biochemical ways from their human hosts. Targeting these biochemical differences allows selective drug action. For example, beta-lactam antibiotics target cell wall synthesis in bacteria, but mammalian cells do not make cell walls. Thus beta-lactam antibiotics can affect pathogenic bacteria but have little direct effect on the tissues of infected patients. The exact mechanism of action of each antibiotic class will be covered in the individual chapters following this introduction, but the most important mechanisms by which antibiotics attack bacteria are summarized in Figure 24-1.

MEASURES OF ANTIBIOTIC EFFECTIVENESS
Bactericidal or Bacteriostatic Drugs

Antibiotics are classified not only by specific biochemical mechanisms but are also broadly divided into two categories. **Bactericidal** drugs directly kill bacteria. For example, antibiotics that block cell wall synthesis may cause the bacterium to explode because the osmotic forces within the cytoplasm can no longer be contained by the impaired cell wall. Likewise, antibiotics that disrupt the bacterial cell membranes allow the cytoplasmic contents of the bacterium to leak out, thus killing it. **Bacteriostatic** drugs halt bacterial reproduction without directly

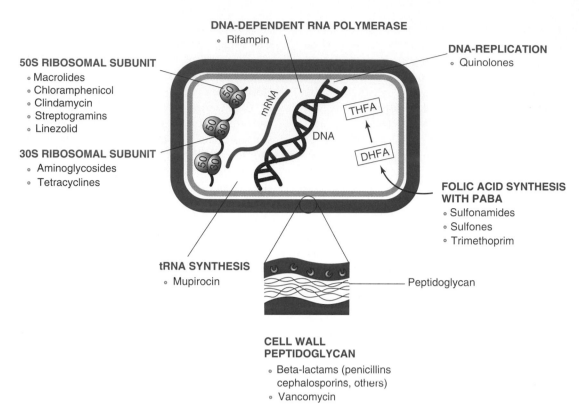

DNA-DEPENDENT RNA POLYMERASE
- Rifampin

DNA-REPLICATION
- Quinolones

50S RIBOSOMAL SUBUNIT
- Macrolides
- Chloramphenicol
- Clindamycin
- Streptogramins
- Linezolid

30S RIBOSOMAL SUBUNIT
- Aminoglycosides
- Tetracyclines

mRNA

DNA

THFA

DHFA

FOLIC ACID SYNTHESIS WITH PABA
- Sulfonamides
- Sulfones
- Trimethoprim

tRNA SYNTHESIS
- Mupirocin

Peptidoglycan

CELL WALL PEPTIDOGLYCAN
- Beta-lactams (penicillins cephalosporins, others)
- Vancomycin

FIGURE 24-1 Targets for antibiotic action. The mechanism of action of antibiotics depends on differences in structures and processes between the bacterial pathogen and the human host. Thus bacterial cell walls are effective targets for antibiotics because similar structures do not exist in humans. Likewise, folic acid synthesis is a good target because bacteria must synthesize the vitamin, whereas humans obtain it preformed. Other targets such as ribosomes or processes related to DNA or RNA are found both in humans and bacteria, but sufficient differences exist to allow the processes to be inhibited in bacteria with minimal effects in the host.

killing the bacteria; bacteria removed from exposure to these drugs can resume growth. The host's immune system must still immobilize and kill the pathogens for therapy with bacteriostatic drugs to achieve a long-term cure. In theory, bactericidal drugs can cure a patient regardless of immune function, but such cures are not easily achieved, especially in immunosuppressed patients. Even in patients with normal immune function and with appropriately prescribed bactericidal drugs, cures of bacterial disease depend strongly on immunologic factors.

To classify a drug as exclusively bactericidal or bacteriostatic may be misleading. Many antibiotics may act in either way, depending on the dose, the site of infection, and the causative organism. For example, sulfonamides are often bacteriostatic for systemic infections, but because of their high concentration in urine, they may be bactericidal for urinary tract infections. Some

microorganisms have greater sensitivity to a certain antibiotic. For the more sensitive organism, the serum and tissue levels achieved with normal dosage may produce bactericidal action, whereas a more resistant organism may simply suffer growth inhibition, a bacteriostatic effect, at that same concentration of antibiotic.

Therapeutic Index

No current drug is a perfectly selective agent for pathogens; at some dosage every antiinfective drug may cause a direct effect on the host. One way to evaluate the degree of selective toxicity that may be achieved with an antimicrobial drug is by means of the therapeutic index (see Chapter 1). The **therapeutic index (TI)** when applied to antibiotics is usually defined as the ratio of the amount of drug that kills 50% of the test animals (lethal dose, or LD) to the amount of that drug that is effective in 50% of the animals (effective dose, or ED); this is expressed as $TI = LD_{50}/ED_{50}$. A drug that is relatively nontoxic may require very large dosages to kill the test animals. If the drug is also potent, it may require only a small dosage to achieve the desired clinical effect, which in this case is to cure the infection. Such a drug would have a large TI and would be considered to display good selective toxicity: it attacks the pathogen at dosages much smaller than those that are dangerous to the host. In contrast, a drug with low TI would not have good selective toxicity. A drug with a TI of 1 would be equally toxic to the bacteria and to the patient.

The TI is derived from studies on laboratory animals. Because correlating animal studies with the clinical effectiveness of a drug is sometimes difficult, other ways of expressing selective toxicity have been used to indicate clinical experience with a drug. For example, the safety margin of a drug is the percentage increase above the standard therapeutic dose that is required to produce serious toxic reactions in a certain percentage of patients. This evaluation is based entirely on clinical experience.

A drug with a large TI and a wide safety margin may be given to patients in larger-than-normal dosages without causing significant toxicity in most patients. The antibiotics gentamicin and penicillin G can be used to illustrate this principle. Gentamicin must be given in carefully controlled doses because it can damage the kidneys if the concentration in the blood becomes too high. Gentamicin has such a low TI and narrow safety margin that increasing the dose by 50% may cause significant toxicity (see Chapter 29). In contrast, penicillin G has a very wide safety margin and a high TI. Direct toxicity with this drug is infrequent, and doses three or four times the standard dose may be administered with little risk of toxic reactions in most patients (see Chapter 25).

Antibiotic Susceptibility Testing

The **antimicrobial spectrum** is the range of microbes against which the drug is effective. Table 24-1 lists common pathogenic microorganisms according to criteria set by microbiologists. A drug effective against only a few of these organisms has a narrow spectrum, such as penicillin G, which is primarily effective against gram-positive bacteria. In contrast, a drug that can be used against several groups of organisms has a broad spectrum, such as tetracycline, which is effective against gram-positive and gram-negative bacteria as well as against obligate intracellular pathogens such as Rickettsia and Chlamydia.

For each antibiotic and microorganism, it is possible to determine in the laboratory the amount of a given drug required to halt the growth of the organism (**minimum inhibitory concentration, or MIC**) and the amount required to kill the organism (**minimum bactericidal concentration, or MBC**). The MIC and the MBC are the lowest concentrations at which growth inhibition or cell death, respectively, can be observed. A consideration of these figures and determination of a safe blood level for an antibiotic help determine an effective therapeutic regimen. For example, a blood concentration above the MBC is desirable, but whether that concentration can be obtained depends on the pharmacokinetic properties governing drug absorption and elimination and the threshold for toxicity produced by the drug in the host.

FACTORS AFFECTING OUTCOMES OF ANTIBIOTIC THERAPY
Microbial Resistance to Antibiotics

Not all microorganisms are sensitive to antibiotics. Resistance to antibiotics may be inherent or acquired. *Inherent resistance* to an antibiotic is a stable genetic trait. For example, *Pseudomonas aeruginosa* is resistant to penicillin G in part because the drug cannot penetrate the cell wall complex of this gram-negative bacteria. This property does not change significantly over time or as a result of exposure to penicillin G.

In contrast, **acquired resistance** represents a genetic change that converts a previously drug-sensitive bacteria to a drug-resistant one. *Staphylococcus aureus* is a good example of the clinical importance of acquired resistance. Strains of this bacteria isolated from clinical infections during the 1940s, before penicillin use became widespread, were almost always sensitive to the drug. However, present-day clinically isolated *S. aureus* strains are mainly resistant. Resistance can also be acquired on a much shorter time scale. An example is the drug ciprofloxacin. When originally introduced, this drug was active against many gram-negative bacteria, including *P. aeruginosa*, and against gram-positive bacteria, including methicillin-resistant *S. aureus*. Within a year, however, some institutions reported widespread resistance to the drug.

One particularly important mechanism for acquiring antibiotic resistance is shown in Figure 24-2. **Plasmids** are small circular pieces of DNA separate from the bacterial chromosome. They may be created by transposons, which are small segments of DNA that move freely in and out of the chromosome. Many different kinds of plasmids exist, and not all bacteria contain them. Plasmids are of concern in medicine because many carry genes for antibiotic resistance and may be rapidly passed between bacterial cells. These two features allow antibiotic resistance to spread quickly through an entire bacterial population. This mechanism for acquired resistance often causes serious therapeutic problems because resistance to several antibiotics may occur at once.

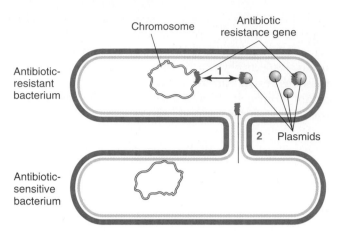

FIGURE 24-2 Transfer of antibiotic resistance. The transfer of genes for antibiotic resistance depends upon the presence of plasmids and upon two processes: (1) transposon carries the antibiotic-resistance gene in or out of the bacterial chromosome, in some cases transferring it to a plasmid with the ability to move from one bacterial cell to another by conjugation; (2) the process of conjugation showing transfer of antibiotic resistance to a previously sensitive bacterium. Plasmids replicate along with the bacteria, assuring that resistance to the antibiotic will be present in the progeny of the originally infected cell.

Microbiologists have recently discovered that plasmids can be shared between distantly related bacteria normally found in the human gastrointestinal (GI) tract. This disturbing fact shows us that if any bacteria is resistant to a drug, the gene for that resistance may be acquired by many bacteria, given enough time and exposure to the drug (Box 24-1).

The mechanisms by which microorganisms achieve resistance to an antibiotic may be divided into three categories. Destruction of the antibiotic by the microorganism usually involves enzymes that chemically alter and thereby inactivate the drug. Examples of this process include penicillinase, which destroys penicillin, and the acetylase, phosphorylase, and adenylating enzymes that inactivate the aminoglycoside antibiotics.

Bacteria may also achieve antibiotic resistance by reducing the uptake of the drug into the bacterial cell. Many antibiotics freely enter and in some cases become concentrated within bacterial cells. Resistance is achieved by blocking this uptake. An example of this type of resistance is tetracycline, which can freely enter sensitive bacteria but not resistant strains.

The third mechanism for resistance involves a mutation or an alteration in the target of the antibiotic in the

| BOX **24-1** | **Are We Losing the Battle Against Infectious Disease?** |

The question of whether we are losing the battle against infectious disease has been posed often in newspapers and magazines in the last few years. The answer is not simple. For most patients receiving antibiotics for acute conditions, therapy is effective. For a small but increasing number of patients, however, therapy fails and often it fails spectacularly. The most worrisome failures are when a well-known organism with a new pattern of resistance causes the infection. For example, *Staphylococcus aureus*, a gram-positive bacterium that causes serious soft tissue infections, first developed resistance to penicillin. Then strains resistant to methicillin, a drug specifically developed to treat *S. aureus*, began to appear and spread. Now in many places, the only antibiotic still effective against *S. aureus* is vancomycin. Vancomycin has also been the last resort for strains of *Enterococcus faecium* or *E. faecalis* that have become resistant to beta-lactam antibiotics, but vancomycin resistance has now appeared in enterococci and other bacteria. Genes for vancomycin resistance are carried on plasmids and are passed between strains of enterococci. It is expected that the genes for vancomycin resistance will in time pass to *S. aureus*, and in the not too distant future, an outbreak of totally drug-resistant *S. aureus* could occur. The appearance of these highly resistant bacteria is driving the development of new drugs that are just beginning to appear (see Chapter 30).

microorganism. For example, methicillin-resistant *S. aureus* and penicillin-resistant *Streptococcus pneumoniae* (see Box 24-1) both produce altered forms of the enzymes that make cell walls. These altered enzymes no longer bind methicillin, penicillin, or related antibiotics. As a result, those drugs no longer inhibit their cell wall synthesis.

Several strategies have been suggested to limit the development of antibiotic-resistant bacteria (Box 24-2). In general, all the strategies are aimed at lessening the selective pressure that causes bacteria to gain antibiotic resistance. Thus antibiotics should be used only for specific, medically justified purposes, and when used for therapy, they should be used at fully effective doses for adequate periods of time. The use of antibiotics for prophylaxis, that is, to prevent infection, is only appropriate in certain clearly defined circumstances, such as when a patient has special risk factors (e.g., immune

| BOX 24-2 | The CDC's Public Health Action Plan to Combat Antimicrobial Resistance |

The Centers for Disease Control and Prevention's Public Health Action Plan to Combat Antimicrobial Resistance was developed by an interagency task force created in 1999. The task force members include the following agencies:

Centers for Disease Control and Prevention
Food and Drug Administration
The National Institutes of Health, which include the following:
  Agency for Healthcare Research and Quality
  Centers for Medicare/Medicaid Services (formerly Health Care Financing Administration)
  Health Resources and Services Administration
  Department of Agriculture
  Department of Defense
  Department of Veterans Affairs
  Environmental Protection Agency

Action Plan

The Action Plan reflects a broad-based consensus of federal agencies on actions needed to address antimicrobial resistance (AR). The plan will be implemented incrementally, depending on the availability of resources. Part I of the Action Plan focuses on domestic issues such as surveillance, prevention, control, research, and product development. Since AR transcends national borders and requires a global approach to its prevention and control, Part II of the plan will identify actions that more specifically address international issues.

Surveillance

Unless AR problems are detected as they emerge, and actions are taken to quickly contain them, the world may soon be faced with previously treatable diseases that have again become untreatable, as in the preantibiotic era. Priority goals and action items in this focus area include the following:

1. Developing and implement a coordinated national plan for AR surveillance
2. Ensuring the availability of reliable drug susceptibility data for surveillance
3. Monitoring patterns of antimicrobial drug use
4. Monitoring AR in agricultural settings to protect the public's health by ensuring a safe food supply as well as animal and plant health

Prevention and Control

The prevention and control of drug-resistant infections requires measures to promote the appropriate use of antimicrobial drugs and prevent the transmission of infections (whether drug resistant or not). Priority goals and action items in this focus area address the following challenges:

1. Extending the useful life of antimicrobial drugs through appropriate use policies that discourage overuse and misuse
2. Improving diagnostic testing practices
3. Preventing infection transmission through improved infection control methods and use of vaccines
4. Preventing and controlling emerging AR problems in agriculture as well as human and veterinary medicine
5. Ensuring that comprehensive programs to prevent and control AR involve a wide variety of nonfederal partners and the public so that these programs become a part of routine practice nationwide.

Research

Basic and clinical research provide the fundamental knowledge necessary to develop appropriate responses to AR emerging and spreading in hospitals, communities, farms, and the food supply. Priority goals and action items in this area focus on the following:

1. Increasing understanding of microbial physiology, ecology, genetics, and mechanisms of resistance
2. Augmenting the existing research infrastructure to support a critical number of researchers in AR and related fields
3. Translating research findings into clinically useful products, such as novel approaches to detecting, preventing, and treating antimicrobial resistant infections

Product Development

As antimicrobial drugs lose their effectiveness, new products must be developed to prevent, rapidly diagnose, and treat infections. The priority goals and action items in this focus area address the following issues:

1. Ensuring that researchers and drug manufacturers are informed of current and projected gaps in the arsenal of antimicrobial drugs, vaccines, and diagnostics and of potential markets for these products
2. Stimulating the development of priority AR products for which market incentives are inadequate, while fostering their appropriate use
3. Optimizing the development and use of veterinary drugs and related agricultural products that reduce the transfer of resistance to pathogens that can affect humans

Health care providers can obtain more information about this vital project from the Centers for Disease Control and Prevention at http://www.cdc.gov/drugresistance/actionplan/html/.

suppression) or during procedures known to have a high risk of infection (e.g., pelvic surgery or repair of a penetrating wound to the abdomen). The use of low doses of antibiotics for prophylaxis in other circumstances favors selection of resistant organisms with little offsetting benefit for the patient. Another factor possibly contributing to the development of antibiotic-resistant bacteria is the use of antibiotics in animals not only to control infections, but also to promote growth. Scientists have long suspected that the widespread use of tetracyclines in farm animals led to increased tetracycline resistance in bacteria found in humans (see Chapter 28). Recently, a specific antibiotic used to promote growth in farm animals in Europe was linked to the appearance of vancomycin-resistant enterococci that were found in meat products for human consumption and then were also found in humans. These enterococci are serious human pathogens because vancomycin has been the only drug effective against enterococci in many circumstances (see Chapter 30). In this case, the antibiotic used to treat the animals was known to produce vancomycin resistance in enterococci, although the drug was not vancomycin. Thus agricultural practices can have significant public health consequences.

Identity of the Organism Causing the Infection

The first step in antimicrobial therapy is to identify the microorganism causing the disease. In some infections, the symptoms are clear enough to allow accurate diagnosis with a physical examination only. In other cases, a culture must be grown to identify the organism. At some institutions, nursing personnel are trained to take specimens for culture, whereas in others laboratory personnel or physicians perform this function.

The second step in treatment is to select the proper antibiotic, a process that depends on knowledge of the pathogen involved. This decision may be based entirely on clinical experience or aided by antibiotic susceptibility testing carried out in the microbiology laboratory on the pathogen isolated from the patient.

Site of Infection

After the proper drug has been selected, there are still several factors that influence the effectiveness of therapy. One factor is the site of infection. For example, meningitis is difficult to treat partly because many antibiotics do not penetrate the blood-brain barrier very well, making an effective drug concentration difficult to achieve at the infection site. Similarly, many abscesses or soft tissue infections are not easily treated, because the areas of infection are poorly perfused, and many

drugs do not penetrate well into these areas. Healing is often hastened by surgical drainage.

Other Drugs

Other drugs the patient is receiving may influence the outcome of antimicrobial therapy. Immunosuppressant drugs, including glucocorticoids, limit antibiotic effectiveness by depressing immune mechanisms that ordinarily assist in clearing the infection. The use patterns of antibiotics can also influence resistance. For example, resistance to ciprofloxacin is more likely in settings where ciprofloxacin or its chemical relatives have been widely used.

Clinical Status of the Patient

A patient's clinical status can alter the outcome of antimicrobial therapy. For example, renal function is important because many antibiotics are excreted by the kidney. If renal function is impaired, drugs eliminated through the kidney may accumulate. Likewise, hepatic disease may cause accumulation of drugs that are eliminated primarily by liver mechanisms. Patients with insufficiencies in these organ systems must be watched closely for signs of drug toxicity, which may occur at dosages lower than normal. Resistance to antibiotics is also more common in patients with certain chronic diseases, such as cystic fibrosis. These patients are likely to have received multiple courses of antibiotic therapy, which also increases the risk of developing antibiotic resistance.

PROBLEMS IN ANTIBIOTIC THERAPY
Direct Toxicity

Each antibiotic should be considered for its potential toxicity to the patient when it is given. The signs of direct toxicity are often highly characteristic for a given class of drugs. For example, any aminoglycoside antibiotic can cause kidney damage and loss of hearing or balance. When any of these drugs are given, the patient should be observed closely for these toxic signs. Even drugs with a high TI sometimes cause direct toxic reactions. For example, at high enough dosages penicillin can have direct effects on the central nervous system (CNS). Health care providers should be alert to these signs. Direct toxic reactions to antibiotics are often dose dependent and would be expected to be more common and serious when high dosages are given or when drug accumulation occurs in patients with renal or hepatic impairment.

Allergic Reactions

Allergies commonly occur with several antibiotics. Allergies develop in patients who have previously been exposed to the antibiotic or compounds chemically related to it. Prior medical use is the most common exposure, but other exposures are possible. Environmental exposure may be direct, as in workers in the antibiotic industry, or more subtle. For example, food animals intended for immediate slaughter may not be treated with antibiotics used in humans, but meat occasionally contains sufficient residues of antibiotics to sensitize some people who consume it.

Allergic reactions range from simple skin reactions such as urticaria (hives) to more serious generalized reactions. Anaphylaxis is an acute, life-threatening allergic reaction that may involve closing of the airway and cardiovascular collapse (see Chapter 1). Beta-lactam antibiotics (see Chapter 25) are known to cause this reaction as well as other allergies, but anaphylaxis is rare.

Superinfections

Superinfections are infections that arise during antibiotic therapy. By definition, they involve microorganisms resistant to the antibiotic originally used; thus superinfections are often serious and difficult to treat. Such infections are more common with broad-spectrum than with narrow-spectrum antibiotics, because broad-spectrum antibiotics eliminate much more of the natural bacterial flora and upset the ecologic controls that normally keep resistant pathogens in check. With tetracyclines, for example, yeasts such as *Candida* are often involved in superinfections.

Antibiotic-Associated Colitis

Broad-spectrum antibiotics and, in particular, antibiotics that destroy anaerobic bacteria in the bowel may upset the balance of organisms and cause diarrhea. When this condition is mild, discontinuation of the antibiotic may be sufficient to control symptoms. Occasionally, however, the destruction of normal bacteria in the bowel leads to the overgrowth of *Clostridium difficile*, an organism that produces a powerful toxin capable of eroding the cells lining the GI tract. This serious condition is a form of pseudomembranous colitis, or antibiotic-associated colitis, and must be treated with specific antibiotics such as metronidazole (see Chapters 30 and 34) or vancomycin (see Chapter 30), to kill *C. difficile* and stop toxin production.

MISUSE OF ANTIBIOTICS
Viral Infections

One common misconception is that antibiotics can cure any type of infectious disease, including those caused by viruses. In fact, no effective drugs yet exist to treat minor viral infections such as colds or sore throats (see Chapter 31). It is not always easy to distinguish these viral infections from bacterial infections that might respond to antibiotics, and patients often request antibiotics for every cold or sore throat they experience. Patients should be reassured that supportive therapy can be the best course of action in the absence of evidence for bacterial infection.

Early Discontinuation of Antibiotics

Many infections resolve quickly once appropriate antibiotics are administered. Thus it is tempting for patients to discontinue the drug as soon as they feel better. This practice is dangerous for several reasons. Antibiotics with bacteriostatic action inhibit growth of bacteria, but the bacteria remain alive, at least until the immune system can eliminate them. Therefore if therapy is stopped too early, these organisms may resume growth and relapse may occur. Not only does this prolong recovery, but it may also make the disease more difficult to treat. The bacteria most resistant to the drugs used are the ones that probably survive longest, and it is these resistant organisms that may cause the relapse. Therapy may therefore be more difficult because some degree of drug resistance has occurred.

One excuse often given when patients stop antibiotic therapy early is that they wish to have the drug on hand in case they ever need it again. This practice is dangerous not only for the reasons just discussed but also because it assumes that patients can diagnose future illnesses accurately. Self-treatment with old, unused antibiotic prescriptions may delay proper medical attention and prolong or worsen the patient's disease. Once drug therapy has been started, culture results become unreliable and proper diagnosis may be impossible. Patients should be discouraged from saving previously prescribed antibiotics to take them just until they can get to the doctor.

Instability of Stored Antibiotics

Many drugs require special storage conditions and do not remain active for long when exposed to the warm, humid environment of most bathroom medicine cabinets (see Chapter 5). For example, tetracyclines tend to be light-sensitive and break down to toxic compounds, making old preparations not only less effective but more likely to cause reactions.

Sharing Antibiotics with Children

Young children may be much more sensitive than adults to certain antibiotics. Thus antibiotics should never be given to children without first consulting a health care provider. By the same token, any antibiotic that remains in the household may be a hazard to children. Proper use and disposal of all drugs is important to protect children from accidental poisoning (see Chapter 5).

APPLICATION TO PRACTICE

ASSESSMENT
History of Present Illness

The patient with an infection typically displays the five cardinal signs and symptoms of infection, which include swelling, redness, pain, heat, and loss of function. If there is a wound, there may be purulent drainage and a foul odor. Although systemic signs and symptoms such as fever and malaise may occur, medical attention is generally sought because the pain has become unbearable or the loss of function has seriously affected the patient's activities of daily living.

Health History

A thorough health history may reveal previous hypersensitivity reactions. The patient should be questioned for clues regarding general health, nutritional status, comorbid disease, living conditions, drug use, hygiene, sexual practices, and environmental exposure to potential pathogens.

Lifespan Considerations

Perinatal. The physiologic changes that occur during pregnancy alter the pharmacokinetics of many drugs, including antimicrobial drugs. Drug dosages may be altered because of the overall increase in body fluids during pregnancy and changes in drug absorption and renal function. When assessing pregnant women, attention should be given to the length of gestation. Many drugs can be safely given only during a specific period.

Pediatric. The immature body systems of the fetus, neonate, and child should be considered when assessing the pediatric patient. Since most drugs are biotransformed in the liver and eliminated through the kidneys, there is the potential for accumulation and toxicity.

Older Adults. The aging process causes the liver and kidneys of older adults to function at a reduced level, similar to that of the immature system seen in pediatric patients. The potential for hepatotoxicity and renal toxicity from drug therapy increase as function decreases. Dosages are adjusted based on results of liver and kidney function tests according to guidelines in the package insert for each drug.

Cultural/Social Considerations

Overall, the cultural and social considerations associated with the use of antimicrobials are minimal. In most cases, infections are short-term, subacute conditions easily treated on an outpatient basis. Hospitalization may be required for serious, potentially life-threatening infections.

Compared with other classes of drugs, many of the antimicrobial drugs, particularly the newer ones, are relatively expensive. The rising cost of antibiotics presents a hardship to many, especially older adults, those who are financially disadvantaged, and those who have pharmacy insurance plans through managed care organizations. Additionally, some of the antimicrobial drugs require expensive laboratory follow-up testing. Because health care insurance systems are in flux and many payment systems are inadequate, the rising cost of antimicrobials, indeed of all drugs, is a major economic concern.

Physical Examination

The physical examination usually reveals signs and symptoms of infection. A thorough examination is particularly necessary to detect any infection traveling indirectly from a distant body site (e.g., a total joint replacement of the hip may fail as a result of a cut finger that became infected). Swelling is usually seen. Although serous fluid is lost initially, protein is lost later, leading to further edema. Pain is felt as fluid exudate causes pressure and subsequent ischemia. Chemical irritation of nerve endings by bradykinins and prostaglandins contributes to the pain of infection. There may be a loss of function of the involved body part as a consequence of swelling and pain. Vital signs may reveal systemic signs (e.g., fever and tachycardia) of infection.

Laboratory Testing

Ideally, before antimicrobial therapy is started, a specimen from the area of infection should be cultured to identify the specific pathogen. The pathogen is then tested for antibiotic sensitivity. Obtaining results of culture and sensitivity testing requires 48 to 72 hours. Other factors, including the drug's ability to penetrate infected tissue, microbial resistance, toxicity, the patient's clinical status, and cost are also used to guide antibiotic selection.

Many antimicrobials have harsh adverse effects on the kidneys, liver, or hearing. Therefore, once drug therapy is started, close monitoring is necessary to reduce the risk of toxicities. Monitoring for nephrotoxicity includes obtaining blood samples for blood urea nitrogen (BUN), creatinine, proteins, and intake and output measurements.

The status of the liver is monitored with liver function tests. Bilirubin and urobilinogen levels provide information about the metabolism and excretion of bile pigments. Albumin and many globulins synthesized by the liver can influence and are influenced by drugs. Blood clotting tests, such as that of prothrombin time

(PT), demonstrate a reduced synthesis of vitamin K–dependent clotting factors by the liver. There are many liver enzymes that are released into the blood when there is liver damage. The ones most commonly used to monitor liver function are alkaline phosphatase, aspartate transaminase (AST), and alanine transaminase (ALT). Alkaline phosphatase is elevated in patients with obstruction of bile flow, as in cholestatic jaundice, although certain drugs can cause this disorder. Ototoxicity is monitored with audiometric tests.

GOALS OF THERAPY

The goals of antimicrobial therapy are to ameliorate the signs and symptoms of infection, to prevent sepsis and death, and to prevent complications associated with therapy. Treatment objectives are achieved through accurate diagnosis, use of the appropriate antimicrobial drug, and close monitoring for adverse effects and toxicities. Although a number of antimicrobials can be considered to treat an infection, the clinical efficacy, adverse effect profile, pharmacokinetic disposition, and cost ultimately guide the choice. Once a drug has been selected, the dosage is based on patient size, site of infection, route of elimination, and other factors such as the likelihood of drug resistance.

Multidrug antimicrobial therapy may be warranted when the infection is known or thought to be caused by multiple organisms. This therapy may also be used for a serious infection in which a combination of drugs would be synergistic. The likely emergence of drug-resistant organisms may also warrant combination therapy. Finally, fever or other evidence that the patient is immunosuppressed may also create a need for this form of therapy. There are, however, disadvantages. There is an increased risk of allergic and toxic reactions, as well as possible antagonism of antimicrobial effects. There may also be an increased risk of superinfection and increased cost. For these reasons, multidrug therapy is employed only when clearly warranted.

INTERVENTION
Administration

Before the first dose of an antimicrobial drug is given, the patient's history should be carefully reviewed for allergies. Try to determine whether any previous events were true hypersensitivity reactions or merely GI irritation that the patient has interpreted as an allergy. Ampicillin, for example, may cause a benign macular skin eruption rather than urticaria. This rash is not a sign of allergy but may be reported as an allergy by the patient. Keep in mind that a negative history of hypersensitivity does not preclude future reactions.

Once the offending organism has been identified, the first dose of an antimicrobial drug may be given. In the case of antibiotics, an initial dose that is larger than usual (called a loading dose) is sometimes given to start the bacteriostatic or bactericidal action against the pathogen. A maintenance dose is used to continue eradication of the pathogens.

Many antimicrobial drugs taken orally cause GI distress. To decrease this distress, some drugs can be taken with food, despite the delay in absorption. Antimicrobial drugs to be taken on an empty stomach should be administered 1 hour before or 2 hours after meals. Acidic fruit juices or beverages should be avoided within 1 hour of taking most drugs. Many drugs differ with regard to route of administration. For example, penicillin G sodium is administered intramuscularly or intravenously; the potassium formulation is given by mouth; benzathine penicillin is given orally or intramuscularly; and procaine formulations are only administered intramuscularly. Before administering the drug, be sure to check carefully that the route ordered is correct for the individual drug.

Intramuscular administration of some antimicrobial drugs results in irritation of local tissues. Warn the patient that the injection may be painful. To help reduce potential tissue irritation, the drug should be reconstituted (when necessary) according to the manufacturer's recommendations. Other measures that can be used to reduce local tissue irritation include the selection of a large muscle site (e.g., dorsal gluteal), rotation of injection sites, and use of the Z-track technique.

Some antimicrobial drugs may cause phlebitis or thrombophlebitis when administered intravenously. To reduce site irritation, the drug is reconstituted and administered in the time frame recommended by the manufacturer. Further, many drugs require properly buffered solutions for stability; thus not all are compatible with common intravenous fluids. The health care provider should check the package insert or ask the pharmacist before adding a drug to any such fluid. The insertion site should be assessed frequently for signs and symptoms of inflammation and the site changed every 3 days or according to agency policy.

The patient should be observed closely for anaphylaxis for at least 30 minutes after the first dose of a parenteral antimicrobial drug is given. Anaphylaxis is most likely to occur with parenteral use and often manifests as nausea, vomiting, pruritus, tachycardia, severe dyspnea, diaphoresis, stridor, vertigo, loss of consciousness, and peripheral circulatory failure. As the process continues, respiration is impaired because of bronchospasm and laryngeal edema. Basic management of the patient with anaphylaxis includes maintenance of a patent airway and intravenous access, oxygen, and administration of epinephrine. If an airway is not maintained and supplemental oxygen is not provided, the patient will die of respiratory failure. Glucocorticosteroids, vasopressors, plasma, and CPR may be required for some patients. The best way to control anaphylaxis is to prevent it from happening in the first place, but this is not always possible.

Monitor patients on antimicrobial therapy for possible superinfection, especially older adults and debilitated patients as well as those receiving immunosuppressants or radiation therapy. Monitor these patients closely, especially for fever. Evidence of superinfection (e.g., diarrhea, vaginal or anal itching, black furry appearance of the tongue) should be reported. Superinfection by *Candida* organisms can usually be managed by discontinuing the antibiotics or by administering an antifungal drug.

Education

Patients should be taught about their drugs. Knowledge is helpful in improving the compliance with the treatment regimen. It is important for patients to understand that antimicrobial drugs are to be taken precisely as prescribed in dosage, frequency, and for the specified time (usually 10 days), even though symptoms may abate before the full course of therapy is completed. For example, if a cephalosporin antibiotic is prescribed every 6 hours, it should be taken as much as possible every 6 hours (not breakfast, lunch, dinner, bedtime), or the drug level in the blood will not be adequately maintained to fight the pathogens. If the blood level of the drug drops because of a late dose or discontinuing the drug too soon, the pathogens have an opportunity to increase in virulence or become resistant to the drug. Oral suspensions of an antibiotic should be refrigerated.

If a dose is missed, it should be taken as soon as remembered unless it is almost time for the next dose. The health care provider should be contacted before other drugs are used to avoid drug-drug interactions. Advise the patient that sharing the antimicrobial with friends or family members, particularly young children, can be dangerous.

Patients should be instructed to report any signs or symptoms of allergic response. Some antimicrobials may initially cause dizziness; thus caution is warranted when driving or operating machinery until the response to the drug is known. Patients with an antimicrobial drug allergy should be advised to wear some form of identification (e.g., medical alert tag or bracelet) to inform health care personnel of the allergy. Carrying the identification in a wallet or purse is usually not helpful if emergency care is needed.

In addition, patients should be taught what signs and symptoms to report to the health care provider. Patients should watch for signs and symptoms of serious adverse effects and toxicities such as nephrotoxicity, neurotoxicity, and hepatotoxicity. Advise the patient to notify the health care provider if GI reactions are severe or persistent.

Because the effects of contraceptives are reduced when taking selected antimicrobial drugs, patients should be advised to use a second form of birth control during treatment and for up to 2 weeks after completing the drug regimen.

Another vital consideration is to educate health care providers about strategies that are underway at the federal level to combat antimicrobial resistance. A number of federal agencies have implemented an incremental action plan addressing antimicrobial resistance (see Box 24-2). Specific information about each of the five action plan areas (i.e., surveillance, prevention, control, research, and product development) can be obtained through the Centers for Disease Control and Prevention website (see Internet Resources).

EVALUATION

Antimicrobial effectiveness is determined by monitoring clinical response and laboratory test results. The frequency of monitoring is proportional to the severity of the infection. Important clinical indicators of effective treatment include a reduction in fever and resolution of the signs and symptoms of infection, vital signs that return to normal, WBC counts that returns to normal limits, and a culture and sensitivity test that is negative for the offending organism. Further proof may include an increase in appetite, energy level, and general sense of well-being.

Bibliography

Gillan J: A prescription for disaster . . . potluck prescribing of antibiotics, *Nurs Times* 95(44):22, 1999.
Gillan J: We must curb antibiotic resistance, *Nurs Times* 96(40):17, 2000.
Nollette KA: Antimicrobial resistance, *J Am Acad Nurs Pract* 12(7):286-299, 2000.

Internet Resources

World Health Organization website on antibiotic resistance. Available online at http://www.who.int/inf-pr-2000/en/pr2000-41.html and http://www.who.int/inf-pr-2000/en/pr2000-43.html.
Merck Manual websites on antibiotic-associated colitis. Available online at http://www.merck.com/pubs/mmanual/section3/chapter29/29a.htm and http://www.merck.com/pubs/mmanual_home/sec9/109.htm.
Centers for Disease Control website on emerging infectious disease. Available online at http://www.cdc.gov/ncidod/eid/index.htm.

Penicillins, Cephalosporins, and Related Drugs

SHERRY F. QUEENER • KATHLEEN GUTIERREZ

 Visit http://evolve.elsevier.com/Gutierrez/ for additional information.

KEY TERMS

Beta-lactam antibiotics, p. 390

Beta-lactamases, p. 390

Cephalosporins, p. 397

Gram-negative bacteria, p. 397

Gram-positive bacteria, p. 393

Methicillin-resistant *Staphylococcus aureus* **(MRSA),** p. 390

Pseudomembranous colitis, p. 392

Repository penicillins, p. 393

OBJECTIVES

- Identify the various classes of beta-lactam antibiotics.
- Explain the specific antibacterial effects of beta-lactam antibiotics.
- Explain how bacteria develop resistance to beta-lactam antibiotics.
- Describe the most common uses for beta-lactam antibiotics.
- Describe the most common adverse effects and toxicities of beta-lactam antibiotics.
- Develop a nursing care plan for a patient receiving one of the drugs discussed in this chapter.

 PATHOPHYSIOLOGY

Bacterial infections trigger a host immune response, which causes local inflammation, fever, chills, and malaise. Beta-lactam antibiotics interrupt these processes by selectively destroying invading bacteria. A full discussion of the pathophysiology of bacterial infections appears in Chapter 24.

DRUG CLASS • Beta-Lactam Antibiotics

MECHANISM OF ACTION

Penicillins, cephalosporins, and all other beta-lactam antibiotics inhibit bacterial cell wall synthesis by irreversibly inactivating a bacterial enzyme called transpeptidase. This enzyme cross-links strands of cell wall material called peptidoglycan. When cross-linking occurs, peptidoglycan becomes rigid and is an effective cell wall. When beta-lactam antibiotics block cross-linking, cell wall synthesis continues, but the unreinforced strands formed cannot resist the osmotic forces within the bacterial cell, possibly causing the bacterium to explode. Because exposed bacteria may be directly killed, beta-lactam antibiotics are classified as bactericidal drugs. However, even at dosages below those required to kill bacteria, penicillins and cephalosporins may disrupt the bacterial cell wall enough to make the bacteria more liable to elimination by the immune system of the host.

Beta-lactam antibiotics prevent the formation of a new, intact cell wall and thus are most effective against actively multiplying bacteria. These drugs cause few adverse effects in patients because the enzyme they target in bacteria does not have a counterpart in mammalian cells that might also be affected by the drugs.

Resistance to penicillins and cephalosporins develops in microorganisms. The most common mechanism for resistance involves enzymes called beta-lactamases. These enzymes are usually referred to as penicillinases or cephalosporinases, depending on which type of drug the enzyme is most effective against. These enzymes destroy the penicillin or cephalosporin molecule, rendering the drug inactive. Some organisms possess these enzymes as part of their normal metabolic makeup and therefore are intrinsically resistant to beta-lactam antibiotics. Other organisms may acquire the enzyme and thus be converted from antibiotic sensitivity to resistance. Clinically important examples of bacteria that have acquired penicillin resistance in the last 25 years are *Staphylococcus aureus* and *Neisseria gonorrhoeae*. In some hospitals, more than 90% of the *S. aureus* strains are resistant.

Although resistance to penicillins is most commonly acquired when bacteria develop beta-lactamase, other important forms of resistance are known. For example, methicillin-resistant *Staphylococcus aureus* (MRSA) achieves resistance by making altered penicillin target proteins. Altered targets are also the basis for resistance of *Streptococcus pneumoniae* to penicillin, which is an increasingly common clinical problem today. These changes in susceptibility influence the clinical use of penicillins.

USES

The large family of beta-lactam antibiotics includes drugs that are effective against most commonly encountered pathogens. The primary clinical uses of the beta-lactam antibiotics are summarized in Table 25-1.

PHARMACOKINETICS

Penicillins and cephalosporins differ widely in their stability when exposed to stomach acid and thus differ in their ability to be effective when administered orally (Table 25-2).

Most penicillins and cephalosporins are excreted by the kidneys, with a combination of glomerular filtration and active tubular secretion. The liver is the secondary route of elimination for most members of the class, although it is the primary route for a few drugs (see later sections on nafcillin and third-generation cephalosporins). There is little hepatic biotransformation of most beta-lactam antibiotics.

Penicillins, cephalosporins, and other beta-lactam antibiotics may accumulate in patients with impaired renal function, therefore their dosage may be reduced. Patients on hemodialysis also need to have their dosages and administration schedules adjusted to compensate for altered excretion of these antibiotics.

Most beta-lactam antibiotics do not readily cross the blood-brain barrier to enter the CNS. Inflammation caused by meningitis increases the passage of drug into the CNS.

ADVERSE REACTIONS AND CONTRAINDICATIONS

Allergy is the most common adverse reaction to penicillins. An estimated 3% to 5% of the general population is allergic to penicillin, but 10% of those who have previously received penicillin may develop allergic sensitivity to the drug. Cross-allergenicity to cephalosporins may develop in 5% to 10% of penicillin-sensitive patients because of the close structural similarity between the two classes of drugs. Cephalosporins are allergens much like penicillins, and many patients experience similar allergic reactions. A medically documented prior allergic response to a penicillin, a cephalosporin, or penicillamine is the only contraindication to the use of most beta-lactam antibiotics. Some patients experience

---

TABLE 25-1

Primary Uses of Beta-Lactam Antibiotics

Organism	Typical Infections	Beta-Lactam Antibiotics Used*
Gram-Positive Bacteria		
Streptococcus pneumoniae penicillin-sensitive	Otitis media, sinusitis, pneumonia, meningitis	amoxicillin, ampicillin, ceftriaxone, PENICILLIIN G
Group A streptococci (e.g., S. pyogenes)	Pharyngitis, impetigo, rheumatic fever	amoxicillin, ampicillin, cephalosporins, piperacillin, PENICILLIN G, PENICILLIN V
Group B streptococci (e.g., S. agalactiae)	Neonatal sepsis, postpartum infections, meningitis	AMOXICILLIN, AMPICILLIN, cephalosporins, MEZLOCILLIN, PENICILLIN G
Enterococci penicillin-sensitive	Endocarditis, urinary tract infections, nosocomial infections	AMPICILLIN, PENICILLIN G
Staphylococcus aureus nonpenicillinase	Endocarditis, meningitis, and infections of bone, skin, and wounds	amoxicillin, ampicillin, CEPHALOSPORINS (first-generation), penicillin G, penicillin V
Staphylococcus aureus penicillinase strains	Endocarditis, meningitis, and infections of bone, skin, and wounds	cephalosporins (first-generation), cloxacillin, dicloxacillin, imipenem, NAFCILLIN, oxacillin
Gram-Negative Bacteria		
Haemophilus influenzae	Pneumonia, tissue infections, otitis media, meningitis	AMOXICILLIN/CLAVULANATE, CEFOTAXIME, CEFTRIAXONE, cephalosporins (second-generation)
Neisseria gonorrhoeae	Gonorrhea, pelvic inflammatory disease	CEFIXIME, CEFPODOXIME, CEFTRIAXONE
Neisseria meningitidis	Meningitis	PENICILLIN G, cefotaxime, CEFTRIAXONE, cefuoxime
Escherichia coli	Diarrhea, wound infections, urinary tract infections	amoxicillin, ampicillin, CEPHALOSPORINS, imipenem, loracarbef, mezlocillin, piperacillin
Klebsiella pneumoniae	Pneumonia, urinary tract infections	ampicillin/sulbactam, aztreonam, CEPHALOSPORINS, (except cefadroxil, cefprozil, cephalexin), imipenem
Pseudomonas aeruginosa	Urinary tract infections, burn infections, wound infections, pneumonia	aztreonam, cefipime, ceftazidime, imipenem, MEZLOCILLIN, PIPERACILLIN, TICARCILLIN
Bacteroides fragilis	Abscesses, infections at anaerobic sites	AMPICILLIN/SULBACTAM, cefoxitin, IMIPENEM, meropenem, TICARCILLIN/CLAVULANATE
Spirochetes		
Treponema pallidum	Syphilis	CEFTRIAXONE, BENZATHINE PENICILLIN G, PENICILLIN G
Borellia burgdorferi	Lyme disease	cefotaxime, CEFTRIAXONE, CEFUROXIME AXETIL

*Primary drugs are set in UPPER CASE; alternative drugs are set in lower case.

TABLE 25-2

Oral Versus Parenteral Penicillins

Oral Use

amoxicillin (Amoxil, Larotid, Trimox)

amoxicillin/K clavulanate (Augmentin)

ampicillin (Omnipen Principen, Totacillin)

bacampicillin (Spectrobid)

carbenicillin indanyl sodium (Geocillin)

nafcillin (Unipen)

oxacillin (Bactocill)

penicillin V (Pen-Vee-K, Uticillin VK, Veetids, generic)

Parenteral Use

ampicillin (Omnipen-N, Principen-N, Totacillin-N)

ampicillin/sulbactam (Unasyn)

mezlocillin (Mezlin)

nafcillin (Nallpen, Unipen)

oxacillin (Bactocill)

penicillin G benzathine suspension (Bicillin L-A, Permapen)

penicillin G potassium (Pfizerpen, generic)

penicillin G procaine suspension (Wycillin)

piperacillin (Pipracil)

piperacillin/tazobactam (Zosyn)

ticarcillin (Ticar)

ticarcillin/clavulanate (Timentin)

BOX 25-1

Patient Problem: Considerations for Using Penicillins and Cephalosporins in Older Adults

The Problem

Most beta-lactam antibiotics are excreted primarily through the kidneys; biliary excretion serves as an alternative route. If renal function is impaired, excretion may be slowed, and the drug can accumulate. Healthy older adult patients may have significantly lower renal function than younger adults and perhaps should be considered as renally impaired.

The Solution

When administering these drugs to older adult patients, it is important to monitor creatinine clearance level. Adjust doses for renal function as prescribed or as described in the package insert.

---

skin rashes or urticaria, but anaphylaxis is a much more dangerous allergic response. Injections of penicillin are responsible for most anaphylactic episodes, but any formulation of penicillin may produce anaphylaxis in sensitive individuals.

Allergic rashes and drug fevers usually appear after several days of therapy, but the onset of anaphylaxis is nearly always within 10 minutes. Anaphylaxis involves profound vasomotor collapse, and patients require resuscitation. Laryngeal edema may complicate resuscitation efforts.

The second most common reaction to beta-lactam antibiotics is GI distress. Oral penicillin or cephalosporin preparations are the most likely to cause this adverse effect. Reactions include irritation and inflammation of the upper GI tract, nausea, vomiting, and diarrhea. Severe reactions may include antibiotic-associated **pseudomembranous colitis.** This condition arises when the normal bacterial flora of the bowel is destroyed by an antibiotic, allowing *Clostridium difficile* to flourish. This anaerobic organism releases a toxin that causes violent, watery diarrhea and sloughing of tissue lining the GI tract (see Chapter 24).

TOXICITY

Direct drug toxicity with penicillins is low; massive doses have been given with no ill effects. The tissue most sensitive to direct effects is the CNS. Intrathecal injection (into the subarachnoid space or cerebrospinal fluid [CSF]) may produce convulsions. Seizures also occur occasionally in patients given high dosages intramuscularly or intravenously, especially if renal impairment exists and the drug accumulates. A relatively high concentration must be achieved in the CSF before seizures occur. This complication could happen in an older adult being treated for a serious infection such as streptococcal endocarditis. This patient may receive 25 to 40 million U of penicillin daily to maintain continuous bactericidal drug concentrations. A healthy person can readily eliminate this large amount through the kidneys, but an older adult may have diminished renal function (see Box 25-1). Therefore the drug may accumulate and penicillin may enter the CNS. The first sign may be loss of consciousness or myoclonic movements; generalized seizures may follow.

Another group of patients with reduced ability to excrete penicillin are newborn infants. Because of this limitation, neonates receive carefully adjusted penicillin dosages based on their body weight and reduced clearance of penicillin.

INTERACTIONS

Probenecid is sometimes used with penicillins to increase their effective duration of action by slowing active tubular secretion in the kidney. However, probenecid can cause toxic reactions that are difficult to distinguish from a penicillin reaction (e.g., chills, fever, rash, GI irritation, and anemia). Probenecid also blocks renal excretion of some, but not all, cephalosporins.

Many penicillins and cephalosporins block excretion of methotrexate because these drugs compete for elimi-

nation by active tubular secretion. If methotrexate accumulates, significant toxicity may result, but monitoring methotrexate levels may allow the dosage to be adjusted to safe levels.

Various penicillins and cephalosporins occasionally have specific interactions with other drugs. These are listed, along with other unique properties of the individual beta-lactam antibiotics, in the following sections.

DRUG CLASS • Narrow-Spectrum Antibiotics

 penicillin G potassium (Pfizerpen, generic)

penicillin G benzathine suspension (Bicillin-LA, Permapen)

penicillin G procaine suspension (Wycillin)

penicillin G sodium (generic)

penicillin V potassium (Pen Vee K, Uticillin VK, Veetids, generic)

USES

Most of the organisms sensitive to narrow spectrum penicillins are **gram-positive bacteria** (see Table 25-2). Common gram-negative organisms normally found in the bowel and those often responsible for urinary tract infections are clinically resistant to penicillin G; however, penicillin G is effective against syphilis.

Penicillin G benzathine and penicillin G suspensions are not appropriate for serious infections when high serum concentrations of drug are required. Rather, these drugs are best used to maintain modest serum levels for relatively long periods, such as when very sensitive organisms are involved in mild to moderately serious infections or when prophylaxis is required.

The use of penicillin V is restricted to conditions in which oral antibiotic therapy is appropriate. Mild to moderately serious infections caused by penicillin-sensitive organisms may be treated with penicillin V; the drug is also appropriate for prophylaxis, especially in patients who have had rheumatic fever. In these patients, penicillin V prophylaxis may prevent recurrent streptococcal infections, which could lead to heart or kidney damage.

Dosages of penicillin G formulations are prescribed in units (1 mg of penicillin G sodium = 1667 units; 1 mg

of penicillin G potassium = 1595 units). Penicillin V formulations are designated with both units and milligrams. All other penicillin formulations are prescribed in milligrams or grams.

PHARMACOKINETICS

Penicillin G, like many other beta-lactam antibiotics, is sensitive to acid. About 30% of an oral dose is absorbed; the rest is destroyed in the stomach or retained in the bowel and destroyed by bacteria in the colon. Because of the incomplete and somewhat variable absorption, oral doses of penicillin G are not recommended. In contrast, penicillin V is more acid stable and thus more efficiently absorbed from the GI tract than penicillin G. Penicillin V should be given 1 hour before or 2 hours after meals, because food can interfere with absorption. Other properties of penicillin V are similar to those of penicillin G.

Penicillin G is rapidly and completely absorbed after intramuscular injection and serum concentration reaches its peak 20 to 30 minutes after injection (Figure 25-1). This peak concentration persists for only a short time, primarily because the kidney so efficiently removes penicillin from the blood and secretes it into the urine. Within 2 to 3 hours after injection, about 60% of the penicillin dose appears in the urine. The drug in urine is unchanged and still possesses antibacterial activity.

Repository penicillins, such as penicillin G benzathine suspension and penicillin G procaine suspension, were designed for slow absorption from intramuscular injection sites, creating a long duration of action. Once the drug is absorbed from depot sites, it is hydrolyzed to release penicillin G. Slower absorption means that the peak concentration is lower and takes

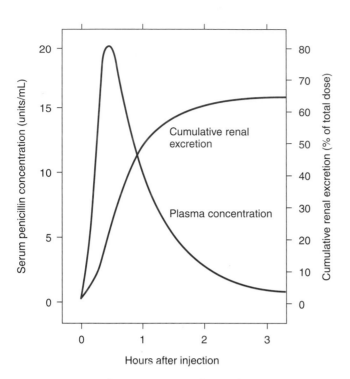

FIGURE 25-1 Serum concentration and urinary excretion of intramuscular (IM) dose of penicillin G. Penicillin G is efficiently and rapidly absorbed after IM injections. Peak plasma concentration appears 20 to 30 minutes after injection. Penicillin G is actively secreted by renal tubules, accounting for rapid elimination half-life of about 20 to 30 minutes. Most of drug dose ends up in urine as unaltered penicillin.

longer to achieve. For example, injections of penicillin G procaine suspension yield a peak concentration in serum 3 to 4 hours later, and a therapeutic serum concentration may persist for 48 hours. A single dose of 300,000 units of aqueous penicillin G gives a peak serum level of 6 to 8 units/mL within 30 minutes of injection, but penicillin G procaine suspension at that same dosage produces peak concentrations of only 1 to 2 units/mL. Penicillin G benzathine suspension is absorbed even more slowly; thus a peak serum level of penicillin G occurs 8 hours after injection with this preparation, and a useful serum level persists for at least 2 weeks. An adult dose of 1.2 million units of penicillin G benzathine suspension produces peak serum levels of only 0.1 to 0.3 units/mL.

Penicillin G is distributed to many tissues, with a high concentration found in blood, liver, kidney, and bile. Very little of the drug is found in brain tissue or cerebrospinal fluid (CSF) in healthy persons. If the meninges are inflamed, as in meningitis, significant amounts of penicillin can enter the CNS.

ADVERSE REACTIONS AND CONTRAINDICATIONS

Penicillin G and penicillin V cause few adverse reactions in most patients, although allergies and GI disturbances are possible, as noted for the whole drug class. Penicillin G procaine suspension is associated with CNS side effects because of the procaine content of the formulation. After injection, procaine may be released in a significant amount into the bloodstream and may produce anxiety, lowered blood pressure, respiratory depression, and convulsions. These CNS reactions to procaine are usually transient, lasting less than 1 hour.

Repository penicillins are intended for deep muscular injections. Both preparations are stabilized suspensions of relatively insoluble forms of penicillin and contain up to about 2% weight/volume of emulsifying agents in addition to buffers. Such preparations should never be given intravenously. Care must be taken on intramuscular injection to prevent the accidental entry of these preparations into blood vessels because occlusion of blood vessels may result.

TOXICITY

Massive doses of penicillin may cause CNS toxicity, including seizures, in susceptible individuals, older adults, or those with renal failure. In addition, potassium or sodium included in drug formulations may cause difficulties for some patients. For example, 1 million units (approximately 600 mg) of penicillin G and penicillin V may contain 1.5 mEq of potassium. Given in high doses for long enough periods, potassium intoxication and cardiac arrhythmia may occur. Some preparations of penicillin G contain high concentrations of sodium, which may cause difficulties in patients with preexisting cardiac or renal dysfunction.

INTERACTIONS

To avoid potassium toxicity, potassium supplements should be discontinued when potassium salts of penicillin G or penicillin V are used.

DRUG CLASS • Penicillinase-Resistant Penicillins

cloxacillin (Cloxapen, Tegopen,✱ Orbenin,✱ generic)

dicloxacillin (Pathocil, generic)

⚠ nafcillin (Nallpen, Unipen, generic)

oxacillin (Bactocill, generic)

USES

These drugs were developed to treat infections caused by penicillinase-producing strains of *S. aureus*. In all other penicillin-sensitive infections, penicillin G is preferred because it is more potent than penicillinase-resistant drugs.

Although these drugs resist penicillinase, other mechanisms of resistance have developed. For example, the use of methicillin, an older drug of this class, led to the selection of resistant strains of *S. aureus* that did not produce penicillinase but instead developed altered targets that rendered the organism tolerant to the drug and all other members of this class (see Chapter 24).

PHARMACOKINETICS

Penicillinase-resistant penicillins are stable in acid and thus may be given orally. Although nafcillin is sometimes given orally, it is not as well absorbed as oxacillin, cloxacillin, and dicloxacillin. With these latter drugs, fasting can approximately double oral absorption, so dosing is normally between meals.

Nafcillin is unique among the penicillins because it is excreted primarily in bile. All other penicillins are excreted primarily by the kidneys.

ADVERSE REACTIONS AND CONTRAINDICATIONS

As with any oral antibiotics, GI tract disturbances may occur with these drugs.

TOXICITY

Hepatotoxicity is associated with cloxacillin, dicloxacillin, and oxacillin more than with other penicillins. Hepatotoxicity may be more prevalent in patients with human immunodeficiency virus (HIV).

DRUG CLASS • Extended-Spectrum Penicillins

 amoxicillin (Amoxil, Larotid, Trimox, generic)

amoxicillin/clavulanate (Augmentin)

ampicillin (Omnipen, Principen, Totacillin, generic)

ampicillin/sulbactam (Unasyn)

bacampicillin (Spectrobid)

USES

The extended-spectrum penicillins penetrate gram-negative cell walls better and are therefore more effective than penicillin G against these organisms. The extended-spectrum penicillins are not resistant to penicillinase and so may not be effective against *S. aureus* strains resistant to penicillin G.

PHARMACOKINETICS

Ampicillin is given orally, but only 35% to 50% of an oral dose is absorbed. Bacampicillin is a prodrug that is more rapidly and completely absorbed than ampicillin and releases ampicillin when broken down in the body. Amoxicillin is more acid stable than ampicillin and therefore is better absorbed orally. Amoxicillin is also more conveniently administered because it can be mixed with a variety of foods or juices, whereas ampicillin must be taken on an empty stomach.

Fixed combinations of ampicillin with sulbactam and amoxicillin with clavulanic acid are available. Sulbactam and clavulanic acid are inhibitors of beta lactamases. Inclusion of these inhibitors in fixed combinations protects the active drugs from destruction, allowing their use against some organisms that would otherwise be resistant.

ADVERSE REACTIONS AND CONTRAINDICATIONS

Ampicillin commonly causes GI upset and is one of the leading causes of antibiotic-associated colitis (see Chapter 24).

TOXICITY

Ampicillin often causes a rash that is not allergic in origin and is referred to as a toxic rash. This rash appears 8 to 10 days after the start of therapy. Incidence of rash is greatly increased in patients with mononucleosis.

INTERACTIONS

Extended-spectrum penicillins may reduce the effectiveness of oral contraceptives by affecting steroid metabolism. Additional birth control measures should be used while taking these antibiotics. Ampicillin and bacampicillin may increase the incidence of rashes in patients receiving allopurinol.

DRUG CLASS • Anti-*Pseudomonas* Penicillins

carbenicillin indanyl sodium (Geocillin)

mezlocillin (Mezlin)

piperacillin (Pipracil)

piperacillin/tazobactam (Zosyn)

picarcillin (Ticar)

ticarcillin/clavulanate (Timentin)

USES

One pathogenic organism that is not sensitive to extended-spectrum penicillins is *Pseudomonas aeruginosa*. This gram-negative bacterium causes certain urinary tract infections (UTIs), bacteremias, infections in burn patients, and pneumonia in patients with cystic fibrosis. This organism is unusually resistant to many antibiotics because of a complex cell wall that effectively excludes many drug classes. Thus the anti-*Pseudomonas* penicillins were developed specifically to penetrate the cell wall and membrane of this organism. Anti-*Pseudomonas* penicillins may be used alone but can also be combined with gentamicin or another anti-*Pseudomonas* aminoglycoside (see Chapter 29) to treat severe infections.

PHARMACOKINETICS

All these drugs except carbenicillin indanyl sodium must be administered parenterally. Although carbenicillin indanyl sodium is intended for oral use, it does not produce a high enough serum level to make the drug effective for most infections. Therefore it is reserved for use in urinary tract infections because the active agent (carbenicillin) accumulates to a high concentration in urine after oral dosage.

ADVERSE REACTIONS AND CONTRAINDICATIONS

Carbenicillin, piperacillin, and ticarcillin often interfere with platelet function. This problem is worse in patients with uremia because they have preexisting platelet dysfunction as a result of their renal disease.

INTERACTIONS

Gentamicin or other aminoglycosides must never be directly mixed in the syringe or IV bottle with any beta-lactam antibiotic, since the two classes of drugs inactivate each other. Flushing the IV tubing between antibiotics is another important way to avoid this type of inactivation.

Anti-*Pseudomonas* penicillins, especially preparations of ticarcillin, contain high concentrations of sodium, which may cause difficulties in patients with preexisting cardiac and renal dysfunction.

DRUG CLASS • Cephalosporins

First Generation

cefadroxil (Duricef)

⚕ cefazolin (Ancef, Kefzol)

cephalexin (Keflex, Keflet)

cephalothin (Keflin)

cephapirin (Cefadyl)

cephradine (Anspor, Velosef)

Second Generation

cefaclor (Ceclor)

cefamandole (Mandol)

cefmetazole (Zefazone)

cefonicid (Monocid)

ceforanide (Precef)

cefotetan (Cefotan)

cefoxitin (Mefoxin)

cefprozil (Cefzil)

cefuroxime axetil (Ceftin)

cefuroxime sodium (Kefurox, Zinacef)

Third Generation

cefdinir (Omnicef)

cefditoren pivoxil (Spectracef)

cefixime (Suprax)

cefoperazone (Cefobid, Claforan)

cefotaxime (Claforan)

cefpodoxime (Vantin)

ceftazidime (Fortaz, Tazicef)

ceftibuten (Cedax)

ceftizoxime (Ceftizox)

⚕ ceftriaxone (Rocephin)

Fourth Generation

cefepime (Maxipime)

USES

The primary usefulness of cephalosporins is based on differences in the antimicrobial spectra of penicillins and cephalosporins. First-generation cephalosporins resemble ampicillin in their effectiveness against gram-negative bacteria. Unlike ampicillin, cephalosporins resist the action of staphylococcal penicillinase and can be used when the organism is resistant to penicillin G. The later-generation cephalosporins are used for specific, serious infections caused by gram-negative bacteria. For example, the third-generation drug ceftriaxone is now considered a first-line drug for treatment of serious cases of pneumonia. Cephalosporins are not effective against enterococci or MRSA.

PHARMACOKINETICS

Several cephalosporins are currently available for oral use (Table 25-3). These preparations are well absorbed and produce effective serum concentrations of antibiotic. Absorption of cephalosporins from the GI tract is slowed by food in the stomach, but about the same amount is ultimately absorbed as in a fasting patient.

Most cephalosporins are given parenterally because they are well absorbed from intramuscular sites. The elimination half-lives of all these drugs are about twice as long as that of penicillin G and are roughly equivalent to those of ampicillin or the penicillinase-resistant penicillins. The first generation cephalosporin cefazolin has a longer half-life than other first-generation drugs and is thus often preferred.

Cephalosporins are distributed in the body in a manner similar to that of penicillins, except that first-generation and most second-generation cephalosporins do not penetrate the CNS well enough to be used in meningitis. The only cephalosporins to achieve adequate concentrations in the CNS are cefotaxime, ceftazidime, ceftizoxime, ceftriaxone, and cefuroxime.

Cephalosporins, with the exception of cefoperazone, cefpodoxime, and ceftriaxone are excreted primarily by the kidneys and are highly concentrated in the urine, making them useful in treating common types of urinary tract infections. With its very long duration of action, ceftriaxone tends to reach a much higher plateau concentration in the blood than other cephalosporins and thus may be preferred for many serious infections (see the Case Study: Soft Tissue Infection).

Most cephalosporins are not biotransformed, except for cefotaxime, cephalothin, and cephapirin, which are biotransformed in the liver to a significant degree. Both metabolites and the unchanged drug are eliminated in urine.

TABLE 25-3

Oral versus Parenteral Cephalosporins and Miscellaneous Beta-Lactam Antibiotics

Common Preparations for Oral Use

First-Generation Cephalosporins
cefadroxil (Duricef)

cephalexin (Keflex, Keflet)

cephradine (Velosef, Anspor)

Second-Generation Cephalosporins
cefaclor (Ceclor)

cefprozil (Cefzil)

cefuroxime axetil (Ceftin)

Third-Generation Cephalosporins
cefdinir (Omnicef)

cefditoren pivoxil (Spectracef)

cefixime (Suprax)

cefpodoxime (Vantin)

ceftibuten (Cedax)

Miscellaneous Beta-Lactam Antibiotics
loracarbef (Lorabid)

Common Preparations for Parenteral Use

First-Generation Cephalosporins
cefazolin (Ancef, Kefzol)

cephalothin (Keflin)

cephapirin (Cefadyl)

Second-Generation Cephalosporins
cefamandole (Mandol)

cefmetazole (Zefazone)

cefonicid (Monocid)

ceforanide (Precef)

cefotetan (Cefotan)

cefoxitin (Mefoxin)

cefuroxime (Kefurox, Zinacef)

Third-Generation Cephalosporins
cefepime (Maxipime)

cefoperazone (Cefobid)

cefotaxime (Claforan)

ceftazidime (Fortaz, Tazicef)

ceftizoxime (Ceftizox)

ceftriaxone (Rocephin)

Miscellaneous Beta-Lactam Antibiotics
aztreonam (Azactam)

ertapenem (Invanz)

imipenem-cilastatin (Primaxin)

meropenem (Merrem)

ADVERSE REACTIONS AND CONTRAINDICATIONS

Many cephalosporins cause pain at the injection site. When given intravenously, these drugs cause phlebitis or thrombophlebitis and pain along the affected vein. Orally administered cephalosporins may cause gastric irritation, nausea, and vomiting. Superinfections may arise when these relatively broad-spectrum drugs are used, the most common being oral or vaginal candidiasis (yeast infections). Allergies to cephalosporins may take the form of rashes, serum sickness, hemolytic anemia, Stevens-Johnson syndrome, or anaphylaxis.

Cefamandole, cefoperazone, and cefotetan have been associated with platelet dysfunction. Patients should be observed for signs of unusual bleeding or bruising. The bleeding time or prothrombin time may require monitoring. Patients with bleeding disorders should not receive these drugs.

Caution should be used if these drugs must be given to patients with hepatic disease or renal impairment, and dosages may require reduction. Patients with GI tract disease may be more likely to develop antibiotic-associated colitis (see Chapter 24).

Overdose of cephalosporins may cause seizures. The drugs should be discontinued if seizures occur; specific treatment for controlling seizure activity may be required.

INTERACTIONS

Interstitial nephritis is sometimes seen with these drugs. There is a danger of synergistic nephrotoxicity when a cephalosporin is given with other nephrotoxic drugs such as an aminoglycoside antibiotic or the diuretics furosemide or ethacrynic acid. In spite of this risk, third-generation cephalosporins such as ceftazidime or cefoperazone may be given with an aminoglycoside such as amikacin, tobramycin, or gentamicin when synergistic activity is required to treat serious infections caused by *P. aeruginosa*.

Probenecid may prolong the persistence of cephalosporins in the body by blocking renal tubular secretion. Probenecid has no effect on the duration of action of cefoperazone, ceftriaxone, or ceftazidime because these three drugs depend less on active tubular secretion for elimination than do the other cephalosporins.

Cefamandole, cefoperazone, and cefotetan all share a chemical feature that may cause excessive bleeding if the drugs are used with anticoagulants or platelet-aggregation inhibitors such as aspirin. These drugs are also more likely than other cephalosporins to cause a disulfiram reaction if alcohol is ingested while the drugs are being taken.

DRUG CLASS • Miscellaneous Beta-Lactam Antibiotic

Monobactams

aztreonam (Azactam)

MECHANISM OF ACTION

Aztreonam inhibits transpeptidase in a way similar to other beta-lactam antibiotics, but unlike most penicillins and cephalosporins, aztreonam acts primarily against gram-negative aerobic bacteria. Aztreonam is ineffective for gram-positive or anaerobic bacteria because the drug fails to bind to critical targets in those organisms.

USES

Aztreonam is given to treat urinary tract infections, septicemia, infections of the lower respiratory tract, intraabdominal or gynecologic infections, and soft tissue infections. Gram-negative aerobic bacteria, including *Pseudomonas*, typically cause these infections.

PHARMACOKINETICS

Aztreonam must be administered parenterally to reach a useful concentration in plasma. The drug is distributed well to many body tissues and fluids but is relatively low in CSF. Excretion is primarily via the kidneys, and only minor amounts of drug are eliminated by hepatic mechanisms.

ADVERSE REACTIONS AND CONTRAINDICATIONS

The principal adverse reactions to aztreonam include pain or phlebitis at the injection site in up to 2.4% of patients. GI tract symptoms (including nausea, diarrhea, or vomiting) occur in up to 1.3% of patients. Rash and other symptoms of allergic reactions occur as with all beta-lactam antibiotics. Caution should be used when the drug must be given to patients with cirrhosis or renal impairment; the dosage may need to be lowered.

DRUG CLASS • Carbapenems

ertapenem (Invanz)
imipenem/cilastatin (Primaxin)
meropenem (Merrem)

MECHANISM OF ACTION

Imipenem/cilastatin and meropenem have broad antimicrobial spectra that include gram-positive, gram-negative, and anaerobic bacteria. The two drugs are remarkably resistant to penicillinases and many cephalosporinases.

USES

Meropenem is used to treat intraabdominal infections and meningitis. Because imipenem/cilastatin has such a broad antimicrobial spectrum, it is used to treat a variety of infections at many sites, including those caused by *P. aeruginosa*. Resistance to imipenem/cilastatin has begun to appear in MRSA, *P. aeruginosa*, and *Enterococcus faecium*. In some cases, unusual beta-lactamases are involved in resistance, but other mechanisms of resistance also occur.

PHARMACOKINETICS

Imipenem is well distributed to many tissues but is low in CSF. Excretion is through the kidneys. When given alone, imipenem is hydrolyzed in the kidneys and excreted as inactive products. The clinical preparation includes cilastatin, an agent chemically related to imipenem but with little antibacterial activity. Cilastatin inhibits destruction of imipenem in the kidneys and allows active imipenem to accumulate in renal tissue and urine.

In contrast to imipenem, biotransformation of meropenem is insignificant: 70% of a given dose appears unchanged in urine. Meropenem distributes to key tissues, including the CNS.

ADVERSE REACTIONS AND CONTRAINDICATIONS

Imipenem/cilastatin is more likely than other beta-lactam antibiotics to cause seizures; dosages greater than 2 g daily further increase the risk. Probenecid is avoided with meropenem because meropenem may accumulate to toxic levels.

DRUG CLASS • Carbacephems

loracarbef (Lorabid)

MECHANISM OF ACTION

Loracarbef is the first member of a new class of drugs called carbacephems, but the group is closely related to cephalosporins and has the same mechanism of action.

USES

Loracarbef is most active against bacteria that cause infections of the throat, ears, and upper respiratory tract. The good distribution of the drug to these sites supports this clinical use.

PHARMACOKINETICS

Over 90% of an oral dose of loracarbef is usually absorbed, although food can delay this absorption. Loracarbef distributes well to middle ear fluid and to soft tissues; for example, the concentration of the drug in tonsils may approach 50% of plasma concentration. The drug is not biotransformed and is eliminated almost entirely by renal mechanisms.

ADVERSE REACTIONS AND CONTRAINDICATIONS

Like other beta-lactam antibiotics, loracarbef can cause allergic reactions. Because it is an oral drug, it can also produce GI disturbances.

INTERACTIONS

Probenecid blocks renal excretion of loracarbef and thus increases the half-life of the drug from about 1 to 1.5 hours.

APPLICATION TO PRACTICE

ASSESSMENT

The general aspects of care for the patient receiving any antimicrobial drug were covered in Chapter 24. In this chapter, only those aspects related specifically to beta-lactam antibiotics are discussed.

History of Present Illness

The patient with an infection typically displays the five cardinal signs and symptoms of infection, which include swelling, redness, pain, heat, and loss of function. Be sure to ask the patient about the location, onset, severity, timing, duration, signs and symptoms, quality, and context of his or her concern as well as anything the patient has tried that improved or worsened these signs and symptoms.

Health History

A thorough health history may reveal previous hypersensitivity reactions. It is important to ask patients who will be taking a beta-lactam drug whether they have ever taken a drug in these classes and if so, whether they developed a skin rash, hives, swelling, or difficulty breathing associated with the drug. Because of the risk of cross-allergenicity with cephalosporins, ask the patient specifically if he or she has ever had an anaphylactic reaction to penicillin. Naming a few of the common penicillins and cephalosporin drugs may help the patient identify previous usage. Be sure to ask about the use of other prescription drugs, herbal remedies, and OTC drugs to minimize the risk of drug-drug interactions.

Inquire if the patient has a history of bleeding disorders. These patients require monitoring for bleeding tendencies with the administration of carbenicillin, piperacillin, ticarcillin, and cephalosporins because they may cause platelet dysfunction or hypoprothrombinemia. Patients with a history of GI disorders, particularly ulcerative colitis and regional enteritis, are more at risk of pseudomembranous colitis as an adverse reaction to penicillins and cephalosporins. Skin rash may occur in 43% to 100% of patients who have an active case of infectious mononucleosis when ampicillin, bacampicillin, and pivampicillin are used.

Lifespan Considerations

Perinatal. Penicillins fall into pregnancy category B and thus are safe to use during pregnancy in nonallergic patients. These drugs are among the most effective and least toxic antimicrobials available. Penicillin G and most of the other penicillins cross the placenta and appear in the amniotic fluid and fetal blood and tissues. Highly protein-bound penicillins reach a much lower level in the fetus and amniotic fluid than do those that are less bound. They do not appear to be teratogenic.

Penicillins appear in breast milk and may cause diarrhea and candidiasis in a nursing infant.

The first- and second-generation cephalosporins are category B drugs and are generally safe to use during pregnancy. Third-generation cephalosporins have broader spectra and different pharmacokinetic properties than the first- and second-generation drugs. Until more experience is accumulated in pregnant women, this generation of cephalosporins should be reserved for use when no other safer antibiotic is available. Cephalosporins cross the placenta and are found in fetal serum and urine as well as in amniotic fluid. No teratogenic effects have been associated with cephalosporins; however, the third-generation drugs have yet to be extensively tested.

Pediatric. Penicillins and cephalosporins are widely used to treat infections in children and are generally considered to be safe. They should be used with caution in neonates because immature kidney function slows their excretion. For infants less than 3 months old, a history of penicillin allergy in the mother should be sought. Dosages should be based on age, weight, severity of infection, and renal function. The use of aztreonam and imipenem/cilastatin in children has not been well studied. Although no children's dosage has been established for these drugs, they have been given to children with various infections caused by *P. aeruginosa*.

Older Adults. Use of penicillins and cephalosporins in older adults is relatively safe, although decreased renal function associated with changes of aging, other disease processes, and concurrent drug therapies increase the risk of adverse effects. With penicillins, hyperkalemia (an elevated serum potassium level) may occur with large intravenous doses of penicillin G potassium, and hypernatremia (an elevated serum sodium level) may occur with ticarcillin. Hypernatremia is less likely to develop with other anti-*Pseudomonas* penicillins such as mezlocillin and piperacillin. Cephalosporins may aggravate renal impairment, especially if other nephrotoxic drugs are used concurrently. The dosage of most cephalosporins must be reduced in the presence of renal impairment, depending on the creatinine clearance values. No guidelines have been established for the use of aztreonam or imipenem/cilastatin in older adults.

Cultural/Social Considerations

Overall, the cultural and social considerations associated with the use of penicillins and cephalosporins are minimal. In most cases, infections are short-term, subacute conditions easily treated on an outpatient basis. Hospitalization may be required for serious, potentially life-threatening infections.

Compared with the other classes of antimicrobial drugs, the penicillins and many of the first-, second-, and third-generation cephalosporins are relatively inexpensive. However, the rising cost of antibiotics, particularly the newer ones, presents a hardship to many, especially older adults, those who are financially disadvantaged, and those who have pharmacy insurance plans through managed care organizations.

Physical Examination

Assess the patient for signs and symptoms of infection. Be sure to include the vital signs and inspection of any wound. A thorough examination is particularly necessary to detect any infection traveling indirectly from a distant body site (e.g., a total joint replacement of the hip may fail as a result of a cut finger that became infected). Evaluate the patient's level of discomfort related to the infection.

Laboratory Testing

Many antimicrobial drugs have harsh adverse effects on other body systems. Therefore, once drug therapy is started, close monitoring is necessary to reduce the risk of toxicity. Monitoring for nephrotoxicity secondary to penicillin includes measurement of electrolytes for evidence of hyperkalemia or hyponatremia. A partial thromboplastin time (PTT) and prothrombin time (PT) should be obtained for patients receiving parenteral carbenicillin, piperacillin, and ticarcillin. To monitor for nephrotoxicity, renal function studies (BUN, creatinine) may be required during prolonged therapy with methicillin, which causes interstitial nephritis in up to 12% of patients. Because of the risk of superinfection in patients receiving a cephalosporin, observe patients, particularly older adults and those who are debilitated, for symptoms of bacterial and fungal overgrowth. Evidence of superinfection (e.g., diarrhea, vaginal or anal itching, black furry appearance of the tongue) should be reported. Superinfection by *Candida* organisms can usually be managed by discontinuing the antibiotics or by administering an antifungal drug.

GOALS OF THERAPY

The desired goals of treatment with penicillins and cephalosporins are to ameliorate the signs and symptoms of infection, to prevent complications associated with therapy, and to prevent sepsis and death.

INTERVENTION
Administration

Before the first dose of a beta-lactam antibiotic drug is given, the patient's history should be carefully reviewed for allergies. Keep in mind that a negative history of hypersensitivity does not preclude future reactions.

Many drugs differ with regard to route of administration. For example, penicillin G sodium is administered intramuscularly or intravenously; the potassium formulation is given orally; benzathine penicillin is given orally or intramuscularly; and procaine formulations are only administered intramuscularly. Before administering the drug, be sure to carefully check that the route ordered is correct for the individual drug.

When administering oral penicillins, remember that they bind to food and are poorly absorbed in acid media. Penicillins to be taken on an empty stomach should be administered 1 hour before or 2 hours after meals. Acidic fruit juices or beverages should be avoided within 1 hour of ingestion, since juices may facilitate decomposition of the penicillin.

Note that most intravenous penicillins are sodium or potassium salts. Significant amounts of these ions can be received when large doses of these drugs are given intravenously. For example, carbenicillin contains 4.7 mEq of sodium per gram and is typically administered in dosages of 30 to 40 g daily for a total of 141 to 188 mEq of sodium per day. A single dose of 20 million units of potassium penicillin G contains 33 mEq of potassium. Fatalities have occurred, particularly in patients with renal failure, because of the toxic effects of these ions on the heart. Additionally, intravenous beta-lactams should be administered intermittently rather than continuously to avoid blood vessel irritation (phlebitis). To reduce site irritation, the drug should be reconstituted and administered in the time frame recommended by the manufacturer. Furthermore, many drugs require properly buffered solutions for stability; thus not all are compatible with common intravenous fluids. Check the package insert or ask the pharmacist before adding a drug to any fluid. The insertion site should be assessed frequently for signs and symptoms of inflammation and the site changed every 3 days or according to agency policy. Perioperative prophylaxis with parenteral cephalosporins is usually discontinued 24 hours after surgery.

Intramuscular administration of cephalosporin antibiotics results in irritation of local tissues. Warn the patient that the injection may be painful. To reduce potential tissue irritation, the drug should be reconstituted (when necessary) according to the manufacturer's recommendations and given into a large muscle mass (e.g., dorsal gluteal). Use of the Z-track technique and rotation of injection sites also help reduce local tissue irritation.

The patient should be observed closely for anaphylaxis for at least 30 minutes after the first dose of a parenteral beta-lactam antibiotic. Anaphylaxis often manifests as nausea, vomiting, pruritus, tachycardia, severe dyspnea, diaphoresis, stridor, vertigo, loss of consciousness, and peripheral circulatory failure. The best way to control anaphylaxis is by preventing it from happening in the first place.

Education

Instruct the patient to take the full course of the antibiotic drug (usually 10 days), even though symptoms may abate and he or she may start feeling better before the full course of therapy is completed. Emphasize the importance of taking evenly spaced doses to maintain a therapeutic blood level. For example, if a cephalosporin antibiotic is prescribed every 6 hours, it should be taken as much as possible every 6 hours (not breakfast, lunch, dinner, bedtime) for the entire 10 days, or the drug level in the blood will not be adequately maintained to fight the pathogens. Prescriptions for any antibiotic should never be shared with others or saved and taken for a different episode of illness.

Because the effects of estrogen-based contraceptives are reduced when taking penicillin or cephalosporin antibiotics, women should be advised to use a second form of birth control during treatment and for up to 2 weeks after completing the drug regimen.

Patients with diabetes mellitus who use the copper sulfate urine glucose test (Clinitest) may have false–positive results while taking amoxicillin, ampicillin, bacampi-

---

CASE STUDY

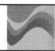

Soft Tissue Infection

ASSESSMENT

HISTORY OF PRESENT ILLNESS

LM is an 82-year-old farmer with complaints of a puncture wound on his right hand sustained when his dog bit him. Initially, he did not notice signs of infection but now reports that his hand is red, swollen, warm, and painful. LM has been unable to work for the past 2 days because of the pain in his hand. He did not seek health care advice at the time of the injury because of transportation issues.

HEALTH HISTORY

LM is allergic to penicillin. He has had Type 1 diabetes mellitus with associated nephropathy and neuropathy for 25 years. He takes 25 units of Humulin NPH insulin bid. He does not remember when he last had a tetanus shot. LM also had a recent myocardial infarction (MI) and is on warfarin therapy. He had a total hip replacement 5 years ago but has done fine ever since the surgery.

LIFESPAN CONSIDERATIONS

LM is at risk for impaired renal function due to the aging process.

CULTURAL/SOCIAL CONSIDERATIONS

LM generally considers himself healthy. He lives alone on his small farm with income from Social Security and occasional financial assistance from his two sons. He has a history of noncompliance with any type of health care treatments. The family has not been informed of his injury. LM is unable to drive and needs assistance to get to the clinic and laboratory for any follow-up medical visits and PT/INR testing.

PHYSICAL EXAMINATION

LM has noticeable edema and warmth on the ring finger of his right hand with induration around the area of the bite. There is palpable right-sided epitrochlear and axillary lymphadenopathy. LM's temperature is 100.2° F, pulse 100, respirations 24, and his blood pressure is 138/85 mm Hg.

Records indicate that the patient does not comply with drug administration schedules.

LABORATORY TESTING

Culture of hand wound reveals *Pasteurella canis* infection. WBC count 18,000; BUN 24 mg/dL; creatinine level 1.9 mg/dL; creatinine clearance level >50 mL/min; HgbA$_{1c}$ 12%; fasting blood sugar 326 mg%.

PATIENT PROBLEM(S)

Infected dog bite, right hand; Type 1 diabetes mellitus with nephropathy and neuropathy; postoperative total hip replacement and MI.

GOALS OF THERAPY

Ameliorate signs and symptoms of infection; prevent sepsis and death; prevent complications such as adverse drug reactions, local extension of infection, tissue necrosis, or bone loss.

CRITICAL THINKING QUESTIONS

1. The health care provider has prescribed 1 g of intravenous ceftriaxone for LM every 12 hours for 10 to 14 days. What is the mechanism of action of this drug?
2. Since ceftriaxone can be given intramuscularly as well as intravenously, what factors in LM's medical history and physical examination contributed to the decision to hospitalize him and give the drug intravenously?
3. What adverse effects should be looked for when ceftriaxone is used?
4. What normal changes of aging predispose LM to the risk of adverse drug effects?
5. LM is also taking warfarin and NPH insulin. What drug-drug interactions with ceftrixone should the nurse watch for?
6. What is the physiologic rationale for giving LM a dose of tetanus toxoid (Td) as well as tetanus immune globulin at this time (TIG)?

cillin, penicillin G, or any of the cephalosporins. Advise the patient to use glucose-enzymatic tests, such as Clinistix or Ketodiastix to monitor their sugar levels.

Caution the patient not to drink alcoholic beverages or take alcohol-containing drugs while taking a cephalosporin antibiotic, because abdominal cramps, nausea and vomiting, hypotension, tachycardia, shortness of breath, sweating, and facial flushing may occur (a disulfiram-like reaction). Advise patients to read labels because many cough and cold remedies contain alcohol.

Instruct patients to contact their health care provider if their condition does not improve in a few days, or if they develop severe diarrhea, rash, fever, or chills, which may indicate a delayed hypersensitivity reaction. Patients with an allergy to penicillins or cephalosporins should be advised to wear some form of identification (e.g., medical alert tag or bracelet) to inform health care personnel of the allergy. Carrying the identification in a wallet or purse is usually not helpful if emergency care is needed.

EVALUATION

The effectiveness of penicillin and cephalosporin therapy is determined by monitoring clinical response and laboratory test results. The frequency of monitoring is proportional to the severity of the infection. Important clinical indicators of effective treatment include a reduction in fever and resolution of the signs and symptoms of infection, vital signs that return to normal for the patient, WBC count that returns to normal limits, and a culture and sensitivity test that is negative for the offending organism. Further proof may include an increase in appetite, energy level, and general sense of well-being.

Bibliography

Braunwald E, Fauci AS, Kasper DL, et al (eds): *Harrison's principles of internal medicine*, ed 15, New York, 2001, McGraw-Hill.

Copstead LC, Banasik JL: *Pathophysiology: biological and behavioral perspectives*, ed 2, Philadelphia, 2000, WB Saunders Company.

Flournoy DJ, Reinert RL, Bell-Dixon C, et al: Increasing antimicrobial resistance in gram-negative bacilli isolated from patients in intensive care units, *Am J Infect Control* 28(3):244-250, 2000.

Horns KM, Gills MB: The NANN pages: neonatal nurse knowledge of penicillin therapy, *J Neonat Nurs* 17:52-55, 1998.

Laliberte R: Is it strep throat? *Parents* 73:42, 44, 1998.

Lewis SM, Heitkemper MM, Dirksen SR: *Medical-surgical nursing: assessment and management of clinical problems*, ed 6, St. Louis, 2003, Mosby.

Mead M: Drugs for: URTIs . . . upper respiratory tract infections, *Pract Nurs* 15:605, 607, 1998.

Presutti RJ: Prevention and treatment of dog bites, *Am Fam Physician* 63:1567-1574, 2001.

Slinger R, Moher D: Best practice. Evidence-based care review: how to assess new treatments, *West J Med* 174:182-186, 2001.

Talan DA, Citron DM, Abrahamian FM, et al: Bacteriologic analysis of infected dog and cat bites, *N Engl J Med* 340:85-92, 1999.

Valyasevi MA, Van Dellen RG: Frequency of systematic reactions to penicillin skin tests, *Ann Allergy Asthma Immunol* 85:363-365, 2000.

Internet Resources

The following sites discuss uses of the class as well as properties of individual drugs.

Merck Manual available online at www.merck.com/pubs/mmanual_home/.

http://www.informed.org/100drugs/penitoc.html.

CHAPTER

26

Macrolides: Erythromycin and Related Drugs

SHERRY F. QUEENER • KATHLEEN GUTIERREZ

 Visit http://evolve.elsevier.com/Gutierrez/ for additional information.

KEY TERMS

Atypical pneumonia, p. 406
Cholestatic hepatitis, p. 409
Enteric coating, p. 406
Macrolides, p. 406
Penicillin substitute, p. 406
Volume of distribution, p. 407

OBJECTIVES

- Explain the common uses for a macrolide antibiotic (e.g., erythromycin).
- Explain why azithromycin may be effectively used in a 5-day regimen as compared with 10-day regimens for comparable penicillins or cephalosporins.
- Describe the common adverse reactions of macrolide drugs.
- Develop a nursing care plan for a patient receiving a macrolide antibiotic drug.

 PATHOPHYSIOLOGY

Bacterial infections trigger immune responses in the host, which produce fever, chills, and malaise as well as local inflammation such as pharyngitis, bronchitis, or otitis media. A full discussion of the pathophysiology of bacterial infections appears in Chapter 24.

DRUG CLASS • Macrolides

azithromycin (Zithromax)

clarithromycin (Biaxin)

dirithromycin (Dynabac)

⚠ erythromycin base (E-Base, E-Mycin, ERYC, Ilotycin, PCE)

erythromycin estolate (Ilosone)

erythromycin ethylsuccinate (E.E.S., EryPed, Erythro)

erythromycin lactobionate (Erythrocin)

erythromycin stearate (Erythrocin, Erythrocot, My-E)

MECHANISM OF ACTION

Macrolides are produced by a species of soil organism called *Streptomycetes*. The antibiotics derived from these large molecules bind to bacterial ribosomes and thus prevent bacterial protein synthesis. At a low concentration this effect is bacteriostatic, but at a high concentration it may be bactericidal.

USES

Macrolides include one widely used older agent (erythromycin) and three newer agents (azithromycin, clarithromycin, and dirithromycin) with somewhat more focused clinical applications. Erythromycin is active against the same gram-positive bacteria usually susceptible to narrow-spectrum penicillins, such as penicillin G, but erythromycin is chemically unrelated to penicillins and is not cross-allergenic with them. Therefore it is a useful substitute in patients who are allergic to penicillins. Because it is active against gram-positive bacteria, erythromycin has been called a **penicillin substitute**, but the correlation is not exact. In addition to being effective against many infections of the throat, ears, respiratory tract, and skin, which are often caused by typical gram-positive bacteria, erythromycin can be used to treat diphtheria (*Corynebacterium diphtheriae*), whooping cough (*Bordetella pertussis*), and pneumonia caused by *Legionella* species or *Mycoplasma pneumoniae*; none of the latter three conditions respond to penicillin.

Gram-positive bacteria may acquire resistance by chemically altering their ribosomes so that the ribosomes no longer bind to erythromycin, thereby preventing inhibition of protein synthesis. This ribosomal change is catalyzed by an enzyme synthesized from genes carried on a bacterial plasmid, which allows resistance to erythromycin to spread rapidly throughout a bacterial population (see Chapter 24). Erythromycin-resistant strains of *Streptococcus pyogenes* have become prominent in some parts of the world, requiring the use of other drugs.

Gram-negative bacteria seem to be relatively impermeable to erythromycin and are therefore intrinsically resistant. The only exceptions are cell wall–deficient variants of *E. coli* and *Proteus mirabilis*, called L-forms, which may be encountered in relapsing urinary tract infections. Because L-form bacteria lack cell walls, they are resistant to penicillins. After penicillin therapy, the L-forms may revert to normal and produce offspring that do have cell walls and the infection may recur. Unlike other gram-negative bacteria, the cell wall–deficient L-forms are permeable and highly sensitive to erythromycin, making this drug useful for eradicating L-forms and preventing recurrence of the infection.

Newer macrolides have additional features that distinguish them from erythromycin. For example, unlike erythromycin, azithromycin is bactericidal against *Streptococcus pyogenes*, *S. pneumoniae*, and *Haemophilus influenzae*, organisms that commonly cause respiratory infections or pharyngitis. This bactericidal action is especially important for pneumonia caused by *H. influenzae*, where azithromycin is a drug of choice, but erythromycin is not.

In general, the newer macrolides are most widely used for genital tract or pulmonary infections caused by *Chlamydia* species or for pneumonias caused by *Legionella pneumophila*, *S. pneumoniae*, or *Mycoplasma pneumoniae*. *M. pneumoniae* causes an **atypical pneumonia**, characterized by generally mild symptoms of fever, chills, headache, and coughing but little sign of bacterial infection.

PHARMACOKINETICS

Erythromycin is sensitive to acid and therefore may be extensively degraded in the stomach. To protect the drug, erythromycin base is often formulated with an **enteric coating**, an acid-resistant shell that allows the drug to pass intact through the stomach and be dissolved and absorbed in the small intestine, where the pH is near neutral (see Chapter 1).

Another way to avoid destruction of the drug in the stomach is to use chemical forms of erythromycin with increased resistance to acid and thus better oral absorption. These compounds are the stearate, ethylsuccinate, and estolate esters of erythromycin. Erythromycin stearate and erythromycin ethylsuccinate are absorbed more rapidly and completely from the gastrointestinal (GI) tract than erythromycin base. Free erythromycin apparently is absorbed from the duodenum with these agents after hydrolysis of the esters. With erythromycin estolate, much better absorption is achieved, and the serum level may be four times higher than with other forms of erythromycin. However, with this form, most of the drug in the serum is actually the ester, and controversy exists regarding whether the ester has biologic activity. Many health care providers prefer erythromycin estolate because of the high tissue and blood levels and note that many tissues and bacteria can hydrolyze the ester form of the drug to release free erythromycin at the infection site.

Oral bioavailability for forms of erythromycin varies from 30% to 65%, depending on which preparation is used (Table 26-1). Food may interfere with the oral absorption of erythromycin base, but enteric preparations or erythromycin estolate, erythromycin ethylsuccinate, and dirithromycin are well absorbed even when food is present. Oral suspensions or tablet forms of azithromycin also yield a higher peak drug concentration when given with food.

Erythromycin readily distributes to tissues, where concentrations of drug may persist well beyond when it can be detected in serum. Erythromycin is especially concentrated in the liver and spleen. It enters fluids of the middle ear and pleural fluids but not cerebrospinal fluid (CSF) unless the meninges are inflamed. The drug crosses the placenta, but fetal blood levels are less than 20% of maternal blood levels. Erythromycin also enters breast milk, producing concentrations equal to that of maternal serum.

Azithromycin, clarithromycin, and dirithromycin are more strongly concentrated in tissues than is erythromycin and therefore persist longer in the body (see Table 26-1). Azithromycin and dirithromycin in particular concentrate in the lungs and other organs. Macrolides generally do not accumulate in normal brain tissue, although this remains to be tested for dirithromycin.

The liver is the major excretory organ for macrolides (see Table 26-1). A large percentage of the orally administered drug is concentrated in bile and excreted in feces. Some reabsorption from the intestine occurs during enterohepatic circulation (see Chapter 1). For erythromycin, most of the dose is inactivated in the liver. Less than 10% of orally administered erythromycin appears as active drug in urine; with intravenous doses, about 14% appears in urine. Clarithromycin also undergoes biotransformation in the liver, but up to 40% of a dose appears unchanged in urine; thus clarithromycin is more dependent on renal function than other macrolides.

Dirithromycin is rapidly converted to its active form erythromycylamine, but the conversion is not dependent on the liver or enzymes. There is little other biotransformation of either the prodrug or the active form. Excretion is almost exclusively biliary (see Table 26-1).

Azithromycin is primarily excreted by the liver, but the process is slow because so much drug is concentrated in the tissue. The half-life of the drug in serum is initially about 14 hours, but after several doses the half-life is as long as 4 days, the same as the tissue half-life. The high concentration of azithromycin in various tissues creates a large **volume of distribution** (Box 26-1). The combination of high tissue concentration and slow excretion from the body allows the drug to be used in 5-day treatment regimens rather than the longer regimens common with drugs that clear rapidly from the body. During treatment, the drug is distributed to various tissues, causing concentrations to rise; when treatment ceases, the drug is

---

TABLE 26-1

Pharmacokinetics of Macrolide Antibiotics

Drug	Bioavailability (%)	V_d	Half-Life	Routes of Excretion
azithromycin	37	2200 L	14 hours-4 days	Biliary: 50% (unchanged drug); liver: 35% demethylated; renal: 5 to 14%
clarithromycin	55	250 L	22 hours	Renal: 40% (unchanged drug); liver: extensive biotransformation
dirithromycin	6-14	800 L	44 hours	Biliary: 97%, no biotransformation*
erythromycin base	30-65	63 L	2 hours	Liver: 90% biotransformed; renal: up to 14% (unchanged drug)

V_d, Volume of distribution.

*Dirithromycin is converted nonenzymatically to its active form, erythromycylamine, almost completely within the body. No further chemical changes have been noted in the body.

BOX **26-1** | **Volume of Distribution**

The volume of distribution, or V_d, is a concept widely used by clinical pharmacologists to compare drugs in terms of their tendency to sequester in tissues. The magnitude of V_d for a particular drug is influenced by its degree of protein binding and its lipid solubility. The simplest way to determine the V_d is as follows:

$$V_d = \frac{\text{Amount of drug administered (mass)}}{\text{Initial serum concentration produced (mass/volume)}}$$

The units are mass divided by mass/volume; thus V_d is expressed in units of volume, such as liters (L).
Although V_d does not represent a real volume within the body, its magnitude is often compared to real volumes to understand the behavior of particular drugs. For example, the plasma volume of an adult is about 5 L, the extracellular fluid is about 10 to 20 L, and the intracellular fluid about 25 to 30 L. Drugs that have a volume of distribution higher than these values are heavily concentrated in tissues so that only a small proportion of the drug remains in plasma. Obviously, a calculated volume of distribution of hundreds or thousands of liters is not a real volume but only the imaginary volume that would be required to dilute the entire body load of the drug to the same concentration found in plasma. For example, azithromycin has a volume of distribution over 2000 L (see Table 26-1), indicating the drug is extensively concentrated in tissues, which can be confirmed by direct measurements. In contrast, many penicillins have a volume of distribution of 20 to 25 L, suggesting that these drugs are largely confined to plasma and extracellular fluid, which can also be confirmed by direct measurements.

DURING THERAPY

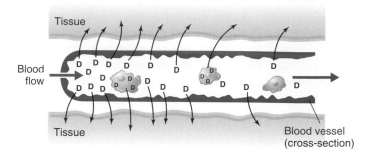

AFTER THERAPY

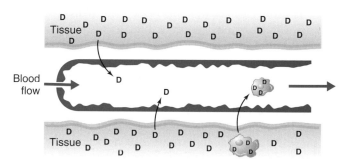

FIGURE 26-1 Tissue distribution of newer macrolide antibiotics. Macrolide antibiotics such as azithromycin, clarithromycin and dirithromycin move readily into white blood cells and tissues during therapy *(upper panel)*. The drug concentration in the blood may be initially high, especially with parenteral administration, but as the cells and the drug move out of the blood vessels into tissues, drug concentration in the blood falls to below tissue levels. After therapy, the drug gradually moves from tissues into the blood and is slowly excreted from the body *(lower panel)*. The long persistence of drug in tissues maintains effective concentrations for a significant period of time after actual dosing has ceased.

slowly released from the tissues and excreted, but effective drug concentrations are maintained well beyond the end of dosing (Figure 26-1).

ADVERSE REACTIONS AND CONTRAINDICATIONS

The most common patient complaint with oral macrolides is some form of GI tract difficulty. Abdominal discomfort and cramping are dose-related reactions to these drugs. Erythromycin probably produces cramping of the stomach because it acts as a agonist at motilin receptors in the stomach, which increases strength of contraction of stomach muscles.

Severe pain and nausea may rarely indicate pancreatitis. At normal dosages, nausea, vomiting, and diarrhea often occur, as with other oral antibiotics. Headache or dizziness may also occur. In addition to these adverse effects, clarithromycin may occasionally cause thrombocytopenia with bruising or bleeding. Azithromycin may cause interstitial nephritis with fever, rash, and joint pain.

Clinical studies suggest that pregnant women have a variable degree of absorption of oral erythromycin, such that many do not achieve an effective serum concentration. Erythromycin estolate also causes hepatotoxicity in about 10% of pregnant women. Therefore erythromycin and especially erythromycin estolate may not be recommended during pregnancy.

Erythromycin lactobionate causes extreme pain if it is infused too rapidly into a vein.

TOXICITY

Rarely, patients who receive more than 4 g of erythromycin daily experience hearing loss that may occur at any time during therapy but is usually reversible.

The most significant toxicity occurs with erythromycin estolate, which damages the liver by direct drug toxicity or an immune reaction. This reaction, called **cholestatic hepatitis,** usually appears 10 to 12 days after therapy is begun but may appear earlier in patients previously exposed to the drug. These patients may experience severe abdominal pain, liver enlargement, fever, and jaundice. In most patients these symptoms rapidly disappear when the drug is discontinued.

INTERACTIONS

Erythromycin is biotransformed in the liver and therefore may compete with other drugs for the limited hepatic metabolic capacity. For example, alfentanil, carbamazepine, cyclosporine, warfarin, valproic acid, and theophylline must be excreted by hepatic mechanisms; when erythromycin is given concurrently, these drugs are excreted more slowly, serum levels rise, and the drugs may accumulate. Because these drugs have dose-related toxicity, an increase in their serum levels also increases the risk of serious toxicity. Clarithromycin also increases serum concentrations of carbamazepine and theophylline. Dirithromycin does not act on hepatic enzymes and therefore shares none of these interactions.

Rarely, erythromycin may cause hepatotoxicity, especially when used at high dosages or for long periods. The risk of liver damage is increased if erythromycin is given concurrently with other hepatotoxic drugs such as acetaminophen (at high dosages), anabolic steroids, androgens, estrogens, isoniazid, ketoconazole, phenothiazines, rifampin, sulfonamides, or valproic acid.

Macrolides can interact in several ways with other antimicrobial drugs. Erythromycin and other macrolides can antagonize the antibacterial effects of clindamycin and chloramphenicol because they share the same target in bacteria and may displace each other. Macrolides should not be used concurrently with these antibiotics. Rifabutin, a drug used to treat *Mycobacterium avium-intracellulare* infections, significantly lowers the serum concentration of clarithromycin. Serum concentration of zidovudine is significantly lowered by clarithromycin; the drugs must be taken at least 4 hours apart to avoid this interaction.

Erythromycin lactobionate or erythromycin gluceptate may be rapidly inactivated if added to fluids below pH 5.5. This sensitivity to pH extremes makes erythromycin incompatible in solution with a number of other drugs. These forms of erythromycin are also incompatible with preservatives sometimes used in sterile water. Before adding erythromycin to any other drug solution, compatibility of the agents should be verified with the pharmacist.

Few interactions have been noted with azithromycin. The major documented interaction involves aluminum and magnesium contained in antacids. These materials partially inhibit absorption of azithromycin and should be taken at least 2 hours before the antibiotic (see the Case Study: *Chlamydia* Infection).

APPLICATION TO PRACTICE

ASSESSMENT

The general aspects of nursing care for the patient receiving any antimicrobial drug were covered in Chapter 24. In this chapter, only those aspects related specifically to macrolide antibiotics are discussed.

History of Present Illness

The patient with an infection typically displays the five cardinal signs and symptoms of infection, which include swelling, redness, pain, heat, and loss of function. Be sure to ask the patient about the location, onset, severity, timing, duration, signs and symptoms, quality, and context of his or her concerns as well as anything the patient has tried that improved or worsened these signs and symptoms.

Health History

A thorough health history may reveal previous hypersensitivity reactions. Determine if the patient has a sensitivity to tartrazine (FDA yellow dye #5), because some erythromycin formulations contain this dye and may provoke an allergic reaction in some patients. It is also important to ask whether he or she has ever taken one of these drugs before and, if so, whether severe abdominal pain, fever, liver enlargement, or jaundice (cholestatic hepatitis) associated with the drug developed. Naming a few of the common macrolide drugs may help the patient identify previous usage. Be sure to ask about use of other prescription drugs, herbal remedies, and OTC drugs so as to minimize the risk of drug-drug interactions.

Determine if the patient has hepatic impairment, in which case erythromycin should be used with caution, particularly erythromycin estolate. Patients with a history of arrhythmia may be at risk for a recurrence with high doses of erythromycin.

Lifespan Considerations

Perinatal. Macrolides fall into pregnancy category B and thus are generally considered safe to use during pregnancy in nonallergic patients. These drugs are safe for the fetus, and they are often recommended to treat syphilis and chlamydia infections in penicillin-allergic pregnant women. However, preparations of the estolate ester should be avoided. In one study, a significant proportion of pregnant women (10% to 15%) who received erythromycin estolate for 3 weeks developed subclinical, reversible hepatic toxicity. The fetal plasma concentration is 5% to 20% of that found in maternal plasma. Macrolide drugs appear in breast milk and may cause diarrhea and candidiasis in the nursing infant.

Pediatric. Macrolides are generally considered safe for use in children.

Older Adults. Use of macrolides in the older adult is relatively safe, although decreased renal function associated with changes of aging, hepatic disease, or other disease processes, and concurrent drug therapies increase the risk of adverse effects.

Cultural/Social Considerations

Overall, the cultural and social considerations associated with the use of macrolides are minimal. In most cases, bacterial infections sensitive to macrolides are short-term, subacute conditions that are easily treated on an outpatient basis.

Compared with the other classes of antimicrobial drugs, the older macrolides are relatively inexpensive. However, the rising cost of antibiotics—particularly the newer ones such as azithromycin—presents a hardship to many, especially older adults, those who are financially disadvantaged, and those who have pharmacy insurance plans through managed care organizations.

Physical Examination

Assess the patient for signs and symptoms of infection. Be sure to include the vital signs and inspect any wound. A thorough examination is particularly necessary to detect any infection traveling indirectly from a distant body site (e.g., a total joint replacement of the hip may fail as a result of a cut finger that became infected). Evaluate the patient's level of discomfort related to the infection.

Laboratory Testing

Many antimicrobials have harsh adverse effects on other body systems. Because of the risk of superinfection in patients receiving a macrolide, observe patients, particularly older adults and those who are debilitated, for symptoms of bacterial and fungal overgrowth. Evidence of superinfection (e.g., diarrhea, vaginal or anal itching, black furry appearance of the tongue) should be reported. Superinfection by *Candida* organisms can usually be managed by discontinuing the antibiotics or by administering an antifungal drug.

GOALS OF THERAPY

The goals of treatment with macrolides are to ameliorate the signs and symptoms of infection, to prevent complications associated with therapy, and to prevent sepsis and death.

INTERVENTION
Administration

Before the first dose of macrolide is given, the patient's history should be carefully reviewed for allergies. Keep in mind that a negative history of hypersensitivity does not preclude future reactions.

The erythromycin base, estolate, stearate, and ethylsuccinate formulations are available for oral use. Erythromycin lactobionate is available as an intravenous formulation, but it can cause extreme pain if it is infused too rapidly into a vein. This form of erythromycin may be rapidly inactivated if added to intravenous fluids with a pH below 5.5. This sensitivity to pH extremes makes erythromycin incompatible in solution with a number of other drugs. Erythromycin is also incompatible with preservatives sometimes used in sterile water. Before adding erythromycin to any other drug solution, compatibility of the drugs should be verified with the pharmacist.

The film-coated formulations of erythromycin base and stearate are absorbed better on an empty stomach, at least 1 hour before or 2 hours after meals. They may be taken with food if GI irritation occurs. Enteric-coated formulations may be taken without regard to meals. Erythromycin ethylsuccinate is best absorbed when taken with meals. Chewable tablets should be crushed or chewed and not swallowed whole. The delayed-release capsules of erythromycin base may be opened and sprinkled on applesauce, jelly, or ice cream immediately before ingestion.

Erythromycin formulations may be administered intermittently or as a continuous intravenous infusion over a period of 4 hours. Caution is warranted in regard to compatibility with other drugs and intravenous fluids.

Topical formulations of erythromycin are available in ointments, gels, or solutions. They should be used only as directed, and the affected area should be cleansed prior to application. The nurse should wear gloves during application.

Education

Instruct the patient to take the full course of the antibiotic drug (usually 10 days) even though symptoms may abate and he or she may start feeling better before the full course of therapy is completed. Emphasize the importance of taking evenly spaced doses to maintain a therapeutic blood level. Missed doses should be taken as soon as remembered; remaining doses should be evenly spaced throughout the day. Prescriptions for any antibiotic should never be shared with others or saved and taken for a different episode of illness.

Also instruct the patient to contact the health care provider if his or her condition does not improve in a few days. The patient should report persistent nausea, vomiting, diarrhea, or stomach cramps or if there is severe abdominal pain, a yellowish discoloration of the skin or eyes, darkened urine, pale stools, or he or she develops unusual tiredness. Have the patient contact the health care provider if evidence of superinfection develops.

Patients with an allergy to a macrolide drug should be advised to wear some form of identification (e.g., medical alert tag or bracelet) to inform health care personnel of the allergy. Carrying the identification in a wallet or purse is usually not helpful if emergency care is needed.

EVALUATION

The effectiveness of macrolide therapy is determined by monitoring the clinical response. The frequency of monitoring is proportional to the severity of the infec-

---

CASE STUDY  Chlamydia *Infection*

ASSESSMENT

HISTORY OF PRESENT ILLNESS

JC is a 20-year-old pregnant woman in for her first prenatal visit. She thinks she is 12 weeks pregnant and is complaining of lower abdominal pain, cramping, and symptoms of urinary tract infection. Her last menstrual period (LMP) was 4 months ago.

HEALTH HISTORY

JC is allergic to penicillins and cephalosporins, which cause a rash. Her history is negative for cardiovascular, respiratory, renal, hepatic, or neurologic disorders.

LIFESPAN CONSIDERATIONS

JC is at risk for premature labor, premature rupture of membranes (PROM), and infant prematurity resulting from the infection. *Chlamydia* infection is the leading cause of conjunctivitis (known as ophthalmia neonatorum) and afebrile pneumonia in neonates.

CULTURAL/SOCIAL CONSIDERATIONS

JC generally considers herself healthy. She lives alone in a small rural community with income from a small food stand supplemented by assistance from the Women, Infants, and Children's (WIC) Program. Predisposing factors that increase likelihood of chlamydial infection are single status, oral contraceptive use, young age, and lower socioeconomic status.

PHYSICAL EXAMINATION

JC's temperature is 98.2° F, pulse 80, respirations 16, and blood pressure is 134/88 mm Hg. The results of her urinal-

ysis are within normal limits; the pregnancy test is positive. She has scant vaginal discharge, no odor; nulliparous cervix is closed, nontender, and mobile; Goodell's and Chadwick's signs are positive; adnexa are negative. The fundus is slightly below the umbilicus (16-week size); linea nigra is present; fetal heart tones (FHT) are 160 beats per minute.

LABORATORY TESTING

Culture is positive for *Chlamydia*, negative for gonorrhea, syphilis, and HIV.

PATIENT PROBLEM(S)

Chlamydia infection during pregnancy.

GOALS OF THERAPY

Ameliorate chlamydial infection, thus reducing the risk of preterm labor and premature birth.

CRITICAL THINKING QUESTIONS

1. Erythromycin base 500 mg po 4 times daily for 7 days has been ordered for JC. What is the mechanism of action of this drug? Is it bacteriocidal or bacteriostatic?
2. What common adverse effects should be watched for when erythromycin is used?
3. Pregnant women have variable absorption of oral erythromycin. What is the outcome of variable absorption?
4. What is the major route of excretion of macrolides?
5. What advantage do the esters of erythromycin have over erythromycin base?
6. What toxic reaction is unique to erythromycin estolate?

tion. Important clinical indicators of effective treatment include a reduction in fever and resolution of the signs and symptoms of infection, vital signs that return to normal for the patient, WBC count that returns to normal limits, and a culture and sensitivity test that is negative for the offending organism. Further proof may include an increase in appetite, energy level, and general sense of well-being.

Bibliography

Farrington E: Macrolide antibiotics, *Pediatr Nurs* 24(5):433-434, 437-438, 1998.

Mead M: Drugs for chest infections, *Pract Nurse* 19(3):126-127, 2000.

Miller D: Using the newer antibiotics wisely, *Patient Care* 33(14):97-108, 1999.

Pinkowish MD: Community-acquired pneumonia: atypical may not be unusual, *Patient Care* 34(2):15, 18-19, 2000.

Self TH: Macrolide-drug interactions: maintaining vigilance reduces risk, *J Crit Illn* 15(2):91-92, 2000.

Zuckerman JM: The newer macrolides: azithromycin and clarithromycin, *Infect Dis Clin North Am* 14(2):449-462, 2000.

Internet Resource

Nurses PDR. Available online at http://www.nursespdr.com/members/database/ndrhtml/azithromycin.html.

Fluoroquinolones and Related Drugs

SHERRY F. QUEENER • KATHLEEN GUTIERREZ

 Visit **http://evolve.elsevier.com/Gutierrez/** for additional information.

KEY TERMS

Community-acquired pneumonia, p. 413

Crystalluria, p. 416

Topoisomerases, p. 414

OBJECTIVES

- Explain the unique mechanism of action of fluoroquinolone antibiotics.
- Discuss the adverse effects that are most common with fluoroquinolones.
- Explain why fluoroquinolones are generally not used in children and should be avoided by patients with a history of seizures.
- Develop a nursing care plan for a patient receiving a fluoroquinolone.

 ## PATHOPHYSIOLOGY

Infections caused by bacteria range from mild local infections to life-threatening systemic diseases (see Chapter 24). Gram-positive bacteria are associated with many infections of the throat and ears as well as soft tissue infections. These bacteria also typically cause community-acquired pneumonia in adults, which is a type of infection acquired outside of the patient-care setting. Gram-negative bacteria are likely to be the cause of urinary tract infections (UTIs). These organisms may also cause pneumonia, especially in hospitalized or chronically ill patients.

DRUG CLASS • Fluoroquinolones

alatrofloxacin (Trovan preservative-free)

⚕ ciprofloxacin (Cipro, Ciloxin)

gatifloxacin (Tequin)

grepafloxacin (Raxar)

⚕ levofloxacin (Levaquin, Quixin)

lomefloxacin (Maxaquin)

moxifloxacin (Avelox)

norfloxacin (Noroxin)

ofloxacin (Floxin, Ocuflox)

sparfloxacin (Zagam)

trovafloxacin (Trovan)

MECHANISM OF ACTION

Fluoroquinolones interfere with DNA replication in bacteria by inhibiting topoisomerases, enzymes involved in handling DNA, which exist in bacteria as a single closed circular chromosome. In gram-negative bacteria, the primary target is a topoisomerase II known as DNA gyrase. This enzyme allows the tightly wound, double strands of bacterial DNA to unwind (relax) so that replication may proceed. In gram-positive bacteria, the primary target may be topoisomerase IV, an enzyme that opens the closed circles of DNA and allows the daughter chromosomes to separate after replication. By interfering with the activity of these enzymes, fluoroquinolones block bacterial reproduction and may cause breaks in double-stranded DNA. These drugs are bactericidal at concentrations achieved in the blood.

Resistance to fluoroquinolones can occur by a variety of mechanisms. Some resistance is carried by plasmids, but resistance also arises spontaneously. For example, mutation of the topoisomerases such that they no longer bind with the antibiotic confers resistance. Increasing transport mechanisms to move the antibiotic out of bacterial cells is another common mechanism for resistance.

USES

The fluoroquinolone antibiotics are potent drugs that act against a variety of bacteria. They are especially useful for infections caused by gram-negative organisms. Thus fluoroquinolones that penetrate adequately into the urogenital tract are used for urinary tract infections, gonorrhea, urethritis, cervicitis, and prostatitis (Table 27-1). In addition, ofloxacin may be used for pelvic inflammatory disease, and gatifloxacin or levofloxacin may be indicated for pyelonephritis. Ciprofloxacin is the most effective of the class against *Pseudomonas aeruginosa*, a gram-negative bacteria that causes serious infections of the urinary tract and other sites.

Intraabdominal infections and even typhoid fever are sometimes treated with ciprofloxacin, but this drug, like most other fluoroquinolones, is not strongly effective against anaerobic bacteria. Thus it may need to be combined with another drug with specific activ-

---

TABLE 27-1

Primary Indications for Fluoroquinolones

Infection	Drug
Primarily Involving Gram-Negative Bacteria	
Urinary tract infections	**ciprofloxacin,** gatifloxacin, **levofloxacin,** lomefloxacin, norfloxacin, ofloxacin
Gonorrhea	**ciprofloxacin,** gatifloxacin, norfloxacin, ofloxacin
Nongonococcal urethritis/cervicitis	ofloxacin
Prostatitis	**ciprofloxacin,** norfloxacin, ofloxacin
Primarily Involving Gram-Positive Bacteria	
Community-acquired pneumonia	gatifloxacin, **levofloxacin,** moxifloxacin, ofloxacin, sparfloxacin
Acute worsening of chronic bronchitis	**ciprofloxacin,** gatifloxacin, **levofloxacin,** lomefloxacin, moxifloxacin, ofloxacin, sparfloxacin
Acute sinusitis	**ciprofloxacin,** gatifloxacin, **levofloxacin,** moxifloxacin
Uncomplicated skin/soft tissue infections	**ciprofloxacin, levofloxacin,** ofloxacin

ity against anaerobic bacteria (see Chapter 30). Newer fluoroquinolones such as moxifloxacin and especially trovafoxacin have better activity against anaerobic bacteria than other fluoroquinolones.

Many fluoroquinolones are well distributed to the lung and other soft tissues. Thus they may be effective against bronchitis, pneumonia, and skin infections caused by susceptible organisms (see Table 27-1). Many of these infections are caused by gram-positive bacteria, which have differing levels of susceptibility to fluoroquinolones. For example, strains of *Staphylococcus aureus* that produce penicillinase can be susceptible to fluoroquinolones, but methicillin-resistant *S. aureus* (MRSA) has become mostly resistant. Likewise, streptococcal pneumonia has sometimes developed or progressed during therapy with ciprofloxacin. Some of the newer fluoroquinolones, such as gatifloxacin or levofloxacin, are more effective against gram-positive bacteria and may become the preferred drugs for infections likely to

involve these bacteria. Ciprofloxacin remains the drug of choice for both cutaneous and pulmonary anthrax (Box 27-1).

Trovafloxacin and its prodrug alatrofloxacin have very restricted uses; they are indicated only for life-threatening infections of the urinary or respiratory tract.

PHARMACOKINETICS

Fluoroquinolones are generally well absorbed when given orally; oral bioavailability ranges from 70% to almost 100%. Persistence in plasma is greatest with the new drugs gatifloxacin, grepafloxacin and sparfloxacin; their half-lives range from 7 to 30 hours. For other fluoroquinolones, the half-lives range from 3 to 12 hours. As a class, the fluoroquinolones penetrate tissues well, and in some cases, tissue concentration exceeds the serum concentration.

Portal circulation carries orally administered fluoroquinolones directly to the liver, where biotransformation occurs. Grepafloxacin, moxifloxacin, and sparfloxacin are extensively biotransformed, partly to glucuronides, which may be excreted renally, and partly to other forms. For ciprofloxacin, norfloxacin, and trovafloxacin, hepatic biotransformation accounts for 20% to 25% of a dose. Gatifloxacin, levofloxacin, lomefloxacin, and ofloxacin undergo little hepatic biotransformation.

Trovafloxacin is given orally, but when intravenous doses are required, the prodrug alatrofloxacin is used. Upon entry into the body, the prodrug is rapidly split to release trovafloxacin.

Gatifloxacin, levofloxacin, lomefloxacin, and ofloxacin rely almost solely on renal mechanisms for elimination, with little contribution by hepatic metabolism or biliary excretion. The amount of an oral dose of one of these drugs that appears unchanged in urine ranges from 60% to 87%. Dosages of these drugs and many other fluoroquinolones may require adjustment in patients with renal impairment, because the kidneys are the primary organ of excretion not only of the active drug but also of metabolites. Typically, doses are cut in half or the dosing interval is doubled when the creatinine clearance level falls below about 50% of normal values.

ADVERSE REACTIONS AND CONTRAINDICATIONS

Fluoroquinolones have two adverse reactions that limit the clinical use of the whole class. The first, which involves the CNS, includes symptoms such as headache, dizziness, tinnitus, insomnia, shakiness, changes in vision, and seizures. These drugs are used cautiously in patients with preexisting CNS disease, such as previous seizure activity, because they can worsen the problem.

BOX 27-1 | **Anthrax: An Old Disease Becomes a Public Health Threat**

Anthrax is an infection caused by *Bacillus anthracis*, a bacterium that persists for years in soil as spores. The spores are consumed by animals, which leads to infection from time to time. In the United States before 2001, anthrax in humans was a rare cutaneous infection largely confined to persons exposed to animals or animal hides, but today both the cutaneous and the more serious, pulmonary forms of the disease are of concern to public health officials because of bioterrorism. Partially purified preparations of the spores have been delivered through the mail, contaminating postal workers as well as infecting the recipients.

Several features of the disease are important to understand when assessing the true level of the health threat. First, a large number of spores is usually required to produce pulmonary disease. Second, the disease does not spread from person to person, so infection depends on exposure to the spores. Third, the disease is treatable. For pulmonary forms of anthrax, it is important that therapy begin soon after exposure to be most effective. For cutaneous forms of the disease, therapy usually begins after symptoms develop but is nevertheless usually effective.

The drug of choice for anthrax is ciprofloxacin. However, many other drugs have also been used effectively, including penicillin G, doxycycline, erythromycin, or chloramphenicol. Thus the tools exist for effective control of this bioterrorist weapon.

The second adverse reaction shared by the whole class of fluoroquinolones is a tendency to damage cartilage. This reaction, which leads to permanent damage and lameness, was observed in young animals during preclinical trials of the first fluoroquinolones. Therefore these drugs are not given to children or adolescents up to age 18 years. Tendinitis, especially of the Achilles tendon, has also been noted occasionally in adults receiving these drugs; thus they are contraindicated in patients with a history of tendinitis or tendon rupture.

In addition to the serious adverse reactions already noted, fluoroquinolones, like many other oral antibiotics, can cause mild to moderate gastrointestinal (GI) tract symptoms, including nausea, vomiting, and diarrhea.

Allergies to fluoroquinolones are uncommon but can be severe. Symptoms include rashes, itching, shortness of breath, serum sickness, and Stevens-Johnson syndrome. Allergy to nalidixic acid or any other fluoroquinolone may be a contraindication for receiving any fluoroquinolone, because cross-allergenicity does exist.

A few individual fluoroquinolones have specific serious adverse reactions. Gatifloxacin, grepafloxacin, moxifloxacin, and sparfloxacin cause a prolongation of the QTc interval on the electrocardiogram. This action may slow the heart rate and produce symptoms, including fainting. Therefore, these drugs are avoided in patients with hypokalemia or other preexisting conditions that prolong the QTc interval. They are also not recommended for patients with a history of atrial fibrillation, bradycardia, congestive heart failure, or myocardial infarction. Because of these serious adverse reactions, grepafloxacin has been withdrawn from the U.S. market by one company that licensed it.

Trovafloxacin has been linked to acute liver failure, which led to death or the need for liver transplantation in 14 patients in early clinical trials. For these reasons, the FDA recommends that this drug, or its prodrug alatrofloxacin, be limited to 14-day therapy for life-threatening situations when other antibiotics are not indicated. If either drug is used, liver enzymes must be monitored to detect early signs of liver toxicity.

TOXICITY

Overdoses may require gastric lavage or induction of emesis. High dosages of any fluoroquinolone may cause signs of CNS toxicity, including tremors or seizures. High dosages of ciprofloxacin or norfloxacin may cause renal difficulties because both drugs are relatively insoluble, especially in alkaline urine. Most people have slightly acidic urine, but strict vegetarians and persons taking certain drugs (see the following discussion) may have alkaline urine. Under these conditions, the drug may crystallize in the urinary tract, causing pain and obstruction. The risk for this complication, called **crystalluria**, can be lessened by acidifying the urine and maintaining an adequate fluid intake.

Overdoses of fluoroquinolones may cause arrhythmias; patients should be carefully observed for any changes in heart rate or rhythm.

INTERACTIONS

Antacids or nutritional supplements (e.g., Ensure) containing aluminum or magnesium compounds can block absorption of fluoroquinolones. Lower plasma and urinary concentrations of the antibiotic and loss of antibacterial effectiveness result. To avoid this interaction, the antibiotics should be taken 2 hours before the antacids. Didanosine, an antiretroviral drug used to combat human immunodeficiency virus (HIV), reduces absorption of ciprofloxacin and possibly other fluoroquinolones because the didanosine preparation contains aluminum. These combinations should be avoided.

Sodium bicarbonate, citrates, carbonic anhydrase inhibitors, and antacids containing calcium may alkalinize urine, which renders ciprofloxacin and norfloxacin less soluble. Avoiding these drugs and maintaining an adequate fluid intake lessen the risk of crystalluria.

Ciprofloxacin and grepafloxacin lower hepatic clearance of the asthma medication theophylline, which can cause this drug to accumulate. As the serum theophylline level increases, so does the risk of CNS toxicity; nausea, vomiting, tremors, restlessness, agitation, and palpitations may occur. Most case reports of seizure activity in patients receiving fluoroquinolones have involved patients who were also receiving theophylline. Caffeine clearance can also be slowed by some fluoroquinolones. Levofloxacin, lomefloxacin, ofloxacin, sparfloxacin, and trovafloxacin have little or no effect on caffeine or theophylline clearance and thus are not subject to this interaction.

Warfarin anticoagulation effects may be increased by ciprofloxacin or norfloxacin and possibly other fluoroquinolones. To avoid episodes of bleeding, prothrombin times should be monitored in patients receiving warfarin and a fluoroquinolone.

Grepafloxacin and sparfloxacin must be avoided in patients receiving drugs such as disopyramide, erythromycin, phenothiazines, and tricyclic antidepressants, because all these drugs can increase the QT interval. These combinations put patients at risk of a potentially fatal ventricular arrhythmia called *torsade de pointes*.

APPLICATION TO PRACTICE

ASSESSMENT

The general aspects of nursing care for the patient receiving any antimicrobial drug were covered in Chapter 24. In this chapter, only those aspects related specifically to fluoroquinolone antibiotics are discussed.

History of Present Illness

In addition to the typical inquiry regarding the onset, precipitating factors (what makes it better, what makes it worse), quality, radiation, severity (how this illness interferes with activities of daily living), and attempts at self-treatment, ask the patient what he or she thinks is producing the illness (Box 27-2).

Health History

Ask the patient if he or she has a history of arrhythmia, bronchitis, pneumonia, urinary tract infections, gonorrhea, urethritis, cervicitis, pelvic inflammatory disease, prostatitis, pyelonephritis, intraabdominal infections, skin infections, tendonitis, or seizure activity. If the patient has end-stage renal disease, be sure to ask if he or she is on dialysis, because fluoroquinolones increase the risk of tendon rupture and CNS toxicity. In addition, ask about the patient's general health, comorbid disease, living conditions, drug use, hygiene practices, sexual practices, travel history, and environmental exposure to potential pathogens.

A thorough health history may reveal previous hypersensitivity drug reactions. Naming a few of the common fluoroquinolone drugs may help the patient identify any previous use. Be sure also to ask about use of other prescription drugs (e.g., theophylline, anticoagulants), herbal remedies, and OTC drugs (particularly antacids or drugs containing iron or zinc) to minimize the risk of drug-drug interactions.

 Dietary Considerations: Fluoroquinolones and Food Consumption

A strictly vegetarian diet produces alkaline urine, which may contribute to fluoroquinolone-induced crystalluria. Ask about the patient's caffeine consumption, dietary preferences, and the use of any dietary supplements or tube feedings.

Milk and yogurt decrease the absorption of ciprofloxacin. Advise the patient not to consume them concurrently with this drug.

Lifespan Considerations

Perinatal. Fluoroquinolones are pregnancy category C drugs and as such should not be used during pregnancy and lactation.

Pediatric. Fluoroquinolones are contraindicated in children and adolescents under the age of 18 years because of the risk of cartilage damage.

Older Adults. Tendinitis, especially of the Achilles tendon, has been noted occasionally in adults receiving fluoroquinolones; thus patients with a history of tendinitis or tendon rupture should avoid these drugs.

Cultural/Social Considerations

In most cases, infections are short-term, subacute conditions easily treated on an outpatient basis. However, in some cases, hospitalization is required for serious, potentially life-threatening infections. The effect of cultural and social variables should be noted, although the considerations associated with fluoroquinolones are overall minimal. These drugs, however, tend to be expensive and are not covered by many pharmacy insurance plans. The cost of fluoroquinolones may present a hardship to many patients, especially older adults and disadvantaged patients.

Physical Examination

The physical examination of a patient with an infection should include vital signs as well as assessment of body systems suspected of harboring the infection (e.g., lungs, kidneys, GI or genitourinary [GU] tract, skin). Because a high dosage of any fluoroquinolone can cause CNS toxicity, be sure to perform a neurologic and mental status examination and watch for tremors or evidence of seizure activity.

Laboratory Testing

Culture and sensitivity tests should be performed to determine the causative organism before starting drug therapy; however, in many cases treatment will be started empirically. High doses of ciprofloxacin or norfloxacin increase the risk of nephrotoxicity. Thus baseline laboratory values for BUN, serum creatinine, proteinuria, azotemia, and intake and output measurement will help determine the onset of nephrotoxicity.

GOALS OF THERAPY

The treatment goals when using fluoroquinolones are to ameliorate the signs and symptoms of infection, to prevent complications associated with therapy, and to prevent sepsis and death. Although a number of different classes of antibiotics can be considered, clinical efficacy, adverse effect profile, pharmacokinetic disposition, and cost considerations ultimately guide the drug choice. Once a drug has been selected, the dosage must be based on patient size, site of infection, route of elimination, and other factors such as the likelihood of drug resistance.

INTERVENTION
Administration

Before the first dose of a fluoroquinolone antibiotic is given, the patient's history should be carefully reviewed for allergies. Keep in mind that a negative history of hypersensitivity does not preclude future reactions. Dosage adjustment of a fluoroquinolone for the older adult based simply on age is not required.

Fluoroquinolones can be administered orally or intravenously. Before administration, the health care provider should check thoroughly that the route ordered is correct for the individual drug. Give the drug as directed at evenly spaced times. Missed doses should be taken as soon as possible, unless it is almost time for the next dose. Do not double doses. Administer norfloxacin, ofloxacin, levofloxacin, lomefloxacin, sparfloxacin, trovafloxacin, and enoxacin with a full glass of water on an empty stomach 1 hour before or 2 hours after meals. If gastric irritation occurs, ciprofloxacin and lomefloxacin may be administered with meals, although food slows drug absorption and may even slightly reduce it. Antacids containing magnesium or aluminum, sucralfate, or iron or zinc preparations should not be taken within 4 hours before and 2 hours after administration.

Fluoroquinolones frequently cause irritation when they are administered intravenously. To reduce site irritation, the drug should be diluted and administered in the time frame recommended by the manufacturer. The insertion site should be assessed frequently for signs and symptoms of inflammation (e.g., redness or tenderness) so that the site can be changed as needed.

To avoid the risk for nephrotoxicity that may result from fluoroquinolones, patients should be kept well hydrated, and the drug therapy should be limited to 14 days or less (in most cases). Monitor for signs and symptoms of nephrotoxicity.

Education

Patients should be taught about their drug; knowledge is helpful in improving compliance with the dosage regimen. It is important that patients understand that fluoroquinolones are to be taken precisely as prescribed in dosage, frequency, and for the specified time, even though symptoms may abate before the full course of therapy is completed. If the blood level of the fluoroquinolone drops because of a late dose or from discontinuing the drug too soon, the pathogens have an opportunity to increase in virulence or to become resistant to the drug.

If a dose is missed, it should be taken as soon as remembered, unless it is almost time for the next dose. To avoid drug-drug interactions, the health care provider should be contacted before other drugs are used. Advise the patient that sharing the antibiotic with friends or family members can be dangerous.

Patients should be instructed to report any signs or symptoms of allergic response. Patients with a fluoroquinolone allergy should be advised to wear some form of identification (e.g., medical alert identification bracelet or necklace) to inform health care personnel of the allergy. Carrying the identification in a wallet or purse is usually not helpful if emergency care is needed.

Teach the patient to increase consumption of breads, cranberries, cereals, cheese, eggs, fish, meats, prunes, plums, poultry, tomatoes, and tomato sauce to help acidify the urine and reduce the risk of crystalluria. Maintaining a daily fluid intake of at least 1.5 to 2 L also helps.

In addition, the patient should be taught what signs and symptoms to report to the health care provider. The patient should watch for signs and symptoms of serious adverse effects and toxicities such as GI discomfort, nausea, vomiting, diarrhea, oliguria, headache, dizziness, agitation, confusion, hallucinations, insomnia, tremors, changes in vision, and heel pain or Achilles discomfort. Advise the patient to notify the health care provider if GI reactions are severe or persistent. Caution the patient to avoid driving or operating hazardous machinery if CNS symptoms develop, and to notify the health care provider immediately if rash, tendon pain, or inflammation occur. The health care provider should also be contacted if symptoms of the illness do not improve within 48 hours, although the time for complete resolution depends on the specific organism and the site of infection.

Photosensitivity may occur with high doses of lomefloxacin and phototoxicity with sparfloxacin. Advise the patient to use sunscreen and to wear sunglasses and protective clothing when taking these drugs and for the 5 days following conclusion of therapy.

Instruct the patient to report signs of superinfection (furry overgrowth on the tongue, vaginal itching or discharge, loose or foul-smelling stools).

EVALUATION

Antibiotic effectiveness is assessed by monitoring clinical responses and laboratory results. The frequency of monitoring is proportional to the severity of the infection. Clinical indicators of effective treatment include a

CASE STUDY  *Community-Acquired Pneumonia*

ASSESSMENT

HISTORY OF PRESENT ILLNESS

TE is a 75-year-old woman who comes to the office today accompanied by her elderly roommate. TE complains of a headache; fever; a sudden onset of chills; pleuritic chest pain; a cough with dark, thick, bloody sputum; increasing shortness of breath; and anorexia. TE had an episode of what appeared to be bronchitis about 5 weeks ago. She seemed to recover for a time but feels she has had a relapse. She has done nothing to treat herself except to increase her fluid intake. She reports a fever as high as 101° F. Her roommate mentions noticing increasing confusion in TE.

HEALTH HISTORY

TE's routine drugs include a multiple vitamin, warfarin sodium, furosemide, enalapril, budesonide inhaler, and albuterol. She refused the pneumonia vaccination and flu shot, stating that it gives her the flu. She has no known allergies. She has a long-standing history of hypertension, heart failure, and chronic obstructive pulmonary disease.

LIFESPAN CONSIDERATIONS

Dosage adjustment based on age alone is not necessary.

CULTURAL/SOCIAL CONSIDERATIONS

TE shares household expenses by living with a woman who is a heavy smoker. TE herself has not smoked in 20 years. She is on a fixed income, a large portion of which goes to pay for her drugs and health care.

PHYSICAL EXAMINATION

TE's temperature is 102.3° F, pulse 100, respirations 32, and blood pressure is 110/60 mm Hg. Her SaO_2 level is 89% at rest on room air, desaturating to 83% with exercise. Blood gas levels: pH, 7.3; pCO_2, 50 mm Hg; and HCO_3, 17 mEq/L.

TE's posteroanterior (PA) and lateral chest x-ray studies show multifocal peribronchial consolidation.

LABORATORY TESTING

Sputum culture reveals *Streptococcus pneumoniae* organisms; leukocytosis is present with an immature shift to the left on the differential. The CBC count, urinalysis, BUN, and creatinine levels are all within normal limits.

PATIENT PROBLEM(S)

Community-acquired pneumonia.

GOALS OF THERAPY

Eradicate lung infection while minimizing adverse effects of drug therapy and effect on comorbid conditions.

CRITICAL THINKING QUESTIONS

1. Levofloxacin 500 mg po daily for 14 days has been ordered for TE. Is this a safe dosage for her?
2. What is the mechanism of action of levofloxacin?
3. Why is it important to know the renal status of a patient receiving a fluoroquinolone antibiotic?
4. Does TE have any contraindications to the use of or factors that warrant cautious use of levofloxacin in treating her bronchopneumonia?
5. Which type of patients are most likely to develop seizures if they receive a fluoroquinolone?
6. Which drug-drug interactions can occur with levofloxacin? Should this drug be taken on an empty stomach?
7. How soon would you expect improvement in TE once levofloxacin is started? What would be the next course of action if she does not respond within this expected time frame?

reduction in fever and resolution of the signs and symptoms of infection, vital signs return to normal for the patient, the WBC count returns to normal limits, and a culture and sensitivity test is negative for the offending organism. Further proof may include an increase in appetite, energy level, and general sense of well-being.

Bibliography

Anonymous: Resistant strep strains continue troubling rise: penicillin on the run; are fluoroquinolones next? Hospital Infection Control 26:147-151, 156, 1999.

Behta M, Khan KM, Hartman BJ: The new fluoroquinolones: a review of their properties, *Emergency Medicine* 33(1):16-26, 2001.

Hardman J, Limbird L: *Goodman and Gilman's pharmacological basis of therapeutics,* ed 10, New York, 2001, McGraw-Hill.

North DS: Common questions about the newer fluoroquinolone antibiotics, *Nurse Practitioner* 24(3):124-127, 1999.

Pau AK, Slone RB: Antibiotics in primary care: focus on fluoroquinolones and other new and investigational antimicrobial agents, *Primary Care Practice* 3(1):39-54, 1999.

Internet Resources

Medline. Available online at http://www.nlm.nih.gov/ medlineplus/druginfo/fluoroquinolones.

http://www.nursefriendly.com/nursing/drugs/antibiotics/ fluoroquinolones.htm.

Micromedex. Available online at http://www.micromedex.com/ products/demoswebready/Professional/Usp_DI/data_005.html.

Sports Medicine. Available online at http://www.esportmed.com/ smu/content/viewsumm.cfm?sid=317.

World Health Organization. Available online at http://www. who.int/emc-documents/zoonoses/whoemcxdi986c.html.

28

Tetracyclines and Chloramphenicol

SHERRY F. QUEENER • KATHLEEN GUTIERREZ

 Visit **http://evolve.elsevier.com/Gutierrez/** for additional information.

KEY TERMS

OBJECTIVES

- Describe how the antimicrobial spectra of tetracyclines and chloramphenicol differ from those of erythromycin (see Chapter 26) and penicillin G (see Chapter 25).
- Name the most common route of administration for tetracyclines and chloramphenicol.
- Explain how doxycycline and minocycline differ from other tetracyclines.
- Describe the common adverse effects of tetracyclines.
- Describe the serious adverse effects of chloramphenicol.
- Develop a nursing care plan for a patient receiving doxycycline or chloramphenicol.

 PATHOPHYSIOLOGY • **Nonbacterial Infections**

Infections caused by bacteria range from mild local infections to life-threatening systemic disease (see Chapter 24), but other organisms can cause diseases with similar symptoms. For example, *Chlamydia trachomatis* causes genitourinary tract infections, and various rickettsiae (small intracellular parasites) cause diseases such as typhus and Rocky Mountain spotted fever. Without treatment, these nonbacterial diseases are serious and potentially fatal.

DRUG CLASS • Tetracyclines

demeclocycline (Declomycin)

⚠ doxycycline (Apo-Doxy,✱ Atridox, Doryx, Doxy, Doxycin,✱ Monodox, Novo-doxylin,✱ Periostat, Vibramycin)

minocycline (Arestin, Minocin, Vectrin)

oxytetracycline (Terramycin)

tetracycline (Achromycin, Novotetra,✱ Sumycin)

tetracycline phosphate complex (Tetrex)

MECHANISM OF ACTION

Tetracyclines block bacterial growth by preventing ribosomes from binding messenger RNA, thereby preventing the start of protein synthesis. Members of this drug family are therefore bacteriostatic rather than bactericidal. The term tetracycline refers to the four chemical rings that form the central structure of all members of this class; tetracycline is thus used to refer to the entire family, but the oldest member of the group also carries the generic name tetracycline.

For tetracyclines to be effective, they must first be transported into bacteria via an energy-dependent transport system. Resistant bacteria lose the ability to take in tetracyclines, and the antibiotic does not come in contact with its target inside the cell. Most tetracycline resistance involves a plasmid (see Chapter 24) transmitted from bacterium to bacterium and may therefore spread rapidly throughout bacterial populations. For example, when a patient is treated on a long-term basis with a low dosage of a tetracycline drug, that patient as well as others who are close household contacts may lose their normal tetracycline-sensitive bacterial flora and gain tetracycline-resistant forms. Cross-resistance between the older tetracycline drugs is complete. Minocycline and doxycycline are two newer drugs that are more lipid soluble than the other drugs and are transported into bacteria by different mechanisms than the older drugs. These newer drugs may therefore penetrate bacterial cells that do not concentrate the older tetracyclines.

USES

Tetracyclines are clinically important because of their wide antibacterial spectrum, but the drugs are no longer used clinically for most common infections caused by gram-positive or gram-negative bacteria. Although most gram-positive organisms remain sensitive to tetracyclines, most infections caused by these organisms are best treated by other drugs because penicillins,

cephalosporins, and erythromycin are equally or more effective against these organisms and are less toxic. Gram-negative bacterial pathogens involved in diseases such as urinary tract infections or pneumonia today are often resistant to tetracyclines; thus these common infections are also better treated with other drugs.

Tetracyclines remain clinically effective for a number of bacterial infections that are relatively rare in the United States, including chancroid (*Haemophilus ducreyi*), rabbit fever or tularemia (*Francisella tularensis*), black plague (*Yersinia pestis*), brucellosis (*Brucella species*), and cholera (*Vibrio cholerae*). Doxycycline is the drug of choice for these infections and is an alternative therapy for anthrax (*Bacillus anthracis*) (see Box 27-1).

Tetracyclines are highly effective for diseases caused by Rickettsiae (tick fever, Rocky Mountain spotted fever, typhus, and Q fever), *Chlamydia* (parrot fever or psittacosis, trachoma, and lymphogranuloma venereum), and *Mycoplasma pneumoniae* (atypical, or "walking," pneumonia). Doxycycline is currently a drug of choice for these infections.

Tetracyclines are useful in treating Lyme disease, relapsing fever, syphilis, and yaws, which are all caused by spirochetes. These drugs may have a useful role in treating amebic dysentery as well.

Tetracyclines are also widely used to treat acne. Relatively low dosages may be prescribed over long periods. Although this treatment is effective for many patients, questions arise as to long-term adverse effects of the drugs and to the contribution this practice makes to the development of tetracycline-resistant bacterial populations.

Various tetracycline preparations are available for use on the skin or for other nonsystemic applications. For example, chlortetracycline, a member of the family not used for systemic infections, is available as an ophthalmic ointment (see Chapter 65). Tetracycline periodontal fibers can be used locally to control inflammation and edema of the periodontal pocket caused by normal bacterial flora of the mouth. Although the fibers are removed after 10 days, the antibacterial effect persists perhaps because tetracycline tends to bind to the tooth surface.

PHARMACOKINETICS

Tetracyclines are most often given orally, usually as a hydrochloride salt to increase solubility and thereby increase absorption. Absorption is influenced by acid lability, water solubility, and lipid solubility. All first-generation tetracyclines are acid labile and are partly destroyed by stomach acid. These tetracyclines are poorly soluble in water, and this solubility may be further reduced by complex formation with metal ions in food or other drugs. In these insoluble forms, drugs are not absorbed but remain in the intestine and are excreted in feces. The second-generation drugs doxycycline and minocycline are different in that they are highly lipid soluble. Therefore both drugs pass freely through gastrointestinal (GI) membranes and are more completely and rapidly absorbed than other tetracyclines (Table 28-1).

Intramuscular use of tetracycline drugs is limited because absorption is poor and it often causes local tissue irritation and pain at the injection site.

Tetracyclines may be used intravenously in serious infections. Oxytetracycline, doxycycline, and minocycline can be obtained in a form suitable for intravenous use. These drugs are not highly water soluble and must be diluted extensively before use by this route. When used intravenously, tetracyclines may cause thrombophlebitis. Improper dilution of the drug or repeated infusion into the same vein increases the likelihood of this complication.

Tetracyclines are well distributed in most body tissues and fluids, appearing in the liver, spleen, bone marrow, bile, and cerebrospinal fluid (CSF), even in the absence of inflammation. The drugs pass the placental barrier and enter fetal circulation in appreciable amounts. Tetracyclines also appear in breast milk.

Differences in lipid solubility among the tetracyclines affect their elimination. The more polar or water-soluble drugs are eliminated through the kidneys in greater amounts than are the lipid-soluble tetracyclines doxycycline and minocycline (see Table 28-1). All tetracyclines enter urine by passive glomerular filtration, but lipid-soluble drugs are more completely reabsorbed from kidney tubules than drugs charged at the acid pH of tubular fluid. This high degree of reabsorption is reflected in the longer elimination half-life for doxycycline and minocycline (11 to 23 hours) than those of less lipid-soluble tetracyclines such as oxytetracycline, tetracycline, and demeclocycline (6 to 14 hours).

The second major route of elimination is by biliary excretion. Tetracyclines are concentrated in the liver and the bile and carried into the intestine, where they may be reabsorbed by enterohepatic circulation. The liver is also the site for biotransformation of several tetracyclines. In general, the more lipid-soluble drugs penetrate liver cells and are more extensively biotransformed. In particular, minocycline is extensively biotransformed. The high lipid solubility of doxycycline and its tendency to form insoluble complexes with intestinal solids account for an unusual mode of elimination for this drug. Doxycycline diffuses directly into the intestine, where it is sequestered by complex formation with fecal material. Because of this unusual mechanism for excretion, doxycycline does not accumulate in patients with renal failure.

ADVERSE REACTIONS AND CONTRAINDICATIONS

Tetracyclines cause a wide variety of adverse reactions. The most common complaint is GI irritation. Many patients experience nausea, vomiting, or pain with oral tetracyclines. Diarrhea may result from irritation by unabsorbed tetracycline remaining in the bowel or from changes in the intestinal flora. Occasionally, the effects of these broad-spectrum drugs on intestinal

TABLE 28-1

Pharmacokinetics of Tetracyclines

| | Oral Absorption | | | Half-Life (hrs) | | | |
	Percent Absorbed	Effect of Food	Dosing Interval	Normal	Anuric	Primary Route of Excretion	Liver Biotransformation
First Generation							
demeclocycline	66	Lower	q6-12h	8-14	40-60	Renal	Minor
oxytetracycline	58	Lower	q6h	6-10	47-66	Renal	Minor
tetracycline	76	Lower	q6h	6-10	57-108	Renal	Minor
Second Generation							
doxycycline	90-100	Minor	q12-24h	12-22	12-22	Biliary	Extensive
minocycline	90-100	Minor	q12h	11-23	11-23	Biliary	Extensive

flora are so extensive that an overgrowth of drug-resistant bacteria occurs. Life-threatening staphylococcal enterocolitis may result, producing bloody diarrhea and extensive damage to the intestinal epithelium. *Candida* infections of the throat, vagina, and bowel also occur occasionally.

Tetracyclines are also commonly associated with CNS effects, causing dizziness or unsteadiness. Allergies to tetracyclines are uncommon, but urticaria, measles-like rashes, and dermatitis can occur, as well as more serious reactions such as asthma, angioedema, and anaphylaxis.

Tetracyclines are not entirely specific for bacterial ribosomes and may inhibit mammalian protein synthesis to a small degree. This may explain their toxic effect on various tissues. For example, kidney function may be impaired by tetracyclines, and the effects may be worse in a kidney already damaged by disease or by trauma. Renal function should therefore be watched carefully in patients receiving these drugs.

Older adults who are extremely debilitated or patients who are recovering from extensive surgery or traumatic injuries may experience negative nitrogen balance when given tetracyclines. This reaction may also result from tetracycline inhibition of mammalian protein synthesis.

Tetracyclines may delay blood coagulation. The exact mechanism for this reaction is unknown, but it may involve binding the calcium required in coagulation.

The ability of tetracyclines to bind calcium also leads to their deposition in bones and teeth. In adults this binding produces little visible effect, but in children less than 8 years of age, the newly formed permanent teeth may be stained irreversibly by the drug. Binding of tetracyclines to bones may detectably slow bone growth in fetuses or young children. Infants may also display increased intracranial pressure with bulging fontanelles when given tetracyclines.

All tetracyclines can be degraded to toxic products by exposure to light, but demeclocycline most commonly causes these reactions. The drug is broken down by the action of ultraviolet light on the skin, and the toxic products released cause an intense sunburn reaction; this reaction is called **phototoxicity.** Because tetracyclines other than demeclocycline can cause this reaction, patients receiving these drugs should be cautioned to limit their exposure to direct sunlight, especially in subtropical or tropical climates.

Ingestion of outdated tetracycline preparations has sometimes led to severe adverse reactions apparently caused by the toxic breakdown products of the drugs. One such reaction is Fanconi syndrome, which involves the loss of amino acids, proteins, and glucose in urine as well as polyuria, polydipsia, acidosis, nausea, and vomiting. These reactions slowly disappear after the drug is discontinued. In other cases, patients show symptoms reminiscent of systemic lupus erythematosus.

Specific tetracyclines may cause unique adverse reactions. For example, minocycline can damage vestibular function, thereby impairing balance. Minocycline may also discolor skin and mucous membranes. Demeclocycline is the tetracycline most likely to induce nephrogenic diabetes insipidus, a disorder marked by weakness, thirst, and increased urination.

TOXICITY

The liver may be sensitive to tetracyclines. Hepatotoxicity may progress to jaundice, fatty liver, and death unless the drugs are discontinued at the first sign of difficulty. Pregnant women are most sensitive to this complication and should rarely if ever be given tetracyclines. These drugs belong to FDA Pregnancy Category D.

INTERACTIONS

Several interactions with other drugs result from the ability of tetracyclines to form insoluble complexes with metal ions. For example, oral tetracyclines often cause gastric irritation; therefore patients may wish to take antacids along with the antibiotic. This practice should be discouraged because common antacids include magnesium and aluminum salts, which complex with tetracyclines and prevent their absorption from the GI tract, reducing the antibacterial effect of the antibiotic. Likewise, iron-containing preparations such as vitamin or mineral supplements may prevent tetracycline absorption. Milk and other dairy products are high in calcium and also impair absorption. Sodium bicarbonate taken with a tetracycline tablet may impede tablet dissolution in the stomach and thereby reduce absorption of the drug.

Food in the stomach impairs absorption of first-generation tetracyclines, but the lipid-soluble second-generation drugs (doxycycline and minocycline) are absorbed well even in the presence of food or milk products in the stomach.

Cholestyramine and colestipol bind tetracyclines and impair oral absorption of the antibiotics. As a result, effective blood concentrations may not be achieved with concurrent use of these drugs.

Several tetracyclines, especially doxycycline and minocycline, are biotransformed to some degree in the liver. Drugs such as barbiturates, which increase hepatic drug-biotransforming enzymes, shorten the duration of action of doxycycline and minocycline, reducing the antibacterial effectiveness of these drugs.

Estrogen-containing contraceptives may be less effective when tetracyclines are used over prolonged periods as a result of their influence on the biotransformation of the estrogen.

The bacteriostatic mechanism of action of tetracyclines leads to specific interactions. For example, penicillin given with a tetracycline drug may be less effective than penicillin given alone. Penicillin drugs are bactericidal and act against actively multiplying bacteria. By inhibiting bacterial growth, tetracycline drugs make the bacteria resistant to the action of the penicillin.

The nephrotoxic effect of tetracyclines may become significant and dangerous when these antibiotics are given with other nephrotoxic drugs (see Appendix B).

DRUG CLASS • Acetamides

chloramphenicol (Chloromycetin, Mychel)

MECHANISM OF ACTION

Chloramphenicol is a very simple synthetic molecule that inhibits late steps in bacterial protein synthesis. Similar to tetracyclines, chloramphenicol is usually bacteriostatic rather than bactericidal. Chloramphenicol is the only member of its chemical class approved for use in the United States.

Bacterial resistance to chloramphenicol usually involves destruction of the drug by bacterial enzymes that may be induced by exposure of potentially resistant bacteria to sublethal dosages. The genes required for synthesizing this enzyme are usually carried on plasmids (see Chapter 24) and thus may be transmitted widely throughout bacterial populations.

USES

Because of the possibility of dangerous adverse reactions, chloramphenicol is used only for life-threatening infections such as bacteremias, brain abcesses, and meningitis when the pathogen has proven sensitive to the drug. The antibacterial spectrum of chloramphenicol is similar to that of tetracyclines and includes gram-negative bacteria, *Rickettsia*, and *Chlamydia*. Although once the drug of choice for treating typhoid fever, chloramphenicol has been replaced by safer, more effective drugs.

PHARMACOKINETICS

Chloramphenicol is nearly completely absorbed from the GI tract after oral administration; peak serum concentrations are similar to oral and intravenous doses. Intramuscular injection produces a lower blood level than oral administration and thus is not recommended. Seriously ill patients should receive chloramphenicol intravenously because oral absorption may be impaired in these patients.

Chloramphenicol is well distributed throughout body tissues and fluids. Effective concentrations of the drug enter the eye, joint (synovial), and pleural fluids. Unlike many other antibiotics, chloramphenicol enters the CSF relatively easily, even when the meninges are not inflamed. Chloramphenicol also crosses the placenta and appears in breast milk.

Most of a dose of chloramphenicol is conjugated in the liver with glucuronic acid to form the inactive chloramphenicol glucuronide. This inactive drug form may be excreted by renal tubular secretion, whereas unaltered chloramphenicol is excreted solely by glomerular filtration. The concentration of active chloramphenicol in urine is high enough to be antibacterial, but the active drug is only a small fraction of the total drug excreted by this route.

ADVERSE REACTIONS AND CONTRAINDICATIONS

The clinical use of chloramphenicol is limited by its potential for bone marrow toxicity. A reversible form of bone marrow depression causes leukopenia and a reduction of reticulocytes. These symptoms usually resolve when the drug is discontinued. Patients receiving chloramphenicol should have routine blood tests performed during therapy to detect early signs of this toxic reaction.

Chloramphenicol may also cause irreversible bone marrow depression, which leads to aplastic anemia, a condition that usually includes pancytopenia (loss of all forms of blood cells). Aplastic anemia may appear weeks or months after chloramphenicol therapy. This time lag between drug administration and the appearance of this disorder complicates accurate calculation of drug-associated risk, especially since most patients have received more than one other drug during the interim between chloramphenicol therapy and development of aplastic anemia. Best estimates suggest that about 1 in 30,000 chloramphenicol-treated patients will develop this disorder. Although this incidence rate is low, the often fatal outcome is sufficient cause to restrict the use of chloramphenicol to the treatment of very serious infections.

Less severe problems also occur with chloramphenicol, including allergies of various types and GI irritation. Long-term therapy has been associated with neuritis, which may involve the optic nerve and occasionally causes blindness. Also occasionally seen are CNS symptoms, including headache, mental confusion, depression, and delirium.

Chloramphenicol crosses the placenta and may concentrate in the fetal liver. Therefore the drug is not given to pregnant women near term.

TOXICITY

Patients with reduced liver function are at risk of severe toxic reactions because of drug accumulation. The liver normally converts more than 90% of administered chloramphenicol, which is toxic, to a glucuronide, which is nontoxic. Therefore any reduction in the ability to form glucuronides may cause accumulation of the toxic drug unless dosages are appropriately reduced. Neonates have an immature liver that lacks the enzyme to form glucuronides, increasing their risk for this complication. When these infants are given a weight-adjusted dosage based on adult doses, many develop gray baby syndrome. Drug accumulation proceeds without symptoms for 3 to 4 days, but then the infant may develop abdominal distension, emesis, progressive pallid cyanosis, and irregular respiration. In a high percentage of cases, vasomotor collapse and death result. If early signs of the condition are noted by alert health care personnel and the drug discontinued, most infants recover.

INTERACTIONS

Chloramphenicol inhibits drug-biotransforming enzymes in the liver. This property may lead to dangerous interactions with drugs that have a low therapeutic index and that are eliminated by microsomal enzymes. Drugs in this category include alfentanil, chlorpropamide, phenytoin, tolbutamide, and coumarin anticoagulants. Chloramphenicol may cause these normally biotransformed drugs to accumulate. As a result, a patient's previously well-controlled conditions may escape control. For example, a patient with well-controlled diabetes may become hypoglycemic, a patient who has successfully undergone anticoagulant therapy may develop spontaneous bleeding, or a patient with epilepsy may develop phenytoin toxicity.

Chloramphenicol competes with erythromycin and clindamycin for binding sites on bacterial ribosomes. As a result, the drugs may be antagonistic with one another and should not be combined (see the Case Study: Lyme Disease).

APPLICATION TO PRACTICE

ASSESSMENT

The general aspects of care for the patient receiving any antimicrobial drug were covered in Chapter 24. In this chapter, only those aspects that are related specifically to tetracycline antibiotics and chloramphenicol are discussed.

History of Present Illness

The patient with an infection typically displays the five cardinal signs and symptoms of infection, which include swelling, redness, pain, heat, and loss of function. Be sure to elicit the location, onset, severity, timing, duration, signs and symptoms, quality, and context of his or her concern as well as anything the patient has tried that improved or worsened these signs and symptoms.

Health History

A thorough health history may reveal previous hypersensitivity reactions. It is important to also ask whether the patient has ever taken one of these drugs before, and if so, whether he or she developed GI irritation associated with it. Naming a few of the common tetracycline drugs may help the patient identify any previous use. Be sure to ask also about use of other prescription drugs (e.g., oral contraceptives), herbal remedies, and OTC drugs to minimize the risk of drug-drug interactions. A number of drugs and food products taken concurrently with tetracyclines may reduce absorption and effectiveness of the drugs (Box 28-1).

Determine if the patient takes antacids containing aluminum or magnesium salts, iron, or sodium bicarbonate preparations which complex with tetracycline drugs, prevent their absorption from the GI tract, and reduce their antibacterial effects.

Lifespan Considerations

Perinatal. Tetracyclines are pregnancy category D drugs and as such are contraindicated during pregnancy and lactation. These drugs cross the placenta

Patient Problem: Food and Drug Interactions with Tetracyclines

The Problem

Certain tetracyclines bind tightly to metal ions such as calcium, magnesium, iron, and zinc. When so bound, these drugs are virtually insoluble and are not absorbed orally. Thus foods, dietary supplements, and other drugs that contain these elements block absorption and prevent the antibacterial effect of orally administered demeclocycline, oxytetracycline, and tetracycline. In contrast, the absorption of lipid-soluble drugs such as minocycline and doxycycline is not affected by food.

The Solution

- Do not consume milk, cheese, yogurt, or other dairy products along with demeclocycline, oxytetracycline, or tetracycline.
- If dietary supplements containing calcium, magnesium, iron, or zinc are used, they should be taken 1 hour before or 2 hours after taking a tetracycline drug.
- If gastric irritation occurs with demeclocycline, oxytetracycline, or tetracycline, the drugs can be taken with small amounts of food, taking care to avoid calcium-enriched products.
- Minocycline and doxycycline may be taken at meals or with milk to avoid gastric irritation.

and are deposited in fetal teeth and bones. Hepatotoxicity in the form of acute fatty liver, leading to death in some cases, has been reported in pregnant women. In addition, chronic low-dose therapy before conception has been reported to result in fetal hepatotoxicity. It is speculated that with chronic use, tetracyclines are deposited in bone and released during periods of bone turnover, including pregnancy, at which time they damage the liver.

Because of adverse effects on fetal organs and the potential for maternal toxicity, other antibiotics should be used in the pregnant woman. The deciduous teeth begin to mineralize at approximately 14 weeks gestation. This process continues until 2 to 3 months after birth. Staining of teeth is most likely when tetracyclines are administered after the twenty-fifth week of pregnancy.

Chloramphenicol is a pregnancy category C drug. If it is given during the last few days of pregnancy or during labor, the drug may cause gray baby syndrome. Infants exposed to this drug should be monitored for failure to feed, abdominal distension, emesis, progressive pallid cyanosis, and irregular respiration.

Pediatric. Young children rapidly form bones and teeth, which are primarily composed of calcium phosphates. As this material is deposited, tetracyclines may be so tightly bound to the calcium in bones and teeth that they cannot be released. Fetal bone growth may be slowed. Fibular growth may be inhibited in premature infants.

Over time, tetracyclines are degraded by light and exposure to chemicals. This process occurs even though the drug is incorporated into the solid matrix of teeth. The degraded tetracyclines appear as brown- or gray-colored permanent stains on the teeth. Thus tetracyclines should be avoided during the last half of pregnancy and in children under the age of 8 years. In addition, there have been some reports that tetracycline exposure during pregnancy has a possible association with infants born with hypospadias, inguinal hernias, limb hypoplasia, and clubfoot.

Older Adults. Use of tetracyclines in the older adult is relatively safe, although decreased renal function associated with changes of aging, hepatic disease or other disease processes, and concurrent drug therapies can increase the risk of adverse effects. The older adult who is extremely debilitated or the patient recovering from extensive surgery or traumatic injuries may experience a negative nitrogen balance when given tetracyclines.

Cultural/Social Considerations

Overall, the cultural and social considerations associated with the use of tetracyclines are minimal. In most cases, bacterial infections sensitive to tetracyclines are short-term, subacute conditions that are easily treated on an outpatient basis.

Compared with the other classes of antimicrobial drugs, tetracyclines are inexpensive. However, the rising cost of antibiotics, particularly the newer ones, continues to present a hardship to many, especially older adults, those who are financially disadvantaged, and those who have pharmacy insurance plans through managed care organizations.

Physical Examination

The patient should be assessed for signs and symptoms of infection, including the vital signs and inspection of any wound. A thorough examination is particularly necessary to detect any infection traveling indirectly from a distant body site. The patient's level of discomfort should be evaluated in relation to the infection.

Laboratory Testing

Many antimicrobial drugs have harsh adverse effects on other body systems. Because of the risk of superinfection in the patient receiving tetracyclines, observe the patient (particularly if an older adult or one who is debilitated) for symptoms of bacterial and fungal overgrowth. Evidence of superinfection (e.g., diarrhea, vaginal or anal itching, or black, furry appearance of the tongue) should be reported. Superinfection by *Candida* organisms can usually be managed by discontinuing the antibiotics or by administering an antifungal drug.

Renal and liver function tests as well as a CBC count should be monitored periodically during long-term therapy with tetracyclines or chloramphenicol. Tetracyclines may cause increased concentrations of aspartate aminotransferase (AST), alanine aminotransferase (ALT), serum alkaline phosphatase, bilirubin, and amylase. All tetracyclines except for doxycycline can also cause an elevated blood urea nitrogen (BUN) level. The serum drug level of chloramphenicol should be monitored.

GOALS OF THERAPY

The desired goals of treatment with tetracyclines or chloramphenicol are to ameliorate the signs and symptoms of infection, to prevent complications associated with therapy, and to prevent sepsis and death.

INTERVENTION
Administration

Before the first dose of tetracycline antibiotic or chloramphenicol is given, the patient's history should be carefully reviewed for allergies. Keep in mind that a negative history of hypersensitivity does not preclude future reactions.

Administer the dose of tetracycline around the clock, at least 1 hour before or 2 hours after meals. Administer with a full glass of liquid at least 1 hour before bedtime to avoid esophageal ulceration. Do not administer a tetracycline within 1 to 3 hours of other drugs, particularly those containing calcium, magnesium, iron, or sodium bicarbonate. Doxycycline and minocycline may be given with milk or food if GI irritation develops. If an oral suspension of a tetracycline is required, administer the drug through a straw to avoid exposure to teeth.

When intravenous doxycycline is administered, the solution should be protected from direct sunlight. Intravenous tetracyclines may cause thrombophlebitis. Rapid administration should be avoided and monitor for signs and symptoms of extravasation. Incompatibilities between drugs, especially those administered intravenously, must be checked and avoided.

Education

Instruct the patient to take the full course of antibiotic therapy (usually 10 days) even though symptoms may abate and he or she may start feeling better before the full course of therapy is completed. Emphasize the importance of taking evenly spaced doses to maintain a therapeutic blood level. Missed doses should be taken as soon as remembered unless it is almost time for the next dose. Do not double doses. Advise the patient to properly discard outdated tetracycline drugs because they may become toxic. Prescriptions for any antibiotic should never be shared with others or saved and taken for a different episode of illness.

Instruct the patient to contact the health care provider if his or her condition does not improve in a few days or if evidence of superinfection develops. Skin rash, pruritus, and urticaria should also be reported. Caution the patient to avoid direct sunlight, especially in subtropical or tropical climates, and to wear sunscreen and protective clothing to avoid photosensitivity reactions. Because minocycline commonly causes dizziness or unsteadiness, caution the patient to avoid driving or other activities requiring alertness until response to the drug is known. Patients with an allergy to tetracyclines or chloramphenicol should be advised to wear some form of identification (e.g., a medical alert tag or bracelet) to inform health care personnel of the allergy. Carrying the identification in a wallet or purse is usually not helpful if emergency care is needed.

EVALUATION

The effectiveness of tetracycline or chloramphenicol therapy is determined by monitoring the clinical response. The frequency of monitoring is proportional to the severity of the infection. Important clinical indicators of effective treatment include a reduction in fever and resolution of the signs and symptoms of infection, vital signs that return to normal for the patient, WBC count that returns to normal limits, and a culture and sensitivity test that is negative for the offending organism. Further proof may include an increase in appetite, energy level, and general sense of well-being.

CASE STUDY *Lyme Disease*

ASSESSMENT

HISTORY OF PRESENT ILLNESS

DD is a 16-year-old girl who complains of an expanding rash, fever, headache, and muscle and joint pains for the past 4 weeks. She remembers finding a tick on her on her lower leg after she returned from a spring camping expedition in the local woods of Minnesota. She was successful in removing the tick. No insect repellent was available to the camp participants. She does not know how long the tick had been present.

HEALTH HISTORY

DD is allergic to penicillins and cephalosporins, which cause a rash. Her current drugs include oral contraceptives. She did not take her contraceptive while at camp because she kept forgetting. Her health history is negative for cardiovascular, respiratory, renal, hepatic, or neurologic disorders.

PHYSICAL EXAMINATION

DD's temperature is 100.2° F, pulse 78, respirations 20, blood pressure 114/68 mm Hg. She has an erythematous macular/papular rash that has expanding borders and an area of central clearing over her lower legs.

LABORATORY TESTING

ELISA test results show elevated IgM and IgG levels and the punch biopsy culture is positive for the spirochete *Borellia burgdorferi*.

LIFESPAN CONSIDERATIONS

DD is at risk for pregnancy because of inconsistent use of contraception.

CULTURAL/SOCIAL CONSIDERATIONS

DD is worried about how long the rash will be present because she has weekend plans with her friends and one boy in particular.

PATIENT PROBLEM(S)

Lyme disease.

GOALS OF THERAPY

DD's infection will resolve without incident.

CRITICAL THINKING QUESTIONS

1. Doxycycline 100 mg po bid for 14 days has been ordered for DD. What is the mechanism of action of this drug? Is it bacteriocidal or bacteriostatic? Is it broad spectrum or narrow spectrum?
2. What adverse effects should be watched for when doxycycline is used?
3. What are the main toxic reactions common to all tetracycline antibiotics?
4. How does the absorption of doxycycline compare with that of other tetracyclines?
5. What are the three main routes of excretion for tetracyclines?
6. How do bacteria become resistant to tetracyclines?
7. What factors limit the intramuscular administration of tetracyclines?
8. What toxicity is associated with outdated tetracycline preparations?
9. Knowing the contraindications to the use of tetracyclines, what nursing action is recommended, given that DD did not take her contraceptives while at camp?

Bibliography

Gurenlian JR, MacAdoo KS: Periomedicine: local drug delivery in periodontal therapy, *Access* 15(2):33-37, 2001.

O'Donoghue MN: Update on acne therapy, *Dermatol Nurs* 11(3):205-208, 1999.

Suggs DM: Pharmacokinetics in children: history, considerations, and applications, J *Am Acad Nurse Pract* 12(6):236-239, 2000.

Internet Resources

http://www.fda.gov/cvm/index/updates/tetraup.html.

Medline Plus. Available online at http://www.nlm.nih.gov/medlineplus/druginfo/tetracyclinessystemic202552.html.

Merck Manual. Available online at http://www.merck.com/pubs/mmanual/section13/chapter153/153e.htm.

http://www.nlm.nih.gov/medlineplus/druginfo/tetracyclinesophthalmic202551.html.

CHAPTER

29

Aminoglycosides

SHERRY F. QUEENER • KATHLEEN GUTIERREZ

Visit **http://evolve.elsevier.com/Gutierrez/** for additional information.

KEY TERMS

Aminoglycoside, p. 432
Neuromuscular blockade, p. 433
Ototoxicity, p. 433
Peak serum drug levels, p. 435
Trough serum drug levels, p. 435

OBJECTIVES

- Explain why aminoglycosides are administered only by parenteral routes.
- Describe the toxicities associated with aminoglycoside use.
- Explain why aminoglycosides are sometimes used along with penicillins for serious infections.
- Develop a nursing care plan for a patient receiving an aminoglycoside.

PATHOPHYSIOLOGY

Aminoglycoside antibiotics are effective only against gram-negative aerobic bacteria. Diseases caused by these bacteria include pneumonia, urinary tract infections, septicemia, and CNS infections (see Chapter 24).

DRUG CLASS • Aminoglycosides

amikacin (Amikin)

gentamicin (Cidomycin,✱ Garamycin)

kanamycin sulfate (Kantrex)

neomycin (Mycifradin, Neo-RX)

streptomycin

tobramycin (Nebcin, TOBI, Tobrax)

MECHANISM OF ACTION

Aminoglycoside antibiotics are composed of three or four amino sugars held together by the same sort of chemical bonds that link simple sugars to form sucrose. Great variability in structure is possible in these component sugars; as a result, several antibiotics of this type exist. All aminoglycosides inhibit early steps in bacterial protein synthesis by binding to bacterial ribosomes. Bacterial protein synthesis may continue in the presence of aminoglycosides but with a greatly increased error rate. Defective proteins formed may damage the bacterial cell. Aminoglycosides also affect bacterial cell membranes. These drugs are bactericidal, unlike many other antibiotics that inhibit bacterial protein synthesis.

Aminoglycosides must be pumped into bacterial cells to reach their site of action. The pump mechanism requires energy and oxygen to function. Thus in anaerobic sites, aminoglycosides do not enter bacteria in sufficient amounts to inhibit protein synthesis. For this reason, aminoglycosides are used only for aerobic bacteria.

Resistance to aminoglycosides occurs as a result of reduced antibiotic uptake, changes in antibiotic binding to ribosomes, or enzymatic destruction of the aminoglycosides. The most common mechanism for resistance involves antibiotic destruction. Bacterial enzymes modify the drugs by adding phosphates or other groups at various sites on the aminoglycoside. Any of these substitutions inactivates the aminoglycoside. At least 13 separate enzymes catalyzing these reactions have been identified. Aminoglycosides differ in susceptibility to degradation, ranging from kanamycin, which is destroyed by at least six different enzymes, to amikacin, which is sensitive to only two enzymes.

USES

The clinical use of these drugs is limited by their toxic potential. In general, the aminoglycosides are reserved for serious infections caused by aerobic gram-negative bacteria or by mycobacteria (see Chapter 33).

Individual drugs in this family differ in specific uses as a result of differences in relative toxicity and antibacterial activity. For example, they differ in their degree of effectiveness against *Pseudomonas aeruginosa*. Amikacin, gentamicin, and tobramycin are most effective against this pathogen (Table 29-1), but kanamycin usually is not effective. Amikacin differs from other aminoglycosides in being less sensitive to common aminoglycoside-degrading enzymes. This drug is therefore effective against some bacterial strains that are resistant to other aminoglycosides.

Streptomycin is most useful today in combination with other drugs to treat infections in which strict bactericidal action is required for most effective therapy. Examples of these infections are bacterial endocarditis and tuberculosis (see Chapter 33).

Neomycin is an aminoglycoside used primarily by topical routes (see Chapter 67) because of its potential for excessive systemic toxicity. Because the drug is essentially not absorbed from the gastrointestinal (GI)

TABLE 29-1	

Clinical Uses of Aminoglycosides

Aminoglycoside	*Primary Clinical Use*
amikacin, gentamicin, tobramycin	Serious infections caused by aerobic, gram-negative bacteria includin *Pseudomonas aeruginosa*
kanamycin	Serious infections caused by aerobic, gram-negative bacteria not including P. aeruginosa
streptomycin	Combined with isoniazid or other drugs to treat tuberculosis; used with beta-lactam drugs for endocarditis
neomycin	Topical use for minor skin infections as well as in otic and ophthalmic preparations; to reduce bacteria in bowel

tract, neomycin can be used orally to prepare the GI tract for surgery, to decrease the number of ammonia-producing bacteria in the gut as part of the management of hepatic encephalopathy, and to treat some forms of infectious diarrhea. Gentamicin and tobramycin may also be used topically as otic or ophthalmic preparations (see Chapters 65 and 66).

PHARMACOKINETICS

Aminoglycosides carry multiple positive charges at physiologic pH. Being charged, these drugs do not readily penetrate mammalian membranes and are not absorbed when given orally. They must therefore be delivered by intramuscular or intravenous routes; such therapy usually involves hospitalized patients who have moderate to severe infections. Absorption of aminoglycosides from intramuscular injection sites is rapid, and peak serum concentrations usually occur within 60 to 90 minutes.

Aminoglycosides do not enter the CNS to any significant extent in most persons, but some of the drug does appear in cerebrospinal fluid (CSF) when meningitis is present. Gentamicin may be given by intralumbar or intraventricular injection to improve the drug level in the CNS. Aminoglycosides enter most other body fluids and tissues. These drugs cross the placenta and achieve significant concentrations in the fetus.

Aminoglycosides are excreted by glomerular filtration in the kidneys. The active drug is concentrated in urine. Because the kidneys are the primary sites for elimination of these drugs, any reduction in renal function may lower excretion enough to cause aminoglycoside accumulation. The approximate half-life for elimination of these drugs is 2 to 4 hours, but in renal failure it may be greatly prolonged. Excretion is also slower in neonates, who have immature kidneys, and in older adults, whose renal function is diminished simply because of age (Box 29-1).

BOX 29-1 Serum Drug Levels of Select Aminoglycosides

Drug	Trough Serum Level	Peak Serum Level
amikacin	<5 mcg/mL	Not to exceed 35 mcg/mL
gentamicin	<2 mcg/mL	Not to exceed 10 mcg/mL
kanamycin	<5 mcg/mL	Not to exceed 35 mcg/mL
streptomycin	—	Not to exceed 35 mcg/mL
tobramycin	<2 mcg/mL	Not to exceed 10 mcg/mL

ADVERSE REACTIONS AND CONTRAINDICATIONS

Because aminoglycosides may be nephrotoxic, renal function must be monitored in patients receiving them (see next section). Serum levels of these drugs are monitored so doses can be adjusted to prevent toxic concentrations from accumulating.

Aminoglycosides must be used with caution in patients with any condition that impairs transmission at the neuromuscular junction or otherwise weakens muscular function. Therefore patients with myasthenia gravis, Parkinson's disease, or infant botulism would normally not receive aminoglycosides; if they do receive aminoglycosides, however, they must be watched carefully for excessive muscle weakness during therapy.

Patients with preexisting renal, auditory, or vestibular damage are not ordinarily given an aminoglycoside if an alternative drug is available. These patients may be more at risk for the dose-related toxicity described in the next section.

Less common adverse reactions include effects on a variety of organ systems. Blood dyscrasias, although rare, may occur with any aminoglycoside. Neurotoxicity is also rare, but may cause headaches, paresthesia, tremor, confusion, and disorientation. The aminoglycosides are also somewhat irritating and may cause pain at the injection site. Allergies to these drugs are possible as well, and a prior allergic reaction to any aminoglycoside is a contraindication to receiving the drugs again.

TOXICITY

The aminoglycosides exert significant dose-dependent toxicity of three major types: **ototoxicity**, renal toxicity, and **neuromuscular blockade**. Ototoxicity may cause hearing loss, loss of equilibrium control, or both. In some patients hearing loss continues even after the drug is discontinued. Loss of equilibrium may be less obvious than hearing loss but it can usually be revealed by appropriate tests. Nausea or dizziness may signal disturbance of equilibrium. Ototoxicity is more severe when peak serum concentrations of aminoglycosides exceed 8 to 10 mcg/mL. The total dose administered may also be a factor; some patients treated over long periods may display these symptoms despite never having excessively high serum levels of the drugs.

Recent genetic studies have suggested that some families have increased sensitivity to aminoglycoside-induced ototoxicity. This increased sensitivity has been traced to a mutation in mitochondrial ribosomal RNA that tends to slow mitochondrial protein synthesis. When these vulnerable mitochondria are exposed to aminoglycosides, mitochondrial protein synthesis apparently falls further, and the cell can no longer function normally. Deafness may result when critical cells in the inner ear are affected.

Aminoglycosides may damage both the tubules and the glomeruli in the kidney, especially when high dosages are given. This toxic potential can cause a rapid clinical deterioration because renal impairment causes the drug to accumulate, which causes further damage to the kidneys. This cycle of accumulation and increasing renal damage can destroy kidney function. Patients who accumulate the drug because of renal dysfunction are also more prone to ototoxicity.

The third characteristic toxic reaction to aminoglycosides is neuromuscular blockade. This reaction is usually observed in surgical patients when an aminoglycoside is used in peritoneal lavage. Neuromuscular blockade usually is manifested by respiratory paralysis because the muscles of the chest involved in breathing are prevented from functioning. Some of the aminoglycosides produce a competitive neuromuscular blockade, which may be reversed by neostigmine. Others, such as kanamycin, produce an irreversible blockade, although calcium may relieve the blockade in some cases. Patients who have recently received muscle relaxants are more prone to neuromuscular blockade with aminogly-

cosides. Patients with myasthenia gravis are also more sensitive to this effect.

INTERACTIONS

The ototoxicity and nephrotoxicity of aminoglycoside antibiotics may be enhanced by a variety of drugs. For example, if a patient receiving an aminoglycoside is also given a nephrotoxic drug such as a cephalosporin, the risk of kidney damage is increased. Likewise, ototoxic drugs such as ethacrynic acid may enhance ototoxicity in a patient receiving an aminoglycoside. All aminoglycosides possess neuromuscular-blocking activity, which has led to the enhancement of neuromuscular-blocking drugs used during surgery.

Gentamicin is commonly combined with an anti-*Pseudomonas* penicillin to treat *P. aeruginosa* infections. Although these drugs may be used in the same patient, they should never be physically mixed, because penicillins chemically inactivate gentamicin in solution.

Aminoglycosides are many times more effective at the slightly alkaline pH of normal serum (pH 7.4) than at the acidic pH of normal urine (pH 5). Therefore, in the treatment of urinary tract infections with these drugs, a therapeutic advantage may be gained by alkalinizing the urine (see the Case Study: Sepsis).

APPLICATION TO PRACTICE

ASSESSMENT

The general aspects of nursing care for the patient receiving any antimicrobial drug were covered in Chapter 24. In this chapter, only those aspects related specifically to aminoglycoside antibiotics are discussed.

History of Present Illness

The patient with an infection typically displays the five cardinal signs and symptoms of infection, which include swelling, redness, pain, heat, and loss of function. Be sure to ask the patient about the location, onset, severity, timing, duration, signs and symptoms, quality, and context of his or her concerns along with anything the patient has tried that improved or worsened these signs and symptoms.

Health History

A thorough health history may reveal previous hypersensitivity reactions. Cross-sensitivity among aminoglycosides may occur as well. It is also important to ask whether the patient has ever taken one of these drugs before, and if so, whether he or she developed unexpected bleeding or kidney problems, hearing difficulties, headaches, paresthesia, tremor, confusion,

disorientation, or excessive muscular weakness associated with the drug taken. Naming a few of the common aminoglycoside drugs may help the patient identify any previous use. Be sure to ask about use of other prescription drugs (e.g., cephalosporins, methoxyflurane, ethacrynic acid), herbal remedies, and OTC drugs to minimize the risk of drug-drug interactions. Find out if the patient has a hypersensitivity to bisulfites.

Lifespan Considerations

Perinatal. Aminoglycosides should be given during pregnancy only when serious gram-negative infections are suspected. If necessary, gentamicin is preferable to amikacin, netilmicin, or tobramycin because it has been more extensively studied. Studies of effects of aminoglycoside administration during labor have not demonstrated toxicity to the fetus.

Kanamycin, tobramycin, and the topical use of other aminoglycosides (e.g., neomycin) are classified as pregnancy category C drugs. Amikacin, gentamicin, netilmicin, and streptomycin are pregnancy category D. Tobramycin and streptomycin may cause congenital hearing loss.

Pediatric. Aminoglycosides have been used in pediatric patients and are generally considered safe, although the immature renal function of infants increases the risk of adverse effects. Because the aminoglycosides are excreted through the kidneys, there is a risk for drug accumulation.

Older Adults. The aging process affects the hepatic and renal systems of the older adult. The potential for nephrotoxicity and hepatotoxicity increases as function decreases.

Cultural/Social Considerations

Overall, the cultural and social considerations associated with the use of aminoglycosides are minimal. Compared with the other classes of antimicrobial drugs, aminoglycosides are expensive. The rising cost of antibiotics, particularly the newer ones, continues to present a hardship to many, especially older adults, those who are financially disadvantaged, and those who have pharmacy insurance plans through managed care organizations.

Physical Examination

Assess the patient for signs and symptoms of infection. Be sure to include the vital signs and to inspect any wound. A thorough examination is particularly necessary to detect any infection traveling indirectly from a distant body site. Evaluate the patient's level of discomfort related to the infection.

Laboratory Testing

Many antimicrobial drugs have harsh adverse effects on other body systems. Evaluate the results of urinalysis, BUN, creatinine, and creatinine clearance, as well as liver function tests such as AST, ALT, serum alkaline phosphatase, bilirubin, and LDH concentrations before starting therapy. Aminoglycosides may cause decreased serum calcium, magnesium, potassium, and sodium concentrations; thus these values should also be evaluated before therapy.

GOALS OF THERAPY

The desired goals of treatment with aminoglycosides are to ameliorate the signs and symptoms of infection, to prevent complications associated with therapy, and to prevent sepsis and death.

INTERVENTION
Administration

Before the first dose of an aminoglycoside antibiotic is given, the patient's history should be carefully reviewed for allergies. Keep in mind that a negative history of hypersensitivity does not preclude future reactions. Be sure to assess vestibular, renal, and hepatic function as well

as hearing acuity and perform a CBC count before and during treatment. Assessing hearing and vestibular function in older adults and premature infants may be difficult; thus these drugs should be used with caution. Note whether the patient has received any other neuromuscular-blocking drugs or whether he or she has any condition such as myasthenia gravis, Parkinson's disease, or infant botulism, which may predispose him or her to respiratory paralysis.

In general the patient should be well hydrated (1.5 to 2 L daily) during treatment. Oral aminoglycosides can be administered without regard to meals. Neomycin is usually used in conjunction with erythromycin, a low-residue diet, and a cathartic or enema to prepare the patient for intestinal surgery.

Most parenteral formulations contain bisulfites and should be avoided by patients with a known intolerance. Products containing benzyl alcohol should not be given to neonates. Intramuscular administration should be deep into a well-developed muscle (i.e., the gluteus maximus) with sites rotated. Follow the manufacturer's instructions regarding administration of intravenous aminoglycosides. Most are administered intermittently and slowly over a minimum of 30 minutes. Too rapid administration can cause neuromuscular blockade. If aminoglycosides must be administered concurrently with penicillins or cephalosporins, do so at separate intravenous sites at least 1 hour apart.

The potential for toxicity with aminoglycosides is monitored with **trough** and **peak serum drug levels.** These levels are typically drawn before and after the third dose is given. The trough level should be drawn just before the third scheduled dose. The peak level should be drawn 1 hour after an intramuscular injection and 30 minutes after an intravenous infusion is completed. Box 29-1 provides an overview of expected trough and peak serum drug levels. Notify the laboratory of the time a dose will be given so that specimens can be obtained at the proper times for accurate calculation of drug levels.

There are no unusual effects on the mother during pregnancy, but serum aminoglycoside levels are usually lower in pregnancy than in nonpregnant patients receiving equivalent doses. Thus it is important to monitor serum levels frequently to prevent subtherapeutic dosing.

Monitor vital signs and auscultate breath sounds. Have a suction machine, neostigmine, an acetylcholinesterase inhibitor, and calcium chloride available when aminoglycosides are used with high-risk patients (e.g., in the operating room, the postanesthesia care unit, and the intensive care unit). Monitor intake and output and obtain the patient's weight daily. Because of the possibility of hypotension or vertigo, keep the siderails up and supervise the patient's ambulation. Assess for increased thirst, nausea, vomiting, anorexia, and an increase or decrease in the frequency of urination. Monitor for vestibular dysfunction (e.g., vertigo, ataxia, nausea, vomiting). Eighth cranial nerve dysfunction is associated with a persistently elevated peak aminoglycoside level. Although streptomycin is used infrequently, be sure to assess for a burning sensation of the face, numbness, and tingling, which may suggest a peripheral neuritis.

Assess the patient for evidence of superinfection (e.g., fever, upper respiratory infection, vaginal or anal itching or discharge, increasing malaise, diarrhea). Report these findings to the health care provider.

Education

Instruct the patient to take the full course of oral antibiotic (usually 10 days) even though symptoms may abate and they may start feeling better before the full course of therapy is completed. Emphasize the importance of taking evenly spaced doses to maintain a therapeutic blood level. Missed doses should be taken as soon as remembered unless it is almost time for the next dose. Do not double doses. Prescriptions for any antibiotic should never be shared with others or saved and taken for a different episode of illness.

CASE STUDY  *Sepsis*

ASSESSMENT

HISTORY OF PRESENT ILLNESS

EA is a 75-year-old man admitted to the ICU with sepsis resulting from a urinary tract infection. He has had an indwelling urinary catheter for 2 weeks while rehabilitating from a hip fracture at the extended care facility. His granddaughter brought him to the hospital emergency room after the nursing supervisor noticed a sudden change in his mental status (i.e., confusion, delirium, agitation).

HEALTH HISTORY

EA has a history of Type 2 diabetes mellitus and has been taking Glucotrol XL daily; otherwise he is considered to be healthy. He has allergies to erythromycin and beta-lactam antibiotics.

PHYSICAL EXAMINATION

EA's temperature is 101.6° F, pulse 120, respirations 28, blood pressure 90/60 mm Hg, and he weighs 150 pounds. His urine output is 300 mL/24 hours; the urine is cloudy and foul smelling. His mucous membranes are dry, and his skin cool and dry.

LABORATORY TESTING

EA's test results show his WBC count is 26,000/mm³, and he has eosinopenia, mild hyperbilirubinemia, and proteinuria. His blood glucose level is 250 mg/dL; his serum creatinine level is 1.7 mg/dL; serum calcium 8.2 mg/dL; serum magnesium 1.2 mEq/L; serum sodium 135 mEq/L; and serum potassium 3.5 mEq/L. His SaO₂ level is 87% on room air; the arterial pH is 7.30; the PaCO₂ level is <32 mm Hg. The results of three blood cultures are postive for *Pseudomonas aeruginosa*; the urine culture is positive for *P. aeruginosa* snd *Escherichia coli*.

CULTURAL/SOCIAL CONSIDERATIONS

EA has been living on Medicare and Medicaid for the past several years. He has no supplemental health care insurance. His granddaughter is concerned about the rising cost of care in the intensive care unit.

LIFESPAN CONSIDERATIONS

EA's only relative is his granddaughter, who holds his durable medical power of attorney. He has a living will that states no heroic measures are to be taken should he have a cardiac or respiratory arrest. The granddaughter has been asked about the use of a ventilator should his respiratory status deteriorate. She agrees that no heroic measures are to be taken per EA's living will.

PATIENT PROBLEM(S)

Sepsis resulting from urinary tract infection.

GOALS OF THERAPY

EA's infection will resolve without serious adverse drug effects.

CRITICAL THINKING QUESTIONS

1. Amikacin 1020 mg IV q12h has been ordered for EA. Is this within a safe dosage range? Why or why not? (Dosage calculated based on 15 mg/kg daily.)
2. What is the mechanism of action of this drug? Is it bacteriocidal or bacteriostatic? Is it broad- or narrow-spectrum?
3. Which adverse effects should be watched for when amikacin is used?
4. What are the expected serum trough and peak drug levels for amikacin?
5. What is the primary route of excretion of amikacin?
6. How fast should EA's amikacin be administered intravenously? Why?
7. How do aminoglycosides affect the neuromuscular junction?
8. Which laboratory tests are necessary (other than trough and peak levels) for EA?
9. Which groups of patients might be more prone to aminoglycoside ototoxicity and nephrotoxicity?

Instruct the patient using a topical aminoglycoside to wash the affected area gently and pat dry. Apply a thin film of ointment. Occlusive dressings may be used if ordered by the health care provider. Teach the patient to assess skin condition and to inform the health care provider if skin irritation develops or the infection worsens. Instruct the patient to contact the health care provider if the condition does not improve in a few days.

The patient with an allergy to an aminoglycoside should be advised to wear some form of identification (e.g., medical alert tag or bracelet) to inform health care personnel of the allergy. Carrying the identification in a wallet or purse is usually not helpful if emergency care is needed.

EVALUATION

The effectiveness of aminoglycoside therapy is determined by monitoring clinical response. The frequency of monitoring is proportional to the severity of the infection. If no response is seen within 3 to 5 days of drug therapy, new cultures should be taken.

Important clinical indicators of effective treatment include a reduction in fever and resolution of the signs and symptoms of infection, vital signs that return to normal for the patient, WBC count that returns to normal limits, and a culture and sensitivity test that is negative for the offending organism. Further proof may include an increase in appetite, energy level, and general sense of well-being. Improved neurologic status should be noted in patients with hepatic encephalopathy. Patients who have undergone intestinal surgery should be free of infection.

Bibliography

Calder JH, Jacobson GP: Acquired bilateral peripheral vestibular system impairment: rehabilitative options and potential outcomes, *J Am Acad Audiol* 11(9):514-521, 2000.

Casano RAM, Johnson DF, Bykhovskaya Y, et al: Inherited susceptibility to aminoglycoside ototoxicity: genetic heterogeneity and clinical implications, *Am J Otolaryngol* 20(3):151-156, 1999.

Fausti SA, Henry JA, Helt WJ, et al: An individualized, sensitive frequency range for early detection of ototoxicity, *Ear Hear* 20(6):497-505, 1999.

Fisman DN, Kaye KM: Once-daily dosing of aminoglycoside antibiotics, *Infect Dis Clin North Am* 14(2):475-487, 2000.

Gerding DN: Antimicrobial cycling: lessons learned from the aminoglycoside experience, *Infect Control Hosp Epidemiol* 21(suppl 9):S12-S17, 2000.

May L, Navarro VB, Gottsch JD: First do no harm: routine use of aminoglycosides in the operating room, *Insight* 25(3):77-80, 2000.

Internet Resources

http://clinweb2.kumc.edu/formulas/aminogly.htm.
http://www.home.eznet.net/webtent/oda.html.

CHAPTER

30

Antibacterial Drugs for Special Purposes

SHERRY F. QUEENER • KATHLEEN GUTIERREZ

 Visit http://evolve.elsevier.com/Gutierrez/ for additional information.

KEY TERMS

Anaerobes, p. 447

Crystallurla, p. 444

Cystitis, p. 440

Iatrogenic, p. 449

Nosocomial, p. 449

Obligate anaerobes, p. 447

Pyelonephritis, p. 440

Sulfonamides, p. 441

Tetrahydrofolic acid (THFA), p. 441

OBJECTIVES

- Describe the common features of drugs used for urinary tract infections.
- List the drugs with special application to anaerobic infections.
- Discuss the treatment of nosocomial infections.
- Develop a nursing care plan for patients receiving drugs that are discussed in this chapter.

PATHOPHYSIOLOGY • Urinary Tract Infections

Bacterial infections of the urinary tract are one of the most common complaints seen by health care providers. **Cystitis** is an infection of the bladder. The symptoms of fever, malaise, and burning pain during urination may be related to the inflammatory response evoked by the presence of bacteria in the normally sterile environment of the bladder. The most common route of infection seems to be fecal contamination of the opening of the urethra (Figure 30-1), which is especially common in female patients because of the anatomical closeness of the anus to the urethral opening and because the female urethra is so short.

Although the lower urinary tract is constantly exposed to pathogenic bacteria, a symptomatic infection requiring treatment may not always result. Several host defense mechanisms protect the bladder from bacterial invasion. Regular, spontaneous voiding with complete bladder emptying promptly clears invading bacteria and is the urinary tract's principal line of defense against in-

fection. Mechanical obstructions such as stones slow the flow of urine and thus predispose the urinary tract to infection. Another important defense is the natural antibacterial action of urine. Extremes in urinary pH, high urine osmolality, and concentrations of urea nitrogen and ammonium are intrinsic factors that inhibit bacterial growth. The presence of specific antibodies (IgA and IgG) and antibacterial enzymes (lysozyme and lactoferrin) in the urine also deter bacteria. An intact mucosal lining of the bladder readily resists bacterial invasion. However, when the mucosa is altered from its normal state by infrequent voiding, repeated overdistention, obstruction, pregnancy, or ischemia, it is more susceptible to bacterial adherence and infection.

Pyelonephritis is an infection within the kidneys. Infections at this site produce systemic symptoms and are potentially much more serious than infections in the bladder. Pyelonephritis usually results from bacteria traveling up the ureters from an infected bladder to the

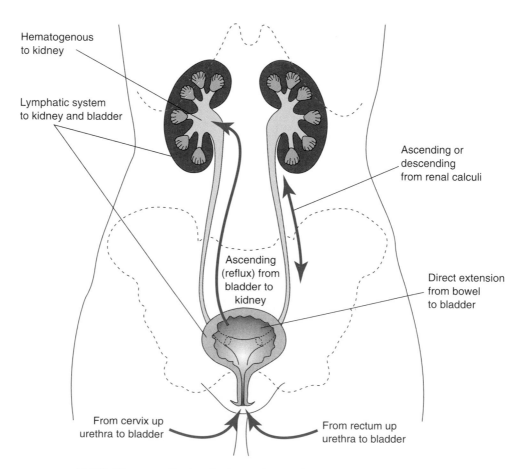

FIGURE 30-1 Routes for bacteria entering the female urinary tract.

kidneys (see Figure 30-1). The migration of bacteria to the kidneys is facilitated by conditions that impair urine flow, such as stones or poor muscle tone in the ureters.

On rare occasions, bacteria can spread to the kidney through the bloodstream from a distant focus of infection such as infections of the teeth, gums, ears, or throat. More unusual, although possible, is the lymphatic spread of bacteria from the large intestine to the kidney.

Pathologic changes that occur with acute pyelonephritis include gross enlargement and yellow abscesses throughout the renal parenchyma. Mucosal surfaces of the renal pelvis and calices become congested, thickened, and covered by exudate. With bacterial persistence, the kidney becomes scarred and pitted. Fibrosis and thinning are evident in portions of the parenchyma. In some instances, glomeruli become fibrotic and the tubules atrophy, destroying function in the affected area of the kidney.

The organisms that cause urinary tract infections (UTIs) are mostly gram-negative bacteria. For example, 80% of bladder infections acquired outside a medical setting (i.e., community acquired) are caused by uropathogenic strains of *Escherichia coli*. These strains of *E. coli* differ from most *E. coli* in the bowel because they have developed mechanisms that allow them to bind to mannose receptors on the epithelial cells lining the urinary tract. Other strains of *E. coli* may bind to different receptors and be more closely associated with pyelonephritis.

Although gram-negative bacteria are the primary cause of UTIs, they are not the only important pathogens to be considered. For example, the second leading cause of community-acquired urinary tract infections in sexually active young women is *Staphylococcus saprophyticus*, which is a species of gram-positive bacteria.

Hospital-acquired UTIs, which often involve patients with catheters or other instrumentation of the urinary tract, present a more complicated array of organisms to be considered. In addition to the organisms noted above for community-acquired infections, organisms such as *Pseudomonas aeruginosa*, enterococci, and even the yeast *Candida* are often involved with hospital-acquired UTIs.

The drugs covered in the section that follows are used either exclusively or primarily to treat UTIs. Drugs with broader clinical uses that may include UTIs were covered in Chapters 25, 26, and 27. Selection of antimicrobial drugs to treat UTIs depends primarily on the organism found in the urine culture and the results of antibiotic susceptibility testing.

DRUG CLASS • Sulfonamides

sulfamethizole (Thiosulfil)

sulfamethoxazole (Gantanol)

sulfisoxazole (Gantrisin)

MECHANISM OF ACTION

Sulfonamides block bacterial synthesis of folic acid, a vitamin required for the synthesis of amino acids and nucleic acids. The metabolically active form of folic acid, **tetrahydrofolic acid (THFA)**, is synthesized in many bacteria from simple precursor molecules (Figure 30-2). Two of the enzymes involved in these conversions have been exploited as targets of antibacterial drugs. Dihydropteroate synthase, which converts paraaminobenzoic acid (PABA) and other small molecules to dihydropteroate, is competitively inhibited by sulfonamides. Sulfonamides are thus selectively toxic to organisms that must form folic acid from PABA. Fortunately, humans are not sensitive to this action because we cannot synthesize folic acid but must absorb it preformed in our diet. Sulfonamides are primarily bacteriostatic drugs.

USES

Sulfonamide drugs are useful against UTIs because they are effective against most of the common pathogens (Table 30-1) and they achieve a high concentration in urine (Table 30-2). Drugs of this class are potentially active against a wide range of gram-positive and gram-negative organisms, as well as *Nocardia*, *Chlamydia*, and *Actinomyces*, but bacterial resistance has limited use for many infections requiring systemic therapy.

Sulfamethoxazole is the most widely used sulfonamide for general infections. This sulfonamide is also combined with trimethoprim for use against UTIs and some systemic infections (Table 30-3). When trimethoprim and sulfamethoxazole are used to treat UTIs, they may be combined with phenazopyridine for symptomatic relief. The sulfonamide and trimethoprim supply antibacterial activity and the phenazopyridine, which is excreted in urine, exerts an analgesic effect on the mucosa of the urinary tract. The added phenazopyridine therefore relieves the pain, burning, and itching associated with UTIs.

Sulfonamides have a variety of other medical uses, and thus several members of the family are covered in other chapters. Sulfadiazine or sulfadoxine are used in combinations to treat malaria (Chapter 34). Sulfapyridine is used for dermatitis herpetiformis, a chronic skin disease associated with severe itching and reddened le-

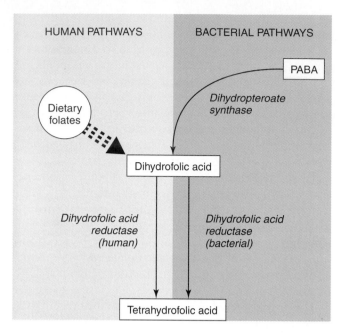

HUMAN PATHWAYS

BACTERIAL PATHWAYS

PABA

Dietary folates

Dihydropteroate synthase

Dihydrofolic acid

Dihydrofolic acid reductase (human)

Dihydrofolic acid reductase (bacterial)

Tetrahydrofolic acid

FIGURE 30-2 Synthesis of tetrahydrofolic acid (THFA) in bacteria and humans. THFA is a vitamin required for nucleic acid and amino acid synthesis. Many bacteria form this vitamin from paraaminobenzoic acid (PABA) and other small molecules. Two enzymes involved in this synthesis have proven useful in chemotherapy: dihydropteroate synthase and dihydrofolic acid reductase. Sulfonamides inhibit dihydropteroate synthase, thereby blocking THFA synthesis in bacteria. Humans are immune to this action because preformed folate and dihydrofolic acid are supplied in the diet. Dihydrofolic acid reductase in bacteria is inhibited by trimethoprim, but the human form of the enzyme is relatively resistant.

TABLE 30-1

Urinary Tract Antimicrobials and Susceptible Organisms

Common Pathogens	Generally Effective Drugs
Escherichia coli, *Klebsiella*, *Proteus*	Cephalosporins, fluoroquinolones, sulfonamides, trimethoprim, urinary tract antiseptics*
Staphylococci, including *S. saprophyticus*	Cephalosporins, fluoroquinolones, sulfonamides, trimethoprim
Enterococci	Beta-lactams (selected), fluoroquinolones (selected), nitrofurantoin
Pseudomonas aeruginosa	Beta-lactams (selected), fluoroquinolones (selected)
Candida	Fluconazole or ketoconazole (see Chapter 32)

*Nitrofurantoin has little activity against *Proteus*.

---

sions (Chapter 67). Sulfasalazine is a poorly absorbed sulfonamide drug used for ulcerative colitis (Chapter 49). Sulfonamides are also available in preparations for vaginal application, but no evidence of effectiveness exists. Moreover, using these drugs may produce sensitization. Finally, topical sulfonamides, such as mafenide and silver sulfadiazine, are used to treat or prevent infections on burned or abraded skin (Chapter 67), and sulfacetamide sodium may be used to treat conjunctivitis (Chapter 65).

PHARMACOKINETICS

Sulfonamide drugs used to treat systemic or urinary tract infections are well absorbed when given orally and well distributed to body tissues. Concentrations of sul-

---

TABLE 30-2

Urinary Levels of Selected Antimicrobial Drugs

Drug	Urinary Excretion* (%)	Urinary Active Antimicrobial Concentration (mcg/mL)
Beta-Lactams (see Chapter 25)		
amoxicillin	60-75	>300
cefixime	50	164
cephalexin	80-90	5000
Fluoroquinolones (see Chapter 27)		
ciprofloxacin	25-50	200
norfloxacin	25-40	168-417
Tetracyclines (see Chapter 28)		
doxycycline	<35	134
Aminoglycoside (see Chapter 29)		
gentamicin	>95	400-500
Antibacterial Drugs Primarily for Urinary Tract Infections (see Chapter 30)		
cinoxacin	50-60	390
methenamine	90	300-3000 (as formaldehyde)
nalidixic acid	5-15	>63
nitrofurantoin	30-40	25-300
sulfamethizole	85	700
sulfisoxazole	50-70	>1000
sulfamethoxazole (SMX)	20-40	100-600
trimethoprim (TMP)	20-60	70-100
co-trimoxazole	25-60	30-165 TMP, 10-133 SMX

*Includes only active unchanged drug or active metabolites.

fonamides in cerebrospinal and other body fluids may approach those of serum. Sulfonamides also pass placental membranes and enter the fetus.

Elimination of sulfonamides involves both the liver and kidneys. The liver converts a portion of the sulfonamide in blood to an acetylated derivative, which is usually bacteriologically inactive. Acetylated as well as free drug are eliminated by the kidneys, primarily by glomerular filtration. Tubular reabsorption is significant for some sulfonamides. Excretion of sulfonamides is favored by alkalinizing the urine. This procedure increases the solubility of these drugs in urine and also converts the drugs to a charged form that does not undergo renal tubular reabsorption.

Sulfamethizole produces a yellow-orange coloration in alkaline urine. This coloration, also observable in skin, is not harmful.

ADVERSE REACTIONS AND CONTRAINDICATIONS

Sulfonamides induce allergic reactions in a significant proportion of patients receiving the drugs. The most common reactions are skin rashes and itching, photosensitivity, and periorbital edema. Photosensitivity is localized to skin exposed to sun or sunlamps, but the redness of the skin may be confused with an allergic reaction. Anaphylaxis has been reported. Because sulfonamides are chemically related to the thiazide diuretics, acetazolamide, and oral hypoglycemic drugs, a patient who becomes allergic to a sulfonamide may also become allergic to one or more of these drugs.

Drug fever and other more serious reactions such as Stevens-Johnson syndrome are uncommon but may occur with sulfonamides. Stevens-Johnson syndrome is a skin and mucous membrane reaction producing macular, bullous, papular, or vesicular lesions in the oral and anogenital mucosa, eyes, and viscera. Constitutional symptoms such as malaise, headache, fever, arthralgia, and conjunctivitis are also seen with this syndrome.

Gastrointestinal (GI) tract disturbances are common with sulfonamides. In addition to nausea, vomiting, and diarrhea, more serious reactions such as pancreatitis, hepatitis, and stomatitis may occur. Central nervous system (CNS) alterations have also been observed, including headache, ataxia, hallucinations, and convulsions.

Deaths from aplastic anemia and other blood dyscrasias, although rare, have been associated with sulfonamide therapy. Sore throat, fever, or pallor may signal a serious blood dyscrasia. Older adults are more likely than younger adults to experience severe blood and skin reactions to sulfonamides. Diuretics, commonly taken to treat high blood pressure, compound the risk.

Patients with preexisting renal or hepatic disease are more prone to develop adverse effects because these organs remove sulfonamides from the body. Patients with a genetic deficiency of glucose-6-phosphate dehydrogenase (G6PD) have greater risk for hemolytic anemia induced by sulfonamides. The highest frequency of G6PD deficiency is observed among African Americans and Mediterranean populations; patients from these groups should be watched carefully for signs of anemia. Sulfonamides may also worsen anemias caused by folate deficiency.

TABLE 30-3

Sulfonamide and Trimethoprim Preparations Used for Urinary Tract Infections

Generic Name	Brand Name	Formulation
sulfamethizole	Thiosulfil	Tablet
sulfamethoxazole (SMX)	Gantanol	Tablet
sulfisoxazole	Sosol	Tablet
sulfisoxazole	Gantrisin	Oral syrup or suspension
trimethoprim (TMP)	Proloprim, Trimpex	Tablet
trimethoprim	Primsol	Oral suspension
sulfamethoxazole/trimethoprim	Bactrim, Septra, Sulfatrim	Injectable; oral suspension
sulfamethoxazole/trimethoprim	Bactrim, Cotrim, Septra, Sulfamethoprim	Tablet
sulfamethoxazole/trimethoprim	Bactrim DS, Cotrim DS, Septra DS, Sulfamethoprim DS	Tablet
phenazopyridine(PNP)/ sulfamethoxazole/trimethoprim	generic	Tablet
sulfadiazine/sulfamerazine/ sulfamethazine	Triple Sulfoid	Tablet

TOXICITY

Renal toxicity with sulfonamides may occur if the drug crystallizes in urine or tubular fluid, a condition called **crystalluria**. These drugs precipitate because their solubility is limited in normal acidic urine. The least soluble sulfonamides in use today are sulfadiazine and the acetylated metabolite of sulfamethoxazole. Patients who receive any sulfonamide drug should consume sufficient fluids to produce at least 1 L of urine daily. The solubility of sulfonamides in urine may be increased by alkalinizing the urine.

INTERACTIONS

Sulfonamides are highly bound to serum proteins and, therefore, may displace other drugs from protein-binding sites. This displacement can occur with oral anticoagulants, sulfonylureas, phenytoin, the antiinflammatory drugs phenylbutazone and sulfinpyrazone, and the antineoplastic drug methotrexate. In newborns displacement of bilirubin by sulfonamides may place the patient at risk for kernicterus, with signs of lethargy, poor feeding, and neurologic changes.

Drugs such as sulfonylureas, primaquine, procainamide, and quinidine increase the risk of hemolysis with sulfonamides.

The urinary antiseptic methenamine releases formaldehyde in acidic urine for antibacterial effect. Sulfonamides can form insoluble complexes with this formaldehyde, resulting in crystalluria.

DRUG CLASS • Dihydrofolate Reductase Inhibitors

trimethoprim (Primsol, Proloprim, Trimpex)

MECHANISM OF ACTION

Trimethoprim inhibits bacterial dihydrofolic acid reductase, thus preventing THFA formation in bacteria (see Figure 30-2). Dihydrofolic acid reductase is needed in humans because much of the folate in mammalian diets is dihydrofolic acid that must be converted to THFA. Fortunately, dihydrofolic acid reductase in humans is relatively resistant to the action of trimethoprim, and the drug may be given at dosages that inhibit this enzyme in bacteria but not in humans; hence the conversion of dietary folates to THFA in patients can proceed normally in the presence of antibacterial concentrations of trimethoprim.

USES

Trimethoprim has a spectrum of antimicrobial activity similar to that of sulfonamides, with some exceptions (see Table 30-1). Trimethoprim is more active against gram-negative bacteria such as *Proteus* and *Klebsiella* but is not useful alone against *Chlamydia* or *Nocardia*. Although trimethoprim is used in the United States most commonly in combination with a sulfonamide, a preparation of trimethoprim alone is available for use in UTIs.

PHARMACOKINETICS

Trimethoprim is most often used in a fixed 1:5 ratio with sulfamethoxazole (see Table 30-2) to exploit the properties of both drugs for therapeutic effect. Both drugs are well absorbed from the GI tract. Serum concentrations of the free drug not bound to serum proteins are usually in a 1:20 ratio of trimethoprim to sulfamethoxazole. At this concentration ratio, the combination is *synergistic*, which means they are more effective in combination than would be expected from the action of either drug alone. Synergy may result because both drugs starve sensitive bacteria for THFA, but the drugs work on two different enzymes in the sequence of reactions leading to THFA. Sequential blockade of this metabolic pathway is much more effective than the blockade of a single step by one drug at high concentrations.

Trimethoprim penetrates tissues better than sulfamethoxazole, with concentrations in breast milk, bile, prostatic fluid, vaginal fluids, liver, spleen, skin, and kidneys usually exceeding plasma concentrations of trimethoprim. Penetration into other tissues, including the CNS, is adequate.

Trimethoprim appears in urine at a concentration approximately 100 times the plasma concentration (see Table 30-2), with most of the drug in the active form. The urinary concentration of sulfamethoxazole is about five times the plasma concentration.

ADVERSE REACTIONS AND CONTRAINDICATIONS

Serious reactions to trimethoprim are rare, but anorexia, diarrhea, headache, nausea, and vomiting sometimes occur.

TOXICITY

Toxicity from trimethoprim is expected only with large overdoses. Treatment of the patient may include acidifying the urine to hasten excretion of trimethoprim and giving leucovorin, a form of folic acid, to overcome its antifolate effects.

INTERACTIONS

Trimethoprim is synergistic with any systemically effective sulfonamide. Sulfamethoxazole was chosen for use in the fixed combination with trimethoprim because the kinetics of elimination of the two drugs are similar, as discussed previously.

Trimethoprim should not be combined with methotrexate, pyrimethamine, or trimetrexate because these drugs have potent antifolate activity. The result could be megaloblastic anemia.

DRUG CLASS   •   Urinary Tract Antiseptics

Quinolone-like Drugs

   cinoxacin (Cinobac)

   enoxacin (Penetrex)

   nalidixic acid (NegGram)

MECHANISM OF ACTION

Cinoxacin, enoxacin, and nalidixic acid are relatives of fluoroquinolone antibiotics and have similar actions on DNA remodeling enzymes (Chapter 27), but these drugs are much less potent than fluoroquinolones. Low potency contributes to frequent development of resistance.

USES

These drugs concentrate in urine and thus may be used for simple urinary tract infections (see Table 30-1). Nalidixic acid and cinoxacin are used exclusively for urinary tract infections, but enoxacin has also been used for gonorrhea. These three drugs are not appropriate for systemic infections because they produce low plasma concentrations.

PHARMACOKINETICS

Nalidixic acid, enoxacin, and cinoxacin rapidly enter the blood after oral administration. Nalidixic acid is the most extensively biotransformed drug of this group, with glucuronide and hydroxylated derivatives being formed during the process. The hydroxylated form of nalidixic acid is biologically active and comprises a significant proportion of the active drug in blood or urine. More than 90% of nalidixic acid in blood is bound to serum proteins. Little enters most body tissues. The only organs in which drug concentration exceeds the plasma concentration are the kidneys. Nalidixic acid has the lowest plasma concentration of any drug in this group.

Cinoxacin and enoxacin are primarily excreted renally. In addition, 40% of a dose of cinoxacin and 20% of enoxacin are biotransformed by the liver, and the metabolites excreted in the urine.

ADVERSE REACTIONS AND CONTRAINDICATIONS

As relatives of fluoroquinolones, these three drugs share the potential for causing cartilage damage in weight-bearing joints (Chapter 27). They also share the potential for producing CNS effects. For nalidixic acid these symptoms may include seizures, mental instability, headache, dizziness, and visual disturbances. Older adults may be more susceptible to the confusion and CNS irritability that this drug produces, especially when cerebral arteriosclerosis is present.

Both nalidixic acid and cinoxacin can cause blood dyscrasias, which may include hemolytic anemia or eosinophilia. All three drugs of this class should be avoided in children. Some health care professionals have used nalidixic acid during the second or third trimester of pregnancy, but the drug should never be used in the first trimester or at term. Enoxacin and cinoxacin are usually avoided during pregnancy.

INTERACTIONS

Nalidixic acid interacts with anticoagulants such as warfarin, causing an increase in the anticoagulant effect because the anticoagulants are displaced from protein-binding sites.

Enoxacin is especially effective at decreasing the biotransformation of caffeine and theophylline, leading to increases in toxicity with these compounds.

The combination of nalidixic acid with other antibacterial drugs is usually avoided because of unpredictable actions. For example, gentamicin seems to act synergistically with nalidixic acid in laboratory tests, but tetracycline or nitrofurantoin antagonize the action of nalidixic acid.

Formaldehyde Generator

   methenamine (Urex, Hiprex)

MECHANISM OF ACTION

Methenamine is bactericidal because it decomposes in urine to produce ammonia and formaldehyde. Bacteria are sensitive to formaldehyde when urinary concentrations rise above 20 mcg/mL, and urinary pH is less than 5.5. The combination of methenamine with an acid salt (hippurate) helps maintain urinary pH in the desired range.

USES

Methenamine is used for long-term prophylaxis or as suppressive therapy for patients at risk for bacterial reinfection. This drug is not appropriate to treat acute, symptomatic infection but instead should be used after the urinary tract infection has been cleared with an effective antimicrobial drug. Methenamine acts against most common gram-negative urinary tract pathogens (see Table 30-1).

PHARMACOKINETICS

Methenamine is absorbed quickly after oral administration, undergoes biotransformation in the liver, and is excreted in urine. The effectiveness of methenamine depends on maintaining an adequate urinary concentration of formaldehyde. Peak urine concentrations of formaldehyde usually occur 2 hours after a single dose of methenamine hippurate. Formaldehyde levels in urine should stabilize at a constant level within 2 to 3 days after treatment begins.

ADVERSE REACTIONS AND CONTRAINDICATIONS

Adverse effects reported with methenamine include nausea, vomiting, cramps, and anorexia. Urinary symptoms such as dysuria, frequency or urgency, hematuria, and proteinuria also may be noted. When taken in large doses, methenamine can cause crystalluria. Methenamine is contraindicated in patients with renal insufficiency, severe dehydration, or severe hepatic insufficiency. Although empirical evidence suggests that methenamine may be safely given to women during the last trimester of pregnancy (Category C), the drug should be used in pregnant women only if clinically necessary.

INTERACTIONS

As noted with sulfonamides, methenamine can form insoluble complexes with formaldehyde and thus lead to crystalluria in acidic urine.

Furantoin

nitrofurantoin (Furadantin, Macrobid, Macrodantin)

MECHANISM OF ACTION

Nitrofurantoin is activated in bacteria to compounds that attack bacterial proteins and interfere with several metabolic processes. Development of resistance to nitrofurantoin is uncommon.

USES

Nitrofurantoin can be used for primary treatment of uncomplicated acute UTIs and is among the few drugs considered safe for such use during pregnancy. It is effective against many common pathogens of the urinary tract (see Table 30-1) but not against *Proteus* or *Pseudomonas* species. In most patients, nitrofurantoin is more effective when used for prolonged treatment of persistent bacteriuria or episodes of reinfection caused by *E. coli* or some strains of *Klebsiella*. Nitrofurantoin is not recommended for treating pyelonephritis or perinephric abscess.

PHARMACOKINETICS

Nitrofurantoin is an effective antibacterial drug in the laboratory but is ineffective when used to treat systemic infections because of its unfavorable pharmacokinetics. The drug is adequately absorbed from the small intestine, especially in the presence of food, but never achieves satisfactory blood levels because the kidneys remove the drug so quickly that it fails to accumulate in blood. Nitrofurantoin is concentrated in the kidneys and achieves bactericidal concentrations in urine.

ADVERSE REACTIONS AND CONTRAINDICATIONS

Gastric irritation with anorexia, nausea, and emesis are common with nitrofurantoin. The large crystal form of the drug (Macrodantin) may cause less irritation than the microcrystalline form. Gastric irritation is lessened by taking the drug with milk or food.

Prolonged use of nitrofurantoin produces rare but potentially serious adverse effects including pulmonary fibrosis, peripheral neuropathy, and acute or chronic hepatic injury. Because of the severity and irreversible nature of these conditions, patients taking nitrofurantoin should be monitored continually and carefully for early signs of adverse reactions. The likelihood of a severe pulmonary reaction is increased in patients with preexisting pulmonary disease.

Nitrofurantoin should be used with caution in patients with peripheral neuropathy because it may worsen the condition. Vitamin B deficiency, common in individuals with alcoholism, may also predispose a patient to peripheral neuropathy. Diabetes mellitus, a disease that may cause peripheral neuropathy, may produce an added risk of neural complications.

As with any drug that is excreted primarily by the kidneys, nitrofurantoin may accumulate in patients with renal failure. Therefore patients with renal failure are more likely to have significant adverse effects of nitrofurantoin therapy. Nitrofurantoin causes the urine to turn brown, but this reaction is harmless.

Rashes, allergies, and reversible blood dyscrasias have been observed with nitrofurantoin. Hemolytic anemia similar to that seen with sulfonamides may also occur. Persons with G6PD deficiency are at increased risk for hemolysis. Infants less than 1 month old have undeveloped enzyme systems that make them especially susceptible to hemolytic anemia induced by nitrofurantoin; therefore the drug is avoided in neonates. Although nitrofurantoin is generally regarded as safe for use during pregnancy, it is contraindicated in pregnant women at term and during labor and delivery (Category B).

TOXICITY

Peripheral neuropathy is one of the most serious toxic effects of nitrofurantoin. If detected early, the condition may disappear after discontinuation of the drug. Damage may be permanent if the drug is continued after signs of peripheral neuropathy have developed.

INTERACTIONS

To avoid excessive risk of hemolysis, nitrofurantoin should not be used with hemolytic drugs such as sulfonylureas, primaquine, procainamide, and quinidine. To avoid excessive neurotoxicity, nitrofurantoin should not be combined with neurotoxic drugs. If nitrofurantoin is used with probenecid or sulfinpyrazone, the effectiveness of nitrofurantoin may be impaired because these drugs block renal secretion of nitrofurantoin. As a result, lower concentrations of the antibacterial drug are achieved in urine.

PATHOPHYSIOLOGY • Anaerobic Infections

Much of the life on earth depends on oxygen, but there are important exceptions. For example, there are many types of bacteria that grow in the absence of oxygen; these bacteria are called **anaerobes**. Some bacterial species can grow in either an aerobic (with oxygen) or an anaerobic (without oxygen) environment. An example of such an organism would be *E. coli*. In contrast to these more adaptable organisms, there are some species of bacteria, called **obligate anaerobes,** that are strictly anaerobic and cannot survive in the presence of oxygen. The most common example of such an obligate anaerobe would be the *Bacteroides* species found in the human colon, where they constitute about 95% of the total bacterial population.

The human body contains several anaerobic sites that favor the growth of anaerobic bacteria. As noted above, the human colon is one example but others include the mouth, sinuses, and genital tract. These sites harbor harmless as well as potentially pathogenic anaerobic bacteria. Anaerobic bacteria take on medical importance most often when there is injury or some condition that introduces these organisms into anaerobic sites that are normally sterile. For example, anaerobic bacteria from the bowel may infect the peritoneal cavity when disease or injury causes a perforation of the bowel. Likewise, anaerobic bacteria carried from the skin or from a contaminated object may infect a penetrating wound and lead to soft tissue infection caused by *Clostridium* species or other organisms. Bone infections can also be caused when injury introduces an anaerobic pathogen onto the broken surface of the bone. Abscesses are considered anaerobic because blood flow to the site is impaired by the infectious process and by the presence of dead or dying tissue. This combination of impaired blood flow and necrotic tissue creates an ideal environment for growth of anaerobic bacteria.

Infections caused by anaerobic bacteria are often difficult to treat because several of our most useful drug classes are less effective against anaerobes than against aerobic bacteria. For example, aminoglycosides depend on oxygen for uptake into bacterial cells and are therefore ineffective at anaerobic sites (see Chapter 29). Likewise, fluoroquinolones have poor activity against most important anaerobic pathogens, including *Bacteroides fragilis* and *Clostridium difficile* (see Chapter 27). Macrolides (see Chapter 26) have marginal activity against these organisms. In contrast, metronidazole and clindamycin have been found to be very effective in anaerobic environments and against anaerobic pathogens.

DRUG CLASS • Nitroimidazoles

metronidazole (Flagyl)

MECHANISM OF ACTION

Metronidazole is active against anaerobic organisms because it is reduced by anaerobic processes to a short-lived metabolite that directly damages DNA and leads to cell death. Production of the cytotoxic metabolite does not occur in aerobic environments.

USES

In addition to being a first-line drug to treat infections and abscesses caused by anaerobic bacteria, metronidazole is a primary drug for the treatment of intestinal amebiasis and tissue abscesses caused by amebae. It has also been used to treat trichomoniasis and giardiasis (Chapter 34).

PHARMACOKINETICS

Metronidazole is well absorbed after oral administration. The drug is biotransformed by various pathways. Both metabolites and unchanged drug appear in urine. Some patients observe a reddish brown discoloration of urine while taking metronidazole. This harmless discoloration is caused by a colored metabolite of the drug.

ADVERSE REACTIONS AND CONTRAINDICATIONS

Metronidazole can produce various GI tract symptoms, including a sharp, metallic taste, as well as nausea, diarrhea, vomiting, epigastric pain, and abdominal cramping. Although annoying, these symptoms rarely require the patient to discontinue use of the drug.

Metronidazole commonly causes dizziness or headache, but other CNS effects such as ataxia (incoordination affecting walking), numbness, and paresthesias are uncommon. These latter symptoms may signal that metronidazole should be withdrawn. Metronidazole may also produce discomfort in the pelvic organs. Dysuria, cystitis, and dryness of the vagina may be noted.

Because of its action on DNA, metronidazole may be mutagenic or carcinogenic in experimental animals. This potential problem precludes routine use of the drug in pregnant women. Metronidazole is also avoided, if possible, in patients with significant CNS disease or blood dyscrasias because the drug may worsen both conditions. Patients with hepatic impairment may accumulate the drug because the liver is the primary organ for elimination of metronidazole; however, reduced dosages may be used.

TOXICITY

High dosages of metronidazole may cause seizures.

INTERACTIONS

Metronidazole causes an alarming reaction when ethyl alcohol is ingested. Patients experience intense flushing, nausea, headaches, and abdominal cramps. This reaction is similar to that experienced by patients taking both disulfiram and ethyl alcohol.

Metronidazole may potentiate the action of warfarin. Patients receiving both drugs should be observed for signs of bleeding.

 DRUG CLASS • Lincosamine

clindamycin (Cleocin)

MECHANISM OF ACTION

Clindamycin inhibits the action of bacterial ribosomes in a manner similar to erythromycin. This drug halts bacterial protein synthesis and may be bacteriostatic or bactericidal, depending on drug concentrations. Bacterial resistance to clindamycin develops in several ways. Some organisms may become impermeable to the drugs, but others alter their ribosomes to prevent binding of clindamycin. With this latter mechanism, organisms may also become resistant to erythromycin or chloramphenicol. In practice, most clinically observed resistance to clindamycin develops in a gradual, stepwise manner.

USES

Clindamycin is effective against several anaerobic organisms, particularly *Bacteroides fragilis*. Infections caused by these organisms are a major indication for clindamycin. Clindamycin is also effective against gram-positive bacteria, although it is not as effective as penicillin against *Neisseria gonorrhoeae* or other gram-negative cocci.

PHARMACOKINETICS

Clindamycin is well absorbed orally, and oral absorption is not significantly impaired by food. Clindamycin palmitate is available as flavored granules to be used in suspension for oral administration. The palmitate is rapidly removed to release active clindamycin.

Clindamycin-2-phosphate may be injected intramuscularly, but local pain may occur. Absorption of drug by this route is good, with serum peaks being achieved 30 to 60 minutes after injection. These drugs are also suitable for intravenous use. By this route, clindamycin-2-phosphate causes pain and phlebitis. Clindamycin-2-phosphate is inactive as an antibiotic but is rapidly converted to clindamycin in the body.

Clindamycin is well distributed to most body tissues, with the exception of the CNS; it does not appear in the cerebrospinal fluid (CSF) even when meningitis is present. Clindamycin appears in the milk of lactating women treated with this drug.

Clindamycin is extensively biodegraded in the body; the liver is the primary site of biotransformation. Because less than 20% of the total drug administered orally shows up as active antibiotic in urine or feces, these drugs are used in normal dosages in patients with renal insufficiency or failure. Clindamycin is not removed by hemodialysis.

ADVERSE REACTIONS AND CONTRAINDICATIONS

The most serious reaction to clindamycin is colitis. Symptoms range from mild diarrhea to the life-threatening condition called pseudomembranous colitis (Chapter 24). Increased frequency of bowel movements or softness of the stools may be reason to discontinue the drug, especially in older adults. Significant diarrhea should prompt discontinuation of the drug and may be relieved by that measure alone. Fluid and electrolyte replacement and other supportive therapy also may be required. Drugs that slow peristaltic action may worsen the condition or prolong it; thus opiates and diphenoxylate with atropine are not appropriate for use in these patients.

In addition to colitis, clindamycin may produce GI tract irritation ranging from nausea and vomiting to glossitis and stomatitis. This drug is usually avoided in patients with significant preexisting GI tract disease.

Allergies to clindamycin range from mild rashes to fever and anaphylactic shock. These reactions may occur in anyone but are more common in those with other drug allergies. The appearance of any allergic response is cause for discontinuing the drug.

Blood dyscrasias and liver dysfunction may occur during clindamycin therapy. Patients with significant preexisting hepatic disease often receive lowered dosages of clindamycin to avoid drug accumulation.

TOXICITY

Direct toxicity of oral doses of clindamycin is low, except for the increased risk of GI tract symptoms arising from alteration of bacterial populations in the bowel. Direct infusion of clindamycin may also affect the cardiovascular system. Clindamycin is normally given in an intravenous solution no more concentrated than 0.6 g/dL at a rate no more rapid than 100 mL/20 min.

INTERACTIONS

Clindamycin is incompatible in solutions with aminophylline, ampicillin, barbiturates, calcium gluconate, magnesium sulfate, and phenytoin. Chloramphenicol and erythromycin antagonize the antibacterial effect of clindamycin.

Because clindamycin has neuromuscular-blocking properties, it may enhance the action of various neuromuscular-blocking drugs and inhalation anesthetics.

The use of kaolin-pectin antidiarrheal drugs given at the time oral clindamycin is ingested significantly lowers the serum concentrations of the antibiotic.

PATHOPHYSIOLOGY • Nosocomial Infections

Distinction has been made in several chapters between community-acquired infections and hospital-acquired infections. This distinction is important because the organisms that may be causing the infections are different. Medicine as it is practiced today is aggressive in prolonging life and many of the processes require invasive procedures. Long-term or repeated use of antibiotics is common. The undesired outcome of these medical advances has been the selection of highly antibiotic-resistant bacteria, which tend to be concentrated in the sites where these very ill patients are treated. The term **nosocomial** infections refers to those infections acquired in a hospital or other health care setting (the meaning of the Greek root words is "taking care of disease"). A related term is **iatrogenic,** which literally means "caused by a physician," but is used to mean a condition caused by medical treatment.

In the 60 years since antibiotics came into wide use, several bacteria have emerged as dangerous pathogens well able to resist common antibiotics. *Staphylococcus aureus* was a bacterial pathogen that commonly caused wound infections, and when penicillin was first tried in patients in 1940 the drug was extremely effective against this organism. Within 2 years, strains of *S. aureus* were discovered that produced penicillinase, which conferred resistance to penicillin (Chapter 25). Nosocomial infections caused by these strains were impossible to treat until additional drugs were developed. Methicillin was a drug developed specifically to resist penicillinase from *S. aureus* and, thus, became useful for these nosocomial infections. Within a few years of its introduction, methicillin also fell victim to the creativity of bacteria under selection pressure: *S. aureus* gained the ability to form different penicillin-binding proteins that no longer bound to methicillin, making it resistant to the drug's action. To make matters worse, methicillin resistance gave resistance to all beta-lactam antibiotics, as well as to other antibiotics because the plasmids that carried methicillin resistance often carried resistance to several classes of antibiotics. Methicillin is no longer distributed in the United States, but the legacy of methicillin-resistant *S. aureus* remains and treatment of this multiresistant organism is a clinical challenge.

Enterococci, including *Enterococcus faecium* and *Enterococcus faecalis*, are another group of bacteria that have become more important pathogens during the age of antibiotics. These gram-positive bacteria were originally sensitive to a few penicillins (but not cephalosporins). Resistance to the penicillins and the few other effective drugs developed readily. As resistance to other drugs became more common, vancomycin (see next section) became the drug of last resort for serious infections caused by these bacteria. Resistance to vancomycin developed slowly, with the first strains of vancomycin-resistant enterococci (VRE) appearing in the United States in 1988, about 30 years after discovery of the drug. Vancomycin is a rapid-acting bactericidal drug, which may partly explain why the low incidence of bacterial resistance to this drug persisted for so many years. Unfortunately, the resistance to vancomycin that has appeared is carried on plasmids that spread readily among strains of enterococci. By 1992 some hospitals reported VRE accounted for 10% of isolates of enterococci. Infections caused by VRE are difficult to treat. Bacteremia (bacteria shed into the blood) caused by VRE has a very high mortality rate.

Clostridium difficile is another important cause of nosocomial superinfections. This organism, which may exist in the bowel without causing symptoms, becomes a clinical problem when antibiotic therapy wipes out other bacteria normally found in the bowel. The highly resistant *C. difficile* is then able to proliferate and produce toxins that cause antibiotic colitis or pseudomembranous colitis (Chapter 24).

The most serious nosocomial infections are caused by the bacteria discussed above, but not all nosocomial infections include these organisms. For example, community-acquired pneumonia is usually caused by *Streptococcus pneumoniae* or *Haemophilis influenzae*; hospitalized patients, especially those on ventilators, are more likely to have pneumonia that involves gram-negative bacteria such as *Pseudomonas aeruginosa* or *Klebsiella pneumoniae*. Likewise, hospital-acquired UTIs are more likely to involve *P. aeruginosa* or enterococci than are community-acquired infections.

In the next section of this chapter, we consider antibiotics that have their most important uses against organisms that have evolved in response to heavy antibiotic use and are thus resistant to most of the first-line antibiotics covered in earlier chapters.

DRUG CLASS • Glycopeptides

vancomycin (Vancocin, Vancoled)

MECHANISM OF ACTION

Vancomycin prevents synthesis of bacterial cell walls by blocking peptidoglycan strand formation. This site of action is different from the sites sensitive to penicillin and other antibiotics that interfere with cell wall synthesis.

USES

Vancomycin is most often used for serious or life-threatening staphylococcal or streptococcal infections, as well as for infections caused by sensitive enterococci. Because the drug is chemically unrelated to penicillins and has a different mechanism of action, it acts against organisms that resist penicillins, including methicillin-resistant *Staphylococcus aureus*. Vancomycin and penicillin are not cross-allergenic; thus vancomycin is useful in patients who are allergic to penicillins. Vancomycin also has special utility in treating antibiotic-induced colitis, which arises from a superinfection with *C. difficile* in the bowel.

PHARMACOKINETICS

Vancomycin is a complex glycopeptide that may be positively or negatively charged, depending on pH. Therefore vancomycin does not easily cross biologic membranes and is not significantly absorbed after oral administration. Vancomycin is most often given by intermittent intravenous infusion but may be given by mouth for intestinal infections. Bactericidal concentrations of drug are not obtained in systemic circulation with oral doses.

Vancomycin is well distributed throughout the body and reaches clinically effective concentrations in various body fluid compartments such as pericardial, synovial, and pleural fluids. It does not penetrate normal CSF but does enter the CNS when the meninges are inflamed.

Active vancomycin appears in very high concentrations in urine. The kidney is the major excretory organ for vancomycin, and nonrenal elimination is limited. In older adults and patients with renal insufficiency, vancomycin may accumulate unless drug dosages are reduced to compensate for loss of excretory efficiency. Serum vancomycin levels should be monitored regularly. In patients who lack kidney function, vancomycin is usually given only once between dialysis treatments. Vancomycin is not cleared from the body by hemodialysis.

ADVERSE REACTIONS AND CONTRAINDICATIONS

Intravenous infusion of vancomycin has produced nausea, flushing, and itching. These reactions are more likely when undiluted vancomycin is dripped directly into a running intravenous line rather than being properly diluted beforehand. The reaction, which is caused by generalized histamine release, is sometimes called red man syndrome because of the intense flushing reactions observed. If vancomycin inadvertently enters tissues around an intravenous site, local necrosis may develop.

TOXICITY

Vancomycin causes deafness in some patients, especially when serum concentrations exceed 80 mg/mL serum. Patients with impaired renal function and older adult patients are more likely than healthy or younger persons to show drug accumulation and should be watched closely for ringing in the ears (tinnitus) or hearing loss. Audiometry testing should be performed before starting vancomycin and repeated periodically during long-term therapy. Some patients have regained some hearing acuity when they stopped taking vancomycin, but for others, hearing loss may persist.

Nephrotoxicity may occur, with symptoms of increased thirst, altered urination, anorexia, or weakness. Blood and protein in the patient's urine occasionally have been noted.

INTERACTIONS

Vancomycin should not be combined with another ototoxic or nephrotoxic drug, such as an aminoglycoside antibiotic, bumetanide, cisplatin, ethacrynic acid, or furosemide. Combining one of these drugs with vancomycin may result in additive toxic effects. Complete loss of hearing or renal failure is possible.

DRUG CLASS • Streptogramins

quinupristin/dalfopristin (Synercid)

MECHANISM OF ACTION

Streptogramins such as quinupristin/dalfopristin have multiple effects on bacterial protein synthesis, mostly affecting functions of the 50S ribosomal subunit. For many bacteria the combination is bactericidal in action.

USES

The fixed combination quinupristin/dalfopristin is used for nosocomial infections caused by vancomycin-resistant *Enterococcus faecium*, for methicillin-resistant *Staphylococcus aureus* or *Staphylococcus epidermidis*, and for drug-resistant *Streptococcus pneumoniae*.

PHARMACOKINETICS

Although oral forms of this drug are available in Europe and Canada, as of this writing this combination is used only by intravenous injection in the United States. The distribution of the drug is adequate for skin and soft tissue infections as well as for systemic infections. The two components of the combination are extensively biotransformed and some of the metabolites are active.

ADVERSE REACTIONS AND CONTRAINDICATIONS

Local irritation at the injection site has been a common complaint with this drug combination. Muscle aches and a general feeling of malaise are also common. Chest pain, arrhythmias, or bloody diarrhea have occurred less often.

Patients with liver disease may be at increased risk with this combination. The drugs tend to elevate liver enzymes, suggesting that they may be hepatotoxic.

INTERACTIONS

Both the streptogramins in this fixed combination are active antibacterial drugs. The 70:30 ratio of quinupristin/dalfopristin has synergistic antibacterial action that justifies use of the combination.

DRUG CLASS • **Oxazolidinone**

linezolid (Zyvox)

MECHANISM OF ACTION

Linezolid, the only member of the oxazolidinone family yet approved, inhibits an early stage in the formation of the initiation complex in bacterial protein synthesis. Much of the drug action is thus on the 50S ribosomal subunit.

Resistance to linezolid is rare, but when it occurs it usually involves a ribosomal mutation that interferes with the binding of linezolid, as well as clindamycin and chloramphenicol, to bacterial ribosomes. This resistance has been noted in enterococci.

USES

The primary indication for linezolid is the treatment of serious infections caused by vancomycin-resistant *Enterococcus faecium*. Linezolid also has activity against other gram-positive pathogens but is generally reserved for use in very serious or life-threatening infections caused by methicillin-susceptible *Staphylococcus aureus* or *Streptococcus pyogenes*. Although the drug has been tested against methicillin-resistant *S. aureus*, it is not yet approved for that indication.

PHARMACOKINETICS

Linezolid is well absorbed orally, producing blood levels equivalent to those produced by intravenous administration. The concentration of drug in blood exceeds the MIC90 for staphylococci, enterococci, and streptococci.

The half-life is about 5 hours in normal adults. The drug is well distributed in the body and appears in breast milk.

Linezolid is biotransformed to two major metabolites, but 35% of a dose appears unchanged in urine. The metabolites are also primarily excreted in urine, but a small amount also appears in feces. In renal failure, the metabolites accumulate but their full toxicity has not been evaluated.

ADVERSE REACTIONS AND CONTRAINDICATIONS

The most common adverse reactions are nausea, headache, vomiting, and diarrhea, but thrombocytopenia has been noted in up to 13% of patients receiving linezolid. Antibiotic-associated pseudomembranous colitis has also been noted (Chapter 24).

Blood pressure should also be monitored in hypertensive patients.

INTERACTIONS

Linezolid is a reversible MAO inhibitor and may have additive effects with other MAO inhibitors such as phenelzine or tranylcypromine; the combination is usually avoided. Linezolid acts with sympathomimetic amines to increase blood pressure. Therefore the drug should not be used with pseudoephedrine, dopamine, epinephrine, or serotonin reuptake inhibitor antidepressants. Foods rich in tyramine should be avoided since they also have a sympathomimetic action (see Box 18-2).

 APPLICATION TO PRACTICE

ASSESSMENT

In the past, terms such as acute, chronic, and recurrent have been commonly used to describe the spectrum of UTIs. These words have been replaced by terminology considered more descriptive of the clinical presentation of a UTI (Box 30-1, Commonly Confused Terms). To enhance drug treatment, the current terminology for classifying UTIs must be understood.

The general aspects of nursing care for the patient receiving any antimicrobial drug were covered in Chapter 24. In this section, only those aspects related specifically to urinary antimicrobials are discussed since UTIs are very common.

History of Present Illness

Urinary frequency, urgency, and dysuria are classic symptoms of acute cystitis. Patients with these symptoms often describe an overwhelming urge to urinate more often than every 2 or 3 hours, and sometimes as frequently as every 15 to 30 minutes. The act of voiding is often associated with suprapubic discomfort or a burning sensation at the start of, during, or at the end of urination. The female patient may describe pain or burning along the entire length of the urethra, whereas the male patient may notice discomfort only in the distal urethra. Reports of fever, chills, a dull ache, or tenderness in the flank, or hematuria may suggest an upper UTI.

Development of a UTI, especially in women, is often related to sexual intercourse within the previous 24 to 48 hours. Careful questioning of the patient may reveal that on the day intercourse occurred, a hectic or unusual schedule caused her to take in fewer fluids and void much less frequently than would be customary. The patient also may report that the act of intercourse itself was more pro-

- *Acute urinary tract infection:* Symptomatic infection caused by a single pathogen. For most persons the occurrence will be their first documented urinary tract infection.
- *Unresolved bacteriuria:* The presence of bacteria in the urine after initial treatment for urinary tract infection is completed.
- *Bacterial persistence:* Recurrence of infection by the same organism several days after antimicrobial therapy has been discontinued and urine culture shows sterile urine.
- *Reinfection:* Recurrence of infection by a different pathogen after a previous infection has been eradicated. It is estimated that 80% to 95% of all recurrent infections are reinfections.
- *Uncomplicated urinary tract infection:* An afebrile infection, usually of the lower urinary tract, in a young, sexually active, nonpregnant, immunocompetent woman with no known structural abnormalities or urinary dysfunction.
- *Complicated urinary tract infection:* Infection occurring in patients who have structural or functional abnormalities of the urinary tract, or who have coexisting illness.

longed or repetitive than usual, and that voiding after intercourse was delayed until many hours afterward.

The health care provider should elicit a sexual history specifically focusing on a new sexual partner, a partner who has a penile discharge, or recent urethritis, mucoid vaginal discharge, or a gradual onset of symptoms. A recent history of chlamydial urethritis, gonorrhea, or exposure to these disorders should also be checked.

Health History

The health care provider should elicit information about the patient's normal voiding patterns (day and nighttime), the type, the amount of fluid typically consumed in a 24-hour period, and previous treatment for any urinary, gynecologic, or GI disorders. Determine also if the patient has a history of hepatic or renal impairment, because urinary tract antiseptics should be used with caution in these patients.

Determine if the patient has a history of blood dyscrasias, G6PD deficiency, or porphyria, since these disorders contraindicate the use of sulfonamides. Information about contraceptive use (specifically the diaphragm, spermicidal gel/foam, and condom), personal hygiene habits (frequency of tub baths, direction of wip-

ing after elimination), tampon use, and information about the type of undergarments usually worn should also be discussed. Elicit from the patient whether he or she is taking a thiazide diuretic, either alone or as a component of other drugs, since these may increase the risk of blood or skin reactions to sulfonamides.

The patient who has a reinfection of the lower urinary tract should be questioned about the length of time between this and the previous episode of acute infection and the number of infections treated within the last year. Detailed information should be obtained about previous drug therapy for UTIs including drug names, duration of treatment, and treatment efficacy. All patients should be questioned about known hypersensitivity or adverse reactions to urinary antimicrobials and related drugs. A thorough drug history is also important, since many drugs cause varying degrees of urinary retention or obstructive, irritative symptoms.

Lifespan Considerations

UTI or cystitis is a common health problem among all age groups. It is estimated that dysuria, urgency, and frequency characteristic of upper and lower UTIs account for more than 6 million patient visits to health care providers annually. It is a particular scourge among women of childbearing age.

Perinatal. UTIs frequently occur in the second trimester of pregnancy and are considered a common complication. Increasing levels of progesterone and an enlarging uterus induce physiologic changes in both the upper and lower portions of the urinary tract, creating an environment that favors the development of bacteriuria. The highest prevalence of UTIs is among women of lower socioeconomic groups who have a high parity, a history of UTI, and sickle cell disease or sickle cell trait.

Asymptomatic bacteriuria, defined as repeated recovery of greater than 10^5 CFU (colony-forming unit)/mL in voided urine, occurs in approximately 5% of pregnancies. Without prophylaxis, 25% to 40% of pregnant women with untreated asymptomatic bacteriuria will develop pyelonephritis. The risk of bacteriuria is greatest between the ninth and seventeenth weeks of gestation.

Untreated asymptomatic bacteriuria can result in preterm labor. Women with bacteriuria are also twice as likely to deliver a low-birth-weight infant. The relative risk of perinatal infant mortality is estimated to be 1 in 6. If a pregnant woman develops an acute UTI, especially one accompanied by a high fever, amniotic fluid infection may develop and retard the growth of the placenta.

Sulfonamides are often used but should be avoided, particularly late in the third trimester. These drugs tend to raise the level of free bilirubin in the serum, thus increasing the risk of kernicterus in the neonate. Sulfonamides should be avoided in infants younger than 1 month of age.

Pediatric. During the first 6 months of life, all healthy children are susceptible to UTIs. This is due in part to their immature immune systems and the intense bacterial colonization of the periurethral area in girls and the foreskin in boys. Uncircumcised infants seem to have significantly more UTIs than circumcised infants. By 4 months of age, UTIs are 10 times more common in girls than in boys. Beyond the newborn and infant periods, the prevalence of UTI in childhood and adolescence is less than 1%. However, the incidence of UTI in girls increases throughout childhood and extends into adulthood.

Children troubled by bacterial persistence or repeated reinfection are thought to have some pathophysiologic predisposition to UTIs. Additionally, congenital conditions such as vesicoureteral reflux, ureteropelvic junction obstruction, megaureter, and spina bifida contribute to the incidence of urinary infection in children. Other factors such as the use of bubble bath and constipation also have been suggested as contributing factors in the development of UTIs. Scientific evidence supporting these factors as causal is limited.

Older Adults. The incidence of asymptomatic bacteriuria is increased in older adults. Long-term use of an indwelling urinary catheter almost guarantees such a situation. Further, there is an increased incidence of bacteremia and death in these patients. Atypical presentations of UTI in older adults are common. Blunted fever response, anorexia, nausea, vomiting, and abdominal pain may be present. Confusion and changes in behavior also are common. Fever, chills, and flank pain in the older adult is considered a medical emergency because septicemia may develop.

Dosage amounts of all antimicrobial drugs may need to be decreased for the older adult because of age-related changes in the glomerular filtration rate. Colonization with Enterobacteriaceae occurs postmenopausally and is believed to account for much of the increased risk of UTI seen in this age group. Estrogen-deficient tissues are more susceptible to colonization by *E. coli*.

Cultural/Social Considerations

Because the onset of symptoms so closely coincides with sexual intercourse, young women with acute postcoital (honeymoon) UTIs are often embarrassed and may be reluctant to seek help. It is important that these patients understand that the development of a UTI is commonly associated with normal sexual activity and does not imply that the patient engaged in unusual or abnormal sexual acts (see the Case Study: Acute Urinary Tract Infection).

Physical Examination

Acute cystitis is unique in that there are no specific physical findings to distinguish the condition. An examination of the patient should begin with a determination of body temperature followed by percussion of the costovertebral angle (CVA) for tenderness. The health care provider may evoke pain or tenderness in the suprapubic region to deep palpation or percussion; however, the absence of such a response in no way rules out the diagnosis of an acute infection.

Patients who complain of dysuria without frequency or urgency, for example, may actually have vulvovaginitis or urethritis. Thus, a pelvic examination may be warranted in patients in whom the possibility of sexually transmitted diseases exists.

Laboratory Testing

A clean-catch, midstream urine specimen should be collected. Female patients may be catheterized to obtain a urine sample, but the clean voided specimen is preferred because it eliminates the risk of contaminating bladder urine with urethral bacteria. When assessing for the presence of bacteria in infants, paraplegics, and adult patients unable to produce a voided specimen, suprapubic bladder aspiration is considered a safe method for obtaining uncontaminated urine.

Nitrite testing for bacteriuria by dipstick has a sensitivity of greater than 90%, but the specificity is variable, ranging from 35% to 85%. Dipstick tests for leukocyte esterase activity as a marker for pyuria are more sensitive (72% to 97%) but less specific (64% to 82%). The finding of pyuria (more than 2 to 5 WBCs per high-power field on examination of spun sediment) is indicative of UTI and predictive of a positive response to antimicrobial therapy. The absence of pyuria suggests a vaginal cause for the symptoms. A urinalysis negative for bacteria does not necessarily mean that the patient is not experiencing an acute inflammation of the bladder any more than the presence of large numbers of microscopic bacteria is always a predictor of a positive urine culture.

Pyuria and hematuria are considered reliable indicators of UTI, especially when they are correlated with complaints of frequency, urgency, and dysuria. If there is no pyuria, the health care provider should question the diagnosis of a UTI until culture results prove otherwise. It is also important to remember that other diseases of the urinary tract can cause pyuria and hematuria without bacteriuria.

A urine culture is considered diagnostic when there are greater than 100,000 (10^5) colony-forming units (CFU) of a single pathogen per milliliter of urine. The urine culture should be considered contaminated when the growth of multiple organisms is reported. Contaminated urine usually contains fewer than 10,000 (10^4) CFU/mL. However, a count of 100 to 10,000 CFU/mL may be clinically significant, especially if a single known organism has been isolated and the patient is symptomatic, because frequent voiding slows the doubling or incubation time for bacteria in the urine.

For initial and infrequent lower UTIs, cultures are not needed as long as treatment is successful. If signs and symptoms persist after initial treatment, repeat urine cultures should be obtained to verify the sensitivity of the offending organism. Follow-up cultures are mandatory in children, pregnant patients with recurrent symptoms of upper UTIs, and patients who are at high risk for renal damage (even if they are asymptomatic) within 1 to 2 weeks of completion of treatment.

Urine collected for culture should be sent to the laboratory or refrigerated immediately. If promptly refrigerated, specimens can be cultured up to 24 hours after collection. Exposure to room temperature for longer than 1 hour after collection allows excessive multiplication of bacteria, contributing to inaccurate results.

Other diagnostic tests, imaging procedures, and cystoscopy are not indicated for patients with a first-time, uncomplicated, acute infection. However, patients with persistent bacteriuria or frequent episodes of reinfection require further assessment.

GOALS OF THERAPY

Treatment goals for all patients with a UTI focus on the prompt eradication of symptomatic infection, the identification and correction of predisposing factors, and the prevention of reinfection and of subsequent ascending progression of the disease to the kidneys.

INTERVENTION
Administration

Adequate fluid intake is extremely important for the patient taking a urinary antimicrobial drug; the patient with a UTI should consume 1.5 to 2 L of fluids daily. A higher fluid intake compromises the efficacy of the prescribed antimicrobial by making the urine too dilute. Water is preferred over other types of beverages, and in most instances a full glass of water should be consumed with each oral dose of the drug.

Drugs that should be taken with food include sulfonamides, methenamine, nitrofurantoin, and sulfonamides. Quinolone-like drugs should be taken at least 2 hours after meals or on an empty stomach. Cinoxacin and trimethoprim may be administered without regard to meal times.

Because most urinary antimicrobial drugs are excreted by the kidneys and have a higher concentration in urine than in serum, attention to renal function is required. Older adults and those with renal insufficiency require either reduced dosages or lengthened dosage intervals to avoid retaining the drug and developing nephrotoxicity.

Monitor for evidence of blood dyscrasias in older adults since sulfonamides may increase their risk of bone marrow depression. Inspect the patient's skin carefully for rash or purpura.

Education

First and foremost, patients should be taught about nondrug approaches that help keep the bladder healthy. Dark, concentrated urine suggests a need for better hydration. Box 30-2 identifies strategies that help to prevent UTIs.

BOX 30-2 **Strategies for Preventing Urinary Tract Infections**

- Make regular urination a habit (i.e., at 3- to 4-hour intervals); avoid long waits.
- Practice good hygiene, including wiping from front to back after urination and bowel movements. Take a shower rather than a bath. Avoid bubble bath, perfumed soap, feminine hygiene sprays, or products containing hexachlorophene.
- Increase fluid intake, especially water, to a minimum of six to eight glasses daily. Drink cranberry, blueberry, or prune juice or other foods and take vitamin C to help acidify the urine and relieve symptoms.
- Avoid bladder irritants such as caffeine, alcohol, and carbonated beverages and Alka-Seltzer and sodium bicarbonate, which alkalinizes the urine.
- Avoid prolonged bicycling, motorcycling, horseback riding, and traveling involving long periods of sitting, which can contribute to irritation of the urethral meatus.
- Be aware that vigorous or frequent sexual activity may contribute to urinary tract infection. Urinate before and after intercourse to empty the bladder and cleanse the urethra. Consider changing from a diaphragm and spermicide for birth control to another method if prone to UTIs.
- Do not ignore vaginal discharge or other signs of vaginal infection.
- Avoid wearing nylon pantyhose, tight slacks, or any clothing that traps perineal moisture and prevents evaporation.
- When an indwelling catheter is required, use the smallest size possible; maintain a closed sterile drainage system and unobstructed urine flow. Change the catheter every 4 to 6 weeks; reevaluate frequently the need for the catheter and remove as soon as feasible. Use Credé's maneuver to facilitate bladder emptying when appropriate.
- Menopausal women may consider estrogen replacement therapy since estrogen-deficient tissues are more susceptible to bacterial colonization.
- Complete prescribed drug regimens even though symptoms are diminished. Do not use drugs left over from previous infections.

Middle-aged and older adults are often fearful of being diagnosed with cancer and need to be reassured that there is no relationship between the classic symptoms of acute UTI and cancer. Help male patients to understand that an underlying condition, such as benign prostatic hyperplasia, may in fact be the cause for infection and that further assessment is required. Because the discomfort associated with an acute UTI resolves quickly once treatment begins, patients of all ages tend to discontinue treatment or engage in self-determined alternative dosing, disregarding information about the prevention of future infections.

Patients should be taught the importance of completing the entire course of treatment. Although shorter treatment regimens have significantly enhanced patient compliance, there is still a tendency to discontinue the drug once UTI symptoms have resolved. Emphasize to patients that the infection may persist and symptoms recur without strict adherence to the treatment regimen. To enhance compliance, explain to the patient or caregiver the premise underlying the action of all urinary antimicrobials, that is, the ability to achieve a therapeutic concentration in the urine.

Patients also should be taught about the potential adverse effects of the prescribed drugs. Signs and symptoms of a hypersensitivity reaction, particularly if a sulfonamide has been prescribed, should be provided along with suggested strategies for managing a hypersensitivity response.

CASE STUDY 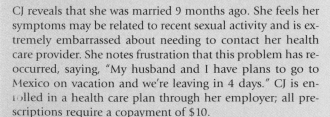 *Urinary Tract Infection*

ASSESSMENT

HISTORY OF PRESENT ILLNESS

CJ is a 25-year-old African-American woman who came to the primary care office with concerns about blood in her urine. She complains of burning when urinating, suprapubic discomfort, and the need to go to the bathroom every 30 to 60 minutes. She has had these symptoms for about 36 hours but they have intensified over the last 24 hours. CJ states she usually voids every 4 to 5 hours during the day, and rarely at night.

HEALTH HISTORY

CJ has had this problem twice before within the last 8 months. She was given antibiotics for both of these episodes. She denies having a history of hospitalizations, surgery, or major trauma. Diaphragm and spermicidal gel are used for contraception. She has no known drug allergies.

LIFESPAN CONSIDERATIONS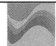

CJ works as a computer operator and describes her job as "very demanding."

CULTURAL/SOCIAL CONSIDERATIONS

CJ reveals that she was married 9 months ago. She feels her symptoms may be related to recent sexual activity and is extremely embarrassed about needing to contact her health care provider. She notes frustration that this problem has reoccurred, saying, "My husband and I have plans to go to Mexico on vacation and we're leaving in 4 days." CJ is enrolled in a health care plan through her employer; all prescriptions require a copayment of $10.

PHYSICAL EXAMINATION

CJ's temperature is 98.8° F, pulse 72, respirations 16, blood pressure 110/60 mm Hg. She weighs 110 pounds. There is palpable suprapubic tenderness but no CVA tenderness. CJ has been in the bathroom three times since arriving for her appointment.

LABORATORY TESTING

CJ's urine is cloudy and foul smelling with a pH of 5.0, a specific gravity 1.030, a small amount of blood, and a large amount of leukocyte esterase and nitrates. All other urinary components were within normal limits. Gram stain shows more than 100,000 colonies of gram-negative bacteria/mL of urine. Her urine was sent for culture and sensitivity testing.

PATIENT PROBLEM(S)

Acute urinary tract infection.

GOALS OF THERAPY

CJ's infection will resolve without sequelae.

CRITICAL THINKING QUESTIONS

1. The health care provider has ordered one tablet of double-strength sulfamethoxazole/trimethoprim (Bactrim DS) to be taken twice daily for 3 days. Why is this combination drug especially useful for treatment of CJ's acute UTI?
2. Is sulfamethoxazole/trimethoprim a bacteriocidal or bacteriostatic drug? Is it broad spectrum or narrow spectrum?
3. What common adverse effects of sulfamethoxazole/trimethoprim should be included in CJ's teaching?
4. Why has phenazopyridine been ordered for CJ in addition to the other two drugs? What common adverse effects of this drug should CJ be alerted about?
5. Before the patient leaves the office the nurse gives her an educational pamphlet with recommendations for preventing UTIs. What key points would you expect the nurse to cover with CJ?

Patients who require long-term suppressive or prophylactic therapy should be taught the importance of taking the drug just before going to bed. Urinary antimicrobial drugs used for this purpose are more effective when they reach peak urine concentration levels during the longest natural period of urinary retention (i.e., while the patient sleeps). Patients taking methenamine for suppressive therapy should be taught to monitor the pH of their urine to ensure the effectiveness of the drug.

Patients taking the urinary analgesic phenazopyridine should be advised that there will be a reddish orange discoloration to the urine and other body fluids, such as sweat and tears, and that it may stain clothing, bedding, and soft contact lenses. A sanitary napkin can be worn to avoid clothing stains. Eyeglasses should be substituted for soft contact lenses during the period that the drug is taken.

EVALUATION

Relief of irritative voiding symptoms, the absence of urine odor, and the return of urine to its characteristic clear, light yellow color provide strong evidence that a UTI has been effectively treated. Nonetheless, a follow-up urine culture should be performed to ensure that the urine has been rendered sterile. The ideal time to perform the "test of cure" culture is 4 to 7 days after the completion of drug therapy.

Urgency, frequency, and dysuria should disappear after 24 to 48 hours if the appropriate therapy has been instituted. If a patient experiences a relapse after a 3-day or 7- to 10-day antimicrobial course, treatment should be reinstituted for 2 weeks. If the patient experiences another relapse after 2 weeks, treatment should be extended for 6 weeks. If the patient experiences relapse after 6 weeks, treatment should continue for 6 months. Patients who continue to have recurrent infections should receive prophylactic therapy for an extended period; treatment lasting 1 to 2 years is not unusual.

Bibliography

Armstrong EP: Clinical and economic outcomes of an ambulatory urinary tract infection disease management program, *Am J Manag Care* 7(3):269-280, 2001.

Byers KE, Anglim AM, Anneski CJ, et al: A hospital epidemic of vancomycin-resistant *Enterococcus*: risk factors and control, *Infect Control Hosp Epidemiol* 22(3):140-147, 2001.

Cook DM: Clinical practice: iatrogenic illness: a primer for nurses, *Medsurg Nurs* 10(3):139-145, 2001.

Ferroni A, Nguyen L, Pron B, et al: Outbreak of nosocomial urinary tract infections due to *Pseudomonas aeruginosa* in a paediatric surgical unit associated with tap-water contamination, *J Hosp Infect* 39(4):301-307, 1998.

Goolsby MJ: Clinical practice guidelines: urinary tract infection, *J Am Acad Nurse Pract* 13(9):395-398, 2001.

Gupta K, Hooton TM, Roberts PL, et al: Patient-initiated treatment of uncomplicated recurrent urinary tract infections in young women, *Ann Intern Med* 135(1):9-16, 2001.

McFarland LV, Surawicz CM, Rubin M, et al: Recurrent *Clostridium difficile* disease: epidemiology and clinical characteristics, *Infect Control Hosp Epidemiol* 20(1):43-50, 1999.

Miller JM, Walton JC, Tordecilla LL: Advanced practice: recognizing and managing *Clostridium difficile*-associated diarrhea, *Medsurg Nurs* 7(6):348-349, 352-356, 1998.

Robert R, Grollier G, Doré P, et al: Nosocomial pneumonia with isolation of anaerobic bacteria in ICU patients: therapeutic considerations and outcome, *J Crit Care* 14(3):114-119, 1999.

Simpson L: Indwelling urethral catheters: reducing the risk of potential complications through proactive management, *Nursing Standard* 15(46):47-56, 2001.

Towers PM: CE forum: urinary tract infections, *J Am Acad Nurse Pract* 12(4):149-157, 2000.

Wallach FR: Infectious disease: update on treatment of pneumonia, influenza, and urinary tract infections, *Geriatrics* 56(9):43-48, 2001.

Yardy GW, Cox RA: An outbreak of *Pseudomonas aeruginosa* infection associated with contaminated urodynamic equipment, *J Hosp Infection* 47(1):60-63, 2001.

Internet Resources

http://www.ahealthyme.com/topic/topic100586425.
http://www.cdc.gov/ncidod/hip/guide/uritract.htm.
http://www.cdc.gov/ncidod/hip/NNIS/@nnis.htm.
http://www.cdc.gov/ncidod/hip/SURVEILL/SURVEILL.HTM.
http://www.merck.com/pubs/mmanual/section13/chapter157/157e.htm.
http://www.niddk.nih.gov/health/urolog/pubs/utiadult/utiadult.htm.
http://www.niddk.nih.gov/health/urolog/pubs/utichild/utichild.htm.
http://www.nlm.nih.gov/medlineplus/urinarytractinfections.html.

CHAPTER

31

Antiviral Drugs

SHERRY F. QUEENER • KATHLEEN GUTIERREZ

 Visit http://evolve.elsevier.com/Gutierrez/ for additional information.

KEY TERMS

Acquired immunodeficiency syndrome (AIDS), p. 461

Highly active antiretroviral therapy (HAART), p. 462

HIV protease, p. 460

Host specific, p. 470

Human Immunodeficiency virus (HIV), p. 459

Nonnucleoside RT inhibitors (NNRTIs), p. 465

Nucleoside RT inhibitors (NRTIs), p. 462

Nucleotide RT inhibitors (NtRTIs), p. 464

Opportunistic infections, p. 461

Postexposure chemoprophylaxis, p. 473

Reverse transcriptase (RT), p. 460

Viremia, p. 460

OBJECTIVES

- Explain the rationale for HAART.
- Explain why acyclovir is selectively active against virus-infected cells.
- Develop a nursing care plan for a patient receiving HAART therapy.
- Discuss the current thinking about HIV postexposure prophylaxis.

PATHOPHYSIOLOGY • Viral Infections

Viruses cause a wide variety of clinical diseases, both chronic and acute. Acute illnesses include the common cold, influenza, and hepatitis A. These illnesses often resolve quickly and leave no latent infections or sequelae. Chronic infections are those in which the disease runs a protracted course with long periods of remission interspersed with reappearance of the disease. For example, herpes infections involve active viral replication in ep-

ithelial cells alternating with latent periods during which the virus remains dormant within sensory neurons. Hepatitis B and hepatitis C, which cause progressive liver disease, and human immunodeficiency virus (HIV), which causes progressive destruction of the immune system, are also examples of chronic viral infections.

Viruses may target specific cells by interacting with unique receptors or cell surface markers. For example, in-

459

fluenza viruses affect only the tissues of the respiratory tract, interacting primarily with the ciliated epithelial cells. Both influenza type A and type B viruses have two distinctive glycoproteins (proteins chemically linked to carbohydrate molecules), neuraminidase and hemagglutinin, that show on their surfaces. Hemagglutinin binds to cells that have *N*-acetylneuraminic acid on their surfaces. Cells in the respiratory mucosa are normally protected by mucus, a secretion also rich in *N*-acetylneuraminic acid. Viruses that bind to this material do not penetrate to the surface of the cells and thus cannot begin to replicate. Influenza viruses overcome this defense mechanism by using their neuraminidase to break down the mucus, leaving the cell open to bind the virus.

Once a virus has bound to the surface of a specific host cell, the virus must genetically reengineer the host cell to make more viruses. As a first step, a virus must deliver its genetic material, either as RNA or DNA, into the host cell. The virus coat, necessary to protect the viral nucleic acid and to target the virus to an appropriate host cell, is shed as the nucleic acid enters the mammalian cell. The viral nucleic acid may either be incorporated into the host DNA or remain independent, but as a result of infection, the host cell begins to make more viral nucleic acid and proteins. These building blocks may be assembled into viruses that are then either shed from the surface of the cell or released upon cell death. In the example of influenza viruses, the targeted columnar epithelial cells form new viruses by budding them off from the cell surface. These cells only survive about 8 hours after virus budding starts. The death and sloughing off of these cells produce the pulmonary symptoms of influenza.

Influenza is a viral disease that remains localized, but not all viral diseases operate this way. Some viruses are shed into the blood in a process called **viremia,** during which tissues throughout the body may be invaded (Table 31-1). Clinical symptoms do not appear in most diseases spread in this manner until the secondary viremia occurs. Some viruses produce infections that are self-limiting at this stage and usually resolve even without medical attention (e.g., varicella [chicken pox] and measles). These viruses very rarely spread to the brain. A different situation exists with poliovirus, which produces few if any symptoms during the early stages of the infection, but in about 1% of infected persons, the virus invades the central nervous system (CNS), causing self-limiting aseptic meningitis or, rarely, paralytic poliomyelitis.

HIV is an example of a virus that attacks specific cells but produces a syndrome that affects the entire body. The initial target of HIV is any cell carrying the CD4 receptor, which includes the T helper lymphocytes, macrophages, monocytes, and follicular dendritic cells in lymph nodes. The CD4 and accessory receptors allow HIV to enter the cell and release the viral RNA (Figure 31-1). A viral enzyme called **reverse transcriptase (RT)** allows this single strand of RNA to be converted into a double strand of complementary DNA (cDNA) that is then integrated into the host genome by the viral enzyme called integrase. The presence of this cDNA copy of the virus within the host genome creates an essentially permanent state of infection. Virus copies will continue to be made under the direction of both host and viral elements, and if the cell should happen to divide, both daughter cells will carry the virus. Viruses released from host cells require maturation to be able to infect a new cell. The action of **HIV protease** is required for this step. This unique protease cuts long protein molecules into the

TABLE 31-1

Viremic Spread in the Mammalian Body

Site	Symptoms
Primary Site of Infection For example, lungs in pox, measles, or mumps; gastrointestinal tract in polio	First wave of replication produces no symptoms
Bloodstream Viruses free or bound to blood cells	Primary viremia produces no symptoms
Secondary Sites of Infection For example, liver, spleen, bone marrow, or lymphoid tissue	Second wave of replication may produce mild symptoms for some viral diseases
Bloodstream Viruses free or bound to blood cells	Secondary viremia may produce fever, rashes, or chills; severity depends on number of viruses released
Central Nervous System	Although rarely involved, infections at this site are serious

shorter forms that carry enyzmatic activity the virus needs for infecting a new cell.

The clinical course of HIV infection is complicated and prolonged. After a mild symptomatic phase following initial infection, the virus disappears from the blood and reproduces in lymphoid tissue but may not cause symptoms for years. Unless treated, however, HIV infection ultimately leads to the loss of CD4 T lymphocytes and failure of the immune system, a condition called **acquired immunodeficiency syndrome (AIDS)**. These patients experience **opportunistic infections**, which are infections caused by organisms that would be unlikely to cause disease in persons with normal immune systems.

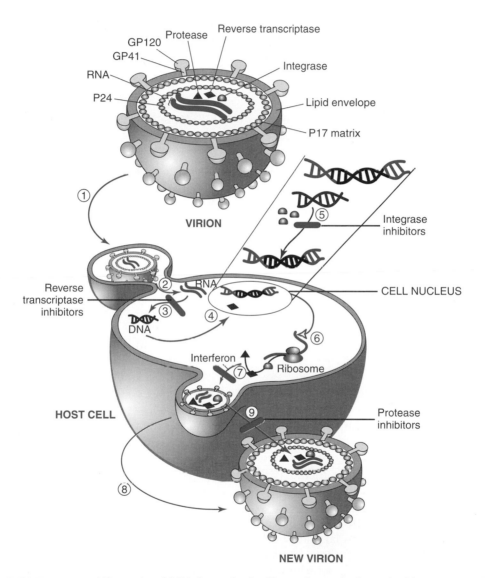

FIGURE 31-1 Life cycle of HIV. Steps in the life cycle are indicated with arrows and linked to the key below by numbers. The action of classes of inhibitors are shown by bars across the steps being blocked. *(1)* The virion (infectious virus particle) attaches and is injected into the host cell. *(2)* The virion uncoats, releasing two copies of viral RNA. *(3)* Reverse transcriptase converts single-stranded viral RNA to double-stranded DNA corresponding to viral genome. *(4)* Viral DNA migrates to host cell nucleus. *(5)* Viral integrase enzyme splices viral DNA into host cell DNA, creating provirus. *(6)* New viral RNA is formed by transcription and subsequent translation into viral protein precursors by host ribosomes. *(7)* Viral proteins are assembled to form immature virus. *(8)* Virus buds and is released. *(9)* Viral precursor protein is cleaved by HIV protease to form fully functional viral proteins, the final step in producing a fully infectious virion.

Therapy of any viral infection is aimed at arresting or delaying replication of the virus to preserve adequate numbers of the target cells. In the case of HIV, the goal is to allow CD4 cells to remain plentiful enough to fight infections. Currently used anti-HIV drugs inhibit either the viral protease or the RT enzyme, which are found in cells infected by retroviruses such as HIV but not in normal mammalian cells. Various other approaches, including blocking specific absorption of the virus to its target cells or attacking HIV integrase, are being explored. The status of these investigational drugs changes quickly. Current information can be obtained by consulting the AIDS sec-

tion at the National Institutes of Health or by consulting current publications devoted to AIDS research.

Control of HIV infection depends on using the available drug classes in combinations, because no single class of drug is effective alone at controlling the disease. Combinations allow better control of adverse effects and, more importantly, help control the development of resistance, which happens quickly if monotherapy is used. The various combinations used for HIV are collectively called **highly active antiretroviral therapy (HAART)** (see the Interventions section later in the chapter).

DRUG CLASS • Nucleoside Reverse Transcriptase Inhibitors (NRTIs) for HIV

abacavir sulfate (Ziagen)

abacavir sulfate + lamivudine + zidovudine (Trizivir)

didanosine or ddI (Videx)

lamivudine or 3TC (Epivir)

lamivudine + zidovudine (Combivir)

stavudine or d4T (Zerit)

zalcitabine or ddC (HIVID)

 zidovudine or AZT (Apo-Zidovudine, Novo-AZT,✶ Retrovir)

MECHANISM OF ACTION

HIV is a retrovirus. Retroviruses use RNA as their genetic material and must therefore convert RNA into DNA within the host cell for viral replication to take place. This unusual process, which does not normally occur in human cells, is catalyzed by the viral enzyme reverse transcriptase (RT). Zidovudine and other members of this class inhibit RT because the drugs are analogs of natural nucleosides; thus this class is referred to as **nucleoside RT inhibitors (NRTIs)**. To be effective inhibitors, NRTIs must be activated by three sequential phosphorylation reactions within cells. The triphosphate forms of the drugs are competitive inhibitors of RT, which means the inhibition is lost as soon as drug levels fall. The fully phosphorylated NRTI not only inhibits RT but also may be incorporated into viral DNA, where it causes premature DNA chain termination. Both actions block viral replication, and these drugs are effective only against replicating viruses. Zidovudine and other members of this class do not cure HIV infection or AIDS, but by slowing the replication of HIV, NRTIs may delay damage to the immune system and lower the incidence of opportunistic infections in these patients.

Resistance to zidovudine or any other member of this class occurs readily if the drug is used alone against HIV. Therefore NRTIs are most commonly combined with at least one other drug or used in HAART.

USES

Zidovudine is a primary drug used to treat HIV infections. It may be used in asymptomatic patients to delay the decline in T cell counts, as well as in patients with more advanced forms of the disease. Zidovudine has been used in HIV-infected children as well. The drug is also effective in lowering the incidence of transmission of HIV from an infected mother to her fetus.

Abacavir is used only in combination with other antiviral drugs for HIV infections. Didanosine is currently used primarily as a substitute for zidovudine in patients who have failed therapy or become intolerant of zidovudine. Lamivudine is used against HIV only in combination with zidovudine or another RT inhibitor, primarily to slow the development of resistance. Lamivudine has also been approved for use against hepatitis B infections. Stavudine is used for advanced HIV disease in patients who already received zidovudine for prolonged periods and can no longer benefit from it. Stavudine is not used as often as other NRTIs. Zalcitabine is used in advanced HIV disease in combination with zidovudine or protease inhibitors.

PHARMACOKINETICS

Absorption of zidovudine from the gastrointestinal (GI) tract is rapid and nearly complete, but the drug is quickly biotransformed to an inactive glucuronide on the first pass through the liver. These factors give zidovudine a half-life of only about 1 hour. This short half-life and the fact that the primary effect of zidovudine is competitive inhibition of RT means that, if used alone, zidovudine must be taken every 4 hours around the clock to maintain virustatic concentrations. When used in combinations, the dosage frequency of zidovudine may be extended to every 8 hours.

Other NRTIs have better bioavailability than zidovudine and persist longer in serum and within cells (Table 31-2). The only member of this class with worse bioavailability than zidovudine is didanosine. Didanosine has a poor bioavailability in most patients because it is destroyed by stomach acid. Current formulations include buffers to improve absorption by reducing acidity and preserving the integrity of the drug. The optimal dosing frequency for didanosine is twice daily.

ADVERSE REACTIONS AND CONTRAINDICATIONS

Nearly all patients experience adverse reactions from NRTIs. Several serious reactions become more likely the longer these drugs are used and may relate to the toxic effects the drugs have on mitochondria. NRTIs are known to contribute to fat loss, primarily in the arms and legs. This fat redistribution is a feature of lipodystrophy syndrome, which is common in patients with AIDS who are undergoing long-term treatment for HIV infections. Other serious long-term effects of NRTIs that may be related to mitochondrial toxicity are lactic acidosis and hepatotoxicity, including hepatic steatosis. Pa-

tients must be watched for signs of increasing liver size and an elevation of the serum lactic acid level so that the drugs may be halted before fatal lactic acidosis occurs.

Zidovudine, like all other NRTIs, can cause fat redistribution, lactic acidosis, and hepatotoxicity with long term use, but the most common reactions to this drug are granulocytopenia and anemia, which typically appear 4 to 6 weeks after therapy starts. Routine blood monitoring is extremely important. A drug holiday from zidovudine may be necessary to allow recovery from drug-induced blood dyscrasias. Didanosine, lamivudine, and stavudine rarely cause anemia.

Peripheral neuropathy is the most common serious adverse effect with didanosine, stavudine, and zalcitabine. Up to 31% of adult patients with AIDS who are receiving zalcitabine experience this adverse effect. Signs include tingling or aching in the legs or feet and diminished reflexes. Some of the effects may be reversed if the drug is stopped quickly. Peripheral neuropathy is more common with higher dosages or with patients in whom the drug accumulates.

Neurotoxicity associated with zidovudine is more likely to cause CNS effects, such as anxiety, headache, irritability, and sleeplessness. Didanosine may also cause these symptoms.

Pancreatitis is a rare adverse effect with most NRTIs but it is more common with didanosine and lamivudine. This disorder develops in 5% to 13% of adults

TABLE 31-2

Pharmacokinetics of Inhibitors of HIV Reverse Transcriptase

Drug	Bioavailability (%)*	Serum Half-Life (hours)	Intracellular Half-Life (hours)	Biotransformation†
Nucleosides				
abacavir	83	0.9-2.1	Not available	Extensive
didanosine	33-37	0.8-2.7	8-24	Extensive
lamivudine	80-88	2-11	11-15	Minimal
stavudine	78-86	1-1.6	3.5	Moderate
zalcitabine	>80	1-3	2.6-10	Minimal
zidovudine	52-75	0.8-1.2	3.3	Extensive
Nucleotide				
tenofovir	25 (fasting) 40 (with food)	12-18	15-50 (resting cells) 10 (dividing cells)	Minimal
Nonnucleosides				
delavirdine	<85	2-11	Not available	Extensive
efavirenz	Not available	40-55	Not available	Extensive
nevirapine	91-93	25-30	Not available	Extensive

* In adults; bioavailability in children tends to be lower.
†Excludes metabolic activation (phosphorylation) required for activity of nucleosides and nucleotide.

treated with didanosine and 14% to 15% of children treated with lamivudine. The signs of the reaction include strong abdominal pain often accompanied by nausea or vomiting. In adults the fatality rate of this adverse reaction is approximately 1 in 300 patients.

Hypersensitivity with fever or skin rash has occurred with abacavir and stavudine. More severe hypersensitivity reactions, including muscle pain, shortness of breath, redness or swelling of the eyes, malaise, and stomach or abdominal distress, occur in 5% of patients receiving abacavir. This reaction may progress to multiorgan failure and death unless abacavir is discontinued.

A hypersensitivity reaction to abacavir is a contraindication for receiving the drug again. There are no absolute contraindications to the use of other NRTIs, but there are specific precautions for individual drugs. Patients with bone marrow depression may be at greater risk for anemia or other blood disorders if they take zidovudine. These patients should be monitored carefully. Patients with hepatic impairment may also be prone to increased risk of drug toxicity. Patients with preexisting peripheral neuropathy or renal function impairment may require lower dosages of didanosine, lamivudine, or stavudine. Patients with peripheral neuropathy should not be given zalcitabine. A history of pancreatitis increases the risk of that reaction with zalcitabine, lamivudine, or didanosine.

TOXICITY

A few patients have taken large overdoses of zidovudine, either by accident or in deliberate suicide attempts. Signs of overdose include anemia, ataxia, fatigue, leukopenia, severe nausea, nystagmus, thrombocytopenia, and vomiting. Seizures are rare. Treatment is supportive only.

INTERACTIONS

Drug interactions may occur with zidovudine and other drugs often used in patients who are immunosuppressed. Ganciclovir and zidovudine combine to produce severe hematologic toxicity. Other bone marrow depressants, including interferon alfa, may also increase zidovudine toxicity. Ribavirin interferes with activation of zidovudine within a virus-infected cell and thereby blocks its anti-HIV effect. Clarithromycin lowers the peak concentration of zidovudine in the blood, which may interfere with anti-HIV activity. Probenecid increases the concentration of zidovudine in the blood and slows its elimination, which increases the risk of toxicity.

Abacavir is partly biotransformed by alcohol dehydrogenase. Thus ethanol can interfere with the biotransformation of abacavir and lengthen the half-life of the antiviral drug.

The buffers in didanosine preparations impair absorption of dapsone, itraconazole, and ketoconazole. Fluoroquinolone and tetracycline antibiotics are chelated by components of the buffering system in didanosine, decreasing absorption of the antibiotics. Didanosine also increases the risk of pancreatitis if given with other drugs that cause this reaction (see Appendix B).

Didanosine, stavudine, and zalcitabine should be avoided by patients also receiving other drugs that cause peripheral neuropathy (see Appendix B).

Zalcitabine should also be avoided, if possible, in combination with other drugs that cause pancreatitis (see Appendix B). Aminoglycosides, amphotericin B, and foscarnet block renal excretion of zalcitabine, thus increasing the risk of toxicity. Antacids block absorption of this drug.

DRUG CLASS • Nucleotide Reverse Transcriptase Inhibitors (NtRTIs) for HIV

tenofovir disoproxil fumarate (Viread, PMPA)

MECHANISM OF ACTION

Nucleoside RT inhibitors, such as zidovudine, require three steps to convert them from a nucleoside to the active triphosphate form. Nucleotide RT inhibitors (NtRTIs), however, have taken one step down the road to activation because they resemble a nucleotide monophosphate and thus require only two further phosphorylations to become fully activated (Box 31-1). These steps are often easier and more rapid than the initial formation of a monophosphate. Thus NtRTIs should in theory be more easily activated in vivo than NRTIs.

USES

Tenofovir is a new drug that has not yet been fully evaluated for all possible uses in treating AIDS. The clinical trials leading to its approval combined tenofovir with several anti-HIV drug classes. These studies suggested that tenofovir contributed to the effectiveness of the combinations and that combinations including tenofovir were adequately tolerated.

PHARMACOKINETICS

Tenofovir disoproxil fumarate is administered orally and is best absorbed if taken with food; fat is helpful in increasing the amount of the drug absorbed (see

---

| BOX **31-1** | **Differences Between a Nucleoside and a Nucleotide** |

DNA contains four different bases that allow genes to carry genetic information: adenine, cytosine, guanine, and thymine. RNA is the same, except uracil is substituted for thymine. To put these bases into long continuous molecules, they must first be linked to a sugar, which is ribose for RNA and deoxyribose for DNA. When the base is linked to a sugar, it is called a nucleoside. Energy is required for the second step in linking these building blocks into DNA or RNA. The cell supplies this energy by adding phosphate groups, three of which are required for full activation. When the first phosphate group is added, the nucleoside becomes a nucleotide.

| | | Nucleotides | | |
Bases	Nucleosides	Monophosphate	Diphosphate	Triphosphate
Adenine (A)	A-ribose	AMP	ADP	ATP
	A-deoxyribose	dAMP	dAMP	dATP
Cytosine (C)	C-ribose	CMP	CDP	CTP
	C-deoxyribose	dCMP	dCDP	dCTP
Guanine (G)	G-ribose	GMP	GDP	GTP
	G-deoxyribose	dGMP	dGDP	dGTP
Thymine (T)	T-ribose	TMP	TDP	TTP
	T-deoxyribose	dTMP	dTDP	dTTP
Uracil (U)	U-ribose	UMP	UDP	UTP
	U-deoxyribose	dUMP	dUDP	dUTP

Table 31-2). Once absorbed, the preparation is rapidly converted to tenofovir, which is the nucleotide analog. Tenofovir penetrates cells and is phosphorylated to its active form. Tenofovir disoproxil fumarate is biotransformed by the kidneys, but there is little biotransformation in the liver.

ADVERSE REACTIONS AND CONTRAINDICATIONS

The most common adverse reactions to tenofovir are gastrointestinal and include diarrhea, flatulence, nausea, or vomiting. Animal studies have suggested a concern with bone damage, but human studies have not yet been reported to confirm or refute the occurrence of this adverse reaction.

Tenofovir is currently contraindicated in pregnancy.

INTERACTIONS

Tenofovir has been in use too short a time to allow a full assessment of possible interactions. One interaction that has been suggested is with didanosine because tenofovir increases this drug's blood level, which may in turn increase the risk of potentially fatal pancreatitis.

DRUG CLASS • Nonnucleoside Reverse Transcriptase Inhibitors (NNRTIs) for HIV

delavirdine mesylate (Rescriptor)

efavirenz (Sustiva)

nevirapine (Viramune)

MECHANISM OF ACTION

Unlike nucleoside or nucleotide RT inhibitors, the non-nucleoside RT inhibitors (NNRTIs) do not require activation. These drugs are not competitive inhibitors of HIV RT and bind at a different site than that occupied by nucleoside or nucleotide RT inhibitors. Because the mechanism of action is different, NNRTIs can have additive or synergistic effects when used in combination with nucleoside or nucleotide RT inhibitors as well as with protease inhibitors.

USES

The NNRTIs should not be used alone because of the rapid development of resistance. Thus they are recommended in combination with at least two other anti-HIV drugs, which may include NRTIs and protease inhibitors.

PHARMACOKINETICS

NNRTIs are adequately absorbed when given orally and may be taken with or without food. All drugs in this group are extensively biotransformed by the CYP3A enzymes in the liver. The metabolites are excreted to variable degrees in feces and urine (see Table 31-2).

ADVERSE REACTIONS AND CONTRAINDICATIONS

The most common adverse reactions to NNRTIs include skin rashes, which occur in 12% to 46% of patients. Severe rashes may indicate a serious reaction and should be reported to the health care provider. NNRTIs also commonly cause diarrhea, headache, and nausea. Efavirenz is also often linked to CNS effects leading to bizarre dreams, dizziness, and sleep disorders. Aggression, depression, paranoia, and suicidal thoughts are also linked to efavirenz but occur in fewer than 2% of patients.

NNRTIs may accumulate when liver function is impaired. Thus these drugs may be used cautiously in patients with mild liver dysfunction but should be avoided if possible in those with moderate to severe liver dysfunction.

INTERACTIONS

NNRTIs inhibit liver enzymes in the CYP3A family, thereby possibly elevating blood levels of drugs normally biotransformed by those enzymes. Drugs to avoid include benzodiazepines, calcium-channel blockers, cisapride, and indinavir.

BOX 31-2 **Efavirenz and St. John's Wort**

St. John's wort consists of the dried flowering tops of *Hypericum perforatum*. The active ingredient is usually believed to be hypericin, but many other chemicals are also present and may contribute to various activities. Extracts of the herb are commonly used for its purported effects on the CNS (see Chapters 8 and 18), which may include reversal of symptoms of mild or moderate depression. In addition to its desired effects, the extracts may also induce CYP3A4, a powerful liver enzyme capable of inactivating efavirenz as well as other drugs. As a result of this effect, the antiviral action of efavirenz may be lost. Patients taking efavirenz should be warned to avoid herbal, vitamin, or food supplement preparations that contain St. John's wort.

Carbamazepine, phenobarbital, and phenytoin reduce the concentration of delavirdine in the blood; therefore these drugs should not be used together. Cimetidine and related drugs lower gastric pH and thus reduce absorption of delavirdine. Both rifabutin and rifampin decrease the absorption of delavirdine, whereas clarithromycin increases it.

Nevirapine lowers the blood levels of estrogens, HIV protease inhibitors, and ketoconazole such that clinical effectiveness may be lost.

Efavirenz interacts with a common herbal preparation, St. John's wort (Box 31-2).

DRUG CLASS • HIV Protease Inhibitors

amprenavir (Agenerase)

indinavir sulfate (Crixivan)

lopinavir + ritonavir (Kaletra)

nelfinavir mesylate (Viracept)

ritonavir (Norvir)

saquinavir (Fortovase)

saquinavir mesylate (Invirase)

MECHANISM OF ACTION

Protease inhibitors bind to the active site of HIV protease, preventing the natural substrate from binding. As a result, the protease fails to separate the HIV precursor protein into the active enzymes the virus needs to mature fully. Thus immature, noninfective viruses are produced. Protease inhibitors act only during viral replication.

Resistance to protease inhibitors develops readily and by several different mutations of the HIV protease. For this reason, these drugs should not be used alone.

USES

Protease inhibitors are used only for HIV infections, usually in combination with NRTIs or in other combinations for HAART.

PHARMACOKINETICS

Protease inhibitors have variable oral absorption, and absolute bioavailability has yet to be measured for some members of the class. It is known that heavy foods can significantly impair absorption of amprenavir and indinavir sulfate, but food increases absorption of other protease inhibitors. Oral bioavailability of saquinavir depends on the formulation used. The original saquinavir mesylate capsules yielded only about 4% bioavailability as a result of poor absorption and an active first-pass effect (see Chapter 1). The newer formulation is a soft gelatin capsule that more than triples absorption, but the total bioavailability is still low.

Serum half-lives vary from short (indinavir, 1.8 hours) to long (saquinavir, 7 to 12 hours; amprenavir, 7 to 11 hours). All protease inhibitors are extensively biotransformed by liver enzymes, particularly CYP3A4. Most of the metabolites are eliminated in feces; only a limited amount is found in urine. Little of the active drug is excreted.

ADVERSE REACTIONS AND CONTRAINDICATIONS

The most common adverse reactions to protease inhibitors are GI disturbances including abdominal pain, diarrhea, nausea, and vomiting. Weakness is also a common complaint. Less common adverse reactions include diabetes or ketoacidosis. Paresthesia (numbness or tingling) has also been noted with retonavir, saquinavir, and amprenavir. Kidney stones occur in about 4% of patients receiving indinavir.

Nelfinavir should be avoided by patients with impaired liver function, and all other protease inhibitors are used with great caution because the liver is the primary route for elimination of these drugs. They may accumulate in patients with impaired liver function, leading to an increase in dangerous adverse reactions.

TOXICITY

Long-term use of dosages higher than 2.4 g daily is associated with a higher risk of developing kidney stones. The effects of very large doses of ritonavir have not been documented, but doses of 1.5 g for 2 days in one patient produced paresthesia that resolved when the drug was stopped. No evidence of toxicity has been documented with overdoses of other protease inhibitors, but charcoal may be used with emesis or gastric lavage to reduce absorption of the drug as a general precaution.

INTERACTIONS

Protease inhibitors may compete for the liver enzyme CYP3A4 and thus interfere with the biotransformation of other drugs normally acted on by CYP3A4. Examples of drugs that might accumulate to dangerous levels include cisapride, clozapine, HMG-CoA reductase inhibitors (see Chapter 42), loratadine, midazolam, pimozide, rifabutin, quinidine, sildenafil, triazolam, tricyclic antidepressants, and warfarin.

Other drugs may induce CYP3A4 and increase the biotransformation of protease inhibitors, which reduces serum concentrations of the antiviral drugs below effective levels. Examples of such drugs include carbamazepine, phenobarbital, phenytoin, and rifampin.

Protease inhibitors may reduce the serum concentration of oral contraceptives, increasing the risk of unwanted pregnancy. Alternative, nondrug forms of contraception should be employed.

Some interactions occur only with one protease inhibitor rather than the entire class. For example, ketoconazole more than doubles the serum level of indinavir, and if the drugs must be used together, the dose of indinavir must be reduced. Indinavir must not be given at the same time as didanosine, because indinavir requires an acid environment for best absorption, but didanosine is given with buffers to elevate gastric pH. If both drugs are being used for the same patient, the doses should be given at least 1 hour apart on an empty stomach.

Delavirdine, indinavir, nelfinavir, and ritonavir can greatly increase the blood level of saquinavir. Dosage adjustments may be required.

DRUG CLASS • Acyclic Nucleoside Analogs for Systemic Viral Diseases Other than AIDS

⚠ acyclovir (generic, Zovirax)

famciclovir (Famvir)

valacyclovir (Valtrex)

MECHANISM OF ACTION

Acyclovir and related acyclic nucleoside analogs are among the most highly selective of the antiviral drugs. These drugs are activated by viral thymidine kinase, an enzyme found only in virus-infected cells. The activated form of the drug preferentially inhibits the viral DNA polymerase present in infected cells, thereby effectively halting virus production. These drugs may also be incorporated into viral DNA, which immediately stops further synthesis of the chain. A much higher concentration is required to halt normal human cell metabolism. Therefore effective doses for antiviral activity are relatively nontoxic to normal host cells.

USES

Acyclovir is used to treat initial lesions or recurrences of genital herpes, mucocutaneous herpes simplex infections either in immunocompromised or immunocompetent patients, herpes simplex encephalitis, and herpes zoster infections (shingles). Acyclovir can also be used for varicella (chicken pox) if started within 24 hours of the appearance of the rash, but this use is usually restricted to patients with special risk factors.

Famciclovir is used for herpes zoster infection in immunocompetent adults or for recurrent episodes of genital herpes. Valacyclovir is used for initial or recurrent episodes of genital herpes or for herpes zoster infections. Penciclovir, a relative of acyclovir, is used as a topical agent for herpetic infections.

PHARMACOKINETICS

Acyclovir sodium is given intravenously. Oral administration of acyclovir leads to incomplete absorption, but this route is effective when used for mild to moderate genital herpes. Topical preparations may be useful in mild herpes infections (see Chapter 67), but parenteral routes are more effective and usually preferred.

Valacyclovir is a oral prodrug form that is rapidly converted to acyclovir in the body. Once absorbed, acyclovir is widely distributed to tissues. Famciclovir is also a prodrug, but the active agent released in the body is penciclovir. This active agent has a mechanism of action similar to acyclovir but persists longer inside virus-infected cells. The half-life of penciclovir within virus-infected cells ranges from 7 to 20 hours, depending on the type of virus present.

Excretion of these drugs is almost entirely by renal mechanisms. Serum half-lives of the prodrugs are very short, as they are rapidly converted to the active drug forms. The active drugs have serum half-lives ranging from 2 to 3 hours in patients with normal renal func-

tion, but the half-life is increased in those with renal failure.

ADVERSE REACTIONS AND CONTRAINDICATIONS

Acyclovir generally causes few adverse reactions. Phlebitis at the injection site may occur with intravenous acyclovir sodium. Rarely, patients receiving parenteral acyclovir may experience confusion, seizures, or tremors, or even fall into coma. Light-headedness, GI disturbances, and malaise are more common.

Famciclovir may cause any of the same adverse reactions as oral acyclovir, but they are less common with famciclovir. Valacyclovir is more likely to cause dysmenorrhea as well as headache and GI disturbances.

None of the acyclic nucleoside analogs should be given at full dosage to patients with renal impairment or to dehydrated patients.

When used at a high dosage for a prolonged period in patients with impaired immune systems, valacyclovir has been associated with a potentially life-threatening condition called thrombotic thrombocytopenic purpura/hemolytic uremic syndrome. Thus patients receiving organ transplants and those with HIV infections should not receive valacyclovir.

TOXICITY

Neuropsychiatric reactions and nephrotoxicity are more common with a high dosage of acyclovir or in patients who accumulate the drug because of poor renal function. Nephrotoxicity, including crystallization of the drug in the renal tubule, can be minimized by giving the drug as a slow infusion rather than as a rapid bolus. Increasing water intake also helps.

INTERACTIONS

Because of the potential for nephrotoxicity, acyclovir should not be given with other nephrotoxic drugs.

DRUG CLASS • Neuraminidase Inhibitors for Influenza

oseltamivir (Tamiflu)
zanamivir (Relenza)

MECHANISM OF ACTION

Neuraminidase inhibitors block one of the key proteins exposed on the surface of influenza viruses (see earlier section on pathophysiology). The main effect of the two drugs currently available may be to alter aggregation of virus particles and their proper release from infected cells. As a result, the viral infection does not spread readily to surrounding cells.

USES

Neuraminidase inhibitors are used only for infections caused by influenza A or B and must be started within 2 days of the onset of symptoms. The clinical effect of these drugs is to reduce the duration of acute illness by about 36 hours. They do not cure influenza nor do they prevent a treated patient from spreading the virus.

PHARMACOKINETICS

Oseltamivir phosphate is rapidly absorbed when given orally. The drug is activated by esterase enzymes to oseltamivir carboxylate. These esterases are located in the liver but are not related to the CYP drug-converting enzymes (see Chapter 1). Oseltamivir is not further biotransformed and is excreted primarily in the urine.

Zanamivir is administered as a dry powder by inhalation. Less than 20% of the inhaled dose is absorbed systemically. The small amount of drug that is absorbed is excreted unchanged in urine.

ADVERSE REACTIONS AND CONTRAINDICATIONS

Because of the low degree of systemic absorption, zanamivir causes few adverse reactions other than those specific to the lung. The most serious reaction includes bronchospasm or other pulmonary symptoms such as wheezing. Allergic reactions, including swelling of the mouth and throat, have also been noted. All of these reactions require immediate medical attention.

Oseltamivir has been most commonly associated with adverse reactions such as nausea and vomiting, which occurred about twice as often in drug-treated patients as it did in those treated with a placebo.

INTERACTIONS

Neither oseltamivir nor zanamivir have been associated with significant drug interactions.

 DRUG CLASS • **Amantidines for Influenza**

amantadine (Endantadine,✴ Gen-Amantadine,✴ Symmetrel)

rimantadine (Flumadine)

MECHANISM OF ACTION

Amantadine and rimantadine block early phases of viral replication, but the exact mechanism is unclear. They are thought to block uncoating of the virus, which prevents release of viral nucleic acid into the host cell. These drugs are effective only against influenza type A.

USES

Amantadine is effective in preventing influenza caused by the type A virus. Prophylaxis is usually limited, however, to older adults or others in whom influenza is likely to lead to life-threatening complications. If used within 24 hours of the onset of symptoms, this drug may be helpful. Amantadine has also been used to treat parkinsonism (see Chapter 23).

Rimantadine is used only for prophylaxis of influenza type A.

PHARMACOKINETICS

Amantadine is well absorbed orally and distributes well to various tissues. The drug concentration in lung tissue may exceed its concentration in serum. The concentration of amantadine that reaches the epithelial surfaces of lung tissues is the determining factor in protecting against influenza type A infections. Nearly all elimination of the drug is carried out by renal mechanisms. The half-life for elimination is about 15 hours in patients with normal renal function, 24 to 29 hours in older adults, and 7 to 10 days in renally impaired patients.

Rimantadine is well absorbed orally but unlike amantadine is extensively biotransformed in the liver. Metabolites are eliminated in urine. The half-life of the drug ranges from 13 to 38 hours. In general, older adults or those with liver impairment eliminate the drug more slowly.

ADVERSE REACTIONS AND CONTRAINDICATIONS

Anorexia and nausea are common adverse effects with amantadine. Anticholinergic effects, including constipation, dry mouth, blurred vision, difficulty in urination, and CNS signs, may also be seen. Because of these effects, the drug should be used cautiously if at all in an older adult with cerebral arteriosclerosis or in any patient with a history of epilepsy.

Adverse effects are more common when amantadine is used for parkinsonism because the dosages are about twice that given for influenza prophylaxis (see Chapter 23).

Rimantadine causes CNS effects less often than amantadine, but headache, insomnia, and fatigue are possible. Anorexia, dry mouth, nausea, and vomiting may also occur.

A patient with a history of seizures may be at risk of increased frequency of seizures with rimantadine. The patients with reduced hepatic function will require a reduced dosage of rimantadine to compensate for slower drug elimination.

TOXICITY

Overdose with amantadine may produce signs of CNS and cardiopulmonary toxicity, such as cardiac arrhythmia, pulmonary edema, toxic psychosis, or convulsions. A single 2-g dose of amantadine has resulted in death.

INTERACTIONS

Alcohol consumption increases the risk of seizure activity with amantadine. Anticholinergic drugs may be dangerously potentiated by the anticholinergic action of amantadine. CNS stimulants and amantadine increase the risk of CNS irritability or seizures. Rimantadine lacks the CNS activity of amantadine, however, and thus is less likely to cause these interactions.

DRUG CLASS • Nucleoside Analog for Systemic Viral Diseases

ribavirin (Rebetol, Virazole)

Ribavirin is a synthetic purine nucleoside that interferes with multiple steps leading to synthesis of nucleic acids in several types of viruses. In the United States, ribavirin is prescribed only for therapy of severe respiratory syncytial virus (RSV) in children, but in other parts of the world, the drug has been used to treat various virus-induced hemorrhagic fevers, including Lassa fever.

Ribavirin is administered as an aerosol to treat respiratory viruses. This way the drug level in the lungs is maximized, but systemic absorption is low, minimizing adverse effects.

Skin rashes can occur with this drug. Health care workers exposed to the drug during administration can experience headaches and eye irritation. Oral or intravenous administration of ribavirin often causes anemia and may cause CNS or GI effects. Little systemic toxicity occurs when ribavirin is given by inhalation.

Because ribavirin blocks phosphorylation of nucleosides, it interferes with activation of zidovudine and therefore should not be given to a patient receiving zidovudine.

DRUG CLASS • Alfa Interferons for Systemic Viral Diseases

interferon alfa-2b, recombinant (Intron A)
interferon alfa-n1l (LNS) (Wellferon)
interferon alfa-n3 (Alferon A)

MECHANISM OF ACTION

Interferons inhibit virus replication in infected cells and in general inhibit cell proliferation (see Chapter 37). They are produced by mammals as part of an immune response. Interferons are host specific and not virus specific, meaning that they induce resistance to several types of viruses at once. However, only human interferons prevent viral disease in humans. Human interferons are produced as drugs by recombinant DNA technology or are harvested from pooled human leukocytes (interferon alfa-n3).

USES

Interferons alfa-2b and alfa-n1 are used to treat active or chronic hepatitis C. Interferon alfa-2b is also used to treat chronic hepatitis B infections. Interferons alfa-2b, alfa-n1, and alfa-n3 may be used by intralesional injection to treat genital warts, which are induced by *Papillo-* *mavirus.* These interferons and others are also used to treat certain cancers (see Chapter 37).

PHARMACOKINETICS

Interferons are proteins that must be administered parenterally. Uptake is good from intramuscular or subcutaneous injection sites.

ADVERSE REACTIONS AND CONTRAINDICATIONS

Adverse reactions are more common when interferons are used systemically to treat hepatitis than when used locally for genital warts. Possible reactions include anorexia, blood dyscrasias (anemia, leukopenia, thrombocytopenia), diarrhea, fatigue, nausea, and vomiting. A flulike syndrome with fever, chills, and headache is common and may physically stress the patient. Patients with cardiac disease, severe diabetes, or pulmonary disease may be unable to cope with this stress.

Interferons should be avoided by patients with autoimmune disease because the immune reactions may increase. In contrast, patients with chicken pox or herpes zoster may have worsened symptoms. The conditions of patients with CNS disease, including psychiatric disorders and seizures, may also be worsened by interferons.

Interferon alfa-2b is contraindicated in patients with impaired thyroid function because this impairment may be worsened.

TOXICITY

Cardiotoxicity has been reported, but this condition is rare.

INTERACTIONS

Blood dyscrasias may be worsened by other drugs producing the same adverse effects as the alfa interferons.

APPLICATION TO PRACTICE

Although there are many viral infections with which the health care provider may come in contact, HIV infections are by far the most serious. In most cases, it is viewed as a chronic viral illness. Therefore assessment should not be restricted to the immediate clinical status of the patient; rather, it should focus on potential problems that may be encountered during the illness trajectory. Thus the following discussion focuses on patients at risk for HIV infection (see the Case Study: HIV Infection with *Pneumocystis carinii* Pneumonia [PCP]).

ASSESSMENT
History of Present Illness

The demographic data to be collected include date, patient's name, age, gender, race or ethnic origin, birthplace, marital status, and occupation. These data provide information relevant to identified risk factors correlated with viral infections and assist in the diagnosis and individualization of a treatment plan specific to meet the patient's needs.

A chronologic record of the reason the patient is seeking care should be obtained. Many patients with an acute retroviral syndrome may be asymptomatic after initial infection, but a significant majority develop abrupt-onset febrile illness resembling acute mononucleosis or influenza. Early HIV infection and acute retroviral syndrome exhibit a wide range of unique clinical features. The patient remains generally healthy, but the most common complaints are fatigue, myalgia or arthralgia, pharyngitis, sore mouth, nausea, vomiting, diarrhea, headache, and weight loss. Complaints of night sweats and low-grade fevers are not uncommon. For many patients these symptoms of early HIV infection go undetected.

Health History

The health history provides information about childhood and adult illnesses (e.g., chicken pox, measles, mumps, mononucleosis, Epstein-Barr virus, tuberculo-

sis, parasitic infections), accidents, injuries, hospitalizations, operations, obstetric history, allergies, and foreign travel. It is important to note any operative procedures that may have included the administration of blood between the years 1977 and 1985, the time before blood was thoroughly tested for diseases. The presence of hemophilia or other blood diseases is significant.

Obtaining a complete sexual health history is critically important. Questions that relate to current sexual partner(s), past sexual partners, number of sexual relationships, types of sexual activity, history of sexually transmitted disease, homosexual or bisexual activity, and sexual relationships with persons who used intravenous drugs are necessary.

The drug history should include information about prescribed and OTC drugs, immunization history (e.g., hepatitis B, DTP, MMR, tetanus, polio), and the use of herbal remedies. The use of any immunosuppressant drugs is critically important to note.

Lifespan Considerations

Perinatal. Various processes are involved in the perinatal transmission of HIV infection to newborns. Virus transmission has been documented in utero by direct transplacental hematogenous spread, by ascending infection of amniotic fluid, iatrogenically by direct invasive methods used for diagnosis (such as scalp monitoring), and through breast-feeding.

Maternal characteristics that may increase risk factors related to transmission include increased maternal viremia, declining maternal health due to advanced disease, and immunosuppression. Asymptomatic women transmit HIV at a much lower rate than women with AIDS. Prolonged or complicated labor, clinical chorioamnionitis, and continued illicit drug use also increase the risk of perinatal HIV transmission.

Intrauterine transmission is believed to be responsible for a significant amount of transmission. The rate of infection may be as high as 50% to 70%. Placental factors include cell susceptibility to viral infection as well as developmental stage and integrity of the placenta. Maternal viral virulence as well as virus phenotype and genotype are also being studied.

Intrapartum factors resulting in HIV infections include extended time from rupture of membranes, invasive fetal monitoring, the route of delivery, birth order in multiple births (the firstborn has a greater risk), and gestational age at delivery. Many infants swallow secretions in the birth process; it is theorized that direct exposure to the virus in blood or secretions during labor and delivery results in a higher risk of infection. Cesarean section is associated with a slightly lower infection rate.

Other factors that affect a newborn's susceptibility to infection include gestational age at birth, the development of the immune system, and breast-feeding. Infants born to HIV-infected mothers before 34 weeks' gestation have an increased risk of infection. HIV has been found in breast milk.

Pediatric. Most new pediatric infections are acquired perinatally. Identification of HIV-infected infants soon after delivery or during the first few weeks following birth provides opportunities for the treatment of primary HIV infection. Initial testing is recommended within the first 48 hours after birth because nearly 40% of infected infants can be identified at this time.

Children depend on caregivers for the administration of drug therapy. The environment as well as the willingness of the caregiver to adhere to the complex multidrug regimen should be evaluated. Absorption of some antiretroviral drugs is affected by food. It can be difficult to juggle drug administration times around infant feedings. The adolescent has developmental issues that are unique as well. Concrete thought processes make it difficult to adhere to a drug treatment regimen when the adolescent generally feels well. Adolescents also do not want to be different from their peers.

Older Adults. HIV infection is often overlooked in older adults because health care providers often do not consider this group to be at risk. Risk factors most often associated with HIV transmission in the older adult include sexual contact, blood transfusions before 1985, and illicit drug use.

Many factors relate to the increased risk of the older adult becoming infected through sexual activity. For example, they often do not use condoms. Pregnancy is no longer an issue, and older adults do not consider themselves at risk for sexually transmitted diseases. Changes occur in the vagina (e.g., reduced lubrication, friable tissues) and immune response that make older women more susceptible to transmission of disease. Older men

who have been with prostitutes are also at risk for disease transmission. Older homosexual men may be at increased risk after the death of a long-term mate or a change to a younger partner.

HIV infection in the older adult has been called the great imitator because it can cause dementia that is mistaken for Alzheimer's disease or other chronic illness. Subtle differences between Alzheimer's disease–related dementias and HIV dementia also make patient assessment difficult. In addition, other symptoms, such as fatigue, weakness, anorexia, and weight loss, occur in many comorbid conditions that the patient may have other than HIV infection.

Cultural/Social Considerations

Social history and prejudices constitute a large portion of what preoccupies HIV-infected people. Health care providers should focus vital information on issues that relate to housing, family and community support, family dynamics, employment, and health insurance. It may be necessary to remove system barriers to treatment in order to stabilize patients' lives before initiating drug therapy.

Economic realities provide a blunt boundary line for this disease. Many people at high risk for HIV infection belong to lower socioeconomic groups. These patients often do not have health insurance or ready access to health care.

Noncompliance seems to be a major impediment to maximal benefit from medical intervention. Many patients are lost to follow-up, and there are as many reasons for those losses as there are patients. Patients often lack transportation or have no permanent address or phone number, suffer from psychiatric illness, use illicit drugs, or may be incarcerated. Some are embarrassed because they are unable to pay bills and purchase the required drugs. Many patients need constant social service intervention to ensure continuity of care. A psychosocial history will uncover problems with coping and stress management. Additionally, the health care provider should determine if the patient has a history of depression, suicidal tendencies, isolation, insomnia, or any other emotional problems. The kind of social support the patient has in place will either facilitate or hinder treatment.

Physical Examination

The physical examination begins with the patient's general overall appearance. Note his or her height and weight. Specific signs of HIV infection include recent weight loss, fever, chills, and night sweats or other signs that may indicate underlying conditions. The baseline physical examination should cover each of the systems most likely to be affected by HIV infection or the opportunistic infections associated with it. These systems include the neuropsychiatric, neurologic, musculoskeletal, cardiorespiratory, GI, genitourinary, and dermatologic systems, as well as the head, eyes, ears, nose, and throat (HEENT). Many patients who complain of no symptoms at baseline will have some abnormalities noted on the physical examination or laboratory evaluation.

Laboratory Testing

The laboratory testing used in the diagnosis of HIV includes enzyme-linked immunosorbent assay (ELISA), Western blot, immunofluorescence assay, and polymerase chain reaction (PCR). ELISA detects antibodies to HIV but does not detect HIV directly. Results are reported as positive, negative, or indeterminate. If the ELISA is positive or indeterminate, a repeat test is done. If the specimen is repeatedly positive, a more specific confirming test such as the Western blot or indirect immunofluorescence assay is done. Blood that is reactive in all three steps is reported as HIV positive.

The Western blot detects HIV antibodies and identifies the individual viral components to which antibodies are reactive. If the ELISA is either positive or indeterminate but the Western blot is negative, the ELISA is considered falsely positive, and the patient is not infected with HIV. The indirect immunofluorescence assay may be used as a substitute for a Western blot and may be able to clarify the results of indeterminate Western blot findings, but it requires significant time, expense, and expertise to perform.

CD4 cell counts indicate the extent of HIV-induced immune damage the patient has sustained. This test is necessary to determine the risk of disease progression and when to initiate or modify antiretroviral treatment regimens. The CD4 count is calculated based on the percentage of CD4 cells in the total lymphocyte count. The normal count is approximately 800 to 1100 cells/mm^3 with a range of 500 to 1400 cells/mm^3, or 40% percent of the total number of lymphocytes. A count of less than 500 is considered abnormally low. A count below 200 is a criterion for diagnosing AIDS in HIV-infected patients. CD4 cell counts less than 22, or less than 14% of lymphocytes, place the patient at risk for developing an opportunistic infection. Patients with AIDS may have a CD4 count as low as 5 to 10 and a percentage of 1% to 2% of all lymphocytes. Both CD4 counts and percentages reflect immune status, not HIV activity.

Viral load testing measures the amount of HIV RNA or genetic material in plasma. Viral load determinations are an important prognostic marker of disease progression and provide a valuable tool in the management of individual patients. In each of the three viral load tests, results are reported in copies per milliliter. Fewer than 10,000 copies/mL indicates a low risk for clinical progression; 10,000 to 100,000 indicates a moderate risk; and more than 100,000 copies indicates a high risk.

GOALS OF THERAPY

The goals of therapy are (1) to maximally suppress viral loads to undetectable levels, (2) to suppress viral replication, (3) to preserve immune function, (4) to prolong health and life, and (5) to decrease the risk of drug resistance caused by early suppression of viral replication. Any patient who has a CD4 cell count of less than 500 or has more than 10,000 (bDNA) or 20,000 (RT-PCR) copies of HIV RNA/mL of plasma and who is committed to lifelong adherence to necessary treatment should be offered therapy. The potential toxicities of therapy, quality of life, and ability to adhere to a complex antiretroviral drug regimen need to be balanced with the anticipated clinical benefit of maximal suppression of HIV replication.

INTERVENTION

One of the most dramatic improvements in anti-HIV therapy occurred when potent combinations of drugs began to be used. This strategy, called HAART, (see pathophysiology section), commonly uses three or sometimes four anti-HIV drugs in combination; care is taken to include drugs with different mechanisms of action (Box 31-3). For example, an NRTI might be combined with a protease inhibitor and an NNRTI. A potent antiviral effect may be achieved by attacking through two independent mechanisms, reducing the chance for resistance. A four-drug regimen might include two NRTIs, a protease inhibitor, and an NNRTI. The rationale for using two NRTIs together is that some combinations of NRTIs seem to limit development of resistance.

Occupational Exposure

The current recommendations for **postexposure chemoprophylaxis (PEP)** to HIV are determined by the type of exposure and the source material. Most occupational exposures do not result in infection transmission, and the potential toxicity of antiretroviral drugs must be carefully considered. Patients with occupational exposures to source patients with unknown HIV status may be candidates for PEP therapy on a case-by-case basis.

For example, PEP is recommended for health care workers with immediate exposure to individuals with a high risk for HIV transmission. For exposures with a lower but nonnegligible risk, PEP should be offered, balancing the lower risk against the potential benefits and adverse effects of the drugs. PEP is not recommended for exposures with negligible risk. Table 31-3 lists the PEP recommendations for persons with occupational HIV exposure.

Health care workers considering PEP should have baseline values for creatinine, CBC with differential,

---

BOX 31-3 | **What's at the Heart of HAART?**

HAART, or high activity antiretroviral therapy, refers to any one of several combinations of anti-HIV drugs that greatly reduce viral loads in patients. HAART reduces viral RNA in blood to below detectable levels in many patients. Other signs of success are weight gain, an elevation in CD4 cell counts, and clearing of some opportunistic infections.

Each of the drugs used in HAART is flawed when used alone. For example, zidovudine used alone must be given every 4 hours, is toxic, and selects for viral resistance. Protease inhibitors alone quickly select for resistant HIV and lose their effectiveness. The same problem exists for NNRTIs used alone. When anti-HIV drugs are used together, many of these problems are lessened. For example, zidovudine is given every 8 hours in combinations, rather than every 4 hours, and combining it with other drugs slows the appearance of drug-resistant mutations. Because the drugs are acting by different mechanisms, there may also be a synergistic antiviral effect.

The bad news is that the HAART regimen must be followed exactly to achieve the desired antiviral effect. If doses are missed, especially with the protease inhibitors, resistance can develop quickly and the effect of the combinations will be lost. Because these combinations include drugs from all categories of anti-HIV drugs, few other options are available when resistance develops.

Why is HAART hard to follow? The reason is partly that each of the three or four drugs must be taken on its own schedule, with or without food as appropriate. Scheduling these doses is difficult because an average AIDS patient may be taking more than 10 different drugs, including prophylaxis drugs for *Pneumocystis carinii* pneumonia (PCP) or for *Mycobacterium avium*. The combination of many drugs and the serious effects of AIDS itself make adverse reactions common. The reactions may force discontinuation of one or more of the drugs.

All of these factors point out the challenge faced by the patient and the health care support team. For best effectiveness, these drugs must be taken continuously as prescribed. Failure for any reason can lead to the development of multidrug-resistant HIV, which will not only complicate subsequent therapy for that patient but also may spread to other contacts and compromise the effectiveness of our best drugs in other patients.

TABLE 31-3

Recommendations for Occupational HIV Exposure Chemoprophylaxis*

	Application	*Drug Recommendation*
Basic	Occupational HIV exposure for which there is a recognized transmission risk	28 days of both zidovudine in divided doses and lamivudine
Expanded	Occupational HIV exposure that poses an increased risk (e.g., larger volume of blood and/or a higher virus titer in blood)	Basic recommendation plus either indinavir q8h on an empty stomach or nelfinavir tid with meals

Information from United States Public Health Service: Guidelines for the management of health care worker exposure to HIV and recommendations for postexposure prophylaxis, *MMWR Morb Mortal Wkly Rep* 47(RR-7):1-28, 1998. Available online: *www.cdc.gov/mmwr/preview/mmwrhtml/0052722.htm*

---

liver enzymes, pregnancy, HIV antibody, and hepatitis B and C done before starting therapy. HIV antibody testing should be done periodically for at least 6 months after exposure. Monitoring for potential drug toxicities is required if PEP therapy is initiated.

Administration

Before initiating antiretroviral therapy, a detailed discussion between the patient and the primary caretaker is necessary to assess the patient's ability and willingness to commit to a complex, costly, and potentially toxic drug regimen. This is very important in asymptomatic patients at an early stage of illness in whom the ability to maintain a long-term adherence to the regimen is a major challenge.

Drug treatment is lifelong and uses multiple classes of drugs. Schedules that require fewer daily doses make life easier for patients. Multidrug therapy should be maintained at recommended dosages; underdosing should be avoided. Antiretroviral drug resistance is less likely to develop when all drug therapy is temporarily stopped than if the dosage is reduced or if one component is withheld.

Education

Psychologists believe that the biggest predictor of adherence to prescribed drug regimens is the amount of chaos in the patient's life. For many, the circumstances are such that he or she has neither the capacity nor the will to comply with drug therapy. It is particularly difficult for patients to adhere to drug treatment when they are asymptomatic, especially if the drugs have adverse effects that interfere with the activities of daily living. The cost of drugs for many patients is significant, a factor which also contributes to nonadherence.

Adequate information enables patients to make informed choices about the lifestyle issues with which they are faced. In the absence of a vaccination, education and behavioral change are the only effective tools for prevention and treatment of HIV infection. Educational messages should be specific to the patient's needs, culturally sensitive, and age specific.

Once the decision has been made to begin therapy, specific information concerning drug administration, expected outcomes, and adverse effects should be discussed with the patient and family. Advise them that antiretroviral drug therapy is not a cure for HIV infection, nor does therapy reduce the risk of transmission of HIV to others through sexual contact, blood contamination, or contact with body fluids.

Instruct the patient to take the drugs exactly as prescribed. In some cases therapy is required around the clock, even if sleep is interrupted. It is often necessary to use a drug box that will conveniently organize the day's or week's medications according to administration times. The importance of not taking more than the prescribed amount and not discontinuing a drug without first consulting with the health care provider must be emphasized. In most cases, missed doses are taken as soon as the patient remembers, unless it is almost time for the next dose. Doses should not be doubled. The patient should be cautioned not to share the drugs with others. The patient should avoid OTC drugs without first contacting the health care provider. Inform the female patient to contact the health care provider if she is taking an oral contraceptive. An alternative, nondrug method of birth control may be required.

The impact of drug therapy on the overall monthly cost of HIV care is significant. The patient should be informed that there are compassionate-use drug programs that have been put in place to offer assistance with the economic realities of care (Box 31-4).

The health care provider must be clear when teaching the patient about the drug regimen. Some drugs must be taken on an empty stomach; others must be taken with water; still others are to be mixed with juice, milk, or formulas (e.g., Ensure, Advera). For example, a patient with achlorhydria requires an acidic beverage when taking delavirdine for maximum benefit. In contrast, a patient using the powdered formulation of didanosine should be advised to mix the powder with wa-

---

| BOX 31-4 | **AIDS Information Resources** |

National Institutes of Health AIDS Clinical Trials Group Information Service
- 1-800-TRIALS-A (874-2572) (English and Spanish)

American Foundation for AIDS Research
- 1-212-719-0033

National AIDS Hotline
- 1-800-342-AIDS (342-2437) (English)
- 1-800-344-SIDA (344-7432) (Spanish)
- 1-800-AIDS-TTY (243-7889) (hearing impaired)

National Pediatric HIV Resource Center
- 1-800-362-0071

Antiretroviral Pregnancy Registry
- 1-919-483-9437
- 1-800-722-9292 x 39437
- FAX 1-929-315-8981

HIV Postexposure Prophylaxis (PEP) Registry
- 1-888-737-4448

---

ter (not fruit juice or an acid-containing beverage). Some drugs, such as retonavir, may be mixed with chocolate milk, Ensure, or Advera to improve the taste. The patient should be instructed on the proper storage of the drugs. Some drugs (e.g., indinavir) are sensitive to moisture; others should be stored in the refrigerator; still others may be kept at room temperature.

Instruct the patient to promptly call the health care provider if adverse effects appear. Some drugs may cause drowsiness and blurred vision (e.g., didanosine); thus the patient should be cautioned to avoid driving or other activities that require alertness until the response to the drugs is known. Frequent oral rinses, sugarless gum or candy, and good oral hygiene help relieve the dry mouth associated with some of the drugs. If dry mouth persists longer than 2 weeks, advise the patient to contact the health care provider or dentist regarding the use of saliva substitutes. Adequate fluid intake, at least 1 to 2 L of water, should be taken daily to reduce the risk of adverse effects (e.g., kidney stones with lamivudine).

Avoidance of temperature extremes is necessary when taking some drugs. The patient should also be advised to change position slowly to minimize the orthostatic hypotension associated with some antiretroviral drugs. Additionally, if diarrhea occurs along with drug therapy, it can usually be controlled with OTC drugs (e.g., loperamide), but the patient should first contact the health care provider before attempting self-treatment.

Patients should also be cautioned to avoid crowds and people with known infections. Teach the patient to use a soft toothbrush, exercise caution when using toothpicks or dental floss, and have dental work performed before therapy, when possible. The importance of regular follow-up examinations and laboratory testing to determine progress and to monitor for adverse effects should be emphasized.

EVALUATION

The effectiveness of drug therapy can be demonstrated by decreasing viral load values, increasing CD4 counts, and general improvement of health status. Treatment failure is identified when (1) viral loads fail to drop tenfold (1 log) within the first 4 weeks of treatment; (2) the viral load fails to drop to undetectable levels within the first 4 to 6 months of therapy; (3) the viral load rebounds after falling to an undetectable level; (4) CD4 counts continue to drop despite antiretroviral therapy; or (5) clinical symptoms continue to progress in the presence of antiretroviral therapy.

CASE STUDY

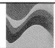

HIV Infection and Pneumocystis carinii *Pneumonia (PCP)*

ASSESSMENT

HISTORY OF PRESENT ILLNESS

JD is a 33-year-old man with a newly diagnosed HIV infection. His symptoms include fatigue, night sweats, dyspnea, and dry cough.

HEALTH HISTORY

JD has no known allergies. He has never received antiretroviral therapy. He follows a vegetarian diet and is a nonsmoker and nondrinker.

PHYSICAL EXAMINATION

JD's temperature is 103.2° F, pulse 128, respirations 32, blood pressure 124/82 mm Hg. He weighs 110 pounds—a loss of 40 pounds over the last 3 months. His O_2 Sat blood level on room air is 90%. He has no skin lesions or masses; his breath sounds are diminished but clear. He has a dry cough. His neurologic examination is negative; cranial nerves II-XII are intact.

LABORATORY TESTING

JD's chest x-ray study reveals diffuse infiltrates. Results of bronchial washings are pending; PPD is negative, CD4 count is 128, WBC count 5.8, RBC count 3.35, hemoglobin 10.6 mg/dL, hematocrit 30 mg/dL, lymph is 15%, viral load results are pending, potassium level is 3.9 mg/dL, blood urea nitrogen (BUN) level is 10 mg/dL, and creatinine level is 0.7 mg/dL.

LIFESPAN CONSIDERATIONS

HIV is primarily a disease of young people. Diagnosis interrupted JD's perceived ability to carry out his developmental tasks.

CULTURAL/SOCIAL CONSIDERATIONS

JD was married but is now divorced and lives alone. He suspects his HIV infection may have been contracted through heterosexual transmission. He is currently on leave from his job as a computer programmer. His support system includes one sister. His present health plan will cover prescriptions; copayment of $25.00 per prescription.

PATIENT PROBLEM(S)

HIV infection; chest x-ray study is consistent with PCP infection.

GOALS OF THERAPY

Maintain immune function as near a normal state as possible. Prevent disease progression and prolong survival. Preserve quality of life by effectively suppressing HIV replication.

CRITICAL THINKING QUESTIONS

1. The following drugs have been ordered for JD: sulfamethoxazole/trimethoprim DS 5 mg/kg IV for 21 days; efavirenz 600 mg po qd with or without food; ritonavir 600 mg po bid with food; and lamivudine 150 mg po bid. What are the mechanisms of action of these drugs?
2. Which adverse effects should be monitored? Are there specific laboratory tests that should be ordered? How frequently should the tests be performed?
3. The nurse is preparing JD for discharge in the next few days. What patient teaching is appropriate in regard to the use of antiretroviral drugs?
4. How is treatment failure defined?
5. Which issues of social justice concern the availability of combination antiretroviral drug therapy?
6. Should requirements for supervised administration of HIV treatment regimens exist for noncompliant patients?
7. Can our society choose to restrict successful therapies to select groups of patients? On an economic basis? On a public health basis?

Bibliography

Brechtl JR, Breitbart W, Galietta M, et al: The use of highly active antiretroviral therapy (HAART) in patients with advanced HIV infection: impact on medical, palliative care, and quality of life outcomes, *J Pain Symptom Manage* 21(1):41-51, 2001.

Burpo RH: Common antiviral agents used in women's and children's care, part 1, *J Obstet Gynecol Neonatal Nurs* 29(2):181-190, 2000.

Carreiro LI: Influenza: an overview, *Physician Assist* 25(9):26-30, 33-34, 2001.

Collura J, Kraus DM: Pediatric pharmacology. New pediatric antiretroviral agents . . . abacavir, efavirenz, and amprenavir, *J Pediatr Health Care* 14(4):183-192, 2000.

El-Sadr W, Oleske J, Agins B, et al: Managing early HIV infection: quick reference guide for clinicians, AHCPR Publication No. 94-0573, Rockville, MD, 1994, Agency for Health Care Policy and Research, Public Health Service, U.S. Department of Health and Human Services.

Public Health Service Guidelines for the Management of Health-Care Worker Exposures to HIV and Recommendations for Postexposure Prophylaxis. *MMWR Morb Mortal Wkly Rep* 47(RR-7):1-28, 1998.

Revised adult treatment guidelines focus on NNRTIs: pediatric guidelines include amprenavir info . . . nonnucleoside reverse transcriptase inhibitors, *AIDS Alert* 15(4):45-46, 48, 2000.

Scott F: Shingles: diagnosis and treatment, *Nurs Times* 96(50):36-37, 2000.

Internet Resources

Haddad M, Inch C, Glazier RH, et al: Patient support and education for promoting adherence to highly active antiretroviral therapy for HIV/AIDS. In *The Cochrane Library* 4, 2001, Oxford, Update Software. Available online at http://www.cochranelibrary.com/enter/.

Jefferson T, Demicheli V, Deeks J, et al: Neuraminidase. inhibitors for preventing and treating influenza in healthy adults. In *The Cochrane Library* 4, 2001, Oxford, Update Software. Available online at http://www.cochranelibrary.com/enter/.

Antifungal Drugs

SHERRY F. QUEENER • KATHLEEN GUTIERREZ

 Visit **http://evolve.elsevier.com/Gutierrez/** for additional information.

KEY TERMS

Azole antifungal drugs, p. 480

Dermatophytes, p. 484

Ergosterol, p. 480

Fungi, p. 480

Liposomes, p. 482

Opportunistic infection, p. 481

Polyene antifungal drug, p. 481

Tinea, p. 489

OBJECTIVES

- Explain the mechanism of action of amphotericin B and azole antifungal drugs.

- Discuss the dose-limiting toxicity of amphotericin B.

- Explain why drugs that are too toxic for systemic use may be used topically for local fungal infections.

- Develop a nursing care plan for the patient receiving one of the parenteral, oral, or topical antifungal drugs discussed in this chapter.

Fungal diseases range from mild infections in localized areas of the skin (Chapter 67) to grave systemic infections. Diseases may be produced by a wide range of fungi; the seriousness of the infection is determined largely by the nature of the infecting organism and the immune status of the host.

Although the fungi that cause disease in humans are single-celled organisms, they resemble human cells more than bacteria in their biochemical properties. Their biochemical similarities to human cells present therapeutic problems. For instance, none of the antibiotics that inhibit bacterial protein synthesis affect that process in fungi because fungal ribosomes resemble human ribosomes and are sensitive to the same drugs. Therefore, selective toxicity cannot be achieved by this mechanism. Moreover, fungal cells do not contain a peptidoglycan cell wall, which renders them resistant to all antibiotics that block peptidoglycan synthesis (e.g., penicillins). For these reasons, the antimicrobial drugs discussed in previous chapters cannot be used to treat fungal diseases.

The design of new antifungal drugs depends on the recognition of biochemical differences between fungal and mammalian cells. The first clinically exploited difference was in the cellular membrane (Figure 32-1). Human cellular membranes contain cholesterol, whereas those of fungi contain the sterol called ergosterol. This unique membrane component of fungi is the direct target of polyene antifungal drugs, whereas azole antifungal drugs inhibit the synthesis of ergosterol. The newest antifungal drugs are aimed at a different target: the enzyme glucan synthetase, which is involved in synthesis of fungal cell walls. Another antifungal drug, griseofulvin, interferes with fungal cell mitosis.

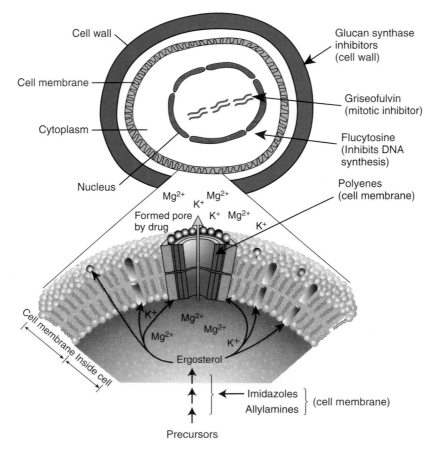

FIGURE 32-1 Sites of action of antifungal drugs. The primary target of most antifungal drugs is the fungal cell membrane. Polyenes bind ergosterol in the membrane, causing pores to form that allow potassium, magnesium, and other cell components to leak out, as shown in the inset. Imidazoles and allylamines block synthesis of ergosterol, which also damages the fungal cell membrane. Other antifungal drugs target cell wall synthesis, mitosis, or DNA synthesis, as shown.

Fungal cells possess many antigens, which ultimately provoke host immune responses. Most fungal infections resolve in this way, many times without the host ever being aware of an active disease. This pattern is especially common with fungal diseases contracted by breathing in spores from contaminated soil. This primary infection may resemble a cold or a mild case of influenza. Examples of diseases of this type are histoplasmosis, blastomycosis, cryptococcosis, coccidioidomycosis, and aspergillosis. Several of these diseases are concentrated in specific geographic areas. For example, coccidioidomycosis is most common, or endemic, in the southernmost portions of California, Nevada, Utah, Arizona, New Mexico, and Texas. Histoplasmosis is endemic in the states bordering the Mississippi and Ohio rivers. Blastomycosis is endemic in isolated areas along the Mississippi and Ohio rivers, around the Great Lakes, along the St. Lawrence River, and in the Carolinas.

Some fungal diseases are spread by contact with soil contaminated with bird droppings. For example, histoplasmosis is associated with soil contaminated with chicken or starling droppings or bat guano. Cryptococcosis may result from exposure to high concentrations of pigeon droppings. Although pulmonary forms of these diseases are usually mild and limited by the development of immunity in the victim, in rare cases the fungus may become disseminated and invade other body tissues. A notorious example is the yeast *Cryptococcus neoformans*, which can cause meningitis, pulmonary disease, and infections at many other sites. The disseminated, or systemic, fungal diseases are most likely to develop in patients with immune systems depressed by disease or drug therapy, especially those treated with glucocorticoids or immunosuppressant antineoplastic drugs.

The yeast *Candida* may cause a range of infections from serious systemic disease to annoying mucous membrane infections. Because *Candida* is normally found on the skin and mucous membranes of healthy persons, the growth of *Candida* leading to disease usually represents an **opportunistic infection**. *Candida* infections are therefore most common in persons receiving broad-spectrum antibacterial drugs such as tetracyclines (Chapter 28) or in persons with suppressed immune systems. Opportunistic infections caused by *Candida* are common in patients with acquired immunodeficiency syndrome (AIDS).

DRUG CLASS • Polyenes

amphotericin B (Amphocin, Fungizone)

amphotericin B cholesteryl complex (Amphotec)

amphotericin B lipid complex (Abelcet)

amphotericin B liposomal complex (AmBisome)

nystatin (Mycostatin, Nilstat)

MECHANISM OF ACTION

Amphotericin B is the only polyene antifungal drug currently used for systemic fungal infections. Polyene antifungal drugs have a greater affinity for ergosterol than for cholesterol and therefore react with ergosterol from fungal cell membranes. This action destroys the integrity of the cell membrane and the cell dies as its cytoplasmic components are lost. This membrane-disruptive effect is not entirely selective, and some of the cholesterol-containing membranes of mammalian cells are also damaged.

USES

Amphotericin B can be used to treat many different systemic fungal diseases, including those caused by *Histoplasma*, *Blastomyces*, *Cryptococcus*, and *Aspergillus* organisms. Amphotericin B may also treat systemic *Candida* and *Coccidioides* infections. Topical use of amphotericin B is not recommended because other topical drugs are more effective. For example, another polyene, nystatin, is used for vaginal infections (Table 32-1).

PHARMACOKINETICS

Amphotericin B has a high affinity for lipids and thus tends to bind to tissues rather than remain in blood. During long-term therapy, only a fraction of the daily dose can be recovered in urine or feces. The unrecovered drug is held in tissues and continues to appear in urine for a long period after therapy is stopped. The tissue-binding properties and the relative water insolubility of amphotericin B prevent the drug from entering body fluids efficiently. Therefore, concentrations of the drug in the cerebrospinal fluid (CSF) or in ocular fluid may be too low to effectively eliminate infections at those sites. To overcome this problem, amphotericin B (Fungizone) may be injected intrathecally (into the CSF) to treat meningitis.

Amphotericin B is usually administered intravenously, although the drug irritates vascular tissue and often causes phlebitis. This lipid-soluble drug may be administered as a colloidal suspension stabilized with a small amount of the detergent deoxycholate. Amphotericin B in this form (Fungizone) must be infused at a concentration of less than 0.1 mg/mL in a 5% dextrose solution; these infusions typically take 6 hours. Higher drug concentrations cause precipitation of the drug in the intravenous (IV) solution and endanger the patient.

TABLE 32-1

Drugs to Treat Vaginal Candidiasis

Generic Name	Brand Name	Dosage Form	Duration of Therapy*
butoconazole	Femstat 3	Cream	3 days
clotrimazole	Gyne-Lotrimin, Mycelex	Cream	6 to 14 days
	FemCare, Gyne-Lotrimin	Tablets	6 to 7 days
	Gyne-Lotrimin 3	Tablets	3 days
	Mycelex-G	Tablet	1 day
miconazole	Femzole-M, Monistat 7	Cream	7 days
	Monistat 7	Suppository	7 days
	Monistat 3	Suppository	3 days
nystatin	Nilstat	Tablet	14 days
terconazole	Terazol 7	Cream	7 days
	Terazol 3	Cream	3 days
	Terazole 3	Suppository	3 days
tioconazole	Monistat 1, Vagistat-1	Ointment	1 day

*In nonpregnant patients with normal immune function.

BOX 32-1	**Patient Problem: Alert for Amphotericin B**

The Problem

Amphotericin B is available in two very different types of formulations. The original formulation (Fungizone) contains amphotericin B solubilized with the detergent deoxycholate. The solubility of this preparation is limited, and it must be extensively diluted before administration. It is also highly toxic, and dosages must be carefully controlled to prevent renal damage, electrolyte imbalance, or death.

The newer formulations of amphotericin B complex the drug with lipids (Amphotec, Abelcet) or enclose it in liposomes (AmBisome). This process increases the solubility of the drug, alters its disposition in the body, and reduces toxicity. Thus, these new formulations can be administered at higher dosages than Fungizone. This difference in dosage has resulted in fatal drug errors when Fungizone was used at dosages intended only for the newer formulations.

The Solution

Carefully note the form of amphotericin B that is ordered for the patient. Question any drug orders outside the following guidelines.

- Fungizone must be diluted to 0.1 mg/mL in 5% dextrose and administered at a rate of 0.1 mg/kg/hour. The daily dose should not exceed 50 mg. Question any concentration, rate of administration, or dosage in excess of these values.
- Amphotec may be infused at a rate of 1 mg/kg/hour; dosages are 3 to 4 mg/kg once daily.
- Abelcet or AmBisome may be infused at rates up to 2.5 mg/kg/hour for dosages of 5 mg/kg once daily.

Recently, other forms of amphotericin have been developed to improve the pharmacokinetics of the drug. Amphotericin B may be complexed with cholesteryl sulfate (Amphotec) or with two phospholipids (Abelcet) to improve the water solubility of the drug. Amphotericin B has also been inserted into **liposomes,** which are lipid structures that maintain a specific form in solution (AmBisome, Box 32-1). In this case the liposomes consist of a bilayer of phospholipids stabilized with alpha-tocopherol (vitamin E). These structures maintain a hydrophobic (i.e., water-repelling, lipid-attracting) region where amphotericin may concentrate, as well as a hydrophilic (i.e., water-attracting) face that is in contact with the solution and maintains solubility. Each of these lipid-containing preparations allows higher concentrations of the drug to be used by improving water solubility. These lipid formulations of amphotericin B have also improved distribution of the drug in the body while lowering toxicity. Care must be taken not to use dosages calculated for the new formu-

---

BOX **32-2** | **Patient Problem: Hypokalemia**

The Problem

An abnormally low level of potassium in the blood, known as hypokalemia, can occur secondary to the use of IV amphotericin B and can occasionally be life-threatening. The common signs and symptoms of hypokalemia include malaise; fatigue; paresthesias; depressed reflexes; muscle weakness and cramps; confusion; delayed thought processes; depression; rapid, irregular pulse; hypotension; shallow breathing; shortness of breath; vomiting; abdominal distension; and polyuria. ECG changes seen with low potassium levels include ST segment depression, flattened T waves, presence of U waves, and ventricular arrhythmias.

Solutions

- Assess for and report immediately signs of hypokalemia.
- Monitor intake and output, watching for polyuria.
- Monitor serum potassium levels in laboratory reports.
- Provide oral potassium supplementation as prescribed. If needed, IV potassium may be given at a rate of 10 to 15 mEq/hour of a solution containing 40 mEq/L. Determine whether the patient has adequate kidney function before administering IV potassium supplements. Carefully label containers to which potassium has been added.

---

lations with the older, more toxic formulation (Fungizone); deaths have resulted (Box 32-1).

ADVERSE REACTIONS AND CONTRAINDICATIONS

Most patients start on low doses of amphotericin B, and the dosage is increased as tolerance to adverse effects develops. Fever, headache, nausea, and vomiting may occur after the first few doses, but these reactions usually subside as therapy continues. Renal damage is related to the total amount of drug given and may become irreversible when the total cumulative amount of amphotericin B administered approaches 4 g. Anemia and electrolyte disturbances, including acidosis and hypokalemia (low blood potassium), also increase during therapy (Box 32-2).

There are no absolute contraindications to the use of amphotericin B for serious systemic fungal infections, but in patients with renal disease the risk of increased nephrotoxicity is significant.

TOXICITY

Amphotericin B therapy must be used for long periods to cure disseminated fungal disease. No firm guidelines

for therapy exist, although health care providers try to limit the total drug dosage to less than 4 g. Even with cumulative doses approaching this limit, cure is not always obtained. For many patients therapy must be discontinued early because of toxicity.

INTERACTIONS

Amphotericin B is incompatible in solution with sodium chloride and with benzyl alcohol. These compounds cause precipitation of the colloidal suspension of amphotericin B used for IV administration.

Because amphotericin B has significant toxicity on its own, it can cause serious interactions with other drugs. Bone marrow depressants and radiation therapy increase the risk of anemia with amphotericin B. Nephrotoxic drugs increase the risk of renal damage with amphotericin B.

Amphotericin B tends to cause hypokalemia. This action increases the risk of toxicity with cardiac glycosides and with potassium-depleting diuretics. The risk of serious hypokalemia is also increased with corticosteroid use.

DRUG CLASS • Antimetabolites

flucytosine (Ancobon)

MECHANISM OF ACTION

Flucytosine is a pyrimidine analog that is converted to the cytotoxic agent 5-fluorouracil in sensitive fungi. Because this metabolite is not freely formed in humans, a degree of selective toxicity is achieved.

USES

A relatively narrow range of fungi are sensitive to flucytosine, including *Cryptococcus, Candida*, and a few other, rarely encountered pathogenic fungi. A significant number of clinically encountered *Candida* strains may have an intrinsic resistance to flucytosine, and resistance to the drug may also be acquired by species of *Cryptococcus* during therapy. This pattern of resistance has limited the drug's usefulness.

Flucytosine is often combined with amphotericin B for treatment of disseminated fungal disease. The rationale for combining these drugs for serious infections is twofold: the combination allows the dose of amphotericin B to be lowered somewhat, thereby reducing toxicity, and resistance to flucytosine is minimized by combination chemotherapy.

PHARMACOKINETICS

Flucytosine is a water-soluble drug that is well absorbed from the gastrointestinal (GI) tract and well distributed into body fluids. Drug concentration in the CSF may be 50% to 70% of the serum level, in contrast to amphotericin B, for which the CSF level is less than 5% of the serum level. More than 90% of an oral dose of flucytosine is renally excreted, producing high concentrations of unchanged drug in urine. The elimination half-life is about 6 hours.

ADVERSE REACTIONS AND CONTRAINDICATIONS

Flucytosine therapy is usually continued for several weeks to months. Nausea and diarrhea appear in roughly 25% of patients. Blood dyscrasias such as anemia and

thrombocytopenia (unusual bruising or bleeding) and transient liver abnormalities have been reported.

The only absolute contraindication to the use of flucytosine is a documented allergy to the drug, but the drug should be used cautiously in patients with impaired renal function or those with bone marrow depression caused by drugs or disease.

TOXICITY

High serum concentrations of flucytosine increase the risk of hematologic toxicity. Hemodialysis may be required to remove the drug from the system, especially in patients with poor renal function.

INTERACTIONS

Because of its effects on bone marrow, flucytosine should not be used with other drugs that also depress bone marrow function.

 DRUG CLASS • **Azole Antifungal Drugs**

fluconazole (Diflucan)

itraconazole (Sporanox)

ketoconazole (Nizoral)

MECHANISM OF ACTION

Azole antifungal drugs inhibit the synthesis of ergosterol. As a result, the function of fungal cell membranes is impaired. *Candida* cells in the body are normally in the yeast phase, with rounded shapes, but in certain conditions the *Candida* may change to a form that produces tubular bodies called hyphae, which are capable of invading tissues and allowing the organism to lodge firmly within the host. Development of invasive hyphae by *Candida* cells may be retarded by azole antifungal drugs, enhancing the ability of the host immune system to eliminate the fungal cells.

USES

Azole antifungal drugs are used to treat a variety of fungal infections. Fluconazole is used for cryptococcal meningitis and for systemic, esophageal, or oropharyngeal candidiasis. Ketoconazole is used against *Histoplasma* and *Paracoccidioides*. It may also be effective in

certain patients with disseminated candidiasis and blastomycosis. Itraconazole is indicated for aspergillosis, blastomycosis, and histoplasmosis. Clotrimazole, miconazole, terconazole, and tioconazole are used for vaginal infections caused by *Candida* (Box 32-3). Other members of this family are used topically to treat tinea infections and other **dermatophytes**, which are fungi primarily restricted to the skin (Chapter 67).

PHARMACOKINETICS

Ketoconazole is adequately absorbed orally, but bioavailability depends on sufficient stomach acidity. Ketoconazole should not be administered within 2 hours of a dose of antacids or H_2-antagonists such as cimetidine. Ketoconazole is poorly distributed to some tissues and is especially low in CSF. Elimination is primarily by the liver, which forms inactive metabolites and excretes the drug into bile. The half-life of the drug is 8 hours.

Fluconazole is well absorbed orally, with a bioavailability of about 90%; absorption does not depend on stomach acidity as much as with ketoconazole. Fluconazole is well distributed to most body tissues, including the CSF. Little hepatic biotransformation of flu-

---

The Problem

The dark, moist environment of the vagina is prone to infection by a variety of organisms. Some chronic health problems such as diabetes mellitus increase susceptibility to vaginal infection. Treatment with some groups of drugs such as antibiotics may increase susceptibility to fungal superinfection. Finally, some invading organisms are transmitted during sexual relations. Treatment of vaginal infections may be messy and difficult. It is difficult to reach all mucosal surfaces. Also, because the woman is upright during most of the day, drugs may drain out because of gravity.

Solutions

- Use prescribed drugs for the full course of therapy; do not stop when symptoms disappear.
- Do not wear tampons during therapy. Wear sanitary napkins to prevent staining of clothing.
- Continue therapy through the menstrual period.
- Wash hands carefully before and after using prescribed drugs.
- Insert the vaginal suppository, cream, or ointment just before going to bed to allow the drug to remain in the vaginal area as long as possible.

- If douching is prescribed, wash douche equipment carefully after each use and dry it.
- Depending on the infecting agent, your sexual partner may also need to be treated; consult the clinician.
- Usually, avoid sexual intercourse during the course of therapy. If this is not possible, your sexual partner should wear a condom.

To Help Prevent Vaginal Infection

- Wear clean underwear daily, preferably of cotton material. Synthetic fabrics do not allow air to circulate as well, thus they keep the vaginal area more moist than normal. Avoid pantyhose for the same reason. Do not wear pantyhose and slacks at the same time.
- Wipe from front to back after voiding or defecating.
- Do not douche unless prescribed by the health care provider. Do not douche between doses of vaginal drugs.
- Avoid bubble baths and soaps that may irritate vaginal mucosa. Wash the vaginal area gently and rinse soap off well. Some women may need to wash with water only, if soap is irritating to the vaginal area.
- Use vaginal water-soluble lubricants, if needed. Avoid oil-based products such as petroleum jelly.

---

conazole occurs, and most of the drug is excreted unchanged in urine. The half-life of the drug in patients with normal renal function is 30 hours.

Itraconazole is relatively lipid soluble and is absorbed after oral administration. Food increases the absorption of oral doses of this drug. Itraconazole concentrates in tissues such as the skin and lungs but does not enter the vitreous humor or CSF adequately to treat infections at those sites. Itraconazole metabolites are formed in the liver and excreted in urine.

ADVERSE REACTIONS AND CONTRAINDICATIONS

Ketoconazole is relatively nontoxic for many patients. Nausea and pruritus occur in less than 5% of treated patients. Dizziness, nervousness, and headache have been reported less often.

Fluconazole may cause adverse effects in up to 13% of treated patients. Gastrointestinal disturbances such as nausea or diarrhea, and headaches are the most common complaints. Thrombocytopenia, which produces unusual bleeding or bruising, and hepatotoxicity are more serious rare effects. Rarely, a patient may develop a dangerous allergic reaction such as Stevens-Johnson syndrome or exfoliative skin disorders.

Itraconazole appears to be associated with less hepatotoxicity than ketoconazole. All azole antifungal drugs are capable of inducing allergic reactions.

TOXICITY

Hepatotoxicity is an idiosyncratic reaction that occurs in about 1 in 10,000 patients receiving ketoconazole. High dosages of azole antifungal drugs inhibit testosterone and cortisol synthesis. This inhibition may produce gynecomastia (enlargement of breast tissue), which has been noted in about 10% of men receiving ketoconazole.

INTERACTIONS

Azole antifungal drugs are subject to a wide array of drug interactions. Pharmacokinetic interactions include those that block absorption of the azoles. For example, antacids or H_2-antagonists that raise gastric pH lower the absorption of ketoconazole and itraconazole because these azoles require strong acidity for absorption. Didanosine is formulated with buffers that raise gastric pH and so it also lowers the absorption of azoles.

Another potentially serious pharmacokinetic interaction arises because azole antifungal drugs, especially ketoconazole and itraconazole, inhibit hepatic biotransformation of a variety of drugs. This action leads to a rise in blood concentrations of drugs such as cyclosporine, digoxin, phenytoin, warfarin, and the sulfonylurea antidiabetic drugs. Increased blood levels of these drugs can produce serious or even life-threatening adverse effects.

Drugs that lower the blood concentrations of azole antifungal drugs and cause failure of therapy include carbamazepine and the antituberculosis drugs rifampin and isoniazid.

Ketoconazole has been linked to hepatotoxic reactions when given with other hepatotoxic drugs or when used in patients who abuse alcohol. Concurrent use of ketoconazole and alcohol may cause a disulfiram-like reaction (facial flushing, tightness in the chest, difficulty breathing).

 DRUG CLASS • Echinocandin

caspofungin

MECHANISM OF ACTION

Caspofungin is a new drug that inhibits an enzyme called glucan synthase, which plays a key role in forming the fungal cell wall. When this enzyme is inhibited, cell wall synthesis is impaired, leading to damage of the fungal cell.

USES

Caspofungin is used for invasive aspergillosis, usually after other drugs have been tried and failed.

PHARMACOKINETICS

Caspofungin must be given by intravenous infusion. The drug tends to be bound in tissues. It also undergoes biotransformation in various tissues and may be ultimately broken down into amino acids. These and other metabolites appear in both urine and feces.

ADVERSE REACTIONS AND CONTRAINDICATIONS

Caspofungin has caused pain and phlebitis at the intravenous infusion site in up to 14% of treated patients. Fever also occurs commonly. In addition to these reactions, a variety of GI symptoms have been reported, including stomach pain, nausea, and vomiting.

INTERACTIONS

Data on drug interactions with caspofungin are limited, but there is a suggestion that drugs such as carbamazepine, dexamethazone, efavirenz, nelfinavir, nevirapine, phenytoin, and rifampin may lower the serum level of caspofungin. Patients receiving one of these drugs as well as caspofungin may have to have the caspofungin dosage raised.

Cyclosporine increases the serum level of caspofungin, requiring that the serum level be monitored if these drugs are used together. Caspofungin lowers the blood level of tacrolimus, requiring that tacrolimus level be monitored.

 APPLICATION TO PRACTICE

ASSESSMENT
History of Present Illness

Initial questions to be elicited from a patient with a dermatologic complaint include when and where the disorder began. Establishing the time of onset helps determine if the problem is acute or chronic or whether a relapse has occurred. Knowledge about the site of the initial lesion and whether there is pruritus may also be helpful. The distribution and development of individual lesions are often characteristic; therefore, information regarding any changes in the lesions should be elicited. Determining if the patient has had any other symptoms helps distinguish systemic from localized problems. Information about what has been done to treat the disorder should be noted, because many fungal infections are altered by therapies—some for the better, some for the worse.

The patient should be asked about the effect of sunlight because several disorders may result from photosensitivity. Questions about possible exposure to others with a similar skin condition helps elicit information about contagious illness. Asking patients what they think may be causing the problem often provides insight into the origin. Often, however, the patient guesses incorrectly.

Other factors to be considered are the patient's profession and home and workplace environments. It is important to understand what the patient comes in contact with and to what extent. For example, does the patient work around chemicals? What is the home environment like? Are there pets, plants, or flowers in the home or workplace? Patient-determined or health care provider–prescribed factors that may have alleviated the condition and the patient's psychologic response to the problem should also be noted.

Health History

Patients should be asked if they have had a similar problem in the past. This question may help reveal a recurrent condition. They should also be asked about the presence of other types of skin lesions or rashes and other illnesses they now have or had in the past. The background check helps the health care provider identify factors that contribute to the antifungal condition and the patient's response to treatment.

Ask about the patient's self-care habits. Determine the frequency with which soaps, lotions, abrasives, and cosmetics are used. Elicit information about drugs in current use. HIV-infected patients may have a long list of such drugs.

Lifespan Considerations

Perinatal. Except for vaginal infections secondary to *Candida*, mycotic infections in healthy pregnant women are uncommon. Disseminated candidiasis, cryptococcosis, aspergillosis, and histoplasmosis occur as opportunistic infections in immunocompromised patients. Vulvovaginal candidiasis is common during pregnancy, and is evidenced by the characteristic curdy, white, itchy discharge.

Neither the incidence nor the severity of cryptococcal or histoplasmal infections is known to be affected by pregnancy. In contrast, coccidioidomycosis can be very severe in pregnancy, and disseminated infections may be fatal if left untreated. Oral candidiasis is common in infants who pass through a birth canal colonized with *Candida*. Fetal loss may be as high as 50% in instances where the fungus invades the placenta. Infants born to mothers with cryptococcosis are without illness, indicating the lack of placental transfer of the fungus. Data on the effects, if any, of maternal histoplasmosis on the fetus are scarce.

Pediatric. Children have an increased risk of systemic toxicity from topically applied drugs for two reasons. First, because of their greater surface area–to-weight ratio, a given amount of applied drug represents a greater dose (in mg/kg) as compared with adults. Second, at least in preterm neonates, the permeability of the skin is increased (Chapter 3).

Older Adults. The physiologic changes of aging affect the skin. Progressive impairment of the peripheral vascular circulation alters the cutaneous response to physical trauma, cold, or infection. Compared with a pediatric patient, the skin of an older adult is less permeable to drugs, perhaps because of the altered lipid content and loss of subcutaneous tissue (Chapter 4). Changes in the CNS modify the perception of itching and pain, and atrophy of the reticuloendothelial system may impair

the immune response. Also, emotional factors are certainly important and may prolong or exacerbate a skin disorder.

Cultural/Social Considerations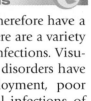

Many fungal infections are visible and therefore have a profound psychologic effect. Further, there are a variety of cultural attitudes toward illness and infections. Visually or physically disabling chronic skin disorders have been associated with chronic unemployment, poor mental health, and even suicide. Fungal infections of the genitourinary tract may suggest inappropriate sexual activity. In light of this, it is best not to assume, based on someone's ethnicity or financial status, that a certain ideal or belief is attached to the illness. Stereotyping inhibits an effective patient–health care provider relationship. It is better to ask the patient how he or she feels about the condition and to individualize care.

Physical Examination

The diagnosis of a superficial fungal disorder is based on one feature—the appearance of the skin lesion. Therefore, inspection, palpation, and measurements are essential in evaluating skin lesions. The examination should compare the left side of the body with the right side using a good light source. Lesions should be inspected for color, size, shape, margin characteristics, location and distribution (localized or generalized), texture, temperature, and odor. The examination should also determine the arrangement (clustered, linear, annular, diffuse, or dermatomal), whether the lesions are primary or secondary (see Chapter 67), and if there is evidence of healing.

Primary lesions develop without any preceding skin changes. In many cases primary lesions are not seen; thus, the health care provider must depend on the patient to describe how the lesion looked when it first appeared. Primary lesions include macules, papules, patches, plaques, nodules, wheals, vesicles, bullae, and pustules. Dermatologic diagnoses rely heavily on these primary lesions.

Secondary lesions result from changes in primary lesions and are influenced by scratching or infection. These changes may be brought about by the patient or the patient's environment and often occur in the epidermal layer of skin. Secondary lesions include scales, crusts, lichenification, keloids, scars, excoriations, atrophy, ulcers, and fissures.

Skin lesions may be observed in the perineal and intertriginous areas. They are usually moist, inflamed, pruritic areas with vesicles and pustules. Vaginal infection causes a cheesy vaginal discharge, burning, and itching. Intestinal infections may appear as diarrhea. Oral lesions appear as white patches that adhere to the buccal (inside cheek) mucosa. The patient with cryptococcosis, coccidioidomycosis, or histoplasmosis often complains of a cough, fever, malaise, and other pulmonary manifestations.

Laboratory Testing

Cultures are used to identify the specific type of fungus. Superficial infections can be diagnosed by microscopy and culture of skin scrapings, plucked (not cut) hairs, or nail clippings. Systemic infections are diagnosed by microscopy and culture of blood, spinal fluid, sputum, urine, feces, exudate, and tissue biopsy. Gram's stain or potassium hydroxide (KOH) testing determines the presence of mycelial fragments, arthrospores, and budding yeast cells. The use of a Wood lamp helps determine the presence of a fungus; in a darkened room, infected hair will fluoresce a bright yellow-green. Serologic testing is available, primarily in specialty laboratories, and helps establish the diagnosis of many mycoses.

GOALS OF THERAPY

The primary goal of treatment with most antifungal drugs is to prevent colonization of new organisms. In addition, treatment aims to control localized symptoms, avoid preventable adverse effects secondary to the use of systemic drugs, and prevent reinfection.

Treatment of fungal infections is related to the type and location of fungi and may include both topical and systemic formulations. Each antifungal drug has a distinct spectrum of antifungal activity and specific therapeutic uses. However, not all generic topical drugs are equivalent to their brand-name counterparts, either in potency or in the presence of ingredients that may cause further irritation or allergy.

INTERVENTION
Administration

Systemic Administration of Amphotericin B. The manufacturer's recommendations for preparation of intravenous amphotericin B should be followed. Use of an in-line IV filter is controversial. If an IV filter is used, it must be at least 1 micron in diameter. Disagreement also exists about the need to cover the IV tubing and fluid reservoir with foil. Agency policy should be followed; most agencies still cover the IV bag with an opaque plastic or paper bag. With the wrapping, the diluted solution is usually stable for 24 hours.

An infusion monitoring device should be used to assist in regulating the IV rate. The patient should not be left unattended for long periods. Too rapid an infusion is associated with arrhythmias. The diluted drug is a suspension; the bag or bottle should be gently agitated regularly during the infusion to promote uniform dilution. The patient should be checked and vital signs should be monitored for evidence of adverse effects. Febrile reac-

tions (fever, chills, headache, nausea) occur in 20% to 90% of patients, usually within 1 to 2 hours of initiation of the infusion and subside within 4 hours after the drug is discontinued. The severity of this reaction usually decreases with continued therapy. Other intravenous drugs should not be administered via the amphotericin B line without flushing well before and after the dose with 5% dextrose and water. If other intravenous drugs are to be administered during amphotericin B infusion, a separate IV access line should be started and maintained. If therapy is interrupted for more than a few days, it may be necessary to resume treatment with a low dosage and increase the dosage gradually to the desired level.

Amphotericin B commonly causes local inflammation or thrombosis at the injection site, particularly if extravasation occurs. Extravasation is more likely to occur in the older adult because of the loss of tissue elasticity. The infusion site should be checked at least every 8 hours or according to agency policy. The risk of thrombophlebitis may be reduced by using a scalp vein needle in the most distal vein possible, by alternating veins, by the addition of heparin or hydrocortisone (as prescribed) to the infusion, and by using alternate-day dosing schedules.

Some health care providers prescribe prophylactic use (e.g., 1 hour before administration) of aspirin or acetaminophen for fever or headache. Codeine or other analgesics may also be used to treat headache. Antiemetics may be given 30 minutes before administration to help prevent nausea and vomiting. Meperidine given intravenously may be used to treat rigors (shaking chills). Mannitol may be administered before and after administration of amphotericin B to reduce nephrotoxic effects. Corticosteroids may be given before and after the drug to help prevent adverse effects.

Keep the health care provider informed of changes in the patient's condition. Monitor the blood count (CBC) and differential, platelet count, blood glucose level, serum creatinine level, BUN level, liver function test results, and the serum electrolyte level. In addition, with amphotericin B cholesteryl complex, monitor the prothrombin time (PT) and the patient for unexplained bruising or bleeding. Monitor intake and output (I&O) and weight. Report immediately oliguria, any change in the I&O ratio or appearance of urine (e.g., sediment, pink or cloudy urine), abnormal laboratory test results, or unusual weight gain or loss. Generally, renal damage is reversible if the drug is discontinued when the first signs of renal dysfunction appear.

Topical Administration of an Antifungal Drug. Consult with the health care provider for instructions for cleansing the lesion(s) before applying antifungal creams and ointments. Wear gloves while applying small amounts of the drug to the affected area. Avoid the use of occlusive dressings unless directed by the health care provider because these dressings increase absorption of the drug.

Shake aerosol powders or solutions well before using. Hold the spray opening 6 to 10 inches from the area to be treated, and spray well. Caution the patient not to inhale the powder or solution and avoid the eyes. Sprinkle powder forms liberally on the affected area. When treating the toes and feet, make certain the drug reaches the area between the toes and the bottom of the feet. Sprinkle or spray the drug onto socks or in shoes as directed by the health care provider.

If a liquid formulation of the drug is to be used orally (e.g., nystatin), the patient may be asked to "swish and swallow" or "swish and spit." Ask the patient to hold the drug in the mouth, swish, and gargle for as long as possible before swallowing or spitting the remaining drug out.

Have the patient dissolve troches or lozenges in the mouth. These formulations are usually designed for slow release over several minutes. The patient should swallow the saliva as needed but should not chew or break the lozenge. Advise the patient to avoid drinking, eating, or smoking until the troche has dissolved. Warn the patient not to permit children younger than 5 years to have lozenges because they may choke on them. For fungus on dentures, instruct the patient to soak the dentures in nystatin solution. In rare instances it may be necessary to have new dentures made.

Vaginal Administration of an Antifungal Drug. In most cases the patient with a vaginal fungal infection self-treats with an OTC antifungal drug. When the nurse administers the drug, the patient should be asked to lie in the dorsal recumbent position or Sims' position. After preparing the drug according to the manufacturer's recommendations and putting on gloves, gently spread the labial folds. The rounded end of the suppository is inserted into the vagina and directed along the posterior wall 5 to 7 cm (2 to 3 inches). If an applicator device is used for administration, it is inserted into the vagina 5 to 7 cm (2 to 3 inches), and the plunger depressed to release the drug into the vagina. Your finger or the device is then withdrawn. The patient is asked to remain on her back for at least 10 minutes.

Azole antifungal drugs for vaginal use may cause the latex in condoms, diaphragms, or cervical caps to weaken and break, so these forms of birth control will be unreliable. The patient should use an alternative method of birth control. Drugs in this group include butoconazole, clotrimazole, econazole, miconazole, terconazole, and tioconazole. Remind women that no drugs, even topical ones, should be used during pregnancy or lactation without prior consultation with the health care provider.

Topical treatment should be discontinued promptly if signs of hypersensitivity, irritation, or worsening of lesions occurs.

Education

The patient and family should be informed that systemic fungal infections are not contagious; however, superficial fungal infections are highly contagious. The importance of handwashing should be emphasized repeatedly. Parents of children with a fungal infection should be taught how to care for the child. In some cases, the child may need to stay home from school until the treatment regimen is established and the child is responding.

Tinea infections can be prevented by educating the patient, especially parents, about the danger of acquiring the infection from infected children as well as from dogs, cats, and other animals. The fungus is transmitted by direct skin-to-skin contact or indirect contact, especially from the backs of theater seats, barber clippers, toilet articles such as combs and hairbrushes, or clothing and hats contaminated with hair from infected persons or animals.

Tinea cruris (jock itch) and tinea corporis (ringworm) infections can be prevented with thorough laundering of towels and clothing with hot water and fungicidal agents. Maintaining general cleanliness in showers and dressing rooms of gymnasiums and frequent hosing and rapid draining of shower rooms may help. Careful attention to drying and ventilation of intertriginous areas can help prevent candidiasis.

The risk of tinea pedis (athlete's foot) may be reduced by advising the patient to carefully dry the feet, especially between the toes, after bathing or showering. Instruct the patient to avoid wearing socks made of materials that hold moisture and to wear clean cotton socks and change them at least daily. Tell the patient to wear sandals or well-ventilated shoes with air holes and to rotate shoes so that they can dry thoroughly between wearings. The patient should be instructed to use an absorbent powder or antifungal powder, but should not apply the powder at the same time as the antifungal creams, lotions, or solutions.

Onychomycosis is transmitted presumably by direct contact with skin or nail lesions of infected persons and possibly from contaminated floors and shower stalls. However, patients need to be advised that there is a low rate of transmission, even to close family members. The patient and family members should be advised that cleanliness and the use of a fungicidal agent for disinfecting floors in common use, and frequent hosing and rapid draining of shower rooms reduce organism growth.

The risk of cryptococcosis can be reduced by wearing masks when working around old pigeon nests and droppings. The risk of histoplasmosis can be reduced by teaching the patient to avoid old chicken houses, caves harboring bats, and starling and blackbird roosts. Rodent burrows are the reservoir for coccidioidomycosis. The fungus can be transmitted to humans, cattle, cats, dogs, horses, burros, sheep, swine, coyotes, chinchillas, llamas, and other animals given the appropriate temperature, moisture, and soil requirements. Thus the patient may be told to avoid dusty occupations, such as road building.

Patients who are immunocompromised should be advised to contact their health care provider as soon as possible for early detection and treatment of oral, esophageal, or genitourinary tract candidiasis to prevent systemic spread. In addition, these patients should be advised to decrease their exposure to environmental fungi. For example, soil-containing plants should be disposed of or removed from the patient's immediate environment. Regular inspection of air-conditioning systems should also be performed.

EVALUATION

Treatment effectiveness can be demonstrated by a decrease in skin irritation and resolution of infection. Early relief of symptoms may be seen in 2 or 3 days. However, for *Candida*, tinea cruris, and tinea corporis, 2 weeks or more of therapy may be needed before improvement becomes evident. For tinea pedis, therapeutic response may take as much as 3 to 4 weeks. Treatment effectiveness for vulvovaginal candidiasis is noted as a decrease in skin irritation and vaginal discomfort. Therapeutic response is usually observed after 1 week. Recurrent fungal infections may be a sign of systemic illness.

The response rate for topical therapy usually decreases with repeated episodes, as evidenced by an increased time needed to achieve symptomatic relief with each new episode as well as a shortening of the symptom-free interval between episodes. In this case, a

---

CASE STUDY    *Vaginal Candidiasis during Pregnancy*

ASSESSMENT

HISTORY OF PRESENT ILLNESS

MR is an 18-year-old woman scheduled for an episodic visit. She states, "I have a vaginal discharge that I want checked out. It is a thick white discharge that makes me really itch, and it burns a little when I urinate. We used condoms most of the time, but I am scared that I might have a sexually transmitted disease. I would like the pill you take one time."

HEALTH HISTORY

MR has no known allergies. She has had no past hospitalizations or surgeries. She has had all childhood immunizations except for hepatitis B.

LIFESPAN CONSIDERATIONS

MR is attempting to develop a personal lifestyle, trying to establish a relationship with her significant other, and trying to form a commitment to something. She is in the stage of identity versus role confusion.

CULTURAL/SOCIAL CONSIDERATIONS

MR's parents divorced when she was 14 years old. She has lived on the streets ever since, supporting herself by panhandling. Her current boyfriend also lives on the streets. She denies knowledge of being pregnant.

PHYSICAL EXAMINATION

MR's temperature is 98.6° F, pulse 74, respirations 20, and blood pressure 136/76 mm Hg. MR is 5'1" tall, weighs 135 pounds, and has a body mass index (BMI) of 26. Her vulva has no lesions or redness; vagina has a moderate amount of white, cottage cheese–like discharge; cervix is nulliparous, with no lesions or negative cervical motion tenderness; her uterus is at 16- to 20-week size; the adnexa is nontender and there is no enlargement bilaterally.

LABORATORY TESTING

Wet prep: negative whiff test; vaginal pH is 4.2; hyphae are present. Urine pregnancy test result is positive. Urine dipstick test result is negative for leukocytes or nitrites.

PATIENT PROBLEM(S)

Vaginal candidiasis in context of pregnancy.

GOALS OF THERAPY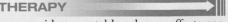

Control symptoms; avoid preventable adverse effects secondary to use of systemic drugs; prevent reinfection.

CRITICAL THINKING QUESTIONS

1. MR is given a sample of 1% clotrimazole vaginal cream (500 mg) for one-time use. The Centers for Disease Control and Prevention recommend a longer regimen for candidiasis in pregnant women. If this is so, why was MR given a one-time dose?
2. MR is disappointed that she cannot take the "one-time pill." What is your response to her disappointment?
3. What is the mechanism of action of clotrimazole?
4. What adverse effects may occur with vaginal clotrimazole?
5. What suggestions can be made that will help MR prevent future vaginal candidiasis infections?

change may be made to systemic antifungal therapy. Systemic therapy may be warranted if persistent symptoms are severe enough to warrant the increased expense and potential risk of adverse effects or drug interactions. A combination of topical and systemic therapy is not recommended, as it usually does not increase efficacy.

Bibliography

Anonymous. Clinical update: practical summaries of recent guidelines. Fungal infections: guidelines for treatment, *J Resp Dis* 22(1):54-58, 2001.

Linc LG, Campbell JM, Kinion ES: Infections in patients receiving cytotoxic chemotherapy, *Medsurg Nurs* 10(2):61-70, 2001.

Maertens J, Vrebos M, Boogaerts M: Assessing risk factors for systemic fungal infections, *Eur J Cancer Care* 10(1):56-62, 2001.

Michaud D: Liposomal amphotericin B for the treatment of severe fungal infection, *Dynamics* 12(1):17-21, 2001.

Shelton BK: Opportunistic fungal infections in the critically ill, *Crit Care Nurs Clin N Am* 12(3):323-340, 2000.

Weller IV, Williams IG: ABC of AIDS: treatment of infections, *BMJ* 322(7298):1350-1354, 2001.

Internet Resource

Medical Letter: Caspofungin (Cancidas) for Aspergillosis. Available online at http://www.medicalletter.com(#108).

CHAPTER

33

Antitubercular and Other Mycobacterial Drugs

SHERRY F. QUEENER • KATHLEEN GUTIERREZ

 Visit http://evolve.elsevier.com/Gutierrez/ for additional information.

KEY TERMS

Directly observed therapy (DOT), p. 502

Leprotic reactions, p. 505

Multibacillary leprosy, p. 505

Multidrug resistance (MDR), p. 496

Mycobacterium avium **complex (MAC),** p. 507

Paucibacillary leprosy, p. 505

Tuberculosis (TB), p. 493

OBJECTIVES

- Explain why drug therapy for mycobacterial diseases must continue for years.
- Describe the uses of isoniazid and identify which patients are most at risk for severe reactions.
- Discuss why drug combinations are commonly used for tuberculosis and leprosy.
- Develop a nursing care plan for a patient receiving drug therapy for tuberculosis, leprosy, or *Mycobacterium avium* complex.

PATHOPHYSIOLOGY • Tuberculosis

Tuberculosis (TB) is an ancient affliction that remained a major cause of death in Europe well into modern times. Most cases were concentrated in cities where human populations were most dense. It is estimated that about 20% of all deaths in London in the eighteenth century were caused by tuberculosis. In the nineteenth century, as many as 33% of deaths in Paris may have been linked to the disease. These high death tolls, more or less matched by those of densely populated cities in the Americas, drove medical and public health authorities to push for better methods of control. By the early twentieth century, public health measures included quarantine of infected individuals and bolstering of the immune system with good nutrition and bed rest. The first effective drugs for tuberculosis were introduced in the 1940s and 1950s.

Public health measures and effective drug therapy led to a decline in cases of tuberculosis in the United States, but by 1986 the decline stalled, and in fact the number of cases once again began to rise. Reported cases in the United States numbered over 16,000 in 2000. Foreign-born persons, though representing a small minority of the population, accounted for 46% of the reported cases of tuberculosis in the United States in 2000, according to the Centers for Disease Control and Prevention (see Internet Resource). Most of those cases occurred in persons described as Hispanic or Asian/Pacific Islander. These numbers suggest that increased immigration from areas where this disease has remained endemic has contributed to its recent rise in the United States.

Another factor contributing to the persistence of tuberculosis in the United States is the epidemic of HIV infection and AIDS. Persons with AIDS are highly susceptible to opportunistic infections, including tuberculosis. Because of the overlap of risk groups, the index of suspicion for tuberculosis should be high in HIV-infected persons. Similarly, the index of suspicion for HIV infection should be high in persons diagnosed with tuberculosis (Box 33-1).

Tuberculosis is produced by *Mycobacterium tuberculosis* or, less commonly, by other mycobacteria harbored by cattle or birds. Two features of *M. tuberculosis* are especially important for understanding how they produce disease in humans. First is the interaction of *M. tuberculosis* with macrophages: rather than being killed by phagocytosis, *M. tuberculosis* resists the acids and enzymes that usually destroy bacteria within macrophages. The macrophages thus transport the bacteria to many organs and sites in the body as well as protect the bacteria from some drugs that poorly penetrate cells. Second, mycobacteria are relatively slow-growing organisms. These organisms grow best in strongly aerobic environments but very slowly in less favorable sites. This slow growth contributes to the difficulty encountered in treating the disease, because it is during active growth that an organism is most susceptible to metabolic interference by drugs.

Tuberculosis may occur in several forms. The initial or *primary infection* usually occurs in the lungs as a result of inhaling droplets containing live *M. tuberculosis*. These infective aerosols are generated when a patient with an active infection coughs or sneezes. The tiny droplets that spread into the air quickly dry out, leaving behind microscopic particles of dust that can remain in the air for hours. The organism is not harmed by drying and may remain alive on the particle unless inactivated by UV irradiation from sunlight or other sources. Once inhaled into the alveoli, *M. tuberculosis* is phagocytized and reproduces within macrophages. Infected macrophages

---

BOX 33-1   **Groups at High Risk for Tuberculosis**

The Centers for Disease Control and Prevention recognizes the following groups as having a higher incidence of tuberculosis in the United States:

• Patients with medical factors that increase their risk of developing active disease (e.g., persons with HIV)
• Racial or ethnic minorities (e.g., Native Americans, Alaskan Natives, Hispanics, African Americans, Asians, and Pacific Islanders)
• Intravenous drug users and those who abuse alcohol
• Immigrants to the United States born in countries where the disease is endemic
• Members of low-income population groups who do not receive routine medical evaluations
• People living in close environments with persons suspected or known to have the disease
• Residents of nursing homes, correctional facilities, mental institutions, and other long-term care facilities
• The homeless population

---

may remain in the lungs or may enter the lymphatic system or the bloodstream and be carried throughout the body. In response to the increasing number of tubercle bacilli in the lungs, a pneumonia-like condition may develop within 4 to 12 weeks. This inflammatory response may continue for a few weeks, but in most people this process is finally halted by the delayed immune reaction provoked by the infection. Lesions within the lungs resolve when infective loci become calcified. Living tubercle bacilli no longer appear in sputum at this stage, and the disease is said to be inactive.

Reactivation may occur months or years after the primary infection. When relapse occurs, localized areas again become sites of active multiplication of tubercle bacilli. Local necrosis develops while the cellular immunity factors attempt to isolate the infection. Necrosis may spread as a result of this inflammatory response and may cause large cavities within the lungs or other tissues (Figure 33-1).

Miliary tuberculosis is a disseminated form of the disease. It is accompanied by lesions in many organs and tissues of the body such as the pleura, brain, kidneys, and bone. Patients usually exhibit a fever of unknown origin. Other possible forms include a type of meningitis and bone or joint infections.

M. tuberculosis, like most bacteria, can acquire resistance to drugs. Development of resistance is common when patients are treated with a single drug. To minimize this complication, multidrug therapy (MDT) is used. The rationale for this therapy is simple: when two drugs with different mechanisms of action are administered to-

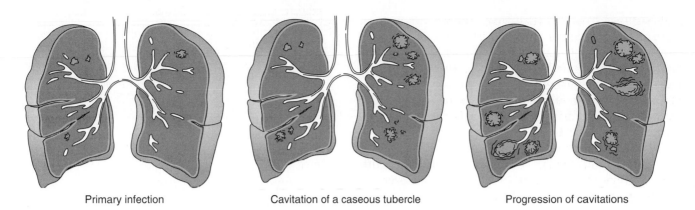

Primary infection   Cavitation of a caseous tubercle   Progression of cavitations

FIGURE 33-1 Tubercular lesions may occur in any lobe of the lung. Lesions in various stages of development and resolution are noted: primary infections, cavitation of a caseous tubercle, and progression of the cavitations with erosion into bronchi. Cavitations are illustrated as open blue areas.

TABLE 33-1

Treatment Regimens for Tuberculosis

Patient Criteria	Treatment Schedule
Option 1 Born in United States; never treated for tuberculosis; low risk of drug-resistant *Mycobacterium*	Isoniazid, rifampin, and pyrazinamide daily for 2 months; then isoniazid and rifampin daily or twice weekly for 4 to 22 months
Option 2 Born in United States; never treated for tuberculosis; risk of drug-resistant *Mycobacterium*	Isoniazid, rifampin, ethambutol, and pyrazinamide daily for 6 to 24 months
Option 3 Non–HIV-infected patient; isoniazid resistance >4% locally; drugs taken under direct observation	Isoniazid, rifampin, pyrazinamide, and streptomycin for 8 weeks; isoniazid and rifampin daily or 2 or 3 times weekly for 16 weeks if bacteria are susceptible
Option 4 Non–HIV-infected patient; drugs taken under direct observation	Isoniazid, rifampin, pyrazinamide, and streptomycin daily for 2 weeks, then twice weekly for 6 weeks; isoniazid and rifampin twice weekly for 16 more weeks
Option 5 Non–HIV-infected patient; drugs taken under direct observation	Isoniazid, rifampin, pyrazinamide, and streptomycin or ethambutol three times weekly for 6 months
Option 6 HIV-infected patient; drugs taken under direct observation	Options 3, 4, or 5 but continued for at least 9 months and at least 6 months beyond culture conversion
Option 7 Known drug-resistant *Mycobacterium*; prior therapy for tuberculosis in culture	Option 5 plus one or two other drugs to include at least 3 drugs demonstrated effective

gether, the organism must acquire two independent mutations to become resistant to both drugs. Because mutations are rare, the likelihood of simultaneously acquiring two specific mutations is small. Using three or more drugs lowers the probability of developing resistance even further. The options for treating tuberculosis use three to six drugs initially and continue for 6 to 24 months (Table 33-1). Treated patients rapidly cease to be infectious, but therapy must be continued for long periods to eliminate most of the dormant tubercle bacilli.

Resistance to individual drugs approaches 10% in both the United States and Canada (Table 33-2). Multidrug resistance (MDR) occurs in 2.2% of tuberculosis cases in the United States, but nearly 50% of those cases occurred in New York City. Multidrug resistance is seen in 1% of tuberculosis cases in Canada, but overall resistance to any tuberculosis drug is 11.2%. Other parts of the world have a greater incidence of multidrug-resistant tuberculosis: Africa, China, Estonia, India, Iran, Latvia, Romania, Russia, and South American countries have an incidence rate of over 3% among primary cases.

The properties and uses of antituberculosis drugs are discussed in the following sections, with the drugs considered in order of their clinical importance.

TABLE 33-2		
Tuberculosis Resistance to Primary Drugs		
	Resistance (% of Total Cases Reported)	
Drug	*United States**	*Canada†*
ethambutol	2.2%	1.4%
isoniazid	8.4%	7.4%
rifampin	3.0%	1.2%
pyrazinamide	3.0%	2.1%
streptomycin	6.2%	5.5%
MDR‡	2.2%	1.0%

*Data from the Centers for Disease Control and Prevention, 1993-1996, as reported in *JAMA* 278:833-837, 1997.
†Data from the Canadian Tuberculosis Laboratory Surveillance System (http://www.hc-sc.gc.ca/hpb/cdc/publicat/tbdrc98)
‡Defined as resistance to at least isoniazid and rifampin.

DRUG CLASS • Primary Drugs Used to Treat Tuberculosis

 isoniazid (Laniazid, Isotamine,✳ Nydrazid, PMS Isoniazid✳)
  isoniazid + rifampin (Rifamate)
  isoniazid + rifampin + pyrazinamide (Rifater)

MECHANISM OF ACTION

Isoniazid is a potent inhibitor of mycolic acids involved in cell wall synthesis and also blocks pyridoxine (vitamin B_6) use in a number of intracellular enzymes. Isoniazid is bactericidal and affects both intracellular (within macrophages) and extracellular mycobacteria.

Mycobacteria rapidly acquire resistance to isoniazid. In early trials when isoniazid was used alone to treat active pulmonary tuberculosis, 11% of the patients carried isoniazid-resistant strains at the end of 1 month of therapy. At the end of 3 months, 71% of these patients harbored resistant mycobacteria. Observations such as these have led to the clinical practice of combining isoniazid therapy with one or more drugs (see Table 33-1).

USES

Isoniazid is considered to be the most useful antituberculosis drug. It is available as a single formulation and in combination with other antituberculosis drugs.

Isoniazid may be used alone for prophylaxis. The drug is prescribed for patients and others with known exposure to tuberculosis or those who have recently converted from negative to positive reactions in the skin test for the disease. These people usually have fewer mycobacteria than would be found in an active, symptomatic case, and for them the use of isoniazid alone may be successful.

PHARMACOKINETICS

Isoniazid is well absorbed after oral administration, achieving a peak serum level in 1 to 2 hours. Bactericidal concentrations are found in most tissues, including pleural fluids and caseous exudates surrounding active loci of infection in lungs.

Isoniazid undergoes several biotransformations in liver, most resulting in an inactive form of the drug, which is excreted primarily by the kidneys. The major metabolite is an acetylated form. The rate of drug acetylation differs significantly among population groups, and two genetically determined types may be distinguished. Rapid acetylators inactivate isoniazid two to three times as rapidly as slow acetylators. As would be expected, rapid acetylators have lower blood levels of the active drug than slow acetylators, but both types of patients respond well to standard therapeutic doses given once daily. Increasing the dosage or frequency of administration in slow acetylators is not wise, because these patients tend to be more prone to adverse effects. Slow acetylators include 45% to 65% of people of northern European descent and African Americans. Asian and Alaskan Native populations contain predominantly rapid acetylators.

ADVERSE REACTIONS AND CONTRAINDICATIONS

Isoniazid reactions occur in a small percentage of patients. The most commonly encountered adverse reaction is peripheral neuropathy. Patients with diabetes or alcoholism and malnourished persons are more prone to this complication than the general population. At least some of these reactions are related to low vitamin B_6 (pyridoxine) levels, which may be prevented by taking the vitamin daily. Peripheral neuropathy is more likely to occur in slow acetylators.

Various other reactions, including allergies, blood dyscrasias, gastric distress, and metabolic acidosis, have occasionally been reported with isoniazid.

TOXICITY

Hepatotoxicity is the most serious adverse effect associated with isoniazid. Fatal liver failure has occurred even among patients receiving the drug for prophylaxis. Hepatitis caused by isoniazid is rare among patients less than 20 years old and occurs in patients 20 to 34 years old at a rate of approximately 3 cases per 1000 patients (0.3%). In patients more than 50 years old, the incidence increases to 23 cases per 1000 patients (2.3%). Patients also have an increased risk of hepatitis if they are rapid acetylators of the drug, if they ingest ethanol daily, or if they also receive the drug rifampin. Liver function should be monitored in all patients receiving isoniazid. Symptoms of hepatitis include anorexia, dark urine, jaundice, nausea, fatigue, or weakness.

INTERACTIONS

Isoniazid may enhance biotransformation, thus reducing the effectiveness of the antifungal drug ketoconazole. In contrast, biotransformation of alfentanil, carbamazepine, and phenytoin is inhibited by isoniazid, and serum concentrations of these drugs may increase when isoniazid is given. Isoniazid should never be given with other hepatotoxic drugs because of the increased risk of hepatic failure.

Rifamycins

   rifampin (generic, Rifadin, Rimactane, Rofact✷)

   rifampin + isoniazid (Rifamate)

   rifampin + isoniazid + pyrazinamide (Rifater)

   rifapentine (Priftin)

MECHANISM OF ACTION

Rifamycins inhibit DNA-dependent RNA polymerase in sensitive organisms. As a result, gene transcription halts, and protein synthesis ceases. Metabolic activity in the bacteria stops, and the bacteria ultimately die or are eliminated by host defenses. Rifamycins are bactericidal both for extracellular bacteria and for bacteria within macrophages and other cells.

Resistance to rifamycins can occur when the drugs are used alone against *M. tuberculosis*. Resistant strains have an altered DNA-dependent RNA polymerase that is no longer inhibited by the drugs.

USES

Rifampin is used as prophylaxis for *Neisseria meningitidis* and as therapy for tuberculosis. Rifampin is as potent as isoniazid against mycobacteria and distributes well to many sites where mycobacteria survive. These advantages have made rifampin a primary drug for combination treatment of tuberculosis.

Rifapentine is a new rifamycin and its use in standard protocols is being explored in clinical trials. One advantage of the drug is that it can be given twice weekly in the early phases of treatment and once weekly in the later stages, whereas rifampin is usually given two or three times weekly throughout therapy.

PHARMACOKINETICS

Rifamycins are adequately absorbed when given orally, regardless of the presence or absence of food. These drugs are relatively lipid soluble, which explains why they are found in higher concentrations in body tissues than in serum. Lipid solubility also explains their ability to penetrate white blood cells and to attack mycobacteria living there.

About 40% of a dose of rifampin is excreted in bile, with less in urine. The drug is also deacetylated by the liver to an active metabolite excreted via bile into feces. Rifapentine is eliminated in similar ways but tends to stay in the body longer than rifampin.

ADVERSE REACTIONS AND CONTRAINDICATIONS

Rifamycins can cause a variety of mild reactions such as gastrointestinal irritation and rashes. These drugs also turn body fluids such as tears, sweat, saliva, and urine an orange-red color, which might be mistaken for blood. This coloration is harmless, but it may stain certain items such as soft contact lenses.

Liver abnormalities may occur with rifampin. Mild abnormalities in liver function may return to normal without discontinuing the drug, but increases in alkaline phosphatase or the appearance of jaundice signals that it should be discontinued.

Intermittent doses of rifampin may cause an immune reaction associated with a variety of symptoms. This flulike syndrome may progress from chills, fever, vomiting, diarrhea, and myalgia to acute renal failure—death has even occurred. Because these symptoms occur when therapy is resumed, patients should be advised not to miss a dose of rifampin, especially if receiving relatively high dosages. Some treatment centers have significantly lowered rifampin dosages for intermittent therapeutic programs and have reduced these immune reactions. Instances of a flulike syndrome are also thought to be more frequent in patients who skip doses of rifapentine.

TOXICITY

Overdoses of rifampin can produce serious reactions, including generalized itching, facial edema, and mental status changes. Activated charcoal may be given orally as a slurry to remove unabsorbed or recirculated rifampin from the system. There has been no experience with overdoses of rifapentine. Neither rifampin nor rifapentine are cleared significantly by forced diuresis or hemodialysis.

INTERACTIONS

Rifamycins induce liver enzymes that biotransform drugs and hormones in humans. This process leads to several drug interactions. Patients receiving coumarin anticoagulants, oral hypoglycemic drugs, delavirdine, zidovudine, theophylline, phenytoin, methadone, various antiarrhythmics, verapamil, or digoxin may require higher doses of these drugs. Rifamycins should not be used with HIV protease inhibitors, because the levels of the antivirals fall below the effective range. Patients receiving oral contraceptives or replacement doses of cortisol may lose the effectiveness of these drugs because rifamycins accelerate breakdown of the steroids. Patients receiving isoniazid along with a rifamycin or patients who regularly use alcohol have an increased risk of drug-induced hepatitis.

Pyrazinamide

pyrazinamide (generic, Tebrazid✲)

MECHANISM OF ACTION

Pyrazinamide (PZA) may be bacteriostatic or bactericidal, depending on the site of infection and the strain of mycobacteria. The mechanism of action or resistance is unknown.

USES

Pyrazinamide is effective only against mycobacteria and is a primary drug for treatment of tuberculosis.

PHARMACOKINETICS

Pyrazinamide is rapidly and completely absorbed when given orally. This drug distributes freely to most tissues, including the brain. In the liver, the drug is converted in part to pyrazinoic acid, which is also active.

The renal elimination half-life for these compounds is 10 to 12 hours in normal persons but 22 to 26 hours when renal function is impaired.

ADVERSE REACTIONS AND CONTRAINDICATIONS

Pyrazinamide often causes joint pain, which may arise from hyperuricemia. Rarely, the drug may cause gouty arthritis or jaundice.

There are no contraindications to pyrazinamide, but the drug should be used cautiously in patients with impaired hepatic function or allergies to ethionamide, isoniazid, or niacin.

TOXICITY

Dosages of 40 to 50 mg/kg body weight daily, if sustained for prolonged periods, may cause hepatotoxicity.

INTERACTIONS

Drugs such as allopurinol, colchicine, probenecid, and sulfinpyrazone may be less effective when pyrazinamide is given because pyrazinamide tends to elevate the uric acid level in the blood.

Ethambutol

ethambutol (Myambutol, Etibi✲)

MECHANISM OF ACTION

Ethambutol (EMB) is most effective against actively dividing mycobacteria, but the precise antibacterial action is unknown. The drug is bacteriostatic. Resistance develops if the drug is used alone in therapy. However, it does not induce cross-resistance to other antituberculosis drugs.

USES

Ethambutol is a primary antituberculosis drug chemically unrelated to other antituberculosis drugs or antibiotics. It is effective only against mycobacteria and not against other bacteria, viruses, or fungi. It has become a first-line antituberculosis drug because of its relatively wide spectrum of activity against species of mycobacteria and because of its relatively low degree of toxicity.

PHARMACOKINETICS

Ethambutol is well absorbed from the GI tract in the presence or the absence of food. The peak serum concentration is observed 2 to 4 hours after an oral dose. This drug is less extensively biotransformed than isoniazid or rifampin, and up to 50% of the drug excreted in urine is in the unaltered active form. Fecal concentrations of the drug represent unabsorbed material as well.

Ethambutol has been detected in cerebrospinal fluid after oral therapy, although the level is below that found in plasma. The drug also concentrates in erythrocytes.

ADVERSE REACTIONS AND CONTRAINDICATIONS

Elevated uric acid levels have been reported in patients receiving ethambutol, potentially causing onset of gouty arthritis. The drug also causes confusion and headaches as well as GI disturbances.

Other reactions to ethambutol appear rarely. Allergic reactions have occasionally been reported. Peripheral neuritis can occur with higher dosages.

TOXICITY

A serious adverse reaction to ethambutol is visual disturbance. Some patients report changes in color vision, whereas others experience a more prominent loss of visual acuity. These signs are sufficient cause to terminate use of the drug. If it is discontinued when visual signs appear, the changes are reversible, although full recovery may take months. These visual changes are caused by optic neuritis and are more common with doses of 25 mg/kg body weight given for 2 months or longer. The drug should not be used in patients with preexisting optic neuritis.

INTERACTIONS

Ethambutol has been associated with few significant interactions but should not be used with other neurotoxic drugs.

Aminoglycoside

streptomycin (generic)

MECHANISM OF ACTION

Streptomycin inhibits protein synthesis in sensitive bacteria (see Chapter 29) and in mycobacteria. The drug is highly effective against most types of pathogenic mycobacteria with the exception of *M. avium*. Resistance develops quickly when the drug is used alone.

USES

The first antituberculosis drug to be discovered, streptomycin is still a reliable drug for initial therapy in multidrug regimens (see Table 33-1). It is commonly discontinued after the number of infective organisms has been greatly reduced (usually after 2 to 4 months), but other drugs are continued. Other aminoglycosides such as kanamycin or amikacin (see Chapter 29) have also been used to treat tuberculosis.

PHARMACOKINETICS

Streptomycin is not absorbed orally and must be given by intramuscular injection for routine clinical use. This route of administration restricts its use to the hospital or to a well-supervised outpatient program.

Streptomycin is well distributed in the body and may be used to treat nonpulmonary tuberculosis. It is excreted almost exclusively by renal mechanisms.

ADVERSE REACTIONS AND CONTRAINDICATIONS

Streptomycin can produce any reaction seen with other aminoglycoside antibiotics (see Chapter 29). Patients with renal insufficiency, older adults, and those receiving long-term therapy are more prone to develop adverse effects or toxic reactions.

TOXICITY

Ototoxicity is the most common reaction in patients with tuberculosis. Careful attention to maintaining the dosage within safe limits (see Chapter 29) prevents this reaction in most patients.

INTERACTIONS

Because streptomycin causes ototoxicity, it should not be combined with other ototoxic drugs, such as the diuretic ethacrynic acid. Patients receiving muscle relaxants along with streptomycin may experience excessive muscle relaxation, because this drug is a weak neuromuscular-blocking agent.

 DRUG CLASS • Miscellaneous Drugs Used to Treat Tuberculosis

aminosalicylate (Sodium P.A.S., Paskalium)
capreomycin sulfate (Capastat Sulfate)
cycloserine (Seromycin)
ethionamide (Trecator-SC)

MECHANISM OF ACTION

Aminosalicylate inhibits folic acid metabolism in mycobacteria. Cycloserine interferes with cell wall biosynthesis. The mechanism of capreomycin and ethionamide are unknown, but they may interfere with bacterial protein synthesis in different ways.

USES

These drugs are included in multidrug regimens when significant resistance to other drugs is expected.

PHARMACOKINETICS

Aminosalicylate, cycloserine, and ethionamide are efficiently absorbed when given orally, but capreomycin must be given intramuscularly. Distribution is adequate to most tissues, but only cycloserine and ethionamide achieve significant concentrations in the CNS. Excretion is primarily renal for all four drugs, but hepatic metabolism of ethionamide forms mostly inactive products.

ADVERSE REACTIONS AND CONTRAINDICATIONS

Most patients receiving aminosalicylate report gastric irritation, which may be relieved by taking the drug with food or antacids. Allergic symptoms, including exfoliative dermatitis and severe organ damage, have also been reported.

Nephrotoxicity is the most common adverse effect of capreomycin. The characteristic reactions to cycloserine include anxiety, confusion, depression, dizziness, irritability, nervousness, mood changes, and thoughts of suicide.

Ethionamide commonly causes anorexia, nausea, vomiting, a metallic taste in the mouth, and orthostatic hypotension. Jaundice, mental status changes, and peripheral neuritis are less common but do occur.

TOXICITY

High dosages or prolonged therapy with aminosalicylate may cause crystalluria or changes in thyroid function. High dosages of capreomycin increase the risk of ototoxicity or nephrotoxicity. High dosages of cycloserine increase the risk and severity of CNS reactions. Neurotoxicity from ethionamide may be reduced by giving pyridoxine (vitamin B$_6$).

INTERACTIONS

Aminobenzoates may block the absorption of aminosalicylate. Risk of nephrotoxicity, ototoxicity, and neuromuscular blockade with capreomycin is increased by aminoglycosides or loop diuretics. Use of cycloserine with alcohol or ethionamide increases the risk of seizures.

APPLICATION TO PRACTICE • Tuberculosis

ASSESSMENT
History of Present Illness

Characteristically, patients with active tuberculosis present with progressive symptoms of fatigue, lethargy, nausea, anorexia, weight loss, irregular menses, low-grade fevers, and night sweats. A cough accompanied by the production of mucoid, mucopurulent, or bloody sputum may also be noticed. Tight, dull, aching chest pain may accompany the cough. The chest pain may also be pleuritic, occurring as a result of inflammation to the parietal pleura. The signs and symptoms have often been attributed to the flu and ignored by the patient. The patient may seek medical attention only after chest pain or hemoptysis appears.

Health History

The patient's and family's health histories provide information helpful in selecting the appropriate treatment for tuberculosis. Ask about the patient's country of origin and any travel to foreign countries in which the disease is endemic. It is also important to note previous testing for tuberculosis and the results of that testing.

It should be determined whether the patient has received the bacillus Calmette-Guérin (BCG) vaccine. This vaccine contains attenuated bacilli and is routinely given in foreign countries to increase resistance to tuberculosis. BCG vaccination of uninfected persons is thought to induce sensitivity in more than 90% of those vaccinated. Recipients of the BCG vaccine have a positive skin test and should get a chest x-ray study to evaluate for tuberculosis. Protection given by the BCG may persist for as long as 20 years.

Lifespan Considerations

Perinatal. All pregnant women with active tuberculosis should receive antitubercular therapy, but it may be prudent to postpone prophylaxis until after delivery. The risks and benefits of antitubercular therapy should be discussed. The expectant mother should understand that problems associated with not treating the disease far outweigh the possible risks to her and her unborn child. Isoniazid, rifampin, and ethambutol have not been shown to have teratogenic effects. Streptomycin, capreomycin, and kanamycin should not be used during pregnancy because of documented fetal ototoxicity. The safe use of pyrazinamide and cycloserine during pregnancy has not been established. Pregnant women who are candidates for antitubercular therapy should not be discouraged from breastfeeding after delivery.

Pediatric. The incidence rate of tuberculosis has risen significantly in children, with a 36.1% increase in children up to 4 years old. A 34.1% rise has been noted in children 5 to 14 years old. These increases have been attributed in part to the many TB-positive persons immigrating to the United States.

Children are susceptible to both *M. tuberculosis* and *M. bovis*. The bovine type is a common source of infection in children in parts of the world where tuberculosis in cattle is not controlled or milk is not pasteurized. The morbidity and mortality rates are higher in girls than in boys, particularly in later childhood and adolescence.

Older Adults. The incidence of tuberculosis is higher among older adults (65 years of age and older) than in any other group except for HIV-positive persons in developing countries. In the older adult population, some persons were infected many years before antitubercular drugs were available. These persons may have been hosts to the dormant bacilli for many years. Tuberculosis among older adults is reactivated by several factors, including diabetes mellitus, poor nutrition, long-term corticosteroid therapy, smoking, alcohol use, and immunosuppression. Older adult residents of long-term care facilities are at greater risk than those in the general population. Careful screening for the disease is required in all long-term care facilities.

Cultural/Social Considerations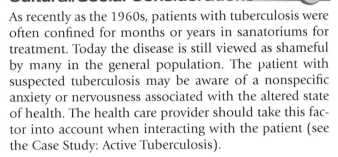

As recently as the 1960s, patients with tuberculosis were often confined for months or years in sanatoriums for treatment. Today the disease is still viewed as shameful by many in the general population. The patient with suspected tuberculosis may be aware of a nonspecific anxiety or nervousness associated with the altered state of health. The health care provider should take this factor into account when interacting with the patient (see the Case Study: Active Tuberculosis).

Physical Examination

The patient with tuberculosis may note a cough and sputum production, hemoptysis, fever, night sweats, malaise, anorexia, and a concomitant weight loss. Lymphadenopathy, pleuritic chest pain, and splenomegaly may also be noted.

Laboratory Testing

An acid-fast bacilli (AFB) stain can give a presumptive diagnosis in most cases. A positive sputum culture confirms the diagnosis of tuberculosis. For suspected pulmonary tuberculosis, at least three morning sputum samples for AFB stain and culture are obtained. Aerosol induction, gastric aspirate (in children), or bronchoalveolar lavage may be needed. Once treatment is started, sputum samples are again obtained to monitor the effectiveness of therapy.

A Mantoux test is useful for screening groups at high risk for developing tuberculosis. The Tine test is not recommended for screening. The purified protein derivative (PPD) is administered intradermally in the forearm, and the site is evaluated 72 hours after injection (Box 33-2). A positive reaction does not suggest active disease, but rather indicates exposure to the bacilli or dormant disease and the development of antibodies. Once a skin test

---

BOX 33-2 | Interpretation of Skin Testing for Tuberculosis and Leprosy

Tuberculosis

An indurated area 15 mm or larger is considered positive in all persons more than 4 years old who have no known risk factors.

A 10-mm or larger area of induration is considered positive in persons in the following higher-risk groups:

- Natives of high-prevalence areas in countries in Asia, Africa, Latin America, and Oceania
- Intravenous drug abusers
- Members of any of the medically underserved, low-income population groups, including high-risk racial or ethnic minorities (African Americans, Hispanic Americans, Native Americans, Eskimo Americans) and the homeless
- Residents of long-term care facilities (e.g., prisons, mental institutions) or congregate living settings
- Those who have medical conditions reported to increase the risk of tuberculosis: silicosis, gastrectomy, jejunoileal bypass, 10% or greater loss of body weight, chronic renal failure, diabetes mellitus, high-dose corticosteroid use, immunosuppressive therapies, hemato-

logic disorders (e.g., leukemia, lymphoma), and other malignancies
- Workers in the health care environment

A 5-mm or greater area of induration is considered positive in patients in the following high-risk groups:

- Those who are known to be HIV positive or who have an unknown HIV status and high-risk factors for infection
- Those who have or have had close or recent contact with patients or persons with confirmed active tuberculosis
- Those who have chest x-ray findings consistent with old, healed tuberculosis lesions

Leprosy

The presence of a nodule and a 3-mm or larger area of induration denotes a positive response in the tuberculoid and borderline tuberculoid forms of leprosy. Lepromatous and borderline lepromatous forms demonstrate a negative response to the lepromin test. With midborderline and indeterminate forms, the results are variable; the response demonstrates the patient's tendency toward either the tuberculoid or the lepromatous end of the immunologic spectrum and is of prognostic value.

is positive, a chest x-ray study or a CT scan of the chest is essential to rule out clinically active tuberculosis or to detect old, healed lesions.

Mycobacterium avium is the organism responsible for tuberculosis in patients with HIV. It is difficult to identify the disease in HIV-positive patients, in whom the skin test may be negative because of a weak immune response. Sputum cultures may also remain negative for acid-fast bacilli.

In the United States, it is mandatory for health care providers to report to the state public health officials all newly diagnosed cases of tuberculosis and situations where patients discontinue treatment prematurely. Detailed treatment records must be kept, including changes in the drug regimen, all bacteriologic reports, and the results of sensitivity testing.

GOALS OF THERAPY

Treatment goals for the patient with tuberculosis include eliminating the infectious state as quickly as possible and maintaining consistently negative sputum cultures thereafter. Preventing drug-resistant strains from forming and avoiding disease reactivation are equally important. To accomplish these goals, treatment is designed to eradicate three replicating populations of bacilli: those in cavitary lesions, those in closed caseous lesions, and those within macrophages.

Active Disease. There are two main principles of antitubercular therapy for active disease. First, treatment must consist of two or more drugs to which the bacilli are sensitive. Second, treatment must continue for at least 3 to 6 months after the sputum becomes negative. This practice sterilizes the lesions and prevents relapse. Because there are three different populations of bacilli, antitubercular drugs differ in their bacteriostatic and bactericidal activity. Furthermore, because *M. tuberculosis* is slow-growing and the disease is often chronic, patient compliance, drug toxicity, and the development of bacterial resistance present special therapeutic problems.

Drug-resistant tuberculosis arises when a health care provider fails to prescribe adequate drug therapy for an infection or the patient fails to take all the drugs as prescribed. One effective strategy for bringing patient compliance to near 100% is **directly observed therapy (DOT)**. This form of treatment requires that another person actually watch the patient as the prescribed drugs are taken. Drug resistance not only is a significant issue for the individual patient but also poses a public health threat, because drug-resistant forms of the disease can spread as readily as the native form.

Prophylaxis. Generally, the benefits of prophylaxis outweigh the risks of hepatotoxicity, the primary form of toxicity with isoniazid. However, prophylaxis is contraindicated in persons who have liver disease or who have had serious adverse reactions to this drug in the past. Persons over age 35 should not be routinely treated, because the risk of isoniazid-induced liver damage increases significantly with age. Prophylaxis should be reserved for TB-positive persons who have other factors placing them at increased risk (e.g., diabetes, leukemia, or drug-induced immunosuppression). Prophylaxis for a pregnant woman should be postponed until after delivery.

INTERVENTION
Administration

Therapy using antitubercular drugs requires special considerations. For example, when isoniazid is prescribed without supplemental pyridoxine (vitamin B_6), the patient should be monitored early for vitamin B_6 deficiency. The signs and symptoms of B_6 deficiency are irritability, seborrhea-like skin lesions, weakness, hypochromic microcytic anemias, impaired immune responses, and seizures (in infants). The prescribed drugs should be taken at the same time each day, and a high fluid intake maintained.

Rifampin, ethambutol, and pyrazinamide should be administered 1 to 2 hours after meals for best absorption and to reduce gastric irritation. If the patient has difficulty swallowing the rifampin capsules, they may be opened and the drug mixed with applesauce or jelly before administration. DOT is recommended in areas where patients do not complete at least 90% of the recommended therapy. This approach is feasible for patients taking their drugs daily, twice weekly, or three times a week. It improves compliance in both rural and urban settings and is cost-effective even though it requires additional resources (see Evidence-Based Practice box).

Education

Patients with tuberculosis should be taught to cover the mouth and nose when coughing or sneezing. Persons in close contact with those who cannot or will not cover their mouths when coughing should wear masks. Patients who have primary tuberculosis or whose sputum is bacteriologically negative but who do not cough and are known to be receiving adequate drug therapy need not be isolated. Hospitalization is necessary only for patients with severe illness and for whom medical or psychosocial circumstances make treatment outside the hospital difficult or impossible.

Most patients need careful instruction to manage their drug regimens properly. Compliance is a key factor in the success of drug treatment for tuberculosis, especially among specific high-risk populations. Patients should be questioned on a regular basis about adherence to drug regimens.

EVIDENCE-BASED PRACTICE
Directly Observed Therapy (DOT)

Setting

This form of therapy is used for two purposes. First, therapeutic compliance is ensured. The population groups at risk for tuberculosis include intravenous drug abusers, the homeless, and foreign-born persons. In these groups, as well as in others, compliance may be a problem. Directly observed therapy (DOT) ensures that the drugs are taken as prescribed so that the patient receives the maximum benefit from them. The second reason has to do with public health. Continuous, effective therapy reduces the period of infectiousness in active cases of tuberculosis, thus lowering the risk of spreading the disease. Noncompliance or early cessation of therapy also fosters the appearance of drug-resistant strains of *Mycobacterium tuberculosis*. Currently, multidrug-resistant *M. tuberculosis* accounts for 2.2% of cases nationwide, but these cases tend to be concentrated in the heavily urban areas of New York and California. Effective programs to identify active cases early and to treat by DOT with effective drug combinations may prevent tuberculosis from becoming an ever greater danger.

Fifty percent of patients with tuberculosis do not complete the treatment regimen. This situation may increase the incidence, morbidity, and mortality of the disease. Strategies to improve compliance with diagnostic regimens and drug therapy are therefore important.

Objective of Literature Review

To assess the success of DOT on cure rates and the rates of completion of treatment regimens in person treated for tuberculosis.

The search was carried out using The Cochrane Controlled Trials Register, the Cochrane Infectious Diseases Group specialized trials register, MEDLINE, EMBASE, and LILACS. In addition, reference lists from the articles were reviewed, and the retrieved studies searched for additional potentially relevant citations. Experts in the field were also contacted.

Criteria for Inclusion of Studies in Review of Literature

Investigators included randomized and quasi-randomized studies that compared self-treatment for tuberculosis with that of directly observed therapy. Outcomes were cure rates and rates for cure plus completion of treatment regimen.

Data Extraction and Analysis

Two reviewers independently performed the extraction and analysis of data and the quality of the studies.

Results of Review

Four studies were included in the review. There was no difference between self-treatment of tuberculosis and DOT on the outcomes of cure or cure plus completion of the treatment regimen. Analysis by the appointed agent (health care provider, lay health worker, family/community member) also revealed no important differences in the outcomes of either treatment strategy. One of the studies, which permitted patients to choose an agent, showed modest benefit for cure and cure plus completion of treatment regimen.

Investigators' Conclusions

There is no evidence that supports DOT as any more successful to the cure rate or the rate of completion of treatment regimen in patients with tuberculosis.

Volmink J, Garner P: Directly observed therapy for treating tuberculosis (Cochrane Review). In *The Cochrane Library*, Issue 2, Oxford, 2002, Update Software.

Spot urine and serum drug level testing and diligent record keeping should be done to validate compliance. Patients are advised to keep clinic appointments for drug dispensing, laboratory testing, and follow-up physical examinations. Public health officials should be notified if appointments are not kept. It may be beneficial to offer incentives for improved compliance, such as taxi fare to and from the clinic, food vouchers, or free day care.

Patients should be taught to recognize the signs and symptoms of drug-induced hepatitis (yellow eyes and skin, nausea and vomiting, anorexia, fatigue or weakness, or dark urine) and optic neuritis (eye pain, blurred and/or loss of vision) as well as hearing disturbances, dizziness, tinnitus, and vertigo. Regular eye examinations aid in the detection and follow-up of optic neuritis. Patients receiving rifampin should be warned that the drug may turn body fluids, including urine, a red-orange color and should be reassured that it is harmless. Patients should wear glasses instead of contact lenses to prevent discoloration of lenses while taking this drug.

EVALUATION

Diminished cough and sputum production, decreased fever and night sweats, amelioration of anorexia with a concomitant weight gain, and fewer bacilli in sputum specimens all constitute evidence of improvement. Successful therapy is further noted as an absence of observable bacilli in the sputum and in sputum cultures. Once sputum cultures are negative, usually in 3 to 6 months, therapy should continue for another 3 to 6 months. The patient's liver function parameters and electrolyte values should remain within normal limits.

Optic neuritis is closely followed through ophthalmologic examinations. Serum uric acid levels should remain within normal limits, and patient records should indicate that the patient is keeping follow-up appointments.

CASE STUDY  *Active Tuberculosis*

ASSESSMENT

HISTORY OF PRESENT ILLNESS

LR is a 47-year-old black woman who has had intermittent, dull chest pain for 2 months; other symptoms include fatigue, night sweats, and bloody sputum. LR has had an unintended 10-pound weight loss in the past 3 months.

HEALTH HISTORY

LR denies allergies to food or drugs. Her only hospitalization was at age 16 for an appendectomy. She has no known allergies. She has been on a 6-month regimen of methotrexate for seropositive rheumatoid arthritis, but denies other drug use. LR's diet is deficient in vitamins C and E.

LIFESPAN CONSIDERATIONS

LR may have less effective hepatic and renal function associated with aging.

CULTURAL/SOCIAL CONSIDERATIONS

LR is currently on active military duty and just returned from a remote 4-year assignment in Southeast Asia. She is single and lives on base in the barracks. She admits to a daily consumption of 16 ounces of alcohol and has a 25 pack/year smoking history. The military health care system provides health care and pharmacy services to patients without cost while on active duty.

PHYSICAL EXAMINATION

LR's blood pressure is 130/80 mm Hg; temperature 100.6° F, pulse 100 bpm, respirations 22 and labored with productive cough and hemoptysis. She weighs 120 pounds.

LABORATORY TESTING

LR's chest x-ray study reveals interstitial infiltrates, hilar enlargement, and cavitation in left upper lobe. Her sputum culture is positive for acid-fast bacilli; the Mantoux (PPD) test result is positive with 12 cm of induration. Results of the liver function tests are within normal limits.

PATIENT PROBLEM(S)

Active tuberculosis.

GOALS OF THERAPY

Render the patient noninfectious; prevent bacilli replication and resistance; and reduce organism count.

CRITICAL THINKING QUESTIONS

1. Isoniazid, rifampin, ethambutol, and pyrazinamide are prescribed for 2 months, then isoniazid and rifampin for 4 months; this is to be continued 3 to 6 months after sputum cultures are negative. Supplemental pyridoxine is also prescribed to minimize the potential for peripheral neuritis. Which factors may make self-administration of this drug regimen difficult for this patient?
2. Which factor in LR's history generally contraindicates the use of isoniazid and pyrazinamide?
3. Which two primary factors contribute to antitubercular drug resistance?
4. Which laboratory tests are required to monitor LR's antitubercular therapy?

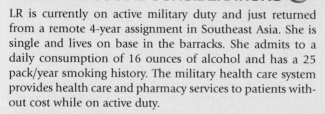

PATHOPHYSIOLOGY • Leprosy

Leprosy (Hansen's disease) is a chronic bacterial infection occurring in approximately 12 million people worldwide. However, 95% of the population have a natural immunity to this disease. In the 5% susceptible to infection, the disease occurs as a result of altered cell-mediated immunity. The areas of the world where leprosy is endemic are South and Southeast Asia, including the Philippines, Indonesia, some Pacific islands, India, Bangladesh, and Myanmar (formerly Burma), as well as tropical Africa. The disease also occurs in the colder climates of Tibet, Nepal, Korea, and Siberia. Between 300 and 500 cases currently occur each year in the United

States, primarily in California, Hawaii, Texas, Florida, Louisiana, New York City, and Puerto Rico. The rise in leprosy in the United States has been attributed to immigration from endemic areas.

Leprosy is caused by *Mycobacterium leprae*, a slow-growing bacillus. Humans are the only significant reservoir. The exact mode of transmission is not clearly understood, but household or prolonged close contact appears to be important. Millions of bacilli are shed daily in the nasal secretions of untreated late-stage patients. Bacilli remain viable for at least 7 days in dried nasal secretions. Cutaneous ulcerations may also shed large numbers of bacilli. In children less than 1 year old, transmission is presumed to have been transplacental. The incubation period for leprosy ranges from 9 months to 40 years.

The World Health Organization classifies leprosy either as **paucibacillary** (if it is characterized by one to five lesions) or as **multibacillary** (in which patients show six or more lesions). The skin lesions range from macular lesions showing loss of hair and alterations in the perception of light touch, pain, and temperature to extensive thickened lesions with sensory loss.

Leprosy is curable with appropriate drug therapy (Box 33-3). **Leprotic reactions** (manifestations of delayed hypersensitivity to *M. leprae*) occur in about 50% of patients during therapy. Type 1 reactions (also called reversal reactions) are seen in tuberculoid forms of leprosy. Type 2 reactions, seen in patients with more extensive disease, are characterized by raised, tender, intracutaneous nodules, severe constitutional symptoms, and high fever. A type 2 reaction is most often associated with therapy but may also be triggered in other situations. It is thought to be an Arthus type of reaction related to release of microbial antigens in patients harboring large numbers of bacilli. Leprotic reactions of either type may be controlled with prednisone or other immunosuppressives that may be used as treatment adjuncts.

BOX 33-3 | Multidrug Therapy of Leprosy

The World Health Organization is spearheading an effort to eradicate leprosy worldwide. That goal has been made possible by Multidrug Therapy (MDT) tailored to the stage of disease in the patient.

Paucibacillary leprosy, also known as tuberculoid disease, is noninfectious and occurs in people who mount strong cell-mediated defenses against the disease. MDT for this form of the disease may be rifampin (also called rifampicin) given once a month in a single supervised dose, along with dapsone given once daily.

Multibacillary leprosy, also called lepromatous leprosy, is infectious and represents a more extensive infection. MDT for this form of leprosy requires three drugs: dapsone and rifampin are used as noted above as well as clofazamine added as a daily dose along with an additional monthly supervised dose.

Standard therapy with MDT has been 24 months, the time thought to be required to eradicate the slow-growing *M. leprae* from the body. Recent clinical data has suggested that 12 months of carefully supervised therapy may be adequate for paucibacillary leprosy.

A further advance has occurred with the advent of single-dose therapy for paucibacillary leprosy in patients who have a single lesion. The drugs used in this combination are rifampin, ofloxacin (see Chapter 27), and minocycline (see Chapter 28).

This form of therapy has been in use worldwide since 1981 and has cured millions of the ancient scourge of leprosy. Directly observed therapy as part of these multidrug regimens is contributing to the success of the worldwide eradication program. Continued success depends not only upon the will to pursue the goal of eradication but also on stable social situations that enable patients to be treated continuously over the relatively long periods of time often required for a cure.

DRUG CLASS • Drugs Used to Treat Leprosy

dapsone (Avlosulfon*)

MECHANISM OF ACTION

Dapsone is an antifolate with actions much like the sulfonamides. The drug is bacteriostatic, and resistance can develop.

USES

Dapsone is used in MDT for treating leprosy (see Box 33-3). It is also used for dermatitis herpetiformis. Combined with trimethoprim, the drug has also been used for prophylaxis of *Pneumocystis carinii* pneumonia in AIDS patients.

PHARMACOKINETICS

Dapsone is slowly but almost completely absorbed when given orally. The drug distributes well to tissues. It is biotransformed in the liver and excreted in urine. Its elimination half-life ranges from 10 to 50 hours.

ADVERSE REACTIONS AND CONTRAINDICATIONS

Dapsone often causes rashes and potentially serious blood dyscrasias such as methemoglobinemia and hemolytic anemia. Symptoms include cyanosis, shortness of breath, bluish coloration to fingernails or lips, anorexia, paleness, and unusual fatigue and weakness.

Dapsone is usually avoided if possible in patients with preexisting anemia or glucose-6-phosphate dehydrogenase (G6PD) deficiency, which increases the risk of hemolytic anemia.

TOXICITY

At higher dosages, dapsone may cause gastric disturbances and CNS toxicity characterized by headache, insomnia, and restlessness. Overdose can lead to death by methemoglobin accumulation. Treatment may include intravenous infusion of methylene blue to preserve oxygenation of tissues.

INTERACTIONS

Dapsone requires an acidic environment for thorough oral absorption. Didanosine may block dapsone absorption because preparations of didanosine include strong buffers to reduce gastric acidity. To avoid unacceptable risk of hemolysis, dapsone should not be combined with other hemolytic drugs.

rifampin (Rifadin, Rimactane, Rofact✱)

Rifampin (RIF), also known as rifampicin, is used in the recommended MDT for leprosy (see Box 33-3). It is probably the single most effective bactericidal drug against *M. leprae*. The properties of rifampin are covered in the earlier section on tuberculosis.

clofazimine (Lamprene)

MECHANISM OF ACTION

Clofazimine is a dye capable of binding DNA in *M. leprae* and may thus block appropriate use of the nucleic acid. The result is a weak bactericidal action. A secondary action of clofazimine is its antiinflammatory effect, which lessens or prevents some of the leprotic reactions that would otherwise occur with effective therapy.

USES

Clofazimine is used in MDT (see Box 33-3) for multibacillary leprosy. Strains of *M. leprae* that acquire resistance to dapsone remain sensitive to clofazimine. The drug was tested in combinations against *M. avium* in AIDS patients, but clinical trial data suggested that the drug actually lowered the survival rate; thus clofazimine is no longer included in multidrug regimens for *M. avium* in AIDS patients.

PHARMACOKINETICS

Clofazimine is adequately absorbed orally and distributes to tissues, where it seems to accumulate. The drug is also excreted in breast milk.

ADVERSE REACTIONS AND CONTRAINDICATIONS

Because clofazimine is a dye, it can produce a strong reddish or brownish discoloration to the skin of individuals treated with the drug. Tears, sweat, sputum, urine, and feces may also be discolored. Gastrointestinal effects have also been noted, including diarrhea, loss of appetite, nausea, and vomiting. Blood in the stool may indicate serious drug-related adverse reactions and should be reported to the health care provider.

Skin rashes may occur with clofazimine, and patients note increased sensitivity to sunlight. Use of a strong sunscreen is recommended in addition to avoiding sunlight when possible.

Clofazimine may be contraindicated in patients allergic to dyes of the same family as the drug. It is also not recommended for patients with liver disease or for use in nursing mothers.

INTERACTIONS

Drug interactions are not usually a major consideration in the use of clofazimine, but care should be exercised if the drug is taken with other drugs that may cause GI damage.

DRUG CLASS • **Miscellaneous Drugs Used to Treat Leprosy**

Alternate drugs for treating leprosy continue to be explored. The antituberculosis drug ethionamide has been used to treat leprosy. Antibiotics such as clarithromycin (see Chapter 26), minocycline (see Chapter 28), and ofloxacin (see Chapter 27) have also been used. Thalidomide is an orphan drug (see Chapter 3) that has also been tried for leprosy; this drug is strongly teratogenic and should never be used in women of childbearing age.

PATHOPHYSIOLOGY • *Mycobacterium avium* Complex

Patients in the latter stages of AIDS are increasingly debilitated from infections not seen in persons with intact immune systems. *Mycobacterium avium* complex (MAC) is one of those infections. *M. avium* and *Mycobacterium intracellulare* are the causative organisms.

M. avium can be inhaled in aerosols, leading to pulmonary infections. In persons with normal immune systems, granulomatous lesions form but gradually heal as the body clears the infection. However, in persons with severely compromised immune function, such as late-stage AIDS patients, granulomas do not form and the disease becomes disseminated. Symptoms may include abdominal pain, anemia, diarrhea, fever, and night sweats. Most organs of the body are involved, although the CNS is rarely included. Patients suffer generalized wasting, and their chance of survival is compromised unless therapy is instituted.

With HAART (see Chapter 31) now widely available for patients with HIV, the number of patients with severe immunosuppression is lower than it was in the past. As a result, the number of cases of disseminated *M. avium* infections is also lower. Effective prophylaxis for *M. avium* has also lowered the incidence rate of the disease.

DRUG CLASS • Drugs Used to Treat *Mycobacterium avium* Complex

rifabutin (Mycobutin)

MECHANISM OF ACTION

Rifabutin is a rifamycin and has a mechanism similar to others of its class, inhibiting DNA-dependent RNA polymerase in *M. avium* and *M. intracellulare*. Cross-resistance can develop with other rifamycins.

USES

Rifabutin is used only to prevent MAC in patients with advanced HIV disease. The drug is administered orally, once daily for life.

PHARMACOKINETICS

Rifabutin is a highly lipophilic drug that is well absorbed following oral administration, but absorption is decreased in about 20% of HIV-positive patients. It is widely distributed to body tissues and fluids and has a half-life of 45 hours. Its onset is rapid; the peak serum level is reached in 2 to 4 hours. The drug is biotransformed by the liver, and less than 5% is eliminated unchanged in the urine.

ADVERSE REACTIONS AND CONTRAINDICATIONS

Rifabutin often causes skin rashes, nausea, and vomiting. The drug also produces a reddish discoloration of body fluids such as urine, tears, sweat, and saliva; this effect is harmless.

Rifabutin should not be given to patients with active tuberculosis, because single-drug therapy is likely to cause development of resistance of *M. tuberculosis* to rifampin, one of the primary drugs for treating tuberculosis.

TOXICITY

Overdosage of rifabutin may cause uveitis, with vision loss and pain in the eye.

INTERACTIONS

Rifabutin may decrease the plasma concentration of zidovudine, but clinical trials have not consistently shown this effect. Rifabutin lowers the plasma concentrations of HIV protease inhibitors, NNRTIs, estrogens, and oral contraceptive drugs. Patients should be counseled to use an alternative, nonhormonal form of contraception throughout therapy with rifabutin.

Macrolides

clarithromycin

Clarithromycin (see Chapter 26) is active against MAC and has been used successfully for therapy as well as for prophylaxis; however, because resistance develops easily, clarithromycin is best used in combinations. A close relative, azithromycin, has also been used for prophylaxis.

APPLICATION TO PRACTICE • Leprosy

ASSESSMENT
History of Present Illness

Elicit from the patient specific information about signs and symptoms related to the skin lesions, any contact with individuals known to have the disease, contact with armadillos (a naturally acquired form of leprosy has been found in armadillos), and immigration from or living for extended periods of time in endemic areas. Specific information to be obtained about the skin lesions includes the time since their appearance, their location, their characteristics, their quantity, and any associated manifestations. The health care provider should ask specifically about loss of sensation, the patient's reaction to the skin lesions, and any use of home remedies.

Health History

The health history provides information about allergies and injuries, hospitalizations not already described, and drug history. Patients with leprosy may have a history of sensorimotor dysfunction leading to deformities, which in turn contributes to accidents or injuries. A detailed family history may identify the source of the infection. A thorough drug history, including allergies, is necessary to determine the appropriate drugs for treating the infection.

Lifespan Considerations

Perinatal. Transmission of leprosy from an untreated infected mother to an infant is common. Pregnancy and the subsequent 6 months of lactation are said to result in an exacerbation in about 33% of patients with the disease. The fetal effects are said to include low birth weight, small placenta, and a high infant mortality rate.

Pediatric. Leprosy can manifest at any age, but it is seldom seen in children less than 3 years old. The physiologic immunodeficiency of the newborn may lead to an early colonization with the bacillus. The age-specific incidence rate peaks during childhood in most developing countries. Up to 20% of cases appear in children less than 10 years old. Because the disease is most prevalent in poorer socioeconomic groups, this figure may simply reflect the age distribution of the high-risk population. The gender ratio of leprosy manifesting during childhood is 1:1, although men predominate by a 2:1 ratio in adulthood manifestation.

Older Adults. The immunosuppression found in the older adult causes infections to be a significant risk factor for this age group. Thymic mass is steadily lost such that serum activity of thymic hormones is almost unde-

tectable. With the decline in T cell activity and the presence of higher numbers of immature T cells in the thymus, cell-mediated immunity significantly declines. Thus T lymphocytes are less able to proliferate in response to *M. leprae.*

Cultural/Social Considerations

The social stigma associated with leprosy has been noted throughout history. The Hebrew word *leper* (from Greek translations) meant someone who was an outcast from society, a person who is "a morally or spiritually harmful influence." Dating back to biblical times, the castigation of persons with leprosy is gradually being replaced with the attitude that leprosy is a disease, not a social stigma. Even today, though, the word *leprosy* has negative connotations. The attitudes of health care providers toward patients with leprosy can influence public opinion.

Physical Examination

Clinical diagnosis of leprosy is based on examination of the skin. All skin areas should be examined, especially the face, ears, and extremities. The skin lesions are characteristically nonpruritic and hypopigmented in dark-skinned persons but erythematous in light-skinned persons. The number, type, location, and characteristics of any lesions must be documented. Any sensorimotor dysfunction, such as loss of sensation, muscular weakness, or deformity, is important to note. The patient should be examined for edema, particularly of the face, hands, and feet. Peripheral nerve trunks (ulnar nerve at the elbow, peroneal nerve at the head of the fibula, and the great auricular nerve) should be examined bilaterally to compare size, extent of softness or hardness, and tenderness.

The patient should also be examined for signs of leprotic reactions. In type 1 reactions, signs of neuritis should be sought. With type 2 reactions, the examiner should watch for signs suggestive of painful skin lesions, fever, inflammation of the eyes, arthritis, lymphadenopathy, and glomerulonephritis.

Laboratory Testing

M. leprae is rarely found in smears made from quiescent lesions but may appear during activity. The bacterium is demonstrable in the lepromatous form of the disorder when Virchow's cells are present.

The lepromin skin test helps identify the form of leprosy a patient has and the prognosis for that patient. Lepromin (a preparation of killed *M. leprae*) is injected intradermally and the reaction is evaluated 4 weeks later (see Box 33-3).

GOALS OF THERAPY

The goal of therapy is to render the patient noninfectious, thereby preventing the spread of the disease. To achieve this objective, the patient should be given the correct dosage and combination of drugs for an appropriate duration and, if necessary, should be supervised to ensure compliance.

The principal treatment for leprosy is drug therapy. Treatment recommendations consist of dapsone, rifampin, and clofazimine. Clinical evidence suggests that in most instances, infectiousness is lost within 3 months of continuous and regular treatment with antileprotic drugs or within 3 days of treatment with rifampin.

Rifampin, in combination with other antileprotic drugs, is recommended for all forms of leprosy. It has a rapid effect, and a single dose has been found to kill 99% of the bacilli, thus rendering the patient noninfectious. The bactericidal effect of ethionamide appears sooner than that of dapsone but later than that of rifampin. The use of combination drug therapy rapidly decreases a patient's infectious state and reduces the likelihood that resistant strains will develop.

Infectious patients need not be hospitalized, providing there is treatment compliance and adequate supervision, the home environment meets specific conditions, and the local public health officer concurs with the disposition of the case.

INTERVENTION
Administration

Efficacy depends on prolonged use. Dapsone should be taken with food if gastric irritation occurs. Dapsone should not be taken if the patient is allergic to sulfonamides.

To maximize absorption, clofazimine should be taken with food or milk. The drug should be protected from moisture and heat. For patients who experience abdominal pain, diarrhea, or colic, the dosage may need to be reduced. If reactional leprosy episodes occur (worsening of leprosy activity related to therapy), the use of other antileprotic drugs, analgesics, corticosteroids, or surgery may be necessary.

The absorption of rifampin is reduced when the drug is taken with food. It should be taken either 1 hour before or 2 hours after a meal, followed by a full glass (240 mL) of water. If gastric irritation becomes a problem, rifampin can be administered with food. Capsules can be opened and their contents mixed with applesauce or jelly for patients who have difficulty swallowing. A pharmacist can compound a syrup for patients unable to swallow the solid formulation.

Education

The patient and family should be given written instructions about all drugs, including the name, the prescribed dosage, the reason for taking the drug, its adverse effects, and when to call the health care provider. The patient should be reminded about the importance of completing the entire drug regimen, which may take years. If the patient misses a dose of antileprotic drugs, the patient should take that dose as soon as possible but should not take a double dose. The adverse effects of the drugs, particularly skin discoloration and serious gastric problems, should be discussed with the patient.

Support and encouragement are warranted to help the patient deal with the changes in skin pigmentation. The health care provider should reassure the patient that skin color changes are usually reversible but may take several months to years to disappear. There have been reports of suicides by patients due to severe depression about the pigmentation effects. The patient should be informed of the support groups available to help with this issue.

EVALUATION

Symptoms that indicate resolution of the infection include improvement of skin lesions and in cell-mediated immunity status. Resolution of skin lesions may take 8 to 12 weeks, depending on the severity of the disease. Determined by the type of leprosy, some treatment regimens may last as long as 10 years and others for life.

Bibliography

Baker T: Tuberculosis returns, *Nurs Times* 97(26):56-57, 2001.
Clinical update: practical summaries of recent national guidelines. Treating latent tuberculosis infection: highlights of the new ATS/CDC recommendations, *J Crit Illn* 16(3):150-152, 2001.
New guidelines offer more nuances, treatment options: extended therapy counseled for some, *TB Monitor* 8(9):101-102, 112, 2001.
Poole J: Leprosy—a growing problem, *J Comm Nurs* 15(6):23-25, 28, 2001.
Scowen P: Tuberculosis in the UK and worldwide: the current picture, *Prof Care Mother Child* 11(3):63-65, 2001.
Update: fatal and severe liver injuries associated with rifampin and pyrazinamide for latent tuberculosis infection, and revisions in American Thoracic Society/CDC recommendations, *MMWR Morb Mortal Wkly Rep* 50(34):733-735, 2001.
Webster KH: Hansen's disease: a modern overview of an ancient illness, *J Contin Educat Top Iss* 2(3):132-136, 2000.

Internet Resource

Centers for Disease Control. Available online at http://www.cdc.gov/nchstp/tb/surv/surv2000/pdfs/t13&14.pdf.

CHAPTER

34

Antiprotozoal and Antihelminthic Drugs

SHERRY F. QUEENER • KATHLEEN GUTIERREZ

 Visit **http://evolve.elsevier.com/Gutierrez/** for additional information.

KEY TERMS

Amebiasis, p. 516

Cestodes, p. 523

Enterobiasis, p. 521

Giardiasis, p. 518

Helminths, p. 521

Malaria, p. 512

Trichomoniasis, p. 519

OBJECTIVES

- Discuss how the site of infestation may affect the success of drug therapy.
- Describe the types of patients in whom specific protozoal or helminthic diseases might be more likely.
- Explain hygienic measures that should accompany drug therapy in controlling pinworm infestations.
- Develop a nursing care plan for the patient receiving one of the drugs discussed in this chapter.

Protozoal and helminthic diseases account for major health problems throughout the world, particularly in developing countries. Health care providers have become more familiar with the diseases as a group because of increased travel and immigration from endemic regions. Although major infestations are commonly associated with tropical climates, outbreaks are becoming universal in distribution.

PATHOPHYSIOLOGY • Malaria

Malaria is a serious protozoal infectious disease transmitted by the bite of *Anopheles* mosquitoes that are infected with one of the four species of *Plasmodium* that produce human disease: *P. falciparum*, *P. vivax*, *P. ovale*, and *P. malariae*.

Plasmodia have a complex life cycle (Figure 34-1). Sporozoites enter human blood, travel directly to the liver, and may persist there for prolonged periods. Clinical malaria results when merozoites, the plasmodial form produced in liver cells, are released into the blood.

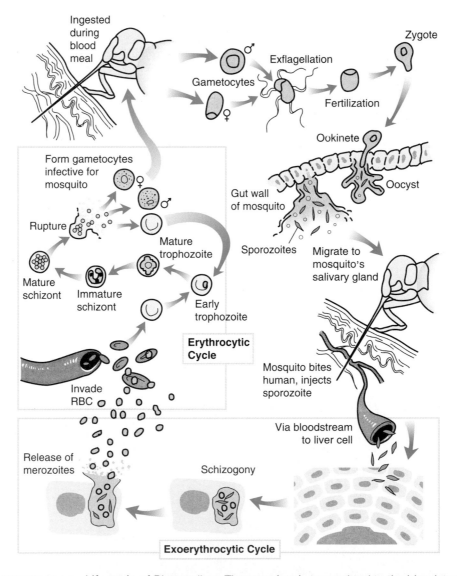

FIGURE 34-1 Life cycle of *Plasmodium*. The organism is transmitted to the bloodstream of humans by the bite of anopheline mosquitoes. The sporozoites migrate to the liver, where they develop and multiply and ultimately invade red blood cells. (From Mahon CR, Manuselis G Jr: *Textbook of diagnostic microbiology*, ed 2, Philadelphia, 2000, Saunders. Used with permission.)

Merozoites attack red blood cells and ultimately cause them to rupture, producing the fever, chills, and sweating characteristic of malaria. A few gametocytes are also formed. Only gametocytes cause a mosquito to become infectious and capable of transmitting the disease. Thus patients at this stage of the disease can transmit parasites to mosquitoes and thence to other human hosts.

Therapy for malaria depends on the stage of the disease and which plasmodial species is involved. *P. falciparum* and *P. malariae* do not produce persistent tissue forms of the parasite; therefore, therapy that destroys blood forms of the protozoan will cure these forms of the disease. With *P. vivax* and *P. ovale*, therapy must include a drug that destroys the persistent tissue forms of *Plasmodium*.

 DRUG CLASS • Antimalarial Drugs

chloroquine (Aralen)

hydroxychloroquine (Plaquenil)

MECHANISM OF ACTION

Chloroquine and hydroxychloroquine are both 4-aminoquinolines. This family of drugs has been the mainstay of antimalarial therapy worldwide since the late 1940s. All effective members of this family bind tightly to double-stranded DNA, thereby altering its physical properties. These drugs may also inhibit metabolic processes in *Plasmodium*.

USES

Chloroquine and hydroxychloroquine are used for suppressive treatment and treatment of acute malaria caused by *P. falciparum*, *P. malariae*, *P. ovale*, and *P. vivax*. Treatment of chloroquine-resistant strains of *P. falciparum* requires the use of a combination of drugs (Table 34-1). Radical cure of *P. ovale* and *P. vivax* requires the addition of primaquine to the drug regimen because chloroquine is not effective against tissue forms of malaria parasites.

TABLE 34-1

Drugs to Treat or Prevent Malaria

Generic Name	Brand Name	Frequency/Duration of Dosing	Indications
atovaquone proguanil HCl	Malarone	Prophylaxis: once daily for 2 days before, each day during, and 7 days after possible exposure Treatment: q24h for 3 days	For treatment or prophylaxis of *P. falciparum* malaria acquired in regions where chloroquine resistance may be present
chloroquine	Aralen	Prophylaxis: once every 7 days Treatment: variable for 2 days	Primary drug for therapy or prophylaxis of malaria
halofantrine	Halfan*	Treatment: q12h for 1 day, then repeat 1 week later	Therapy for acute malaria caused by chloroquine-resistant *P. falciparum*
hydroxychloroquine	Plaquenil	Prophylaxis: once every 7 days Treatment: variable for 2 days	Primary drug for therapy or prophylaxis of malaria
mefloquine	Lariam	Prophylaxis: once every 7 days Treatment: single dose	Prophylaxis or therapy of malaria, including disease caused by chloroquine-resistant *P. falciparum*
primaquine	Generic	Treatment: q24h for 14 days	Primary drug for radical cure of malaria (*P. vivax*, *P. ovale*); kills gametocytes of *P. falciparum*
proguanil	Paludrine*	Prophylaxis: q24h while exposed	May be used with chloroquine or with atovaquone
pyrimethamine + sulfadoxine	Fansidar	Treatment: used as single dose, but in regimens that may include other drugs	Used in combinations to treat malaria caused by chloroquine-resistant *P. falciparum*
quinine	Generic	Treatment: q8h for 3-7 days	Used with other drugs to treat chloroquine-resistant *P. falciparum*

*Not commercially available in the United States.

PHARMACOKINETICS

Chloroquine phosphate and hydroxychloroquine sulfate are satisfactorily absorbed from the gastrointestinal (GI) tract. Chloroquine hydrochloride is available for intramuscular (IM) injection when oral dosage is not possible.

Drugs in the 4-aminoquinoline family become strongly concentrated in the liver, spleen, kidneys, and lungs. More important to their therapeutic usefulness, the drugs also become concentrated in red blood cells. Infected red blood cells may contain concentrations up to 1000 times higher than plasma.

4-Aminoquinolines may be biotransformed by hepatic microsomal enzymes; some of the metabolites retain antiplasmodial activity. The drug and its metabolites are eliminated by the kidneys. Renal excretion is enhanced by acidifying the urine, which converts the drug to a charged form that is not reabsorbed.

ADVERSE REACTIONS AND CONTRAINDICATIONS

Therapeutic dosages of chloroquine and hydroxychloroquine can produce nausea and other GI tract symptoms. The symptoms may be minimized by taking the drugs with meals.

Visual changes may also occur with 4-aminoquinolines; ciliary muscle impairment may be minor but persistent, or more severe changes in vision may signal overdosage (see next section).

Chloroquine and hydroxychloroquine are relatively safe drugs if care is taken to avoid overdosage, prolonged use, or use in sensitive patients. Patients with glucose-6-phosphate dehydrogenase (G6PD) deficiency are more likely than normal patients to experience hemolysis when treated with these drugs. Patients with liver disease or retinal damage are also at greater risk of severe toxic reactions.

Children are more sensitive than adults to 4-aminoquinolines; death has resulted after a child swallowed a small amount of chloroquine. Severe reactions and sudden death have also been reported in children following parenteral use of chloroquine.

TOXICITY

The toxic reactions to 4-aminoquinolines are greatly increased when the drugs are used for prolonged periods, such as with long-term malaria prophylaxis. Signs of overdosage include cardiovascular symptoms (e.g., arrhythmias, cardiovascular collapse, hypotension), CNS toxicity (e.g., drowsiness, excitability, headache, seizures), and visual disturbances (e.g., blurred vision). Blurred vision may signal reversible impairment of accommodation, but retinal or corneal changes are irreversible. Patients reporting misty vision, patchy vision, or foggy patches in the visual field may be developing serious eye damage.

INTERACTIONS

The 4-aminoquinolines should not be used with penicillamine because they may cause excessive accumulation and toxicity of penicillamine.

---

primaquine (generic)

MECHANISM OF ACTION

Primaquine is an 8-aminoquinoline drug. The mechanism of action may be different from the related 4-aminoquinolines, but exactly how primaquine kills certain forms of plasmodia is unknown.

USES

Primaquine keeps gametocytes of *P. falciparum* out of the blood, thereby preventing the transmission of malaria to the mosquito and hence to human hosts. In addition, primaquine is used to produce a radical cure of *P. vivax* and *P. ovale* infections. By destroying the tissue-bound forms of the pathogen, primaquine prevents relapses.

PHARMACOKINETICS

Primaquine is well absorbed when given orally. Drug concentrations in plasma peak within 6 hours of taking the dose, but the drug is extensively biotransformed and rapidly cleared from blood.

ADVERSE REACTIONS AND CONTRAINDICATIONS

Normal therapeutic dosages of primaquine cause little toxicity. Abdominal cramps or epigastric distress can occur, but these symptoms can usually be avoided by taking the drug with meals.

Primaquine may damage red blood cells. The drug blocks production of an intracellular reducing agent, NADPH (reduced nicotinamide adenine dinucleotide). In normal cells this deficit is made up by glucose metabolism and the cell continues to function normally, but patients with reduced levels of G6PD cannot use glucose rapidly enough to make up the deficit. Red blood cells in these patients accumulate oxidized products such as methemoglobin, which is not an efficient oxygen carrier. Cyanosis may result. Ultimately, these red blood cells may rupture. Hemolysis can be severe and signals that the drug dosage should be reduced or that treatment should be stopped. One sign of hemolysis that may be seen easily is darkening of urine.

Primaquine adverse effects are more severe in patients lacking G6PD. The lack of G6PD is genetically determined and exists in high proportions of certain populations such as Sardinians, Sephardic Jews, Greeks, and Iranians. African Americans are less prone to this deficiency than these groups but have a higher incidence than the U.S. white population. Patients with increased sensitivity to primaquine may be given lower dosages of the drug.

TOXICITY

High dosages of primaquine cause methemoglobinemia and other blood dyscrasias.

INTERACTIONS

Primaquine is not routinely used with other bone marrow suppressants because the risk of leukopenia is too great. Quinacrine is also avoided with primaquine because of excessive toxicity with the combination.

 DRUG CLASS • **Drugs Used Primarily to Treat Chloroquine-Resistant Malaria**

atovaquone + proguanil (Malarone)

Proguanil is an older antimalarial drug that seems to interfere with folic acid metabolism in malaria parasites, and atovaquone is a newer drug that blocks energy production. Either drug alone may select resistant parasites, but when they are used together resistance is minimized. This combination of two effective antimalarial drugs is used for prophylaxis or therapy of uncomplicated malaria caused by *P. falciparum* (see Table 34-1). The combination is also recommended for malaria acquired in regions where chloroquine-resistant strains of *P. falciparum* exist. Proguanil is well absorbed when given orally, but the oral absorption of atovaquone is more variable. Both drugs have long half-lives. Atovaquone is almost exclusively eliminated in feces, but proguanil is primarily eliminated in urine. At dosages used for prophylaxis, the most common adverse reactions to this combination are abdominal pain, headache, nausea, and vomiting.

halofantrine (Halfan)

Halofantrine is not commercially available in North America but is used elsewhere to treat acute malaria caused by chloroquine-resistant *P. falciparum* (see Table 34-1).

Halofantrine may interfere with the digestion of hemoglobin by the organism. Oral doses should be taken on an empty stomach; fatty foods may promote a rapid uptake that can produce cardiotoxicity. Halofantrine appears unchanged in feces. Gastric distress and rashes are the most common adverse effects. Cardiovascular toxicity is rare but potentially fatal. Therefore, halofantrine is avoided in patients with a history of cardiac arrhythmias. The drug is also avoided in patients receiving mefloquine because the risk of cardiovascular toxicity is increased.

mefloquine (Lariam)

Mefloquine is used for prophylaxis or therapy of malaria caused by chloroquine-resistant *P. falciparum* or for malaria caused by *P. malariae, P. ovale,* or *P. vivax* (see Table 34-1). For radical cure of *P. ovale* or *P. vivax,*

primaquine must be added to the regimen. Mefloquine is often considered as an alternative to its chemical relative quinine. Mefloquine, like quinine, acts only against the bloodborne forms of *Plasmodium*. Its exact mechanism of action is unknown.

Oral absorption of mefloquine is usually in excess of 85%. The drug distributes well to many tissues, including the cerebrospinal fluid (CSF) and the brain. Mefloquine is concentrated in red blood cells, which may contribute to its effect against the organisms harbored there.

Mefloquine is biotransformed to a variable degree in the liver. Elimination is slow, with the drug remaining in the body for up to 1 month. This long elimination half-life allows the drug to be given as a single dose to treat malaria.

Mefloquine may cause gastric distress, including vomiting. At higher doses it may also cause CNS effects such as dizziness, headache, anxiety, confusion, and seizures. Visual disturbances have also been noted. Slowing of the heart rate (bradycardia) is a rare adverse effect. Mefloquine is not combined with chloroquine so as to avoid excessive CNS toxicity or with quinidine or quinine to avoid excessive cardiovascular toxicity.

proguanil (Paludrine)

Proguanil was once widely used as a single drug for prophylaxis, but resistance has become widespread (see Table 34-1). The most common use of the drug today is in combination with atovaquone (see above). Proguanil is biotransformed in the liver to cycloguanil. In certain Asian and African populations, some individuals do not carry out this reaction adequately, and for these persons proguanil is ineffective.

pyrimethamine + sulfadoxine (Fansidar)

A combination of pyrimethamine with quinine and sulfadoxine is used to treat chloroquine-resistant *P. falciparum* (see Table 34-1). Pyrimethamine is also used as a primary treatment for toxoplasmosis (see later section of this chapter for a full discussion of pyrimethamine).

Sulfadoxine is a sulfonamide (see Table 34-1). Other sulfonamides have also been used against malaria. For a full description of the properties of sulfadoxine and other sulfonamides, see Chapter 30.

Pyrimethamine, as it is normally used in treating chloroquine-resistant malaria, produces few adverse effects.

---

quinine (Quinamm, Novo-Quinine✱)

Quinine may be active against all four forms of *Plasmodium* and is used today primarily for drug-resistant malaria (see Table 34-1). Quinine should be combined with pyrimethamine and sulfadoxine for best effect.

Quinine is rapidly absorbed when given orally. The drug is generally well distributed throughout the body, although it does not enter CSF to a significant degree. Quinine is extensively biotransformed and eliminated in the urine. Elimination is enhanced in acidic urine.

Quinine can produce cinchonism (quinine comes from cinchona bark). Symptoms include ringing in the ears (tinnitus), altered hearing acuity, headache, blurred vision, and diarrhea. At the dosages used today, these symptoms are usually mild. If the dosage is increased or if the patient is hypersensitive, severe cinchonism can arise. Various blood dyscrasias may occur as well.

PATHOPHYSIOLOGY • Amebic Disease

Amebic infections are caused by microscopic, single-celled protozoans called *Entamoeba histolytica*. This common human pathogen is passed from host to host by oral ingestion of fecally contaminated food or water. The organism is ingested as cysts, which have thick walls that resist the action of stomach acids. In the intestine the nonmotile cyst changes to a motile, sexually active form called a trophozoite. Trophozoites produce active disease as they reproduce and invade tissues.

Amebiasis may be restricted to the intestinal lumen and cause few symptoms, even though cysts may be shed in feces. In other cases, intestinal symptoms range from mild to severe. The greatest risk comes when trophozoites invade the intestinal lining in the course of the disease and penetrate the intestinal wall. Once outside the intestinal tract the amebae may create abscesses in other tissues and organs. The liver and lung are most commonly affected in this way.

DRUG CLASS • Drugs Used to Treat Amebic Disease

chloroquine (Aralen)
diloxanide (Entamide,✱ Furamide✱)
iodoquinol (Diodoquin,✱ Dioquinol, Yodoxin)
metronidazole (Flagyl, Protostat, Trikacide✱)
paromomycin (Humatin)

MECHANISM OF ACTION

Metronidazole is most effective against anaerobic organisms, being reduced in those organisms to a form that directly damages DNA. Paromomycin is presumed to act on protein synthesis, since it is related to the aminoglycoside family of antibiotics (see Chapter 29), but its exact action on *E. histolytica* is not understood. The mechanism of action of diloxanide, iodoquinol, and chloroquine on *E. histolytica* is unknown.

USES

The choice of drug for treating amebic disease depends on the stage of the disease (Table 34-2).

Several of these drugs also have other uses. Chloroquine is a primary drug for malaria, metronidazole is

the primary drug for anaerobic invasive bacterial infections (Chapter 30), and paromomycin is also used to treat giardiasis.

PHARMACOKINETICS

Chloroquine, diloxanide, and metronidazole are given orally and are well absorbed by that route. Excretion is primarily renal but metabolites of metronidazole are formed by the liver.

Iodoquinol given orally is poorly absorbed from the intestine. The level of iodine in the blood becomes increased, which suggests that some drug is absorbed or that iodine is absorbed after breakdown of the drug in the gut.

Paromomycin is very poorly absorbed from the intestine and is thus effective only as a luminal amebicide.

ADVERSE REACTIONS AND CONTRAINDICATIONS

The most common adverse effects with all of these drugs are gastrointestinal. Diarrhea, esophagitis, flatulence, nausea, or vomiting may occur. Other effects of

TABLE 34-2

Drugs to Treat Amebic Infestations

Generic Name	Brand Name	Frequency/ Duration of Therapy	Indications
chloroquine	Aralen	q6h for 2 days; q12h for up to 3 weeks	Alternative drug used in combinations for amebic liver abscesses
diloxanide	Entamide,* Furamide*	q8h for 10 days	Alternative drug for symptomatic intestinal disease; primary drug for asymptomatic patients shedding cysts
iodoquinol	Diodoquin,* Diquinol, Yodoxin	q8h for 20 days	Alternative drug for asymptomatic intestinal disease; may be used with metronidazole for symptomatic intestinal disease
metronidazole	Flagyl, Protostat	q8h for 5-10 days	Primary drug for intestinal or extraintestinal amebiasis
paromomycin	Humatin	q8h for 5-10 days	May be used with metronidazole for symptomatic intestinal disease

*Not commercially available in the United States.

chloroquine are noted in the previous section on malaria.

Other adverse effects of iodoquinol may include allergic reactions, fevers, and chills. This drug contains significant iodine, and so may also cause the thyroid gland to enlarge. This iodine content also makes iodoquinol potentially dangerous for patients with hepatic or renal failure.

In addition to GI distress, metronidazole also commonly causes dizziness or headache. Other reactions are described in Chapter 30.

Paromomycin may cause dizziness, edema, headache, hearing loss, ringing of the ears, or skin rash. These symptoms may signal serious reactions and should be reported to the health care provider.

TOXICITY

Under most circumstances these drugs are used at dosages well below toxic levels. Prolonged high dosages of iodoquinol may produce optic neuritis or atrophy and other signs of neuropathy. High dosages of metronidazole may cause seizures. At extremely high dosages or if unusual intestinal absorption of the drug occurs, paromomycin may cause hearing loss or renal damage.

INTERACTIONS

Iodoquinol causes persistent interference with thyroid function tests because the iodine level may be high in the blood. Metronidazole may cause a disulfiram-like reaction if taken with alcohol. Metronidazole may also potentiate the action of warfarin. Patients receiving both drugs should be observed for signs of bleeding.

PATHOPHYSIOLOGY • Selected Parasitic Diseases

The diseases discussed in this section ordinarily occur in a small number of patients. The diseases may be related to travel (giardiasis), occur as opportunistic infections mostly in immunosuppressed hosts (cryptosporidiosis, pneumocystosis, toxoplasmosis), or be passed from host to host (trichomoniasis).

CRYPTOSPORIDIOSIS AND MICROSPORIDIOSIS

Cryptosporidia and microsporidia are protozoans that infect microvilli of host intestinal cells and cause diarrhea in several species of animals and in humans. The most com-

mon infections in humans are caused by *Cryptosporidium parvum*. The disease is passed from host to host by ingestion of thick-walled cysts; but within a single host, thin-walled cysts can release sporozoites that invade surrounding host cells. This recycling autoinfection is more common in severely immunocompromised patients.

Cryptosporidium has spread as a waterborne infection when the highly chlorine-resistant thick-walled cysts contaminate water supplies. Runoff from feedlots where large numbers of cattle are maintained may pose a risk of contaminating human water supplies unless these facilities are kept well away from the watershed area of the water supply. Animals, including calves, puppies, kittens, and rodents, harbor *Cryptosporidium* and may pass it to humans.

Patients with acquired immunodeficiency syndrome (AIDS) may have chronic, debilitating diarrhea in the late stages of their disease; for many of these patients, infection with *C. parvum* or a microsporidium is a contributing factor to the diarrhea. Patients with intact immune systems generally recover well with only supportive therapy to maintain fluid and electrolyte balance. No effective therapy for these infections exists, although several drug classes have been tried.

GIARDIASIS

Giardiasis is an intestinal infection caused by the protozoan *Giardia lamblia*. This disease, which is passed between human hosts by ingestion of fecally contaminated food, may be asymptomatic in many patients. For others it may be much more severe, producing diarrhea, GI distress, and malabsorption. Quinacrine or metronidazole are primary drugs for the treatment of giardiasis in adults (Table 34-3).

LEISHMANIASIS

Leishmaniasis is the name applied to several related diseases that are transmitted to humans by insect bites. *Leishmania donovoni* causes visceral leishmaniasis (kalaazar), which may affect most internal organs. Symptoms include enlarged lymph nodes, fever, splenomegaly, emaciation, and pancytopenia. Other species of *Leish-* *mania* cause mucocutaneous disease that may be self-limiting in most cases. Treatment of leishmaniasis is difficult and may include amphotericin B (see Chapter 32), paromomycin (see Chapter 33), or a heavy metal compound called meglumine antimoniate that is not available in the United States.

PNEUMOCYSTOSIS

Pneumocystis carinii has been recognized as an opportunistic pathogen for several decades, but knowledge of the life cycle is incomplete. Although the organism is closely related to fungi, the clinically effective drugs are antiprotozoal drugs. *P. carinii* seldom causes disease in healthy humans, but it can produce severe pulmonary disease in patients receiving immunosuppressive drugs or in patients with AIDS. Young, malnourished children are also susceptible. Unless treated, as many as half of the patients who acquire this disease may die. Patients receiving immunosuppressive cancer chemotherapy or those receiving immunosuppressive drugs to prevent rejection of a transplanted organ usually respond well to the fixed combination of sulfamethoxazole and trimethoprim for prophylaxis or therapy (see Chapter 30).

Sulfamethoxazole and trimethoprim may be used to treat *P. carinii* pneumonia in AIDS, but AIDS patients have an unusually high incidence of serious reactions to these drugs. Pentamidine is also effective against *P. carinii* pneumonia but it, too, causes serious toxicity. Alternative therapy for *P. carinii* pneumonia in AIDS patients includes atovaquone, clindamycin with pri-

---

TABLE 34-3

Drugs to Treat Selected Parasitic Diseases

Generic Name	Brand Name	Frequency/ Duration of Dosing	Indications
amphotericin B	AmBisome	21 or 38 days, discontinuous	Leishmaniasis
atovaquone	Mepron	q12h for 21 days	*Pneumocystis carinii* pneumonia
furazolidone	Furoxone	q6h for 7-10 days	Giardiasis
meglumine antimoniate	Glucantim*	q24h for 20-28 days	Leishmaniasis
metronidazole	Flagyl	q24h for 3 days q8h for 7 days	Giardiasis Trichomoniasis
pentamidine	Pentam, Nebupent	q24h for 21 days	*P. carinii* pneumonia
pyrimethamine	Daraprim	q24h for life, with sulfonamide	*Toxoplasma gondii* encephalitis in AIDS
quinacrine	Atabrine	q8h for 5-7 days	Giardiasis
sulfamethoxazole + trimethoprim	Bactrim	q8h for 14 days	*P. carinii* pneumonia
trimetrexate	Neutrexin	q24h for 21 days	*P. carinii* pneumonia

*Not available in the United States.

maquine, dapsone with trimethoprim, and trimetrexate with leucovorin.

TOXOPLASMOSIS

In the United States, toxoplasmosis is primarily acquired from ingestion of the oocyte of *Toxoplasma gondii*. The most common source of infection is cat feces. In adult humans the disease is usually mild and transitory, with symptoms resembling those of mild mononucleosis. Occasionally, the disease may involve the eyes or nervous system in adults, but congenital toxoplasmosis is usually fatal, causing severe damage to the eyes, brain, and other organs of the fetus. Because of the dangers this disease poses to fetuses, many obstetricians suggest that pregnant women not handle used cat litter and avoid close contact with cats. Pyrimethamine and sulfadiazine are used in combination to treat this disease (see Table 34-3).

Toxoplasmosis is common in AIDS patients, and it can produce encephalitis that may result in death. Ag-

gressive therapy with pyrimethamine and sulfonamides is usually attempted; for patients who cannot tolerate sulfonamides, other drugs such as clindamycin may be combined with pyrimethamine. Alternative drugs include atovaquone and piritrexim.

TRICHOMONIASIS

Vaginal infections caused by *Trichomonas vaginalis* are common. Trichomoniasis is marked by a watery discharge from the vagina and signs of tissue irritation. *Trichomonas* may go unnoticed in the urinary tract and in the rectum, but these sites can serve as sources of infection.

Vaginal trichomoniasis may be treated with locally applied drugs such as gels or douches. Complete cure of the sites other than the vagina and of infections in the male urinary tract may require a systemic drug. Metronidazole is the drug of choice (see Table 34-3).

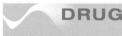

DRUG CLASS • Primary Drugs Used to Treat Selected Parasitic and Opportunistic Diseases

metronidazole

Metronidazole has become a primary drug for the treatment of giardiasis and trichomoniasis (see Table 34-3). A full discussion of the drug appears in Chapter 30, where it is discussed as a primary drug for anaerobic bacterial infections. Metronidazole is also a primary drug for amebiasis.

pentamidine (Nebupent, Pentam, Pentacarinat✱)

MECHANISM OF ACTION

The action of pentamidine against *P. carinii* (see Table 34-3) is not completely understood but involves an interference with DNA function.

USES

Pentamidine is the primary drug for *Pneumocystis* pneumonia in patients who cannot tolerate trimethoprim and sulfamethoxazole.

PHARMACOKINETICS

Pentamidine is given intravenously for therapy. For prophylaxis of *P. carinii* pneumonia, pentamidine may be aerosolized. When properly administered by this route, the drug is carried into the lungs in droplets small

enough to be deposited into the alveoli where *P. carinii* lodges. High concentrations are thereby achieved at the site of infection, but because systemic absorption from lungs is low, whole body toxicity is minimized. Unfortunately, with this type of prophylaxis *P. carinii* infections at other sites occur because the systemic concentration of drug is low.

Pentamidine is concentrated in renal tissue and is excreted primarily in urine. Complete elimination from the body is slow, with drug appearing in urine as long as 8 weeks after therapy stops.

ADVERSE REACTIONS AND CONTRAINDICATIONS

Patients receiving pentamidine intravenously may experience acute hypotension, arrhythmias, and death. Hypoglycemia may be severe. Long-term effects may include hyperglycemia or diabetes mellitus. Nephrotoxicity and blood dyscrasias can also develop. The incidence of adverse effects can vary depending on the patient being treated. In general, AIDS patients experience more of the major and minor reactions to pentamidine than do other patients.

Pentamidine is contraindicated in patients who have had allergic reactions to either parenteral or inhaled pentamidine. Pentamidine worsens bone marrow depression, diabetes mellitus, heart disease, hypoglycemia, and renal impairment.

TOXICITY

High dosages of pentamidine given rapidly by intravenous infusion cause dangerous hypotension.

INTERACTIONS

Pentamidine worsens the effects of drugs that cause bone marrow depression and nephrotoxic drugs. The risk of pancreatitis is worsened with didanosine. Foscarnet and pentamidine significantly alter calcium and magnesium levels in blood.

---

pyrimethamine (Daraprim)

MECHANISM OF ACTION

Pyrimethamine inhibits the enzyme dihydrofolate reductase in susceptible organisms, thereby blocking the formation of tetrahydrofolic acid (THFA), a cofactor required for several metabolic transformations. The blocked enzyme normally converts dihydrofolic acid (DHA) to THFA. The formation of DHA may be blocked by sulfonamides. Combining pyrimethamine and a sulfonamide is an example of the synergistic effect produced by two drugs acting in the same metabolic pathway. Another example is trimethoprim and sulfamethoxazole (Chapter 30).

USES

Pyrimethamine in combination with sulfadiazine is used to treat or suppress toxoplasmosis. Clindamycin may substitute for sulfadiazine if the patient cannot tolerate sulfonamides. Pyrimethamine is an alternative drug for malaria, and is used with sulfadoxine for chloroquine-resistant *P. falciparum* malaria.

PHARMACOKINETICS

Pyrimethamine is well absorbed when given orally. The drug concentrates in blood cells and tissues, including the liver, where it is biotransformed. Metabolites are excreted in urine. Pyrimethamine appears in breast milk.

ADVERSE REACTIONS AND CONTRAINDICATIONS

As it is normally used in treating chloroquine-resistant malaria, pyrimethamine produces few adverse effects. At higher dosages, such as those used to treat toxoplasmosis, the drug may impair host folic acid metabolism, leading to megaloblastic anemia and various other blood dyscrasias. Treatment with leucovorin (a folinic acid supplement) may be required.

Pyrimethamine is usually avoided in patients with anemia, bone marrow depression, or a history of seizures.

TOXICITY

Large doses of pyrimethamine may produce nausea and vomiting. Excitability and signs of CNS overstimulation, including seizures, may occur within 2 hours of taking the drug. Very high dosages may produce respiratory depression or circulatory collapse and death.

INTERACTIONS

Pyrimethamine is avoided if possible in persons also receiving other folate antagonists or bone marrow depressants to avoid excessive actions of these drugs.

DRUG CLASS • Miscellaneous Drugs Used to Treat Selected Parasitic and Opportunistic Diseases

atovaquone (Mepron)

Atovaquone is an oral drug used to treat *P. carinii* pneumonia in patients who cannot tolerate trimethoprim and sulfamethoxazole. The drug is also active against *T. gondii* in AIDS patients.

Atovaquone is absorbed poorly, and the amount of drug absorbed varies greatly from patient to patient. The half-life of the drug is between 2 and 3 days. There is little biotransformation, with most of the drug slowly eliminated in feces.

Adverse effects of atovaquone observed in AIDS patients include allergic reactions (fever, skin rash) and GI tract symptoms (diarrhea, nausea, vomiting). Coughing, headache, and insomnia have also been reported.

furazolidone (Furoxone)

Furazolidone is a nitrofuran similar in action to those used to treat urinary tract infections (see Chapter 30). The drug is given orally to treat infections of the bowel. Like other nitrofurans, it does not reach high serum concentrations.

Furazolidone is biotransformed by the liver. One of the breakdown products is a potent inhibitor of monoamine oxidase (MAO). Inhibition of this enzyme lowers elimination of catecholamines, which may cause hypertension. In addition, this action makes drugs such as adrenergics (e.g., ephedrine, phenylephrine), MAO inhibitors (e.g., pargyline), or foods rich in tyramine (e.g., cheese, beer, wine) unsafe for patients receiving furazolidone.

Furazolidone may produce hemolytic reactions, especially in patients who have G6PD deficiency. Allergies and GI tract symptoms may also occur. Patients receiving furazolidone who also drink alcohol may exhibit a disulfiram-like reaction with flushing, difficulty breathing, and a feeling of constriction in the chest.

quinacrine (Atabrine)

Quinacrine has been used to treat giardiasis, malaria, and helminthic infestations but is no longer available in the United States. Quinacrine has multiple metabolic effects but its exact action is unknown. The drug is well absorbed from the GI tract, but when given orally, induces vomiting in many patients because of its bitter taste. Quinacrine binds strongly to tissues. Patients may notice a yellow discoloration of the skin. The reaction is not a sign of jaundice but illustrates the distribution of this yellow-colored drug to the skin.

Quinacrine causes few serious adverse effects when used for short-term treatment. The most common reactions to quinacrine are headache, nausea, and vomiting. Quinacrine crosses the placenta and should not be used in pregnant patients. The drug is also avoided in patients with psychosis or psoriasis because these conditions may be worsened. Use of high dosages of quinacrine or prolonged use of the drug may cause aplastic anemia, corneal edema, hepatitis, or retinopathy. Life-threatening overdose is characterized by seizures, hypotension, and arrhythmias followed by cardiovascular collapse.

Quinacrine may increase primaquine concentrations in blood, resulting in toxicity. This rise in blood levels may result from lowered biotransformation of primaquine and displacement of primaquine from tissues.

sulfamethoxazole + trimethoprim (Bactrim, Septra, Co-trimazole)

Sulfamethoxazole and trimethoprim are used together to treat pneumocystosis. For a full description of these drugs, see Chapter 30.

trimetrexate (Neotrexin)

Trimetrexate is an alternative drug for *P. carinii* pneumonia. Trimetrexate acts in the same way as pyrimethamine but is a much more potent inhibitor of dihydrofolate reductase and therefore does not require concurrent administration of a sulfonamide; however, trimetrexate requires coadministration of leucovorin, a form of folic acid that rescues mammalian cells from the antifolate effects of trimetrexate.

Trimetrexate is administered intravenously. Hepatic biotransformation of the drug produces several metabolites, including a glucuronide. The drug and metabolites are eliminated by the kidneys.

The most common adverse effect with trimetrexate is neutropenia, with fever and sore throat. Other blood dyscrasias, such as thrombocytopenia or anemia, may also occur; signs include unusual bleeding, bruising, or tiredness. Less common adverse effects are confusion, itching, and GI tract symptoms.

PATHOPHYSIOLOGY • Diseases Caused by Helminths

Helminths include flukes, tapeworms, and roundworms that can cause disease.

ASCARIASIS

Ascariasis, also called roundworm infestation, is caused by ingesting the eggs of *Ascaris lumbricoides*. This common disease is spread by ingestion of fecally contaminated food and water. Larvae and adult worms migrate through the lungs, liver, gallbladder, or other organs and may cause severe damage. *Ascaris* infestations may be treated effectively with several drugs, including albendazole, mebendazole, piperazine, and pyrantel (Table 34-4).

ENTEROBIASIS

Enterobiasis is pinworm infestation. Pinworms are freely passed between people living close together. Infestation is caused by the direct transfer of eggs from the anus to the mouth by the hands (Figure 34-2). Constant reinfection occurs because huge numbers of eggs are passed and adhere to clothing, towels, and hands. The disease is usually mild, but some patients may experience pruritus ani, pruritus vulvae, or more serious symptoms.

Because pinworms tend to stay within the intestinal tract, treatment of the disease is relatively simple. Albendazole, mebendazole, and pyrantel are all nearly 100% effective after a single dose. Piperazine is also effective, but therapy continues over several days (see Table 34-4).

WHIPWORM INFESTATION

Whipworm infestation is usually asymptomatic, although large numbers of worms in small children may produce diarrhea, anemia, and cachexia. Whipworm infestations are effectively treated with mebendazole (see Table 34-4).

TABLE 34-4

Drugs to Treat Diseases Caused by Helminths

Generic Name	Brand Name	Frequency/Duration of Dosing	Indications
albendazole	Albenza	q24h for 3-10 days, depending on helminth	Alternative drug for helminthic infestations
ivermectin	Stromectol	Single dose; may repeat in 1 year	Threadworm
mebendazole	Vermox	Single dose; may repeat in 2-3 weeks q12h for 3 days; may repeat in 2-3 weeks	Enterobiasis Ascariasis, hookworm, or whipworm
niclosamide	Niclocide	q24h for 1-7 days	Tapeworm
piperazine	Entacyl*	2 days 7 days	Ascariasis Enterobiasis
praziquantel	Biltricide	q8h for 1 day	Alternative drug for infections caused by flatworms; primary drug for schistosomiasis
pyrantel	Antiminth	Single dose; may repeat in 2-3 weeks	Ascariasis, enterobiasis
thiabendazole	Mintezol	q12h for 2-7 days	Hookworm, threadworm, or trichinosis

*Not available in the United States.

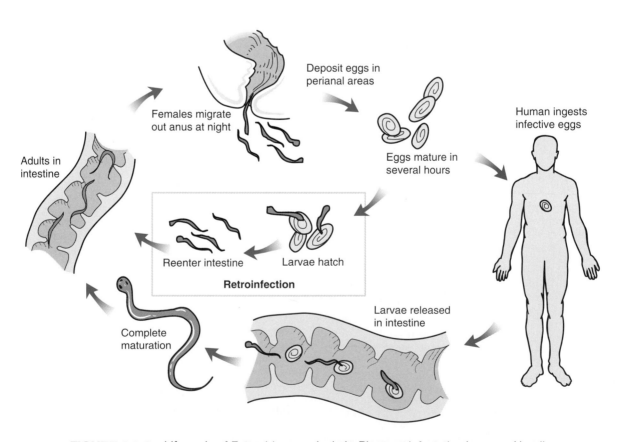

FIGURE 34-2   Life cycle of *Enterobius vermicularis*. Pinworm infestation is caused by direct transfer of infective eggs by hand from the anus to the mouth of the same or another person. Larvae from ingested eggs hatch in the small intestine. Young worms mature in the cecum and upper portions of the colon. (From Mahon CR, Manuselis G Jr: *Textbook of diagnostic microbiology,* ed 2, Philadelphia, 2000, Saunders. Used with permission.)

THREADWORM INFESTATION

Threadworm infestation, also called strongyloidiasis, is more serious than many infestations because the worms may reproduce in humans. Larvae migrate from the intestinal wall into systemic circulation and then return to the intestine to mature and further increase the numbers of worms in the host. Malabsorption syndrome, diarrhea, and duodenal irritation may occur.

Most drugs used to treat helminthic infections are ineffective against threadworms because they live within intestinal tissue. Thiabendazole is well distributed to the tissues where this parasite lives and thus eliminates infestation. Ivermectin, a drug developed to treat river blindness and filariasis in tropical regions, is also useful against threadworms (see Table 34-4).

HOOKWORM INFESTATION

Hookworm infestation, called necatoriasis, occurs in the southern United States. Although two species of hookworms are known, most infestations encountered in the United States are caused by *Necator*. Therefore most patients are treated with mebendazole or pyrantel. Another type of hookworm from dogs and cats produces a cutaneous lesion called creeping eruption, or cutaneous larva migrans. Thiabendazole, either applied topically or given orally, may kill the parasites and limit allergic responses, which cause itching, burning, and skin damage (see Table 34-4).

TRICHINOSIS

Trichinosis, or pork roundworm infestation, is uncommon today. Ingested cysts from raw or improperly cooked meat develop into adult worms in the intestine. Larvae are released into the circulation and enter muscle to form cysts. Patients experience GI tract upset, fever, muscle aches, and eosinophilia.

Trichinosis cannot yet be effectively treated. Most patients receive therapy to minimize symptoms rather than produce a cure (most patients survive the disease and carry the quiescent worms encysted in skeletal muscle for the rest of their lives). Thiabendazole, albendazole, and mebendazole have been used in some cases to try to prevent the migration of worms to muscles (see Table 34-4).

TAPEWORM INFESTATION

Tapeworms, or **cestodes**, of several types can infest humans. Beef, pork, fish, and dwarf tapeworms are all sensitive to niclosamide. Praziquantel, a drug used primarily in the tropics for schistosomiasis, may also be effective against tapeworms (see Table 34-4). All detected infestations are treated, even though they are mostly asymptomatic. Pork tapeworm infestations may become serious if reflux of eggs from the intestine allows them to reach the stomach and hatch into larvae that invade tissues.

 DRUG CLASS • Drugs Used to Treat Diseases Caused by Helminths

ivermectin (Mectizan,✱ Stromectol)

Ivermectin blocks chloride channels in muscles and nerves of certain helminths. This action and effects on gamma-aminobutyric acid (GABA) receptors in helminths interfere with function of the nervous system in threadworms and other parasites. The paralyzed worms may die.

Ivermectin is given as a single oral dose that is effective for up to 1 year. The drug concentrates in the liver and fatty tissues. Elimination is primarily in feces, with little drug being found in urine.

Ivermectin may cause dizziness, fever, headache, arthralgia, myalgia, and swollen lymph nodes. Postural hypotension is rare.

mebendazole (generic, Vermox)

MECHANISM OF ACTION

Mebendazole is an effective broad-spectrum antihelminthic drug that causes microtubules in helminths to disintegrate. This action blocks glucose uptake in sensitive helminths. Because these worms must take up glu-

cose to maintain energy levels, blockade of glucose absorption destroys them.

USES

Mebendazole is an excellent drug against a variety of helminthic diseases, including ascariasis and enterobiasis, as well as infestations caused by hookworms or whipworms (see Table 34-4).

PHARMACOKINETICS

Mebendazole is given orally for its action against intestinal helminths. Very little drug is absorbed into systemic circulation. The small amount of drug that enters the blood is biotransformed by the liver and excreted in urine. If liver function is impaired, the small amount of drug absorbed may accumulate and cause toxicity. Fatty foods favor absorption of mebendazole.

ADVERSE REACTIONS AND CONTRAINDICATIONS

Mebendazole produces few toxic reactions. Abdominal discomfort and diarrhea may result, especially when large masses of worms are expelled.

INTERACTIONS

Few interactions with mebendazole exist, but patients taking mebendazole often have higher-than-normal liver enzyme (alanine aminotransferase [ALT], aspartate aminotransferase [AST]) and blood urea nitrogen (BUN) levels.

niclosamide (Niclocide)

Niclosamide is effective against tapeworms that are limited to the intestinal tract. It is not effective for cysticercosis, in which tapeworm larvae live in the intestinal wall. Segmented flatworms are killed by a single dose of niclosamide. The dead worm segments are often digested by proteolytic agents in the gut. Therefore, a cathartic may be given 1 or 2 hours after the drug has been taken to allow the dead but still intact worm parts to be identified in feces. This purge is required when the infestation is caused by the pork tapeworm. With this organism, digestion of the dead worm segments releases living eggs, which can develop in humans and cause more serious, invasive disease. The purge removes the worm segments before they rupture and prevents this complication.

Niclosamide is not absorbed from the bowel and exerts all of its actions within the lumen of the bowel. For this reason, the drug has few adverse reactions. Some patients have mild GI tract symptoms on the day of therapy. There are no contraindications other than a possible history of allergy to the drug.

piperazine (Multifuge)

Piperazine is effective against *Ascaris* and pinworm infestations. The drug apparently blocks the action of acetylcholine on the muscles of these parasites. As a result, the worms are paralyzed and eliminated alive from the bowel by normal peristaltic flow.

Piperazine is well absorbed after oral administration. A portion of the drug is biotransformed to various inactive products. The kidney is the primary route for excretion. Patients with impaired renal or hepatic function may be more sensitive to piperazine than other patients.

Piperazine occasionally causes GI upset or skin rashes. Transient neurologic signs ranging from headache and dizziness to ataxia, paresthesias, or convulsions have been seen, but severe reactions are more common with overdoses. The more severe reactions also occur in patients with renal dysfunction, who tend to accumulate the drug, and in patients with seizure disorders, who are more sensitive to the CNS effects of the drug.

praziquantel (Biltricide)

Praziquantel interferes with muscle function in flukes and other helminths and can cause local destruction of the integument of these organisms. The drug is well absorbed after oral administration but undergoes extensive first-pass biotransformation in the liver (see Chapter 1). The metabolites formed are eliminated by the kidneys.

Praziquantel often causes mild and transient effects on the CNS. Common symptoms are headache, dizziness, and malaise. Most patients also report GI tract distress. The drug can cause immediate gagging or vomiting if the tablets are chewed instead of being swallowed whole.

pyrantel (Antiminth, Combantriln✱)

Pyrantel is a depolarizing neuromuscular blocker, similar in action to succinylcholine. Pyrantel causes spastic paralysis and contraction of the muscle in worms. The parasites are eliminated from the body by normal peristalsis. Pyrantel is effective, when given in short courses, against a variety of worms, including roundworms (ascariasis) and pinworms (enterobiasis). Purges are not necessary adjuncts to therapy with this drug.

Pyrantel is not absorbed from the GI tract to any great extent. The small amount absorbed is eliminated by the kidneys. Pyrantel produces its desired effects entirely within the lumen of the bowel.

Because pyrantel is not well absorbed when given orally, few systemic adverse reactions occur. Headache, muscle twitching, and dizziness may result from CNS effects of this drug. More commonly the drug causes mild GI tract upset and transient changes in liver function tests.

Piperazine may antagonize the action of pyrantel; they are not used together.

thiabendazole (Mintezol)

Thiabendazole is believed to attack a metabolic process essential in helminths but not found in humans. Thiabendazole is used for cutaneous or visceral larva migrans caused by hookworm and other agents, for threadworm infections, and for trichinosis. The drug must be taken as soon as possible after ingestion of meat infected with *Trichinella spiralis* to lessen subsequent infection in host muscle. Thiabendazole has no effect on larvae encysted in muscle.

Thiabendazole is well absorbed when given orally, and peak blood levels occur within 1 hour of ingestion. Most of the drug is eliminated by hydroxylation and conjugation, the metabolites being the predominant forms of the drug excreted in urine. Very little unchanged drug appears in feces.

Thiabendazole can cause a wide variety of transient, dose-related reactions. The most common adverse reactions are anorexia, dizziness, nausea or vomiting, and numbness in the extremities. A few patients have more severe GI tract symptoms or CNS effects such as drowsiness, headache, or giddiness. Rarely, tinnitus, abnormal sensations in the eyes, or metabolic derangements occur. Although these symptoms may incapacitate a patient, it is rare for reactions to persist beyond 48 hours, and most subside much sooner.

Thiabendazole alters liver function in some patients. Therefore, patients with preexisting liver disease should be carefully observed for progressive liver damage.

Patients often report a strong, unpleasant odor to their urine after thiabendazole therapy. Patients may be reassured that this odor is caused by a metabolite of thiabendazole and is harmless.

Thiabendazole overdoses can cause significant GI tract and CNS symptoms. No specific antidote exists, but emesis or gastric lavage may help limit reactions.

Thiabendazole significantly lowers clearance of theophylline, causing theophylline to accumulate to dangerously high concentrations in blood. Serious CNS toxicity may arise.

APPLICATION TO PRACTICE

ASSESSMENT
History of Present Illness

Geographic. The history provides valuable information about potential exposures to protozoan, parasitic, and helminthic infections. A history of travel to, residence or work in, or immigration from areas of the world in which various protozoans, parasites, and helminths not endemic in the United States are encountered offers a clue to possible etiologies of the patient's infectious disease. Some infestations manifest after a traveler's return home from the endemic area.

For the patient with a history of recent travel, the onset of GI symptoms only after return suggests protozoal diseases characterized by a 1- to 2-week delay between acquisition and appearance of symptoms—notably giardiasis and cryptosporidiosis. These infestations produce GI symptoms lasting longer than a week. Diseases such as strongyloidiasis can manifest years after an individual leaves an endemic region. Information regarding exposure to mosquitoes, the use of mosquito netting when sleeping, and the application of mosquito repellents should be noted.

For the individual who has never been out of the United States, trichomoniasis, strongyloidiasis, giardiasis, cryptosporidiosis, and pinworm are among the parasitic infestations endemic within the United States. Fecal contamination of soil or other environmental sites increases the risk for hookworm, ascariasis, amebiasis, and strongyloidiasis. Walking barefoot on soil contaminated with parasitic larvae predisposes residents of such areas as well as travelers to acquisition of cutaneous larva migrans, hookworm, and strongyloidiasis.

Dietary History. If several patients develop similar symptoms in a given situation, a common source, such as water- or foodborne diseases, such as giardiasis and cryptosporidiosis, should be considered. Waterborne infections are more likely to be acquired from surface water supplies, ranging from mountain streams to municipal reservoirs. Patient reports of eating raw or exotic meats (e.g., walrus, seal, moose) and fishing or swimming in snail-infested locations, such as swamps or undrained ponds, should alert the health care provider to the potential for infestation. Ingestion of undercooked fish predisposes the patient to infection with fish-dwelling nematodes, tapeworms, or flukes. Consumption of ground-grown vegetables, including those from fields contaminated with human feces, provides an opportunity to ingest nematode eggs of *Ascaris lumbricoides*.

Other Exposures. Residence in an institutional setting where fecal/oral hygiene may be less than fastidious raises the possibility of giardiasis, cryptosporidiosis, strongyloidiasis, and pinworm. Child care centers provide opportunities for young children and their families to acquire these infections. Trichomoniasis is transmitted sexually; giardiasis, cryptosporidiosis, amebiasis, and strongyloidiasis can be transmitted during anal intercourse or oral-anal contact.

Health History

It is important to note any preexisting conditions or drugs taken by the patient that influence the choice of drug treatment—specifically, a history of myasthenia gravis, thrombocytopenic purpura, arrhythmias, G6PD deficiency, psoriasis or porphyria, seizure disorders, and blood dyscrasias. In a patient with any of these disorders, specific antiprotozoal, antiparasitic, and antimalarial drugs may be contraindicated or at least will need to be used with caution. A thorough drug history should be obtained to minimize the potential for drug interactions.

Lifespan Considerations

Protozoal, parasitic, and helminthic infections can occur in any age group.

Malaria in the perinatal and pediatric populations requires special considerations. Many of the antimalarial drugs are contraindicated in children who are less than 3 years old or weigh less than 30 pounds.

Pinworm infestations are more common in preschool or school-age children. If neonatal infestation is identified, a neonatologist or pediatrician should be consulted before treatment. The neonate's systems are still developing, and competition for nutritional substrates by the helminth can cause severe complications. In such a circumstance, the family must be considered the source of infestation, their living conditions scrutinized, and large-scale treatment considered. Most anthelminthic drugs are contraindicated for children less than 30 pounds or younger than 3 years.

Cultural/Social Considerations

The primary cultural/social implication of an infestation is embarrassment if the condition becomes public knowledge. Use of public facilities to toilet, bathe, or wash clothes may be limited or nonexistent for homeless, indigent, or mentally troubled wanderers who present with symptoms. Investigations of the patient's home, family members, and living conditions (e.g., institutional living), such as laundry, cleanliness, personal habits, food preparation, and elimination facilities, must be conducted with tact and consideration. Use of public health departments and other public resources can be invaluable for support and education of an individual with an infestation.

Patients who have infestations are often reluctant to discuss the problem. They may have used home remedies for a long time before seeking professional help, and they are often socially unacceptable in behavior and attitude. They may not divulge personal information that would assist in their treatment and in the prevention of additional infestations.

About 10% of African Americans, and 5% to 10% of Sephardic Jews, Greeks, Iranians, Chinese, Filipinos, and Indonesians have G6PD deficiency. There is evidence that G6PD is essential for metabolism in the plasmodia, so persons with this genetic deficiency are believed to have some natural immunity to malaria (see the Case Study: Malaria).

Physical Examination

Most persons with amebiasis are asymptomatic or have minimal diarrhea complaints. *E. histolytica* is divided into pathogenic and nonpathogenic strains. The pathogenic strains commonly cause invasive infection, whereas the noninvasive strains cause only asymptomatic intestinal infection (90%). In a few patients, invasive intestinal or extraintestinal (e.g., liver, and less commonly the kidneys, bladder, genitalia, skin, lung, or brain) infection results. Signs and symptoms of invasive amebiasis include abdominal pain and tenderness, rectal pain, bloody diarrhea, fever, and systemic toxicity. Amebic abscess of the liver may develop during the

acute attack or 1 to 3 months later. Symptoms can be abrupt or insidious. Extraintestinal infection produces a fever, systemic toxicity, right upper quadrant tenderness and pain, nausea and vomiting, diarrhea, hematuria, dysuria, and urinary frequency and urgency.

If the patient has been in a region of the world where malaria is endemic (even for a brief time, such as an airport layover), fever mandates a consideration for malaria, whether or not malaria prophylaxis has been used. The patient with malaria usually presents with a history of headache, malaise, fever and chills, and nausea 48 hours after exposure to *P. vivax* or *P. ovale*, or 72 hours after exposure to *P. malariae*. Dormant parasites may remain in the liver, causing relapse months after the initial infection. By contrast, the incubation period for patients infected with *P. falciparum* is usually 12 to 14 days, with subsequent high fevers every 48 hours within 2 months of the infection. Diarrhea is a common complaint among children with *P. falciparum* infection.

In addition to a general physical examination, ophthalmic and neurologic examinations should be performed. The findings will be used, in part, as a baseline for drug monitoring. Attention should be given to signs and symptoms of dehydration and electrolyte imbalance.

Laboratory Testing

Diarrheal stool from the patient with amebiasis should be examined immediately for trophozoites in addition to fixed stool specimens (e.g., white blood cells, culture). Serologic tests are done in patients with idiopathic inflammatory bowel disease to rule out amebiasis. Amebae and/or cysts may be found in the urine.

Identification of plasmodia in serial blood smears is definitive for malaria. It is best to obtain blood during or immediately after a fever spike. If the health care provider suspects a drug-resistant strain of *P. falciparum*, the laboratory order forms should be marked accordingly. A commercial kit is available for the diagnosis. The identification of the type of plasmodium is important for therapy. In some cases, the patient is infected with more than one strain of plasmodia. The liver function test results may be elevated and thrombocytopenia, anemia, and leukopenia may be present. Malaria causes hemolysis. Baseline laboratory tests, including electrolytes, G6PD measurement, platelet counts, and renal function tests should be performed before the start of drug therapy.

The perianal "scotch tape" test can be used to check for ova in patients with *E. vermicularis* (pinworms) and occasionally for other helminthic infections. Collection of pinworms is best accomplished during the night, when they tend to migrate to the anal surface. Examination of stool specimens may reveal ascariasis (roundworm), whipworm, *Strongyloides*, and hookworm infestations.

GOALS OF THERAPY

The primary goal of treatment for infestations is to kill or destroy the offending organism. The key to eradication of an infestation is to use drug(s) that interfere with the life cycle of the organism. Most antiprotozoal, antiparasitic, and antihelminthic drugs are highly effective against specific organisms; thus the organism must be accurately identified before treatment is started. Antibiotics are not appropriate for the treatment of infestations. Many of the drugs used in treatment are not routinely available in the United States. In some cases, the drugs are available only through the Parasitic Disease Drug Service at the CDC. Consultation with a pharmacist, public health department, and/or the CDC will be helpful.

INTERVENTION
Administration

The drug regimen for specific infestations must be followed closely for treatment to be successful. The half-lives of some drugs are increased when they are taken with fatty foods. Further, for many of the drugs, gastric irritation can be minimized if the drugs are taken with food. Depending on the specific drug, the formulation may be crushed and mixed with applesauce or other food for administration.

Prophylaxis. A malaria vaccine is not available, although it is hoped that this goal will ultimately be achieved. Because the three major parasitic stages of malaria in humans are antigenically distinct, a successful vaccine will likely need to contain at least three parasite antigens (sporozoite, merozoite, and gametocyte). A vaccine that limits the magnitude of parasitemia could have a marked effect on survival, even if it had no effect on the incidence of infection, because severe morbidity and mortality are associated with high parasitemias.

A calendar can be prepared for the patient taking antimalarial drugs for prophylaxis, with the drug administration days identified. Mefloquine, for example, should be taken the same day each week, with food and a full 8-ounce glass of water, beginning 1 week before exposure and continuing for 4 weeks after the traveler has returned to a malaria-free area. The drugs should be taken with meals to minimize GI distress. Updated recommendations on malaria prophylaxis may be obtained 24 hours a day, 7 days a week through the Centers for Disease Control and Prevention.

Pyrimethamine should be started 1 week before departure for endemic areas, and continued during the travel period and for 6 to 10 weeks following return. Regular blood tests will be necessary during therapy.

Treatment. Regardless of the drug chosen for treatment of malaria, compliance with the regimen is important. Patients should be instructed to take the drug exactly as prescribed. Sustained-release drug forms should not be crushed or chewed. Most antimalarial drugs should be taken with food to minimize GI upset. Ophthalmic examinations should be scheduled when the drugs are used for long periods of time.

Education

The compliance and dependability of the person being treated are crucial factors for successful elimination of the parasites. Careful instructions must be given for timing of return visits, for submission of specimens, and for taking of medications.

The importance of meticulous hygiene—that is, washing hands before eating and after toileting, and keeping hands or objects away from the mouth—should be emphasized. Toilet facilities should be disinfected daily. The patient should be instructed to take frequent showers rather than baths, and to change clothing, bed linens, and towels daily to prevent reinfection. The importance of follow-up with the health care provider cannot be stressed enough.

Because niclosamide, praziquantel, pyrantel pamoate, and thiabendazole may cause drowsiness and dizziness, the patient should be advised not to drive a motor vehicle or operate machinery until his or her reaction is known. The patient should also be warned that oxamniquine causes a harmless reddish-orange discoloration of the urine.

Travelers must be cautioned regarding the reservoir for helminths when they are visiting other countries. This is particularly important if their travel takes them to underdeveloped areas with primitive facilities for elimination, eating, or drinking.

Because of growing drug resistance, greater emphasis is placed on reducing exposure to the *Anopheles* mosquito, especially in hyperendemic areas such as Africa. Strategies that are successful and should be considered include the application of insect repellents that contain DEET (diethyltoluamide) and the use of netting impregnated with pyrethrin (insecticide) over the bed for protection during sleep. DDT (dichlorodiphenyltrichloroethane) is no longer effective in most regions of the world because of widespread resistance. Exposed nonimmune persons should be advised to consider malaria prophylaxis, to use insect repellents, and otherwise to reduce their exposure to the *Anopheles* mosquito.

Persons who harbor the sexual forms of plasmodia are called carriers. It is from the carriers that mosquitoes receive the forms of the parasite that perpetuate the disease. Carriers should be advised to avoid giving blood, because it is possible that the recipient of their blood will contract malaria or become a carrier. A growing number of malaria cases have been associated with the transfusion of infected blood. Any person who has had malaria or has been exposed to the disease by visiting a region where it is prevalent must be disqualified as a blood donor.

EVALUATION

Treatment effectiveness is identified by the absence of clinical signs and symptoms, by negative cultures, and by lack of adverse drug reactions. Untreated invasive amebiasis is frequently fatal. With treatment, improvement usually occurs within a few days. Some patients with amebic colitis have irritable bowel symptoms for weeks after successful treatment. Relapses are possible.

If fever persists after adequate antimalarial therapy, the diagnosis must be reevaluated.

For most patients with helminthic infestation, three stool samples examined after the completion of therapy should be negative. After roundworm infestation, the patient's stool samples should be free of ova, larvae, or worms 2 to 3 weeks after completion of therapy. Specimens from a patient with flukes should be negative for several months before the patient is considered cured. For pinworm infestation, perianal swabs should be negative for 7 days.

CASE STUDY    *Malaria*

ASSESSMENT

HISTORY OF PRESENT ILLNESS

JD is a 26-year-old woman, a missionary trainee, who returned 1 week ago from a 6-month stay with the Klong tribes of Thailand. She has faithfully taken the mefloquine provided for malaria prophylaxis. She is complaining of general malaise, sporadic occurrence of fevers as high as 103° F, headaches, intermittent cold sensations, myalgia, and diarrhea. Her symptoms started about 3 weeks ago, resolved, and have now returned. She thinks she may have a bad flu, because some of her companions have the same symptoms.

HEALTH HISTORY

JD's general health is good; she passed a full physical examination before the church appointment 9 months ago. She denies history of diabetes, hypertension, or cancer. Her family health history is benign; her mother and father are alive and well, as are two siblings.

LIFESPAN CONSIDERATIONS

JD is hoping to marry soon and have her first child within the next year.

CULTURAL/SOCIAL CONSIDERATIONS

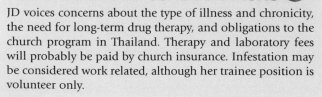

JD voices concerns about the type of illness and chronicity, the need for long-term drug therapy, and obligations to the church program in Thailand. Therapy and laboratory fees will probably be paid by church insurance. Infestation may be considered work related, although her trainee position is volunteer only.

PHYSICAL EXAMINATION

JD's blood pressure is 110/76 mm Hg, her temperature is 102.6° F with chills lasting 20 to 36 hours, her pulse is 110, and respirations are 32. Her skin is intact, pink, and clear; she is diaphoretic. Her abdominal examination is unremarkable; bowel sounds are present; and her lungs are clear to auscultation.

LABORATORY TESTING

Suspect malarial parasite from travel history; blood tests reflect presence of *P. falciparum*; organism is sensitive to atovaquone + proguanil, resistant to chloroquine.

PATIENT PROBLEM(S)

P. falciparum malaria.

GOALS OF THERAPY

Cure infestation; reduce risk of reoccurrence.

CRITICAL THINKING QUESTIONS

1. Discuss the life cycle of the *Plasmodium* organism.
2. JD's health care provider orders atovaquone + proguanil. What is the mechanism of action of these drugs?
3. Why did JD's health care provider not use chloroquine to treat the malaria?
4. To what adverse effects of atovaquone and proguanil should JD be alerted?
5. By what route(s) are atovaquone and proguanil eliminated?

Bibliography

Anonymous: Atovaquone/proguanil (Malarone) for malaria, *Med Lett Drugs Ther* 42(1093):109-111, 2000.

Anonymous: Availability and use of parenteral quinidine gluconate for severe or complicated malaria, *MMWR Morb Mortal Wkly Rep* 49(50):1138-1140, 2000.

Bastow V: Identifying and treating PCP. . . *Pneumocystis carinii* . . . including commentary by Wilkinson J, *Nurs Times* 96(37 NTplus):19-20, 2000.

Glatt A: In consultation. *Pneumocystis carinii* pneumonia: how to treat and prevent in the era of HAART, *J Crit Illness*, 15(4):186-187, 2000.

Lynch JS: Malaria—always a possibility in the febrile traveler or immigrant, *JAAPA* 13(9):61-62, 65-66, 68, 2000.

Martin J: Malaria, *Nurs Stand* 15(26):47-52, 54-55, March 14-20, 2001.

Mead M: The complaint threadworms, *Pract Nurse* 20(3):169-170, 2000.

Weller IV, Williams IG: ABC of AIDS: treatment of infections, *BMJ*, 322(7298):1350-1354, 2001.

Internet Resources

Centers for Disease Control and Prevention. Available online at http://www.cdc.gov/ncidod/dpd/parasites/listing.htm.

Medscape: antihelminthic drugs. Available online at http://www.medscape.com/viewarticle/434844.

CHAPTER

35

Immunizing Drugs

SUSAN SCIACCA

 Visit http://evolve.elsevier.com/Gutierrez/ for additional information.

KEY TERMS

Acquired immunity, p. 532

Antibodies, p. 532

Antigens, p. 532

Antisera, p. 534

Antitoxins, p. 539

Attenuated, p. 533

Humoral immunity, p. 532

Innate immunity, p. 532

Immunoglobulins, p. 532

Toxoid, p. 534

Vaccine, p. 533

OBJECTIVES

- Distinguish between active and passive immunity.
- Describe the actions of vaccines, toxoids, antisera, and antitoxins.
- Identify the current recommendations for infant, child, and adult immunizations.
- Describe the adverse effects of vaccines, toxoids, antisera, and antitoxins.
- Identify patients for whom a vaccine, serum, or other immunizing drug may be contraindicated.
- Explain the nursing responsibilities for proper administration of vaccines, toxoids, sera, and antitoxins, including patient health history, vaccine storage, patient record keeping, patient education, and monitoring and reporting of adverse effects.

PHYSIOLOGY • Immunostimulation

The immune system allows us to live in a world full of dangerous organisms that can invade the body and cause disease. The immune system offers both innate protection and the ability to acquire immunity in response to new challenges. **Innate immunity** is a nonspecific type of immunity derived from all of the elements with which a person is born. Each varies in duration and effectiveness, depending on how it developed.

Innate Immunity

Innate immunity is a natural, nonspecific immunity that is provided through receptors encoded in a person's germline. It is always available on short notice to protect the body from challenges by foreign materials, and prior exposure is not required to mount a defense. The mechanisms of innate immunity are based on recognition of molecular patterns shared by pathogens but not found in the host. For example, phagocytosis, which is ingestion and destruction of foreign particles, such as bacteria, by individual cells of the immune system, may be trigged by receptors on macrophages that recognize the mannose on the surface of a bacteria as foreign. These nonspecific defense mechanisms work against any foreign agent that contains the pattern of mannose on its surface. Thus, the protection is general, acting against many common pathogens.

Acquired Immunity

In addition to innate immunity, the body has the ability to develop specific immunity against individual foreign agents such as bacteria, viruses, toxins, and even foreign tissues from other people or animals. This is called **acquired immunity,** and unlike innate immunity, acquired immunity is not present at birth but develops as the individual encounters various foreign agents.

Acquired immunity is not fully exhibited until the person has had two sequential exposures to the same foreign agent. Each foreign agent contains one or more specific compounds in its makeup that make it different from all other agents. In general, these are proteins, large polysaccharides, or lipids found on the surface of cells. These substances, called **antigens,** initiate the acquired immunity response when they are attacked by lymphocytes, which are the primary providers of acquired immunity.

Two types of lymphocytes originate from the stem cells in bone marrow: T lymphocytes (T cells) and B lymphocytes (B cells) (see Chapter 36). When an antigen is first introduced into the body, it is phagocytized by a macrophage, which then presents the antigen to a vast array of T cells that contain randomly generated recognition sites. T cells within this population that contain a receptor for that specific antigen are selected and become activated. Both the macrophage and the activated T cells secrete chemicals that stimulate replication of the activated T cells. Some of these activated T cells, called killer T cells, destroy cells with the antigen.

The T cells that provide long-term acquired immunity are called *memory T cells.* These cells recognize the specific antigen that triggered the initial response and stimulate a faster and more intense response if the same antigen is encountered again.

B lymphocytes (B cells) are responsible for **humoral immunity.** Similar to T cells, each type of B cell responds to only one specific type of antigen. Unlike T cells, however, B cells do not act directly on the antigen. Instead, they produce soluble proteins called **antibodies** that react with the antigen. Antibody-mediated immunity is most effective against bacteria, viruses that are outside body cells, and toxins.

When an antigen enters the body, a macrophage will engulf and process it, then present it to B cells and helper T cells (see Chapter 36). The B cells and helper T cells that have receptors for that specific antigen become activated. The activated helper T cells secrete substances that stimulate the activated B cells to rapidly replicate in a process called clonal expansion that produces populations of plasma cells and memory B cells. The plasma cells produce antibodies that are transported in the blood and lymph to the site of the infection, where they inactivate the antigens. This initial action is called the primary response (Figure 35-1). After the antigens are destroyed, macrophages clean up the debris and suppressor T cells decrease the immune response. Memory B cells remain dormant in lymphatic tissue until the same antigen again enters the body. At that time the memory cells recognize the antigen and launch a rapid and intense response called a secondary response. The purpose of vaccination is to provide an initial exposure so that memory cells are available at subsequent exposure to the antigen.

In general, all antibodies have a similar amino acid structure, but one portion of the molecule is different. That component makes each antibody capable of reacting with a specific antigen. Antibodies belong to a class of proteins known as globulins. Because they are involved in the immune response they are known as **immunoglobulins.**

There are five classes of immunoglobulins: IgA, IgD, IgE, IgG, and IgM. Each class has a specific role in immunity. IgM is the first antibody produced during a primary immune response, and it is distributed primarily in the intravascular space. IgM activates complement and is efficient in agglutinating antibodies. Immunoglobulins of the IgG class are called *gamma globulins.*

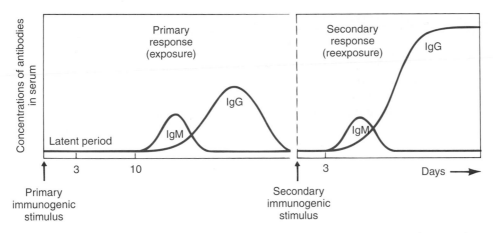

FIGURE 35-1 Time course of antibody release on first exposure versus subsequent exposure. KEY: *IgG*, immunoglobulin G; *IgM*, immunoglobulin M.

Immunoglobulin G, the most abundant immunoglobulin in serum, is found in the intravascular and extravascular spaces. It is responsible for most responses to antigens, including activation of complement, sensitization of target cells for destruction by killer cells, neutralization of toxins and viruses, and immobilization of bacteria. *IgA* is the most common antibody found in secretions, where it protects mucous membranes. It is also found in the intravascular space. *IgE* mediates hypersensitivity and allergic reactions and protects against parasite infections. It is found on basophils and mast cells as well as in saliva and nasal secretions. *IgD* is located on the surface of B lymphocytes with a trace found in the serum. It serves as an antigen-specific receptor on B cells and is thought to be involved in differentiation of B lymphocytes.

TYPES OF IMMUNITY
Natural Immunity

Active Natural Immunity. A person can achieve active natural immunity in two ways. The first is by having the disease. For example, the body of a child with chicken pox responds to the specific pathogen by developing antibodies. After the first exposure the child does not get chicken pox again, because the immune system has a ready supply of antibodies and memory cells that respond quickly to the second exposure to the chicken pox virus. Because the body produced the antibodies, this type of naturally acquired immunity is called active natural immunity. Active immunity usually persists for years.

Passive Natural Immunity. The second way to acquire immunity is by receiving antibodies from the mother. The fetus is protected from bacterial and viral infections as well as from microbial toxins by maternal IgG antibodies, which pass to the fetus through the placenta. IgG is the only antibody that crosses the placenta. The mother developed this antibody in response to the pathogens she encountered throughout her lifetime. Because the child's immune system did not produce these antibodies (having received them from the mother), this type of immunity is called passive natural immunity. The mother's antibodies afford protection to the infant for about the first 6 months of life. Breast milk contains IgA antibodies, which may extend the length of immunoprotection. Unlike active immunity, which often lasts a lifetime, passive immunity provides protection as long as the antibodies remain in the blood and are active, which is usually a period of a few weeks.

Acquired Immunity

Active Acquired Immunity. Active acquired immunity can be achieved by deliberately administering a specific vaccine or toxoid. A **vaccine** is an antigen-containing substance injected into a person in an attempt to stimulate antibody production. The vaccine usually consists of **attenuated** (weakened), inactivated, or dead pathogens or their toxins. The antigens still stimulate the immune system but are altered so they do not produce symptoms of the disease. Because the use of a vaccine stimulates the body to produce its own antibodies, vaccines induce active immunity.

A vaccine can also be prepared from the toxin secreted by a pathogen. The toxin is altered to reduce its harmfulness, but it still acts as an antigen to induce an immune response. The altered toxin is known as a **toxoid.** Because a toxoid also incites antibody production, it produces active immunity.

Passive Acquired Immunity. Passive acquired immunity results when antibodies that developed in another person (or animal) are injected to an individual. **Antisera** is the general term used for the formulation that contains the antibodies. Antisera may contain antibodies that act against microorganisms, bacterial toxins, or venoms. Antisera are usually obtained from animals that received the antigen, either by injection into the tissues or blood or by infection. Passive acquired immunity provides immediate but short-lived protection against the injurious antigen.

An immunoglobulin differs from a vaccine in that it is obtained from a donor (human or animal) and contains antibodies. The antibodies are formed in the donor in response to a specific antigen. These preformed antibodies are taken from the donor and injected into the recipient, thereby conveying passive immunity.

DRUG CLASS • Vaccines and Toxoids

MECHANISM OF ACTION

All vaccines contain similar major constituents. The antigenic substance may be in one of four forms: (1) *dead bacteria*, as in typhoid fever immunization; (2) *dead viruses*, as in the Salk poliovirus vaccine; (3) *live attenuated virus*, as in the smallpox vaccine; and (4) *toxoids*, as in immunization against tetanus and diphtheria. The antigenic component is contained in a suspension, usually normal saline, or in water. Trace amounts of chemicals serve as preservatives, stabilizers, and antimicrobial agents. Additives (e.g., aluminum compounds) may be used to increase the antigenicity of the vaccine and to prolong its immunostimulatory effects. Identification of these components is necessary so that potential hypersensitivity can be identified before immunization. Table 35-1 identifies the indications, formulations, efficacy, and duration of action of available vaccines and toxoids.

Live, attenuated bacterial vaccines stimulate the production of various antibodies. Those antibodies that play a protective role are directed against antigens on the surface of the bacterial cell or its exotoxin. Coating the bacterial surface with antibodies either renders the organisms susceptible to phagocytosis, lysis, and aggregation or interferes with the function of critical bacterial surface structures. Polysaccharide vaccines provide long-term protection, usually after a single dose (except in children less than 2 years old). Bacterial vaccines are prepared from any of the following sources:
- Whole bacteria (e.g., pertussis vaccine)
- Purified products of whole-cell vaccine (e.g., acellular pertussis vaccine)
- Purified capsular polysaccharides of certain bacteria (e.g., pneumococcal and meningococcal vaccines)
- Purified polysaccharides conjugated to protein carriers to improve immunogenicity (e.g., *Haemophilus influenzae* type B vaccine)

Vaccines containing live, attenuated viruses produce a mild or subclinical infection that results in long-term active immunity. Repeated dosing of the vaccine is required since replication of the virus in the host is necessary to induce immunity. In contrast, inactivated, nonliving, whole viral vaccines must contain a sufficient amount of antigen to induce the desired immune response, because the organisms in these preparations cannot replicate in the host. Repeated dosing is usually necessary to provoke long-term immunity. Viral vaccines are prepared from any of the following sources:
- Live, attenuated viruses (e.g., measles, mumps, rubella)
- Dead whole-cell viruses (e.g., influenza, rabies, inactivated poliovirus vaccines)
- Antigenic components of the virus particle (e.g., influenza "split-virus" vaccine, hepatitis B vaccine)

Vaccines are antigens and not antibodies, and therefore generate an active immune response. Toxoids, like vaccines, stimulate active immunity without causing disease. During preparation of a toxoid, the original toxin's pathogenic quality is destroyed, but its antigenic properties remain. Some toxoids are precipitated or absorbed with chemicals that cause them to remain in the tissues longer. The absorbed formulation increases the production of antibodies, making the response long-lasting. Nevertheless, toxoids can produce painful, localized reactions. The adverse effects, which are more pronounced in adults and older children, may necessitate the use of smaller initial doses.

USES
Childhood Immunizations

A number of infectious diseases are almost completely preventable through routine childhood immunizations. The recommended childhood immunization schedule in the United States begins soon after birth so that the infant can mount an effective immune response when the maternal antibodies lose their effectiveness. The recommended childhood immunizations include he-

Text continued on p. 538

TABLE 35-1

Drugs for Active Immunity

Drug	Indications	Formulation	Efficacy/Duration	Implications
Vaccines				
Bacillus Calmette-Guérin (TICE BCG)	Tuberculosis in adults and children with negative Tb skin tests who reside in high-risk house-holds; for health care workers exposed to resistant TB; travelers to endemic areas	Live attenuated/live vaccine	Protection variable; duration variable	Avoid persons who have active TB for 6-12 weeks after immunization
Cholera	Only for persons traveling to countries where cholera is endemic or vaccination is required	Inactivated whole cell bacterial vaccine	50% immunity when two doses are received; 6 months; booster required	Administer yellow fever vaccine at least 3 weeks apart from cholera since it may decrease antibody formation
Diphtheria-tetanus (DT)	For primary immunization of a child who has a contra-indication to pertussis vaccine	Toxoid	10 years; booster required	Do not administer to a child with a fever or to a child who has a history of neurologic or severe hyper-sensitivity reaction to a previous dose
Diphtheria-tetanus-acellular pertussis (DTaP, Acel-Immune, Tripedia, Infanrix)	Children 2 months to 7 years; decreases serious adverse effects associated with whole-cell vaccine	Toxoid	High; 10 years; boosters required for tetanus toxoid component	Do not administer to a child with fever or history of severe reaction to an earlier DTP
Haemophilus influenzae type B polysaccharide (HibTiter, PedvaxHIB, ProHibit)	Children to 6 years of age; for all children whose spleens have been removed	Inactivated bacteria	Unknown duration, probably 1.5-3 years	Three conjugate vaccines are available; be sure to check formulation used; contraindicated in febrile illness or active infection
Hepatitis A (Havrix, VAQTA)	Hepatitis A prophylaxis for persons at high risk, including military personnel and travelers to endemic areas	Inactivated virus	80%-98%; 10 years; booster dose after 6-12 months	Can give along with other vaccines without interfering with immune responses; contraindicated in patients who have bleeding disorders or febrile illness
Hepatitis B (Energix B, Heptavax B, Recombivax HB)	Hepatitis B prophylaxis for infants, young children, persons with environmental or lifestyle risk, including those who have hemophilia or are receiving hemodialysis	Inactivated virus	96% in children, 88% in adults; duration un-known but at least 5 years; booster needed if antibody level <10 million units/mL 1-2 months after third dose	Dialysis patients receive a special formulation

Continued

TABLE 35-1

Drugs for Active Immunity—cont'd

Drug	Indications	Formulation	Efficacy/Duration	Implications
Vaccines—cont'd				
Influenzae (Fluzone, FluShield, Fluvirin, Influenza Virus)	Influenza prophylaxis for adults over age 65 years, persons with asthma or other respiratory conditions and health care providers	Inactivated virus	60%-75% ; 1 year	Contraindicated in patients allergic to eggs, egg protein, chickens, bisulfites, or thimerisol, and those with a history of Guillian-Barré syndrome
Japanese encephalitis (Je-Vax)	Prophylaxis for adults and children traveling to or residing in areas endemic for disease	Inactivated virus	78% after second dose, 99% after third dose; duration at least 2 years after three doses	Do not travel within 10 days of vaccination
Lyme vaccine (Lymerix)	Prophylaxis in persons age 15-70 years residing in high-risk areas	Recombinant lipoprotein	Unknown at this time	Safety and efficacy dependent on administration of second and third doses several weeks before onset of *Borrelia* transmission season
Measles-mumps-rubella (M-M-R II)	Children to age 12 years	Live attenuated virus	95%; years to life; second dose recommended on entry to grade school, middle school, or high school	Combination drug preferred over single formulations; contraindicated in persons with allergies to eggs or neomycin
Measles (rubeola) (Attenuvax)	Children and adults born after 1956 without a history of measles or live virus vaccination on or after their first birthday	Live attenuated virus	95%; years to life	Usually given with mumps and rubella vaccines; may invalidate TB test if given within 6 weeks of immunization
Measles-Rubella (M-R-Vax II)	Susceptible persons over 12 years who have immunity to mumps	Live attenuated virus	8 years	
Meningococcus (Menomune A/C/Y/W)	For military personnel, persons without spleens or who are immunosuppressed, and those with household, institutional, or travel contact with the disease	Inactivated bacteria	90% in adults, variable in young children; effectiveness drops to 67% after 3 years	Not for routine immunization
Mumps (Mumpsvax)	Adults born after 1956 without a history of mumps or live virus vaccine on or after their first birthday	Live attenuated virus	Permanent immunity in 75%-90% of patients; 10 years	
Mumps-Rubella (Biavax III)	All susceptible persons over age 12 years, except pregnant women	Live attenuated virus	Permanent immunity	Used less often than MMR

TABLE 35-1

Drugs for Active Immunity—cont'd

Drug	Indications	Formulations	Efficacy/Duration	Implications
Vaccines—cont'd				
Plague	Laboratory personnel working with *Yersinia pestis*, persons in contact with rodents or fleas, and persons in endemic areas	Inactivated bacteria	Three booster doses at 6 month intervals; then every 1-2 years	Contraindicated in persons with sensitivity to beef protein, soy, casein; use of vaccine increases chances of recovery in epidemic situations; continue drug regi-men as long as danger of exposure exists
Pneumococcus (Pneumovax 23, Pnu-Immune 23)	Adults over age 65 years and persons at risk including people with weakened immune systems, cancers, organ transplants, or chronic diseases	Inactivated bacteria	Years	Available as heptavalent conjugate or polysaccharide; check formulation before using; contraindicated in hypersensitivity to phenol or thimerisol
Pneumococcal 7 valent (Prevnar)	Universal immunization of children 2 to 23 months and high risk children ages 24-59 months	Inactivated bacteria	92%-100%; unknown duration	Requires a series of four injections
Poliovirus (Salk) (IPV, IPOL)	Children 6 weeks to adulthood and adults at high risk	Inactivated whole virus	90%; booster required	Although a protective immune response cannot be assured in an immuno-compromised individual, IPV is still recommended because the vaccine is safe and some protection may result from its administration
Rabies, human diploid cell (HDCV, Imovax, Imovax Rabies ID)	Precxposure prophylaxis for persons at risk through animal handling; post-exposure prophylaxis	Inactivated virus	Boosters recommended	Rabies immunoglobulin admin-istered at same time as initial dose of HDCV vaccine
Rabies (absorbed) (RVA)	Postexposure prophylaxis in adults	Inactivated virus	2 years	Check antibody levels after 2 years; give booster if necessary
Rabies (purified chick embryo cell culture) (RabAvert)	Preexposure prophylaxis for persons at risk through animal handling; postexposure prophylaxis	Inactivated virus	2 years; check antibody levels after 2 years; give booster if necessary	Complete preexposure prophylaxis does not eliminate need for rabies vaccine after an exposure.
Rubella (Meruvax II)	Persons over age 12 years, nonpregnant women, postpartum women with no history of immunization, and persons traveling to endemic areas	Live attenuated virus	95%; 6-15 years; booster not recommended	Contraindicated in pregnancy, immunosuppression, allergy to neomycin
Smallpox (calf lymph) (DryVax)	Preexposure and postexposure smallpox prophylaxis	Live virus	Unknown	The vaccine take rate is >90% for current stockpile of drug

Continued

TABLE 35-1

Drugs for Active Immunity—cont'd

Drug	Indications	Formulation	Efficacy/Duration	Implications
Vaccines—cont'd				
Tetanus-diphtheria (adult) (Td)	Adults and susceptible children over 7 years	Toxoid (absorbed)	10 years; booster required every 6-10 years	Contraindicated in those with allergy to thimerisol
Tetanus-diphtheria (pediatric) (DT)	Adults and routine administration for children up to 6 years in whom pertussis vaccine is contraindicated	Toxoid	10 years	Do not administer to a child with a fever or to someone with a history of neurologic or severe hypersensitivity reaction to a previous dose
Varicella (Varivax)	Healthy adults and children with no history of chicken pox	Live attenuated virus	95%-97% ages 1-12 years; 79% ages 13-17 years	Can be given along with MMR using separate syringes and injection sites
Toxoids				
Tetanus toxoid	All children and adults	Toxoid	High; 10 years; booster required	Available as fluid and absorbed formulations containing different concentrations of tetanus toxoid
Typhold (Ty2 S. typhi)	Military personnel and persons in or traveling to endemic areas	Inactivated bacteria	70%-90%; 3 years; booster may be given when needed	Avoid concurrent use with antibiotics or within 7 days of an antibiotic; has more troublesome adverse effects than oral formulation
Typhoid oral TY21a (Virotif Berna)	Persons in or traveling to endemic areas	Live, attenuated virus	5 years; booster required	Avoid concurrent use with antibiotics or within 7 days of an antibiotic
Varicella (Varivax)	Persons over age 1 year, including adolescents and adults with no history of chicken pox	Live virus	Unknown; a new vaccine; booster required	Contraindicated in patients who are immunosuppressed, have active untreated Tb, active febrile infection
Yellow fever (YF-Vax)	Persons over age 9 years who are living in or traveling to areas of South America or Africa where yellow fever is endemic	Live attenuated virus	100% after 7-10 days; 10 years	Cautious use in persons allergic to chicken or egg products; contraindicated in patients who are immunosuppressed, in children under 6 months, and during pregnancy

patitis B (Hep B), diphtheria-tetanus-pertussis (DTaP), *Haemophilus influenzae* type B (Hib), inactivated poliovirus (IPV), measles-mumps-rubella (MMR), chicken pox (varicella zoster virus [VZV]), and pneumococcal (PCV).

Adult Immunizations

Adults who have no history of disease or active immunization against measles, mumps, rubella, or chicken pox should be immunized for these diseases because they are more severe in adults than in children. Most adults in the United States have been immunized against poliovirus. A booster for tetanus and diphtheria (Td) should be administered every 10 years throughout life. Adults more than 65 years old are advised to have an annual influenza vaccination and at least one pneumococcal vaccination.

Special Populations

Women of childbearing age who do not have rubella immunity should be immunized when they are not pregnant, preferably during the immediate postpartum period. Travelers (especially those visiting underdeveloped regions), military personnel, and health care providers should be immunized against hepatitis A and hepatitis B. Immunization against hepatitis B is also recommended for individuals living in the same household as an infected person, for individuals with multiple sex partners, and for intravenous drug users. Immunization against pneumococcal pneumonia is recommended not only for those over age 65 years but also for those with chronic disease or weakened immunity, persons who abuse alcohol, organ transplant recipients, and those over age 50 years who are living in group homes. Vaccination against influenza is recommended not only for those over age 65 years but also for nursing home residents as well as those who have chronic disease, weakened immunity, or contact with high-risk persons.

Special immunizations are recommended for those at specific risk for diseases such as cholera, meningococcal meningitis, plague, rabies, typhoid, or yellow fever.

Currently available drugs are identified in Table 35-1. Postexposure prophylaxis should be provided for individuals exposed to *H. influenzae* type B, meningococcal infection, hepatitis A, hepatitis B, tuberculosis, and rabies.

PHARMACOKINETICS

Because vaccines stimulate the immune system to respond actively rather than passively, protection persists after the injected drug has disappeared. The duration of protection is usually 1 to 10 years. Because vaccines are antigens and not antibodies, they are taken up and processed by antigen-presenting cells for the generation of immune responses. Some of the injected drug is biotransformed in this manner. Once antibodies have been produced, any remaining injected drug can be complexed with the antibodies and cleared by phagocytosis.

ADVERSE REACTIONS AND CONTRAINDICATIONS

In general, vaccines should not be administered when the individual has a fever or febrile illness. Live and attenuated viral vaccines should not be used in patients receiving immunosuppressive therapy and those with AIDS or other immune system diseases such as leukemia or lymphoma, because these vaccines can cause progressive disease in immunocompromised patients. Live-virus vaccines are also contraindicated in pregnant women because such vaccines can damage the fetus. Live-virus vaccines stimulate a mild infection in the host with limited symptoms of disease. Examples of these vaccines include the bacillus Calmette Guérin (BCG) vaccine for tuberculosis (see Chapter 33) as well as measles-mumps-rubella (MMR), typhoid, varicella (chicken pox), and yellow fever vaccines.

Most adverse effects are localized reactions at the injection site, including swelling, redness, warmth, and pain. Less common systemic adverse effects include myalgias, malaise, headache, fever, chills, and anorexia. Anaphylaxis and seizure are rare reactions. Individuals with an allergy to eggs or egg proteins may experience adverse reactions to viruses grown in eggs, such as those found in the influenza, MMR, and yellow fever vaccines.

INTERACTIONS

All immunosuppressive drugs interfere with the generation of active immunity induced by vaccines and toxoids. Corticosteroids, azathioprine, cyclosporine, and some drugs used in antineoplastic therapy fall in this category.

 DRUG CLASS • **Antisera and Antitoxins**

MECHANISM OF ACTION

Passive acquired immunity involves administration of preformed substances such as antisera that can immediately combine with the foreign agent to which they are directed. Antisera and antitoxin antibodies are obtained by injecting an animal, such as a horse, with a purified antigen. After antibodies have had time to develop, blood is withdrawn from the animal and prepared for clinical use. **Antitoxins** contain specific antibodies produced in response to the presence of a toxin; they neutralize pathogenic toxins but have no effect directly on the pathogens. The passive immunity offered by immune sera, antibodies, or globulins lasts only weeks.

Human serum vaccine is a sterile, concentrated protein solution (15% to 18%) composed primarily of the immunoglobulin fraction with trace amounts of IgA or IgM. It contains specific antibodies in proportion to the infection and immunization experience of the population from which it is derived.

USES

Antitoxins are used when an individual has been exposed to an organism that secretes exotoxins, such as tetanus, botulism, diphtheria, gas gangrene, and rabies. They are used for both prophylaxis and treatment to provide temporary passive immunity against pathogenic organisms, microbial exotoxins, and snake or insect venoms. Immune globulin is indicated as replacement therapy for patients with antibody deficiency disorders or hepatitis A and for measles prophylaxis. Table 35-2 provides an overview of selected antisera and antitoxins.

PHARMACOKINETICS

Intramuscular injection is the usual route of administration of the antitoxins, antisera, and immune globulins. Oral administration is usually impossible with these drugs because the degradative processes in the GI tract render them inactive before they can be absorbed. Distribution is fairly rapid after intramuscular injection, but if very rapid therapy is required, these drugs can be given intravenously, resulting in immediate distribution. Peak serum levels of antibodies are achieved 48 to 72 hours after inoculation. The immunity provided by antitoxins, antisera, and immune globulins generally last from 1 to 6 weeks. Once injected, the antibodies interact with the entire organism against which they were generated, thus facilitating phagocytosis of the organism by monocytes or macrophages and polymorphonuclear neutrophil leukocytes (PMNs). Antibodies made against toxins of pathogenic microorganisms form complexes with the toxin; phagocytes also clear these immune complexes. Immunity is lost when the injected antibodies have been cleared from the system.

ADVERSE REACTIONS AND CONTRAINDICATIONS

Many adverse reactions to these drugs are dose related. There may be pain at the injection site, mild chest pain, and chills. Less common adverse reactions include malaise, headache, nausea and vomiting, dyspnea, syncope, and back pain. Hepatitis B immune globulin can also cause urticaria and angioedema. Varicella zoster immune globulin injections can cause a mild rash, usually observed 10 to 14 days after immunization.

TOXICITY

Antisera, especially those compounded from nonhuman proteins, can cause anaphylaxis in individuals with a history of hypersensitivity reactions to immune globulin injections. This serum sickness develops as massive immune complex formation occurs, followed by deposition of these complexes in the kidney and circulatory system, leading to nephritis and arteritis. The deposited immune complexes also initiate mediator release from platelets, basophils, and PMNs. This massive mediator release can be life threatening. Local deposition of insoluble immune complexes at an injection site can produce an Arthus reaction, in which redness and edema occur near blood vessels. Other signs of serum sickness include arthralgias, lymphadenopathy, and pruritus. In serious cases, abdominal pain, fever, headache, and malaise may occur. Use of antisera is generally contraindicated in patients with thrombocytopenia because excessive bleeding may occur at the injection site.

INTERACTIONS

There are no known drug interactions associated with the use of passive immunostimulants.

TABLE 35-2				
Drugs for Passive Immunity				
Drug	*Indications*	*Formulation*	*Efficacy/Duration*	*Comments*
Antisera				
Cytomegalovirus human immune globulin (CMV-IVIG, Cytogam)	Cytomegalovirus infection	Antisera	Weeks to months	May interfere with immune response to live virus vaccines; wait 3 months before administering
Hepatitis B immune globulin (H-BIG, Hyper-Hep, Hep-B-Gammagee)	Postexposure prophylaxis	Antisera	70%-80% after second dose; 94%-98% after third dose; 2 months	Not for treatment of fulminant acute or chronic active hepatitis B

```
TABLE 35-2
```

Drugs for Passive Immunity—cont'd

Drug	Indications	Formulation	Efficacy/Duration	Comments
Antisera—cont'd				
Immune serum globulin (gamma globulin, ISG, Gammar, Gamastan)	Primary immunodeficiency states, idiopathic thrombo-cytopenia, bone marrow transplant, pediatric HIV	IgG with trace amounts of IgA and IgM	Adequate serum levels of IgG in 2-5 days	Routine use in early pregnancy is not recommended
Immune serum globulin (IVIG, Gamimune, Sando-Globulin)	Primary immunodeficiency states, idiopathic thrombo-cytopenia, bone marrow transplant, pediatric HIV	IgG with trace amounts of IgA and IgM	May be given more often or dosage increased if clinical response or serum level of IgG is insufficient	May interfere with immune response to live virus vaccines; wait 3 months before administering
Rabies immune serum globulin (RIG, Hyperab, Imogam)	Part of postexposure prophylaxis of persons with rabies exposure who lack a history of preexposure or postexposure prophylaxis with rabies vaccine	Antisera	21 days	It is preferable to give with the first dose of vaccine, but it can be given up to 8 days after vaccination; one-half of the dosage may be infiltrated around the wound
Rh₀ human immune globulin (Rh₀Gam, Gamulin Rh, HypRh₀-D)	Obstetric use; transfusion mishap	IgG-antiD (Rh1)	12 weeks	Consult package insert for blood typing and drug administration procedures
Tetanus human immune globulin (TIG, Hyper-Tet)	Tetanus prophylaxis in patients whose immunization status is incomplete or uncertain	IgG	21 days	Preferred to tetanus antitoxin because it is less likely to cause allergic reactions and has longer duration of action; tetanus toxoid should be given at same time to initiate active immune response
Varicella zoster human immune globulin (VZIG)	Varicella zoster in children younger than 15 years and adults with significant risk factors on an individual basis	Antisera	21 days	Not for immunocompromised persons; most effective given within 72 hours of exposure; no evidence that drug modifies established infection
Antitoxins				
Botulism antitoxin	Botulism	Equine antitoxin	100% with 3 doses; unavailable	Available from the CDC; test for hypersensitivity to horse serum before giving
Diphtheria antitoxin	Diphtheria	Equine antitoxin		Used in conjunction with antibiotics to eliminate bacteria but does not eliminate bacterial toxins according to ACIP there currently is no evidence to support any additional benefit of diphtheria antitoxin in persons who have received appropriate antibiotic prophylaxis; skin test before administering
Tetanus antitoxin	Tetanus	Equine antitoxin		Rarely used; tetanus immune globulin is used if available

ACIP, Advisory Committee on Immunization Practices.

APPLICATION TO PRACTICE

ASSESSMENT
History of Present Illness

For routine immunizations, a patient's history of present illness is irrelevant. In most cases, these are considered well-person visits.

For persons exposed to infectious disease, determine the extent of exposure and when it occurred, whether it was related to household contacts or to a brief, casual contact with the infected animal or individual. For persons with wounds, determine how and when the wound was sustained and what was done for treatment.

For persons traveling internationally who may be exposed to disease, ask about the destination (i.e., urban or rural), the geographic itinerary, planned activities, month, and duration of travel in each country. Vaccine recommendations for persons residing in the United States are formulated by the Advisory Committee on Immunization Practices (ACIP). The Centers for Disease Control and Prevention (CDC) provides recommendations and position statements on immunizations required for international travel. The World Health Organization (WHO) regulates vaccine requirements for entry into member countries. The International Certificate of Vaccination (a shot record), a document in booklet form, validates the immunization status of international travelers.

Health History

The person should be asked to bring the immunization record to the appointment. Because some immunizations should not be given in close proximity to others, attention should be paid to the dates previous immunizations were received. For example, an immune globulin should not be given 3 months before or 2 weeks after a live viral vaccine.

Because many parents are unaware of the exact name and date of each immunization their child has received, the most reliable source of information is the immunization record, hospital, clinic, or health care provider record. All immunizations should be listed there, including the name of the specific vaccine, number of injections received, the dosage (sometimes lesser amounts may be given if a reaction is anticipated), the ages when the drug was administered (for children), and the occurrence of any reaction following the administration.

Determine whether the patient has any allergies. Information about allergies to sulfites, thimerosal, neomycin, or other components of an immunizing drug should be elicited from the patient. Inquire about previous administration of any horse or other foreign serum, recent administration of gamma globulin or blood transfusion, and anaphylactic reactions to neomycin, chickens, eggs, or egg proteins.

Ask about a history of immunosuppression. Many vaccines are not administered to a patient with an acute infection or to anyone who is immunosuppressed. Furthermore, female patients should be questioned about the possibility of pregnancy because some vaccines are contraindicated during pregnancy (e.g., varicella vaccine). In addition, persons who may be at risk for disease exposure should be identified.

Lifespan Considerations

Perinatal. Infection is still a major cause of morbidity and mortality during the perinatal period. The health care provider's goal is to prevent infection in the woman, as well as in the fetus and newborn infant. Evaluation of the pregnant woman should include information about the hepatitis B surface antigen (HBsAg) to identify newborns that require immunoprophylaxis for the prevention of perinatal infection and to identify household contacts who should be vaccinated.

Women who have not received the influenza vaccine risk pneumonia and exacerbation of chronic cardiovascular and other disorders. The general risk to a pregnant woman who is not up-to-date on her mumps vaccination includes unilateral sensorineural hearing loss, deafness, meningitis, pancreatitis, oophoritis, and death. There is no significant risk to the fetus directly related to maternal mumps infection. Abortion, stillbirth, prematurity, and low birth weight have been associated with measles infection in pregnant women. The infant of a mother who contacts measles is likely to have been transplacentally infected with measles and has an increased risk of other infections. Rubella, which is asymptomatic in up to 50% of pregnant women is neither more severe in pregnancy nor a cause for maternal complications in pregnancy but is associated with arthralgias, neuritis, thrombocytopenia purpura, and meningoencephalitis. Placental infection can lead to spontaneous abortion, stillbirth, or congenital defects. Passive immunity may modify the risk of a varicella zoster infection, although the woman should be tested for antibody status before being immunized.

Pediatric. Although many of the immunizations can be given to individuals of any age, the recommended primary schedule begins during infancy, and with the exception of boosters, is completed during early childhood. The risk of receiving childhood immunizations is most often offset by the benefit they provide. Immunization of children and older adults who have chronic illnesses should be provided but with an awareness as to the potential adverse effects.

An immunization update is an important part of adolescent preventive care. As teenagers move through adolescence, they are able to assume increasing responsibility for their own health, including immunizations. Parents should respect their teenager's independence and move toward the role of consultant about health issues while maintaining some level of parental involvement in the immunization process. In response to changes in adolescent morbidity and mortality, the American Medical Association developed the *Guidelines for Adolescent Preventive Services* (GAPS), which provides a framework for health care providers to use in clinical practice. The guidelines include information about specific topics and recommendations related to screening, guidance, and immunizations.

Older Adults. Influenza in the older adult is associated with high rates of hospitalization and death. Because the older adult is at risk for developing influenza, immunization is advocated. The CDC has immunization recommendations for all persons over age 65 years and for persons of any age who have chronic diseases that increase their risk of influenza. Influenza vaccination programs offered at a nominal cost or no cost to senior center participants could ultimately decrease the influenza rate significantly.

Cultural/Social Considerations

The benefits of immunization range from partial to complete protection against the consequences of the infection. The risks vary from common, minor, and inconvenient effects to rare, severe, and life-threatening conditions. Physical, cultural, social, and economic barriers and risks must be considered to achieve optimal protection against infectious diseases.

The health care provider should suspect that a child might not have been properly immunized if one or both parents have less than a high school education or if there are three or more siblings. Members of families who are economically disadvantaged or who seek health care at public clinics also may not have full immunization.

Physical Examination

The patient's temperature should be taken before administration of an immunizing drug. The presence of a fever may preclude vaccination; however, a mild, acute, afebrile illness (e.g., diarrhea or a minor upper respiratory tract illness, including otitis media) does not ordinarily contraindicate an immunization. Mild to moderate local reactions or low-grade fever following a prior dose of the vaccine, premature birth, breast-feeding, or recent exposure to an infectious disease also do not contraindicate vaccination.

Laboratory Testing

No true laboratory testing is required before immunization. However, certain antigenic constituents of vaccines (e.g., eggs, egg protein, neomycin) and antisera may cause hypersensitivity reactions.

An intracutaneous skin test preceded by a conjunctival test must be performed before injection of any animal serum, regardless of whether the patient has previously received the serum species. A negative conjunctival or skin test, however, does not guarantee hypersensitivity is absent. It only suggests that sensitivity is probably lacking. Test results can be false in the presence of antihistamines.

In the patient whose pregnancy status is questionable, a pregnancy test should be done before immunizations are given. For a pregnant women not known to be immunized against rubella, the serum antibody titer should be measured to determine resistance or susceptibility to the disease.

GOALS OF THERAPY

The long-term goal of immunization programs is eradication of disease. The immediate goal is prevention of disease in individuals and groups. National Health Objectives for the Year 2010 include achieving an 80% primary immunization rate for children younger than 3 years and a 90% immunization rate for influenza and pneumococcal vaccines in adults aged 65 years and older. To achieve these goals, participation in immunization programs must be a high priority for people of all ages—children, adolescents, and adults—and factors interfering with these goals must be addressed.

Recommendations for vaccinating infants, children, and adults are based on characteristics of immunobiologics, scientific knowledge about the principles of active and passive immunity, and the epidemiology of diseases. In the United States, the Advisory Committee on Immunization Practices (ACIP) of the Centers for Disease Control and Prevention, and the Committee on Infectious Diseases of the American Academy of Pediatrics (AAP) govern the recommendations for immunization policies and procedures. In Canada, the recommendations come from the National Advisory Committee on Immunization under the authority of the Minister of National Health and Welfare. The policies of each committee are *recommendations*, not rules, and they change based on advances in the field of immunology. There may be some differences between committee recommendations and those of the ACIP in its journal, *Morbidity and Mortality Weekly Report* (MMWR). Box 35-1 provides information as to how to keep current on vaccine recommendations.

For routine immunizations, combined antigenic preparations are preferred (e.g., DTaP, MMR). Single

---

BOX 35-1 | **Keeping Up to Date on Immunization Recommendations**

Morbidity and Mortality Weekly Report (MMWR)

The *Morbidity and Mortality Weekly Report* (MMWR) is a publication of the CDC. It contains comprehensive reviews of the literature as well as important background data, regarding vaccine efficacy and adverse reactions. To receive an electronic copy, send an e-mail message to *listserv@listserv.cdc.gov*. The body content should read: SUBscribe mmwr-toc. Electronic copy also is available from the CDC's website or from the CDC's file transfer protocol server at *ftp.cdc.gov*. To subscribe for a paper copy contact the Superintendent of Documents; U.S. Government Printing Office; Washington, DC 20402; (202) 512-1800. The CDC may be contacted at:

Centers for Disease Control and Prevention
1600 Clifton Road, Northeast
Atlanta, GA 30333
Available online at *www.cdc.gov*
National Immunization Program at CDC: www.cdc.gov/nip
Information Hotline: (800) 232-2522 or (800) 232-7468
International Travel Hotline: (877) 394-8747
Spanish Hotline: (800) 232-0233

Report of the Committee on Infectious Diseases (Redbook)

The *Report of the Committee on Infectious Diseases*, known as the *Redbook*, is produced by the AAP and is an authoritative source of information on vaccines and other important pediatric infectious diseases. It lacks, however, an in-depth review and reference list of controversial issues. The recommendations in *Redbook* appear first in the journal *Pediatrics* or the *AAP News*. Typically, the most recent immunization schedule appears in the January issue of the journal. The AAP may be contacted at:

American Academy of Pediatrics
141 Northwest Point Boulevard
P.O. Box 747
Elk Grove Village, IL 60009
Available online at *www.aap.org*
Information: (888) 227-1770
FAX: (847) 228-1281

Vaccine Information Statements (VIS)

Vaccine Information Statements are available by calling your state or local health department. They can also be downloaded from the Immunization Action Coalition's website at *www.immunize.org/vis/* or the CDC's website at *www.cdc.gov/publications/vis*. Some translations are available.

Immunization Gateway: Your Vaccine Fact-Finder

Your Vaccine Fact-Finder at *www.immunofacts.com* provides direct links to all of the best vaccine resources on the Internet.

---

antigenic formulations are recommended when other components in the formulation are contraindicated. Immunization for adults should be individualized based on age, physical health, and possible allergic reactions. For example, pertussis immunization is inappropriate in an adult because the risk of reaction to the vaccine outweighs the protection it provides, particularly in older adults. Live attenuated viral vaccines (e.g., MMR, varicella) should not be given to people who are immunocompromised (e.g., those with HIV infection, leukemia, or lymphoma) or who are taking corticosteroid or antineoplastic drugs. If such a patient is exposed to varicella, immune globulin or varicella-zoster immune globulin may be given for passive immunization.

INTERVENTION
Legal Implications of Immunizations

Benefits and risks of vaccines should be explained before the administration of a vaccine, sera, or other immunizing drug. All immunization providers are required by law, before administration of each dose of certain vaccines, to provide a copy of the most current Vaccine Information Statement (VIS) to either the adult vaccinee or to the child's parent/legal guardian. VISs are developed by the CDC and discuss the benefits and risks associated with specific vaccines. Patient understanding of the major benefits and rare adverse effects of immunizations is crucial to the safety of the patient and the success of immunization programs. Signature sheets reflecting informed consent should be used.

On the other hand, several years ago there was a serious shortage of Td and DTaP vaccines because drug manufacturers were fearful of product liability suits. The federal government intervened and now accepts responsibility under the National Childhood Vaccine Injury Act of 1986. The 1986 Act requires that a Vaccine Adverse Event Report (Figure 35-2) be filed whenever an immunization recipient experiences any of the adverse reactions identified in Table 35-3 (Law 42 USC 300aa-25).

Under this legislation, provisions are made for a one-time payment to families of children who experience significant adverse reactions following the administration of vaccines (as an alternative to civil litigation under the

VACCINE ADVERSE EVENT REPORTING SYSTEM
24 Hour Toll-free information line 1-800-822-7967
P.O. Box 1100, Rockville, MD 20849-1100
PATIENT IDENTITY KEPT CONFIDENTIAL

For CDC/FDA Use Only

VAERS Number _____

Date Received _____

Patient Name:

Last   First   M.I.

Address

City   State   Zip

Telephone no. (_____)_____

Vaccine administered by (Name):

Responsible Physician _____

Facility Name/Address

City   State   Zip

Telephone no. (_____)_____

Form completed by (Name):

Relation to Patient □ Vaccine Provider □ Patient/Parent □ Manufacturer □ Other

Address *(if different from patient or provider)*

City   State   Zip

Telephone no. (_____)_____

1. State
2. County where administered
3. Date of birth / / mm dd yy
4. Patient age
5. Sex □ M □ F
6. Date form completed / / mm dd yy

7. Describe adverse event(s) (symptoms, signs, time course) and treatment, if any

8. Check all appropriate:
□ Patient died (date ___/___/___ mm dd yy)
□ Life-threatening illness
□ Required emergency room/doctor visit
□ Required hospitalization (_____ days)
□ Resulted in prolongation of hospitalization
□ Resulted in permanent disability
□ None of the above

9. Patient recovered □ YES □ NO □ UNKNOWN

10. Date of vaccination / / mm dd yy AM Time_____ PM

11. Adverse event onset / / mm dd yy AM Time_____ PM

12. Relevant diagnostic tests/laboratory data

13. Enter all vaccines given on date listed in no. 10

Vaccine (type)	Manufacturer	Lot number	Route/site	No. previous doses
a.				
b.				
c.				
d.				

14. Any other vaccinations within 4 weeks prior to the date listed in no. 10

Vaccine (type)	Manufacturer	Lot number	Route/site	No. previous doses	Date given
a.					
b.					

15. Vaccinated at:
□ Private doctor's office/hospital □ Military clinic/hospital
□ Public health clinic/hospital □ Other/unknown

16. Vaccine purchased with:
□ Private funds □ Military funds
□ Public funds □ Other /unknown

17. Other medications

18. Illness at time of vaccination (specify)

19. Pre-existing physician-diagnosed allergies, birth defects, medical conditions (specify)

20. Have you reported this adverse event previously?
□ No □ To health department □ To doctor □ To manufacturer

Only for children 5 and under
22. Birth weight _____ lb. _____ oz.
23. No. of brothers and sisters

21. Adverse event following prior vaccination (check all applicable, specify)

	Adverse event	Onset age	Type vaccine	Dose no. in series
□ In patient				
□ In brother or sister				

Only for reports submitted by manufacturer/immunization project
24. Mfr. / imm. proj. report no.
25. Date received by mfr. / imm. proj.
26. 15 day report? □ Yes □ No
27. Report type □ Initial □ Follow-Up

Health care providers and manufacturers are required by law (42 USC 300aa-25) to report reactions to vaccines listed in the Table of Reportable Events Following Immunization. Reports for reactions to other vaccines are voluntary except when required as a condition of immunization grant awards.

Form VAERS -1

FIGURE 35-2 Vaccine Adverse Event Report, Food and Drug Administration (Law 42 USC 300aa-25) requires that a report be filed whenever a recipient of an immunization experiences an adverse reaction to vaccines listed in Table 35-1. (From Vaccine Adverse Event Reporting System: *The reportable events table*, Rockville, Md, 2002.)

TABLE 35-3

Reportable Events

Event	Interval Between Immunization and Event
DTaP, Pertussis, Combined DTP/Poliovirus	
Anaphylaxis or anaphylactic shock	7 days
Bacterial neuritis	28 days
Encephalopathy or encephalitis	7 days
Any sequelae of above events (including death)	Not applicable
Events described in manufacturer's package insert as contraindications to additional doses of vaccine	See package insert
Measles, Mumps, Rubella (In Any Combination: MMR, MR, M, or R)	
Anaphylaxis or anaphylactic shock	7 days
Chronic arthritis	42 days
Acute complications or sequelae of above events (including death)	Not applicable
Events described in manufacturer's package insert as contraindications to additional doses of vaccine	See package insert
Hepatitis B (Hep B)	
Anaphylaxis or anaphylactic shock	7 days
Any sequelae of the above event (including death)	Not applicable
Events described in manufacturer's package insert as contraindications to additional doses of vaccine	See package insert
***Haemophilus influenzae* type B**	
Early onset Hib disease (polysaccharide or conjugate)	7 days
Events described in manufacturer's package insert as contraindications to additional doses of vaccine	See package insert
Pneumococcus	
Events described in manufacturer's package insert as contraindications to additional doses of vaccine	See package insert
Varicella (Chicken Pox)	
Events described in manufacturer's package insert as contraindications to additional doses of vaccine	See package insert

Data from Vaccine Adverse Event Reporting System: *The reportable events table,* Rockville, Md, 2002.

---

traditional tort system). A report of the adverse reaction must be submitted and an agreement not to pursue litigation made before payment.

Storage

Immunizing drugs are stored according to manufacturer's directions to maintain efficacy of vaccines and other biologic preparations. Most are stored in the refrigerator (but not on the refrigerator door) at temperatures ranging from 35.6° to 46.4° F (2° to 8° C). Vaccine stock should be rotated so the oldest vaccines are used first, and vaccines should never be administered after the expiration date. Some vaccines (e.g., MMR) re-

quire protection from light. If immunizing drugs are to be transported, ice packs and polystyrene foam containers should be used. Poliovirus vaccines should be transported in dry ice only.

Administration

The health care provider should read the package insert before administering any immunization. There are a number of proposals before the FDA regarding delivery route for the immunizing drug (Box 35-2).

Most immunizing drugs are mixed just before use. The vaccine and diluent should be inspected for particulate matter or discoloration. The solution should be

BOX 35-2 **On the Horizon**

Most current immunizing drugs are administered by injection. Current research is aimed at new methods for vaccine delivery. An influenza vaccine administered by nasal spray is being tested. Vaccine contained in slowly soluble microspheres may be injected to release small doses over a long period, eliminating the need for booster injections. It may be possible to administer DNA-encoding antigenic material for incorporation into the body's own cells. The antigenic protein would be made over a long period and induce a strong, long-lasting immunity. Antigen material may be genetically engineered into plants such as bananas or potatoes, to induce protective immunity when eaten.

The most successful immunization programs are for those viral diseases in which few pathogenic strains exist and with which antigenic properties do not change. The vaccine for poliovirus fits these criteria. However, immunization against rhinoviruses has not been feasible because there are approximately 100 strains. Each strain induces a separate antibody in humans and the antibodies are not cross-reactive. Influenza vaccines are of value for a limited time because the viruses shift antigenic properties every few years, leaving the old vaccines ineffective.

discarded if precipitate or discoloration is present. Vaccines should not be mixed in a single syringe unless approved for mixing by the Food and Drug Administration (FDA).

All needed vaccines should be administered during the same visit to increase the likelihood that full immunization is achieved. When multiple vaccines are administered simultaneously, each drug should be given at a different site, using separate needles and syringes. If two injections are administered in the same limb, the injection sites are separated by 1 to 2 inches so that local reactions do not overlap.

In general, patients are instructed to wait 30 minutes after the vaccination so they may be observed for allergic reactions. Signs of serious allergic reaction to vaccines include difficulty breathing, hoarseness or wheezing, urticaria, paleness, weakness, and tachycardia. Epinephrine and equipment to support breathing should be readily available.

Timing of Administration

Some vaccines require more than one dose for development of an adequate antibody response. Others require periodic reinforcement (booster doses) to maintain protection. The ACIP recommends the interval between administration of doses and vaccines. Administering doses of a vaccine or toxoid at less than the recommended minimum intervals may decrease the antibody response and should be avoided. When administered too frequently, some vaccines increase the risk of local or systemic reactions in some recipients (e.g., DTaP). Longer than recommended dosage intervals do not reduce antibody concentrations. The health care provider should take care to maintain good record keeping and to follow recommended immunization schedules to avoid administration of extra doses of vaccines.

Killed vaccines can be administered simultaneously at separate sites. Local or systemic reactions can be accentuated when killed vaccines are administered simultaneously. Live and inactivated vaccines may be administered simultaneously. Simultaneous administration of routine vaccinations does not interfere with the immune response to these vaccines.

Inactivated vaccines generally do not interfere with the patient's immune response to other inactivated vaccines or to live vaccines. Yellow fever and cholera vaccines are exceptions to this rule. Immune response to one live virus vaccine might be impaired if it is administered within 30 days of another live virus vaccine. Children receiving routine vaccinations for varicella virus and MMR should have the drugs administered at the same time, at separate sites, and with separate syringes. When not administered at the same visit, varicella and MMR vaccines must be given 30 days apart.

Administration of immune globulin inhibits the immune response to live vaccines for 3 months or more. Therefore, MMR or its individual components should be administered 3 months after the administration of immune globulin. Immune globulin formulations interact less with inactivated vaccines and toxoids than with live vaccines. Therefore, they can be administered simultaneously or at any interval between. They should be administered at different sites and using the standard recommended dose of corresponding vaccine.

It is not unusual for a health care provider to encounter people without adequate documentation of immunizations. Immunizations should not be postponed for lack of records. Such persons should be considered susceptible and an appropriate immunization schedule initiated.

Immunization Records

Health care providers who administer one or more of the vaccines covered by the National Childhood Vaccine Injury Act of 1986 must ensure that the recipient's permanent medical records include the date the vaccine was administered, the vaccine manufacturer, the vaccine lot number, the name, address, and title of the person administering the vaccine, the date that the VIS was given and the publication date of the VIS. The ACIP recommends that this information be kept for all vaccinations. In addition, it is recommended that a permanent immunization record be kept and that it be continually updated.

Education

Many people think certain diseases have been eradicated and are no longer a threat, so it is not unusual for patients or parents to resist immunization recommendations. Others fear serious adverse effects, are deterred by the cost of the vaccine, or say they do not have the time for successive vaccinations or boosters. Children without health insurance coverage, all those enrolled in Medicaid, and American Indians and Alaskan Natives are eligible for free vaccinations through a federal program, Vaccines for Children. Barriers to adult immunization include not knowing immunizations are needed, misconceptions about the efficacy of immunization, and lack of recommendations from health care providers. Public education is vital so that people understand the need for prevention and the reasons for seeking health care in the event of injury, animal bite, or potential exposure to contagious diseases.

Vaccine recipients should be advised that adverse reactions have been reported for all vaccines. The reactions are usually local and transient, but they can be systemic, and either immediate or delayed. Local inflammatory reactions at the injection site are the most common. Fever, rash, and hypersensitivity are rare. Most reactions resolve within 48 hours and can usually be effectively managed with symptomatic treatment. This information is also transmitted through VIS and patient education materials.

Travel Immunizations

The increased risk of contracting infectious diseases during international travel results from two primary factors: the close proximity of individuals in transportation and exposure to exotic infectious agents through contact with foreign populations and natural environments. The number and kind of immunizations needed are determined by the patient's itinerary. The health care provider must consider the geographic location, accommodations, and planned activities when determining which immunizations are needed. The patient's age, prior immunization history, allergies, general health, efficacy and adverse reactions of vaccines must be taken into account.

Individuals traveling to high-risk areas should be instructed to contact their health care provider, health department, and/or travel clinic for guidance regarding required immunizations. Information about vaccinations is also available from the CDC via the Internet (see Box 35-2). In addition, patients traveling in areas where there is serious endemic disease (e.g.,

cholera) should be cautioned to not drink untreated water or eat raw fish or uncooked or unpeeled fruits and vegetables.

EVALUATION

Evaluation of the benefits of immunization is difficult to ascertain directly. Data gathered in 1998 indicates 73% of children less than 3 years old had received all vaccines on the recommended immunization schedule. Statistics regarding immunizations recommended for adults aged 65 years and older reveal that influenza immunization rates are 64% and pneumococcal immunization rates approximately 46%, falling far short of the National Health Objectives goal of 90% for both vaccines.

If universal immunization of infants is successful, there will be a dramatic decline in the transmission of infectious diseases. Greater attention to the vaccination of high-risk individuals would minimize the decline. Compliance with recommended immunization regimens helps in identifying the patient's understanding of the importance of immunizations. Cultural barriers, religious or philosophic objections, adverse effects, and contraindications must be considered when designing an effective immunization campaign.

Bibliography

Boyd T, Linkins R: Immunization registry use and progress—United States 2001, *MMWR Morb Mortal Wkly Rep* 51(3): 53-56, 2002.

Centers for Disease Control: Combination vaccines for childhood immunization, *MMWR Morb Mortal Wkly Rep* 48(5): 1-15, 1999.

Centers for Disease Control: Notice to readers: recommended childhood immunization schedule–United States 2002, *MMWR Morb Mortal Wkly Rep* 51(2):31-33, 2002.

Centers for Disease Control: Notice to readers: update on the supply of tetanus and diphtheria toxoids and acellular pertussis, *MMWR Morb Mortal Wkly Rep* 50(10):1-2, 2002. htm. Accessed February 20, 2002.

Centers for Disease Control: Public health dispatch: acute flaccid paralysis associated with circulating vaccine-derived poliovirus–Philippines 2001, *MMWR Morb Mortal Wkly Rep* 50(40):874-875, 2001.

Centers for Disease Control. Recommendations for the use of Lyme disease vaccine recommendations of the advisory committee on immunizations practices (ACIP). *MMWR Morb Mortal Wkly Rep* 48(7):1-17.

Chan-Tack K: Influenza and pneumococcal immunization rates among a high-risk population, *South Med* 94(3):323-324, 2001.

Estrada B: An update on hepatitis B immunization, *Infect Med* 18(3):127-130, 2001.

Estrada B: MMR and autism: suspect or superstition? *Infect Med* 18(4):183, 2001.

Halperin S: Should all adolescents and adults be vaccinated against pertussis? *Infect Med* 18(10):473-475, 2001.

LaForce F: Use of nonroutine vaccines: hepatitis A, rabies, typhoid, and meningococcal vaccines, *Infect Med* 18(8):22-26, 2001.

Martin M, Weld L, Tsai T, et al: Advanced age a risk factor for illness temporally associated with yellow fever vaccination, *Emerg Infect Dis* 7(6):1-10, 2001.

Phelan D, Jacobson R, Poland G: Current adult and pediatric vaccine recommendations, *Infect Med* 18(8):6-14, 2001.

Raj V: Treatment of hepatitis B, *Clin Cornerstone* 3(6):24-36, 2001.

United States Department of Health and Human Services: *Healthy people 2010*, Washington DC, 2000, US Department of Health and Human Services.

Watson B: Vaccines in the pipeline–an overview, *Infect Med* 18(8):27-32, 2001.

Internet Resources

Centers for Disease Control: Adult immunization schedule. Available online at http://www.cdc.gov/nip/recs/adult_schedule.htm. Accessed February 20, 2002.

Centers for Disease Control: How do vaccines work? Available online at http://www.cdc.gov/nip/publications/fs/gen/howvacswork.htm. Accessed February 20, 2002.

Centers for Disease Control: Immunization schedule modifications for international travel. Available online at http://www.cdc.gov/travel/child-vax.htm. Accessed March 6, 2002.

Centers for Disease Control: Overview of vaccine safety. Available online at http://www.cdc.gov/nip/vacsafe/default.htm. Accessed February 20, 2002.

Centers for Disease Control: Recommended childhood immunization schedule, United States, 2002. Available online at http://www.cdc.gov/nip/acip. Accessed February 20, 2002.

Centers for Disease Control: Six common misconceptions about vaccination and how to respond to them. Available online at http://www.cdc.gov/nip/publications/6mishome.htm. Accessed February 20, 2002.

Centers for Disease Control: Ten things you need to know about immunizations. Available online at http://www.cdc.gov/nip/publications/fs/gen/shouldknow.htm. Accessed February 20, 2002.

Centers for Disease Control: Vaccine fact sheets. Available online at http://www.cdc.gov/od/nvpo/fs_tableIII_doc1.htm. Accessed February 20, 2002.

Centers for Disease Control: Vaccine safety: the providers role. Available online at http://www.cdc.gov/nip/vacsafe/providers_role.htm. Accessed February 20, 2002.

Centers for Disease Control: Vaccine side effects. Available online at http://www.cdc.gov/nip/vacsafe/concerns/side-effects.htm. Accessed February 20, 2002.

Centers for Disease Control: Vaccines: the safe choice. Available online at http://cdc.gov/nip/vacsafe/vacsafe-parents.htm. Accessed February 20, 2002.

Vaccine Adverse Event Reporting System: Table of reportable events following vaccination. Available online at http://www.vaers.org/reportable.htm. Accessed March 5, 2002.

Biologic Response Modifiers

SHERRY F. QUEENER • KATHLEEN GUTIERREZ

 Visit **http://evolve.elsevier.com/Gutierrez/** for additional information.

KEY TERMS

OBJECTIVES

- Describe the clinical uses of biologic response modifiers.
- Discuss the pharmacology of cyclosporine.
- Describe the types of patients who might receive an immunostimulant.
- Develop a nursing care plan for a patient receiving a biologic response modifier.

PATHOPHYSIOLOGY • Immune System Dysfunction

The human immune system is a highly complex network of cells and molecules that interact to protect our bodies from foreign agents. Foreign agents may be invading microorganisms, but can also include virus-infected cells and certain malignant cells as well as foreign tissue such as transplanted organs or tissues. Thus modern medicine must modulate the immune system to achieve successful transplantation, and may take advantage of new im-

munologic strategies for dealing with virus infections and cancer. The term **biologic response modifier (BRM)** refers to several types of drugs used to influence the function of the immune system to achieve a medical goal. To understand the role of these modifiers, it is first necessary to review normal immune function.

The bone marrow in adults produces stem cells from which the active cells of the immune system, including

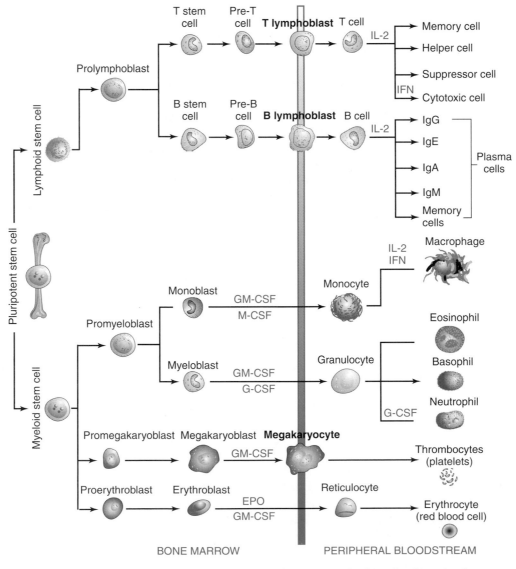

FIGURE 36-1 Differentiation of blood cells and immune cells. Blood cell production occurs in the liver and spleen of the fetus, but it occurs in the bone marrow in the adult. Each cell type is derived from a stem cell that undergoes mitosis in response to specific biochemical signals. The action of key BRMs is shown associated with the process influenced. Only BRMs currently used clinically are shown. (KEY: *GM-CSF,* Granulocyte-macrophage colony-stimulating factor; *G-CSF,* granulocyte colony-stimulating factor; *M-CSF,* macrophage colony-stimulating factor; *IFN,* interferon; *EPO,* erythropoietin.

leukocytes (white blood cells), evolve. There are two stem cell lines: (1) the *myeloid stem cells* that produce granulocytes and monocytes, and (2) the *lymphoid stem cells* that produce T lymphocytes (T cells) and B lymphocytes (B cells) (Figure 36-1).

There are three different types of granulocytes: neutrophils, eosinophils, and basophils. The *neutrophils*, also referred to as polymorphonuclear leukocytes, make up 60% of the circulating leukocytes. They are responsible for phagocytosis and are essential for the nonspecific immune response or innate immunity (see Chapter 35). *Eosinophils* make up 1% to 4% of the white blood cells and cause allergic reactions by evoking histamine release from mast cells and basophils. Eosinophils also participate in the destruction of parasitic organisms by phagocytosis. *Basophils* make up 1% of the total leukocyte count and participate in both allergic and inflammatory responses.

Lymphocytes and monocytes are sometimes referred to as agranulocytes. Monocyte and macrophage receptors recognize foreign agents and respond quickly. Any foreign agent or altered host component capable of evoking an immune response is called an antigen. Macrophages are monocytes that leave the circulation to reside in the tissues. They aid white blood cells in phagocytosis and chemotaxis, and also process and present antigens, which, in turn, activate the T and B lymphocytes. The lymph nodes, alveoli, spleen, tonsils, and liver accumulate significant quantities of agranulocytes.

Lymphocytes are subdivided into the thymus-derived lymphocytes (T lymphocytes) and the bone marrow-derived cells (B lymphocytes). The B lymphocytes produce antibodies, which generate the **humoral immune response** (discussed in Chapter 35). T lymphocytes are subdivided into helper T cells and cytotoxic T cells. Helper T cells assist B lymphocytes in responding to an antigen and mediate delayed hypersensitivity. Cytotoxic T cells reject grafts and destroy virus-infected cells. The ratio of helper cells to cytotoxic cells normally ranges from 1.2:1 to 2:1. In the acquired immunodeficiency syndrome (AIDS), this ratio is usually reversed and can be as low as 0.2 (1:5).

Organs of the immune system are classified as primary or secondary. The primary lymphoid organs are the thymus and the bone marrow. Maturation of lymphocytes occurs in these structures. The spleen, lymph nodes, and Peyer's patches are the secondary lymphoid organs. Peyer's patches are clusters of lymphocytes spread throughout the lining of the intestinal wall, tonsils, and appendix. Secondary lymphoid tissues trap and concentrate foreign substances and are the main sites of antibody production and generation of antigen-specific T lymphocytes.

The preceding discussion illustrates that the immune system is a complex and diffuse system involving many cell types. The success of the immune system depends on an efficient and reliable way for these cells to communicate and to act collectively and in harmony. This fine level of coordination is achieved through the release of various **cytokines,** which are soluble factors released by one immune cell to influence the action of another immune cell. Key cytokines are presented in Figure 36-2 and the discussion that follows, but they are by no means the only ones important for immune function.

Interleukins are a diverse series of cytokines allowing one type of leukocyte to influence the function of other leukocytes. Some of these mediators can act on or be produced by cells outside of the immune system.

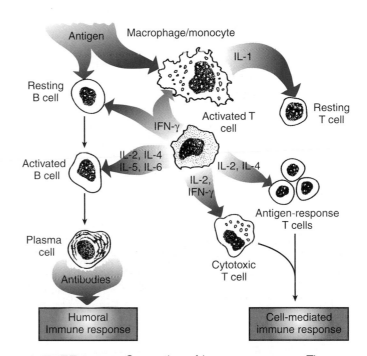

FIGURE 36-2 Generation of immune response. The appearance of antigen evokes both humoral and cell-mediated immune responses. Activation of T lymphocytes requires antigen-presenting cells such as macrophages. T lymphocytes are activated by interaction with the complex of processed antigen and histocompatibility antigen on the surface of the antigen-presenting cells. B lymphocytes are activated by interacting directly with unprocessed antigen via antibody molecules on their surface. Once activated, T and B lymphocytes express receptors for growth factors synthesized and released primarily by activated helper T cells. In response to these growth factors, T and B cells proliferate. Having undergone proliferation, B and T cells can then respond to other soluble mediators secreted by activated helper T cells and will differentiate into functional effector cells. B lymphocytes differentiate into antibody-secreting plasma cells. T lymphocytes differentiate into cells capable of mediating delayed hypersensitivity or into cytotoxic cells.

The **interferons** are a group of cytokines originally identified by their antiviral activity. Interferon-gamma (IFN-gamma) is produced mainly by the TH1 subset of activated T cells and natural killer cells to promote a cellular inflammatory response. IFN-gamma activates other immune cells and promotes inflammation. IFN-gamma is implicated in the pathogenesis of several autoimmune and chronic inflammatory conditions, including lupus and type 1 diabetes mellitus.

Tumor necrosis factor (TNF) is the principal cytokine produced in response to gram-negative bacteria. TNF-alpha is a mediator of both natural and acquired immunity and is also an important link between specific immune responses and acute inflammation. However, the overproduction of TNF-alpha leads to shock. Activated monocytes and macrophages are the major source of TNF-alpha, whose activities include enhanced proliferation of activated T cells and B lymphocytes and expression of adhesion molecules on endothelial cells. TNF-alpha mediates several diseases, including septic shock syndrome, cachexia, and certain autoimmune diseases, such as Crohn's disease or rheumatoid arthritis. The role of TNF-beta is less clear, but it may play a role in the development of peripheral lymphoid organs.

Colony-stimulating factors control the differentiation of hematopoietic stem cells to produce new leukocytes. Figure 36-1 shows the major colony-stimulating factors and the cells that develop from their action. The development of some immune cells can be directed by more than one of these factors. Other growth factors influence production of platelets and erythrocytes. For example, erythropoietin stimulates production of erythrocytes.

As with any body system, the immune system can exhibit pathologic changes and abnormal responses. Hypersensitivity, or allergy, refers to a pathologic, exaggerated reaction to a foreign substance (see Chapter 53). Autoimmune diseases, in which the immune system manufactures T cells and antibodies directed against the body's own cells, are a more serious concern. These T cells and autoantibodies contribute to such diseases as diabetes (see Chapter 58), rheumatoid arthritis (see Chapter 14), systemic lupus erythematosus, myasthenia gravis (see Chapter 23), multiple sclerosis, and Graves' disease (see Chapter 56).

Disorders in the development of immune cells during the generation of immune responses or in the synthesis of the products of the immune system may also cause immunologic disorders ranging in severity from mild to fatal. B cell deficiencies can result in the absence of one or all immunoglobulin classes. Persons with B cell deficiencies mainly experience recurrent bacterial infections. Although immunoglobulin replacement therapy may maintain these patients for as long as 20 to 30 years, the prognosis is poor and many succumb to chronic lung disease.

T cell deficiencies affect not only cell-mediated immune responses but also synthesis of antibodies because T cells contribute to most antibody responses. Patients with T cell disorders are extremely susceptible to fungal, viral, and protozoal infections.

Severe combined immunodeficiencies result from defects in both T and B lymphocytes. These disorders are very serious. Untreated infants rarely survive beyond 1 year of age. Patients with combined immunodeficiencies are susceptible to every type of infection. Treatment with drugs alone is ineffective, but infants can be cured by bone marrow transplants, provided the transplant is done before irreversible complications of the disease arise.

Secondary immune deficiencies occur as complications of other diseases. The most common cause of these disorders is the deliberate immune suppression associated with the use of antineoplastic drugs in cancer treatment or the immunosuppressive drugs used to prevent rejection of transplanted organs. The best known secondary immune deficiency is AIDS. This disease is caused by infection with human immunodeficiency virus (HIV). The immune deficiency associated with AIDS is largely caused by the loss of helper T cells. Patients with secondary immune deficiencies from any cause experience severe recurrent infections from opportunistic organisms that are normally not pathogenic.

Several neoplastic diseases arise from abnormal proliferation of B lymphocytes and plasma cells. These diseases are called **gammopathies.** Multiple myeloma is the most common of the gammopathies, resulting from the malignant proliferation of plasma cells. It is characterized by the synthesis of large amounts of a given isotype of immunoglobulin and may be accompanied by the production of free light chains (called Bence Jones proteins). Multiple myeloma involves multiple organ systems; it results from an infiltration of these systems by malignant plasma cells. Patients are susceptible to recurrent bacterial and viral infections because of suppression of the synthesis of normal antibodies.

DRUG CLASS • Colony-Stimulating Factors

filgrastim (Neupogen)

pegfilgrastim (Neulasta)

sargramostim (Leukine, Prokine, GM-CSF)

MECHANISM OF ACTION

Colony-stimulating factors increase the numbers of various immune cells. Filgrastim (a recombinant human granulocyte colony-stimulating factor) and pegfilgrastim (a covalent conjugate of filgrastim and polyethylene glycol) bind to receptors on specific progenitor cells in bone marrow, causing them to increase production of neutrophils. Because neutrophils play a key role in phagocytosis, treatment with filgrastim or pegfilgrastim promotes the return of cell-mediated immunity.

Sargramostim (a recombinant granulocyte-macrophage colony-stimulating factor) binds to receptors on a less differentiated progenitor cell than filgrastim; therefore production of more than one type of cell is promoted. The most important cell types that increase in response to sargramostim are neutrophils and monocyte-macrophages.

The natural colony-stimulating factors are present in the body in very small amounts, but recombinant DNA technology allows unlimited quantities of these human proteins to be manufactured. Filgrastim and pegfilgrastim are produced by recombinantly engineered *Escherichia coli* bacteria. Sargramostim is produced by a similar technology in yeast cells.

USES

The primary use for filgrastim and pegfilgrastim is to shorten the period of febrile neutropenia induced by myelosuppressive antineoplastic drugs in patients with nonmyeloid cancers. This strategy lessens the risk of infection. Sargramostim was originally used to promote myeloid engraftment after bone marrow transplantation and to improve the yield of progenitor cells. More recently it has been used to reverse antineoplastic drug–induced neutropenia, especially in older adults with acute myelogenous leukemia or patients with non-Hodgkins lymphomas.

Filgrastim is also approved for use in patients who have acute myeloid leukemia.

PHARMACOKINETICS

Both filgrastim and sargramostim are rapidly absorbed from subcutaneous sites and achieve peak concentrations within hours. The effect of filgrastim on neutrophil production can be seen usually within a day, whereas the effects of sargramostim on leukocyte production occur over several days. Pegfilgrastim is not cleared by the kidneys as readily as is filgrastim. Pegfilgrastim, therefore, persists longer in the body than filgrastim.

ADVERSE REACTIONS AND CONTRAINDICATIONS

The most common adverse reaction to filgrastim, pegfilgrastim, or sargramostim is bone pain. This pain seems to correlate with recovery of the bone marrow and increased production of neutrophils.

Patients who have a significant number of leukemic myeloid blasts are at risk for further leukemic progression when treated with colony-stimulating factors because these drugs may promote proliferation of the precursor cells. Filgrastim has also been noted to induce crises in patients with sickle cell anemia.

Allergic reactions to filgrastim occur and may include anaphylaxis, rash, and urticaria. Patients who are sensitive to proteins derived from *E. coli* are more likely to show signs of an allergy to filgrastim or pegfilgrastim, which are made by recombinant *E. coli* cells.

Rupture of the spleen has been seen in patients receiving filgrastim, but it is rare. Adult respiratory distress syndrome (ARDS) has also been noted, most commonly in patients with sepsis. Filgrastim must be discontinued while the ARDS is treated.

Sargramostim may cause capillary leak syndrome. Symptoms include peripheral edema, pleural effusion, and shortness of breath. Patients may also react to the first dose of sargramostim with an episode of flushing, hypotension, and syncope. This reaction usually does not recur with subsequent doses. Sargramostim may also cause pain at the subcutaneous injection site; sites should be rotated.

TOXICITY

Capillary leak syndrome and fever are dose-related responses to sargramostim. Overdosage can therefore lead to serious or life-threatening reactions.

INTERACTIONS

Filgrastim or pegfilgrastim should be avoided in the 14 days before and 24 hours after radiation therapy. Lithium can stimulate release of neutrophils, thus altering the response to filgrastim or pegfilgrastim; neutrophil counts should be closely monitored.

DRUG CLASS • Growth Factors that Stimulate Platelet or Erythrocyte Production

darbepoetin alfa (Aranesp)

epoetin alfa (Epogen, Eprex,✱ Procrit)

oprelvekin (Neumega)

MECHANISM OF ACTION

Growth factors are normally produced in various tissues to promote or sustain production of critical components of blood. Human erythropoietin is produced by renal tissue and released into the blood when hypoxia occurs; in response to erythropoietin, more erythrocytes are formed from precursor cells (see Figure 36-1). Epoetin alfa is a recombinant protein that is the same as the growth factor normally produced in the body and acts in the same way. Darbepoetin alfa, also a recombinant protein, differs from the native growth factor in the type of carbohydrate attached to the protein, but the mechanism of action is the same.

Oprelvekin is closely related to interleukin 11 (IL-11), and acts as a growth factor that stimulates precursor cells to form platelets (see Figure 36-1).

USES

Epoetin alfa and darbepoetin alfa are used to control anemia related to renal failure, a condition in which endogenous production of erythopoietin may be impaired (see Chapter 47). The drugs may also be recommended for use in certain other types of anemia, such as those related to drug therapy.

Oprelvekin is used to prevent thrombocytopenia after myelosuppressive therapy in patients with non-myeloid cancers. The alternative is platelet transfusions (see Chapter 45).

PHARMACOKINETICS

Epoetin alfa and darbepoetin alfa may be administered either intravenously or subcutaneously. Although darbepoetin alfa has a longer elimination half-life than epoetin alfa, both drugs produce their peak effects on erythrocyte production 2 to 6 weeks after the start of therapy. As proteins, these drugs are cleared from the blood as native erythropoietin.

Oprelvekin is administered subcutaneously and is cleared after biotransformation by the kidneys. The effects of the drug persist for up to a week after the end of therapy.

ADVERSE REACTIONS AND CONTRAINDICATIONS

Common adverse reactions with epoetin alfa and darbepoetin alfa include hypertension, which is observed in about 25% of all patients who receive the drugs, as well as chest pain, edema, headache, and altered heart rhythm; an increased tendency to clot or excess viscosity of the blood may be noted. Less serious adverse reactions include GI symptoms, muscle pain, weakness, and skin reactions at the injection site. An increased risk of infection has been noted with darbepoetin. These drugs are contraindicated for patients who have uncontrolled hypertension or in those allergic to albumin, which is present in the product.

Similar adverse reactions occur with oprelvekin, but the most notable are edema, tachycardia, palpitations, atrial flutter, visual blurring, shortness of breath, and oral yeast infections. Although the drug is not contraindicated except for documented allergies, it must be used with great care in patients with hypokalemia; patients who were hypokalemic have died suddenly when given oprelvekin.

INTERACTIONS

Because epoetin alfa and darbepoetin alfa may increase blood pressure, they can interfere with adequate control of blood pressure, requiring changes in drug regimens.

Oprelvekin should be used with caution in patients who may be at risk of hypokalemia because of therapy with thiazide or loop diuretics (see Chapter 46).

DRUG CLASS • Interleukins

aldesleukin (Proleukin)

MECHANISM OF ACTION

Aldesleukin is a recombinant form of interleukin-2 (IL-2), one of the major cytokines regulating function of the immune system (see Figure 36-2). Multiple effects of aldesleukin contribute to stimulation of cell-mediated immunity.

USES

Aldesleukin is indicated for metastatic renal cell carcinoma and metastatic melanoma. The very high risk of adverse reactions limits its use for other indications.

PHARMACOKINETICS

Aldesleukin is given only by intravenous routes. The drug distributes well to many sites. Elimination involves hydrolysis of this protein into amino acids in the kidneys. The biologic effect of aldesleukin on immune function may persist for months.

ADVERSE REACTIONS AND CONTRAINDICATIONS

Aldesleukin causes a wide array of potentially serious adverse reactions. Central nervous system (CNS) effects include agitation, confusion, depression, dizziness, and fatigue. Pulmonary symptoms may include lung congestion, edema, and shortness of breath. Patients with anemia may require blood transfusions. Arrhythmias are usually transient but may occasionally be life threatening.

A skin rash with redness, itchiness, and peeling commonly appears 2 or 3 days after the start of treatment and begins to resolve only after the drug is discontinued. Blisters on the skin may signal a more dangerous condition, exfoliative dermatitis, which can be fatal. Dizziness, nausea, and vomiting almost always occur.

Aldesleukin is contraindicated for patients with preexisting impairment of cardiac or pulmonary function. The drug is also avoided in patients with metastatic cancer in the CNS. Aldesleukin is not used in patients with transplanted organs because the immune system stimulation produced by the drug may prompt organ rejection.

TOXICITY

Capillary leak syndrome is more likely at higher dosages. Symptoms of capillary leak syndrome include peripheral edema, pleural effusion, and shortness of breath. This condition may be fatal.

INTERACTIONS

Drugs like daunorubicin or doxorubicin may cause dangerous additive cardiotoxicity with aldesleukin. Likewise the toxicity of bone marrow depressants, hepatotoxic drugs, and nephrotoxic medications may be worsened by aldesleukin. Corticosteroids may antagonize the actions of aldesleukin.

 DRUG CLASS • Interleukin Receptor Blockers and Other Immunosuppressant Antibodies

anti-thymocyte globulin [rabbit] (Thymoglobulin)

basiliximab (Simulect)

daclizumab (Zenapax)

lymphocyte immune globulin (Atgam)

muromonab-CD3 (Orthoclone OKT3)

MECHANISM OF ACTION

Daclizumab and basiliximab are monoclonal antibodies that bind to IL-2 receptors on lymphocytes. As a result of this binding, the response of lymphocytes to IL-2 is impaired. Without IL-2 activation of lymphocytes, cell-mediated immune reactions are diminished.

Anti-thymocyte globulin and lymphocyte immune globulin both interact with various T cell antigens. This binding interferes with T cell function, resulting in suppression of cell-mediated immunity. Muromonab-CD3 is a monoclonal antibody that binds to the CD3 receptor on human helper T cells. The binding of the drug prevents the cell from responding to signals from activated macrophages or monocytes. As a result, T cell function is inhibited and cell-mediated immune responses are blunted.

USES

These drugs are currently used to prevent acute rejection of transplanted kidneys or other organs. The drugs are used in combination with other immunosuppressants such as cyclosporine and corticosteroids.

PHARMACOKINETICS

Because these immunosuppressant drugs are proteins, they are administered intravenously. Recombinant antibodies persist in the body for up to a month, which is about the same as for natural antibodies. Muromonab-CD3 binds directly to helper T cells; therefore its action is almost immediate. The number of fully functional CD3 cells usually returns to normal within a week after muromonab-CD3 is discontinued.

ADVERSE REACTIONS AND CONTRAINDICATIONS

Adverse reactions to daclizumab include chest pain, edema, gastric distress, shortness of breath, pain in the joints, and slow wound healing. In addition to these effects, basiliximab may cause headache, insomnia, dizziness, and tremor. The only absolute contraindication to these drugs is a documented allergy to the proteins.

Drugs such as muromonab-CD3 may provoke release of cytokines. Symptoms that can occur during infusion include chills, diarrhea, dizziness, fainting, spiking fever, headache, malaise, muscle or joint pain, nausea, and vomiting. These symptoms may progress to more serious signs such as arrhythmias, chest pain, shortness of breath caused by pulmonary edema, trembling, and weakness. The cytokine release reaction usually appears 30 minutes to 48 hours after injection. Anaphylaxis may also produce similar symptoms but usually appears within 10 minutes of injection.

Many adverse effects on the CNS may also occur with these antibodies. These effects may include confusion, headache, hallucinations, sensitivity to light, and sleep changes. More serious reactions include coma or seizures.

Monoclonal antibodies are usually avoided in patients who have fluid overloads or heart failure because of the excessive risk of potentially fatal pulmonary edema. These antibodies may also trigger arrhythmias. These drugs should not be given to patients with fever or infections. Many of the drugs have profound immunosuppressant effects that may impair the ability to fight off infections.

Muromonab-CD3 is a mouse protein. Patients with strong allergies to mice should not receive the drug because the risk of a serious allergic reaction is increased.

TOXICITY

Most of the reactions to muromonab-CD3 are caused by the release of cytokines in the body. The effects may worsen with increases in dosage of this drug and others of its class.

INTERACTIONS

When immunosuppressive BRMs are combined with other immunosuppressants, the risk of severe immune suppression is increased. Immune function should be monitored and dosages of both drugs adjusted as necessary. Patients should also be monitored for signs of infections.

Immunosuppressants should not be used with live virus vaccines because the immune suppression caused by the drugs may allow an uncontrolled proliferation of the virus. Serious generalized disease may result.

 DRUG CLASS • Cytokine Release Inhibitors

⚠ cyclosporine (Sandimmune, Neoral)
tacrolimus (Prograf)

MECHANISM OF ACTION

Cyclosporine interferes with the synthesis and release of IL-2 and other cytokines from activated helper T cells. This action inhibits induction of cytotoxic T lymphocytes (see Figure 36-2). As a result, cell-mediated immunity is suppressed. Tacrolimus is much more potent than cyclosporine, but has a similar effect on cell-mediated immunity.

USES

Because cell-mediated immune reactions are the key elements of transplant rejection reactions, and drugs such as cyclosporine and tacrolimus block cell-mediated immunity, these drugs are widely used for prevention of organ rejection after transplantation. They are often combined with corticosteroids (see Chapter 57).

PHARMACOKINETICS

Oral absorption of the original preparation of cyclosporine (Sandimmune) is variable, and bioavailability is only about 30%. The drug is now also available as a microemulsion (Neoral) that is more readily absorbed and produces higher blood levels.

Cyclosporine is extensively biotransformed by the liver. The half-life of the drug is long in adults, ranging from 10 to 27 hours but tends to be shorter in

children. Elimination of the drug is through bile into the feces.

Tacrolimus may be absorbed orally or may be used by intravenous infusion. Oral absorption is highly variable and may be diminished by food. Tacrolimus is biotransformed by the CYP3A enzyme systems in the liver (see Chapter 1). Very little of the drug is eliminated renally.

ADVERSE REACTIONS AND CONTRAINDICATIONS

Both cyclosporine and tacrolimus cause nephrotoxicity and neurotoxicity, and may induce diabetes. Nephrotoxicity can lead to electrolyte imbalances, in particular alterations in serum potassium levels that may lead to confusion, paresthesias, shortness of breath, and muscle weakness. Neurotoxicity caused by cyclosporine may involve tremors or paresthesias, but tacrolimus may produce confusion, headaches, or convulsions as well as tremors.

Hepatotoxicity has been noted with cyclosporine. The drug is also associated with excessive hair growth (hirsutism) and gingival hyperplasia. Tacrolimus is more often associated with anorexia, diarrhea, nausea, weight loss, and vomiting.

Because cyclosporine and tacrolimus suppress part of the immune system, the risk of serious infection is increased with these drugs. Their use should also be avoided in patients with active infections, which may be worsened by the drug.

TOXICITY

Several of the reactions to cyclosporine and tacrolimus are dose related. Irreversible nephrotoxicity or diabetes may occur with persistently high dosages. Tremors are another dose-related symptom that may signal overdose.

INTERACTIONS

Many drugs that are biotransformed in the liver may interfere with the breakdown of cyclosporine and therefore cause accumulation, leading to serious adverse reactions.

Drugs that may act in this way include androgens, cimetidine, danazol, diltiazem, erythromycin, estrogens, and imidazole antifungal drugs. The risk of hyperkalemia is increased when drug preparations containing potassium are used. Other drugs such as potassium-sparing diuretics and succinylcholine may also increase the risk.

Live-virus vaccines should not be used with cyclosporine or tacrolimus because the immune suppression caused by these drugs may allow an uncontrolled proliferation of the virus. Serious generalized disease may result.

DRUG CLASS • Interferons

interferon alfa-2b (Intron A)

interferon beta-1a (Avonex)

interferon gamma-1b (Actimmune)

MECHANISM OF ACTION

Interferon gamma promotes the formation of reactive forms of oxygen in phagocytes. This and other actions improve phagocytosis. Interferon beta has complex actions on several types of cells. Alpha interferons also have multiple effects, but clinically they are most commonly used to treat viral diseases (see Chapter 31).

USES

Interferon gamma-1b is used in chronic granulomatous disease, a condition in which oxidative functions of phagocytic cells are impaired. Thus the direct actions of the drug tend to reverse the genetically induced defect, resulting in improved immune function. Interferon gamma-1b has also been used for osteopetrosis, a rare inherited disease related to altered osteoclast function.

Interferon beta-1a is used in treating relapsing forms of multiple sclerosis. The drug slows the progression of physical disability, but its exact mechanism of action in this disease is unclear.

Interferon alfa-2b is approved for use in follicular lymphoma, along with antineoplastic therapy. This drug is also used to treat viral hepatitis and is discussed more fully in Chapter 31.

PHARMACOKINETICS

The absorption of interferon gamma-1b from injection sites is slow but relatively efficient. Peak concentrations in blood occur in 4 to 7 hours. Mechanisms for biotransformation or elimination may involve both the liver and kidneys.

Interferon beta-1a may be given either intramuscularly or subcutaneously, but the two routes are not equivalent and should not be interchanged. Interferon beta-1a is eliminated with a half-life of about 10 hours, but biologic effects persist for at least 4 days following a single injection. Patients with multiple sclerosis typically receive one injection weekly.

ADVERSE REACTIONS AND CONTRAINDICATIONS

Interferons may cause a flulike syndrome. Symptoms include achiness, chills, fever, headache, and joint pain. Diarrhea, nausea, and vomiting are also common and may contribute to weight loss. Rashes and dizziness may occur. Interferon gamma-1b commonly causes leukopenia, but symptoms are rare.

Interferons also stress the cardiovascular system, and may cause additional symptoms, especially in patients with preexisting cardiovascular disease. Patients with CNS disease may also be at greater risk for serious reactions with the use of interferons. Seizure activity and suicidal thoughts are two serious reactions that have occurred.

A history of allergic reactions to *E. coli*–derived products may indicate an increased risk with recombinant interferons, which are produced in *E. coli*.

TOXICITY

Leukopenia, CNS effects, and GI tract adverse effects are dose-related reactions to interferon gamma. These reactions are therefore worse with very high dosages.

INTERACTIONS

Any drugs that interfere with bone marrow function can influence the activity of interferon gamma-1b. Few interactions have been noted with interferon beta-1a.

DRUG CLASS • Antagonists of Tumor Necrosis Factor (TNF-alpha)

drotrecogin alfa, activated (Xigris)

etanercept (Enbrel)

infliximab (Remicade)

MECHANISM OF ACTION

All members of this drug class interfere with the action of tumor necrosis factor alpha (TNF-alpha), but do so in different ways. Drotrecogin alfa inhibits production of TNF-alpha by monocytes, along with several other antiinflammatory and profibrinolytic actions (see Chapter 43). Etanercept binds to TNF-alpha and prevents it from interacting with its receptors on cells, thus exerting strong antiinflammatory effects. The drug is designed to bind two molecules of TNF-alpha. Infliximab also binds to TNF-alpha and prevents the cytokine from acting on target cells.

USES

Drotrecogin alfa is recommended for use in cases of severe sepsis, when organ function is compromised. The antiinflammatory effects and profibrinolytic activities all contribute to improved survival.

Etanercept is used for several types of severe or advanced arthritis, such as in patients with progressive structural damage in active rheumatoid arthritis, psoriatic arthritis, or in those with severe disease who have not responded to one of the disease-modifying antirheumatic drugs (see Chapter 14).

Infliximab was originally recommended for Crohn's disease, a chronic inflammatory condition of the bowel in which TNF-alpha plays a role. More recently, infliximab was also approved for use in patients with severe rheumatoid arthritis who have not responded to methotrexate.

PHARMACOKINETICS

Drotrecogin alfa and infliximab are given intravenously. Drotrecogin alfa is infused over 96 hours during the period when effects of sepsis are most severe. There is no information on effects of repeated doses. Infliximab infusions may be repeated at 4- or 8-week intervals for arthritis or, more frequently, for Crohn's disease. Etanercept is administered by twice-weekly subcutaneous injections.

The half-life of infliximab is 8 to 9.5 days and this drug remains primarily within the vascular compart-

ment. The level of drotrecogin alfa falls quickly after infusion of the drug is stopped. Etanercept has a plasma half-life of 102 hours. As proteins, these drugs are cleared by normal mechanisms for removing other proteins from the blood.

ADVERSE REACTIONS AND CONTRAINDICATIONS

Drotrecogin alfa commonly causes bleeding, which can be at various sites and can be severe. Intracranial bleeding has been observed, although it is rare. The most common sites are skin (ecchymoses) and GI bleeding. Drotrecogin alfa is contraindicated in patients with active internal bleeding, those who have had a hemorrhagic stroke within the past 3 months, in patients with an epidural catheter, or when there is evidence of intracranial mass lesion. Head trauma or surgery within the spinal column or cranium within the past 2 months are also reasons to withhold the drug.

Etanercept causes reactions at the injection site in about 37% of patients. Symptoms include redness, swelling, itching, and pain. Patients who receive etanercept are at an increased risk to develop autoantibodies. The incidence of headache, nausea, abdominal pain, and vomiting are also increased for these patients. Infections seem to be increased in patients receiving etanercept, and the drug is contraindicated in patients with sepsis.

Infliximab causes an infusion reaction in about 20% of treated patients. Symptoms include fever, chills, changes in blood pressure, dyspnea, skin rash, or itch. Anaphylaxis, convulsions, and hypotension occurred rarely in patients, especially in those with proven antibodies to infliximab. Lupus-like syndrome has also been noted with infliximab. Respiratory symptoms, including infections, also occur in 6% to 33% of patients. Infliximab is contraindicated in patients with known allergies to mouse proteins.

INTERACTIONS

Drug interactions with this class of drugs has not yet been adequately evaluated. Drotrecogin alfa should be used cautiously with other drugs that affect hemostasis. It is recommended that live vaccines not be given to patients taking etanercept.

DRUG CLASS • Biologic Response Modifiers Targeted to Cell-Specific Markers

See Table 36-1 for a listing of drugs in this class.

MECHANISM OF ACTION

Most of the BRMs in this category are monoclonal antibodies, which are designed to specifically attack a single target (Figure 36-3). The result of the attachment of the monoclonal antibody can be quite varied. For example, alemtuzumab attaches to the CD52 receptor on both malignant and normal B or T lymphocytes and induces lysis. Denileukin diftitox contains elements of IL-2 and of the diphtheria toxin; as a result, the fused protein binds to cells with IL-2 receptors, which are then directly exposed to the cytotoxic action of diphtheria toxin. Gemtuzumab ozogamicin is an antibody linked to a cytotoxic agent, calicheamicin; the antibody is designed to bind to CD33 antigen

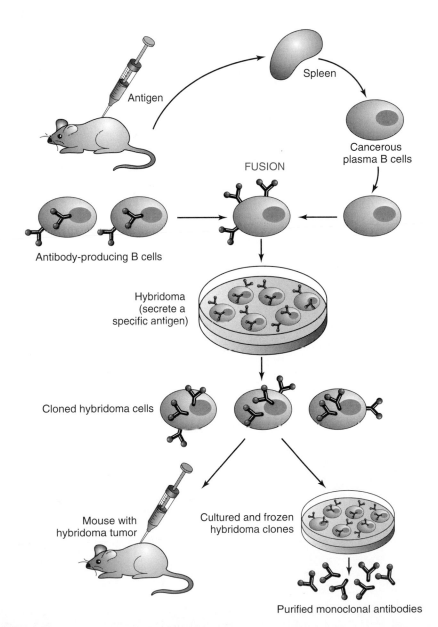

FIGURE 36-3 Hybridoma technology. Monoclonal antibodies may be produced by hybridizing B cells from the spleens of mice that have been injected with a specific antigen with B cells from a plasma cell tumor. The result is a hybridoma that is both antigen-specific and capable of indefinite proliferation.

on leukemic myeloblasts and expose them directly to the attached calicheamicin. Thus, BRMs of this category may be effective anticancer agents.

Monoclonal antibodies have also been linked to markers such as technetium-99 and indium-111 to allow better detection of specific cancer cells. Examples include arcitumomab, imciromab pentetate, nofetumomab merpentan, and satumomab pendetide (Table 36-1).

USES

The clinical uses of these drugs are linked to the targeted antigen and the cells affected. Uses include antineoplastic therapy, antiviral therapy, and diagnostic applications (see Table 36-1).

PHARMACOKINETICS

As proteins, these drugs are usually given intravenously and tend to be proteolytically degraded by various organs, including the kidneys. The rate of degradation is usually similar to that for normal antibody molecules, so effects tend to persist.

ADVERSE REACTIONS AND CONTRAINDICATIONS

Any drug in this category may cause acute hypersensitivity reactions. Some of them must be administered after premedicating the patient with acetaminophen and diphenhydramine to reduce the hypersensitivity response.

TABLE 36-1

Biologic Response Modifiers Targeted to Cell-Specific Markers

Drug	Brand Name	Target Antigen	Cells Affected	Clinical Use
alemtuzumab	Campath	CD52	Lymphocytes; macrophage/monocytes; cytotoxic cells; male reproductive tissues	B-cell chronic lymphocytic leukemia, after failure of first line drugs
arcitumomab	CEA-Scan	CEA	Colorectal cancer cells	Diagnostic agent for colorectal cancer
capromab pendetide	ProstaScint	Tumor antigen	Prostate cells	Linked to indium (^{111}In) for diagnosis of metastatic prostate cancer
denileukin diftitox	Ontak	CD25	Activated B lymphocytes; activated T lymphocytes; activated macrophages	Persistent or recurrent T cell lymphoma, when the cells express the CD25 antigen
gemtuzumab ozogamicin	Mylotarg	CD33	Leukemic myeloblasts; immature myeloid precursors	Acute myeloid leukemia (CD33 positive) in a patient over 60 years old, in first relapse, not a candidate for cytotoxic antineoplastic therapy
ibritumomab tiuxetan	Zeralin	B cell antigens	B lymphocytes	In combinations to treat B-cell non-Hodgkins lymphoma
imciromab pentetate	Myoscint	Myosin	Damaged cardiac cells	Imaging drug with ^{111}In to show myocardial injury after suspected heart attack
nofetumomab	Verluma	Tumor antigen	Small-cell lung cancer	Diagnostic aid to show disease progression
palivizumab	Synagis	RSV protein	Respiratory syncytial virus	To prevent infection with RSV by inactivating the virus
rituximab	Rituxan	CD20	B lymphocytes	To treat B-cell non-Hodgkins lymphoma
satumomab pendetide	Oncoscint	TAG-72	Cells in adenocarcinomas; ovarian carcinoma cells	Diagnostic aid to identify metastatic spread
trastuzumab	Herceptin	HER2	Breast cancer cells	To treat metastatic breast cancer in tumors expressing HER2

Hematologic adverse reactions are significant for several of these drugs. Anemia, neutropenia, or thrombocytopenia were common with alemtuzumab, gemtuzumab ozogamicin, and trastuzumab. Infusion-related adverse reactions noted for these same three drugs include fever, nausea, vomiting, hypotension, rash or itching, dyspnea, headache, or diarrhea.

Vascular leak syndrome, characterized by hypotension and hypoalbuminemia has been noted with denileukin diftitox.

Trastuzumab has been linked to heart failure and other signs of cardiotoxicity. The drug is avoided in patients with preexisting cardiac disease.

INTERACTIONS

Drug interactions are not fully evaluated for most of these agents, but alemtuzumab, gemtuzumab ozogamicin, and trastuzumab should be used with caution with other drugs that cause anemia or other blood dyscrasias. Trastuzumab should not be used with other cardiotoxic drugs.

DRUG CLASS • Miscellaneous Modulators of Immune Function

levamisole (Ergamisol)

mycophenolate mofetil hydrochloride (CellCept)

pegademase (Adagen)

Several types of drugs other than those discussed above influence immune function. Immunosuppressants include mycophenolate (discussed below), azathioprine (see Chapter 14), methotrexate (see Chapter 37), and the corticosteroids (see Chapter 57). Immunostimulants include a general agent, levamisole (discussed below), and pegademase (p. 564), a specific replacement therapy for severe combined immunodeficiency disease (SCID).

---

levamisole

MECHANISM OF ACTION

Levamisole returns leukocyte function to normal levels after antineoplastic therapy or surgery. T cells, monocytes, macrophages, and neutrophils are influenced.

USES

Levamisole is used as an adjunct for surgery and antineoplastic therapy for patients with primary colorectal carcinoma. Metastatic disease does not respond.

PHARMACOKINETICS

Levamisole is easily absorbed orally and undergoes extensive biotransformation in the liver. The drug persists in blood for several hours. Metabolites of levamisole are primarily eliminated in urine.

ADVERSE REACTIONS AND CONTRAINDICATIONS

Gastric effects such as nausea and diarrhea are common with levamisole. Blood dyscrasias can also occur but usually cause no symptoms. A flulike syndrome may be related to the onset of serious blood dyscrasias.

CNS impairment is rare but can include ataxia, blurred vision, confusion, mental changes, paresthesias, seizures, tardive dyskinesia, or tremors. Bone marrow depression or infections may be worsened by levamisole; patients with these conditions should be carefully watched for serious reactions.

TOXICITY

Many of the potentially serious effects of levamisole are allergic or idiosyncratic reactions and are therefore not dose related.

INTERACTIONS

Levamisole is often used in combination with fluorouracil; the drugs may have additive effects on blood cell counts. Leukopenia is usually transient with levamisole alone, but when combined with fluorouracil, leukopenia may persist or develop into agranulocytopenia.

---

mycophenolate mofetil

MECHANISM OF ACTION

Mycophenolate inhibits inosine monophosphate dehydrogenase, an enzyme required for synthesis of the guanine nucleotides needed for DNA synthesis. Both T and B lymphocytes must maintain synthesis of DNA to proliferate normally. Therefore the result of treatment with mycophenolate is to block proliferation of T and B lymphocytes, thereby impairing cell-mediated immune responses that might promote rejection of transplanted organs.

USES

The current indications for mycophenolate are to prevent rejection of allogeneic cardiac, hepatic, or renal transplants. The drug is combined with cyclosporine and glucocorticoids.

PHARMACOKINETICS

Mycophenolate mofetil, the prodrug form that is actually administered, is adequately absorbed orally, and the prodrug is rapidly converted in the body to mycophenolic acid, the active metabolite. If the drug is taken with food or cholestyramine, the blood level may be decreased; therefore the drug is taken on an empty stomach. The drug is highly bound to plasma proteins and has a half-life of 17 to 18 hours. It appears to undergo extensive enterohepatic circulation (see Chapter 1). The liver forms inactive metabolites, including a glucuronide that is eliminated renally.

ADVERSE REACTIONS AND CONTRAINDICATIONS

Gastric symptoms are common and include abdominal pain, constipation or diarrhea, heartburn, nausea, and vomiting. Headache and general weakness are also common. Common reactions that are more serious include anemia, blood in urine, chest pain, edema, hypertension, and neutropenia. Neutropenia, which exposes the patient to increased risk of infection, peaks 1 to 6 months after transplantation and the start of immunosuppression.

Mycophenolate should be used with caution in patients who have serious GI tract disease because the drug may increase the risk of hemorrhage or perforation. Patients with renal impairment may require lower dosages.

TOXICITY

Overdoses have not been reported. Cholestyramine might be expected to assist in such cases by sequestering mycophenolate and promoting fecal excretion.

INTERACTIONS

Mycophenolate is used cautiously in combination with other immunosuppressants; the risk of excessive immunosuppression or development of lymphomas may be increased.

pegademase

MECHANISM OF ACTION

Pegademase is bovine adenosine deaminase, an enzyme required for the removal of toxic metabolites of adenosine. Without this enzyme, lymphocytes die. The absence of this enzyme is the cause of SCID.

USES

Pegademase is used only for adenosine deaminase deficiency or SCID.

PHARMACOKINETICS

The design of pegademase is such that the adenosine deaminase is covalently linked to a larger molecule that allows the material to remain in the circulation for several days. The onset of action on immune function is gradual, and significant clinical improvement may not occur for as long as a year.

ADVERSE REACTIONS AND CONTRAINDICATIONS

Adverse reactions are rare with pegademase but may include headache or pain at the site of injection. Pegademase is avoided in patients with thrombocytopenia because of the risk of bleeding.

TOXICITY

Toxicity has not been documented with doses below 30 mg/kg.

APPLICATION TO PRACTICE

ASSESSMENT
History of Present Illness

The history of the patient's present illness should be obtained with attention to the integrity of the patient's immune system. Particularly note any treatment with antineoplastic drugs, other immunosuppressants, immuno-stimulating drugs, or radiation therapy. An affirmative response may suggest prior organ injury or circumstances that contribute to chronic fatigue or nutrition problems.

Health History

The patient's health history should include other medical conditions for which the patient has received treatment as well as concurrent conditions that may make the patient more susceptible to adverse effects of BRMs. A history of cardiac disease, GI disorders, renal disease, alcohol abuse, liver disease, or mood swings and depression indicates a higher risk for severe adverse effects of BRMs. Ask the patient about allergies, including food, drugs, insect, or pollen sensitivities. Determine how the allergies affect the patient and what measures are ordinarily used to diminish the allergic response. Ask specifically about sneezing, sniffling, rhinitis, nasal stuffiness, itching of the throat, wheezing, and frequent cough.

Lifespan Considerations

Perinatal. BRMs are generally not recommended during pregnancy or lactation because the effects are unclear. To prevent undesirable complications to the fetus or neonate, determine whether the patient is pregnant or nursing before administering BRMs.

Pediatric. BRMs are ordinarily not given to patients less than 18 years old. However, if the patient is an infant, ask if the child is breast-fed or bottle-fed. Breast-feeding introduces antibodies to the infant's GI tract, conferring some immunity. For all children, determine which immunizations they have received (e.g., measles, mumps, pertussis) (see Chapter 35).

Older Adults. Changes caused by increasing age place the older adult at a greater risk for the constitutional, cardiovascular, and neurologic adverse effects of BRMs.

Cultural/Social Considerations

Determine potential sources of infections in the home. Ascertain the age of all household members. Does anyone in the home have a chronic, low-grade infection (e.g., bronchitis)? Is the home generally free of major allergens? Ask about the patient's workplace environment. Is the patient exposed to substances that affect the immune system?

Lifelong compliance by the patient is necessary with most immunosuppressant treatment regimens. Unfortunately, these drugs often cause undesirable clinical responses that contribute to the patient discontinuing drug use or to reducing the dosage. Early detection of noncompliance may allow alterations in the type or amount of drug prescribed and contribute to improved compliance.

Determine the patient's social network and support system. Quality of life is a great issue with BRM therapies and cannot be ignored. There is a significant incidence of adverse effects because BRM therapy often continues for months to years, and fatigue is a significant adverse effect of many BRMs. Fatigue diminishes the patient's ability to work and participate in activities of daily living, even though the person is still able to perform self-care. Increased tumor response and survival do not directly correlate with enhanced quality of life.

The use of BRMs has raised many economic issues because these drugs go beyond current applications for reimbursement. A major economic consideration in the use of BRMs is their investigational status; some BRMs are FDA approved, but many more are used in clinical trials. FDA indications are usually narrow, whereas clinical applications can be quite broad. Reimbursement is frequently refused when the use is outside approved FDA indications.

BRM drugs are expensive. Prices are established to offset the high cost of years of research and development. The technology used to produce the products (hybridoma and recombinant DNA) is expensive as well. For example, one hospitalization for 14 doses of IL-2 therapy can easily exceed $30,000; one course of an antineoplastic drug with

the additional support of a TNF can increase the cost of treatment by $2500. The cost of sargramostim to the pharmacist alone is more than $4000.

Many of the BRM injections are self-administered. This method is generally not covered by insurance, because it assumes the patient can be taught to give the drug. However, not all patients are able and willing to administer the drug to themselves, nor do they have another person who can assist. In addition, many patients are too ill to reliably take the drug but not sick enough to be hospitalized.

Physical Examination

BRMs can affect every organ system in the body. Adverse reactions can be acute (anaphylaxis) or chronic (fatigue), constitutional (fever, chills), or system specific (hypotension). Therefore, a complete physical examination is required before beginning BRM therapy. The examination should emphasize those systems expected to benefit from BRM therapy. Inspect all lymph node regions. Look for visible nodal enlargement or color abnormalities. Palpate superficial lymph nodes of the head and neck, axilla, and inguinal and popliteal regions. Blood pressure should be assessed in both lying and standing positions to rule out hydration problems that may be magnified by the effects of certain BRMs. Intake and output measurements provide insight into the possibility of fluid deficit or excess.

Laboratory Testing

Common laboratory testing includes a CBC count, RBC indices, a WBC count with differential, a platelet count, activated partial thromboplastin time, and immunoelectrophoresis. In some cases, a bone marrow aspiration may be performed. Results of a chest x-ray study and electrocardiogram help establish a baseline for pulmonary and cardiac function (Box 36-1). In some cases, arterial blood gas sampling may be required.

BOX 36-1 | Recommended Baseline Testing for Patients Receiving BRMs

- Complete blood cell (CBC) count, differential, and platelet count
- Prothrombin time (PT) and partial thromboplastin time (PTT)
- Blood urea nitrogen (BUN) and creatinine levels
- Sodium, potassium, chloride, and carbon dioxide levels
- Serum albumin level
- Alkaline phosphatase, lactate dehydrogenase (LDH), serum glutamic-oxaloacetic transaminase (AST), serum glutamic-pyruvic transaminase (ALT), and bilirubin levels
- Urinalysis
- Arterial blood gases (for selected patients)

GOALS OF THERAPY

Treatment goals for the patient receiving BRMs depend on the reason for use of the drug. In general, the major goal is to decrease the risk of organ toxicities and constitutional adverse effects of the BRMs while improving the patient's immune status. For example, for patients receiving granulocyte-stimulating drugs, the objective is to abate the risk of infection by accelerating the recovery of neutrophils after high-dose antineoplastic therapy. For patients taking granulocyte-macrophage stimulating drugs, the goal is to hasten myeloid recovery in patients who have received an autologous bone marrow transplant subsequent to high-dose antineoplastic therapy. The goal for the patient receiving interleukins may be to reduce the size of the tumor. Patients who receive epoetin alfa hope for the restoration and maintenance of red blood cell counts.

INTERVENTION
Administration

For all patients receiving BRMs, early detection and treatment of infection (should it occur) are paramount. Be sure to check the results of laboratory testing before administering a BRM. Assess patients who are at high risk for organ or drug toxicities. Be sure to assess the patient closely throughout therapy for adverse effects.

Administration of BRMs includes all the usual factors: knowledge of the route, correct dosage, drug formulation, storage, and transport. The unique characteristics of BRMs are considered as well. Dosages vary according to the disease being treated and the expected therapeutic effects. Because dosage units are not necessarily standardized, different formulations are not interchangeable unless approved by the health care provider and pharmacist.

Remain with the patient for at least 30 minutes after administration of a BRM to monitor for adverse effects. Headache, fever, chills, fatigue, malaise, and weakness are more pronounced in older adult patients. BRM therapy ordinarily involves the use of many other drugs to reduce or minimize the adverse effects of the biologic drug. For example, using meperidine helps reduce shaking chills (rigors); histamine-2 antagonists (e.g., ranitidine) or proton pump inhibitors (e.g., lansoprazole) can be used for prophylaxis of gastric irritation and bleeding; antiemetics for nausea; and antidiarrheal drugs for diarrhea. The patient taking monoclonal antibodies may require premedication with an antihistamine, acetaminophen, and glucocorticoids to alleviate adverse reactions.

In general, BRMs are less stable than chemical drugs. Most require refrigeration and tolerate room temperatures only for short periods after reconstitution. They are more difficult to reconstitute and may need to be administered more quickly after reconstitution. This has implications for home use because improper storage may mean administration of an inactive drug; as a result, there may be no tumor response, biologic activity, or expected adverse effects.

To preserve their biologic activity, the drugs should not be shaken during preparation. Be aware of which BRMs require skin testing before administration.

BRMs can be administered orally, intravenously, intramuscularly, or subcutaneously. Some BRMs can be taken with food, but others cannot; check the package insert for information. Drugs to be given on an empty stomach should be taken 1 hour before or 2 hours after a meal. Further, some oral formulations (e.g., cyclosporine) must be measured with a dropper and then diluted in a glass container. It is important to use proper technique when preparing the drug for administration and to know which drug formulations can be crushed, which can be chewed, which can have the capsule opened, or which must be taken whole.

Drugs given intravenously should be infused through a large vessel and the site must be closely monitored for extravasation. Drug monographs should be checked for proper administration times and requirements for an in-line filter. A drug given intramuscularly should be administered in a large muscle. Intramuscular and subcutaneous injection sites should be rotated.

Education

Patients receiving BRMs have the same educational needs with regard to their drug therapy as do other patients. Information and the ability to participate in self-care activities increase self-esteem and enhance coping ability. Teach the patient about the basic function of the immune system, the mechanism of action of the specific drug taken, and the desired therapeutic results. The expected adverse effects, both of the specific BRM and the combination therapy (e.g., BRM plus antineoplastic drug, or more than one BRM), and administration techniques also should be covered. The importance of laboratory testing and follow-up with the health care provider cannot be overemphasized. Be sure the patient and family know when to contact the health care provider. Patients also should be advised to avoid driving or operating hazardous machinery if blurry vision or drowsiness occurs. The female patient should be taught to use contraceptive measures during BRM treatment and for 12 weeks after ending therapy.

The family must be considered a resource for the patient. The patient often needs a partner and coach to tolerate the physical and emotional strain of BRM therapy. Teach the family to identify and report adverse effects that the patient may be unable to recognize (e.g., neurologic changes).

Because the patient is at risk for infection while taking immunosuppressing BRMs, teach the patient and family to monitor specifically for signs and symptoms of infection. The patient should be taught how to take his or her temperature. Advise the patient to avoid persons who have just received immunizations containing live vaccine. Some immunocompromised patients may need to avoid exposure to house plants and animals, and in some cases, may need to be isolated to reduce the risk of contracting an infection. Conscientious hand washing is required of all who come in contact with the patient.

Patient and family knowledge about what constitutes adequate nutrition is vital. Encourage the patient to consume high-quality dietary nutrients and to avoid as much as possible "empty" calories. Use of supplemental vitamins and minerals or protein supplements may be needed.

EVALUATION

The effectiveness of BRM therapy is specific to the disorder under treatment. For example, therapeutic effectiveness may be demonstrated by immunosuppression of an autoimmune disorder or the absence of graft rejection for patients who have undergone transplantation. Tumor regression and decreased spread of a malignancy can be noted as early as 4 weeks after completion of the first course of interleukin therapy and may continue for up to 12 months after the start of therapy. The patient taking interleukins for relapsing-remitting multiple sclerosis may see a decrease in the frequency of relapse, further providing evidence of drug effectiveness.

Normalized blood parameters provide evidence of therapeutic response. The time to hematopoietic response is related to the interval required for immature cells to become fully mature and to be released into the peripheral circulation. Available iron stores, baseline hematocrit, and the presence of comorbid disorders influence the rate and extent of hematopoietic response.

Bibliography

Bush WW, Bartucci MR, Cupples SA: Overview of transplantation immunology and the pharmacotherapy of adult solid organ transplant recipients: focus on immunosuppression, *AACN Clin Issues* 10(2):253-269, 1999.

Kher U: Autoimmune diseases: new ways to intervene when the body attacks itself, *Time* 157(2):76, 79, 2001.

Mihich E: Historical overview of biologic response modifiers, *Cancer Invest* 18(5):456-466, 2000.

Reed JC, Kitada S, Kim Y, et al: Modulating apoptosis pathways in low-grade B-cell malignancies using biological response modifiers, *Semin Oncol* 29(1 Suppl 2):10-24, 2002.

Weaver AL: Etanercept and other biologic response modifiers for RA: new therapies more effective in arresting disease, *J Musculoskelet Med* 17(9):521-524, 526-528, 533-534, 2000.

Internet Resources

http://www.bccancer.bc.ca/pg_g_03.asp?PageID=518&Parent ID=2.

http://www.fda.gov/cber/advisory/brm/brmchart.htm.

http://www3.mdanderson.org/~oncolog/06_Biological_Ther. html.

37

Antineoplastic Drugs

SHERRY F. QUEENER • KATHLEEN GUTIERREZ

 Visit http://evolve.elsevier.com/Gutierrez/ for additional information.

KEY TERMS

OBJECTIVES

- Explain what is meant by the term *cancer*.
- Explain how the cell cycle affects antineoplastic therapy.
- Relate the mechanism of action of classes of anticancer drugs to selective toxicity.
- Explain the characteristic adverse reactions of classes of anticancer drugs.
- Develop a nursing care plan for the patient with depressed white blood cell production, bleeding tendencies, or stomatitis.

PATHOPHYSIOLOGY • Cancer

Cancer develops when normal cells are transformed by chemicals, viruses, or radiation and thereby become resistant to appropriate regulation of cell division. The public thinks of cancer as a single disease, but it is a large family of related diseases that differ from one another in characteristic disease patterns. For example, skin cancer runs a different clinical course than lung cancer. Skin cancer, lung cancer, and many other forms of cancer may affect diverse types of patients, but other cancers such as Wilms' tumor, Kaposi's sarcoma, and choriocarcinoma tend to strike a certain age and gender of patient (Table 37-1).

Cancers may be more formally grouped and categorized according to the cells or tissue of origin (Table 37-2). For example, carcinomas all arise from epithelial cells, but because epithelial cells are found in many organs or sites in the body, carcinomas likewise can be found in many sites, including the breast, prostate, lungs, liver, or kidneys. This classification scheme also allows subdivisions within the categories. For example, leukemias can arise from any of the various cells within bone marrow. Therefore myelogenous leukemias (arising from myeloid tissue in the marrow), lymphocytic leukemias (arising from cells that form lymphocytes), and other forms of the disease exist.

One reason for thinking of cancer in terms of its cell of origin is that cancerous cells may retain some properties of the parent cells. For example, carcinomas of the breast or of the prostate may retain some of the hormone receptors normally present in the cell of origin. Antineoplastic therapy may thus be directed to these cancerous cells by using the retained hormone receptors as targets. Likewise, lymphomas may retain receptors that recognize glucocorticoid hormones; thus these hormones may suppress lymphomas in the same way as normal lymphoid tissue.

Common Properties of Cancer

The clinical course of many cancers illustrates some unique properties of cancer cells. For example, cancer cells lose the normal property of contact inhibition. **Contact inhibition** prevents normal cells from dividing when they are crowded together, but cancer cells continue to divide even when the pressure of the surrounding cell mass is considerable. In certain tissues, as the cancer proliferates, it forms a solid mass and crowds surrounding normal tissue as the mass, or tumor, grows. In other tissues, such as bone marrow, growth of neoplastic cells is more diffuse, but ultimately normal tissue is overwhelmed and crowded out by the uncontrolled proliferation of the cancerous tissues.

A second unique property of cancers is their ability to spread far from the original site. In this process, cancer cells separate from the original mass and move directly or are carried by blood or lymph to distant sites. There the cells lodge in healthy tissue and begin to divide,

---

TABLE 37-1

Selected Neoplastic Diseases

Disease	Characteristics
Burkitt's lymphoma	Rapidly growing tumor of lymphoid tissue; highly responsive to chemotherapy
Choriocarcinoma (gestational trophoblastic tumors)	Rapidly growing tumor of embryonic cells; seeded in mother during abortion, childbirth, or after hydatidiform mole; highly responsive to chemotherapy
Ewing's sarcoma	Rapidly growing tumor most often found in children; responsive in early stages to combination of surgery, radiation, and chemotherapy
Hodgkin's disease	Tumor of lymph nodes, spleen, and other lymphoid tissue; highly responsive to chemotherapy
Kaposi's sarcoma	Highly malignant, metastasizing tumor usually noted on skin of extremities; although characteristic of AIDS patients, tumor is also seen in older men without HIV/AIDS
Lymphocytic leukemia	Cancer of lymphoid tissue causes excess lymphocytes or lymphoblasts in blood; response to therapy is best in acute form of disease
Myelogenous leukemia	Cancer of myeloid tissue leads to excess granular polymorphonuclear leukocytes in blood; response to therapy not as good as in lymphocytic leukemia
Wilms' tumor	Rapidly growing tumor of children; highly responsive to combination of surgery, radiation, and chemotherapy

AIDS, Acquired immunodeficiency syndrome.

thus producing a **metastasis** (secondary tumor). Tumors have been produced in experimental animals with a single cancer cell. This property of cancer cells explains why cure of malignancies may require destruction of every cancer cell in the body.

The single defining property of cancer cells is that they are no longer responsive to appropriate signals controlling cell proliferation. An injured liver may regenerate to replace lost tissue, but the process is self-limited and stops after a certain amount of tissue is replaced. In contrast, a liver tumor proliferates continuously to the point of crowding out and destroying normal surrounding tissue. The proliferation of these cancerous cells is not self-limited and will continue so long as the host survives. The next section discusses normal cell proliferation and explains how cells can escape from normal regulation of this process.

Regulation of Cell Division

The **cell cycle** is a programmed sequence of events that occurs during cell division. The cycle is divided into several segments according to the processes that occur during that phase. The first phase of the cycle, termed G_1, involves primarily RNA synthesis (Figure 37-1). This phase is crucial to the fate of the cell and is regulated by extracellular signals. Up to a certain point in G_1, if these external signals are removed, the cell reverts to the resting phase (G_0) and does not divide. At some time late in G_1, cells pass a control point and become committed to cell division, even if the external signals are withdrawn. This transition from G_1 is regulated by proteins called **cyclins**, which act on cyclin-dependent protein kinases (CDKs). The activation of these proteins increases the activity of several enzymes crucial for DNA synthesis. This process sets the stage for the next phase in the cell cycle, the S phase, during which DNA synthesis occurs. DNA is the nucleic acid that contains the genetic information for the cell. When DNA synthesis is complete, the cell contains twice the amount of DNA found in a

TABLE 37-2	
Tissue of Origin for Types of Cancer	
Cancer	*Tissue of Origin*
Carcinoma	Epithelial cells (e.g., skin and mucous membranes of lung and GI tract)
Leukemia	Blood-forming organ (e.g., bone marrow or lymphoid tissue)
Lymphoma	Lymphoid tissue
Melanoma	Pigmented skin cells
Myeloma	Bone marrow
Sarcoma	Connective tissue (e.g., bone, cartilage)

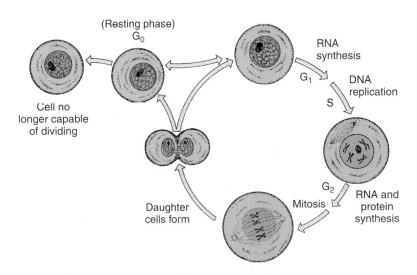

FIGURE 37-1 Proliferative cycle of mammalian cells. In actively dividing cells, metabolic processes required for cell division take place at different times during the cycle. DNA synthesis precedes messenger RNA and protein synthesis; these processes must be complete before mitosis, or cell division, can occur. Because of metabolic differences, cells at different phases of cycle have different sensitivities to many drugs used to control cancer.

nondividing cell. At this point RNA and protein synthesis increase, and the cell enters the G_2 phase. At the end of this phase the cell contains enough material to form two complete cells, and mitosis begins.

Mitosis is a process that begins with the condensation of DNA to form chromosomes and ends with the production of two daughter cells. As mitosis begins the cell has two copies of each chromosome. To separate these pairs so that one copy of each chromosome goes into each daughter cell, the cell forms microtubules that are organized into the mitotic spindle. Without the mitotic spindle to pull the chromosomes into opposite ends of the cell, reproduction would halt. Once the chromosomes have been successfully segregated into two complete sets, closing of the cell membrane, which divides the mother cell into two daughter cells, completes division.

Once cell division is complete a cell may immediately reenter the reproductive cycle or it may become temporarily nonreproductive. In this nonreproductive phase, called G_0, the cell only repairs existing DNA and synthesizes only the RNA and protein needed for maintenance of the cell. A cell in the G_0 phase may become altered so that it is no longer capable of dividing, or after some time, it may enter phase G_1 and divide again.

The control point between G_1 and the S phase is regulated by cyclins and CDKs, as noted previously. This transition point is also the focus of another regulatory system that serves as a brake to the cyclin system that drives proliferation. This braking or checkpoint system involves a gene called p53. This gene seems not to be required for cell division but becomes necessary when the cell's DNA is damaged. Under these conditions p53 interferes with the signals that would drive the cell through the G_1-S phase transition point, so the cell becomes arrested at the G_1 phase. This delay gives the cell time to repair its DNA before it is replicated. If the DNA is too badly damaged, p53 may induce **apoptosis**, or programmed cell death. Thus, the overall action of p53 is to protect the accuracy of gene replication during cell division and ensure that only healthy cells with intact genomes survive and divide. Because of its function to remove genetically damaged cells, which may of course include cancer cells, the p53 gene is sometimes called a **tumor suppressor gene.**

Origin and Molecular Basis of Cancer

Carcinogenesis is the process by which a normal cell is transformed into a cancerous cell. Agents called carcinogens may start this transformation by causing mutations or chromosomal translocations. Cells at this stage may divide, die, or remain in the resting state.

Tumor promoters are agents that do not necessarily affect the DNA of a cell but in some other way influence the fate of a transformed cell. For example, some chemicals promote division of the altered cell and may cause it to become fully malignant.

Cell division in cancer is perturbed so that cells seem to divide independent of any external signal. Significant genetic changes are associated with this property, including the expression of oncogenes. **Oncogenes** are genes that are activated in human cancers, override normal regulation of gene expression, and drive cell proliferation. These genes are very similar to normal genes encoding proteins that transmit growth stimulatory messages. The oncogenes code for altered forms of these regulatory proteins so that the message to divide is powerful and constant in a cancer cell.

More than 100 oncogenes have been recognized in human cancers. Some of these oncogenes involve positive regulators such as Ras and Myc. *Ras* is a protein that occurs early in the cascade that ultimately increases the formation of cyclin D1, which drives cells through the G_1-S phase transition. *Myc* is a protein from the latter stages of that same pathway. If Ras or Myc are altered so that the signal to produce cyclins is continuous, the cell may be driven to divide continuously.

Oncogenes may also involve tumor suppressor genes. For example, some disruption of the function of p53 has been noted in up to half of all human cancers, making these mutations the most common in human disease. In some specific types of cancer, such as lung cancer or colon cancer, the percentages showing altered p53 are even higher, ranging from 60% to 70%. The mutated **tumor suppressor gene** acts as an oncogene because the normal action of p53 to monitor transition into the cell cycle or to induce apoptosis in damaged cells may be lost, allowing altered cells to proliferate and generate cancer.

The p53 system may also interact with telomeres differently in normal versus cancer cells. Telomeres are the repetitive ends of linear chromosomes, such as those found in humans. Under normal conditions, each cell division shortens the telomere until at some point the shortened telomere triggers the action of p53 protein and apoptosis is induced. Cancer cells may overproduce an enzyme, telomerase, which maintains the length of the telomeres so that even after many generations they are not short enough to trigger apoptosis. Thus one of the normal mechanisms to limit proliferation is lost in cancer cells.

How Can Cancer be Controlled?

Host Responses. In theory, one cancer cell left alive after therapy can cause recurrence of cancer. In contrast, antibacterial therapy can be successful if bacteria are stopped from growing long enough for the immune system to attack and eliminate the invaders. With cancer the immune system is much less effective. One reason for this difference is that cancer cells are not easily recognized as foreign by the host immune system. Another factor that seems to lower immune responses to cancer is that as tumors become massive, they produce a specific immune tolerance. Modulation of the immune system is possible, and there are now strategies allowing the immune system to be recruited to combat cancer. In one approach, cytotoxic drugs target tumor cells by linking the drugs to antibodies that specifically bind to cancer cells (see Chapter 36). Even more sophisticated strategies may eventually induce a cancer to produce an antigen that will attract other factors that will cause the cancer cell to undergo apoptosis. One variation of this strategy would apply to cancer cells that overproduce

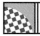

Dietary Considerations for ANTIOXIDANT AND ANTICANCER ACTIVITY

Green Tea

Tea is traditionally made from the leaves of the Asian plant *Camelia sinesis*. This beverage, which has been made for thousands of years in China, may fall into three categories depending on how the tea leaves are handled both before and after picking. Black tea, which is common in the United States, is made from fermented tea leaves. This tea tends to have a high content of tannins, which accounts for the dark color and the astringency of the brew. Oolong tea is made from semifermented leaves and tends to have less tannin than black tea. Green teas are brewed from leaves that are harvested and dried without any fermentation. Some forms of green tea leaves are taken from plants that are protected from the sun for several days, whereas others come directly from plants growing openly in the field. On average, green teas contain less tannin and more proteins or amino acids than black or oolong teas. The color of green tea is a light green or light tan.

The benefit of tea, and especially green tea, is related to the complex mixtures of chemicals in the leaves that act as antioxidants. This protective effect from the destructive action of oxygen can be demonstrated in laboratory tests with isolated cells. In animal trials, green tea seems as effective as vitamin E as an antioxidant under many conditions. One of the most interesting claims for green tea is that its antioxidant effects may protect against development of cancer. Such action has been seen in several animal trials and tests in humans are under way.

No matter what the outcome of the trials for anticancer effects, green tea with its low tannin and moderate caffeine content is a beverage that has comforted people for thousands of years and no doubt will continue to be enjoyed throughout the world.

p53 protein because these cells present fragments of p53 on their cell surface, in theory allowing cytotoxic T lymphocytes to target these cells.

Antineoplastic Therapy. Antineoplastic therapy often involves the use of **cytotoxic** drugs, drugs that are designed to cause cell death. Obviously, such drugs must be used with caution because they can kill normal cells as well as cancer cells. The issue with these drugs, as with all drugs, is one of selectivity of action.

Rapidly growing cells are more sensitive to cytotoxic drugs than are resting cells. Thus, some selective drug action can be generated because most normal tissues have very few cells actively reproducing at any one time, whereas in many cancers there is a derangement in regulation of growth so that the cancer cells divide continuously.

It must be remembered that normal cell types with rapid, noncancerous growth will be targeted by cytotoxic anticancer drugs, right along with the cancerous tissues. Tissues at risk because of high rates of cell division include bone marrow, which is the site for formation of blood cells, and lymphoid tissue, which is the site for formation of lymphocytes and monocytes. The intestinal lining, testes, ovaries, endometrium, and hair follicles are all additional sites of rapid cell division. Thus, these cytotoxic drugs predictably cause bone marrow toxicity, gastrointestinal (GI) distress, depression of spermatogenesis, and hair loss as common adverse effects. The action of so many cytotoxic drugs on the bone marrow also explains why antineoplastic therapy for cancers is often followed by autologous bone marrow transplantation to replace the blood-forming cells destroyed by the drugs.

Understanding regulation of the cell cycle and the biology of individual cancers led to the beginnings of cancer-specific drug therapy. For example, one form of chronic myeloid leukemia is associated with a chromosomal abnormality referred to as the Philadelphia chromosome, referring to the place the first example was discovered. This chromosomal abnormality is now known to generate an abnormal growth factor, called Bcr-Abl tyrosine kinase, which is produced continuously in affected cells. A new drug called imatinib mesylate inhibits this enzyme and thus blocks proliferation as well as induces apoptosis in the leukemic cells. Selectivity is not yet perfect because the drug also inhibits the tyrosine kinase receptors for platelet-derived growth factor and others. Nevertheless, this drug is an example of a new strategy to use much more specific targets than is possible with cytotoxic drugs.

Receptors other than tyrosine kinases have long been used to advantage for antineoplastic therapy of certain tumors. The sex steroids (androgens, estrogens, and progestins) are used in cancer therapy because the presence (or absence) of these hormones regulates growth and function of many reproductive tissues. These steroid hormones enter sensitive cells and, complexed with specific receptor proteins, are transported to the cell nucleus. Within the nucleus they alter RNA and protein synthesis, thereby changing the function of the cell. The rationale behind all forms of this therapy is that tumors of reproductive tissues tend to retain some dependence on hormones. Thus the use of these drugs in cancer antineoplastic therapy depends on knowledge of the hormone dependence of specific tissues. For example, the prostate gland depends on androgens; without these hormones the gland shrinks and loses function. Carcinoma of the prostate gland retains a degree of this hormonal control, and suppressing androgen production or function can often produce tumor regression. Suppression of production may be with surgical castration to remove the major source of endogenous androgens or may be with a luteinizing hormone–releasing hormone (LH-RH) analog that suppresses androgen synthesis. Antagonists that block binding to androgen receptors may diminish androgen function; estrogens and drugs such as flutamide act in this way.

Suppression of tumor growth in many breast carcinomas can likewise be achieved by treating them with estrogens, antiestrogens, or androgens; the choice of drug is determined by the receptor pattern of the particular tumor. For estrogen-responsive tumors, the strategy may be to antagonize estrogen effects with excess androgenic steroids or by the use of antiestrogens such as tamoxifen. Alternatively, compounds may be used that block aromatase, an enzyme required for the conversion of certain adrenal steroids to estrogen. These strategies are most effective in postmenopausal women. In these women the ovaries no longer produce estrogens, and most of the estrogen in their bodies is produced by the action of aromatase on steroids from the adrenal glands.

Gene therapy or therapy aimed at reversing the effects of oncogenes are in the future for cancer. In general, the trials that have been performed have highlighted the difficulty in getting the new gene into enough cells to overcome the disease, but several new strategies are under development.

Classifications of Drugs Used Against Cancer

Scientists and clinicians have classified antineoplastic drugs in many ways. One widely used scheme is based on the chemical properties and origins of the drugs (Table 37-3). In this scheme, an antibiotic is a chemical made by a fungus, bacteria, or streptomycete and has an action on mammalian cells. Alkylating drugs are synthetic, highly reactive chemicals that change DNA and other substances by adding a carbon-containing substituent to certain sites. Antimetabolites mimic normal metabolites and block one or more enzymes in the metabolic pathway.

One drawback of this classification scheme is that it is based on properties far from clinical experience. The system is also old and does not reflect the current level of understanding of mechanisms of the drugs. Therefore, in this text the cytotoxic drugs are grouped according to the site in the cell cycle where the drug acts (Figure 37-2).

Combinations of Antineoplastic Drugs

Few of the antineoplastic drugs discussed in this chapter are used alone. Experience has demonstrated that combinations of these drugs are much more effective than single drugs. Several reasons for this increased success exist. First, combinations of drugs acting by different mechanisms are less likely to cause drug resistance. Like microbial cells, cancer cells can adapt and become drug resistant. The degree and type of resistance depends on the blood supply and nutrients available to the tumor, the bioavailability of the drug, and the presence of tumor in sanctuary sites relatively inaccessible to drugs. This process occurs easily if only a single drug is used. If several are used, the cancer cell

---

TABLE 37-3

Classification of Selected Cytotoxic Antineoplastic Drugs Based on Source and Chemistry

Classification	Drugs
Alkylating drugs	busulphan, chlorambucil, cyclophosphamide, dacarbazine, nitrogen mustards (mechlorethamine), nitrosoureas, procarbazine
Purine and pyrimidine analogs	cytosine arabinoside, fludarabine, 5-fluorouracil, gemcitabine, 6-mercaptopurine
Antibiotics	bleomycin, dactinomycin, daunorubicin, doxorubicin
Antifolates	methotrexate
Vinca alkaloids	vincristine, vinblastine

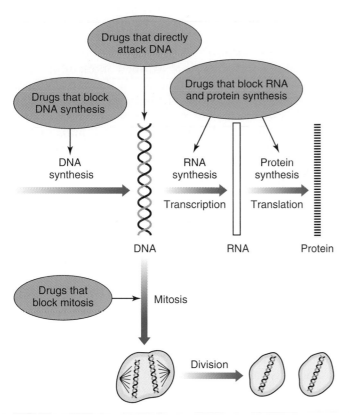

FIGURE 37-2 Molecular processes targeted by antineoplastic drugs. RNA and protein synthesis take place in every cell, although the processes will be stimulated in cell division. Likewise, the DNA is used for transcription in resting as well as dividing cells. Drugs targeted at these processes can therefore affect resting or dividing cells. Drugs that target DNA synthesis or mitosis tend to be most effective against dividing cells.

has greater difficulty in developing simultaneous resistance. Simultaneous resistance is not impossible, however, if the cancer cells acquire the multidrug resistance pump, a system that effectively removes many drugs from inside cells.

Second, drug combinations allow the health care provider to select drugs that produce different patterns of toxicity and thereby reduce the damage directed at any one organ system. Many antineoplastic drugs cause bone marrow suppression. Combining these suppressive drugs with drugs such as bleomycin or vincristine, which do not damage bone marrow, allows more anticancer effect to be achieved with no added damage to bone marrow.

Third, combining antineoplastic drugs that act at different stages of the cell cycle allows for more tumor cells to be killed than would occur with the use of one drug that would affect only one stage of the cycle. For example, a drug such as procarbazine is specific for the S phase of the cell cycle. Therefore tumor cells that pass into that phase while exposed to procarbazine die, but cells in resting phase survive. If an alkylating drug is added to the treatment regimen, a percentage of the cells that survive procarbazine treatment are expected to be killed by the second drug. Adding a third drug with yet a different mechanism of action, such as vincristine, further reduces the number of surviving cancer cells.

Finally, if it is possible to add a tissue-specific drug or an immune modulator to the regimen, an even greater anticancer effect may be gained. Examples of such combination therapies used for various types of cancer are shown in Table 37-4.

TABLE 37-4

Combination Chemotherapeutic Regimens

Regimen	Drugs Included	Disease
ABVD	doxorubicin (**A**driamycin), **b**leomycin, **v**inblastine, **d**acarbazine	Hodgkin's disease
BCVPP	carmustine (**B**iCNU), **c**yclophosphamide, **v**inblastine, **p**rocarbazine, **p**rednisone	Advanced Hodgkin's disease
CMF	**c**yclophosphamide, **m**ethotrexate, **f**luorouracil	Breast carcinoma
CVP	**c**yclophosphamide, **v**incristine, **p**rednisone	Non-Hodgkin's lymphoma
MOPP	**m**echlorethamine, vincristine (**O**ncovin), **p**rocarbazine, **p**rednisone	Hodgkin's disease
POMP	**p**rednisone, vincristine (**O**ncovin), **m**ethotrexate, mercaptopurine (**P**urinethol)	Acute lymphocytic leukemia
TAD	**t**hioguanine, cytarabine (**A**ra-C), **d**aunorubicin	Acute myeloid leukemia
VIP	etoposide (**Ve**Pesid), **i**fosfamide, cisplatin (**P**latinol)	Testicular cancer

Why Don't Drugs Cure All Cancers?

A primary difficulty in treating neoplastic diseases is that cancer cells offer fewer targets for selective toxicity than do bacterial cells, for example. This similarity in structure and metabolic processes reminds us that cancer cells are derived from host cells. Some differences between normal and cancerous cells can be identified, but they are mostly quantitative rather than qualitative. Thus nearly all the effective drugs have a **dose-limiting toxicity**, which is an adverse effect that limits the dose of drug that can be given. If the drugs were given at high enough concentrations to kill all the cancer cells, so many normal cells would also be killed that the patient could not survive. Thus most anticancer drugs have a low therapeutic index and a narrow safety margin (see Chapter 1).

Another primary difficulty may lie within the mutations accumulated by the cancer cells. For example, many cytotoxic drugs like fluorouracil and cisplatin actually induce apoptosis in sensitive cells. However, if the targeted cancer cells contain a mutated p53 that does not support apoptosis, then the cells will be resistant to the drugs. Other changes are linked to different forms of drug resistance. For example, cells that produce a specific pump mechanism called MDR (multidrug resistance) become resistant because anticancer drugs are effectively pumped out of the cancer cell, before they can damage the cell.

Antineoplastic therapy is also at a disadvantage because diagnosis often occurs late in the course of the disease. A single transformed cell after 10 cycles of cell division can produce at most 1024 cells, a mass far too small to be noticed. By the time the tumor weighs about 1 g, it will have gone through about 30 division cycles. A 1-g tumor is approximately the size of a small grape. In many locations within the body, a tumor this size may easily escape detection, yet in just 10 more cell divisions this tumor could exceed a mass of 1 kg (2.2 lb). Most tumors do not grow nearly as rapidly as the theoretical example just cited, in which it was assumed that every cell formed immediately reentered the reproductive cycle, but no matter how long it takes, the result of this process is a large mass containing more than 1 billion cells. Treatment at this stage with a drug that killed 99.99% of these cells, which would be an exceptionally effective drug, would still leave 100,000 cells that could eventually regrow.

The example in the preceding paragraph reminds us that earlier detection could give a therapeutic advantage for antineoplastic therapy since there would be fewer cancer cells to fight. For several diseases, early detection is being made possible by the use of molecular markers of disease. For example, prostatic cancer can be detected in a blood test far earlier than it might be detected in a physical examination because this type of cancer releases into the blood a protein called prostate-specific antigen (PSA).

DRUG CLASS • Cytotoxic Drugs that Directly Attack DNA

 cyclophosphamide (Cytoxan, Neosar, Cytoxan,✻ Procytox✻)

For other drugs in this class see Table 37-5.

MECHANISM OF ACTION

The genetic information necessary for cell reproduction resides in DNA. Damage to the DNA of many normal cells is undetectable because those cells rarely divide and they have effective mechanisms for DNA repair. In contrast, cancer cells have rapid rates of replication and more limited DNA repair mechanisms, thus making them more vulnerable to being killed by damage to their DNA. This rationale explains the use of a large group of antineoplastic drugs that chemically modify DNA.

Alkylating drugs may attack DNA in its double-stranded form, attaching various compounds to one strand or the other. Other drugs may form cross-links, or chemical bonds, between the strands. Because the strands must unwind and separate during replication, **cross-linking** effectively blocks replication. Induction of DNA strand breaks is also common with drugs of this class. Whether produced by direct drug action or by inhibition of one of the topoisomerases, DNA strand breaks are eventually lethal to the cell. The specific action of individual drugs of this class is noted in Table 37-5.

Cyclophosphamide, the prototype drug of this class, is biotransformed into several metabolites by microsomal enzymes in the liver. At least one of these metabolites is a potent alkylating drug with activity similar to that of nitrogen mustard. Because the drug as administered is not active, it does not possess the strong vesicant activity (direct blistering and damage of tissues) seen with other nitrogen mustard alkylating drugs.

USES

The clinical uses of antineoplastic drugs that directly attack DNA are summarized in Table 37-5.

PHARMACOKINETICS

Many drugs of this class are rapidly destroyed in the body. A few drugs such as cisplatin, busulfan, mechlorethamine,

TABLE 37-5

Antineoplastic Drugs that Directly Attack DNA

Generic Name	Brand Name	Indications	Class/Mechanism	Distinguishing Characteristics
altretamine	Hexalen, Hexstat✷	Ovarian carcinoma	Alkylates DNA, after activation	Neurologic toxicity with anxiety, confusion, awkwardness, dizziness, numbness in limbs, or seizures; interacts with MAO inhibitors, causing orthostatic hypotension
arsenic trioxide	Trisenox	Acute promyelocytic leukemia	Heavy metal, fragments DNA	May cause potentially fatal differentiation syndrome, with fever, dyspnea, lung infiltrates, pleural or pericardial effusions
bleomycin	Blenoxane	Lymphomas, squamous cell carcinomas, testicular or ovarian carcinomas, malignant pleural effusions	Antibiotic, causes strand breaks in DNA	Unlike other drugs of this class, bleomycin does not cause bone marrow suppression
busulfan	Myleran	Chronic myelocytic leukemia	Alkylsulfonate; alkylates DNA	May elevate uric acid and interacts with probenecid and sulfinpyrazone
carboplatin	Paraplatin, Paraplatin-AQ✷	Recurrent ovarian carcinoma	Platinum complex; cross-links DNA	Ototoxicity and peripheral neurologic toxicity are common
carmustine	BiCNU	CNS tumors, lymphomas, and myelomas	Nitrosourea; alkylates DNA	Penetrates blood-brain barrier well; lung fibrosis may occur
carmustine	Gliadel	Recurrent glioblastoma multiforme	Nitrosourea; alkylates DNA	Wafer is implanted during surgery to remove tumor
chlorambucil	Leukeran	Lymphocytic leukemias and lymphomas	Nitrogen mustard; alkylates DNA	Slowest acting and least toxic nitrogen mustard alkylating agent; may raise uric acid levels
cisplatin	Platinol, Platinol-AQ✷	Testicular cancer and carcinomas in many tissues	Platinum complex; crosslinks DNA	Renal toxicity, ototoxicity, and neurologic toxicity are dose-limiting
cyclophos-phamide	Cytoxan	Lymphomas, solid tumors, leukemias, and myelomas	Activated to nitrogen mustard; alkylates DNA	Prototype drug of this class; may raise uric acid levels
dacarbazine	DTIC,✷ DTIC-Dome	Malignant melanoma, lymphomas	Alkylating agent	Causes severe pain at injection site
etoposide	Etopophos Toposar, VePesid	Refractory testicular tumors and small-cell lung carcinoma	Inhibits topoisomerase II; induces DNA strand breaks	Highly protein bound and excreted slowly by renal mechanisms
ifosfamide	IFEX	Germ cell testicular tumors	Activated to nitrogen mustard; alkylating agent	Causes dose-related CNS effects and hemorrhagic cystitis
irinotecan	Camptosar	Colorectal carcinoma refractory to first-line drugs	Inhibitor of topoisomerase I; induces strand breaks in DNA	May cause severe diarrhea; use with diuretics may cause dehydration
lomustine	CeeNU	CNS tumors, lymphomas, and myelomas	Nitrosourea; alkylates DNA	Penetrates blood-brain barrier well; lung fibrosis may occur

Continued

TABLE 37-5

Antineoplastic Drugs that Directly Attack DNA—cont'd

Generic Name	Brand Name	Indications	Class/Mechanism	Distinguising Characteristics
mechloreth-amine	Mustargen	Hodgkin's disease and other lymphomas; solid tumors and their effusions	Nitrogen mustard; alkylates DNA	Strong immunosuppressant; known to induce malignancies; germinal tissue damaged; raises uric acid levels
melphalan	Alkeran	Multiple myeloma and ovarian carcinomas	Nitrogen mustard; alkylates DNA	May raise uric acid levels
mitomycin	Mutamycin	GI tumors	Antibiotic; activated to alkylate DNA	May cause renal failure with hemolysis, liver toxicity, or lung damage
procarbazine	Matulane, Natulan ✽	Hodgkin's lymphoma	Alkylating agent	MAO inhibitor; involved in many drug interactions
temozolomide	Temodar	Refractory astrocytoma	Alkylates DNA	Used after failure of nitrosourea and procarbazine
teniposide	Vumon	Childhood acute lymphocytic leukemia and neuroblastoma	Inhibits topoi-somerase II; induces DNA strand breaks	Highly protein bound; interacts with drugs such as salicylates that displace it from protein sites
thiotepa	Thiotepa	Lymphomas, carcinomas, and malignant effusions	Nitrogen mustard; alkylates DNA	Toxicity limited by direct application to tumor; raises uric acid levels
topotecan	Hycantin	Ovarian carcinoma or small-cell lung cancer after first-line drugs fail	Inhibits topoisomerase I; induces DNA strand breaks	Distributes to the CNS

✽ Available only in Canada.

and melphalan are hydrolyzed or destroyed by nonenzymatic mechanisms in many fluids and tissues. Other drugs such as altretamine, bleomycin, carmustine, chlorambucil, cyclophosphamide, and lomustine are rapidly biotransformed in the liver. Biotransformation lowers the activity of most of these drugs, but altretamine, cyclophosphamide, ifosfamide, and lomustine are either activated by biotransformation or their metabolites retain significant activity.

Bleomycin is degraded by enzymes in many tissues, except for skin and lungs; therefore the drug tends to concentrate at those sites and produce toxic reactions. Tumors tend not to inactivate bleomycin, so the drug is also concentrated in that tissue.

Carmustine penetrates the blood-brain barrier better than most drugs of this class. Carmustine has also been used in an implantable form for insertion into the cavity left by surgical removal of a brain tumor called glioblastoma multiforme (see Table 37-5). This implant, which is made from a biodegradable polymer, raises the concentration of drug at the site and prolongs the action.

The duration of action of this class of drugs is variable and does not always match the kinetics of elimination. For example, drugs such as mechlorethamine are destroyed within seconds of administration, but the biologic effect may persist for weeks.

Renal excretion is the most common route of elimination for these drugs. Some, such as chlorambucil and lomustine, are eliminated as metabolites; others, such as ifosfamide and bleomycin, are excreted largely unchanged.

ADVERSE REACTIONS AND CONTRAINDICATIONS

All cells will undergo attack by these drugs, although the action is lethal primarily when cells attempt division. Therefore tissues with high percentages of dividing cells are most sensitive. Clinical symptoms to be expected when these drugs attack normal, rapidly dividing tissues include bone marrow suppression that produces leukopenia (low white blood cell counts), thrombocytopenia (low platelet counts), or other blood dyscrasias; mucocutaneous reactions, including stomatitis or other signs; and gastrointestinal (GI) toxicity, including acute or delayed nausea and vomiting. These adverse reactions are discussed in more detail in the Application to Practice section.

Alkylating drugs chemically alter DNA and are thus mutagenic. Therefore this class of drugs can induce cancers of various types that may show up years after exposure to the drug. Not every patient will develop a second cancer as a result of therapy, but for patients exposed to alkylating drugs, the risk is increased many times over the normal, low incidence rate.

Some of these drugs have immunosuppressive activity. This action is especially strong with cyclophosphamide but is also observed with chlorambucil, melphalan, and mechlorethamine.

Bleomycin often causes skin and mucous membrane changes, fever, chills, anorexia, and vomiting. Pulmonary reactions occur in 10% to 40% of treated patients, and 1% may die. Lung toxicity begins as pneumonitis and progresses to pulmonary fibrosis. Pulmonary toxicity is both age and dose dependent. Pulmonary fibrosis may also be an insidious adverse effect with carmustine and lomustine. Shortness of breath or cough should be investigated quickly for cause.

Cisplatin is toxic to renal tubules and may cause serious damage with high dosages or too frequent administration. A drug called amifostine is used to protect the kidneys from damage by cisplatin. Amifostine generates free thiols, metabolites that concentrate in tissues and protect against free radicals and other damaging byproducts of cisplatin. Cisplatin also causes hearing loss in the upper frequency ranges and ringing in the ears (tinnitus). Ototoxicity tends to progress with repeated doses. Peripheral neuropathies may occur with either carboplatin or cisplatin.

Ifosfamide causes dose-related CNS effects and hemorrhagic cystitis. Administering the drug mesna at 20% of the ifosfamide dosage can control cystitis; mesna is given intravenously at the time ifosfamide is administered, then again 4 and 8 hours later.

TOXICITY

The dose-limiting toxicity with many of these drugs is bone marrow suppression, which increases as dosage increases. In addition to these expected effects on bone marrow, which are reflected in lower numbers of various cells in the blood, some of these drugs also have dosage-related effects on other organs. For example, bleomycin and carmustine cause pulmonary toxicity, whereas cyclophosphamide causes cardiac toxicity. At high doses, chlorambucil can also cause pulmonary fibrosis or liver toxicity.

INTERACTIONS

All drugs of this class except bleomycin may have significant interactions with bone marrow suppressants or radiation because the combinations profoundly depress production of blood cells. Live-virus vaccines must be avoided in patients who receive any of these drugs because generalized viral infections may occur as a result of the immunosuppression these drugs produce.

Drugs of this class that raise uric acid levels (see Table 37-5) may interact with probenecid or sulfinpyrazone because probenecid and sulfinpyrazone block reabsorption of uric acid from renal tubules. As a result, renal toxicity from uric acid deposits may occur.

Bleomycin also makes lung tissues more susceptible to damage by oxygen. As a result, general anesthetics may provoke a rapid deterioration in pulmonary function.

Cisplatin shows additive renal toxicity or ototoxicity with other drugs sharing these adverse effects.

Procarbazine inhibits monoamine oxidase. Therefore patients should not receive both procarbazine and drugs that elevate biogenic amine levels (e.g., sympathomimetics, tricyclic antidepressants, phenothiazines, tyramine-containing foods). Procarbazine can produce a disulfiram-like reaction with ethyl alcohol. Procarbazine can also cause significant interactions with anesthetics, drugs with anticholinergic effects, antidiabetic drugs, MAO inhibitors, CNS depressants, dextromethorphan, fluoxetine, levodopa, meperidine, methyldopa, and methylphenidate.

DRUG CLASS • Drugs that Block DNA Synthesis

⚠ **cytarabine**

⚠ **methotrexate**

For other drugs in this class see Table 37-6.

MECHANISM OF ACTION

Drugs may block DNA synthesis in several ways. Some of the drugs discussed in this section are specific enzyme inhibitors and prevent the action of an enzyme required for DNA synthesis. Other drugs chemically very similar to the natural purines and pyrimidines used to form DNA may be incorporated into DNA but make the DNA unstable and nonfunctional. The enzyme DNA polymerase is a common target of drugs of this type, being inhibited by various activated forms of these drugs. Cytarabine acts in this way. DNA polymerase may also contribute to instability of formed DNA by recognizing activated drugs of this class as substrate and inserting them into DNA in place of the normal bases. Cladribine and gemcitabine act in this way.

Methotrexate is commonly described as a folic acid antagonist because it prevents the regeneration of the metabolically active form of folic acid, tetrahydrofolate (THF). Without THF, cells cannot carry out carbon-transfer reactions, and normal biotransformation is blocked at several points. One of these blockades prevents the formation of thymidylic acid, and another arrests adenine and guanine nucleotide synthesis at an early stage. Without these precursors, DNA synthesis halts. Methotrexate is therefore specific for the S phase of the cell cycle.

A drug that inhibits DNA synthesis will not damage a cell that is not forming DNA. Therefore nonproliferating cells or cells in resting phase are relatively insensitive to these drugs. These drugs are called cycle-specific or phase-specific drugs because most affect primarily cells in S phase.

The property of phase specificity explains why S-phase inhibitors must be given on a repeating schedule. In a single treatment, only the fraction of cells in the tumor that are growing will be affected. A recovery period with no drug given allows normal tissues with many dividing cells such as bone marrow to return to normal function. During this recovery period, many cells in the cancerous tissue will move from G_0 phase into the reproductive cycle. Other cells that were not in S phase during treatment continue to proliferate, and the tumor continues to grow. Repeated, widely spaced doses of the drug give the maximum opportunity for the drug to catch the dividing cells in S phase when they will be sensitive.

USES

The clinical uses of antineoplastic drugs that block DNA synthesis are summarized in Table 37-6. In addition to its use as an anticancer drug, methotrexate is used for rheumatoid arthritis because the drug also has potent immunosuppressive actions (see Chapter 14).

Pharmacokinetics

Many S-phase inhibitors must be activated before they exhibit antineoplastic activity. Some are activated in the liver, but others are activated in cells of many types. Biotransformation and renal excretion are the major routes of elimination from the body.

Cytarabine must be injected, either subcutaneously, intrathecally, or intravenously. Subcutaneous injections are used only to maintain remissions and are given once or twice a week. Cytarabine does not easily pass into the cerebrospinal fluid (CSF). If it is administered intrathecally, it may persist in CSF for several hours because that

fluid has little of the deaminating enzyme that inactivates cytarabine.

Methotrexate may be administered orally, intramuscularly, intravenously, intraarterially, or intrathecally. For many patients the oral route is satisfactory because effective serum concentrations are reached within 1 hour. Parenteral administration results in a slightly faster absorption rate. The intrathecal route is required to treat patients with leukemias that have penetrated the CNS. Methotrexate does not pass from the blood into CSF in useful amounts but is otherwise well distributed in the body and may accumulate in some tissues. Liver cells seem especially able to bind the drug for long periods, and it also persists in the kidneys. These tissue sites of drug accumulation normally account for a small fraction of the total dose of methotrexate. Most of the drug is excreted directly in urine. Little degradation of methotrexate occurs, and the excreted drug is unchanged.

The route of administration of floxuridine determines its metabolic fate and its effectiveness. Floxuridine given intravenously by rapid injection is broken down into fluorouracil and then into the normal breakdown products of fluorouracil. When floxuridine is given slowly by intraarterial infusion, biotransformation to fluorouracil is reduced and most of the drug is converted to floxuridine monophosphate. The intraarterial route requires a lower dosage, yet it is more effective than intravenous administration.

Gemcitabine must be given by IV infusion. Distribution of the drug in the body is influenced by the rate of infusion and the patient's age and gender. Slow infusion favors distribution of drug into the tissues. Because gemcitabine is eliminated almost entirely by the kidneys, the normal age-related decline in renal function causes corresponding decline in clearance of the drug. Female patients of all ages eliminate gemcitabine less efficiently than male patients of the same age.

ADVERSE REACTIONS AND CONTRAINDICATIONS

Because the specificity of S-phase inhibitors is toward any active DNA synthesis, many normal cells will be sensitive. At highest risk of toxicity are those tissues with high numbers of dividing cells. Bone marrow depression and suppression of lymphocyte formation are characteristic adverse effects of these drugs. Lowered lymphocyte formation reduces the ability of the patient to fight infection, which may reduce the patient's chance for survival. Gastric mucosa also has a high growth fraction and is a target of serious toxic reactions to these drugs. Nausea, vomiting, and stomatitis are observed. In addition to these adverse reactions, cytarabine may cause CNS toxicity in up to 10% of treated patients.

TABLE 37-6

Anticancer Drugs that Block DNA Synthesis

Generic Name	Brand Name	Indications	Specific Mechanism	Distinguishing Characteristics
capecitabine	Xeloda	Metastatic colorectal or breast cancer	Prodrug of 5-fluorouracil; antimetabolite	Activated by three enzymes found in both normal and cancerous tissues
cladribine	Leustatin	Hairy cell leukemia	Adenosine analog; antimetabolite	Selective for S phase but affects cells in all phases; raises uric acid levels
cytarabine	Cytosar	Induce or maintain remissions in leukemias and lymphomas	Cytidine analog; antimetabolite	Raises uric acid levels
cytarabine, liposomal	DepoCyt	Lymphomatous meningitis	Cytidine analog; antimetabolite	Directly injected intrathecally, drug effects are maintained for 2 weeks
floxuridine	FUDR	Solid tumors not treatable by other means	Uracil analog; antimetabolite	GI adverse effects are dose limiting; may include bowel perforation
fludarabine	Fludara	Chronic lymphocytic leukemia	Adenine analog; antimetabolite	Raises uric acid levels; may cause fatal damage with pentostatin
fluorouracil	Adrucil, Efudex, Fluoroplex	Solid tumors not treatable by other means; topical for multiple actinic keratoses	Uracil analog; antimetabolite	GI adverse effects are dose limiting; may include bowel perforation
gemcitabine	Gemzar	Pancreatic carcinoma, advanced non–small-cell lung cancer	Pyrimidine analog; antimetabolite	Strong immunosuppressant; may cause adverse pulmonary and cardiovascular reactions
hydroxyurea	Hydrea	Melanoma, myelocytic leukemia, carcinomas	Inhibits ribotide reductase, thus halting synthesis of DNA precursors	Raises uric acid levels
mercaptopurine	Purinethol	To induce remissions in leukemia	Adenine analog; antimetabolite	Immunosuppressant; may also affect liver function
methotrexate	Folex, Mexate	Choriocarcinoma, lymphomas, lymphocytic leukemia, carcinomas	Strong inhibitor of dihydrofolate reductase; antifolate	Antifolate action blocks DNA synthesis
mitoxantrone	Novantrone	Refractory prostatic carcinoma, acute nonlymphocytic leukemias	Inhibits DNA and RNA synthesis	Cardiac toxicity a risk, especially above total dose of 140 mg/kg; colors urine blue-green
thioguanine	Lanvis✱	Myelocytic leukemia	Guanine analog; antimetabolite	Immunosuppressant

✱ Available only in Canada.

TOXICITY

Bone marrow suppression is often a dose-related adverse effect. Therefore very high dosages may have profound effects on the bone marrow.

INTERACTIONS

S-phase inhibitors all may produce serious interactions with bone marrow suppressants or radiation because the combinations significantly depress production of blood cells. The immunosuppression these drugs produce also puts patients at risk of generalized viral infections if they are given a live-virus vaccine during or shortly after receiving an S-phase inhibitor.

Mercaptopurine toxicity may be greatly increased by concomitant treatment with allopurinol. Allopurinol blocks uric acid synthesis and is often used to prevent toxic accumulation of that substance after extensive tumor cell destruction by antineoplastic therapy, but allopurinol also inhibits the biotransformation of mercaptopurine. Therefore, when the drugs are combined, more mercaptopurine persists in blood and in tissues for longer periods and greater toxicity results.

Cytarabine elevates uric acid levels and may change the dosage of probenecid or sulfinpyrazone needed to control hyperuricemia. Cytarabine with cyclophosphamide increases the risk of cardiac toxicity.

Salicylates (e.g., aspirin) may increase methotrexate toxicity by displacing methotrexate from plasma proteins. The increase in free plasma methotrexate often produces toxicity. Acyclovir may increase the risk of CNS effects when methotrexate is injected intrathecally. Alcohol or other hepatotoxic drugs increase the risk of liver damage. Asparaginase may block the action of methotrexate. Nonsteroidal antiinflammatory drugs (NSAIDs) may increase bone marrow effects of methotrexate.

Methotrexate acts by blocking regeneration of THF (tetrahydrofolate). Thus it is possible to prevent the action of the drug by supplying the body with THF. This use has been exploited for treating methotrexate overdose. Tumors such as osteosarcoma are treated with massive doses of methotrexate that would destroy the bone marrow and be lethal, but if the patient receives intravenous leucovorin, a drug containing THF and other forms of folic acid, the bone marrow can be protected. This type of therapy is called leucovorin rescue.

DRUG CLASS • Drugs that Block RNA or Protein Synthesis

 dactinomycin

For other drugs in the class, see Table 37-7.

MECHANISM OF ACTION

Drugs that block RNA formation can inhibit the rapid proliferation of cancer cells. Many of these drugs have this action because they bind very tightly to DNA and prevent reading of genes. These drugs are not highly specific for cancer cells but rather interfere with RNA and protein synthesis in any rapidly dividing tissue. Most, but not all drugs in the class, are most effective in the S and G_2 phases of the cell cycle.

Asparaginase and pegaspargase have different mechanisms that give some selectivity for cancer cells. Asparaginase is an enzyme that converts the amino acid asparagine to aspartic acid; pegaspargase is a chemically modified form of asparaginase. The therapeutic effect of these drugs arises because many types of cancer cells cannot form asparagine fast enough to support their growth. The enzyme destroys circulating asparagine, starving the cancer cells for asparagine. Normal cells are spared because they can form asparagine internally. To be most effective, asparagine starvation should occur in the G_1 phase of the cell cycle. If asparagine levels are kept low during that period, the asparagine-dependent cancer cell will be unable to carry out protein synthesis, and ultimately, RNA and DNA synthesis will cease. If asparagine starvation occurs later in the cell cycle after many critical proteins and nucleic acids have been formed, the cell may not die.

USES

The clinical uses of these drugs are summarized in Table 37-7.

PHARMACOKINETICS

Drugs of this class are not well absorbed orally and may be highly irritating to skin and soft tissues; therefore they must be given intravenously. The drugs are widely distributed to many tissues and organs, but rapid and extensive biotransformation occurs in the liver. Active and inactive metabolites are formed. Most drug elimination occurs through the liver. These drugs do not readily enter the CNS.

Liposomal preparations with rather different pharmacokinetics than the standard preparations are available for both daunorubicin and doxorubicin. In the liposomal formulations the drugs tend to stay in the blood rather than enter normal tissues and are protected from metabolic breakdown. The liposomal preparations do enter tumors, where the active drug is slowly released.

TABLE 37-7

Antineoplastic Drugs that Block RNA or Protein Synthesis

Generic Name	Brand Name	Indications	Specific Mechanism	Distinguishing Characteristics
asparaginase	Elspar, Kidrolase ✱	Acute lymphocytic leukemia	Enzyme depletes asparagine, thus slowing protein synthesis	Elicits severe allergic reactions; has anticoagulant effects
dactinomycin	Cosmogen	Choriocarcinoma, sarcomas, carcinomas	Antibiotic prevents DNA-dependent RNA synthesis	Highly corrosive to tissues
daunorubicin	Cerubidine	Leukemias	Antibiotic prevents DNA-dependent RNA synthesis	Cardiac toxicity occurs especially when total doses approach 500 mg/m²
daunorubicin, liposomal	DaunoXome	Kaposi's sarcoma	Antibiotic prevents DNA-dependent RNA synthesis	Liposomal preparation stays in blood longer than free compound
doxorubicin	Adriamycin, Rubex	Leukemias, lymphomas, sarcomas, carcinomas	Antibiotic prevents DNA-dependent RNA synthesis	Cardiac toxicity occurs especially when total doses approach 500 mg/m²
doxorubicin, liposomal	Doxil	Kaposi's sarcoma, metastatic ovarian cancer	Antibiotic prevents DNA-dependent RNA synthesis	Liposomal preparation stays in blood longer than free compound
epirubicin	Ellence, Pharmorubicin ✱	Carcinomas, lymphomas	Antibiotic prevents DNA-dependent RNA synthesis	Cardiac toxicity may occur
idarubicin	Idamycin	Acute myelocytic leukemia	Antibiotic prevents DNA-dependent RNA synthesis	Cardiac toxicity may occur
pegaspargase	Oncaspar	Acute lymphoblastic leukemia	Enzyme depletes asparagine, thus slowing protein synthesis	Persists in blood longer than asparaginase, so has longer action
plicamycin	Mithracin	Testicular carcinoma, metastatic bone tumors	Antibiotic prevents DNA-dependent RNA synthesis	Most useful to control hypercalcemia associated with malignancy
valrubicin	Valstar	BCG-refractory carcinoma of the bladder	Antibiotic prevents DNA-dependent RNA synthesis	Used inside the bladder rather than systemically

✱ Available only in Canada.

Asparaginase is a protein and must therefore be administered parenterally. The original form of asparaginase persists in the blood for 1 to 2 days; the modified form (pegaspargase) persists much longer, allowing this form to be used every 2 weeks. Neither form enters CSF in useful amounts. Excretion is mostly by nonrenal mechanisms.

Dactinomycin is rapidly cleared from the blood, entering the liver and other tissues. The drug does not cross the blood-brain barrier in effective amounts. Excretion of dactinomycin is mainly into bile, with smaller amounts of unchanged drug also appearing in urine.

ADVERSE REACTIONS AND CONTRAINDICATIONS

These inhibitors of RNA and protein synthesis attack all rapidly dividing tissues and therefore produce the expected array of adverse effects: bone marrow suppression, leading to lower production of various blood cells; damage to the epithelial layer of the GI tract, producing symptoms ranging from nausea to stomatitis; and damage to the hair follicles, causing hair loss. The exception is asparaginase, a drug whose different mechanism for inhibiting protein synthesis leads to a different array of adverse effects. Because the drug is a protein, it is an effective antigen and may provoke severe allergic reactions. The modified version of the protein in pegaspargase is less antigenic. Renal and hepatic function may be impaired, and some patients have bleeding episodes because the drug suppresses various clotting factors. Hyperglycemia or hypoglycemia has also been observed. Many patients show signs of CNS toxicity, including depression, lowered consciousness, and coma.

All members of the anthracene family (daunorubicin, doxorubicin, epirubicin, idarubicin, and valrubicin) have the potential to cause cardiac toxicity. Preexisting heart disease, prior irradiation to the region of the heart, or prior use of the cardiotoxic drugs cyclophosphamide, mitomycin, or dactinomycin may greatly increase the likelihood for heart damage with these drugs.

Dactinomycin is extremely toxic and must be administered with great care. The highly corrosive nature of the drug requires that intravenous injection be given properly, with no leakage of drug into tissues that surround the vein. Such leaking, or **extravasation,** can cause extensive tissue damage. Patients receiving dactinomycin may experience extreme nausea and vomiting within hours of drug administration. Phenothiazine antiemetics may be required to control vomiting. Dactinomycin also irritates the lining of the entire GI tract. Patients commonly report lip inflammation (cheilitis), difficulty in swallowing (dysphagia), mouth sores (ulcerative stomatitis), inflammation of the pharynx (pharyngitis), abdominal pain, and anal inflammation (proctitis).

TOXICITY

Bone marrow suppression tends to be a dose-dependent adverse effect. Therefore high dosages cause more profound suppression in more patients.

Because cardiac toxicity is dose-related with the anthracene family (daunorubicin, doxorubicin, epirubicin, and idarubicin), total doses of more than 550 mg/m² may produce irreversible toxicity to the heart, including electrocardiographic (ECG) changes and heart failure.

INTERACTIONS

Inhibitors of RNA and protein synthesis, with the exception of asparaginase, may produce serious interactions with bone marrow suppressants or radiation because the combinations significantly depress production of blood cells. The immunosuppression these drugs produce also puts patients at risk for generalized viral infections if they are given a live-virus vaccine during or shortly after receiving one of these drugs.

Treatment with an inhibitor of RNA and protein synthesis often causes an elevation in uric acid in the blood. Therefore dosages of drugs such as probenecid or sulfinpyrazone may need to be changed to prevent hyperuricemia or gout.

Asparaginase toxicity is increased by vincristine or prednisone. Nevertheless, these drugs are cautiously used together in certain combination treatment regimens. The antineoplastic effects of methotrexate may be diminished by asparaginase or pegaspargase. Pegaspargase interferes with normal clotting mechanisms and thus may have dangerous interactions with anticoagulants, aspirin and other salicylates, or NSAIDs (see Chapter 14).

Dactinomycin may cause reddening of the skin (erythema) and signs of inflammation, especially in an area also receiving irradiation.

DRUG CLASS • Drugs that Prevent or Arrest Mitosis

 vincristine

For other drugs of this class, see Table 37-8.

MECHANISM OF ACTION

To segregate chromosomes, a dividing cell must form a mitotic spindle composed of microtubules. Microtubules normally function as part of the cytoplasmic transport systems in cells and are required for certain types of cell movement. The major component of microtubules is the protein tubulin.

Substances that bind to tubulin and cause it to be released from microtubules or cause the tubulin to be held in nonfunctional aggregates can disrupt the structure of microtubules. These alterations of microtubular structure may not be lethal to a cell unless it is in the process of forming the mitotic spindle. Cells exposed at this stage of division are arrested at that point, and reproduction cannot proceed. Ultimately, these cells die. Substances that act in this way are called *mitotic inhibitors.*

USES

The clinical uses of mitotic inhibitors are summarized in Table 37-8.

PHARMACOKINETICS

The compounds in this class have relatively long half-lives that range from a few hours to longer than 2 days. Most of the compounds are biotransformed by the liver and eliminated in bile, but renal mechanisms may

TABLE 37-8

Antineoplastic Drugs that Block Mitosis

Generic Name	Brand Name	Indications	Specific Mechanism	Distinguishing Characteristics
docetaxel	Taxotere	Primary or metastatic breast cancer, non–small-cell lung cancer	Promotes formation of nonfunctional microtubule bundles	Patients must be premedicated to lessen hypersensitivity reactions during infusion
paclitaxel	Taxol	Ovarian or breast carcinoma, non–small-cell lung cancer, AIDS-related Kaposi's sarcoma	Promotes formation of nonfunctional microtubule bundles	Patients must be premedicated to lessen hypersensitivity reactions during infusion
vinblastine	Velban, Velbe, ✲ Belsar	Lymphomas, carcinomas, sarcomas	Vinca alkaloid that disrupts microtubule assembly	Blood dyscrasias are the most common dose-limiting toxicity
vincristine	Oncovin, Vincasar	Acute leukemia, lymphomas, sarcomas, Wilms' tumor	Vinca alkaloid that disrupts microtubule assembly	Vinca alkaloid least likely to cause bone marrow suppression
vindesine	Eldisine✲	Acute lymphocytic leukemia	Modified vinca alkaloid that disrupts microtubule assembly	Not available in the U.S.
vinorelbine	Navelbine	Non–small-cell lung carcinoma	Modified vinca alkaloid that disrupts microtubule assembly	Vinca alkaloid least likely to cause neurologic toxicity

✲ Available only in Canada.

also operate. Paclitaxel and docetaxel are eliminated through biotransformation in the liver by CYP3A enzymes (see Chapter 1).

The vinca alkaloids (vinblastine, vincristine, vindesine, and vinorelbine) must be administered intravenously. They do not cross the blood-brain barrier well enough to combat CNS spread of leukemia but are well distributed to other tissues. They are rapidly cleared from the blood, at which point they concentrate in the liver. The drugs are excreted primarily in bile, with little drug appearing in urine. Biliary obstruction or liver impairment can dangerously impede elimination of these drugs and the dosage will need to be adjusted.

ADVERSE REACTIONS AND CONTRAINDICATIONS

The effects of these drugs are most pronounced on actively dividing cells; therefore adverse effects can be expected to be related to normal rapidly dividing tissues. Bone marrow suppression with anemia, leukopenia, neutropenia (lowered neutrophils), or thrombocytopenia is a common feature with these drugs, the exception being vincristine. Immunosuppression is also common. Alopecia (hair loss) is especially common with this group of drugs. Gastric symptoms, including nausea and vomiting, also occur. The adverse reactions are discussed in more detail in the Application to Practice section.

Peripheral neuropathies with numbness or tingling in the limbs are common with docetaxel and paclitaxel; peripheral neuropathy is the dose-limiting toxicity with vincristine. These effects occur with the inhibitors of microtubule function because microtubules are involved in neurotransmission. Many symptoms of nerve dysfunction may be observed, but loss of the Achilles tendon reflex is viewed as the first sign of neuropathy. Vinblastine produces neurologic toxicity similar to that produced by vincristine. Vinorelbine has the lowest affinity for tubulin in nerve cells within this group of drugs and thus at normal dosages causes less neurologic toxicity than other vinca alkaloids.

The vinca alkaloids may be extremely irritating if they are allowed to escape from the vein into surrounding tissues during administration. Severe pain is produced, and necrosis may develop in the exposed tissue.

Vinblastine produces significant bone marrow suppression, primarily leukopenia. Leukopenia normally progresses to a low point 4 to 10 days after the dose, but recovery usually occurs within 7 to 14 days.

TOXICITY

Neurologic toxicity is the dose-limiting effect for vincristine, but for vinblastine it is bone marrow suppression. Docetaxel overdosage may cause either of these reactions, as well as mucositis; bone marrow suppression may be partially offset by administration of an appropriate colony-stimulating factor (see Chapter 36). The dose-limiting toxicities for other members of this class are extensions of any one of the characteristic adverse reactions for the drugs.

INTERACTIONS

All drugs of this class increase the risk of severe generalized viral disease if the patient receives a live-virus vaccine. Bone marrow suppressants also cause excessive depression of the bone marrow if used with any of these antimitotic drugs. In addition, inhibitors of CYP3A, such as erythromycin, ketoconazole, and androgens can block biotransformation of docetaxel and lead to increased toxicity. Probenecid and sulfinpyrazone should be avoided in patients receiving vincristine or vinblastine.

Because vinca alkaloids work by different mechanisms than most cytotoxic drugs for cancer, they are commonly combined with two, three, or four other drugs to treat a variety of cancers (see Table 37-4). Certain combinations are to be avoided, however. For example, mitomycin seems to predispose patients to pulmonary reactions with vinorelbine. Likewise, doxorubicin is avoided with vincristine because the risk of excessive myelosuppression is increased. Vincristine is used only cautiously with asparaginase because of the risk of excessive neurologic toxicity.

Tissue-Specific Anticancer Drugs

The drugs discussed in the first part of this chapter are all cytotoxic and can damage any growing cell. Modern antineoplastic therapy is moving toward the use of drugs that can be targeted to specific enzymes that support cancerous cells, specific oncogene products that are found only in cancer cells, or to specific receptors required to maintain the cancer cell. The following section describes the many drugs of this expanding category.

DRUG CLASS • Androgens and Anabolic Steroids

testolactone (Teslac)

nandrolone (Deca-Durabolin)

MECHANISM OF ACTION

For estrogen-dependent tissues, androgens often interfere with estrogen function, causing involution of these tissues. This action forms the basis for the use of androgens to control some forms of breast cancer in postmenopausal women. Results of this form of therapy usually do not become evident until after 8 or more weeks of treatment. Anabolic steroids may share this action because of their androgenic activity.

USES

Testolactone is used almost exclusively for breast cancer (Table 37-9). Other androgens, used primarily in replacement therapy, may occasionally be used to treat specific cancers (see Chapter 62).

Nandrolone, as an anabolic steroid, may be used to treat certain anemias; the androgenic effects are of use in breast cancer.

PHARMACOKINETICS

Androgens are in general not well absorbed orally, but testolactone is an exception. Nandrolone, the anabolic steroid most often used for breast cancer, must be given by injection; this oil-soluble substance is slowly absorbed from intramuscular sites. Androgens are biotransformed in the liver.

ADVERSE REACTIONS AND CONTRAINDICATIONS

An advantage of testolactone is that it does not cause as much virilization in women as other androgens. Adverse effects include peripheral neuropathy with numbness or tingling in the face or limbs, anorexia, diarrhea, nausea, or vomiting. Water retention with swelling of feet and ankles may also occur.

Nandrolone may cause a degree of virilization in women. Anemia, edema, and varying signs of liver toxicity are also possible. Nandrolone should not be given to men with breast cancer or prostate cancer because androgenic compounds may promote these diseases.

Patients with hypercalcemia should not receive testolactone or nandrolone because of the risk of increasing the already high calcium levels. Patients with hepatic or renal disease may also be at risk.

TOXICITY

Hypercalcemia may arise from rapid destruction of tumors caused by testolactone. Nandrolone at high dosages may cause liver toxicity.

INTERACTIONS

Anticoagulant effects may be increased; dosage adjustment may be required with either testolactone or nandrolone. Nandrolone may also cause additive liver toxicity when given with other hepatotoxic drugs.

TABLE 37-9

Selected Tissue-Specific Antineoplastic Drugs

Generic Name	Brand Name	Indications	Class/Mechanism	Distinguishing Characteristics
anastrozole	Arimidex	Breast cancer	Aromatase inhibitor	Prototype drug of the class
BCG	Pacis	Bladder carcinoma	Biologic response modifier	Localized use for non-invasive tumors
bexarotene	Targretin	Cutaneous T-cell	Retinoid	Activates retinoid X receptors
bicalutamide	Casodex	With LH-RH analog	Androgen receptor antagonist for prostatic cancer	Like others of class, used with LH-RH analogs
buserelin	Suprefact ✽	Prostatic carcinoma	LH-RH analog	Lowers androgens to castration levels
diethylstilbestrol	Honvol ✽	Prostatic carcinoma	Synthetic estrogen	Associated with long-term effects on fetuses
estramustine	Emcyt	Prostatic carcinoma	Estrogen linked to cytotoxic	Highly localized in prostate
exemestane	Aromasin	Advanced breast cancer	Aromatase inhibitor	Oral absorption increased by fatty meal
flutamide	Euflex, ✽ Eulexin	With LH-RH analog	Androgen receptor antagonist	Prototype drug of the class for prostatic cancer
goserelin	Zoladex	Prostatic carcinoma	LH-RH analog	May also be used as implant
imatinib	Gleevec	Chronic myeloid leukemia	Tyrosine kinase inhibitor	Prototype drug of the class
letrozole	Femara	Breast cancer	Aromatase inhibitor	Oral absorption independent of food
leuprolide	Lupron	Prostatic carcinoma	LH-RH analog	Prototype drug of the class
leuprolide implant	Viadur	Prostatic carcinoma	LH-RH analog	Titanium implant allows slow release of drug
medroxyprogesterone	Depo-Provera	Breast cancer	Progestin	Other uses covered in Chapter 59
megestrol	Megace	Endometrial or breast carcinomas	Estrogen	Other uses covered in Chapter 59
mitotane	Lysodren	Adrenal cortical carcinoma	Adrenal antagonist	Specifically attacks adrenal tissue
nandrolone	Deca-Durabolin	Metastatic breast cancer	Anabolic steroid	Full discussion in Chapter 62
nilutamide	Nilandron	Prostatic cancer	Androgen receptor antagonist	May interact with alcohol to cause flushing reaction
prednisone	Deltasone	Leukemias, lymphomas	Lympholytic glucocorticoid	Also used as anti-inflammatory
streptozocin	Zanosar	Pancreatic tumors	Pancreatic beta-cell antagonist	Lowers insulin production
tamoxifen	Nolvadex, Tamofen ✽	Breast cancer; prevent breast cancer in high-risk patients	Estrogen receptor antagonist	Prototype drug of class
testolactone	Teslac	Breast cancer	Androgen	Can be used orally

LH-RH, Luteinizing hormone–releasing hormone.
✽ Available only in Canada.

Continued

TABLE 37-9

Selected Tissue-Specific Antineoplastic Drugs—cont'd

Generic Name	Brand Name	Indications	Class/Mechanism	Distinguishing Characteristics
toremifene	Fareston	Breast cancer	Estrogen receptor antagonist	Used in post-menopausal women
tretinoin	Vesanoid	Acute promyelocytic leukemia	Retinoid	Activates retinoid A receptors
triptorelin	Trelstar	Advanced prostatic cancer	LH-RH analog	Newest member of the class

---

DRUG CLASS • Antiandrogens

flutamide (Eulexin, Euflex✹)

For other drugs of this class, see Table 37-9.

MECHANISM OF ACTION

Bicalutamide, flutamide, and nilutamide are not steroids, but they bind to androgen receptors inside cells and prevent the normal action of androgenic steroids. Thus these drugs act as receptor antagonists. Because of the effects of their actions, these drugs are called *antiandrogens*.

USES

Bicalutamide, flutamide, or nilutamide are combined with one of the LH-RH analogs (see next section) for metastatic carcinoma of the prostate, a tumor that often depends on androgens for its growth. The combination of antiandrogens with two different mechanisms very effectively eliminates any androgen contribution to tumor growth.

PHARMACOKINETICS

Bicalutamide, flutamide, and nilutamide are well absorbed orally but undergo extensive biotransformation in the liver. Metabolites are excreted both renally and in the bile.

ADVERSE REACTIONS AND CONTRAINDICATIONS

When given with an LH-RH analog, bicalutamide, flutamide, and nilutamide reduce testosterone levels to those expected in castrated men. Many of the adverse effects patients experience are the result of low testosterone levels. Hot flashes are common. Most patients report reduced libido or impotence. Gynecomastia occurs in about 9% of patients. In addition to symptoms arising from testosterone suppression, these drugs may also cause GI disturbances, edema, or peripheral neuropathy.

Nilutamide and bicalutamide are usually avoided in patients with liver disease because biotransformation of the drugs may be impaired.

TOXICITY

Most of the adverse effects of bicalutamide, flutamide, and nilutamide are related to the very low levels of testosterone they induce. Therefore higher dosages may not produce adverse effects that are significantly worse than with regular dosages.

INTERACTIONS

The combination of bicalutamide, flutamide, and nilutamide with one of the LH-RH analogs produces a desired interaction in that these drugs prevent the full activity of androgens and the LH-RH analogs lower the production of androgens. The result is an almost complete abolition of androgen action.

Undesirable interactions with these drugs are unusual, but nilutamide may cause a flushing reaction if taken with alcohol. Nilutamide may also interfere with the biotransformation of anticoagulants, phenytoin, and theophylline because these drugs are biotransformed by the same systems.

DRUG CLASS • LH-RH Analogs

 leuprolide (Lupron)

For other drugs of this class, see Table 37-9.

MECHANISM OF ACTION

Leuprolide, buserelin, triptorelin, and goserelin are synthetic analogs of LH-RH. These LH-RH analogs tend to increase testosterone levels during the first week of therapy, but when given continuously, they begin to suppress secretion of gonadotropin-releasing hormone, resulting in a lower synthesis and release of testosterone. These drugs ultimately produce the same low levels of male sex steroids produced by surgical castration.

USES

LH-RH analogs are used for prostatic cancer to lower circulating androgens that might stimulate the tumor. LH-RH analogs are nearly always combined with bicalutamide, flutamide, or nilutamide (see previous section).

PHARMACOKINETICS

These drugs are peptides and therefore cannot withstand the acidic environment of the stomach, but they are absorbed from subcutaneous or intramuscular injection sites. Buserelin is available in Canada as a nasal spray; the peptide is adequately absorbed across the nasal membranes for use in maintenance therapy.

ADVERSE REACTIONS AND CONTRAINDICATIONS

Buserelin, triptorelin, and goserelin may cause an initial flare of the disease, with pain and swelling, difficult urination, and possibly weakness. Approximately 10% of patients taking goserelin experience disease flare, but only about 1% of patients taking buserelin have this reaction. These early reactions may be related to the initial increase in testosterone produced by these drugs. Later effects such as hot flashes and decreased sexual desire are symptoms caused by the lowering of testosterone levels. Anorexia, breast tenderness, edema, nausea, and vomiting are also possible. In addition, goserelin may cause cardiovascular effects, including arrhythmias, strokes, or infarctions. Goserelin may also be associated with chronic obstructive pulmonary disease or heart failure.

Leuprolide causes all of the adverse effects associated with low testosterone levels mentioned previously. In addition, it may be associated with cardiac arrhythmias or other cardiac symptoms, especially in men. In women the drug suppresses menstrual cycles. Both men and women may show blurred vision, dizziness, edema, headache, insomnia, nausea, numbness in hands or feet, or vomiting.

TOXICITY

Overdoses of these drugs have not been studied, but because most effects of the drugs are related to changes in testosterone levels, symptoms may be similar to clinical doses.

INTERACTIONS

The LH-RH analogs are used with bicalutamide, flutamide, or nilutamide for a desired interaction: greater suppression of androgen effects on tumors. Undesirable interactions with other drugs have not been noted.

DRUG CLASS • Estrogens

estramustine (Emcyt)

megestrol (Megace)

MECHANISM OF ACTION

For androgen-dependent tissues, estrogens often interfere with androgen function. Estrogens can therefore cause involution of these tissues. This action forms the basis for the use of estrogens to control prostatic carcinoma. Some breast cancers also respond to exogenous estrogen therapy, especially those in postmenopausal women.

Estramustine combines estradiol with a nitrogen mustard. The rationale for the combination is that the drug will be most concentrated in estrogen-sensitive tissues, including tumors. In those tissues the antineoplastic effects of the estradiol and the nitrogen mustard may be focused. Toxicity of the drug is largely caused by the estrogen component because release of the active nitrogen mustard into blood is low.

USES

Many of the estrogens discussed in Chapter 59 may be used in palliative therapy for prostatic cancer, but megestrol is primarily used for this indication. Estramustine is indicated only for prostate cancer because of the cytotoxic component in the preparation.

PHARMACOKINETICS

Natural steroid estrogens are not absorbed orally, but several of the synthetic, nonsteroidal estrogens may be given successfully by this route. Estrogens are biotransformed by the liver. Patients with significant liver impairment may accumulate these compounds.

Estramustine is concentrated in the prostate gland because the drug binds to specific protein in that tissue. This concentration of the drug contributes to the tissue-specific action.

ADVERSE REACTIONS AND CONTRAINDICATIONS

Estrogens increase the risks of thromboembolic disease. Estrogens also increase salt and water retention, alter mood in some patients, decrease glucose tolerance, elevate calcium levels, produce nausea and vomiting, and cause breast tenderness and abdominal cramps. Of these adverse reactions, thromboembolic disease, hypercal-

cemia, and edema are the most threatening for cancer patients.

Estramustine and estrogens are usually avoided in patients with thrombophlebitis or other thromboembolic diseases.

TOXICITY

When estrogens are used at high dosages in men with prostatic or breast carcinoma, the risk of heart attack, pulmonary embolism, and thrombophlebitis is increased.

INTERACTIONS

Neither estramustine nor other estrogens should be used with other potentially hepatotoxic drugs because the risk of liver damage is increased. Cardiovascular adverse effects are more common in patients who smoke.

 DRUG CLASS • Antiestrogens

tamoxifen (Nolvadex, Tamofen✸)
toremifene (Fareston)

MECHANISM OF ACTION

Tamoxifen and toremifene are called antiestrogens because they block estrogen binding at receptor sites in cells. This action prevents estrogens from supporting the growth of estrogen-dependent cells. Thus, these drugs are most useful for breast carcinoma in which estrogen dependence of the tumor has been established.

USES

Antiestrogens are indicated for breast carcinoma. They are more likely to benefit women whose tumors contain estrogen receptors. Tamoxifen has also been approved for use to prevent breast cancer in women at high risk for the disease.

PHARMACOKINETICS

Tamoxifen and toremifene are administered orally. Both drugs are extensively biotransformed and handled similarly by the body. Metabolites enter the blood slowly, with peak concentrations occurring 3 to 7 hours after an oral dose. However, the drug and metabolites persist in the blood for days as a result of enterohepatic circulation (see Chapter 1). Elimination is primarily in feces. The kidney contributes little to the excretion. The full antineoplastic effect of antiestrogens may take months to develop.

ADVERSE REACTIONS AND CONTRAINDICATIONS

Tamoxifen and toremifene may produce cancer and birth defects in animals, but it is unknown whether they produce these effects in humans. The most common re-

actions to antiestrogens are nausea, vomiting, and hot flashes.

Patients who begin tamoxifen or toremifene therapy sometimes report an increase in pain at the tumor site and within metastases in bone. Tumor metastases within soft tissue may temporarily increase in size, and the surrounding tissue may become inflamed. This reaction, sometimes called disease flare, may occur even when therapy is effective.

TOXICITY

High dosages may increase the incidence of dizziness, headache, or nausea. The antiestrogenic effects such as hot flashes may be more profound. At higher dosages, the weak estrogenic adverse effects of these drugs may become more noticeable, most commonly as vaginal bleeding.

INTERACTIONS

Interactions are generally of minor importance for tamoxifen. Antacids or histamine H2-receptor blockers may disrupt the enteric coating on tamoxifen tablets, leading to loss of some tamoxifen activity. Estrogens may antagonize the effect of tamoxifen.

Toremifene may block hepatic biotransformation of anticoagulants, leading to more profound effects of those drugs. Phenobarbital and phenytoin may increase biotransformation of toremifene by inducing CYP3A4 enzymes in the liver (see Chapter 1).

DRUG CLASS • Aromatase Inhibitors

⚠ anastrozole (Arimidex)

For other drugs in this class, see Table 37-9.

MECHANISM OF ACTION

Anastrozole and letrozole are nonsteroidal compounds that reversibly inhibit an enzyme called aromatase. Exemestane is a steroidal compound that irreversibly inhibits the same enzyme. Aromatase normally converts androstenedione, a steroid from the adrenal gland, to estrone. Estrone has some estrogenic activity but is further converted by other enzymes to estradiol, a powerful natural estrogen. In postmenopausal women, this pathway produces most of the estrogens that circulate in the blood. If this pathway is blocked with an aromatase inhibitor, the result is a profound lowering of circulating estrogen levels. Withdrawal of estrogen effects from estrogen-dependent tumors causes an involution of that tissue and is the basis of the anticancer effects.

USES

These drugs are used only for breast cancer in postmenopausal women, most often after their cancer failed to respond to tamoxifen. The most recent clinical data show anastrozole used alone is equal or superior to tamoxifen in postmenopausal women with early stage breast cancer. Anastrozole may also suppress subsequent development of tumors in the remaining breast tissue.

PHARMACOKINETICS

Letrozole is completely absorbed orally, with or without food, but the oral absorption of anastrozole may be lowered by food. Absorption of exemestane may be increased by a fatty meal. These drugs are extensively biotransformed in the liver, primarily by CYP3A4 or CYP2A6 (see Chapter 1). The elimination half-lives of these drugs average about 2 days in most patients. Because of these long half-lives, it takes 1 to 6 weeks for steady-state levels to be reached in blood. Both renal and hepatic mechanisms contribute to elimination of the drugs.

ADVERSE REACTIONS AND CONTRAINDICATIONS

Common reactions to these drugs include nausea, chest pain, edema, and shortness of breath. A variety of other effects on the GI tract or nervous system may be noted, but the most dangerous other possibility is a thromboembolism.

TOXICITY

Anastrozole at very high dosages may show more GI disturbances in animals, but its effect in humans is unknown. Letrozole may cause cardiovascular effects at very high dosages in animals, but no effects have been seen in humans.

INTERACTIONS

Inducers of CYP3A4 could, in theory, lower the plasma concentrations of these drugs, but the clinical relevance is unknown.

DRUG CLASS • Progestins

⚠ medroxyprogesterone (Depo-Provera)

MECHANISM OF ACTION

Progestins normally establish secretory function in the estrogen-primed endometrium (see Chapter 59). When used as anticancer drugs, progestins may be effective by blocking tissue responses to other steroid hormones such as estrogens, androgens, or glucocorticoids.

USES

The use of progestins as antineoplastic drugs has been limited primarily to palliative therapy in endometrial carcinoma, but renal, breast, or prostatic carcinomas may also be susceptible.

PHARMACOKINETICS

Medroxyprogesterone used for cancer is usually given as a depot to prolong action. Progestins are biotrans-

formed primarily in the liver; derivatives of progestins appear in urine.

ADVERSE REACTIONS AND CONTRAINDICATIONS

Patients should be observed for signs of thromboembolic disease or sudden changes in vision. Fluid retention and disruption of normal menstrual cycles may also occur.

TOXICITY

High dosages of progestins are associated with greater risk of thromboembolism.

INTERACTIONS

Drugs such as carbamazepine, phenobarbital, phenytoin, rifabutin, and rifampin induce liver enzymes that biotransform progestins. As a result, these drugs may interfere with the action of progestins.

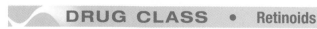

DRUG CLASS • Retinoids

bexarotene (Targretin)
tretinoin (Vesalen)

MECHANISM OF ACTION

Retinoids, which are derivatives of vitamin A, bind to several types of nuclear retinoid receptors and thus influence repression of specific genes involved with cell maturation or differentiation. Retinoids also seem to promote degradation of cyclins, which would be expected to lower the drive to proliferate. Tretinoin, an all-trans retinoic acid (ATRA), is highly specific for a subtype of acute promyelocytic leukemia caused by a chromosome translocation called t(15;17). This altered chromosome causes a fused regulatory protein to be formed, which prevents normal cell maturation and thus serves as an oncogene. In this type of leukemia, tretinoin overcomes the effects of this oncogene and causes the leukemic promyelocytes to mature. Normal cells gradually reappear in the bone marrow and blood.

USES

Tretinoin is used for acute promyelocytic leukemia and has brought long-term remission rates above 60% in most studies. Bexarotene is used for cutaneous symptoms of cutaneous T-lymphocyte lymphomas. Retinoids are also used in the treatment of acne (see Chapter 67).

PHARMACOKINETICS

Tretinoin is taken orally and biotransformed by the liver. Plasma steady-state levels stabilize about 1 week after therapy starts, but full clinical remission may take 6 to 7 weeks. The drug is eliminated by both renal and biliary routes. Bexarotene is eliminated primarily by biliary and hepatic mechanisms.

ADVERSE REACTIONS AND CONTRAINDICATIONS

Retinoids cause many adverse effects, including bone pain, dry skin or membranes, fever, headache, mucositis, nausea, pruritus, sweating, and visual changes. In addition, tretinoin causes retinoic acid–acute promyelocytic leukemia (RA-APL) syndrome in about 25% of treated patients. Symptoms include difficulty breathing, chest pain, bone pain, fever, and weight gain. Other GI, cardiovascular, and pulmonary symptoms are also common. Visual disturbances and CNS effects can also occur.

Bexarotene causes similar adverse reactions to other retinoids but is more likely to cause hyperlipidemia than other drugs of this class. The incidence of this adverse reaction is nearly 80%. Hypothyroidism is also noted with bexarotene. Acute pancreatitis, subdural hematoma, and liver failure each caused one death in clinical trials with this drug.

All retinoids are contraindicated in pregnancy because of the great risk of severe injury to the fetus.

INTERACTIONS

Inducers or inhibitors of hepatic drug metabolizing enzymes may alter retinoid biotransformation, but the effects of these interactions have not been fully documented. Gemfibrozil is known to elevate plasma concentrations of bexarotene, probably because of effects on biotransformation; the drugs should not be used together.

DRUG CLASS • Tyrosine Kinase Inhibitor

imatinib mesylate (Gleevec)

MECHANISM OF ACTION

Imatinib inhibits the enzyme tyrosine kinase that is the receptor for several growth factors, including platelet-derived growth factor (PDGF), stem cell factor (SCF), and others. The clinical use of the drug arises because a particular chromosomal abnormality (Philadelphia chromosome) associated with chronic myeloid leukemia creates an altered enzyme called Bcr-Abl tyrosine kinase produced constantly by leukemic cells. By blocking this enzyme activity, imatinib slows proliferation and induces apoptosis of leukemic cells. The drug may have use in other tumors by blocking other tyrosine kinases, such as c-kit, which binds to stem cell factor, and also serves as a histopathologic marker for GI stromal cell tumors.

USES

Imatinib is used for chronic myeloid leukemia, when the Philadelphia chromosome alteration is present. The drug is also used for GI stromal tumors when the tumors are known to overproduce c-kit.

PHARMACOKINETICS

Imatinib is well absorbed orally, with a bioavailability of about 98%. The drug is biotransformed in the liver, primarily by CYP3A4, and the major metabolite retains activity. The elimination half-life for the parent drug is about 18 hours and about 40 hours for the active metabolite. The drug is slowly removed from the body and is excreted primarily in feces

ADVERSE REACTIONS AND CONTRAINDICATIONS

Imatinib commonly causes edema, which can become so severe that patients suffer ascites, pericardial effusion, pleural effusion, or pulmonary edema. If not halted, these reactions can be fatal. Hematologic toxicity is also noted in some patients, but may be influenced by the stage of the leukemia being treated. GI irritation and occasional hemorrhage may occur.

Liver toxicity may occur, requiring monitoring of liver function before and during therapy. Kidney toxic-

ity and immunosuppression was noted in animal studies but has not yet been confirmed in human trials.

INTERACTIONS

Imatinib can inhibit CYP3A4, which may increase the concentration of drugs such as cyclosporine, pimozide, or simvastatin. Drugs such as the azole antifungal drugs (see Chapter 32) or macrolide antibiotics (see Chapter 26) may inhibit CYP3A4 and significantly increase the plasma concentration of imatinib. Drugs or other agents that induce CYP3A4 activity, such as benzodiazepines, barbiturates, anticonvulsants, rifampicin or St. John's wort, may significantly decrease plasma concentrations of imatinib.

DRUG CLASS • Lympholytic Drugs

⚖ prednisone (Deltasone)

Glucocorticoids such as prednisone affect lymphoid tissue because that tissue contains specific receptors for glucocorticoids. Prednisone is an effective anticancer drug because it is lympholytic; that is, it causes regression of lymphoid tissue (see Chapter 57). When used in various combinations, prednisone is effective against lymphoid tumors and lymphoblastic leukemias, especially in children.

Prednisone is the glucocorticoid most commonly used as an anticancer drug, although several of these drugs are used for symptomatic relief.

Prednisone is effectively absorbed orally and is biotransformed to the active form of the drug, prednisolone. Liver disease may impair this process and thus interfere with the effectiveness of prednisone.

Prednisone may produce all the well-known signs of glucocorticoid excess if given long enough at high dosages. These symptoms are outlined in Chapter 57.

DRUG CLASS • Tissue-Directed Drugs and Isotopes

mitotane (Lysodren)

sodium iodide I-131 (^{131}I)

sodium phosphate P-32 (^{32}P)

streptozocin (Zanosar)

Mitotane, a derivative of the insecticide DDT, causes atrophy of the two inner layers of the adrenal cortex where the glucocorticoid cortisol is formed (see Chapter 57). Mitotane is not cell-cycle specific and is not a generally cytotoxic drug. Because of its unusual tissue selectivity, mitotane is used to treat adrenal cortical carcinoma. The drug is satisfactorily absorbed when given orally and biotransformed by the liver before elimination. If liver function is impaired, the drug may accumulate and toxic reactions may increase. Mitotane causes anorexia, nausea, and vomiting in almost every patient. Nearly half of those treated experience lethargy or dizziness as a result of adrenal insufficiency. Der-

matitis occurs in 20% of patients. Less common but serious reactions include abnormalities of the eye, changes in blood pressure, and hemorrhagic cystitis. Higher dosages are associated with more severe adverse effects. CNS depressants are usually avoided when patients receive mitotane to prevent excessive depression of CNS function.

The use of radioactive isotopes is generally considered palliative therapy for cancer. These drugs act by releasing ionizing radiation. Sodium phosphate P-32 (^{32}P) enters forming DNA, so it tends to be concentrated where that process is highest. Clinically, the use of this drug is to attempt to control proliferation of blood cells in polycythemia vera or in myelocytic leukemia. The use of sodium I-131 (^{131}I), a radioactive isotope of iodine, to destroy thyroid tissue is discussed in Chapter 56.

Streptozocin resembles alkylating drugs, but cells other than pancreatic beta cells are relatively insensitive to the drug. Because of its strong tissue specificity, streptozocin is used to treat insulin-secreting islet cell tumors of the pancreas. Because streptozocin destroys beta cells, insulin production may cease. The drug is unstable and must be given intravenously. It is biotransformed by the liver. Both metabolites and unchanged drug are excreted in urine. Nausea and vomiting often occur. The drug shows dose-dependent toxicity to the kidneys. At high dosages renal function can be fatally compromised. Streptozocin should not be combined with other nephrotoxic drugs. Live-virus vaccines may cause a generalized disease if used in a patient receiving streptozocin. Phenytoin may interfere with the action of streptozocin in pancreatic cells.

DRUG CLASS • Photosensitizing Drugs

methoxsalen (UVADEX)

 porfimer (Photofrin)

Methoxsalen is a natural product found in certain plants. The compound has long been known to sensitize skin to UV irradiation. The original use was to treat psoriasis, but the drug has been shown to be carcinogenic, inducing a variety of skin cancers, including melanoma. Methoxsalen is currently used to control skin problems associated with T-cell lymphomas. To limit adverse reactions, the blood is exposed to UV light outside the body, in a process called photopheresis. Even with this precaution, the eyes and skin remain highly sensitive to sunlight or other sources of UV irradiation for at least 24 hours after therapy.

Porfimer is a polymeric form of the pigment porphyrin. This material is concentrated in skin, liver, and spleen but also concentrates in tumors. The presence of porfimer makes the tissue sensitive to light. By selectively irradiating the tumor with light of 630-nanometer wavelength, selective tumor destruction may be achieved. This technique is used for esophageal cancer and for bronchial invasion by non–small-cell tumors of the lung. A variety of cardiovascular, GI, and pulmonary adverse reactions occur as a result of inflammation of tissues surrounding the site of therapy. Some of these reactions may be serious and include cardiac arrhythmias, pleural effusion, and pneumonia. About 20% of treated patients experience photosensitivity of the skin, with exaggerated sunburn reactions.

APPLICATION TO PRACTICE

ASSESSMENT

Before initiating antineoplastic therapy, it is important that a comprehensive history be obtained, focusing on the patient's physical, psychologic, and emotional status. Antineoplastic therapy is rigorous and may cause many toxic and adverse reactions. To provide safe and effective therapy, patients must be screened for any pre-existing organ disease, physical, or psychosocial concerns that would have an impact on their ability to tolerate therapy.

History of Present Illness

Assessment data includes when the present illness was diagnosed, as well as any symptoms that led to the diagnosis. Any surgeries, diagnostic studies, or previous treatment for the illness should also be recorded in detail. If possible, ask the patient to request records from other institutions where treatment may have been provided.

Health History

Detailed information regarding the patient's health history must be obtained. Surgeries, infectious diseases, chronic illnesses, and medical conditions must be listed in detail in the patient's records. Chronic illnesses unrelated to the neoplastic process may lead to or cause impaired organ function, requiring changes in dosages or treatment protocols. Information regarding all drugs used on a routine basis should also be listed because of the potential for adverse drug interactions. Instances of anaphylaxis have been reported; thus it is important to ask about prior sensitivity. Furthermore, information about previous drugs used or drug therapies received is important because second malignancies have developed in some patients treated with antineoplastic drugs, especially alkylating drugs. Additionally, the patient's medical history may hold clues to the present illness, because many cancers are found following some nonmalignant disorders.

Lifespan Considerations

Perinatal. Malignant diseases that occur in pregnancy, in order of decreasing frequency, include breast cancer, hematopoietic malignancy, melanoma, gynecologic cancer, and bone tumors. The glandular hyperplasia of the breast that accompanies pregnancy makes recognition of suspicious breast masses difficult. However, when matched for age and stage of cancer, survival rates of breast cancer found during pregnancy are no different from the nonpregnant state. Survival is generally not improved by terminating the pregnancy. However, it may be appropriate to avoid the risk of fetal exposure to either antineoplastic drugs or radiation therapy. Treatment recommendations for pregnant women will vary but depend on the location of the cancer, stage of the disease, gestational age of the pregnancy, and maternal health in general. Consult a medical-surgical or oncology text for information regarding the other disorders.

Pediatric. A comprehensive baseline assessment is particularly important for the pediatric patient. Childhood cancers are the second leading cause of death in children ages 1 to 14 years. For children in all pediatric age groups, leukemia is the most frequent type of cancer. Probably the most significant aspect of childhood cancer is the improved prognosis during the last 30 years. Currently, more than 70% of all children with neoplasms treated at major cancer centers will now survive more than 5 years. Abnormal physical examination findings should be thoroughly investigated and reported to the health care provider for further evaluation.

Children ages 1 to 14 are expanding their world with new experiences. Peer group pressure increasingly influences behavior. Physical, cognitive, and social development increase while the child gains increased competence in communication. The pediatric patient's self-concept can be dramatically affected by a diagnosis of cancer and its subsequent treatment. This further adds to the patient's and family's stress level, especially in the face of conflicts. Be sure to evaluate the family's and patient's support systems.

Older Adults. Older adults may suffer from impaired communication ability, sensory deficits, and decreased cognitive function. There is an increased incidence of organ damage as a result of changes associated with age and chronic disease. Obtaining a comprehensive health history may be difficult, particularly if the patient is a poor historian. In this instance, a comprehensive physical examination and evaluation are imperative to avoid an excessively toxic therapeutic regimen.

Cultural/Social Considerations

Patients who are faced with a potentially fatal illness exhibit a wide array of coping behaviors. It is the responsibility of the health care provider to determine which patients exhibit ineffective or harmful coping mechanisms that require psychologic intervention and coun-

seling and to identify available support systems. Social support as well as coping skills have been well documented as important factors in the successful completion of treatment regimens.

A diagnosis of cancer may have a devastating economic effect on the patient and family members. Inability to work may lead to loss of insurance coverage, which then jeopardizes the patient's access to life-saving medical care. Basic insurance coverage may be insufficient to cover the cost of cancer therapy, placing the patient's home, savings, and financial earnings at risk. Most patients with a diagnosis of cancer can benefit from a referral to social services for assistance with financial affairs.

Physical Examination

The person with cancer may appear to be in perfect health, with only mild signs and symptoms, or may be diagnosed in a later stage of the disease, with local and systemic alterations. A comprehensive baseline physical examination is important before initiating antineoplastic therapy. The data obtained must be recorded in the patient's permanent record, where it serves as a basis for comparison and further evaluation after the patient begins a treatment regimen.

Laboratory Testing

Laboratory testing is initially directed toward obtaining a diagnosis and determining the extent and spread of the patient's cancer. During the initial evaluation period, the patient may require biopsies, surgery, radionucleotide scans, and radiologic studies. After the diagnosis is obtained, further diagnostic testing will be directed toward assessing the patient's ability to tolerate drug therapy without suffering lethal consequences.

Depending on the nature of the drug or drugs and anticipated toxicities, a CBC count and serum chemistry panel are obtained as a part of the screening process. Evaluation of cardiopulmonary, hepatic, and renal systems are also done.

GOALS OF THERAPY

Choices of antineoplastic therapies are guided by the most realistic and achievable treatment objectives. The three major goals of antineoplastic therapy are *cure*, *control*, and *palliation*. An increasing number of cancers are curable, particularly if they are identified and treated before metastasis has occurred. Although survival is defined in terms of "cure," biologic cure is not absolute because it is not possible to definitively complete eradication of all cancer cells, and late recurrences do occur. The definition of cure includes: (1) cessation of therapy, (2) continuous freedom from clinical and laboratory evidence of cancer, and (3) minimum to no risk of relapse, as determined by previous experience with the disease. The time that must elapse before a patient clinically free of cancer is considered cured varies with the type of cancer but typically ranges from 2 to 5 years. Cure must not be achieved, however, at the cost of a poor quality of life or disabling treatment-related symptoms.

Control of the disease is the next objective. When the disease is found to be incurable, prolongation of quality life becomes the objective. Given the variety of drugs and treatment options available, it is often possible to control metastatic disease for many months or years while providing an optimal quality of life for the patient.

Palliation is the third and final objective. **Palliation** is defined as providing relief of distressing symptoms (e.g., pain, hypercalcemia) and maintaining function as near normal as possible when it is no longer possible to achieve a remission. When cure or control is not possible, relief of symptoms can still be achieved by antineoplastic therapy, particularly if doses are adjusted to minimize toxicities.

INTERVENTION

When planning an antineoplastic treatment regimen, the health care provider considers variables such as the type, size, and stage of the tumor, growth rate, cell types involved, the heterogeneity of the tumor, and the degree of cellular differentiation. Many solid tumors have micrometastatic disease and are considered systemic diseases incurable by surgery alone. This fact justifies the use of antineoplastic therapy in combination with surgery or radiation therapy. Administration of antineoplastic therapy is therefore based on the biologic behavior of certain cancers that metastasize early in the course of the disease.

Tumors that are poorly differentiated (that is, display the least number of normal cellular characteristics) tend to grow more rapidly, spread more readily, and impose greater lethal consequences for the patient. Because of cellular characteristics, poorly differentiated tumors tend to be more responsive to drug therapy in the short term than slow-growing, well-differentiated cancers. The growth fraction of the tumor, or number of cells that are actively growing at any given time, will also affect how the tumor responds to therapy.

Almost all antineoplastic drugs are given in relatively high doses on an intermittent or cyclic schedule. This appears to be more effective than low doses given continuously or massive doses given only once. It also causes less immunosuppression and provides for drug holidays, during which normal tissues can repair themselves from drug-induced damage. Fortunately,

normal cells repair themselves more quickly than neoplastic cells. Subsequent doses are usually administered as soon as tissue repair becomes evident, usually when leukocyte and platelet counts return to acceptable levels.

Drug Preparation

For the most part, all antineoplastic drugs are carcinogenic, teratogenic, and mutagenic. For the health care provider, the primary exposure routes are through the skin, by inhalation, and by ingestion via contaminated food and surfaces. The effects of exposure may be short-term or long-term. Short-term effects are usually seen at the time of exposure or within hours or days afterward. These include dermatitis and hyperpigmentation of exposed skin areas. Long-term effects may develop months or years after exposure to the antineoplastic drug. Although there is concern about chromosomal abnormalities and carcinogenicity after long-term exposure, there have been no conclusive findings to support the notion that exposure to these drugs is harmful. However, only specially trained health care providers should prepare and administer antineoplastic drugs. These individuals should be familiar with the Occupational Safety and Health Administration (OSHA) guidelines, Oncology Nursing Society (ONS) guidelines, and individual agency policies.

Preparation of antineoplastic drugs should occur in a low traffic area away from patients. Work surfaces should be covered with plastic-backed, absorbent pads. Nonabsorbent gowns, with long sleeves, elastic cuffs, and back closures, and thick, powder-free, disposable, latex gloves should also be worn. The gloves should be changed regularly (i.e., every hour) and immediately after a puncture, tear, or drug spill. Be sure to wash your hands before putting on the gloves. When removing gloves, avoid skin contact, properly dispose of the gloves, and again wash your hands.

Antineoplastic drugs are prepared under a Class II biologic safety cabinet containing a vertical laminar airflow system. If a biologic safety cabinet is not available, a respirator with a high-efficiency filter should be worn. No eating, drinking, or application of makeup is permitted in this area. The drugs should be prepared and stored following the manufacturer's guidelines regarding solution compatibility, sensitivities, and stability.

Use precautions to avoid skin contact during times when leakage of drug may occur, such as during removal of air from syringe or tubing containing the antineoplastic drug, during injection of the drug into an IV bottle, bag, or tubing, or when connecting or disconnecting the IV unit. Syringes, tubings, and connectors used to prepare and administer the drugs should contain Luer-Loks at points of attachment. Whenever possible, blunt cannulas or protected needles should be used to draw up the drug or to flush the IV line to prevent accidental needle sticks.

When opening ampules, clear all fluid from the neck of the ampule before opening. Wrap a sterile gauze or alcohol pad around the neck of the ampule and tilt the ampule away from yourself before opening. Use a syringe that will be no more than three-fourths full when the desired amount is drawn up. Inject excess solution from the ampule into a sealed waste vial or dispose of according to agency policy.

To prevent aerosol generation of the vial of an antineoplastic drug, use an 18- or 19-gauge needle and a 0.2 micron hydrophobic filter or dispensing pin. Create negative pressure in the vial by aspirating a volume of air slightly larger than the volume of diluent added. Add the diluent slowly, allowing it to run down the inside wall of the vial. Perform final dose measurement before removing the needle from the vial. Clear the drug from the needle and the hub of the syringe, and allow air pressure to equalize from the vial back into the syringe before removing the needle from the vial.

Should accidental exposure occur, follow agency policies regarding self-care and reporting. Wash the involved area thoroughly with soap (not a germicidal agent) and water. Accidental exposure to the eyes involves holding the involved eyelid(s) open and irrigating the eye(s) with water or an isotonic eye wash for at least 5 minutes. See your health care provider as soon as possible but specifically after exposure to a cytotoxic drug. Document the incident according to established agency policies.

Administration

Selecting the administration site is an important aspect of giving antineoplastic drugs. In the ideal situation, perform a fresh venipuncture for administering antineoplastic therapy. Otherwise determine that the infusion line to be used is patent. Regional administration routes for antineoplastic drugs include topical, intrathecal, intracavitary, and intraarterial routes. Although intra-arterial routes pose some risk, major organs or tumor sites receive maximal exposure with limited serum drug levels, resulting in limited systemic adverse effects.

Central venous access devices (e.g., Hickman or Groshong single-lumen catheters, Port-A-Cath Dual-Lumen Venous Access System, OmegaPort, Infusaid Microport) are recommended. Because the termination site is in a large central vein, hyperosmolar solutions can be safely administered and rapid dilution and dispersion of irritating drugs will occur. Constant monitoring of the central venous catheter sites for placement and evidence of extravasation is vital.

When a central venous catheter line is not available, administer the antineoplastic drug in the larger veins of the arm, midway between the wrist and elbow. If a drug extravasates in this area, there is maximum soft tissue coverage to prevent functional impairment. Vesicants (e.g., dactinomycin) and irritants (e.g., etoposide) should not be administered through veins in the hands, in the antecubital fossa, or over bony prominences. Extravasation in these areas can lead to destruction of nerves and tendons, resulting in loss of function. Veins that are damaged or sclerosed and sites that have been damaged by burns, grafts, surgery, amputation, and mastectomy should be avoided. Blood return and infusion site should be constantly monitored before, during, and after drug administration for placement and evidence of extravasation.

Intervention for Extravasation. Orders for the treatment of extravasation of an antineoplastic drug should be written before the infusion is begun. An extravasation kit containing agency-approved antidotes should be kept at the patient's side, particularly when the patient is receiving a vesicant drug. If extravasation does occur, discontinue the drug immediately, leaving the IV cannula in place. Follow agency policies for managing the situation. A typical procedure would be to remove residual drug and blood via the IV tubing. If you are unable to aspirate the residual drug, remove the IV cannula. Administer a glucocorticosteroid subcutaneously in the area of extravasation or via the infusion catheter that is still in place. Cover the area with a topical steroid and an occlusive dressing. Apply a cold pack to the area for 15 minutes four times daily to localize the drug and prevent further tissue damage. Avoid applying pressure to the area, but elevate the affected arm for 48 hours. Notify the health care provider of the extravasation and observe the site regularly for pain, erythema, induration, or tissue necrosis. Document the incident including the date and time, size and type of IV needle or cannula used, insertion site, drug administered, sequence of antineoplastic drugs used (if any), approximate amount of drug involved, subjective symptoms reported by the patient, nursing assessment of the site and nursing interventions undertaken, health care provider notification, instructions given to the patient, and any follow-up measures used. Be sure to sign the note. In some cases a photograph of the site may be required. Follow agency policies. Use a fresh venipuncture site for infusion of any remaining antineoplastic drug.

Education

Patient education is essential to antineoplastic therapy. In the past, patients with cancer could rely on health care professionals to monitor their health status. Drug administration, however, is quickly becoming the domain of outpatient and home settings, and it is imperative that patients know how to monitor their own health status. Furthermore, with proper education, many patients in the home are able to self-administer the drugs and adjunctive therapies (e.g., antiemetics, antidiarrheals) and properly identify significant adverse reactions. Instruction sheets for most antineoplastic drugs are available from the National Cancer Institute in English, Spanish, and other languages.

Patients should be given a complete explanation of their treatment regimen, including adverse reactions, before informed consent is obtained for antineoplastic drug administration. Care should be taken to mention not only the life-threatening and pathology-producing adverse effects, but also the adverse reactions that produce discomfort and embarrassment.

Myelosuppression. **Myelosuppression** is a general term used to describe the suppressive effects of cytotoxic drugs on bone marrow. It is a common and often dose-limiting effect of most antineoplastic drugs. Myelosuppression has a greater effect on the bone marrow than it does on the peripheral blood count. When stem cells are affected, all cell lines will be suppressed. **Granulocytopenia**, or a deficiency of granulocytes (neutrophils, basophils, and eosinophils), is a major consequence of the myelosuppressive effects of antineoplastic drugs. As a consequence, patients experience leukopenia, thrombocytopenia, and anemia to varying degrees. Patients should become familiar with what constitutes a normal cell count and learn to monitor their own cell counts.

Leukopenia, a reduction in the number of total circulating white blood cells (granulocytes, lymphocytes, and monocytes), below 4000/mm^3 is a common adverse effect. A normal leukocyte count is 4000 to 10,000 cells/mm^3. Granulocytes are the body's first line of defense against infection. Because the life span of the leukocyte is very brief (12 hours), leukopenia occurs frequently.

The time after antineoplastic drug administration when the white blood cell or platelet count is at the lowest point is known as the **nadir**. For most myelosuppressive drugs, the nadir occurs 7 to 14 days after drug administration. Knowledge of the nadir helps the health care provider predict when the patient is at greatest risk for infection and bleeding.

An absolute neutrophil count (ANC) is calculated by multiplying the WBC count by the percentage of neutrophils in the differential (ANC = WBC × % neutrophils). For example, if the WBC count is 1200 cells/mm^3 and the neutrophil count is 34%, the ANC is 408 cells/mm^3. A patient is considered to have **neutropenia** if the ab-

solute neutrophil count is less than 1000 cells/mm^3. The frequency of infection increases as the ANC falls below 500 cells/mm^3 and the longer the patient remains neutropenic. Neutropenia is often associated with a high mortality rate, secondary to systemic bacterial and fungal infections, in the immunocompromised patient. An inadequate number of white blood cells of any type may aggravate an existing or developing infectious process. Be sure to wash your hands meticulously before caring for patients with suppressed WBC counts.

Avoid putting patients with low WBC counts into multibed rooms where other patients with diagnoses of infection reside. If possible, admit the patient to a private room. Use protective isolation only if necessary because this environment isolates the patient from family and friends; rather, screen visitors and do not permit visits from persons with obvious colds, bronchitis, chicken pox, herpes simplex or herpes zoster, childhood infectious diseases, or any other infections. Avoid the use of rectal thermometers. Carefully assess patients who are also receiving glucocorticosteroids because these drugs may mask symptoms of infection. Monitor the CBC count and differential, hematocrit, hemoglobin, and platelet counts.

If a period of bone marrow suppression is anticipated with each course or dose of drug, find out when the nadir of bone marrow suppression will occur. The risk of infection can be reduced by teaching patients to avoid potential sources of infection (e.g., live plants and flowers [sources of microscopic fungus, bacteria, and insects], fresh fruits and vegetables [unless carefully washed]). Instruct patients to wash hands carefully after using the bathroom and after contact with other persons. Ask family members to wash hands carefully before coming in contact with the patient.

Patients should be advised against receiving live-virus vaccines until months after antineoplastic therapy has been discontinued. In addition, persons in close contact with the patient should not receive live-virus vaccines since the person receiving it excretes the virus, and it can then be transmitted to the patient. Additionally, patients need to understand the importance of reporting the early signs and symptoms of infection (low-grade fever, sore throat, cough). The single most important practice that can be undertaken to prevent infection, however, is for all health care workers, patients, families, and friends to practice strict hand washing.

Thrombocytopenia increases the patient's risk of bleeding if the platelet count falls below 20,000 cells/mm^3. A normal platelet count is 140,000 to 440,000 cells/mm^3. Fatal CNS hemorrhage or massive GI bleeding can occur when the platelet count falls below 10,000 cells/mm^3. Some controversy exists as to whether patients should receive prophylactic transfusions when their platelet count falls below a certain level or when the patient is actively bleeding. Most health care providers will transfuse the patient to keep the platelet count above 20,000 cells/mm³.

Thrombocytopenia is a risk factor for bleeding. The potential for bleeding can be minimized by teaching patients to avoid aspirin and other OTC drugs that prolong clotting times, to substitute electric shavers for razors (decreases the risk of nicks and cuts), refrain from using suppositories (may cause tears to rectal tissue), hold pressure over cuts and venipuncture sites for 5 to 10 minutes, and avoid intramuscular injections as much as possible. Some patients may require activity restrictions or bed rest to decrease the risk of injury. Most importantly, patients need to understand the signs and symptoms of internal bleeding and report these symptoms immediately. Blood counts must be scrutinized closely before a patient undergoes surgery or any invasive procedure.

Anemia is present in patients with cancer (more often as a result of the disease process), but may be related to or aggravated by the myelosuppressive effect of antineoplastic drugs on developing RBCs. Anemia leads to tissue hypoxia secondary to impaired oxygen-carrying capacity and is manifested by a drop in hemoglobin, hematocrit, or RBC count. Dehydration may raise the hematocrit, thus masking an anemia. A normal hemoglobin is 13 to 16 g/dL in men and 12 to 15 g/dL in women. The patient is anemic if the values fall below 13 or 12 g/dL, respectively. Severe anemia can result in hypotension and myocardial infarction. One unit of blood will usually raise the hemoglobin 1 g/dL.

Patients are able to tolerate varying degrees of anemia or may be reluctant to accept transfusions. However, packed RBCs may be required to relieve anemia that is producing symptoms. Erythropoietin, a naturally occurring growth factor, stimulates RBC production in response to the body's needs. It may be ordered to elevate or maintain the RBC level and decrease the need for transfusions (see Chapter 45). Patients receiving erythropoietin note an increase in hematocrit, improved energy, and less fatigue. Other favorable outcomes include improvements in cardiovascular status and cognitive function, exercise tolerance, and quality of life.

Gastrointestinal Effects. Antineoplastic therapy can cause nausea, vomiting, diarrhea, stomatitis, oral mucositis, aversion to food, changes in taste and smell, diarrhea, and constipation. The emetic potential of a particular antineoplastic drug regimen depends on the drugs given, the dose, and route of administration, and the patient's susceptibility to emesis. Uncontrolled nausea and vomiting can result in anorexia, malnutrition,

dehydration, metabolic imbalances, psychologic depression, and reduced immunity.

Three patterns of nausea and vomiting are associated with antineoplastic therapy. Once the patient has experienced nausea and vomiting, anticipatory nausea and vomiting may occur before the next treatment session. Patients who experience four or more of the following characteristics have been reported to be at risk for anticipatory nausea and vomiting:

- Age younger than 50 years
- Nausea or vomiting after last antineoplastic session
- Posttreatment nausea described as moderate, severe, or intolerable
- Posttreatment vomiting described as moderate, severe, or intolerable
- Feeling warm or hot all over after the last antineoplastic therapy session
- Susceptibility to motion sickness
- Sweating after last antineoplastic session
- Generalized weakness after last antineoplastic session

Anticipatory nausea and vomiting develops rapidly, often appearing after only one infusion and escalating in severity during subsequent treatments. Patients typically are apprehensive about the first treatment session and most have heard stories about the horrors of antineoplastic therapy. However, most patients find the first infusion to be much easier than they expected. Nevertheless, as treatment continues, patients begin to notice anticipatory nausea and vomiting.

Acute posttherapy nausea and vomiting occur within the first 24 hours after drug administration. The onset may take place minutes after the drug is administered, but usually occurs 2 to 6 hours after administration. It usually lasts up to 24 hours.

Delayed nausea and vomiting persists or develops 24 hours after drug administration. Its pathophysiology is unclear, but may be the result of residual drug or its metabolites. It is more common in patients receiving high-dose cisplatin or in persons who experience nausea on the day of antineoplastic therapy.

The health care provider responsible for drug administration must be thoroughly familiar with antiemetic drugs and adjunct measures that can be used, because control improves the patient's sense of well-being and aids in maintaining good nutrition. Many antiemetic drugs are available, including relatively new drugs such as granisetron and ondansetron, as well as older drugs such as phenothiazines (see Chapter 50).

Assess the patient's fluid balance and nutritional status, including height and weight, intake and output, eating habits, skin turgor, serum albumin, and total lymphocyte count. Minimize stimuli (sights, sounds, odors) that may stimulate nausea and vomiting. When possible, provide fresh air to minimize odors. Arrange for small frequent meals and include dietary supplements as necessary. Encourage the family to provide favorite foods, as tolerated, but avoid highly sweetened, greasy or fried foods, heavily spiced foods, and foods with strong odors. Offer cool (not cold) liquids.

Teach the patient to identify and use interventions that have relieved nausea during prior illnesses or stressful situations. Use general behavioral techniques such as relaxation therapy, visual imaging, or distraction. When vomiting does occur, empty the emesis basin as promptly as possible, ventilate the room, and perform mouth care.

Stomatitis or oral mucositis is a consequence of delayed cell renewal caused by antineoplastic drugs. What is seen in the mouth is present throughout the GI tract. The drugs most commonly associated with stomatitis are the antimetabolites, the antitumor antibiotics, and the mitotic inhibitors (i.e., vinca alkaloids). The oral lesions may be so severe that patients are unable to eat, drink, speak, or swallow their own oral secretions. Severe stomatitis may be a dose-limiting toxicity for the patient.

If possible, have the teeth professionally cleaned and dental caries repaired before the start of antineoplastic therapy. If toothbrushing is irritating, teach the patient to use swabs to clean the mouth. Avoid flossing when stomatitis is severe. Use water spraying oral-care devices on low setting only. Rinse the mouth after each meal with a mild solution of baking soda and water; baking soda, salt, and water; or hydrogen peroxide and water. Try painting the inside of the mouth with a substrate of magnesia up to four times daily. Allow the milk of magnesia to settle to the bottom of the bottle. Pour off the liquid portion at the top of the bottle, and paint the mouth with the white pasty portion remaining. If a special mouthwash has been prescribed, teach the patient to use it as ordered. Many mouthwashes are effective only when used regularly throughout the day. Because many OTC mouthwashes contain alcohol, they may be irritating.

If chewing and swallowing are painful, switch to a liquid diet, including milkshakes and ice cream. If discomfort is severe, try to maintain an intake of clear liquids of at least 2000 mL per day to prevent dehydration. Advise the patient to try chilling food before eating it. Adding sauces and gravies to foods may help lubricate foods. Avoid alcoholic beverages, spicy foods, and foods with hard crusts or edges. Wear dentures or bridgework only while eating, and remove them at other times to reduce irritation.

If the patient craves a specific food item, it is usually acceptable for the patient to have it. The alternative may be a missed meal. If food preparation is tiring to patients, suggest that they prepare and freeze small portions on days they feel better so that when not feeling well, it is necessary only to thaw and eat the food. Also encourage interested friends and family to prepare individual servings for the patient. Although a microwave oven is not a necessity, the patient may find it helpful to have one to quickly heat food.

Some patients may find that a small glass of wine or sherry before dinner will stimulate their appetite. Encourage snacking and nibbling during the day. Encourage the patient to keep available in the refrigerator high-protein beverages or snacks that may be appealing (e.g., yogurt, milkshakes, eggnog, ice cream). Obtain recipes for high-calorie snacks from dietitians, the American Cancer Society, or the health care provider's office. Some patients may choose to use commercially prepared high-protein supplements that may be consumed as a drink or frozen and eaten as ice cream.

Xerostomia, or dryness of the oral mucosa, is the result of decreased production of saliva. This may cause alterations in taste, difficulty in chewing or swallowing, and poor fit of dentures. Xerostomia may be exacerbated by concomitant radiation therapy to the head and neck. Teach the patient to use lubricating agents, such as artificial saliva, antibacterial moisturizing gels, and lip balm. Using oral rinses before meals, sucking on ice chips or salivary stimulants such as hard candies may help with dryness. The local vasoconstriction caused by cold may decrease the severity of stomatitis.

Mucositis is caused by an inflammation of epithelial cells in response to antineoplastic drugs. This may affect membranes that line the oral, GI, and female reproductive tracts. For anal irritation, avoid suppositories, enemas, and rectal thermometers. Advise the patient to sit in a tub of warm water several times daily. After bowel movements, clean the anal area completely. Some patients may prefer to use a babywipe because of its cool feeling. If vaginal irritation is a problem, teach the patient to keep the vaginal area clean and dry, wipe from the front to back, avoid soaps in the vaginal area, and pat dry after bathing. Avoid douching or using tampons. Advise the patient to notify the health care provider if vaginal discharge develops or if a change in the color, consistency, odor, or amount occurs. Suggest that the patient use a commercially available water-soluble lubricant to decrease irritation during intercourse. Tell the patient to avoid hand lotion or petroleum jelly for this purpose.

Diarrhea is most often associated with antimetabolite drugs. Vinca alkaloids are often responsible for constipation as a result of paralysis of the autonomic nerves that control intestinal motility. Other causes of constipation include opioid use, immobility, decreased fluid and fiber intake, tumor invasion of the GI tract, and depression. This symptom may appear within 24 to 48 hours of receiving the drug or may be delayed for

5 to 10 days. Instruct the patient to switch to a clear-liquid diet or a low-residue diet high in protein and calories. The goal is to maintain a fluid intake of at least 2000 to 2500 mL/day. Caution the patient to avoid foods known to be irritating to the GI tract, such as fruit, fruit juices, spicy foods, raw vegetables, corn, and coffee.

Teach the patient that diarrhea can lead to electrolyte imbalance. In severe cases the patient may need to be admitted to the hospital for intravenous replacement of fluids and electrolytes. Review possible clear-liquid food the patient may like, such as broth, gelatin, tea, iced pops, soft drinks, and water. The patient may be able to tolerate chicken noodle soup. Although electrolyte-containing drinks such as Gatorade are not required, they may provide a pleasant-tasting alternative that is less irritating than fruit juice. If anal irritation occurs, suggest that the patient shower or sit in a warm tub of water several times per day. Wash the anal area with mild soap and water, and pat the area dry gently after each loose bowel movement. Some patients may find it easier or more comfortable to wash the area with baby-wipes or with preparations such as Tucks.

Dermatologic Effects. Dermatologic toxicities of antineoplastic drugs include alopecia, skin and nail hyperpigmentation, and onycholysis of the nails. Toxicities and adverse effects gradually resolve with cessation of treatment. The extent of hair loss, **alopecia**, depends on the specific drug, dosage, and route of administration. Point out that alopecia may involve eyebrows, eyelashes, nasal hair, and pubic hair, although hair loss may be patchy rather than total in these areas. Drugs that cause only mild alopecia or sporadic thinning of hair include bleomycin, carmustine, fluorouracil, lomustine, and melphalan. Drugs causing a moderate degree of alopecia include etoposide, floxuridine, irinotecan, methotrexate, and mitomycin. Still others typically cause complete baldness. These drugs include cyclophosphamide, daunorubicin, docetaxol, doxorubicin, ifosfamide, paclitaxel, teniposide, vinblastine, and vincristine. However, alopecia is temporary. Hair regrowth often occurs before antineoplastic therapy ends, although the hair color and texture may change.

Before starting antineoplastic therapy, inform patients about the possibility of alopecia. Some patients may wish to invest in a wig resembling their own hair color and style before hair loss begins. In some communities the American Cancer Society has a wig bank from which cancer patients can borrow wigs during periods of alopecia. Explore this possibility with the patient. In addition, some insurance companies may reimburse patients for the cost of wigs.

During alopecia, instruct the patient to wash hair every 2 to 4 days. Use a mild shampoo, but not necessarily baby shampoo. The patient's barber or hairdresser may be able to recommend a specific product. Refrain from the use of permanent wave or hair dyes. Instruct the patient to use a cream rinse or conditioner. If the scalp is dry, tell the patient to apply a thin layer of baby oil, mineral oil, or A and D ointment. Brush and comb hair gently. Avoid the use of curling irons; instead use a blow dryer on a cool, gentle setting. Caution the patient to avoid direct exposure to the sun, either by wearing a hat or by using a maximum-protection sunscreen when out of doors (SPF 15 or greater). During cold weather, advise the patient to wear a hat when out of doors. Suggest that patients use satin pillow covers.

Sometimes the patient's head may be cooled with cold compresses before intravenous therapy. This approach is used to cause vasoconstriction to the area, thus reducing contact between the drug and epithelial cells with the hope that less of the drug will reach the scalp and alopecia will be less severe. Inform patients that hair loss will probably occur even with the use of cold compresses. This approach is rarely used today, owing to the risk of creating a sanctuary site for metastatic disease.

Hyperpigmentation of the nail bed, mouth, gums, or teeth, and along veins used for intravenous therapy is not uncommon. The hyperpigmentation usually occurs 2 to 3 weeks after therapy and continues for 10 to 12 weeks following discontinuance. Photosensitivity may result in acute sunburn after just a short exposure to the sun. Instruct the patient to avoid exposure to sunlight and other forms of ultraviolet light by wearing protective clothing over face, arms, and other exposed areas. Use a suncreen with SPF 15 or higher on skin areas exposed to sunlight.

Radiation recall may occur in patients who received radiation therapy weeks or months before the administration of antineoplastic drugs. Skin effects occur in the area previously radiated and range from redness, shedding, or peeling, to blisters and oozing. Once the skin heals, it is permanently darkened.

Genitourinary Effects. The renal system is affected by antineoplastic therapy drugs. Hyperuricemia is a common occurrence with myeloproliferative disorders (e.g., leukemias, lymphomas, multiple myelomas) and disseminated metastatic cancers, and may be precipitated or aggravated by antineoplastic therapy. It is the result of increased production or decreased elimination of uric acid, or both. Uric acid can severely damage kidney cells if it is allowed to increase unchecked. Allopurinol may be needed when large tumor masses are quickly destroyed by antineoplastic therapy, releasing many breakdown products, including uric acid. Allopurinol inhibits the formation of uric acid and therefore can prevent this complication. Allopurinol is also used to treat gout (see Chapter 14).

Adequate hydration before, during, and after antineoplastic therapy is imperative when administering nephrotoxic or bladder toxic drugs. A few drugs are now available that have been designed to directly offset a specific toxicity of a cytotoxic drug. For example, ifosfamide and cyclophosphamide produce toxic metabolites, including acrolein, that cause bladder damage (hemorrhagic cystitis). Mesna binds these toxic metabolites and protects the bladder from injury. Likewise, amifostine is biotransformed to a thiol, which protects the kidneys by binding toxic free radicals produced by cisplatin. Additional measures that may be taken to reduce renal toxicity include administering a diuretic before cisplatin, alkalinizing the urine to a pH of 7.0 or higher before high-dose methotrexate, and administering citrovorum rescue (leucovorin) until methotrexate reaches nontoxic concentrations.

Neurologic Effects. Neurologic toxicity is most commonly seen with administration of vinca alkaloids. The patient with peripheral neuropathy may exhibit paresthesias of the hands or feet, pain along the facial trigeminal nerve, loss of deep tendon reflexes, and motor weakness. The motor weakness is usually more prominent in the lower extremities and is evidenced by foot drop, a slapping gait, and wrist drop. The neuromuscular effects of vincristine frequently develop in sequence. Initially, only sensory impairment and paresthesias may occur. With continued treatment neuritic pain and, later, motor difficulties may appear. Pyridoxine may be administered concurrently with altretamine in an effort to minimize peripheral neuropathy.

Pulmonary Effects. Pulmonary toxicity may be caused by some cytotoxic drugs. The onset of pulmonary toxicity may be acute or chronic, developing within days, months, or years after therapy. High risk factors include age over 60 years, history of smoking, preexisting pulmonary disease, prior or concurrent radiation therapy to the chest, high-dose oxygen therapy, and renal dysfunction. Dyspnea is the cardinal symptom of pulmonary toxicity. Other findings may include a dry nonproductive cough, fatigue, fever, low exercise tolerance, crackles or rhonchi, restlessness, tachypnea, and confusion. There is no specific method for treating pulmonary alterations associated with antineoplastic drugs, thus the nursing responsibility lies in identifying and assessing the high-risk patient to detect problems at an early stage.

Cardiac Effects. Cardiac toxicity may occur with the administration of anthracycline antibiotics (e.g., daunorubicin and doxorubicin) and to a lesser extent with se-

lected other antineoplastic drugs. Patients at risk for cardiac toxicity are children, adults over age 50, persons with preexisting cardiac disease, and those who have received or are receiving chest or mediastinal radiation. Evidence of early cardiac alterations such as heart failure, hypotension, and arrhythmias must be reported as soon as they are recognized. Many cardiotoxicities appear immediately after the last dose or up to 30 months later, with the peak onset at 3 months. Heart failure develops weeks, months, or years after therapy. Cardiomyopathy may appear 5 years or more after anthracycline therapy. Should heart failure develop, the patient may be put on a low-sodium diet with or without fluid restriction, diuretics and potassium (see Chapter 46). Hypotension may be ameliorated by hydrating the patient before therapy. The patient should be taught to move slowly when changing from sitting to lying or from lying to standing positions. Digoxin or other cardiac drugs may be administered if arrhythmias develop.

Reproductive Effects. The effects of antineoplastic therapy on gonadal function and reproduction capacity can be temporary or permanent. The effects on gonadal function vary with respect to the patient's age at the time of therapy, the drugs administered, and total dosage. Azoospermia, oligospermia, sterility, decreased libido, retrograde ejaculation, gynecomastia, and breast tenderness have been documented in men. Amenorrhea, sterility, manifestations of menopause, and osteoporosis have been noted in women. Encourage the patient to discuss his or her feelings regarding gonadal dysfunction. Assist in identifying available interventions and resources to prevent or manage alterations in gonadal function (e.g., donor egg programs, hormonal replacement therapy, artificial vaginal lubricants, sperm banking, sexual dysfunction clinics, drugs to reverse retrograde ejaculation, and support groups). Contraceptives should be used for birth control during therapy and for up to 2 years following completion of therapy.

Hypercalcemia. Hypercalcemia can be a dangerous adverse effect of cancer therapy, especially when tumor metastases exist in bone. Hypercalcemia may occur with androgens, estrogens, and antiestrogen therapy; however, it is more commonly seen as a complication of cancer. Interventions will vary with the extent of hypercalcemia. When possible, the underlying cause is corrected; however, several drugs are available to protect patients from this complication. Etidronate, pamidronate, zoledronic acid, and gallium nitrate block overproduction of calcium (see Chapter 56). Plicamycin helps with this symptom and it also has anticancer activity. Other interventions include encouraging physical activity and ambulation and maintaining hydration.

Pain and Discomfort. Because pain and discomfort associated with advanced cancer can be severe, hospitals and hospices specializing in care for dying cancer patients have a policy of liberal use of opioid analgesics (see Chapter 13). Frequent dosing and large doses may be needed to control pain. Fear of dependency should not prevent adequate pain control in patients with terminal cancer.

Psychologic Stress. A child or other family member diagnosed with cancer places extraordinary stressors on the family unit. The health care provider must be prepared to give the extra time needed to provide patient and family teaching and emotional support. It is particularly important that parents understand the potential for late effects of antineoplastic drugs, including sterility, hypogonadism, growth retardation, and cognitive impairment. Encourage the patient and family to accept counseling or to go to support groups.

EVALUATION

The success of antineoplastic therapy is evaluated based on the patient's response to treatment. Relatively standardized criteria have been developed to evaluate the efficacy of antineoplastic therapy. The criteria include survival rates, degree of response or remission, duration of response, and degree of toxicity. Complete response generally refers to the complete disappearance of all evidence of disease for 1 month or longer following completion of therapy. Partial response is usually defined as a reduction in measurable tumor mass of 50% or more of its original size for 1 month or more. Moreover, there should be no evidence of new disease, and the patient's general well-being should be subjectively improved. Improvement refers to a reduction in measurable tumor mass by 25% to 50% of its original size with subjective improvement in patient status. Stable disease is tumor regression of 25% or less with or without subjective patient improvement. Disease progression refers to clinical evidence of advancing disease during antineoplastic therapy. Assuming that an adequate trial of antineoplastic therapy has been conducted, disease progression indicates a treatment failure.

These anticipated outcomes vary significantly, depending on the patient's physical status, specific diagnosis, and extent of disease. The ultimate goal of antineoplastic therapy is to achieve a cure without unreasonable toxicities and adverse reactions. When cure is impossible, antineoplastic drugs are a valuable tool in prolonging life and minimizing the suffering associated with a diagnosis of cancer. The health care provider must be knowledgeable about the range of antineoplastic drugs and their toxicities to ensure the patient's safety, minimize adverse effects, and assist the patient in coping with a life-threatening illness.

Bibliography

Anastasia PJ: Effectiveness of oral 5-HT3 receptor antagonists for emetogenic chemotherapy, *Oncol Nurs Forum* 27(3):483-493, 2000.

Barrick MC, Mitchell SA: Multiple myeloma: recent advances for this common plasma cell disorder, *Am J Nurs* 101(Suppl):6-12, 49-50, 2001.

Barse PM: Issues in the treatment of metastatic breast cancer, *Semin Oncol Nurs* 16(3):197-205, 2000.

Beaulieu NJ: In the med room: review of antiemetic therapy in adjuvant breast cancer regimens, *Innovations Breast Cancer Care* 5(2):39-43, 51-54, 2000.

Christy P, Oberleitner MG: Brain cancer: emerging treatments require advanced knowledge of oncology and neuroscience, *Am J Nurs* 100(Suppl):4-8, 52-54, 2000.

Conklin KA: Dietary antioxidants during cancer chemotherapy: impact on chemotherapeutic effectiveness and development of side effects, *Nutr Cancer* 37(1):1-18, 2000.

Ganz PA: Late effects of cancer and its treatment, *Semin Oncol Nurs* 17(4):241-248, 2001.

Held-Warmkessel J: Treatment of advanced prostate cancer, *Semin Oncol Nurs* 17(2):118-128, 2001.

Irwin M, Klemm P: Drug interactions in oncology patients: decreasing the undesirable side effects of etoposide, antidepressants, azole antifungals, and steroids, *Am J Nurs* 101(Suppl):23-26, 49-50, 2001.

Keating GM, Goa KL: Management of advanced breast cancer: defining the role of anastrozole, *Dis Manage Health Outcomes* 9(7):385-402, 2001.

Lamson DW, Brignall MS: Antioxidants and cancer therapy II: quick reference guide, *Altern Med Rev* 5(2):152-163, 2000.

Mackey HT, Klemm P: Leukemia: aggressive therapies predispose patients to a host of side effects, *Am J Nurs* 100(Suppl):27-31, 52-54, 2000.

Reddy P, Chow MSS: Safety and efficacy of antiestrogens for prevention of breast cancer, *Am J Health Syst Pharm* 57(14):1315-1325, 2000.

Shagam JY: Principles of chemotherapy, *Radiat Ther* 10(1):37-56, 2001.

Smith IE, Lipton L: Preoperative/neoadjuvant medical therapy for early breast cancer, *Lancet Oncol* 2(9):561-570, 2001.

Sweeney MP, Bagg J: Pain and symptom management: the mouth and palliative care, *Am J Hospice Palliative Care* 17(2):118-124, 2000.

Internet Resources

http://www.cancer.ca/.
http://www.cancercare.org/.
http://www.cancer.gov/cancer information/.
http://www.cancer.gov/clinical_trials/.
http://www.cancer.org/.
OncoLink. Available online at www.oncolink.com.

CHAPTER

38

Drugs Used to Treat Heart Failure

JOSEPH A. DiMICCO • KATHLEEN GUTIERREZ

 Visit http://evolve.elsevier.com/Gutierrez/ for additional information.

KEY TERMS

OBJECTIVES

- Explain why heart failure produces symptoms of edema, shortness of breath, and rapid heart rate (tachycardia).

- Explain the concepts of preload and afterload.

- Explain how angiotensin-converting enzyme (ACE) inhibitors and other vasodilators might slow the progression of heart failure and improve survival.

- Explain how cardiac glycosides relieve symptoms of heart failure.

- Explain how beta-adrenergic drugs and diuretics relieve symptoms of heart failure.

- Develop a nursing care plan for a patient receiving a cardiac glycoside.

PATHOPHYSIOLOGY • Heart Failure

The heart acts as a pump whose purpose is to maintain the pressure required to drive the blood through the circulation. The pumping action of the heart depends on an appropriately timed contraction of adequate force to deliver blood from the ventricles into the arteries. The right ventricle delivers blood to the capillaries in the lungs where oxygen is picked up and carbon dioxide is removed. The left ventricle delivers this oxygenated blood into the arterial tree that supplies the rest of the body. Normally the impulse that causes the contraction of cardiac muscle begins with the firing of a cell in the **sinoatrial (SA) node**. Cells in the SA node have the property of **automaticity**, which means that they fire automatically and spontaneously. Other cells in the heart may be automatic, but because the cells in the SA node have the fastest spontaneous rate, they normally drive the rest of the cells in the heart and determine heart rate. Because of this, these cells are called **pacemakers**.

The impulse that originates in the SA node normally spreads from cell to cell through the rest of the heart in a specific and organized way that maximizes the efficiency of the heart as a pump. The rate at which this impulse moves from cell to cell in the heart, called the **conduction velocity**, varies in different heart regions. First, the impulse spreads rapidly through the atrial muscle, causing the cells of the atria to contract in a coordinated way (see Chapter 40, Figure 40-1). This impulse will not pass directly from the atrial muscle cells to muscle cells in the ventricles because a ring of nonconductive tissue separates them except in one region. This region, called the **atrioventricular (AV) node**, transmits the impulse from the atria to the ventricles but does so relatively slowly. The slow conduction velocity through the AV node provides an important delay that allows the contracting atria to fill the still-relaxed ventricles with blood. Only then does the impulse emerge again from the AV node, at which point it spreads very rapidly through the ventricles, triggering their contraction.

The amount of blood flow required by different tissues varies under different circumstances (e.g., with stress and exertion) and the normal heart adjusts its pumping activity appropriately. The **Frank-Starling law** defines the way the heart regulates its output to meet these variable demands. This principle of physiology states that the force of muscular contraction is directly related to the stretch of the muscle; the more the muscle is stretched, within mechanical limits, the stronger its subsequent contraction. This principle applied to the heart means that when the ventricles are stretched by being filled with larger-than-normal volumes of blood, they contract with greater-than-normal force to deliver the extra blood to the arteries. As a result, blood does not normally accumulate in the veins, and all the blood coming into the heart is pumped out. If cardiac muscle fibers are stretched beyond their mechanical limits, however, the strength of contraction decreases and cardiac output falls. The amount of stretching of the ventricular cardiac muscle just before contraction begins is called the **preload**.

The ability of the heart to pump blood into the arteries is also determined by the resistance against which the heart works, called **afterload**. Afterload is represented by the pressure in the arteries against which the heart must pump. The greater the afterload, the less blood each beat of the heart will be able to deliver to the arteries.

Although changes in preload and afterload cause some adjustment in the performance of the heart, these changes cannot provide the immediate increases necessary under extreme conditions, such as intense exercise. Under such conditions, the body can increase **cardiac output**—the total amount of blood the heart pumps in a given period of time—through the autonomic nervous system. Specifically, the heart is heavily innervated by the sympathetic nervous system; norepinephrine is released from sympathetic nerve endings acting at the beta receptors on cardiac cells to affect three key features of cardiac activity. First, and most importantly for increasing cardiac output, sympathetic activity increases cardiac **contractility**. Contractility, also called inotropy, refers to the strength of the muscular contraction of the heart. Therefore, sympathetic nerve stimulation is said to have a positive **inotropic** effect. The second important effect of sympathetic stimulation of the heart is to increase the rate of firing of pacemaker cells in the SA node. The result is an increase in heart rate, called a positive **chronotropic** effect. The positive inotropic effect of sympathetic stimulation means that the heart beats more forcefully and therefore pumps more blood with each beat, while the positive chronotropic effect means that the heart beats more times in a given time interval. The peak efficiency of the heart under these conditions is reached at about 150 to 175 beats per minute. Faster rates result in incomplete filling of the ventricles and reduce the overall efficiency of the pump. The third important effect of sympathetic nerve activity on the heart occurs at the AV node to increase conduction velocity through the region. The parasympathetic innervation of the heart through the vagus nerve acts mainly in the nodes. Stimulation of the vagus nerve releases acetylcholine, which makes the cells less excitable. In the SA node, this action decreases the rate of firing of pacemaker cells, which reduces heart rate. Stimulation of the vagus nerve also decreases conduction velocity through the AV node. In response to exercise and stress, the activity of the vagus nerve is reduced.

If the heart is subjected to chronic demands for increased output, the ventricles may enlarge. This condition is called **ventricular hypertrophy** and may be a normal response to chronic stress or athletic training. For example, long-distance runners and tennis players may have enlarged hearts. In other instances the enlargement of the heart may signal a pathologic process.

One such pathologic process is **heart failure**, which is a complex pattern of symptoms and changes whose original cause is the failure of the normal strength of the heart (Figure 38-1). As a result of the failure of the heart as a pump, cardiac output eventually falls below the minimum level required to deliver adequate blood flow

to the tissues. At this point, normal regulatory mechanisms come into play as the body tries to compensate. Sympathetic nervous system activity is increased to raise heart rate and contractility and thus cardiac output. Decreased perfusion of the kidneys leads to sodium and water retention, resulting in increased cardiac preload (because of the increased fluid volume). Cardiac hypertrophy may also occur as the body seeks to increase the efficiency of the pump.

A key role in the compensatory response to impaired cardiac performance is also played by the renin-angiotensin system. **Renin** is an enzyme synthesized and released by cells around the blood vessels in the kidneys when blood flow to the kidneys is reduced. This enzyme catalyzes the transformation of a circulating

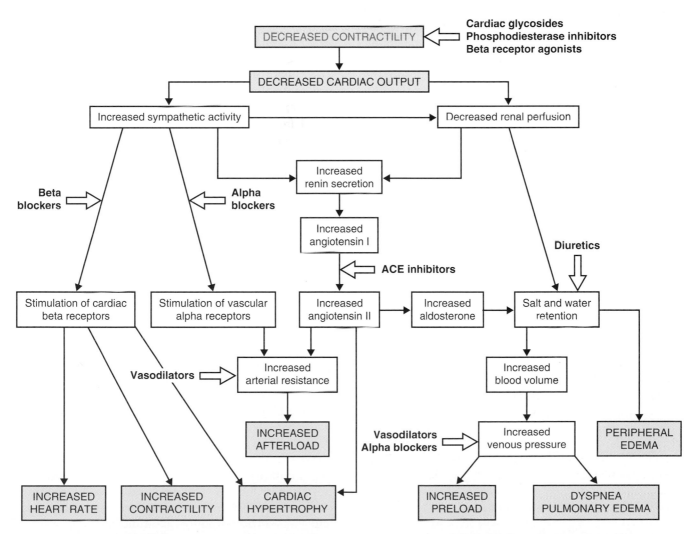

FIGURE 38-1 Compensatory mechanisms associated with heart failure. *ACE,* angiotensin-converting enzyme. Drug classes are shown in bold and their point of action in the disease process is shown by open arrows (⇨).

peptide called angiotensinogen into angiotensin I. Any angiotensin I in the circulation is quickly biotransformed to a much more active substance, angiotensin II (AII), by angiotensin-converting enzyme (ACE). Angiotensin-converting enzyme is found in especially high concentrations in the blood vessels of the pulmonary circulation. Angiotensin II acts at receptors called AT1 receptors (see Chapter 41), causing many important effects aimed at increasing renal perfusion. First, angiotensin II increases arterial pressure by constricting arterioles and enhancing the release of norepinephrine from sympathetic nerve endings. Second, angiotensin II also stimulates the adrenal cortex to increase the production and secretion of aldosterone. Aldosterone is a steroid hormone that causes the kidneys to retain more sodium and water, increasing the extracellular fluid volume in the body. Third, angiotensin II—and perhaps aldosterone as well—may act directly on the heart to cause structural changes, similar in some ways to the hypertrophy that is the normal response to regular athletic training.

In many cases, in the absence of acute demands on the heart, these mechanisms enable a weakened heart to maintain sufficient output. Therefore patients in the early stages of heart failure may have few symptoms, but when examined may have an enlarged heart and increased heart rate. However, heart failure is a progressive disease, meaning that the performance of the heart continues to deteriorate over time. In fact, some of the adaptive changes made by the body to compensate for the decrease in cardiac performance lead to further problems and may actually play a role in the progression of the disease. Eventually, the heart—especially the left ventricle—is unable to pump all the blood delivered to it, leading to symptoms caused by congestion in the pulmonary and venous blood vessels. The symptoms arise directly from insufficient cardiac output and indirectly from the body's attempts to adapt to reduced cardiac output. Blood pooled in the veins increases venous pressure. Excessive venous pressure stretches cardiac muscle fibers beyond their limits. As predicted by the Frank-Starling law, this excessive preload causes a further reduction in the strength of contraction. Chronic activation of the sympathetic nervous system causes systemic vasoconstriction, meaning an increased afterload, and a further reduction in renal blood flow. Reduced blood flow to the kidneys triggers more sodium and water retention, which further worsens symptoms. Moreover, the fall in renal perfusion causes the release of even more renin, resulting in further increases in circulating angiotensin II and aldosterone.

All of these effects increase the filling pressure caused by venous tone (preload) and the pressure against which the heart works as it forces blood into the arteries (afterload), further impairing cardiac output. Edema of the lungs and periphery develops as fluid leaks into tissues from the capillaries. The typical patient who has heart failure is therefore short of breath, has a rapid resting pulse resulting from sympathetic stimulation of the heart, obvious swelling of the hands and feet and sometimes the abdomen, and an enlarged heart. Although heart failure cannot be cured, drug therapy can prolong the patient's life by slowing the progression of the disease and improve the quality of life by reducing symptoms.

DRUG CLASS • Angiotensin-Converting Enzyme (ACE) Inhibitors

benazepril (Lotensin)

⚠ captopril (C apoten)

enalapril (Vasotec)

fosinopril (Monopril)

lisinopril (Prinivil, Zestril)

moexipril (Univasc)

perindopril (Aceon)

quinapril (Accupril)

ramipril (Altace)

trandolapril (Mavik)

MECHANISM OF ACTION

All drugs in this class act as competitive inhibitors of ACE, resulting in decreased conversion of angiotensin I to angiotensin II. The ACE inhibitors may also produce effects on the vasculature, including improvement of coronary artery blood flow, by inhibiting the breakdown of bradykinin. Bradykinin is a peptide with vasodilator actions. Although the circulating level of bradykinin is known to be elevated by ACE inhibitors, the role that this peptide plays in therapeutic response to these drugs is unknown.

USES

ACE inhibitors are now considered first-line drugs for heart failure and left ventricular dysfunction. Inhibiting the production of angiotensin II decreases both preload and afterload and produces an immediate improvement in cardiac performance. Limiting the formation of angiotensin II may also inhibit the structural changes in the heart that are largely responsible for the progression of the disease. Several large clinical trials have confirmed that ACE inhibitors not only improve cardiac function in these patients—and therefore the quality of life—but also reduce mortality from heart failure. Because these drugs block the harmful adaptations to lowered cardiac output, the ACE inhibitors can and should be used early in the process to slow development of heart failure.

The ACE inhibitors are also valuable in the treatment of hypertension (see Chapter 41).

PHARMACOKINETICS

All ACE inhibitors are effective when given orally, although absorption varies widely from 60% or more (captopril, enalapril, perindopril, and quinapril) to only about 10% (trandolapril). With the exception of captopril and lisinopril, all ACE inhibitors are administered as prodrugs and are active only after biotransformation to their corresponding active metabolites (e.g., benazepril to benazeprilat, enalapril to enalaprilat [which is also available for intravenous injection], fosinopril to fosinoprilat). Consequently, plasma half-lives for the prodrugs are typically very short (e.g., 5 to 6 hours for ramipril or trandolapril, 2 hours or less for all the rest), but half-lives of the active metabolites are much longer, typically 10 hours or more. Plasma half-lives of captopril and lisinopril are 3 and 10 hours, respectively. With the exception of captopril, which has a duration of action of about 6 hours, all the other drugs have effective durations of action of about 24 hours. All ACE inhibitors are eliminated primarily by the kidneys, although significant fecal elimination also occurs with all but benazepril, captopril, and lisinopril.

ADVERSE REACTIONS AND CONTRAINDICATIONS

The most common adverse effect of the ACE inhibitors when used in the treatment of heart failure is excessive hypotension, although blood pressure usually recovers after the initial dose. Sodium depletion or volume depletion worsens this reaction. Another common adverse effect is a persistent dry cough that may be especially troublesome at night.

Because of the risk of induction of angioedema with ACE inhibitors, these drugs should not be given to patients with a history of this disorder. The drugs should also be avoided in patients with renal impairment, renal artery stenosis, hyperkalemia, or sodium depletion.

TOXICITY

The main effect of overdosage is severe hypotension. Thus treatment consists of expanding plasma volume to correct hypotension.

INTERACTIONS

Potassium-containing supplements, low-salt milk, or salt substitutes containing large amounts of potassium may lead to hyperkalemia when combined with ACE inhibitors. Diuretics or other drugs causing a decrease in blood pressure may worsen hypotensive reactions to ACE inhibitors.

DRUG CLASS • Cardiac Glycosides

 digoxin (Lanoxicaps, Lanoxin)
digitoxin (Crystodigin)

MECHANISM OF ACTION

Cardiac glycosides inhibit sodium-potassium-ATPase in all cells, reducing intracellular potassium and increasing the level of intracellular sodium. In cardiac muscle cells, this change promotes the accumulation of calcium used for contraction. The increased calcium level directly increases contractility, which increases cardiac output, improves blood flow to the kidneys and periphery, reduces venous pressure, and allows excess fluid to be excreted as edema clears. The diuretic effect of cardiac glycosides results from these actions on the heart.

Cardiac glycosides also have effects in other tissues where sodium-potassium-ATPase is important, including the nervous system. One of the consequences of its action on the nervous system is to increase the activity of the vagus nerve innervating the heart, thus slowing heart rate and slowing conduction velocity through the AV node.

USES

Digoxin is used to treat systolic heart failure because it is, for all practical purposes, the only orally effective drug that directly improves the strength of the heart muscle, elevating cardiac output. Numerous clinical trials have attempted to assess the outcome of digoxin therapy in heart failure. Most studies suggest that optimal effects are seen when digoxin is combined with diuretics, vasodilators, or ACE inhibitors. The most clear-cut effect of digoxin is an improvement in exercise tolerance and hemodynamics; there is no documented improvement in long-term survival with digoxin. Digitoxin is still available and produces the same therapeutic effect (and potential for adverse effects) as digoxin, but it is infrequently used because of its less favorable pharmacokinetics (see below).

Cardiac glycosides are also used in the treatment of certain types of arrhythmia (see Chapter 40).

PHARMACOKINETICS

Digoxin, the most commonly used cardiac glycoside, has a half-life of 32 to 48 hours and is eliminated primarily through renal excretion. Digitoxin has a much longer half-life (5 to 7 days) and is eliminated by hepatic biotransformation. Because the drug is so slowly removed from the system, toxicity may persist for days after digitoxin is stopped. Therefore this drug is used much less frequently than digoxin.

Because of their long half-lives, the use of cardiac glycosides often requires loading doses (known as **digitalization**). With repeated equal doses of any drug, the plateau of drug concentration in blood is achieved after about four elimination half-lives (see Chapter 1). For cardiac glycosides, which have half-lives of 2 to 7 days, the desired therapeutic concentration would not be achieved for weeks after therapy starts. To avoid such long delays, cardiac glycosides are often given first in a loading dose designed to raise the concentration in blood rapidly to the therapeutic range. After the loading dose or doses, a smaller dosage is given on a regular schedule. This smaller dosage, the maintenance dosage, holds the drug concentration in the therapeutic range; adjustments may be needed if the patient's condition changes.

ADVERSE REACTIONS AND CONTRAINDICATIONS

Because the blood levels of cardiac glycosides needed for a therapeutic effect are so close to toxic levels, most patients taking these drugs experience drug-related difficulties. The symptoms may be neurologic, visual, cardiac, or psychiatric. Some of these symptoms are vague and easily confused with those of heart failure.

The neurologic or CNS actions of cardiac glycosides cause many of the characteristic adverse effects, such as weakness, fatigue, and fainting. Visual disturbances such as dimness of vision, double vision, blind spots, flashing lights, or altered color vision also occur. Anorexia, nausea, and vomiting are possible. Psychiatric disturbances range from mood alterations to psychoses or hallucinations.

Patients receiving cardiac glycosides must be checked often for the appearance of extra heartbeats or other arrhythmias. Although bradycardia is the most common sign of cardiac glycoside–induced rhythm problems, other changes in heart rate are possible. Therefore any change in heart rate or rhythm should be noted and reported.

Cardiac glycosides are avoided in patients with any sign of prior toxicity to these drugs or in ventricular fibrillation. Risk of arrhythmia may be increased by hyperkalemia, myxedema, pulmonary disease, or cardiac disease. Risks also rise in the older adult patient.

TOXICITY

Toxicity to cardiac glycosides can be life threatening and is relatively common, occurring in 10% to 20% of patients receiving the drug. The overall incidence of toxicity is uncertain, but it has been estimated that approximately 25% of hospitalized patients taking a cardiac glycoside show some signs and symptoms.

The toxic reactions caused by cardiac glycosides are dose related (see Chapter 1). Bradycardia (slow heart rate) may be an early sign of rising cardiac glycoside blood concentrations and is usually not a serious problem in itself. However, as concentrations continue to rise, other, more dangerous arrhythmias appear; eventually, tachycardia and ultimately ventricular fibrillation and death may occur. Blood levels of cardiac glycosides are routinely monitored to aid in diagnosing drug toxicity.

With digoxin overdose, patients continue to be at risk during the lengthy period required to eliminate these long-acting drugs. If arrhythmia or hyperkalemia becomes life threatening, digoxin-immune Fab (Digibind) can be used to neutralize free drug rapidly. Such treatment can reverse digoxin-induced arrhythmia and electrolyte imbalance within 30 minutes. The inotropic effect of cardiac glycosides persists for several hours longer.

INTERACTIONS

Because therapeutic levels are so close to toxic levels, pharmacokinetic interactions with the cardiac glycosides are of potential importance. Administration of quinidine, amiodarone, or propafenone—antiarrhythmic drugs given often to patients with heart disease—may double the plasma levels of digoxin. The potential for toxicity and elevated plasma levels of cardiac glycosides that were previously well tolerated in a given patient may be increased by treatment with other drugs. Potassium-depleting diuretics such as thiazides or loop diuretics (see Chapter 46) may predispose a patient to toxicity because a low intracellular potassium level increases the likelihood of arrhythmia. Sympathetic agonist drugs also increase the risk of arrhythmia in a patient taking digoxin. A combination of beta blockers or calcium channel blockers with digoxin may result in complete AV block. Many of the calcium channel blockers also appear to interfere with the renal clearance of digoxin, resulting in an increase in the steady-state plasma level.

DRUG CLASS • Phosphodiesterase Inhibitors

amrinone (Inocor)

milrinone (Primacor)

MECHANISM OF ACTION

Amrinone and milrinone inhibit phosphodiesterase, causing an increase in cellular concentrations of cyclic adenosine monophosphate (cAMP); thus the drugs increase the same second messenger that is elevated by stimulation of beta-adrenergic receptors (see Chapter 10). These drugs also act as vasodilators in the periphery. Therefore they increase cardiac output by both increasing cardiac contractility and reducing left ventricular afterload.

USES

Amrinone and milrinone are used for short-term intravenous treatment of heart failure when response to other drugs has been poor. These drugs rapidly increase cardiac output and are usually given to patients also receiving diuretics and digitalis.

PHARMACOKINETICS

Amrinone and milrinone are given only by intravenous injection or infusion. Amrinone has a plasma half-life of about 3 hours in healthy patients and 5 to 8 hours in patients with heart failure. Milrinone has a shorter half-life (about $2\frac{1}{2}$ hours), and both drugs are eliminated primarily by the kidneys.

ADVERSE REACTIONS AND CONTRAINDICATIONS

Phosphodiesterase inhibitors increase the risk of arrhythmia probably by increasing the effects of beta receptor stimulation and may also provoke hypotension. In rare cases, either drug may cause thrombocytopenia. Phosphodiesterase inhibitors are contraindicated in patients with aortic or pulmonary valvular disease.

INTERACTIONS

These drugs may cause additive hypotension if given with other drugs that tend to lower blood pressure.

DRUG CLASS • Diuretics

Diuretics control the pulmonary edema that accompanies severe systolic heart failure. They may also produce a beneficial effect by decreasing preload in those patients where it has caused excessive stretching of the heart muscle. Therapeutic guidelines suggest that diuretics be added if ACE inhibitors alone do not control volume overload or other cardiovascular symptoms. The major consideration limiting the use of diuretics in heart failure is the risk of electrolyte or fluid imbalances, which may be especially dangerous to patients in heart failure. Volume depletion or excessive dehydration must be avoided. Patients receiving digoxin should be carefully observed to prevent complications, because diuretics tend to alter potassium concentration in the blood. Commonly used drugs include furosemide, bumetanide, and torsemide; other diuretics may also be effective. Diuretics are discussed in detail in Chapter 46.

DRUG CLASS • Vasodilators

Vasodilators achieve their most important therapeutic effect in heart failure by decreasing afterload. They reverse the persistent vasoconstriction in late chronic heart failure resulting from long-term compensatory sympathetic nervous system stimulation. Sympathetic nervous system stimulation may support a failing heart, but it constricts peripheral blood vessels, thereby reducing cardiac output and increasing the workload of the heart. Vasodilators reduce afterload, the resistance against which the left ventricle must force blood. Cardiac output is thus increased, and workload is reduced.

Several classes of vasodilators are used in heart failure. Nitroprusside can be used for short-term intravenous therapy in severely ill patients. Hydralazine and isosorbide are more commonly used together as an oral therapy. This combination has been shown to improve the chance of survival, although the effects were not as great as with the ACE inhibitors, which in addition to being vasodilators also have other beneficial effects in heart failure. Vasodilating drugs are discussed in detail in Chapter 39.

DRUG CLASS • Alpha Antagonists

As with vasodilators, drugs that block alpha₁-adrenergic receptors are useful in patients with heart failure primarily because they reduce afterload, decreasing the workload of the heart and improving its ability to pump blood into the systemic arteries. Alpha blockers may also produce a beneficial effect in some patients by reducing preload where venous pressure is so high as to cause excessive stretching of the ventricular walls. Prazosin is the alpha blocker most commonly employed in heart failure. Alpha blockers are discussed in detail in Chapter 12.

DRUG CLASS • Beta Agonists

As described above, the body compensates for the failing heart by elevating sympathetic nervous system activity to increase the stimulation of cardiac beta receptors. Drugs that stimulate beta receptors on the heart to increase cardiac contractility are of limited value in the acute management of patients with severe heart failure. Those used most commonly for this purpose are dobutamine and dopamine, both of which must be given intravenously and have very short durations of action. Despite producing short-term improvement in patients with severe heart failure, these drugs also increase the risk of arrhythmia and do not decrease mortality. The pharmacology of these drugs is discussed in greater detail in Chapter 12.

DRUG CLASS • Beta-Adrenergic Antagonists (Beta Blockers)

The newest approach to the treatment of heart failure employs beta-adrenergic receptor blockers. As discussed above, one of the important ways that the body compensates for a failing heart is to increase activity of the sympathetic nervous system, which stimulates cardiac beta receptors. Therefore health care providers predicted that beta-blockers would make heart failure worse and avoided them in these patients for many years. Then, in a large clinical trial, the relatively new beta blocker, carvedilol, was shown to reduce risk of hospitalization in chronic heart failure and also to reduce risk of mortality from the disease, presumably by preventing arrhythmia arising from excess sympathetic stimulation. At first it was believed that some unique feature of carvedilol unrelated to beta-receptor blockade was responsible for the beneficial response to this drug. However, it now appears that blocking beta receptors in patients with heart failure gradually improves cardiac function. Although the precise mechanism is not known, the benefit derives at least in part from their ability to prevent and perhaps reverse the structural changes that develop over the course of progressive heart failure. As a result, beta-blockers are now widely used in the treatment of heart failure. To avoid acute decompensation that might result from sudden removal of sympathetic activity supporting the heart, treatment typically begins with a low dose increased gradually over time. Beta blockers are discussed in detail in Chapter 12.

APPLICATION TO PRACTICE

ASSESSMENT
History of Present Illness

The most common symptoms of heart failure are shortness of breath, often exertional at first and progressing to orthopnea, paroxysmal nocturnal dyspnea, and resting dyspnea. A more subtle and often overlooked symptom is a chronic nonproductive cough. Patients may also complain of fatigue, weakness, memory loss and confusion, palpitations, anorexia, and insomnia. With right-sided failure, the patient may complain of weight gain, peripheral edema, abdominal distension, gastric distress, anorexia, or nausea (Table 38-1).

Health History

The health history helps reveal the lifelong health record of the patient. The patient should be asked about child-

---

TABLE 38-1

Summary of Clinical Manifestations of Heart Failure

Parameter	Signs and Symptoms
Decreased cardiac output	Decreased blood pressure, pulse pressure, pulsus alternans Tachycardia Supraventricular arrhythmias, presence of S_3 gallop Anxiety, fear, irritability, fatigue, decreased exercise tolerance Chest pain Dizziness, syncope
Pulmonary congestion (left-sided ventricular failure)	Orthopnea, paroxysmal nocturnal dyspnea Cough with frothy sputum Tachypnea Bibasilar crackles Nocturia Increased PADP, PAWP
Systemic congestion (right-sided ventricular failure)	Nausea, vomiting, indigestion, abdominal distension, ascites Weakness Peripheral and sacral edema Hepatosplenomegaly Increased RAP

PADP, Pulmonary artery diastolic pressure; *PAWP*, pulmonary artery wedge pressure; *RAP*, right arterial pressure.

hood and infectious diseases, major illnesses, and hospitalizations. A drug history should be done with attention to the use of antihypertensives, diuretics, vasodilators, cardiac glycosides, anticoagulants, bronchodilators, oral contraceptives, and steroids. Corticosteroids cause hypertension and increase fluid retention. Oral contraceptives increase the risk of thrombophlebitis. Noncardiac drugs can also have profound effects on cardiovascular performance. For example, tricyclic antidepressants and other psychoactive drugs can potentiate arrhythmia. Cocaine increases the heart rate, contractility, blood glucose level, and peripheral vasoconstriction. It also potentiates the effects of circulating catecholamines.

Several other factors can predispose the patient to heart failure or may worsen its state. Elicit information from the patient regarding any history of anemia, thyrotoxicosis, pulmonary disease, and excessive sodium intake. Anemia requires increased cardiac output to meet the body's need for oxygen. Thyrotoxicosis increases the metabolic needs of the body, accelerating the heart rate and the workload of the heart. Pulmonary disease (e.g., chronic airway limitation, pulmonary emboli, primary pulmonary artery hypertension) increases pressure in the pulmonary system, producing sizeable resistance to the emptying of the right ventricle. An excess in circulating blood volume can result from poor renal function, cardiac disease, drugs (e.g., corticosteroids), or excessive sodium intake. Overadministration of parenteral fluids may aggravate preexisting heart failure. Infections and fever increase the oxygen demands of body tissues, and prolonged physical and emotional stress increase sympathetic nervous system tone and release of catecholamine. Stress increases heart rate, myocardial contractility, and blood pressure. Additionally, past myocardial infarction, arrhythmia, and rheumatic carditis also increase the workload of the heart.

Lifespan Considerations

Perinatal. The incidence of heart disease in pregnant women ranges from 0.5% to 2%; however, heart failure still ranks high among the causes of death during pregnancy. Rheumatic fever, once responsible for 88% of cardiac disease seen during pregnancy, is now on the decline, responsible for only about 50% of cardiac disease cases in pregnancy. Congenital disease now plays a more prominent role. Because of increases in total body water and changes in cardiovascular, renal, and hormonal function, a pregnant woman with a preexisting disorder has an increased risk of heart failure, thromboembolism, palpitations, and fluid retention. Although digoxin crosses placental membranes, it does not affect fetal cardiac function. However, this passage into fetal circulation can reduce maternal concentrations and require dosage adjustment. It should also be kept in mind that, just as myocardial contractility is increased, uterine contractility can be affected, leading to preterm labor. Thus the benefit of inotropic drugs should be balanced with the potential for harm to the mother and the fetus.

Pediatric. Heart failure in the pediatric population is most often the result of a surgically correctable structural abnormality. For example, septal defects can cause large left-to-right shunts, resulting in a volume load on the right ventricle. An obstruction to flow from the left ventricle, such as coarctation (narrowing) of the aorta, can cause increased pressure inside the ventricle. Heart failure can also be caused by arrhythmia, anemia, myocardial disease (e.g., myocarditis), sepsis, or hypertension. In addition to the usual symptoms of heart failure, the child may exhibit failure to thrive and feeding difficulties.

Older Adults. Heart failure in the older adult is a fairly common occurrence that increases with age. The physical changes of aging and comorbid diseases such as hypertension, coronary artery disease, bronchitis, and pneumonia influence the incidence of heart failure. Associated peripheral edema, shortness of breath, orthopnea, and weight gain reduce activity tolerance. Age-related changes, such as reduced elasticity and lumen size of vessels as well as an increase in blood pressure interfering with the blood supply to the heart muscle, make the heart work harder. The decreased cardiac reserves of the older adult limit the heart's ability to withstand the effects of disease or injury. Symptoms of heart failure in older patients include confusion, insomnia, wandering during the night, agitation, depression, anorexia, nausea, and weakness.

Cultural/Social Considerations

The psychosocial impact of heart failure on the patient should be assessed. If the patient smokes, inquire about the duration of the smoking habit and the number of cigarettes smoked daily. Cigarette smoking increases the risk of coronary artery disease, worsens hypertension, and contributes to heart failure.

Ask about the intake of caffeine or alcohol, even though there is no conclusive evidence that these substances increase the risk of heart disease. Nevertheless, caffeine increases the heart rate and blood pressure, both of which raise the myocardial workload and can precipitate heart failure. As heart failure worsens, patients may find that their activities of daily living and social activities are restricted because of dyspnea, chest pain, or peripheral edema. Furthermore, the social isolation that results may significantly affect the patient's ability to cope with his or her disease (see the Case Study: Chronic Heart Failure).

Physical Examination

The patient with acute-onset heart failure appears acutely ill but is usually well nourished. In severe failure, peripheral pulses may be weak and thready, and the extremities cool. Patients may exhibit air hunger (gasping for air) when lying flat. The patient with chronic heart failure often appears malnourished and sometimes even cachectic.

Physical examination findings of patients with heart failure include decreased blood and pulse pressures, pulsus alternans, tachycardia, and supraventricular ECG rhythms. The classic physical examination findings of left-sided heart failure include an S_3 gallop, tachypnea, bibasilar crackles, and an increase in pulmonary arterial diastolic and wedge pressures.

Characteristic findings of patients with right-sided heart failure include vomiting, jugular vein distension, peripheral and sacral edema, hepatosplenomegaly, ascites and abdominal distension, and increased right atrial pressure. Crackles are absent in right-sided failure.

Laboratory Testing

Several tests are useful in evaluating the patient with heart failure. Electrocardiography, exercise electrocardiography (stress testing), echocardiography, chest x-ray studies, ventriculography (multigated blood pool imaging [MUGA] scan), and cardiac catheterization are sometimes useful. Echocardiography provides information about chamber size and functional ability. A chest x-ray film may reveal prominent pulmonary vasculature, evidence suggestive of interstitial edema (Kerley B lines), pleural fluid in fissures, and evidence of pleural effusion.

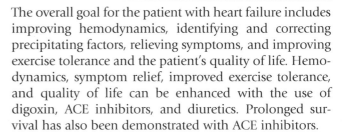

GOALS OF THERAPY

The overall goal for the patient with heart failure includes improving hemodynamics, identifying and correcting precipitating factors, relieving symptoms, and improving exercise tolerance and the patient's quality of life. Hemodynamics, symptom relief, improved exercise tolerance, and quality of life can be enhanced with the use of digoxin, ACE inhibitors, and diuretics. Prolonged survival has also been demonstrated with ACE inhibitors.

INTERVENTION

Intervention for the patient with heart failure begins by treating the underlying cause. If arrhythmia precipitated the failure, the arrhythmia should be treated accordingly. When the underlying cause is hypertension, antihypertensive drugs are helpful. Surgery may be required if valvular or septal defects are the contributing factors.

Treatment of acute heart failure begins with positioning of the patient. A high Fowler's position with the legs maintained in a dependent position as much as possible reduces pulmonary venous congestion and relieves dyspnea. Note that, although the legs may be edematous, elevation increases venous return to the heart, thus adding to its workload.

Oxygen administration by mask or cannula relieves hypoxia and dyspnea and improves oxygen–carbon dioxide exchange. Physical and emotional rest allow the patient to conserve energy and decrease the need for additional oxygen. The amount of rest needed depends on the severity of the heart failure. Bed rest with limited activity is most often prescribed for a patient with severe heart disease. A patient with mild heart failure may be ambulatory with restrictions placed on strenuous activities. For both mild and severe failure, rest periods should be planned between activities.

Administration

Drug labels should be read carefully when preparing a dose of any cardiac glycoside. Because of name similarity, especially between digoxin and digitoxin, care must be taken to avoid giving one drug for another. Dosage and potencies differ.

Oral cardiac glycoside formulations can be administered without regard to meals. However, if gastric irritation occurs, they can be taken with food or milk. Tablets can be crushed and administered with food or fluids if the patient has difficulty swallowing. A calibrating measuring device should be used for liquid formulations. Do not alternate between dosage forms. The bioavailability of capsules is not equal to that of tablets or an elixir.

Intramuscular administration of a cardiac glycoside is not recommended; however, when necessary, it should be given into the gluteal muscle and the area massaged well to reduce painful local reaction.

Rapid digitalization is reserved for the patient in acute distress. It is best accomplished in controlled environments equipped for continuous assessment of cardiac function and prompt treatment of serious arrhythmia. With rapid digitalization, drug toxicities become quickly evident. Intravenous administration may be particularly hazardous. Before administering the initial loading dose, determine if the patient has taken any cardiac glycoside preparation in the preceding 2 to 3 weeks. Intravenous formulations should be administered immediately after mixing and given over at least 5 minutes with the patient on a cardiac monitor. The excipient (i.e., propylene glycol) used in the diluent has a toxic effect on cardiac conduction if given too rapidly.

Slow digitalization may be accomplished on an outpatient basis with therapeutic levels gradually established over a period of 1 to 2 weeks. This period equates somewhat to the fourth half-life of the drug.

The patient's apical and radial pulse should be taken for 1 full minute before administering each dose of cardiac glycoside. Bradycardia is an adverse effect and an indication of toxicity. A slowing of the pulse rate is to be expected, and this alone does not warrant withholding the dose. However, a marked changed in the apical pulse rate, accompanied by changes in rhythm, warrants withholding the dose until consultation with the health care provider can take place. Guidelines may vary according to institution or provider. If bradycardia is present, the drug is ordinarily omitted and the health care provider notified when the pulse rate (taken before a scheduled dose) is less than 60 beats per minute, over 110 (under 90 in children), or unusually irregular.

Monitor intake, output, daily weight, vital signs, and heart and lung sounds. Assess for jugular vein distension. Use data from central venous or arterial lines if available. Assess for dependent edema in the sacral area and in the feet and ankles. Monitor serum drug levels of cardiac glycosides and for ECG changes. A long P-R interval (indicating depressed AV conduction rate), a shortened Q-T interval, and an altered P wave require evaluation before giving another dose of a cardiac glycoside. It is important to note, however, that not all rhythm disturbances are associated with high serum or tissue concentrations of cardiac glycosides and are not necessarily manifestations of toxicity. A low plasma concentration of a cardiac glycoside, though, does not preclude the possibility of drug-induced arrhythmia. Serum concentrations provide a crude, although useful, guide to the likelihood of efficacy and toxicity. A good rule of thumb when evaluating a new rhythm disturbance in a patient receiving a cardiac glycoside is to assume it is drug induced until proven otherwise.

When toxicity is diagnosed, the drug is discontinued. If the toxicity is severe, the timely administration of antigen-binding fragments of digoxin-specific antibody (Digibind) may be appropriate. This antibody, produced in sheep, acts antigenically to unbind the cardiac glycoside, decreasing the concentration of free drug available to interact with myocardial membranes. Total plasma concentration of the cardiac glycoside rises markedly because of binding to the antibody, but the fraction of free drug in the plasma is reduced to an extremely low level. Digibind is readily eliminated in the urine.

Monitor serum electrolyte levels, particularly potassium, calcium, and magnesium. Cardiac glycoside toxicity is aggravated by hypokalemia, and hyperkalemia and hypercalcemia can contribute to glycoside-induced arrhythmia. Recall that vomiting, chronic diarrhea, nasogastric suctioning, and alkalosis contribute to hypokalemia, as can administration of potassium-depleting diuretics, long-term corticosteroid or glucose therapy, and amphotericin B.

Monitor the platelet count in patients taking the phosphodiesterase-inhibitor drugs amrinone and milrinone. The dosage of amrinone may need to be reduced in the presence of thrombocytopenia. These drugs are used only in the acute-care environment. Be sure to keep the patient and family informed of the patient's condition.

Education

Patients should be taught the name of the drug, the dosage, and the reason for its use. Instruct the patient to take cardiac glycosides with meals or snacks to lessen gastric irritation. A large amount of fiber, however, may interfere with the absorption of the cardiac glycoside. Patients should be advised to take the drug at the same time each day to maintain more consistent blood levels and to assist in remembering to take the drug. If a dose is missed, it should be taken as soon as remembered; the dosage should not, however, be doubled. The health care provider should be contacted if dosages for 2 or more days are missed. Also advise the patient to avoid concurrent use of other drugs without first checking with the health care provider and to avoid taking antacids or antidiarrheal drugs within 2 hours of the glycoside.

The patient should be instructed not to mix digoxin tablets in pill containers with other drugs. Accidental poisoning of children with cardiac glycosides can occur. Patients who are around small children should be warned of the danger drugs pose to curious toddlers. Advise the patient to wear a medical identification tag or bracelet indicating that they are taking cardiac glycosides.

If appropriate for the patient's abilities, resources, and medical condition, instruct him or her to monitor and record the apical pulse and blood pressure regularly. Advise

---

CASE STUDY — *Chronic Heart Failure*

ASSESSMENT

HISTORY OF PRESENT ILLNESS

MB is a 70-year-old black man admitted for evaluation of increasing fatigue and ankle edema. Until recently he was able to remain active. During the past month, the persistent dyspnea confined him to his home. He reports that the dyspnea awakens him at night, and he sits by an open window to catch his breath. He reports he has lost his healthy appetite. He feels that the drugs he started 6 weeks ago are not working. Records indicate previous nondrug therapies have failed.

HEALTH HISTORY

MB had an acute MI 5 years ago with subsequent development of chronic heart failure. Since then he has had occasional premature ventricular contractions. Although he has a history of coronary artery disease, he attributes an otherwise healthy state to the fact that he never drank alcohol or smoked cigarettes and he always eats nutritious meals, including salads. "They are easy to fix and easy for my wife and me to eat. They are also cheaper than some other things." Current drugs: benazepril 20 mg po bid, furosemide 20 mg po qd.

LIFESPAN CONSIDERATIONS

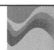

Age-related changes in cardiovascular, GI, and renal function; MB reports he is "simply waiting for [his] turn to meet God."

CULTURAL/SOCIAL CONSIDERATIONS

MB retired 3 years ago after 40 years as a railroad mechanic. On several occasions he has expressed concern that he will become a burden to his wife, who is 74 years old and physically unable to assume the responsibility for his care. He feels that if he needs changes in his drugs, he wants to go to once-daily dosing so he will remember to take it. MB has one son and one daughter who live nearby. They visit their parents regularly and help with transportation to the grocery store, medical appointments, and so forth. MB is covered by Medicare and a railroad supplemental insurance policy that includes pharmacy coverage. He and his wife live on his railroad retirement income.

PHYSICAL EXAMINATION

Height 5'8"; weight 135 pounds (up 9 lb from usual weight); blood pressure 130/70 mm Hg; respirations 28; temperature 98.6° F. Bibasilar breath sounds within normal limits on auscultation. 1+ pitting edema of ankles, liver enlargement present. Skin is pale, but no evidence of cyanosis. An S_3 gallop is present.

LABORATORY TESTING

Chest x-ray study reveals left ventricular enlargement with congestion of pulmonary vasculature (Kerley B lines), fluid level more prominent on right side than left. ECG reflects atrial fibrillation with apical rate of 124 beats per minute. Eight premature ventricular contractions per minute were noted. Sodium 131 mEq/L, potassium 3.8 mEq/L, chlorine 91 mEq/L, BUN 35 mg%, creatinine 1.6 mg%; thyroid-stimulating hormone (TSH) within normal limits.

PATIENT PROBLEM(S)

Heart failure.

GOALS OF THERAPY

Identify and correct precipitating factors; enhance cardiac performance; relieve symptoms; minimize adverse effects of drugs.

CRITICAL THINKING QUESTIONS

1. The health care provider's orders include increasing MB's dosage of benazepril to 40 mg po qd, keeping furosemide at 20 mg po qd, and adding digoxin 0.125 mg po qd with titration to effect. MB is already taking an ACE inhibitor. Why has the health care provider also ordered digoxin for MB?
2. What are the mechanisms of action for the drugs MB is taking?
3. Of which adverse effects should MB and the nurse be aware?
4. Should MB be increasing the potassium in his diet? If not, why not? Which potassium-containing products should MB be cautioned to avoid?
5. Which nursing actions are indicated before the administration of MB's drugs?
6. Which patient teaching is required for MB receiving these three drugs?

the patient to report a weight gain greater than 2 pounds (1 kg) per day or 5 pounds (2 kg) per week.

There are many drug interactions with the drugs used to treat heart failure. Remind patients to keep all health care providers informed of all drugs being taken and to avoid OTC drugs without first consulting with the health care provider.

Evaluate the patient's diet. Patients with heart disease may need instruction about sodium-restricted, weight-reduction, and low-cholesterol diets. Refer the patient to a dietitian as appropriate. Discuss the importance of maintaining an adequate potassium intake when taking cardiac glycosides. Review sources of dietary potassium (see Chapter 46). Many of the drugs used in the treatment of heart failure (e.g., diuretics, ACE inhibitors) may contribute to electrolyte disturbances, whereas other drugs (e.g., cardiac glycosides) are more toxic in the presence of abnormal electrolyte levels. Patients who are taking ACE inhibitors should not take potassium supplements.

One of the most common causes for exacerbation of heart failure is noncompliance with a low-sodium diet, even though control of excessive salt and water retention can be achieved through salt restriction. In the average American diet, sodium usually far exceeds the recommended daily allowance of intake. Approximately 4 g of sodium is contained in the average 10 g of table salt consumed daily. A 4-g sodium diet can be achieved by having the patient avoid salty foods and not add salt at the table. For people with more severe disease, a 2-g sodium diet may be prescribed that requires food be prepared without salt. It is unusual to restrict fluid intake except when severe heart failure with dilutional hyponatremia results. Patients should also be advised to check with their health care provider before using salt substitutes.

EVALUATION

The evaluation of therapy for heart failure is based on a comparison of the information obtained from the patient database and clinical findings. The desired effects of therapy include a decrease in pulse rate; slower, less labored respirations; diuresis accompanied by weight loss; less coughing; less distended neck veins, and better tolerance for exertion. Generally the evaluation criteria also include sufficient knowledge of the disease process and treatment regimen on the part of the patient to actively participate in the plan of care; maintenance of therapeutic blood levels; reduction in symptoms; compliance with dietary modifications; and an understanding of, and compliance with, an exercise regimen.

Bibliography

Hood WB Jr, Dans A, Guyatt GH, et al: Cochrane reviews: digitalis for treatment of congestive heart failure in patients in sinus rhythm, *Nurs Times* 97(34):40, 2001.

Kearney K: Emergency: digitalis toxicity, *Am J Nurs* 100(6):51-52, 2000.

Kim SD: Measurement of the renin-angiotensin system in heart failure, *Biol Res Nurs* 1(3):210-226, 2000.

Levine BS: Intermittent positive inotrope infusion in the management of end-stage, low-output heart failure, *J Cardiovasc Nurs* 14(4):76-93, 2000.

Newton JL, Johnson TW: Detecting digoxin toxicity, *Nursing* 30(12):49, 2000.

Piano MR, Kim SD, Jarvis C: Cellular events linked to cardiac remodeling in heart failure: targets for pharmacologic intervention, *J Cardiovasc Nurs* 14(4):1-23, 119-120, 2000.

Pinkowish MD: Beta-blockers and ACE inhibitors: new data, old myths, *Patient Care Nurse Pract* 3(7):36-38, 40, 43-44, 2000.

Rose SR: What's wrong with this patient?. . . digoxin toxicity, *RN* 63(2):31-33, 2000.

Tedesco C, Reigle J, Bergin J: Sudden cardiac death in heart failure, *J Cardiovasc Nurs* 14(4):38-56, 2000.

Internet Resources

http://www.emedicine.com/EMERG/topic108.htm.
http://www.heartpoint.com/congheartfailure.html.
http://www.nhlbi.nih.gov/health/public/heart/other/hrtfail.htm.

CHAPTER

39

Antianginal and Other Vasodilating Drugs

LYNN ROGER WILLIS • KATHLEEN GUTIERREZ

 Visit http://evolve.elsevier.com/Gutierrez/ for additional information.

KEY TERMS

Afterload, p. 622

Angina pectoris, p. 620

Atherosclerosis, p. 620

Classic angina, p. 621

Levine's sign, p. 630

Preload, p. 622

Unstable angina, p. 621

Variant angina (Prinzmetal's angina), p. 621

OBJECTIVES

- Discuss the role of coronary circulation in balancing oxygen demand and oxygen supply.
- Describe the causes of ischemic heart disease.
- Discuss the relationship between ischemic heart disease and angina pectoris.
- Identify the mechanism of action of drugs used in the treatment of ischemic heart disease.
- List and describe the adverse reactions caused by drugs used for the treatment of ischemic heart disease.
- Develop a nursing care plan for a patient using an antianginal drug.
- Explain the concepts of nitrate tolerance and nitrate toxicity.

PATHOPHYSIOLOGY • Angina Pectoris

CARDIAC ISCHEMIA AND ANGINA PECTORIS

The heart requires large amounts of oxygen and nutrients to meet its metabolic needs. The coronary circulation normally meets those needs by delivering oxygenated blood throughout the myocardium (Figure 39-1). Factors such as heart rate, ventricular wall tension, and ventricular contractility determine the need, or demand, of the heart muscle for oxygen. Because the heart extracts most of the available oxygen from the blood under normal resting conditions, an increase in oxygen demand, such as with exercise, requires the delivery of additional oxygen to the cardiac tissue via an increase in coronary blood flow. The increase in blood flow is mediated by dilation of the coronary vessels.

Angina pectoris, which literally means a choking of the chest, is the sensory response to a temporary insufficiency of oxygen (ischemia) in the heart. Cardiac ischemia occurs when the demand of the myocardium for oxygen exceeds the ability of the coronary vessels to supply that oxygen. The classic cause of cardiac ischemia is coronary artery disease, which prevents dilation of the coronary arterioles in response to increased oxygen demand by the myocardium. The resulting ischemia precipitates an attack of angina pectoris.

Approximately 1 of every 50 American adults develops coronary artery disease associated with **atherosclerosis,** a condition characterized by the accumulation of fatty deposits within the lining of the coronary arteries (Figure 39-2). As the deposits accumulate, the arterial lumen narrows such that resistance to blood flow through the affected arteries increases. Not only do atherosclerotic deposits in coronary arteries restrict blood flow, they also make it difficult for the affected arteries to dilate when they should. An inability to dilate and increase coronary blood flow sets the stage for an increase in oxygen demand by the heart to go unmet. To adjust for the gradual narrowing and reduction of coronary blood flow induced by atherosclerosis, new blood vessels (collateral circulation) will often develop to bypass the affected vessels and maintain adequate perfusion. However, if blood flow is compromised in a large enough area of the heart muscle, ischemic episodes can occur regardless of such adjustments and will precipitate attacks of angina pectoris.

Patients commonly describe attacks of angina pectoris as involving heavy, pressing (crushing) substernal discomfort, often radiating to the left shoulder. The dis-

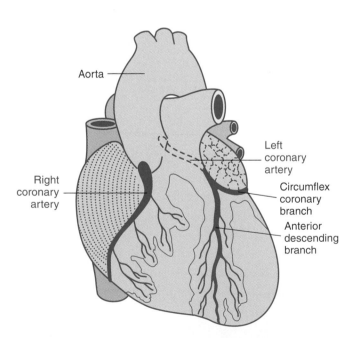

FIGURE 39-1 Coronary arteries. The three major coronary arteries are the right coronary artery and the two branches of the left coronary artery, the circumflex and the anterior descending branches. These arteries supply blood to the heart muscle. Occlusion of one or more of these arteries can cause angina.

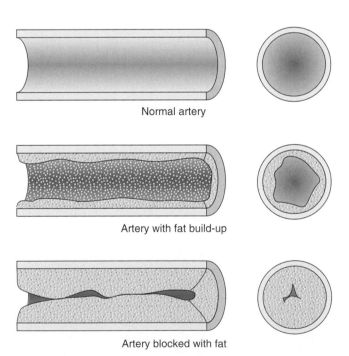

FIGURE 39-2 Schematic drawing of the stages of atherosclerotic plaque formation. Cross section of a normal artery and an artery altered by disease. The affected artery is obstructed by a mass of platelets, red blood cells, and cholesterol plaques and is indicative of coronary heart disease. With progressive disease the artery becomes almost completely obstructed.

comfort may also extend into the neck, jaw, teeth, arms, or elbows. An anginal attack gradually subsides when the victim stops the precipitating activity, thereby permitting the oxygen demand to come into balance with the oxygen supply.

Types of Angina

Classic angina is often called stable angina or exertional angina. In classic angina the large coronary arteries are obstructed by atherosclerosis to the point that blood flow cannot increase to supply more oxygen required by increased work. Coronary atherosclerosis is the most common cause of classic angina.

Variant angina (also called Prinzmetal's angina) has a different origin than classic angina: this form is caused by spasms of the large coronary arteries during which blood flow through the constricted arteriole is reduced. The coronary spasms have no relationship to exercise and may occur at rest. Variant angina often has a daily rhythm, with episodes often occurring more frequently in the morning. Many patients with variant angina also have coronary atherosclerosis and therefore are also susceptible to angina attacks associated with exertion.

Unstable angina refers to angina that has a changing intensity. Attacks of angina pectoris come at decreasing levels of exertion and often at rest. Unstable angina seems to involve rupture of atherosclerotic plaques, with accompanying formation of thrombi. Patients who progress to unstable angina are the most likely to have a heart attack. Consequently, the therapy for patients with unstable angina extends beyond the usual therapy for stable and variant angina and is discussed below.

The treatment of angina begins with recognition that the supply of oxygen to the heart no longer meets the demand. Accordingly, therapy aimed at decreasing oxygen demand may include control of factors known to affect coronary oxygen supply and demand (i.e., smoking, overweight, hypertension, arrhythmia, anxiety, anemia, and lack of regular exercise). The major risk factors for the progression of atherosclerosis are cigarette smoking, hypertension, and a high serum cholesterol level. Evidence confirms the view that reducing or altering these risk factors prolongs life in patients with angina related to coronary atherosclerosis.

The major drugs used to treat angina are the nitrovasodilators, beta blockers, and calcium channel blockers. All of these drugs restore the balance between myocardial oxygen supply and demand by dilating the coronary vasculature or by reducing the workload of the heart by reducing heart rate, left ventricular wall tension, or contractility. Additional drugs for use in patients with atherosclerosis include antiplatelet drugs, such as aspirin (see Chapter 43), to prevent the formation of platelet thrombi, and lipid-lowering drugs (see Chapter 42) to slow the progression of atherosclerosis.

When long-standing atherosclerosis causes severe and frequent angina, coronary artery bypass surgery may be indicated. In this type of surgery, one or more of the main coronary vessels is bypassed with a graft from the aorta to the lower end of the vessel. Replacement of vessels severely narrowed by atherosclerosis greatly improves coronary blood flow. About 70% of patients have no further angina, and another 20% have markedly reduced angina.

Percutaneous transluminal coronary angioplasty is a nonsurgical procedure for opening a coronary artery narrowed by atherosclerosis. The tip of a balloon catheter is inserted into a peripheral artery and threaded into the narrowed coronary artery. Inflation of the balloon disrupts the atherosclerotic deposit, widens the constriction, and permits greater blood flow through the vessel. This procedure is most effective in patients with severe angina who have only one severely narrowed coronary artery.

The treatment of angina pectoris aims at relieving or preventing acute attacks of angina. Organic nitrates primarily offer acute relief of attacks. Beta blockers offer long-term prevention of attacks in classic angina. Calcium channel blockers are especially effective in relieving and preventing the arteriolar spasms of variant angina, but they are also used in the treatment of classic angina.

The ideal antianginal drug would establish a balance between coronary blood flow and the metabolic demands of the heart. It would produce local effects by acting directly on coronary vessels rather than on other organ systems and promote oxygen extraction by the heart from arterial circulation. The drug would be effective when taken orally and would have sustained action. The ideal drug would also not build tolerance. No drug currently meets these ideals.

DRUG CLASS • Organic Nitrovasodilators

isosorbide dinitrate (Isordil, Sorbitrate, Dilatrate-SR, ISDN, Iso-Bid, Isordil, Sorbitrate SA, Apo-ISDN,✳ Cedocard-SR,✳ Coronex✳

isosorbide mononitrate (Imdur, Ismo, Monoket)

⚠ nitroglycerin (Nitrostat, Nitro-Bid IV, Nitrolingual, Nitroglyn, Nitrodisc, Transderm-Nitro, Nitro-Dur)

MECHANISM OF ACTION

Of the general mechanisms by which nitrates may relieve an attack of angina pectoris, their ability to reduce myocardial oxygen demand appears to be the most important. At low doses, nitrates preferentially cause dilation of veins over arterioles, resulting in a pooling of blood in the periphery, which in turn reduces venous return to the heart, left end-diastolic pressure, and left end-diastolic volume (preload). Reduced filling (i.e., volume) of the left ventricle reduces the workload of the heart because less force must be generated to eject the smaller amount of blood. The heart therefore requires less oxygen to do its work, and the anginal discomfort is relieved. Nitrates do not directly change the force of myocardial contraction (inotropy) or heart rate (chronotropy).

At high doses, nitrates dilate arteriolar tissue as well as venous smooth muscle. Arterioles control the vascular resistance to flow, depending on their state of contraction, and it is this resistance (from which is derived the diastolic pressure or afterload) that the ventricles must overcome to eject the cardiac output. Accordingly, arteriolar relaxation induced by the nitrates will, by reducing afterload, reduce the work required of the ventricles to eject blood. A reduction of workload reduces oxygen demand. Unfortunately, arteriolar dilation may reduce afterload (diastolic blood pressure) to the point that autonomic cardiovascular reflexes are activated. The resulting reflex stimulation of the heart (increased heart rate, increased force of contraction) may increase myocardial oxygen demand to the point that the anginal pain is not relieved.

The mechanism by which nitrates relax vascular smooth muscle involves the metabolic conversion of the nitrates to nitric oxide, which activates guanylate cyclase and leads to an increase of cyclic guanosine

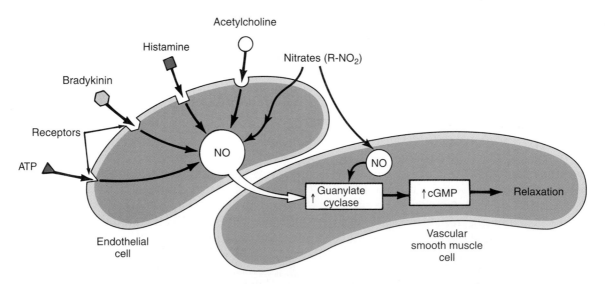

FIGURE 39-3 Nitric oxide (NO) is a very potent vasodilator. Endothelial cells produce nitric oxide from arginine, an amino acid, in response to various substances such as acetylcholine, histamine, bradykinin, and adenosine triphosphate (ATP). Nitrates are also broken down to nitric oxide in endothelial and vascular smooth muscle cells. Nitric oxide stimulates the enzyme, guanylate cyclase, which produces a second-messenger cyclic guanosine monophosphate (cGMP); cGMP activates intracellular events that result in vasodilation.

monophosphate (cGMP) within the smooth muscle cells and subsequent relaxation (Figure 39-3).

USES

For more than 100 years nitroglycerin, an ester of nitric acid, has been the drug of choice for treating attacks of angina pectoris. Today nitroglycerin and the other nitrates remain the major drugs for relieving acute attacks of angina and for preventing attacks. Nitrates are also effective and inexpensive drugs of choice for patients with heart failure or impaired left ventricular function (i.e., ejection fraction less than 40%). The nitrates can be used alone or with beta blockers and calcium channel blockers. Nitrate products may also be used to increase the exercise capacity of patients with coronary artery disease. They can be used in such patients even when mitral valve regurgitation is present. Nitrate products are also used as first-line drugs for patients with angina who also have chronic obstructive pulmonary disease, diabetes mellitus, and intermittent claudication. They are second-line drugs for patients with hypertension and Raynaud's phenomenon.

Oral nitrates have a long history of safety and effectiveness as well as low cost. Because they lack serious adverse effects, they are often used in patients in whom beta blockers are ineffective or are not tolerated.

PHARMACOKINETICS

The preferred drug for rapid relief of the symptoms of angina pectoris is nitroglycerin because the onset of action occurs within 1 to 3 minutes when it is administered as a sublingual or buccal tablet. Isosorbide dinitrate can also be administered by the sublingual or buccal routes with nearly as rapid an onset (2 to 5 minutes). Isosorbide mononitrate is not available for sublingual or buccal administration.

Although oral absorption of the nitrates is effective, oral bioavailability is essentially zero for nitroglycerin and approximately 20% for isosorbide dinitrate (Table 39-1). Hepatic reductases readily remove nitrate groups from these molecules and account for the extensive first-pass biotransformation and short elimination half-lives of these drugs. In contrast, the oral bioavailability of isosorbide mononitrate is nearly 100% because the mononitrate is not a good substrate for the hepatic reductases. Isosorbide mononitrate, in fact, is the active metabolite formed by the biotransformation of isosorbide dinitrate.

The low degree of bioavailability notwithstanding, oral extended-release dosage forms are available for both nitroglycerin and isosorbide dinitrate. Attaining a desired serum concentration in the blood by oral administration of a drug with low bioavailability simply requires a dose that is high enough to overwhelm the hepatic enzymes responsible for the first-pass biotransformation of the drug. Accordingly, extended-release tablets of nitroglycerin contain more of the drug per tablet than would be necessary in sublingual or buccal tablets. By comparison, higher oral versus sublingual doses of isosorbide dinitrate are not required, because the product of the first-pass biotransformation of the dinitrate is the mononitrate, which itself is active and capable of relieving the symptoms of angina pectoris. Extended-release forms of these drugs are designed to be taken every 8 to 12 hours.

Nitroglycerin is also available as an aerosol; the drug is sprayed in a metered dose on or under the tongue. The aerosol provides an alternative to sublingual tablets in the short-term relief of an anginal attack.

Because of its very high degree of lipid solubility, nitroglycerin may also be administered through the skin in an ointment or in a transdermal adhesive patch. Both dosage forms provide sustained absorption of the drug for several hours at a time and are intended to provide continuous protection from the symptoms of an anginal attack.

ADVERSE REACTIONS AND CONTRAINDICATIONS

In general, the adverse effects of nitrates are almost all secondary to their action on the cardiovascular system. The decreased afterload produced by arteriolar dilation causes hypotension. The reduced preload and cardiac output may cause hypotension, which is most noticeable when the patient assumes an upright position. Transient episodes of syncope (dizziness, weakness, and other symptoms of postural hypotension) may develop particularly when the patient stands immobile. However, even with the most severe syncopal episode, positioning and other strategies that facilitate venous return to the heart usually are the only therapeutic measures needed.

Approximately 50% of patients receiving nitrates for acute attacks of angina experience flushing of the face and neck as well as a pounding headache soon after administration. This headache is probably caused by dilation of meningeal blood vessels. Such headaches usually disappear after several days of continued treatment and often can be effectively controlled through reduction of the nitrate dosage. They occur less commonly with long-term prophylaxis therapy.

Other adverse reactions of the nitrates are blurred vision, dry mouth, and peripheral edema. Methemoglobinemia (a condition in which more than 1% of hemoglobin in the blood is oxidized to the ferric form) may occur if large, continuous doses of nitrates are administered. The principal sign of methemoglobinemia is

TABLE 39-1

Pharmacokinetics of Selected Antianginal Drugs

Drug	Route	Onset	Peak	Duration	PB (%)	$t_{1/2}$	BioA (%)
Nitrates*							
amyl nitrate	Inh	30 sec	UK	3-5 min		UA	UA
isosorbide dinitrate, isosorbide mononitrate	SL or chewable	2-5 min	30-60 min	1-2 hr		50 min, 5 hr†	22
	po	15-40 min	UK	4-6 hr		UA	100‡
	SR	Slow	3-4 hr	8-12 hr		UA	UA
nitroglycerin	SL	1-3 min	3-5 min	30-60 min	60	1-4 min	12-64
	IV	1-2 min	UK	3-5 min			100
	Buccal	2-4 min	UK	3-5 hr			UA
	Ointment	30-60 min	UK	2-12 hr			52-92
	TD	30-60 min	UK	18-24 hr			52-92
	po/SR	40-60 min	3-4 hr	4-8 hr			<1
	TL	2 min	UK	30-60 min			UA
Nonselective Beta Blockers§							
nadolol	po	>5 days	2-4 hr	24 hr	30	16-18 hr	29-39
propranolol	po	30 min	60-90 min	6-12 hr	90	3.4-6 hr	16-36
	po/ER	UK	6 hr	24 hr	90	3.4-6 hr	UA
	IV	2 min	1 min‖	4-6 hr	90	3-6 hr	100
Selective Beta Blockers§							
atenolol	po	60 min	2-4 hr	24 hr	<5	6-9 hr	26-86
metoprolol	po	30-60 min	90 min	24 hr	12	3-7 hr	24-52
	IV	Immediate	20 min	5-8 hr	12	3-4 hr	100
Calcium Channel Blockers							
amlodipine	po	UK	UK	24 hr	UA	30-50 hr	64-90
bepridil	po	8 days¶	UK	24 hr	UA	42 hr**	UA
diltiazem	po	30 min	2-3 hr	4-8 hr	70-85	3-5 hr	UA
felodipine	po	60 min	2-4 hr	Up to 24 hr	99	11-16 hr	UA
isradipine	po	<2 hr	2-3 hr	12 hr	95	8 hr	64-90
nicardipine	po	20 min	0.5-2 hr	8 hr	>95	2-4 hr	UA
nifedipine	po	20 min	30 min	2.5-3 hr	92-98	2-5 hr	UA
verapamil	po	30 min	1-2 hr	4-8 hr	83-92	3-7 hr	UA
	SR	UK	5-7 hr	24 hr	83-92	4-12 hr	UA

BioA, Bioavailability; *ER*, extended release; *Inh*, inhaled; *IV*, intravenous; *NA*, not applicable, *PB*, protein binding; *po*, by mouth; *SL*, sublingual; *SR*, sustained release; $t_{1/2}$, elimination half-life; *TD*, transdermal patch; *TL*, translingual spray; *UA*, unavailable; *UK*, unknown.
*Cardiovascular effects of nitrates.
†Half-life values for isosorbide dinitrate and isosorbide mononitrate, respectively.
‡Bioavailability calculations from single doses, because systemic clearance may be reduced with long-term use of isosorbide formulations.
§Because beta blockers are not used for relief of acute anginal pain, their onset of action is difficult to measure.
‖Antianginal effects of propranolol are manifest at 15-90 mcg/mL to achieve a 50% decrease in exercise-induced cardioacceleration.
¶Onset of steady-state antianginal effects with long-term dosing of bepridil.
**Half-life of bepridil following cessation of multiple dosing.

cyanosis, which occurs because the oxidized hemoglobin is unable to transport oxygen.

Organic nitrates occasionally produce a rash. Rashes caused by isosorbide mononitrate are reported less often than rashes caused by isosorbide dinitrate. There is also less facial flushing and halitosis with the mononitrate formulation of isosorbide.

Patients with recent head trauma should not take nitrates because of the increase in cerebrospinal fluid pressure. Patients for whom hypotension is a risk, espe-

---

BOX **39-1**	**Patient Problems**

The Problem: Nitrate Tolerance

Long-term, repeated exposure to high-dose nitrates leads to a decrease in the magnitude of most of the drug's effects, even if the dosage is progressively increased. Patients appear to develop tolerance not just to specific nitrates but to the entire class of drugs. Furthermore, the therapeutic implications of this phenomenon (i.e., the loss of the drug's effectiveness) are likely to proliferate as increasingly higher dosages of oral and transdermal formulations are used.

The Solution

To minimize tolerance, nitrate therapy should be individualized by using the lowest effective dose and an intermittent dosing schedule. Drug holidays—brief periods of no therapy—may be sufficient to avoid the development of tolerance. Although such actions may minimize tolerance, there is a disadvantage to nitrate-free periods. The shortest drug-free period that fosters nitrate effectiveness is unknown. Thus, in some patients, symptoms may worsen toward the end of the drug-free interval. Tolerance has not been reported with buccal forms of nitroglycerin, possibly because of the drug-free interval at night.

The Problem: Nitrate Toxicity

Nitrate toxicity causes dose-dependent hypotension and reflex tachycardia. A simultaneous increase in oxygen demand and a decrease in oxygen supply contribute to myocardial ischemia and the possibility of a MI. Severe hypotension, although rare, may cause cerebral ischemia and stroke.

The Solution

Proper management includes temporarily stopping the nitrate, because the drug's short duration of action usually allows blood pressure to rise in a relatively short period. If an intentional overdose was taken orally, induced emesis and other measures to decrease drug absorption may be indicated. Vasopressors may be given to correct excessive hypotension. However, they should be used with caution to avoid coronary artery vasoconstriction that can further aggravate angina. Epinephrine should not be used, because it may reduce myocardial blood flow and oxygen supply by reducing diastolic pressure and because it almost always increases oxygen demands by causing tachycardia. Oxygen therapy improves saturation and assists in meeting tissue oxygenation needs. It also helps relieve the dyspnea associated with ischemic episodes.

---

cially after a myocardial infarction (MI), should not take these drugs.

TOXICITY

Severe hypotension associated with the use of nitrates is usually transitory (Box 39-1). This hypotension is often accompanied by a reflex increase in heart rate, which increases the workload of the heart and may worsen or precipitate anginal attacks.

INTERACTIONS

Alcohol, beta blockers, calcium channel blockers, and antidepressants enhance the hypotensive effects of nitrates. Patients taking drugs with an anticholinergic action may have a dry mouth that delays dissolution of sublingual and buccal preparations.

DRUG CLASS • Beta Blockers

Nonselective

labetalol (Normodyne, Trandate)

nadolol (Corgard, Syn-Nadolol✳)

pindolol (Visken, Novo-Pindol,✳ Syn-Pindolol✳)

propranolol (Inderal, Inderal LA, Apo-Propranolol✳)

Selective

acebutolol (Sectral, Monitan✳)

atenolol (Tenormin, Apo-Atenolol,✳ Novo-Atenolol✳)

metoprolol (Lopressor, Toprol-XL, Betaloc,✳ Betaloc Durules,✳ Lopresor,✳ Lopresor SR,✳ Novometoprol✳)

MECHANISM OF ACTION

Beta-blocking drugs (see Chapter 12) do not dilate the coronary or systemic vasculature, but they are highly effective in the management of angina pectoris. They are effective because they decrease the oxygen requirements of the heart by reducing heart rate, blood pressure, and myocardial contractility. There is no evidence that any particular beta blocker is better than another in the management of angina, but patients with asthma, diabetes, or peripheral vascular disease are better able to tolerate the selective beta$_1$ blockers.

USES

Beta blockers effectively reduce the severity and frequency of exertional attacks of angina and constitute an effective treatment for angina pectoris second only to nitrates. Patients taking a beta blocker for angina usually note improved exercise tolerance and report a decrease in the number and severity of attacks. Beta blockers are often used as first-line therapy in conjunction with sublingual nitroglycerin for patients with angina who have no comorbid conditions. They can also be used as first-line drugs in patients who have hyperthyroidism, intermittent claudication, or migraine headaches. Other uses for these drugs are discussed in Chapters 12, 40, and 41.

PHARMACOKINETICS

Beta blockers are administered orally or by injection. The frequency of administration depends on the drug.

Beta blockers are generally well absorbed after oral administration and, with the exceptions of nadolol (which is eliminated unchanged in the urine) and esmolol (which is hydrolyzed in plasma), are biotransformed in the liver. Metabolites of the beta blockers are generally eliminated in the urine, although some metabolites are excreted in the feces through the biliary system. The pharmacokinetic properties of the beta blockers are listed in Table 39-1.

ADVERSE REACTIONS AND CONTRAINDICATIONS

Adverse reactions to beta blockers occur most commonly at the start of treatment. Hypotension, bradycardia, and bronchospasm are potentially harmful. Because of the negative inotropic effect and possible increase in preload produced by beta blockers, heart failure may be precipitated or exacerbated. The rapid discontinuance of a beta blocker in susceptible patients may precipitate an anginal attack, hypertension, arrhythmia (especially atrioventricular block), or an acute MI.

Adverse effects of the beta blockers centered in the CNS include dizziness, fatigue, lethargy, confusion, depression, and decreased libido. The gastrointestinal reactions—nausea, vomiting, and diarrhea—are usually transient.

Significant bronchoconstriction may result from blockade of beta receptors. Although this reaction is more likely to occur with the nonselective beta blockers (e.g., nadolol and propranolol), it can also occur with high doses of the beta$_1$-selective drugs (e.g., atenolol and metoprolol).

Beta blockers are contraindicated in patients with variant angina. The deleterious effect of beta blockers on variant angina probably results from an increase in coronary resistance caused by the unopposed effects of catecholamines on alpha receptors.

Nonselective beta blockers are also contraindicated in patients with acute bronchospasm, some forms of valvular heart disease, bradyarrhythmia, and heart block. The drugs should be used cautiously in pregnant and lactating women because they may cause fetal bradycardia and hypoglycemia.

INTERACTIONS

Excessive hypotension may occur when beta blockers are given with calcium channel blockers.

DRUG CLASS • Calcium Channel Blockers

amlodipine (Norvasc)

bepridil (Vascor)

diltiazem (Cardizem, Cardizem SR, Cardizem CD, Dilacor XR)

felodipine (Plendil)

isradipine (DynaCirc)

nicardipine (Cardene, Cardene SR)

nifedipine (Adalat, Adalat CC, Procardia, Procardia XL)

verapamil (Calan, Calan SR, Isoptin, Isoptin SR, Verelan)

MECHANISM OF ACTION

The contractile response of vascular smooth muscle and cardiac cells is mediated by calcium ions that enter through calcium channels opened in response to depolarizing stimuli. Calcium channel blockers prevent the contractile response by binding to the calcium channels and preventing the flow of calcium into the cells. The net effect of this blockade in blood vessels and heart muscle is to relax vascular smooth muscle (a desired effect) and reduce myocardial contractility (an undesirable action). Calcium channel blockers also depress the calcium current in cardiac pacemaker cells (the sinoatrial node) and conductive tissue (the atrioventricular node), slowing both heart rate and AV conduction.

Calcium channel blockers dilate coronary arteries more selectively than they inhibit cardiac contractility. Without this selective preference, the calcium channel blockers would be clinically less useful because they might overly compromise cardiac function. The various drugs of this class differ in the degree of selectivity for causing coronary vasodilation or decreased cardiac contractility (see Chapter 40).

USES

Calcium channel blockers are useful additions to antianginal therapy if nitrates and beta blockers are ineffective. Calcium channel blockers provide long-term prevention of anginal attacks, particularly those associated with variant angina, principally by reducing the workload of the heart. Although the greatest usefulness for these drugs lies with the treatment of variant angina, varying degrees of coronary spasm occur even in classic angina. Consequently there also is a place for them in the treatment of classic angina. Patients with asthma, diabetes mellitus, and peripheral vascular disease who cannot tolerate beta blockers often benefit from calcium channel blockers. Calcium channel blockers are also cur-

rently used in the treatment of certain types of arrhythmia (see Chapter 40) and hypertension (see Chapter 41).

In patients with stable angina who are inadequately controlled with nitrates and beta blockers, the use of a calcium channel blocker with a beta blocker may provide some improvement, but only the dihydropyridines (nicardipine, nifedipine) should be used in conjunction with a beta blocker. The beta blocker lessens the reflex tachycardia caused by the nifedipine. During exercise, the combined use of nifedipine and propranolol achieves a lower heart rate and blood pressure than are observed when either drug is taken alone.

PHARMACOKINETICS

Calcium channel blockers are effective when given orally. They are subject to significant first-pass effect, are highly bound to plasma proteins, and are all subject to extensive hepatic biotransformation. In most cases the metabolites, most of which are inactive, are eliminated in the urine. All of the calcium channel blockers have a relatively rapid onset of action, reaching peak serum levels in 1 to 2 hours. Specific information on these pharmacokinetic parameters is given in Table 39-1.

ADVERSE REACTIONS AND CONTRAINDICATIONS

Because calcium channel blockers decrease afterload and the force of ventricular contraction, they sometimes cause hypotension. Arrhythmia (e.g., bradycardia or tachycardia) and chest pain can occur as the result of inhibition of sinoatrial (SA) and atrioventricular (AV) nodes, particularly with verapamil and diltiazem. The depressant action on myocardial contractility can contribute to the onset or worsening of heart failure. Peripheral edema is possible and is more likely to occur with amlodipine and nifedipine because of the greater tendency for these drugs to reduce arterial pressure and renal perfusion pressure, which promotes the retention of sodium and water.

The vasodilating effect of calcium channel blockers predictably causes dizziness, tachycardia, headache, flushing, and weakness, especially with nicardipine and nifedipine. Other possible adverse effects of calcium channel blockers are dry mouth, anorexia, dyspepsia, nausea (especially with bepridil), vomiting, constipation, diarrhea, and abnormal liver function values. Some patients complain of weight gain, muscle cramps, and joint stiffness associated with these drugs.

A rash or dermatitis, pruritus, and urticaria have been reported with calcium channel blockers, particularly nifedipine, but are less likely to occur with verapamil. Stevens-Johnson syndrome, a rare reaction characterized by severe rash and fever, may be fatal.

Contraindications to the use of calcium channel blockers include hypersensitivity, sick sinus syndrome (severe sinus tachycardia and/or bradycardia with or without AV block), and second- or third-degree heart block (unless a pacemaker is in place). Patients whose systolic blood pressure is less than 90 mm Hg should avoid bepridil, diltiazem, and verapamil. A recent MI or the presence of pulmonary congestion contraindicates diltiazem. Verapamil is contraindicated in patients with heart failure, severe ventricular dysfunction, cardiogenic shock, severe bradycardia, or hypotension.

Calcium channel blockers should be used with caution in patients with severe hepatic or renal dysfunction or those with a history of serious ventricular arrhythmia or heart failure. The safe use of these drugs during pregnancy and lactation has not been established.

INTERACTIONS

Calcium channel blockers may interact with several other drugs. Beta blockers and calcium channel blockers, if given concurrently, may block conduction or cause arrhythmia and hypotension. Diltiazem and verapamil may inhibit the hepatic biotransformation of several drugs, including carbamazepine, cyclosporine, quinidine, theophylline, and valproate, causing potentially toxic concentrations of such drugs to accumulate. Cardiac glycosides such as digoxin may also accumulate to toxic levels in the presence of calcium channel blockers.

 DRUG CLASS • Other Vasodilating Drugs

diazoxide (Hyperstat, Proglycem)

fenoldopam (Corlopam)

hydralazine (Apresoline)

minoxidil (Loniten, Rogaine)

sildenafil (Viagra)

sodium nitroprusside (Nitropress)

MECHANISM OF ACTION

All of the drugs within this class, though chemically diverse and acting through different mechanisms of action, dilate vascular smooth muscle. Hydralazine relaxes arteriolar smooth muscle by an unknown mechanism, but it has no effect on venous smooth muscle. Minoxidil and diazoxide open ATP-modulated potassium channels in arteriolar smooth muscle cells. Potassium ions diffuse through these channels out of the cells, thereby hyperpolarizing the cells, suppressing the contractile mechanism, relaxing the smooth muscle, and dilating the blood vessels. These drugs have no apparent effect on venous smooth muscle.

Sodium nitroprusside is biotransformed in endothelial cells to the powerful vasodilator, nitric oxide, which dilates arterial and venous smooth muscle through the generation of cGMP (as discussed under organic nitrates). Sodium nitroprusside is not an organic nitrate; indeed, the enzymes that convert it to nitric oxide are different from those that generate nitric oxide from the organic nitrates. The end result, in either case, is vasodilation.

Fenoldopam relaxes arteriolar smooth muscle by stimulating the D_1 (dopamine) receptor subtype. The drug is indicated for the short-term intravenous management of severe hypertension (see Chapter 12).

Sildenafil inhibits an enzyme, phosphodiesterase, that catalyzes the metabolic breakdown of cGMP, which is a mediator of nitric oxide–induced vasodilation. Accordingly, sildenafil enhances and prolongs the vasodilating effect of cGMP. In the penis, this effect translates into an enhanced and prolonged erectile response in patients with erectile dysfunction.

USES

Hydralazine and minoxidil are effective when given orally and are used for long-term management of hypertension, although they are not first-line drugs for this purpose and are only used in combination with other antihypertensive drugs, such as diuretics. Hydralazine has also been used as an adjunct in the treatment of severe heart failure, where it reduces afterload (see Chapter 38). Topical minoxidil has also proven profitable as an aid to the treatment and prevention of male pattern baldness.

Diazoxide, nitroprusside, and fenoldopam are administered parenterally and find widest usage in the management of hypertensive emergencies.

Sildenafil has no real utility in the management of hypertension; instead, it has assumed a unique niche in the treatment of male erectile dysfunction.

PHARMACOKINETICS

The pharmacokinetics of these drugs is summarized in Table 39-2. Hydralazine is well absorbed via the GI tract but undergoes extensive first-pass biotransformation in the liver, thus accounting for its low degree of bioavailability. The major pathway for biotransformation of hydralazine involves acetylation, which exhibits bimodal distribution among the population (i.e., patients are ei-

TABLE 39-2

Pharmacokinetics of Selected Direct-Acting Peripheral Vasodilators

Drug	Route	Onset	Peak	Duration	PB (%)	$t_{1/2}$	BioA (%)
diazoxide	IV	Immediate	5 min	3-12 hr	>90	21-45 hr	100
fenoldopam	IV	Immediate	NA	20-30 min	NA	5 min	100
hydralazine	po	45 min	2 hr	3-8 hr	87	2-8 hr	UA
	IM	10-30 min	1 hr				UA
	IV	10-20 min	15-30 min				100
minoxidil	po	30 min	2-3 hr	2-5 days	0	4.2 hr	UA
nitroprusside	IV	Immediate	Rapid	1-10 min	UA	2 min	100
sildenafil	po	30 min	1-2 hr	2 hr	96	4 hr	40

BioA, Bioavailability; *NA*, not available; *PB*, protein binding; $t_{1/2}$, elimination half-life; *UA*, unavailable.

ther fast or slow acetylators of hydralazine). Dose for dose, fast acetylators will show a lower degree of bioavailability, shorter half-lives, and reduced efficacy for hydralazine than will slow acetylators. Conversely, slow acetylators are more likely to experience adverse effects and toxicity from accumulation of the drug unless the dosage is reduced. Most persons are fast acetylators of hydralazine.

Minoxidil is biotransformed to active metabolites, a process which prolongs the duration of the antihypertensive effect of the drug to approximately 24 hours. The principal active metabolite is minoxidil sulfate. Topical use of minoxidil for promotion of hair growth on the scalp results in very little systemic absorption of the drug (1% to 4%). That which is absorbed undergoes renal elimination within 4 days. Up to 4 months of twice-daily application of the lotion is required before significant hair growth occurs. The hair growth stops and the new hair falls out if daily use of the drug is discontinued.

Diazoxide is well absorbed orally, but it is used clinically by the intravenous route for hypertensive emergencies. Up to 50% of an administered dose is eliminated unchanged in the urine.

Nitroprusside is administered only by intravenous drip and lowers blood pressure within seconds of being infused. The drug is rapidly biotransformed to cyanide and nitric oxide. The cyanide is converted to thiocyanate by hepatic rhodanase and is eliminated in the urine. The rapid rate of biotransformation for nitroprusside gives it a short duration of action; blood pressure returns to pretreatment values within 1 to 10 minutes after the infusion is stopped.

Fenoldopam is administered as an intravenous drip. Its antihypertensive action is immediate and persists for about half an hour after the infusion is stopped (the drug's half-life is 5 minutes). These pharmacokinetic characteristics dictate that the initial infusion rate be low and then be titrated upward until the desired reduction of blood pressure is attained.

Sildenafil is rapidly absorbed after oral administration, but food in the stomach can delay the onset of action of the drug by up to an hour. The drug is demethylated to an active metabolite with properties similar to the parent drug. The half-life for both is 4 hours, and both molecules undergo further biotransformation to inactive products. Most of the drug is eliminated as the metabolite; 80% of the metabolites are eliminated in the feces.

ADVERSE REACTIONS AND CONTRAINDICATIONS

Adverse effects common to all of the vasodilator drugs include, to varying degrees, reflex tachycardia, palpitations, dizziness, postural hypotension, and retention of salt and water. All of these reactions are directly the result of systemic vasodilation, which activates compensatory mechanisms intended to restore the blood pressure to the pretreatment value. The tachycardia and palpitations reflect the reflex activation of sympathetic nerves, and the dizziness and postural hypotension reflect the pooling of blood in the lower extremities when the patient assumes the upright posture. The sodium and water retention occurs because systemic vasodilation reduces renal perfusion pressure, which reduces glomerular filtration and activates the renin-angiotensin-aldosterone axis. Retention of sodium and water normally creates medical problems for patients only after the vasodilator drugs have been administered for a long time (days or weeks). Combination therapy with a thiazide diuretic can neutralize or minimize this adverse effect.

Hydralazine may cause a reversible lupuslike syndrome or a more serious but less common serum sickness or drug fever. These effects appear to have an immunologic basis. The incidence rate of adverse effects is low with usual doses of hydralazine but rises substantially in slow acetylators of the drug. Contraindications to the use of hydralazine include coronary artery disease, allergy to the drug, and mitral valve disease such as that associated with rheumatic fever (the drug may elevate pulmonary artery pressure in these patients).

Long-term systemic therapy with minoxidil causes hair to grow (hypertrichosis) in all patients. The hair grows on the face, back, arms, and legs and may create an inconvenient or unpleasant situation for some patients, especially women. When the treatment is discontinued the hair growth stops and the new hair falls out. Topical minoxidil, which is used specifically to promote hair growth on the scalp, may irritate the skin and, in susceptible patients, produce symptoms of systemic vasodilation.

Diazoxide inhibits insulin release from the pancreas. The resulting hyperglycemia may prove problematic in patients with preexisting renal insufficiency or diabetes mellitus.

Sildenafil causes flushing of the face, head, and neck in about 10% of patients, undoubtedly related to vasodilation. Dyspepsia, or acid indigestion, occurs in about 7% of cases. Blurring of vision, sensitivity to light, and changes in color perception affect 2% of patients.

TOXICITY

Hydralazine toxicities are most common in slow acetylators of the drug owing to accumulation of the drug after multiple dosing if the diminished ability to biotransform the drug goes unrecognized.

The most serious toxicity associated with nitroprusside occurs with the accumulation of cyanide. In most cases, the toxicity results from overdose but in rare instances, when it occurs early in treatment, it may reflect a patient's diminished ability to detoxify cyanide because of disease or heredity. The administration of sodium thiosulfate as a sulfur donor aids the metabolism of cyanide.

INTERACTION

Diuretics are commonly used in combination with vasodilator drugs in the long-term management of hypertension because the sodium and water excretion caused by the diuretics tends to offset the sodium and water retention caused by the vasodilators. If not counteracted, the sodium and water retention will expand the blood volume, raising arterial pressure and canceling the desired antihypertensive effects of the vasodilators.

Sildenafil may cause a serious, potentially fatal interaction with organic nitrates in patients being treated for angina pectoris. The interaction causes precipitous reduction of arterial pressure and has produced several fatal heart attacks.

APPLICATION TO PRACTICE

ASSESSMENT
History of Present Illness

The patient with angina may experience pain anywhere in the chest, neck, arms, or back. The most common location is the retrosternal region. The pain, lasting 3 to 5 minutes, commonly radiates to the left arm but may also radiate bilaterally, to the mandible, or to the neck (Figure 39-4). Patients often demonstrate Levine's sign—a clenched fist placed over the sternum—to explain the location of their discomfort. The patient should be asked to rate the chest discomfort on a scale of 1 to 10. In many cases, the discomfort is commonly mistaken for indigestion.

The health care provider should ask about the patient's perception of the pain, including the sensation, location, radiation, and duration. For example, does the chest pain occur with exertion or rest? How long does the pain last? What makes the discomfort better and what makes it worse? Does the patient take nitroglycerin or other drugs for relief?

Health History

If the chest pain is present at the time of the interview, further history-taking activities are delayed until pain relief is initiated. When the patient is more comfortable, information regarding possible stress-related symptoms, such as chest pain, rapid pulse, palpitations, hyperventilation, diarrhea, constipation, anorexia, and diaphoresis, is obtained. Information about drug history, family history, and modifiable risk factors for coronary artery disease (CAD) is also obtained. Eating habits, lifestyle, and physical activity levels should also be documented.

The health care provider should determine preexisting conditions that may require cautious use of a ni-

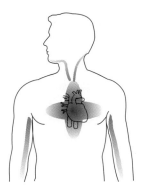

Upper chest or epigastric radiation to neck, jaw, and arms

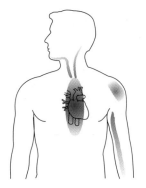

Beneath sternum radiation to neck and jaw or radiation down left arm

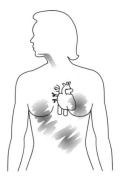

Nausea, shortness of breath, or vague discomfort in upper abdomen or jaw

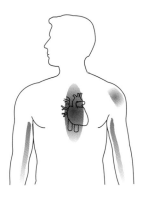

Epigastric or left shoulder radiating down both arms

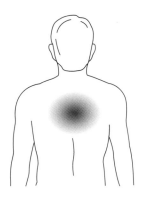

Intrascapular

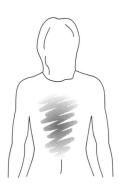

Discomfort in back

FIGURE 39-4 Common sites of anginal pain (shaded areas). The locations of the pain are similar in men and women.

trate, beta blocker, or calcium channel blocker. Such preexisting conditions include asthma, heart block, dehydration, low systolic blood pressure, pregnancy, and lactation. Determine if the patient is taking any other drugs, including OTC or illicit drugs as well as alcoholic beverages.

Lifespan Considerations

Perinatal. Pregnancy is normally accompanied by significant physiologic changes in the maternal cardiovascular system—blood volume, cardiac output, pulse, blood pressure, and peripheral vascular resistance (see Chapter 2). In the majority of patients, these changes present no significant risk to maternal or fetal well-being. However, certain patients experience a sudden decompensation of heart function during pregnancy.

Both the myocardium and the myometrium of the uterus possess alpha and beta receptors. The smooth muscle of the uterus contracts in response to alpha stimulation and relaxes with beta stimulation. Secondary uterine effects should be considered in patients treated with cardiac drugs that cause either type of stimulation. Furthermore, there is controversy regarding the safety of beta blockers in pregnancy. There is some evidence that propranolol may lower umbilical blood flow. An increased incidence of growth retardation, delayed neonatal respiration, bradycardia, hypoglycemia, and blunting of accelerations of intrapartum fetal heart rate have been reported with beta blocker use. Whether these phenomena are related to dose or to the underlying cardiac disease is unclear. No clear evidence exists to suggest that beta blockers are teratogenic.

Pediatric. Each year an estimated 400,000 babies are born with congenital heart disease in the United States. Of these, about one third become critically ill during their first year of life; one third develop problems later in childhood or as young adults; and one third never experience serious handicaps. Management of heart disease in children is primarily surgical.

Older Adults. Physiologic changes in the cardiovascular system manifest in a variety of ways in the older adult. The efficiency and contractile strength of the myocardium declines, resulting in a 1% annual reduction in cardiac output. Stroke volume is thought to decrease by 0.7% yearly. The systolic and diastolic phases of the myocardial cycle are prolonged. Ordinarily, older adults adjust to these changes without much difficulty. However, when unusual demands are placed on the heart (e.g., shoveling snow, running to catch a bus), the changes become more evident. Pulse rates may not reach the levels of younger persons, and tachycardia lasts longer. There is some disagreement among health care providers as to when the normal elevation becomes hypertension. In some older adults, the blood pressure may remain stable while tachycardia progresses to anginal episodes and heart failure.

Resistance to peripheral blood flow increases by 1% each year. Decreased elasticity of the arteries is responsible for vascular changes to the heart. Because of the rigidity of vessel walls and narrowing of lumens, more force is required to move blood through the vessels, increasing the risk of angina. These changes also lead to a higher diastolic blood pressure. Furthermore, there is a decrease in the ability of the aorta to distend, in turn raising systolic pressure. Vagal tone increases, and the heart becomes more sensitive to carotid sinus stimulation. Reduced sensitivity of the baroreceptors potentiates orthostatic hypotension.

Cultural/Social Considerations

Denial is a common early reaction to the chest discomfort associated with angina. On average, the patient with an acute MI waits more than 2 hours before seeking care. Thus the patient's perceived susceptibility to anginal pain, and perhaps to an MI and its subsequent limitations, influences the overall plan of care. Furthermore, the likelihood of compliance with a plan of care is also determined by the ratio of perceived benefits of compliance versus risks of nonaction.

Fear, anxiety, and anger are common reactions of patients and family members to this situation. The health care provider must assess behavioral patterns that stem from these reactions (see the Case Study: Angina Pectoris).

Physical Examination

Diaphoresis, dyspnea, vomiting, dizziness, weakness, palpitations, and pallor may accompany anginal pain. However, the presence of these manifestations without chest pain is still significant. Chest pain may be mild or even absent in 15% to 25% of patients with an MI.

High-priority assessments for the patient with suspected angina or MI are blood pressure and apical pulse measurements. Skin color, temperature, turgor, jugular vein distention, heart rate and rhythm, heart sounds, and peripheral pulses should also be noted, and a respiratory assessment performed. If angina or an uncomplicated MI is occurring, the skin will be warm, with peripheral pulses palpable. In patients with complicated angina or MI, cardiac output may be reduced, manifesting as cool, diaphoretic skin.

An S_3 gallop may be present, often indicating heart failure, a serious and common complication of MI. The presence of an S_4 heart sound is a common finding in patients who have had a previous MI or who have hypertension. Respiratory rate and rhythm should be noted. Auscultation of breath sounds may reflect crackles, rhonchi, or wheezes in the presence of heart failure.

Laboratory Testing

No laboratory tests can confirm a diagnosis of angina. Serum enzyme determinations are not helpful in assessing angina. An MI can be confirmed by the presence of abnormally high levels of cardiac enzymes and isoenzymes. Enzymes that assist in the diagnosis and monitoring of cardiac status include lactate dehydrogenase (LDH) and creatine kinase (CK). Creatine kinase is the most sensitive and reliable indicator of an MI. Troponin I has been shown to be a specific indicator of myocardial infarction. It appears 3 to 6 hours after the onset of the MI, peaks at 16 hours, and decreases in 9 to 10 days. An elevated white blood cell count appears on the second day after an MI.

Other diagnostic testing for the patient with angina may include a stress test. Exercise tolerance testing (stress testing) to assess for ECG changes consistent with angina may also be done. Thallium is a radioisotope used to assess for ischemia.

GOALS OF THERAPY

The primary goal in the treatment of angina is to restore the balance between myocardial oxygen supply and demand. This goal can be accomplished by reducing the duration and intensity of symptoms, preventing attacks, and improving work capacity (even though angina may occur). The ultimate outcome is to prevent or delay the onset of an MI. Diseases or conditions that predispose an individual to angina should be treated as part of a comprehensive therapeutic program.

The choice of antianginal drug and route of administration is made with consideration of the desired goal, onset of therapeutic effects, the suitability of various routes of administration for the particular patient, the need for stable drug concentration, comorbid conditions, and the likelihood of tolerance or toxicity.

INTERVENTION
Administration

The patient's blood pressure and pulse should be taken before administering an antianginal drug and then again at the onset of drug action. Assess breath sounds and heart sounds, rate, and rhythm as well as the intensity, duration, location, and quality of pain.

Buccal Formulations. Buccal extended-release formulations are placed between the cheek and upper gum, or between the lip and upper gum, and allowed to dissolve over 5 hours. When eating or drinking, the patient should place the dose between the upper lip and gum. Tell the patient not to use chewing tobacco while using this drug form. Replace the tablet if it is accidentally swallowed. Tell the patient not to go to sleep with a tablet still in the mouth. Sublingual isosorbide dinitrate and nitroglycerin tablets may also be administered buccally.

Sublingual and Lingual Sprays. Sublingual nitroglycerin tablets and lingual sprays should be left at the bedside of hospitalized patients so they can be used immediately, if needed. An adequate supply should be available to the patient, who should be told to notify the health care provider when a dose has been required. A record should be kept of the time and the dosage administered.

Review the patient instruction leaflet supplied by the manufacturer for proper use of lingual aerosol formulations. To use, remove the cover. Do not shake the container. Hold the container upright, close to the patient's mouth. Administer 1 or 2 sprays (as prescribed) under the tongue. Close the mouth and instruct the patient to avoid swallowing for 1 or 2 minutes. This drug may be used like nitroglycerin tablets: when an attack of angina occurs, the patient should administer a dose as prescribed. If no relief is obtained in 5 minutes, the patient should repeat the dose. If there is no relief in another 5 minutes, dose should be repeated. If no relief occurs after a total of 3 doses in 15 minutes, the patient should seek medical attention.

Tablets and Capsules. For a chewable tablet, instruct the patient to chew it well, then hold it in the mouth for at least 2 minutes before swallowing. The patient should not drink, smoke, eat, or chew tobacco while using this form. Instruct him or her to swallow extended-release capsules whole, without chewing, crushing, or breaking.

Transdermal Formulations. Review the patient instruction leaflet supplied by the manufacturer of transdermal formulations. Do not trim or cut the adhesive patch (Figure 39-5). Remove the previous patch before applying a new dose. Rotate sites to avoid skin irritation. Apply the patch to an area that is clean and dry with little

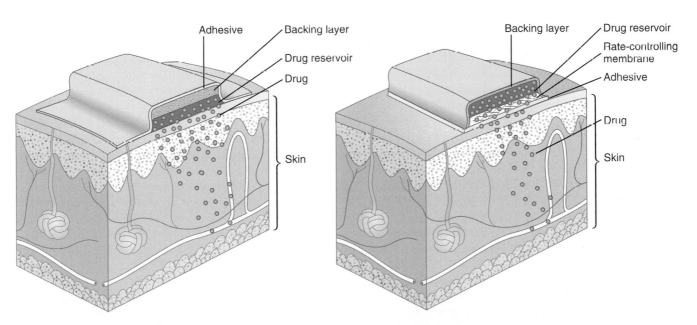

FIGURE 39-5 Schematic drawing of transdermal drug delivery systems. *Left*, in matrix formulations, the drug is slowly dispersed through the polymer matrix to the absorption site. *Right*, in reservoir delivery systems, the drug migrates to the absorption site through a rate-controlling permeable membrane.

or no hair. Avoid scratches, scars, and areas of existing skin irritation. If the patch loosens or falls off, replace it with a new one. Tolerance to this therapy may be lessened if the patches are not used continuously; some health care providers may prescribe a patch-free period each day (e.g., during the night). Transdermal forms should not be used to treat an acute attack of angina.

Review the patient instruction leaflet supplied by the manufacturer for topical ointments. Paste formulations come in a tube, much like toothpaste, with a specially designed paper applicator. The drug is measured (by the inch) onto the paper applicator and then applied to the skin surface. Remove the ointment remaining from a previous dose before applying a fresh dose. Measure the prescribed amount of ointment, using the measuring paper supplied by the manufacturer. Gently spread the ointment over a small area of the paper using a small applicator (not your fingertips). Wear gloves to avoid exposing yourself to the drug. Do not massage the ointment into the skin. Cover the area with plastic kitchen wrap or other dressing if ordered by the health care provider. If a dressing is prescribed, it should be used each time the drug is applied. If a dose is missed, apply it as soon as remembered unless it is within 2 hours of the next dose, in which case the usual dosing schedule should be followed. Do not use more ointment than ordered and do not double up for missed doses.

Both the reservoir and matrix patch systems offer steady-state plasma levels within the therapeutic range over 24 hours, thus making only one application per day necessary (see Figure 39-5). The disadvantage of the reservoir system is the so-called "dose dumping" if the seal is punctured or broken. Dose dumping does not occur with the matrix system. Both systems achieve a plasma steady-state level in approximately 2 hours. However, transdermal nitroglycerin formulations (i.e., paste or patches) must be applied at the same time each day and removed at the same time each evening, allowing for a 10- to 12-hour period each day without the drug to avoid development of tolerance (tachyphylaxis). When oral and topical preparations are used concurrently, the patient is encouraged to stagger administration times to minimize the possibility of additive hypotension and headache. Patients using long-acting antianginal drugs should have a sublingual dosage form on hand at all times.

Intravenous Formulations. Intravenous nitroglycerin should be diluted according to the manufacturer's instructions, and the dosage titrated as needed. Blood pressure and pulse should be checked every 5 to 15 minutes during dose titration and every hour thereafter. The flow rate should be adjusted according to the patient's

response—a drop in systolic blood pressure of 20 mm Hg or relief of pain.

It should be noted, however, that intravenous nitroglycerin binds to the polyvinyl chloride plastic used in most intravenous solution bags and infusion sets. So much drug can bind to the plastic that very little reaches the patient's circulation. Anticipate the need for a dosage increase if polyvinyl chloride infusion sets are used. The tubing that comes with intravenous nitroglycerin from the manufacturer is made of special plastic with which the drug does not bind and should be used when possible. Nitroglycerin solutions should be stored in a glass bottle and used within 24 hours.

Nitroprusside is unstable, decomposing rapidly in the presence of light. Fresh solutions must be prepared for each administration of the drug, and the administration device containing the solution to be infused must be wrapped in aluminum foil to avoid exposure to light. Monitor the blood pressure, heart rate, ECG changes, and pulmonary capillary wedge pressure (PCWP) for patients receiving intravenous nitroglycerin. Administer intravenous formulations only in settings where drugs and experienced personnel to treat cardiovascular emergencies are available.

Calcium Channel Blockers. Monitor the blood pressure, pulse, intake, output, and weight for patients taking calcium channel blockers. Signs of fluid retention are peripheral edema and subjective complaints of tight shoes and rings. Monitor for signs of heart failure, including dyspnea on exertion, distended jugular veins, orthopnea, or moist crackles on pulmonary auscultation. If calcium channel blockers are prescribed for hypertension, see the general guidelines for patients receiving antihypertensives in Chapter 13. The administration of beta blockers was discussed in Chapter 12.

Education

Encourage the patient who has angina to make all recommended lifestyle changes. The patient should be advised to stop cigarette smoking at once. Smoking cessation lowers the risk of CAD by 37%. Smoking raises carboxyhemoglobin levels in the blood, reducing the amount of oxygen available to the myocardium and possibly precipitating an anginal episode. Patients who are exposed for 2 hours to cigarette smoke not only suffer elevations in carboxyhemoglobin concentrations but also experience shortened exercise time and increased heart rate and blood pressure. Second-hand smoke (so-called passive smoking) should also be avoided.

Patients with angina should lose excess weight. They should be encouraged to eat small meals, avoid high-calorie and high-cholesterol foods, abstain from gas-forming foods, and to rest for short periods after eating.

In addition, a high-fiber diet is recommended; it not only prevents constipation and other GI ailments but also decreases the number and severity of anginal episodes. Diets high in fiber also lower serum cholesterol and triglyceride levels. Patients with a high intake of dietary fiber develop CAD less frequently than those with a low intake.

Patients who lead active, hectic lives should be advised to reduce activities to below the level that precipitates anginal episodes. They should try brief rest periods throughout the workday, an earlier bedtime, and longer or more frequent vacations. Relaxation exercises and other stress reduction techniques may be used to reduce the incidence of angina. Help patients who are anxious and nervous to understand the importance of counseling.

Assist the patient and family in identifying activities that trigger anginal pain, such as having increased stress, eating a heavy meal, engaging in strenuous physical activities, lifting heavy objects, being exposed to cold weather, and having sex.

Strenuous exercise is known to precipitate an anginal attack but may be effectively managed with appropriate exercise limitations and patient education. Have the patient check with the health care provider before starting an exercise regimen. Exercise does enlarge heart volume and mass, increase capillary vascularity, and decrease heart rate—all of which may protect the myocardium from the effects of ischemic damage. However, the patient with documented evidence of ischemic heart disease should be cautioned against engaging in strenuous exercise, because it raises myocardial oxygen demand.

Despite compliance with nondrug therapies, some patients continue to experience angina and require frequent monitoring. Antianginal drugs are most often taken on an outpatient basis, so the patient should be instructed to record the number and severity of anginal episodes, along with the effectiveness and total number of nitroglycerin tablets taken daily. Information from the patient is important to monitoring therapeutic and adverse effects of drug therapy.

The patient should also be instructed as to proper storage of antianginal preparations. Sublingual formulations are effective for a period of 5 to 6 months when stored in the original container in a dark, cool location. Tablets are inactivated by light, heat, air, and moisture; they should be stored at room temperature in an amber glass container with a tight-fitting lid. Patients should be advised not to transfer the drug to other containers and to discard unused nitroglycerin tablets 6 months after opening the container. Lingual sprays remain potent for up to 3 years.

For many years, the tingling, burning sensation caused by the sublingual formulation was used as an indicator of the drug's freshness. This sign cannot be regarded as an indicator it will be effective. Older adults may not experience the tingling, even with new nitroglycerin tablets. Patients who doubt the potency of their drug should have their prescription refilled and discard the old drug.

The patient and family should be reminded that antianginal drugs should be taken only as prescribed. Family members should be kept informed about the location and proper use of the drugs in case the patient needs help taking them. The dosage of these drugs is individualized to maximize therapeutic effects and minimize adverse reactions.

Encourage the patient and family to notify the health care provider of any changes in the frequency, intensity, duration, location of the pain or changes in the patient's response to the antianginal drugs. Instruct the patient to avoid alcoholic beverages, because they potentiate the hypotensive effects of vasodilating drugs. Remind the patient to keep all health care providers informed of all drugs used, because diuretics, antihypertensives, CNS depressants, opioids, and sedative-hypnotics may potentiate the hypotensive effects.

To prevent an attack of angina, instruct patients to take the prescribed drug before engaging in the activity expected to produce anginal pain. For sublingual or chewable forms, this may be 5 to 10 minutes before engaging in such activities; for extended-release forms, patients may need to take the drug several hours before the activity. For specific patient needs, consult the health care provider. Abrupt discontinuance of antianginal drugs has been associated with increases in anginal episodes and possible MIs.

If a headache occurs regularly when antianginal drugs are taken, it may indicate too high a dosage. For some patients it may be necessary to use mild analgesics (e.g., acetaminophen) with antianginal therapy. Have the patient discuss this problem with the health care provider.

Storage. These drugs should be kept out of the reach of children and not stored in the bathroom, near the kitchen sink, or in other damp areas. Check expiration dates and replace drugs as needed. For sublingual nitroglycerin, follow the previous instructions and keep tablets in the original glass container. Once the bottle is opened, remove the cotton and do not replace it. Replace the cap tightly and quickly each time the bottle is opened. Do not put other medicines in the same bottle with the nitroglycerin. When a tablet is needed, pour one or more tablets into the lid of the bottle, take the dose out, and return remaining tablets to the bottle. Avoid replacing tablets from the palm of the hand into the bottle. Do not carry the container too close to the body because body warmth may cause the pills to lose their strength.

EVALUATION

The patient with effective antianginal therapy should report a decrease in the frequency and severity of anginal attacks along with improved activity tolerance. If the nitrates were administered for heart failure, the patient should demonstrate a clearing of peripheral edema and lung fields as well as improvement in urinary output and blood pressure. Pulmonary artery and pulmonary capillary wedge pressures should be within normal limits.

The patient using beta blockers and calcium channel blockers to treat angina should also have a decrease in the frequency and severity of anginal attacks. Beta blockers have been shown to prevent recurrent MI. The use of calcium channel blockers is thought to reduce the need for nitrate therapy.

The patient should be able to correctly identify his or her drug, the proper administration technique, and the dosage. The patient should also understand the signs and symptoms of hypotension, ways to minimize orthostatic changes, and the importance of keeping follow-up appointments.

CASE STUDY *Angina Pectoris*

ASSESSMENT

HISTORY OF PRESENT ILLNESS

JS is a 49-year-old man who comes to the clinic accompanied by his wife. He complains of chest pain after shoveling snow this morning but is in no acute distress at this time. During the attack, he complained of being dizzy and anxious. He reports that the pain radiated to his jaw and left arm. It was relieved with rest and two nitroglycerin tablets. His wife noticed he was breathing rapidly and that he looked pale.

HEALTH HISTORY

JS first experienced nonradiating chest pain 3 years ago. A stress test showed ischemic ST wave changes with exercise, and was diagnosed with exercise-induced angina. He was prescribed nitroglycerin tablets, 0.3 mg SL prn chest pain. He reports taking the nitroglycerin two or three times during the past year. He has been on a low-cholesterol diet and taking atorvastatin 40 mg daily for his elevated cholesterol. He uses an albuterol inhaler prn for the reactive airway disease he has had since childhood. JS smokes cigarettes, half a pack per day. He has a strong family history of CAD and hypercholesterolemia.

LIFESPAN CONSIDERATIONS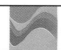

JS has three children under the age of 10. The 7-year-old boy is developmentally disabled and has been having behavioral difficulties at school recently. JS's wife does not work outside the home.

CULTURAL/SOCIAL CONSIDERATIONS

JS is a self-employed accountant who has been spending long periods at the office during tax season. He is an active coach for the local basketball team. He sees his family as upper-middle-class with no unusual financial stressors. The family has health and pharmacy insurance through a local PPO.

PHYSICAL EXAMINATION

BP 188/90 mm Hg, apical pulse 94 and irregular, respirations 26, temperature 98° F. Dyspnea and diaphoresis noted. Breath sounds are clear bilaterally. PMI palpable at fifth ICS, MCL; $S_1 > S_2$ at the apex; no murmur, S_3, or S_4 heart sounds noted on auscultation. Peripheral pulses strong bilaterally. No carotid, aortic, renal artery, or femoral artery bruits noted. No hepatosplenomegaly.

LABORATORY TESTING

CBC count is within normal limits; cardiac enzyme/isoenzyme levels are unremarkable; cholesterol is 260 mg/dL; HDL is 35 mg/dL; triglycerides 220 mg/dL. ST segment shows elevation on ECG.

PATIENT PROBLEM(S)

Classic angina pectoris brought on by exertion.

GOALS OF THERAPY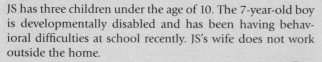

Enhance cardiac performance; decrease the duration and intensity of anginal attacks; improve work capacity.

CRITICAL THINKING QUESTIONS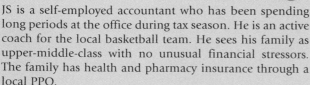

1. The health care provider orders nitroglycerin 0.3 mg SL tablets prn for chest pain × three tablets. If no relief, health care provider should be contacted. What is the mechanism of action of nitroglycerin?
2. The health care provider also ordered atenolol 50 mg po qd, titrating the dose to patient response in 3 to 7 days. What concerns do you have about JS using this drug?
3. What adverse effects can the nitroglycerin cause that JS should be warned about?
4. The health care provider considered using a calcium channel blocker for JS but changed his mind. How do calcium channel blockers relieve angina?
5. What instructions are necessary for patients for whom a nitrate has been prescribed?

Bibliography

Hatzichristou DG, Pescatori ES: Current treatments and emerging therapeutic approaches in male erectile dysfunction, *BJU Int* 88(Suppl)3:11-17, 2001.

Loh E: Overview: old and new controversies in the treatment of advanced congestive heart failure, *J Card Fail* 7(2)(Suppl)1:1-7, 2001.

Motro M, Shemesh J, Grossman E: Coronary benefits of calcium antagonist therapy for patients with hypertension, *Curr Opin in Cardiol* 16(6):349-355, 2001.

O'Connor CM: Raynaud's phenomenon, *J Vasc Nurs* 19(3):87-92, 2001.

Staniforth AD: Contemporary management of chronic stable angina, *Drugs Aging* 18(2):109-121, 2001.

Internet Resources

http://www.docguide.com/news/content.nsf/PatientResAll Categ/Angina.

http://www.nhlbi.nih.gov/health/public/heart/other/angina.htm.

CHAPTER

40

Antiarrhythmic Drugs

JOSEPH A. DiMICCO • ELIZABETH KISSELL

 Visit http://evolve.elsevier.com/Gutierrez/ for additional information.

KEY TERMS

OBJECTIVES

- Explain how normal heart rhythm is maintained.
- Describe the four phases of the cardiac action potential and the ion movements responsible for each phase.
- Describe the four classes of antiarrhythmic drugs.
- Explain how each class of antiarrhythmics suppresses arrhythmias.
- Discuss the cardiotoxicity of antiarrhythmic drugs.
- Develop a nursing care plan for a patient receiving an antiarrhythmic drug.

PHYSIOLOGY • Normal Cardiac Function

The normal beating of the heart is caused by the highly coordinated contraction of individual cardiac muscle cells. This coordinated mechanical activity that makes the heart a highly efficient pump results from electrical changes that take place in cardiac cells, or cardiac electrophysiology. To understand the basic principles of cardiac electrophysiology, it is important to understand the function and movement of three positively charged ions: sodium, potassium, and calcium. Like other cells, cardiac cell membranes contain a number of active transporters, pumps, and channels for these ions. Pumps and transporters keep these three ions at different concentrations inside and outside the cell. The concentration of potassium is relatively high inside the cell and low outside the cell, whereas the opposite is true for sodium and calcium ions.

Because of the concentration differences, these ions would tend to rapidly diffuse across the membrane (potassium from inside to outside, sodium and calcium from outside to inside). However, their electrical charges keep them from moving through the membrane itself. Instead, they can only move through open pores, or ion channels, in the membrane. Different types of channels exist in cardiac cells, but a given channel will allow the passage of only one kind of ion. Furthermore, different channels are only open under certain conditions. In a typical cardiac cell under resting (unstimulated) conditions, only potassium channels are open, meaning that only potassium ions are able to diffuse across the membrane. Because the concentration of potassium is much higher inside the cell than outside, potassium ions have a strong tendency to move rapidly from inside the cell to the outside. Furthermore, because potassium ions are positively charged, this rapid movement leaves the inside of the membrane with less negative charge and the outside of the cell membrane with more. Therefore, the cell membrane is charged at rest, with the inside more negative (and the outside more positive) because of the passive diffusion of potassium ions. This difference in charge across the membrane, called the resting membrane potential, is about −90 mV in most cardiac cells.

Cardiac Action Potential

Contraction of a ventricular or atrial cardiac muscle cell is triggered by depolarization, or reduction in the difference in charge across the membrane. When the cell is depolarized to a critical point or threshold (usually caused by the firing of an adjacent cell), a series of specific events take place that involves the opening and closing of different ion channels, and results in a cardiac **action potential** (Figure 40-1). First, some of the voltage-gated (fast) sodium channels begin to respond. Recall that these channels open briefly in response to depolarization and then close again. Opening these channels allows sodium to move into the cell, causing more depolarization, which results in more sodium channels opening. If the response is too weak, the threshold will not be reached, the sodium channels that have opened will rapidly close again, and the membrane will return to its resting potential. However, if the initial depolarization is strong enough to reach the critical threshold, the chain reaction that results leads to the explosive opening of all the available sodium channels. The sudden rush of sodium into the cell triggers the rapid and complete depolarization of the cell (called *phase 0*), even to the point of a reverse of the original charge on the membrane. Because these sodium channels close quickly, membrane potential is reversed only briefly and begins to move toward negative levels again during *phase 1*. The sodium channels are now closed and are said to be inactive, meaning they cannot open again until the membrane voltage returns to its original hyperpolarized state.

If no other channels opened, the continuing movement of potassium ions out of the cell would return the membrane to its original resting membrane potential of −90 mV. However, the rapid depolarization of the cell in phase 0, caused by the opening of the sodium channels, has caused another type of channel to open. These are the voltage-gated (slow) calcium channels. Similar to the sodium channels, the calcium channels open temporarily when the membrane becomes depolarized, but a major difference is that these channels open and close much more slowly. Consequently, they are sometimes called slow calcium channels. While they are open, calcium moves into the cell, and this movement of positive charge to the inside of the membrane keeps it from returning to its resting potential even though all the sodium channels have now closed and potassium still has a strong tendency to move out of the cell. This prolonged plateau of the action potential, during which the calcium channels are open and calcium is moving across the membrane into the cell, is termed *phase 2*. It is the movement of calcium into the cell during phase 2 that triggers contraction of the cardiac muscle cell.

As the calcium channels close and calcium can no longer move into the cell, the movement of potassium continues and even intensifies as different potassium channels open. Without the opposing effect of calcium ions moving in the opposite direction, the movement of potassium drives the membrane quickly to its resting potential. The rapid return of the membrane potential

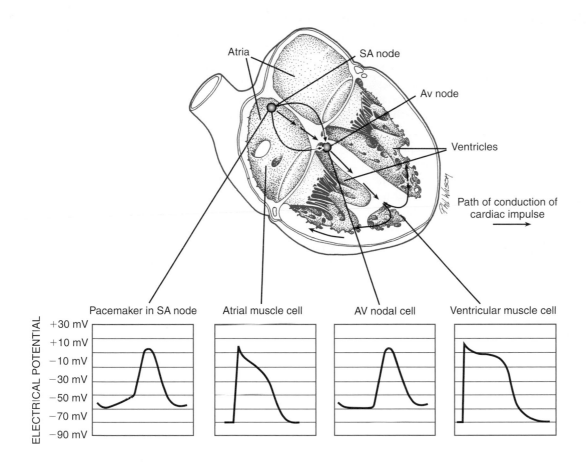

FIGURE 40-1 The normal path of conduction of the cardiac impulse from its origination in the SA node, through the atrial muscle, the AV node, and finally to the ventricles; and action potentials characteristic of different types of cardiac muscle and nodal cells.

to its original resting state is termed *phase 3*. As the cell returns to its resting potential, the fast sodium channels reset and are ready to respond to the next stimulus. *Phase 4* is the period during which the cell is once again at rest, where it will remain until it is stimulated (depolarized). During phase 1, phase 2, and most of phase 3, stimulation of the cell will not cause another action potential because voltage-gated channels have not reset and are still inactivated. This period of inexcitability is called the **refractory period.**

SA and AV Nodes

The sequence of events just described occurs in almost every cell of the heart and is repeated with each heartbeat. However, in cells in two regions of the heart, the sinoatrial (SA) node and atrioventricular (AV) node, the cardiac action potential is very different (see Figure 40-1). First, cells in the nodes have few, if any, fast sodium channels. Therefore, the only voltage-gated channels involved are the slow calcium channels, and

so the ion moving through the membrane during phase 0 is mainly calcium. Because these calcium channels open and close very slowly, phase 0 in nodal tissue is not the rapid and steep upstroke seen in other cardiac cells. Furthermore, there is no phase 1 or 2, but only a slow phase 3, as these same channels gradually close. Because of this characteristic of action potentials in nodal cells, they are termed slow responses, and the nodes are said to be **slow response tissue.** In contrast, cells elsewhere in the heart are called **fast response cells** because of the very rapid depolarization that occurs during phase 0. The upstroke of phase 0 of the cardiac action potential determines the conduction velocity, or the speed with which a cardiac impulse spreads through tissue (see Chapter 38). The slow upstroke of phase 0 in nodal tissue means that an impulse spreads from cell to cell relatively slowly, whereas the fast upstroke seen in atrial and ventricular muscle cells means that transmission is very rapid in most of the heart.

Certain nodal cells in the SA node also differ from other cardiac cells in another important way. These cells do not have a stable membrane potential during phase 4. Instead, they depolarize spontaneously until they reach threshold and fire an action potential (see Figure 40-1). This property is called **automaticity** and these automatic cells are responsible for the normal beating of the heart. In fact, the heart rate is determined by the automatic cell in the SA node with the fastest rate, and this cell is called the **pacemaker.** Activity of the sympathetic nervous system increases the automaticity of the SA node. As a result, phase 4 on the action potential curve is steepened and shortened, phase 0 is triggered sooner, and the heart beats more rapidly. In contrast, activity of the vagus nerve slows the heart rate. This action occurs because acetylcholine from the vagus nerve decreases the automaticity of the SA node. Automaticity is also seen in some specialized ventricular cells, but their rates are so slow that no evidence of this is seen under normal conditions.

Conduction of Cardiac Impulse

As shown in Figure 40-1, the normal heartbeat results from the spread of the cardiac impulse from cell to cell in a specific order, because the action potential in each cell triggers an action potential in the next cell. This wave of excitation begins when the pacemaker cell fires in the SA node. The impulse then spreads through the atria, depolarizing each muscle cell and triggering its

contraction. The spread of the action potential through the atrial muscle is rapid because of the rapid depolarization of each cell in phase 0. However, before the impulse can reach the ventricles, it must pass through the AV node. Because the AV node consists of slow response cells where phase 0 of the action potential rises slowly, the impulse spreads from cell to cell relatively slowly, providing a delay so that the contracting atria can fill the ventricles with blood while they are still completely relaxed. Activity of the autonomic nervous system can markedly alter the speed of conduction through the AV node. Sympathetic nervous system activity increases the conduction speed of the cardiac impulse through the AV node, whereas parasympathetic activity slows AV conduction. Once the impulse emerges from the AV node, it enters the ventricles and is rapidly conducted through the ventricular muscle cells, by way of a specialized conducting system, to trigger a coordinated contraction.

In the clinical setting, this normal sequence of events is recorded on an **electrocardiogram (ECG),** which provides important information about the function of a patient's heart (Figure 40-2). Different parts of the ECG tracings are related to the different phases of the action potentials in various parts of the heart. The change in action potential marked in Figure 40-2 as P (the P wave) is produced by the initial depolarization of atrial cells (phase 0 of the action potential). Very shortly after this wave of depolarization, the atrium contracts to com-

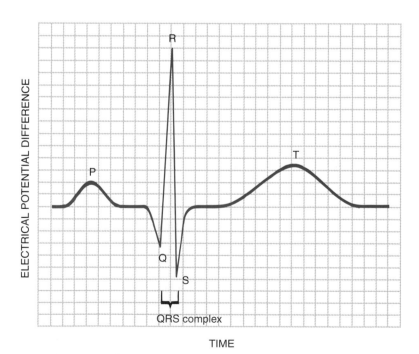

FIGURE 40-2   Electrocardiographic (ECG) tracing showing pattern typical of normal cardiac function.

plete the filling of the ventricles. The waves marked Q, R, and S (QRS complex) result from depolarization of the ventricles. Repolarization of the atria occurs at this time but is masked by the large changes produced by depolarization of the ventricles. The distance between the P wave and the QRS complex, called the P-R interval, is an indication of the time it takes for the impulse to travel across the AV node. Ventricular contraction occurs between the QRS complex and the midpoint of the T wave. The T wave represents repolarization (primarily phase 3 of the action potential) of the ventricles. The distance between the QRS complex and the T wave, called the Q-T interval, is a measure of action potential duration in the ventricular muscle cells.

PATHOPHYSIOLOGY • Cardiac Rhythm Disturbances

Arrhythmias

Arrhythmias (also called dysrhythmias) are defined as changes from the normal rate or pattern of heartbeat. Heart rates that are too slow (bradycardia), too fast (tachycardia), or irregular are included in this classification. Sinus rhythms, the rhythm of the normal beating heart, are those where all the cells of the heart are excited only by impulses arising from a pacemaker in the SA node that follows the normal conduction pathway through the heart. Sinus bradycardia, a slow heart rate originating from a pacemaker in the SA node, is usually of minor importance and is not treated unless it is associated with reduced cardiac output. Sinus tachycardia, a rapid but otherwise normal heart rate, may likewise be harmless. Sinus tachycardia may be produced in healthy persons by anxiety; ingestion of coffee, tea, or other caffeinated products; ingestion of alcoholic beverages; or cigarette smoking. Sympathetic nervous system agonists, anticholinergics, or phenothiazines may also induce transient sinus tachycardia.

More serious arrhythmias occur when (1) cells other than the normal pacemakers in the SA node trigger action potentials that spread to other parts of the heart, or (2) cardiac impulses spread through the heart in abnormal sequences or by abnormal pathways. Many arrhythmias involve a combination of these two basic mechanisms. Abnormal pacemakers, called ectopic pacemakers, may develop when the heart is damaged or diseased (as a result of myocardial infarction or heart failure) or after treatment with certain drugs (e.g., digoxin or high doses of catecholamines). For example, a cell that is normally not automatic may develop automaticity when it is damaged or sick, and the impulses that result may spread from heart cell to heart cell, producing abnormal beats. The movement of sodium or calcium seems to be important in causing this abnormal automaticity. In other cases, a normal action potential may trigger an extra impulse in a nonautomatic muscle cell. These abnormal triggered impulses may occur when the normal action potential is abnormally prolonged, an effect sometimes seen when some of the potassium channels that are responsible for phase 3 repolarization are blocked by certain drugs (see below). Triggered impulses may also occur when the cell is loaded with excessive amounts of calcium, which may happen after treatment with digoxin or during excessive stimulation of cardiac beta receptors by sympathetic nerve activity or catecholamines.

Disorders of conduction arise from various causes. One danger is that conduction of the cardiac impulse may actually fail in a particular region. This may occur in any part of the heart when cells are injured or ischemic (deprived of oxygen) but is especially common in the AV node. Here, conduction is so slow under normal conditions that any further decrease may cause some or all of the impulses entering from the atria to die out altogether, a condition known as AV block, or simply heart block. Impulses will also tend to die out in the AV node when atrial rates are very high, a property called refractoriness. AV refractoriness is enhanced by anything that further slows conduction through the region. During arrhythmias, AV refractoriness may protect the ventricles from high atrial rates so that they can still pump enough blood to maintain blood pressure.

Arrhythmias may also involve conduction of the cardiac impulses through abnormal pathways. For example, it is now known that some hearts have a physical connection between the atria and ventricles that allows the conduction of an impulse to the ventricles, not only through the AV node but also through this accessory pathway. This anatomic abnormality gives rise to an arrhythmia because the impulse passes rapidly through the accessory pathway but slowly through the AV node; thus, the impulse from the node may arrive at the accessory pathway just at the end of the refractory period of those rapidly conducting cells. A wave of depolarization may then pass from the ventricles through this pathway back into the atria, which may trigger a premature beat. An example of this type of anatomically defined arrhythmia is called the Wolff-Parkinson-White syndrome.

A similar situation may exist without an anatomically defined separate pathway, especially if a section of tissue has been damaged by ischemia, such as occurs with a myocardial infarction. The damaged area not only may fail to contract but also may fail to conduct an action potential properly. In some cases, this may lead to a situation where an impulse that has been slowed in such a region emerges to find cells on the other side that have already been excited by the original impulse, which was conducted by a faster route. If conduction is slow enough, these cells encountered by the re-emerging impulse may be past their refractory period and excitable again. Therefore, the original impulse can now reenter this tissue, leading to an extra beat. If a circular or continuous path is available for the impulse, the same impulse may chase itself around and around this pathway, generating a regular rhythm that may be very rapid. This phenomenon is called **reentry**. Reentry is thought to be responsible not only for the Wolff-Parkinson-White syndrome but also for most **supraventricular tachyarrhythmias**, arrhythmias that originate above the ventricles and involve a high atrial rate, as well as for many ventricular tachyarrhythmias. Examples of supraventricular tachyarrhythmias include **atrial flutter** (a very rapid, rhythmic pattern) and **atrial fibrillation** (a disorganized pattern that fails to produce a productive contraction), and **paroxysmal supra-ventricular tachycardia** (a rapid rhythm that begins abruptly with a premature atrial or junctional beat).

The causes of many arrhythmias are not well understood. For example, **premature ventricular contractions (PVCs)** occur occasionally even in healthy persons. The ECG pattern shows a normal QRS complex following a P wave, plus an abnormal QRS complex that does not follow a P wave. If PVCs are infrequent, they are ordinarily not treated. Abstaining from coffee, tea, caffeine, and cigarettes may control the condition.

Today, surgical ablation of the point of origin of a stable arrhythmia is sometimes used. Ablation may involve surgical interruption of the tissue that forms accessory pathways between the atria and ventricles, or it may involve the use of high-energy radio waves delivered by means of a catheter to a site that has been mapped and shown to be the source of the arrhythmia. These surgical techniques are often curative. Drug therapy is usually less ambitious, being intended only to bring an acute arrhythmia under control. Long-term therapy with antiarrhythmic drugs does not necessarily improve survival and is often associated with risks of secondary arrhythmias from the drugs themselves (see below).

Drugs used to treat cardiac arrhythmias act by interfering with one or more of the processes described previously. The drugs are grouped according to their principal action on ion channels or receptors. The classification system, although useful, is imperfect because drugs within a category are now known to differ in significant ways, and many drugs have actions that could place them in more than one category. Table 40-1 lists the major antiarrhythmic drugs by class, along with a summary of the overall effects of each drug on the various channels and receptors that are important for regulating cardiac function.

TABLE 40-1

Mechanisms Responsible for Activity of Antiarrhythmic Drugs

| | Channels | | | | | Receptors | | | |
| | Sodium | | | | | | | | |
Drug	Fast	Medium	Slow	Potassium	Calcium	Alpha	Beta	M	P
Class I-A									
disopyramide		X		X				X	
moricizine		X							
procainamide		X		X					
quinidine		X		X		X		X	
Class I-B									
lidocaine	X			0					
mexiletine	X								
tocainide	X								
Class I-C									
flecainide			X	(X)					
propafenone			X						

Alpha, alpha receptors; *Beta*, beta receptors; *M*, muscarinic receptors; *P*, purinergic (adenosine) receptors; *X*, blocks, primary effect; *(X)*, blocks, secondary or weak effect; *0*, activates, directly or indirectly.

TABLE 40-1

Mechanisms Responsible for Activity of Antiarrhythmic Drugs—cont'd

| | Channels | | | | | Receptors | | | |
| | Sodium | | | | | | | | |
Drug	Fast	Medium	Slow	Potassium	Calcium	Alpha	Beta	M	P
Class II									
propranolol							X		
Class III									
amiodarone		X		X	(X)	(X)	(X)		
bretylium				X		X	X		
dofetilide				X					
ibutilide				X					
sotalol				X			X		
Class IV									
diltiazem					X				
verapamil					X				
Unclassified									
adenosine	—								X
digoxin	—							0	

DRUG CLASS   •   Sodium Channel Blockers (Class I Antiarrhythmics)

Class I-A drugs

quinidine (Quinaglute, Quinidex, Apo-Quinidine,✳ Novoquinidin✳)

disopyramide (Norpace, Rhythmodan,✳ Rhythmodan-LA✳)

moricizine (Ethmozine)

procainamide (Procan SR)

Class I-B drugs

⚠ lidocaine (Lidopen, Xylocaine)

mexiletine (Mexitil)

tocainide (Tonocard)

Class I-C drugs

⚠ flecainide (Tambocor)

propafenone (Rhythmol)

MECHANISM OF ACTION

Class I drugs all share the ability to block voltage-gated sodium channels. Their major effect is to slow the rate of conduction of the cardiac impulse through atrial and ventricular muscles (where phase 0 of the action potential depends on these channels) and also to suppress abnormal automaticity of ectopic pacemakers. Slowing conduction may prevent or terminate a reentrant arrhythmia by changing a one-way block into a complete block in a damaged or diseased region.

The three subclasses of Class I antiarrhythmic drugs differ in the rate at which the drug molecule unbinds or dissociates from the sodium channel. As discussed for the action of local anesthetics in Chapter 16, these drugs bind to the channels when they are open and dissociate when the channel is in the resting state. Class I-B drugs dissociate so quickly that at concentrations used therapeutically, almost all the drug has time to unbind from sodium channels between beats at a normal heart rate. As a result, by the time the cell is stimulated by the next impulse, all the sodium channels are available to open in phase 0 so that the drug has little effect. However, the same concentration could produce marked effects at the high heart rates seen in serious arrhythmias because the drug does not have time to dissociate from all the sodium channels in the shorter time intervals between beats. In contrast to Class I-B drugs, Class I-C drugs dissociate so slowly that they produce equal effects at all heart rates. Class I-A drugs are intermediate between the other two, so they produce only slightly greater effects at higher heart rates.

In addition to their effect on sodium channels, Class I drugs have other important effects that differ between the subclasses. For example, most of the Class I-A drugs and Class I-C drugs also block potassium channels that are responsible for the repolarization of the atrial and ventricular muscle cells during phase 3. As a result, these drugs tend to prolong the duration of the action potential. In contrast, lidocaine, a Class I-B drug, stimulates the opening of a potassium channel, resulting in faster repolarization and shortening action potential duration.

Some drugs in this class also have potentially important activities that are unrelated to cardiac ion channels. Quinidine and disopyramide are antagonists at muscarinic cholinergic receptors. Quinidine also blocks alpha receptors, resulting in vasodilation and decreased blood pressure. Propafenone is a weak antagonist of beta receptors.

USES

In the past, Class I antiarrhythmic drugs were widely used to prevent more serious arrhythmias in patients with mild or asymptomatic arrhythmias or in patients who were thought to be at risk for serious arrhythmias. Today, these drugs are rarely used for prevention of arrhythmias and are not recommended for use in the treatment of less serious arrhythmias (see later section on Adverse Reactions and Contraindications). Instead, their use is generally restricted to the treatment of life-threatening ventricular arrhythmias. Quinidine and procainamide are also used in the treatment of atrial arrhythmias.

PHARMACOKINETICS

Most of the Class I drugs are effective when given orally. The exception is lidocaine, which is cleared too rapidly and erratically by first-pass biotransformation in the liver to be useful. Therefore, lidocaine is used primarily as a continuous intravenous infusion in the treatment of arrhythmias. First-pass biotransformation also significantly limits the bioavailability of moricizine (to 38%) and propafenone (to only 10%). All Class I drugs are extensively biotransformed by the liver, in some cases to active substances. A metabolite of procainamide, N-acetylprocainamide (NAPA), is a potent potassium-channel blocker that can accumulate to toxic levels in patients with renal failure (see next section). Most Class I drugs have relatively short half-lives ranging from 2 to 6 hours. Exceptions are mexiletine and tocainide, which have half-lives of 10 to 15 hours, and flecainide with a half-life of 20 hours. The half-life of propafenone is from 2 to 10 hours in most patients, but about 10% of people are missing the enzyme responsi-

ble for biotransforming the drug. In these individuals, the half-life of propafenone may be almost 3 days. From 20% to 50% of each dose of quinidine, disopyramide, or tocainide is eliminated unchanged in urine, and the drugs may accumulate in patients who are in renal failure.

ADVERSE REACTIONS AND CONTRAINDICATIONS

Ironically, the most serious adverse reaction of Class I antiarrhythmic drugs is their ability to provoke or worsen existing arrhythmias. At one time, Class I antiarrhythmic drugs were widely used in the treatment of patients who were thought to be at risk for serious cardiac arrhythmias. These included individuals who had only occasional PVCs, without any symptoms, because it was thought that suppressing this mild form of arrhythmia would reduce the risk of more serious ones. However, in two large clinical studies (Cardiac Arrhythmia Suppression Trials—CAST I and CAST II), treatment with Class I antiarrhythmic drugs was found to increase deaths, probably by causing the very serious arrhythmias they were intended to suppress. This effect, termed **proarrhythmia**, is now thought to be a potential consequence of treatment with most of the Class I antiarrhythmic drugs, which is why they are used much less frequently. Clinical data suggests that flecainide and moricizine, in particular, are prone to cause serious arrhythmias.

The use of quinidine or procainamide is specifically associated with a potentially deadly arrhythmia called **torsades de pointes.** This arrhythmia consists of ventricular tachycardia at rates so fast that the blood pressure falls sharply, resulting in fainting. Although these periods of ventricular tachycardia usually last only a few seconds, they may progress to ventricular fibrillation, a rapidly fatal arrhythmia in which the ventricular contractions are so fast and disorganized that cardiac output is impaired. It is now believed that torsades de pointes may be provoked by drugs that block potassium channels and, thus, prolong action-potential duration. Procainamide is biotransformed to the potent potassium channel blocker NAPA (see earlier pharmacokinetics section), and NAPA may accumulate to toxic levels in patients with renal failure, therefore use of procainamide should be avoided in these patients.

All Class I drugs should be avoided in patients with any degree of AV heart block, and any of these drugs may produce heart failure in susceptible patients. Again, flecainide is particularly troublesome in this regard and its use should be avoided in patients with structurally damaged hearts.

Antimuscarinic adverse effects are common in patients taking disopyramide and quinidine, and may include dry mouth and difficulty in urination. The anticholinergic effects of quinidine may cause serious complications in treating atrial fibrillation. In this arrhythmia, the rate of the atrial beats is very high. However, because the AV node can only conduct a fraction of the atrial beats to the ventricles (see previous discussion), the ventricles are protected. Quinidine is administered to slow the atrial rate, but the ventricular rate may initially soar dangerously high because of an anticholinergic action that speeds conduction through the AV node.

Quinidine also produces cinchonism, a syndrome including symptoms of blurred vision, dizziness, headache, and ringing in the ears. Quinidine commonly causes diarrhea, stomach pain, and loss of appetite, and may produce hypotension (dizziness or fainting) or fluid retention (heart failure) in some patients.

The most striking adverse effect with long-term use of procainamide is a syndrome resembling lupus erythematosus, with symptoms such as arthritis, arthralgia, myalgia, fever, and pericarditis. Procainamide also commonly causes GI disturbances such as diarrhea, stomach pain, and loss of appetite.

Lidocaine may cause anxiety, dizziness, drowsiness, nervousness, numbness, or the sensation of being hot or cold. Reactions seldom persist after the infusion is discontinued, because the half-life of lidocaine is so short. Mexiletine may produce heartburn, nausea, and vomiting, usually within 2 hours of administration. CNS effects include dizziness, trembling, nervousness, and unsteady gait. The most common adverse effects of tocainide include dizziness, loss of appetite, and nausea. Blisters, peeling skin, or skin rashes may signal a rare but dangerous allergic reaction that can culminate in Stevens-Johnson syndrome. After several weeks of therapy, pulmonary damage can occur, heralded by coughing and shortness of breath. Allergic reactions or pulmonary damage can be fatal.

Moricizine may cause dizziness and other CNS effects. Blurred vision and dizziness are common adverse effects of flecainide; trembling, chest pain, and arrhythmias can also occur. Propafenone may produce dizziness and other CNS effects with long-term use, and many patients treated with this drug also report a change in their sense of taste.

TOXICITY

Overdose with any of the Class I drugs can produce fatal arrhythmias. Usually these arrhythmias are first signaled by a widening of the QRS complex and, in the case of drugs that also block potassium channels, an increased Q-T interval. Apnea, loss of spontaneous respirations, and coma may sometimes precede death from cardiovascular collapse.

Lidocaine is prone to cause CNS reactions ranging from muscle twitching and drowsiness to paresthesia,

respiratory depression, convulsions, and coma. These reactions may be dose dependent. At serum lidocaine concentrations of 6 to 8 mg/mL, blurred vision, double vision, nausea, ringing in the ears, tremors, twitching, and vomiting may occur. When serum concentrations of lidocaine exceed 8 mg/mL, patients may experience bradycardia, difficulty breathing, dizziness, fainting, and seizures. Toxic reactions to lidocaine are more common in patients with reduced hepatic function, because the drug may accumulate in these patients.

Shaking and trembling are early signs of toxicity from tocainide. Overdoses may cause respiratory depression or seizures.

INTERACTIONS

Generally, any of the Class I drugs may worsen the patient's conduction and are more likely to produce arrhythmias in patients who have received other arrhythmic drugs. Such interactions with the drug pimozide are especially common. Other arrhythmic drugs, phenothiazines and rauwolfia alkaloids may have additive cardiac effects with quinidine. Disopyramide should be avoided for 48 hours before and 24 hours after a dose of verapamil; deaths from conduction blockade have occurred. Mexiletine and tocainide, in particular, may worsen cardiac function and impair contractility if combined with beta blockers. Flecainide should not be used with other antiarrhythmic drugs because such combinations may lead to fatal arrhythmias.

Class I drugs are also involved in many potentially important interactions with other drugs that patients with a cardiac disorder are likely to take. Quinidine may double plasma digoxin levels, an interaction of great significance because of digoxin's relatively low therapeutic index. The serum level of quinidine rises when the urine becomes alkaline, because renal reabsorption of the drug is enhanced; therefore drugs that alkalinize the urine, such as antacids, citrates, and carbonic anhydrase inhibitors, must be used with care.

Antihypertensives may produce hypotension if used with quinidine or procainamide, especially in older adults. Actions of anticoagulants and neuromuscular blockers are enhanced by quinidine. Antimyasthenic drugs are antagonized by procainamide, but the effects of neuromuscular blocking drugs are enhanced. Mexiletine may decrease the biotransformation of theophylline, increasing the risk of CNS toxicity. Moricizine may hasten the biotransformation of theophylline. If the drugs must be used together, theophylline concentrations should be monitored in blood, and dosages should be adjusted accordingly to maintain effective control of pulmonary disease. Cimetidine slows the clearance of moricizine. Propafenone interferes with biotransformation or elimination of digoxin and warfarin and can significantly increase serum concentrations of these drugs. Dosages may need to be reduced, and serum concentrations must be monitored when propafenone is also being given.

When administering lidocaine, it is important to remember that the drug has two separate and distinct clinical uses and is packaged differently for each. When intended for use as a local anesthetic, lidocaine is often packaged in solution with epinephrine (e.g., Xylocaine or other trade names with epinephrine). When used with the local anesthetic, epinephrine acts as a vasoconstrictor to reduce local blood flow and prolong the action of the anesthetic (see Chapter 16). If lidocaine with epinephrine were inadvertently used to treat an arrhythmia, the epinephrine might trigger a severe arrhythmia. Lidocaine intended for use in cardiac emergencies is labeled "Xylocaine preservative-free" or "lidocaine for continuous intravenous infusion."

DRUG CLASS • Beta Blockers (Class II Antiarrhythmics)

Beta blockers have an important place in the treatment of many arrhythmias because of their ability to block the effects of sympathetic nervous system activity and catecholamines on the heart. Stimulation of beta receptors increases automaticity in ectopic pacemakers as well as in the SA node, and produces other effects that may cause or support serious arrhythmias. Most importantly, these drugs do not have the ability to cause arrhythmias, as is seen in other antiarrhythmic drug classes. Because of this and the fact that they have few troublesome adverse effects, beta blockers can be used for the long-term prevention of serious ventricular tachyarrhythmias in patients thought to be at risk, such as in those who have suffered a myocardial infarction. However, beta blockers may cause or worsen AV block or precipitate heart failure in susceptible patients. Beta blockers are discussed in detail in Chapter 12.

DRUG CLASS • Drugs Prolonging Action Potential Duration (Class III Antiarrhythmics)

 amiodarone (Cordarone, Pacerone, Cordarone✤)

bretylium (Bretylol, Bretylate✤)

dofetilide (Tikosyn✤)

ibutilide (Corvert)

sotalol (Betapace, Sotacor✤)

MECHANISM OF ACTION

Class III antiarrhythmic drugs prolong action potential duration, usually by blocking potassium channels responsible for repolarization. In this way, they increase refractoriness, or the length of time during which the cell is inexcitable, and may terminate reentrant arrhythmias in this way. As with Class I drugs, however, individual Class III drugs have other actions that play significant roles in their antiarrhythmic effects.

Amiodarone also blocks sodium channels and calcium channels, and has weak but significant blocking activity at both beta receptors and alpha receptors.

Bretylium enters sympathetic nerve endings and disrupts the storage of norepinephrine, ultimately reducing its release. In the heart this would produce an antiarrhythmic effect by reducing the stimulation of beta-adrenergic receptors. However, in rare instances, bretylium may cause some initial release of norepinephrine, resulting in a brief period of increased stimulation of beta receptors in the heart and alpha receptors in blood vessels.

Ibutilide activates sodium channels during phase 3 in addition to potassium channels; the inward movement of sodium that results is also thought to delay repolarization.

Finally, sotalol is an effective beta blocker in addition to blocking potassium channels during phase 3 repolarization.

USES

Amiodarone and bretylium are used in the prevention and treatment of serious ventricular arrhythmias. Ibutilide and dofetilide are used to treat atrial flutter or fibrillation. Sotalol is used in the treatment of both atrial and ventricular arrhythmias.

PHARMACOKINETICS

Oral absorption of amiodarone is variable, and most patients absorb less than half the administered dose. Amiodarone is highly lipid soluble and concentrates in adipose tissue, as well as other sites. As a result antiarrhythmic activity is not seen for days or even months after beginning treatment. The duration of action is also greatly prolonged, partly because of an active metabolite (desethylamiodarone). Amiodarone may be detectable in plasma up to 9 months after its use has been discontinued.

Bretylium is poorly and erratically absorbed after oral administration and so is given only by intravenous or intramuscular injection. The onset of antiarrhythmic effect is usually within 20 minutes by either route, and the duration of action is 6 to 8 hours. Most of the drug is eliminated unchanged by the kidneys.

Dofetilide and sotalol are both well absorbed when given orally and have average plasma half-lives in the range of 10 to 12 hours. Most of a dose of either drug is eliminated unchanged by the kidneys. Dosages should be adjusted in patients who have renal impairment or failure, to reduce the risk of torsades de pointes.

Ibutilide is subject to extensive first-pass biotransformation by the liver and so is not effective when given orally. It is eliminated primarily by the liver, with a variable plasma half-life ranging from 2 to 12 hours.

ADVERSE REACTIONS AND CONTRAINDICATIONS

Because Class III drugs all prolong action potential duration, they may provoke the arrhythmia called torsades de pointes, described earlier. The arrhythmia is a potential problem with dofetilide, ibutilide, and sotalol, but is seen much less frequently with amiodarone or bretylium.

The most common adverse effect of amiodarone is neurotoxicity, characterized by trembling, unsteadiness in walking, numbness, weakness, or tingling of extremities. These effects may resolve slowly after use of the drug is stopped, and the effects are reversible. Chronic therapy with amiodarone is associated with a relatively high incidence of potentially fatal pulmonary fibrosis, and this limits its long-term use. Therefore, it is important to look for and recognize the early signs of pulmonary fibrosis (cough, slight fever, painful breathing, shortness of breath) in patients. Amiodarone is also known to sensitize the skin to ultraviolet light, making the patient highly susceptible to sunburn.

The major adverse effect associated with dofetilide and ibutilide is torsades de pointes, with a reported incidence of 1% to 6%. Arrhythmias produced by ibutilide may be particularly serious and may require immediate cardioversion.

The most common adverse effect associated with the use of bretylium is hypotension resulting from impairment of norepinephrine release from sympathetic nerve endings in blood vessels. Rarely, bretylium may produce initial signs of sympathetic stimulation because of an acute release of norepinephrine. This release may cause or worsen existing arrhythmias and increase blood pressure briefly before blood pressure eventually falls.

Sotalol may cause torsades de pointes, especially when renal function is impaired. Other adverse effects of sotalol are the same as for other beta blockers (see Chapter 12).

TOXICITY

Overdose with amiodarone may result in hypotension, cardiovascular distress, and bradycardia. Because the drug has such a long duration of action, the patient may require monitoring or treatment for weeks after the use of amiodarone is discontinued.

Torsades de pointes is the major toxic reaction associated with dofetilide, ibutilide, and sotalol.

INTERACTIONS

Amiodarone interferes with the biotransformation of many drugs, including coumarin-type anticoagulants, and increases plasma digoxin levels. Because of this, reduction in the dosage of anticoagulant is usually required after initiation of treatment with amiodarone.

The effects of dofetilide, ibutilide, and sotalol are additive with those of any other drugs that prolong the Q-T interval (i.e., increase action potential duration), such as Class I-A antiarrhythmics, tricyclic antidepressants, and phenothiazenes.

The initial sympathetic nervous system effect of bretylium may enhance the possibility of digoxin toxicity.

DRUG CLASS • **Calcium Channel Blockers (Class IV Antiarrhythmics)**

 verapamil (Calan, Isoptin, Verelan, Novo-Vermil,✱ Nu-Verap✱)

 diltiazem (Cardizem, Dilacor, Tiazac, Apo-Diltiaz,✱ Novo-Diltiazem,✱ Syn-Diltiazem✱)

Although several drugs that block calcium channels are available, only diltiazem and verapamil are widely used in the treatment of arrhythmias, primarily for their effects on slow-response cells in the SA node and AV node. Recall that cells at these sites differ because the cardiac action potential represents the movement of calcium and not sodium. Therefore, blocking calcium channels will slow conduction through the AV node. By doing this, these drugs enhance AV block, an effect that may terminate reentrant arrhythmias that involve a pathway through the AV node. Enhancing AV block may also protect the ventricles from high atrial rates during atrial tachyarrhythmias. These drugs also reduce the rate of firing of pacemakers in the SA node, thus lowering the heart rate. The pharmacology of all the calcium channel blockers is discussed in detail in Chapter 41.

 DRUG CLASS • **Adenosine Receptor Agonists**

 adenosine (Adenocard, Adenoscan)

MECHANISM OF ACTION

Adenosine stimulates specific adenosine receptors in the heart, resulting in effects that resemble those caused by stimulating the vagus nerve. Thus, adenosine decreases automaticity in the SA node and slows conduction through the AV node, thereby enhancing AV block.

USES

Adenosine is given intravenously in the acute treatment of supraventricular tachyarrhythmias.

PHARMACOKINETICS

Adenosine has a plasma half-life of only seconds because of its rapid uptake and biotransformation, mostly by the endothelial cells lining blood vessels. Because of this, the drug must be given by rapid intravenous push to produce any effect at all. Typically, the drug will stop the heart for several seconds when it is used effectively.

ADVERSE REACTIONS AND CONTRAINDICATIONS

A major advantage of adenosine is that its effects last only seconds. Rarely, adenosine may cause atrial fibrillation or bronchospasm. Adenosine can lower blood pressure when given by constant infusion. Adenosine is avoided or used with caution in patients with asthma, existing AV block, or unstable angina.

INTERACTIONS

Dipyridamole interferes with the uptake of adenosine and, so, may greatly enhance its effects. Alternatively, caffeine and theophylline antagonize the actions of adenosine, requiring an increase in the dosage to achieve the desired effect.

 DRUG CLASS • **Cardiac Glycosides**

Cardiac glycosides (digoxin and rarely digitoxin) are used in the treatment of supraventricular tachyarrhythmias primarily because they increase the activity of the vagus nerve. This action results in decreased automaticity of pacemakers in the SA node and slowed conduction through the AV node. The slowed AV conduction may either terminate an arrhythmia that involves a reentrant pathway through the region or enhance AV block to protect the ventricles from a high atrial rate. The pharmacology of the cardiac glycosides is discussed in detail in Chapter 38.

APPLICATION TO PRACTICE

ASSESSMENT

History of Present Illness

The reason for the hospitalization or clinic visit should be determined. The patient's perception of the problem, its onset, recent stressors, life changes, or other precipitants should be elicited. When interviewing a patient with a suspected or confirmed arrhythmia, obtain information related to history of heart failure, CAD, rheumatic fever, congenital defects, cardiac arrest, and use of cardiac drugs, diuretics, or potassium supplements. Identify conditions or risk factors that may precipitate arrhythmias, including hypoxia, electrolyte imbalances, acid-base imbalance, ischemic heart disease, valvular heart disease, respiratory disorders, excessive ingestion of caffeine-containing beverages, cigarette smoking, emotional upset, and febrile illness.

Subjective information that should be elicited includes any episode of chest pain, palpitations, shortness of breath, dizziness, syncopal episodes, confusion, and diaphoresis. If the symptoms were experienced before this encounter, the patient should be queried as to the onset, duration, frequency, and intensity of each episode. Mild arrhythmias may be perceived by the individual as palpitations or skipped beats. More severe manifestations may reflect decreased cardiac output and other hemodynamic changes. An estimate of urinary output should be obtained because oliguria from decreased renal blood flow is possible with arrhythmias.

Health History

Include in the query of the patient's health history any allergies and the physiologic response to the allergen, concomitant diseases or illnesses, and drug history, including prescription and OTC drugs. Obtain the patient's history related to alcohol intake (hypomagnesemia is related to excessive alcohol intake). Information from the patient about signs and symptoms of hypoxia related to an underlying respiratory disorder, history of hypertension, thyrotoxicosis, obesity, and diabetes mellitus should also be elicited.

Lifespan Considerations

Perinatal. Pregnancy is normally accompanied by significant physiologic changes in the maternal cardiovascular system. Pregnancy-related changes in blood volume, cardiac output, pulse, blood pressure, and peripheral vascular resistance are discussed in Chapter 2. In the majority of women these changes pose no significant threat to maternal or fetal well-being and are well tolerated. Even in women with preexisting rheumatic heart disease and with most forms of congenital heart disease, the physiologic changes of pregnancy do not result in a significant threat. However, sudden cardiac decompensation may occur in some women, including those with previously diagnosed cardiac dysfunction and those who demonstrate decompensation for the first time during pregnancy. It is important to have a clear understanding of the normal changes of pregnancy so that patient complaints or concerns can be distinguished from cardiac disorders. Symptoms that suggest significant underlying cardiac dysfunction can then be recognized as early as possible.

Pediatric. Antiarrhythmic drugs are needed less often in children than in adults. Supraventricular tachycardias are the most common arrhythmias in children. The onset of supraventricular tachycardia is often sudden, and the duration variable. Infants and young children with this arrhythmia may be unable to communicate the rapid heart rate, and the clinical course can progress to heart failure. Important signs of arrhythmia in the infant and young child include poor feeding, extreme irritability, and pallor.

Older Adults. During the third and fourth decades of life, the number of pacemaker cells decreases whereas myocardial fat, collagen, and elastin fibers increase. This change affects the SA node, which shows evidence of acceleration through the sixth decade. The number of SA cells at age 75 is 10% of what existed at age 20 years. Similarly, the AV node and the bundle of histidine (His) lose conductive cells as the body goes into the fourth decade of life, and the left bundle branch shrinks between the fifth and seventh decades. Alteration in the excitation and contraction mechanisms is an adaptive rather than a degenerative change because they maintain contractile function of the aging heart. The majority of rate irregularities in the older adult are attributed to myocardial damage.

Cultural/Social Considerations

A patient's psychologic response to an arrhythmia is determined by the severity of symptoms and the impact of the arrhythmia on lifestyle. Chronic or recurrent arrhythmias often cause the patient to fear incapacitation or even death if the arrhythmia recurs or cannot be effectively managed. For this reason, the patient's compliance with the plan of care is often enhanced.

Significant short-term emotional distress occurs in patients with ventricular fibrillation and subsequent cardiac resuscitation. The distress manifests as sleep disturbances, restlessness, irritability, and a strong identification with having been dead. Long-term emotional disturbances are rare. The patient's perceived vulnerability and powerlessness can complicate the plan of care. For some patients, the sense of vulnerability is alleviated by surgery (e.g., coronary artery bypass graft) because it is perceived as curative, or by their ability to attribute the arrhythmia to a specific correctable cause (e.g., potassium imbalance). The sense of powerlessness stems from real and perceived losses. These losses may include a loss of employment and financial security, role status, physical or social independence, and short-term memory or a lack of control over their illness (see the Case Study: Atrial Fibrillation).

Physical Examination

The physical examination should include an assessment of vital signs. Severe arrhythmias may produce manifestations that reflect decreased cardiac output and other hemodynamic changes. These manifestations can include hypotension, bradycardia, tachycardia, and irregular rhythm (e.g., pulsus alternans, bigeminal pulse, pulse deficit). Shortness of breath, dyspnea, and cough should be noted. The patient may demonstrate mental confusion from reduced cerebral blood flow.

Physical examination findings may also reveal an apical heart rate below 50 beats per minute (bpm) or above 140 bpm, an extremely irregular heart rate, a first heart sound (S_1) that varies in intensity, the signs and symptoms of heart failure, and a slow regular heart rate that does not change with activity or drug therapy. Arrhythmias that compromise cardiac output are reflected in part as a change in the characteristics of peripheral pulses.

Laboratory Testing

Electrolyte levels, acid-base balance, serum drug levels, and ECG changes should be evaluated. The key to arrhythmia interpretation is the analysis of the form and relationships among the P wave, the P-R interval, and the QRS complex. The ECG tracing should be analyzed with regard to the rate and rhythm, the site of the dominant pacemaker, and the configuration of the P wave and QRS complex. ECG findings should be correlated with clinical observations of the patient. ECG changes reflective of severely compromised cardiac output should be reported immediately before presenting signs and symptoms cause further deterioration of the patient's condition.

Blood drawn for routine serum drug levels is done approximately 30 minutes to 1 hour after the administration of an antiarrhythmic drug for a peak level and immediately before the administration of the next dose for a trough level. Any electrolyte abnormality or acid/base imbalance should be corrected since most antiarrhythmic drugs are less effective in the presence of these imbalances or electrolyte disturbances, particularly those related to potassium.

GOALS OF THERAPY

There are three general goals for the management of arrhythmias. These include abolishing the abnormal rhythm, restoring normal sinus rhythm, and preventing a recurrence of the arrhythmia. Overall desired outcomes of antiarrhythmic therapy include maintained cardiac output, increased activity tolerance, and reduced patient fear and anxiety.

There is a general consensus among health care providers that appropriate management of arrhythmias also includes treating the underlying disease processes contributing to the arrhythmia. These disease processes include cardiovascular (i.e., MI) and noncardiovascular (i.e., chronic pulmonary disease) disorders. Other conditions that predispose the patient to arrhythmias (i.e., hypoxia, electrolyte imbalance) should be prevented or treated. Education related to the hazards of smoking, overeating, excessive coffee intake, and other habits that may cause or aggravate arrhythmias is essential.

INTERVENTION

Administration

Intervention using an antiarrhythmic drug is appropriate when the patient has an acute arrhythmia that is producing life-threatening rhythm disturbances. The patient should be hospitalized in a coronary care unit and placed on telemetry.

Check the blood pressure and apical pulse before the administration of every dose of antiarrhythmic drug. If marked changes are noted in rate, rhythm, or quality of pulses, withhold the dose and contact the health care provider. Hypotension and bradycardia are most likely to occur when therapy to treat arrhythmia is being initiated or the dosage or frequency is altered. These signs are more likely to occur with intravenous drug formulations than with the oral form and may indicate the need for dosage adjustment. Continuous cardiac monitoring should be maintained during intravenous administration of antiarrhythmic drugs.

Intravenous formulations are given through a free-flowing peripheral vein with attention to drug concentration, administration time, drug-drug interactions, and patient response. The majority of intravenous antiarrhythmics should be given via an infusion pump. Be sure to read package labeling carefully. Use only solutions labeled "for cardiac arrhythmias," and do not use solutions that also contain epinephrine. Lidocaine solutions containing epinephrine are used for local anesthesia only. These solutions should never be given intravenously in the management of arrhythmias because the epinephrine can aggravate or cause new arrhythmias. Furthermore, rapid injection (less than 30 seconds) produces transient blood levels several times higher than therapeutic range limits, increasing the risk of toxicity without a concomitant increase in therapeutic effectiveness.

With the exception of adenosine, intravenous antiarrhythmics should be administered in a peripheral vein to allow mixing with blood. Injection into a central line is hazardous because a high drug concentration develops locally within the heart.

When changing from another antiarrhythmic therapy to mexiletine, give the first dose 6 to 12 hours after the last dose of quinidine, 3 to 6 hours after the last dose of procainamide, or 8 to 12 hours after the last dose of tocainide. When changing from parenteral lidocaine, decrease the lidocaine dose, or discontinue the lidocaine 1 to 2 hours after administration of mexiletine, or administer lower doses of mexiletine.

It is recommended that oral antiarrhythmic drug formulations be administered with food to decrease GI irritation. In addition, these drugs should be given at evenly spaced intervals to maintain adequate blood levels.

Knowledge as to when peak plasma levels are reached for the various antiarrhythmic drugs may be helpful in determining when therapeutic effects are most likely to appear. However, there are many other factors that influence therapeutic effects, including the dosage, frequency of administration, presence of conditions that alter drug biotransformation, arterial blood gas values, serum electrolyte levels, and myocardial status. Serum drug levels must be interpreted in light of the patient's clinical response to therapy. Antiarrhythmic drugs can accumulate in patients with renal or hepatic dysfunction, so these patients should be carefully monitored for signs and symptoms of increasing renal impairment. Drug dosages may need to be adjusted based on these data.

Be alert for the development of new arrhythmias because some of these drugs have proarrhythmic effects. For example, a torsades de pointes arrhythmia may develop in patients who receive quinidine, procainamide, disopyramide, amiodarone, or sotalol. Women are more at risk for torsades de pointes than men, especially during administration of cardiovascular drugs that prolong depolarization. Liquid protein diets and electrolyte disturbances (e.g., hypokalemia, hypomagnesemia) may also precipitate the development of this arrhythmia. By prolonging the Q-T interval, certain noncardiac drugs such as some antihypertensives, antibiotics, diuretics, antihistamines, tricyclic antidepressants, and phenothiazines may also set the stage for torsades de pointes. This arrhythmia may manifest as unexplained syncope. This arrhythmia and other proarrhythmic events often occur within a few days of initiating antiarrhythmic therapy, but they may also develop unexpectedly later in the course of long-term treatment.

Education

As with all drugs, antiarrhythmics should be taken as prescribed, with the dosage regimen individualized to maximize therapeutic effects and minimize adverse reactions. The patient and the family should be taught the name of the drug, the dosage, and the reason it is needed. Patients should also be taught a proper administration technique for the drug form they are receiving. Abrupt discontinuance of antiarrhythmic drugs has been associated with reappearance of arrhythmia. Encourage the patient not to miss a dose and to carry information in written form regarding the prescribed drugs. For patients taking several drugs, the health care provider should stress the risks of multidrug therapy, such as the potential for drug-drug interactions, altered drug responses, and increased risk of adverse effects. The patient should also wear a form of medical alert identification.

Teach the patient and family members to recognize and report signs and symptoms of bradycardia, hypotension, arrhythmia, heart failure, pulmonary and peripheral embolism, and cardiac arrest. Teach the patient to avoid sudden changes in position to reduce the severity of postural hypotension. Blood pressure should be monitored according to the health care provider's instructions, particularly in patients with known ventricular dysfunction or hypertrophy. The antiarrhythmic drug may need to be discontinued if severe hypotension occurs. The patient's intake, output, and weight should be monitored weekly for indications of heart failure (i.e., shortness of breath, edema, weight gain, intake greater than urinary output, fatigue).

Advise patients to notify their dentist or health care provider of their drug regimen before dental treatment or surgery and to avoid concurrent use of other drugs (including OTC drugs). In addition, advise patients to avoid alcoholic beverages, cigarette smoking, excess sodium intake, caffeine, and sunlight (for those on amiodarone). They should be cautioned to avoid hazardous activities until the effects of the antiarrhythmic drug are known. Encourage patients to keep follow-up appointments with their health care provider.

EVALUATION

The data required for evaluating the therapeutic effectiveness relate to cardiac output, activity tolerance, fear and anxiety, tissue perfusion status, compliance or lack of compliance with the treatment regimen, and absence of complications resulting from antiarrhythmic therapy. Criteria that may be used to evaluate the therapeutic outcome of antiarrhythmic therapy include the following: (1) the impulse is generated at the SA node; (2) conduction occurs within a uniform, normal time period; (3) contraction takes place at regular, equally spaced intervals at a rate of 60 to 100 bpm in an adult and 130 to 160 bpm in a newborn; and (4) AV and intraventricular conduction take place via the appropriate conduction tissues. The drug's effectiveness can also be evaluated by the nurse by noting improvement in the rate, rhythm, and quality of the pulse.

As with the patient who takes cardiac glycosides or antianginal drugs, the perceived susceptibility to disease and its seriousness influences patient compliance. Because many of the antiarrhythmic drugs have unpleas-

ant or undesirable adverse effects, the likelihood of compliance is an important consideration. It is necessary to work with the patient and family members, when appropriate, to ensure their cooperation. Once the importance of continued medical treatment and follow up is understood, the majority of patients are usually compliant. The fact that the patient is often recovering from a life-threatening event, such as an MI, also motivates compliance.

CASE STUDY   *Atrial Fibrillation*

ASSESSMENT

HISTORY OF PRESENT ILLNESS

BG is an 82-year-old white man in moderate distress with complaints of increasing dyspnea and fatigue. The dyspnea has progressively worsened over the past month, and he is now confined to home. He previously walked 1 mile per day. He sleeps with two pillows but awakens at night with complaints of dyspnea, sitting by the open window to catch his breath. He follows a 1500-mg sodium diet.

HEALTH HISTORY

BG denies allergies to food or drugs. He had a mitral valve replacement at age 64 and an MI at age 75 without sequelae. His last ECG was 2 weeks ago. He denies having a history of other hospitalizations, illness, consumption of alcohol, or smoking. Current drugs: digoxin 0.25 mg po qd; furosemide 20 mg qd; K-lor 15 mEq po qd.

LIFESPAN CONSIDERATIONS

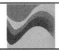

BG is likely to have age-related physiologic changes of the cardiac, renal, and GI systems. He lives on social security and retirement benefits and has Medicare parts A and B. He uses AARP pharmacy mail services for routine drugs. BG will need to obtain the new drug from a local pharmacy until his response to therapy is determined; therefore his cost is greater than what he pays through AARP.

CULTURAL/SOCIAL CONSIDERATIONS

BG retired at age 75. He visits his health care provider only when necessary and takes little preventive care. He believes in natural foods and always eats nutritious meals. On several occasions he has expressed concern that he will become a burden to his 74-year-old wife, who is physically unable to assume responsibility for his care. They have an adult son and daughter who live six blocks away.

PHYSICAL EXAMINATION

BG is 5'9" tall and weighs 155 lbs (9 lbs more than usual); blood pressure 160/70 mm Hg; respirations 28, increasing to 32 with minimal exertion; apical pulse 120 bpm resting

and 130 to 140 bpm with exertion; radial pulse 104 bpm. Bibasilar fine crackles are found on auscultation. Diaphragmatic excursion is 4 cm. Gallop rhythm noted on auscultation of the heart with variation in intensity of S_1. Liver is 5 cm below costal margin. Skin is pale without cyanosis.

LABORATORY TESTING

Chest x-ray study reveals left ventricular enlargement and fluid at both bases and congestion of the pulmonary vasculature. ECG shows atrial fibrillation with a rate of 124 bpm and occasional PVCs. Electrolyte levels: Na^+, 130 mEq/L; K^+, 3.6 mEq/L; Cl^-, 92 mEq/L; BUN, 34 mg/100 mL; creatinine, 1.3 mg/100 mL.

PATIENT PROBLEM(S)

Atrial fibrillation; hypertension.

GOALS OF THERAPY

Restore normal sinus rhythm; prevent development of other arrhythmias; prevent or reduce frequency of recurrent episodes of atrial fibrillation; maintain adequate tissue perfusion and cardiac output.

CRITICAL THINKING QUESTIONS

1. The health care provider leaves the following drug orders: continue digoxin but decrease dosage to 0.125 mg po qd; continue furosemide at 20 mg qd; add diltiazem SR 60 mg bid and warfarin 5 mg qd. What is the mechanism of action of these four drugs?
2. Which of the drugs identified in the previous question is used primarily to reduce the risk of thromboembolic complications associated with BG's atrial fibrillation?
3. What nursing assessments are indicated for BG?
4. What is the therapeutic dosage range for digoxin? Should serum levels of the other drugs BG is taking be measured? If so, what drug and what tests?
5. What findings on the ECG indicate the presence of atrial fibrillation? What findings indicate therapeutic response to drug therapy?

Bibliography

Anonymous: Ventricular arrhythmia: preventing sudden death, *Nurses Drug Alert* 24(2):13, 2000.

Beattie S: A portrait of postop a-fib, *RN* 63(3):26-30, 2000.

Bubien RS: A new beat on an old rhythm, *Am J Nurs* 100(1):42-51, 2000.

Diaz AL, Clifton GD: Considerations in drug therapy. Dofetilide: a new class III antiarrhythmic for the management of atrial fibrillation, *Prog Cardiovasc Nurs* 16(3):126-129, 2001.

Evans-Murray A: Wolff Parkinson White (WPW) syndrome: what the critical care nurse needs to consider when administering antiarrhythmics, *Aust Crit Care* 14(1):5-9, 2001.

Kern LS: Management of postoperative atrial fibrillation, *J Cardiovasc Nurs* 12(3):57-77, 1998.

Owens SG: Nursing management of arrhythmias after cardiac surgery, *AACN News* 17(2):11-12, 2000.

Tedesco C, Reigle J, Bergin J: Sudden cardiac death in heart failure, *J Cardiovasc Nurs* 14(4):38-56, 2000.

Wooten JM, Earnest J, Reyes J: Review of common adverse effects of selected antiarrhythmic drugs, *Crit Care Nurs Q* 22(4):23-38, 2000.

Internet Resources

http://lysine.pharm.utah.edu/netpharm/netpharm_00/druglist/dl_arr.htm.

http://www.med-edu.com/patient/arrhythmia/arrhythmia-treatments.html.

http://www.xagena.it/einthoven/eint0014.htm.

CHAPTER

41

Antihypertensive Drugs

JOSEPH A. DiMICCO • ELIZABETH KISSELL

 Visit http://evolve.elsevier.com/Gutierrez/ for additional information.

KEY TERMS

Angiotensin-receptor blockers (ARBs), p. 663

Angiotensin II, p. 663

Angiotensin-1 (AT$_1$) receptor, p. 658

Essential hypertension, p. 659

Left ventricular hypertrophy, p. 660

Preeclampsia, p. 660

Renin, p. 658

Renin-angiotensin system, p. 658

OBJECTIVES

- Discuss the factors that control blood pressure.
- Discuss the classes of drugs that may be used for initial drug therapy for hypertension.
- Discuss the rationale for combination therapy with drugs from different classes.
- Describe modifications in antihypertensive therapy that may be needed for special populations, such as African Americans, older adults, pregnant women, and patients with coexisting cardiovascular disease.
- Create a nursing care plan for a patient receiving antihypertensive drugs.

PATHOPHYSIOLOGY • Hypertension

Arterial pressure is the driving force for delivery of blood to all the tissues of the body. Because of this important function, arterial pressure is normally kept within relatively narrow limits by a number of mechanisms, the most important of which are (1) renal mechanisms that regulate the circulating blood volume through adjustments of body salt and water (see Chapter 46), (2) neural mechanisms that influence the activity of the heart and blood vessels (see Chapter 12), and (3) hormonal mechanisms, most notably the renin-angiotensin system (see Chapter 38), that may affect both renal function and the cardiovascular system.

The kidneys maintain normal blood volume by regulating salt and water balance, as is discussed in detail in Chapter 46. A person may take in varying amounts of salt and water from day to day. The kidney adjusts the amount of each that it excretes in the urine, retaining more when intake is low and eliminating the excess when intake is high. The result is that the extracellular fluid volume and salt concentration remain constant, and this means that the volume of blood in the body is also held constant.

Although the regulation of blood volume by the kidney is vital for the long-term regulation of arterial pressure, moment-to-moment adjustments are made by the sympathetic nervous system (see Chapter 12). Arterial pressure is maintained by the sympathetic nerves constantly releasing norepinephrine, causing contraction of vascular smooth muscle. Because this action narrows the small blood vessels, resistance to flow is increased and arterial pressure is maintained. Baroreceptors in the aorta and carotid sinus constantly monitor blood pressure and send the information to the brain. The brain integrates this information and adjusts the heart rate and resistance of the blood vessels, largely through the sympathetic nervous system, to fine-tune blood pressure. The center in the brain that controls blood pressure by regulating the activity of the autonomic nervous system is located in the medulla. As the principal neurotransmitter of the sympathetic nervous system, norepinephrine raises blood pressure by stimulating (1) the beta$_1$ receptors of the heart to increase cardiac output and (2) the alpha$_1$ receptors on blood vessels, causing constriction and increasing resistance to blood flow. In contrast, in the CNS, norepinephrine acts at alpha$_2$ receptors to decrease sympathetic nerve activity to the cardiovascular system, resulting in reduced blood pressure.

The renin-angiotensin system influences both the heart and blood vessels directly as well as the renal mechanisms that control salt and water balance. Renin is an enzyme released by certain cells in the kidney when blood pressure falls. The release of renin is also stimulated by the sympathetic nervous system acting through beta receptors. This enzyme acts on a protein in the blood to produce the peptide angiotensin I. Angiotensin I is rapidly transformed by angiotensin-converting enzymes (ACE) into angiotensin II, a small peptide. Angiotensin II (AII) produces actions important for blood pressure regulation at one specific subtype of AII receptor called the **angiotensin-1 (AT$_1$) receptor**. These actions cause (1) vasoconstriction leading to increased blood pressure and (2) secretion of aldosterone from the adrenal cortex. Aldosterone is the mineralocorticoid hormone that causes the kidney to decrease the excretion of sodium and increase potassium excretion. The resulting sodium retention expands the volume of plasma and extracellular fluid, which contributes to the elevation of blood pressure. When these physiologic regulatory mechanisms become unbalanced, blood pressure rises to an abnormally high level, producing hypertension. Table 41-1 provides an overview of the stages of hypertension. Classifications of hypertension are discussed in the following sections.

TABLE 41-1

Classification of Blood Pressure Stages*

Stage	Systolic (mm Hg)	Diastolic (mm Hg)
Optimal†	<120	<180
Normal	<135	<85
High normal	130-139	85-89
Hypertension†		
Stage 1	140-159	90-99
Stage 2	160-179	100-109
Stage 3	>180	>110

From Joint National Committee on Detection, Evaluation, and Treatment of High Blood Pressure. The sixth report of the Joint National Committee on the Prevention, Detection, Evaluation, and Treatment of High Blood Pressure, *Arch Intern Med* 157(21): 2417, 1997.
*Based on an average of two or more readings taken at each of two or more visits following an initial screening in adults over age 18. The patient is not taking antihypertensive drugs and is not acutely ill.
†Optimal blood pressure with respect to cardiovascular risk is less than 120/80 mm Hg. However, unusually low values should be evaluated for clinical significance. When systolic and diastolic pressures fall into different categories, the higher category should be used to classify the patient's blood pressure status. For example, a reading of 182/102 mm Hg would be classified as Stage 3 hypertension.

ESSENTIAL HYPERTENSION

In the United States it is estimated that essential hypertension (also known as primary hypertension) affects 43 million persons (Box 41-1). The cause of essential hypertension is unknown, although a variety of physiologic mechanisms are under investigation for their role in high blood pressure. The renin-angiotensin system, aldosterone, and their mechanisms controlling sodium elimination are of particular interest. This system is usually activated in response to low renal perfusion and causes retention of sodium and water, which increases vascular volume, renal perfusion, and blood pressure. About 15% of patients with hypertension have high levels of renin activity. Hypovolemia and sodium deficiency stimulate renin activity, thus causing sodium and water retention as well as vasoconstriction.

In contrast, 30% of patients with hypertension, including African Americans, have low renin levels. The low renin level is linked to excess sodium, which reduces renin activity. However, as in patients with high renin activity, these patients have increased vascular volume and elevated blood pressure.

Aldosterone is released when the renin-angiotensin system is stimulated. In response to aldosterone, the kidneys retain sodium ions and excrete potassium ions. The possibility of reducing blood pressure by increasing potassium intake rather than by restricting sodium is being evaluated.

Vascular endothelium is now thought to produce a variety of vasoactive substances, some of which are powerful local vasodilators. A deficit of these substances may contribute to high blood pressure.

The role of vasopressin (see Chapter 55) in the development of primary hypertension has also been explored. A heightened sensitivity to vasopressin has been identified in African Americans. This knowledge may help in part to explain some of the ethnic variability in blood pressure.

Type 2 diabetes mellitus has been recognized as a risk factor for primary hypertension. The prevalence of hypertension in these patients is as high as 50%. Obesity in patients with type 2 diabetes explains part of the increased risk of hypertension. Type 2 diabetes, obesity, and hypertension may be accompanied by insulin resistance and hyperinsulinemia. Hypotheses being explored for the hypertensive mechanisms of insulin resistance include increased release of norepinephrine, sodium retention, and increased vascular tone. The increased vascular tone may be related to sodium transport mechanisms in the blood vessels. Blood pressure declines in African-American patients who have diabetes as their blood sugar levels are reduced (independent of antihypertensive drugs).

SECONDARY HYPERTENSION

Secondary hypertension affects less than 5% to 10% of persons with high blood pressure. It is related to an identifiable cause and usually develops in persons less than 35 years old or more than 55 years old. The elevation in both systolic and diastolic blood pressure can be related to coarctation of the aorta, Cushing's syndrome, diabetes mellitus, pheochromocytoma, and a wide variety of drugs and chemicals (e.g., nasal decongestants, oral contraceptives, sympathomimetics,

---

BOX 41-1   Types of Hypertension

Primary (essential) hypertension	Hypertension characterized by a slow, progressive elevation in blood pressure over several years; cause unknown
Secondary hypertension	Hypertension related to underlying renal or endocrine cause; known causes (e.g., coarctation of the aorta, pheochromocytoma, etc.)
Resistant hypertension	Diastolic blood pressure readings consistently above 90 mm Hg while under treatment with antihypertensive drugs
Refractory hypertension	Hypertension that fails to respond to therapy
Malignant hypertension	Diastolic blood pressure over 140 mm Hg associated with papilledema—a medical emergency
Isolated systolic hypertension	Systolic blood pressure above 160 mm Hg in patients over the age of 60
Complicated hypertension	Arterial hypertension of any cause where there is evidence of cardiovascular damage related to blood pressure elevation
White-coat hypertension	Blood pressure that is elevated when taken by health care provider but normal when measured outside of the health care environment
Preeclampsia	Blood pressure elevation 15 mm Hg above normal pressure during pregnancy, accompanied by albuminuria and edema

antidepressants, erythropoietin). The elevation of blood pressure in these patients is treated by focusing on its underlying cause.

ISOLATED SYSTOLIC HYPERTENSION

Isolated systolic hypertension is defined as systolic blood pressure greater than or equal to 140 mm Hg with diastolic blood pressure less than 90 mm Hg. It occurs in approximately 10% of people 65 to 74 years old and in 24% of patients more than 80 years old. As arteriosclerosis progresses with age there is reduced distensibility of the aorta and large arteries. This reduced distensibility causes an elevated systolic blood pressure without an increase in diastolic blood pressure.

MALIGNANT HYPERTENSION

Malignant hypertension is a rapidly progressing, potentially fatal form of hypertension. In this form of hypertension, the diastolic pressure exceeds 120 mm Hg. Approximately 1% of all patients with hypertension develop this form. If the condition is left untreated, the 1-year mortality rate for malignant hypertension is almost 90%. Men, middle-aged adults, and African Americans are most likely to develop this form of hypertension. The most common mechanism of the disorder is bilateral renal artery stenosis. Severe emotional stress, excessive salt intake, or abrupt discontinuance of antihypertensive drug therapy may trigger a hypertensive crisis. Furthermore, any disease or condition that produces high blood pressure can result in this accelerated form of hypertension.

PREECLAMPSIA

Preeclampsia, which is an acute form of hypertension occurring in pregnant women after 24 weeks of gestation, is also characterized by proteinuria and edema. Several theories have been proposed for the cause of preeclampsia. An increased sensitivity to AII, hormonal changes that increase vasoconstriction, and a tendency toward reduced calcium intake during pregnancy may combine to cause a hypertensive state. Generalized vasospasm, perhaps caused by an imbalance in the production of thromboxane A_2 (a vasoconstrictor) and prostacyclin (a vasodilator), may contribute to high blood pressure.

EFFECTS OF HYPERTENSION

A patient with essential, secondary, or isolated systolic hypertension may have no symptoms of the disease but will have an increased risk for stroke, blindness, and heart and renal disease after 10 years or more of sustained high blood pressure that produces vascular

and organ damage. One of the changes that often occurs over time is **left ventricular hypertrophy,** a condition that results from the heart having to pump against abnormally high arterial pressure. Left ventricular hypertrophy is one of the pathophysiologic changes that develops early in heart failure (see Chapter 38). Hypertension is seen more often in older adults than in younger adults, is more common in men than in women during young adulthood and early middle age, but more common in women than men from middle age onward. African Americans, those from the southeastern United States, and economically disadvantaged and less educated individuals also have a higher rate of hypertension.

Effective drug therapy for patients with hypertension has been available for almost 30 years. Over this period, for patients controlling their hypertension with drug therapy, mortality from coronary heart disease has decreased by 50% and from stroke by 57%.

SUMMARY OF DRUG THERAPY FOR HYPERTENSION

Table 41-2 lists those classes of drugs that have a role in the treatment of essential hypertension. These include drugs that act on the kidney to promote salt and wa-

---

TABLE 41-2

Drug Classes Used in the Treatment of Essential Hypertension

First-line drugs*	Diuretics (hydrochlorothiazide, furosemide)
	Beta blockers (propranolol, metoprolol)
	ACE inhibitors (captopril, lisinopril)
	Angiotensin receptor blockers (losartan, valsartan)
Alternative first-line drugs†	Alpha$_1$ blockers (prazosin, terazosin)
	Calcium channel blockers (verapamil, felodipine)
Second- or third-line drugs‡	Centrally acting drugs (methyldopa, clonidine)
	Adrenergic neuron blockers (reserpine, guanadrel)
	Direct-acting vasodilators (hydralazine, minoxidil)

*May be used alone (as monotherapy) or in combination with any other drugs.
†Usually used in combination with a diuretic.
‡Used only in combination therapy after failure to achieve adequate control with other drugs or in special circumstances.

ter excretion, drugs that reduce the activity or effect of the sympathetic nervous system, drugs that interfere with the renin-angiotensin system, and drugs that act directly on vascular smooth muscle to cause vasodilation. Initial drug therapy generally begins with the adminis-

tration of a single drug from one of several drug classes. Diuretics and beta blockers are the preferred classes because of their proven effectiveness in many clinical trials; however, other drug classes may be used, especially when beta blockers and diuretics are ineffective.

DRUG CLASS • Diuretics

chlorothiazide (Diuril)

hydrochlorthiazide (Esidrix, Microzide, Oretic)

hydroflumethiazide (Diucardin, Saluron)

methylclothiazide (Enduron, Aquatensen)

polythiazide (Renese)

trichlormethiazide (Metahydrin, Naqua)

MECHANISM OF ACTION

Traditionally, the most common choice for initial therapy of hypertension has been an oral diuretic, usually a thiazide or thiazide-like drug. Diuretics are especially effective as monotherapy for African-American patients with hypertension. These drugs inhibit renal tubular reabsorption, causing diuresis that leads to reduction of body salt and water (extracellular fluid). The loss of extracellular fluid is associated with reduced arterial blood pressure, but the exact mechanism of this hypotensive action is unknown. This effect is not seen in patients who do not have hypertension. The volume depletion also produces a reduction in plasma volume, although it is not clear that this reduction persists after the first month of therapy.

In addition to their use as monotherapy, diuretics are commonly used in combination with other classes of antihypertensive drugs. The antihypertensive effect of many of the drugs (see below) is often limited by fluid retention, which is the body's normal response to a sudden drop in blood pressure, even when the blood pressure is abnormally elevated. By reducing or preventing fluid accumulation, a greater therapeutic effect can be achieved. This approach is so popular that many of the drugs discussed below are formulated with a thiazide diuretic into a single pill (Table 41-3). Diuretics are discussed further in Chapter 46.

TABLE 41-3

Fixed-Dose Combinations of a Thiazide Diuretic with Another Antihypertensive Drug

Generic Drugs	*Brand Name*
Beta Blocker with Diuretic	
atenolol + chlorthalidone	Tenoretic
bisoprolol + hydrochlorothiazide	Ziac
metoprolol + hydrochlorothiazide	Lopressor HCT
nadolol + bendroflumethiazide	Corzide
pindolol + hydrochlorothiazide	Viskazide
propranolol + hydrochlorothiazide	Inderide LA
timolol + hydrochlorothiazide	Timolide
ACE Inhibitor with Diuretic	
benazepril + hydrochlorothiazide	Lotensin HCT
captopril + hydrochlorothiazide	Capozide
enalapril + hydrochlorothiazide	Vaseretic
lisinopril + hydrochlorothiazide	Zestoretic
moexipril + hydrochlorothiazide	Uniretic
quinapril + hydrochlorothiazide	Accuretic
Angiotensin II Blocker with Diuretic	
candesartan + hydrochlorothiazide	Atacand HCT
losartan + hydrochlorothiazide	Hyzaar
telmisartan + hydrochlorothiazide	Micardis HCT
valsartan + hydrochlorothiazide	Diovan HCT
Alpha Blocker with Diuretic	
prazosin + polythiazide	Minizide
Centrally Acting Antihypertensive with Diuretic	
clonidine + chlorthalidone	Combipres
methyldopa + chlorothiazide	Aldoclor
methyldopa + hydrochlorothiazide	Aldoril
Direct-Acting Vasodilator with Diuretic	
hydralazine + hydrochlorothiazide	Apresazide

DRUG CLASS • Beta Blockers

⚠ propranolol (Inderal)

acebutolol (Sectral)

atenolol (Tenormin)

betaxolol (Kerlone)

bisoprolol (Zebeta)

carteolol (Cartrol)

labetalol (Trandate)

metoprolol (Lopressor, Toprol)

nadolol (Corgard)

penbutolol (Levatol)

pindolol (Visken)

timolol (Blocadren)

MECHANISM OF ACTION

Instead of a diuretic, a beta blocker may be given as the first-line drug. Hypertensive individuals with high plasma renin levels are especially responsive to beta blockers and generally unresponsive to diuretics, because beta blockers inhibit the release of renin from the kidney. In general, however, hypertensive whites in the younger age groups have high renin levels, whereas older African-American adults with hypertension have low renin levels.

A beta blocker is also indicated for patients who have coronary artery disease (CAD). Beta blockers have been shown to have a protective effect against sudden death in individuals who have had a heart attack, whereas diuretics may, by reducing potassium levels, increase the vulnerability of the compromised heart to sudden failure.

Beta blockers that may be of particular use in some patients with hypertension include labetalol and pindolol. Labetalol also blocks alpha receptors, an effect that further lowers blood pressure. Pindolol is a partial agonist at beta receptors (i.e., it has intrinsic sympathomimetic activity) and so may reduce vascular resistance by stimulating these receptors on blood vessels (which are not normally activated except under normal conditions of exercise or stress).

The combination of a beta blocker and a thiazide diuretic has proved so popular that a number of such preparations are available (see Table 41-3). Although these formulations may be more convenient for the patient, fixed-dose combinations do not permit modification of the dosage of one drug independent of the other, which is often necessary to optimize antihypertensive therapy when more than one drug is involved. Beta blockers are discussed further in Chapter 12.

DRUG CLASS • Angiotensin-Converting Enzyme (ACE) Inhibitors

benzapril (Lotensin)

⚠ captopril (Capoten)

enalapril (Vasotec)

fosinopril (Monopril)

lisinopril (Prinivil, Zestril)

moexipril (Univasc)

perindopril (Aceon)

quinapril (Accupril)

ramipril (Altace)

trandolapril (Mavik)

MECHANISM OF ACTION

ACE inhibitors are effective in treating most forms of hypertension and in recent years have become one of the most popular choices for initial therapy suitable for all age groups. ACE inhibitors block the formation of AII, a potent vasoconstrictor, and stimulate aldosterone secretion. The ACE inhibitors are more effective in whites than in African-American patients, but the resistance seen in the latter group can be partly overcome by combining the ACE inhibitor with a diuretic drug. The antihypertensive response is not associated with an increase in heart rate or cardiac output. ACE inhibitors appear to limit the damage to the renal blood vessels typically seen in diabetic patients and in certain other renal disorders. Although their adverse effect profile is generally very good, ACE inhibitors should be avoided in patients with a history of angioedema and should not be taken during pregnancy. ACE inhibitors are also important drugs in the treatment of heart failure and are especially indicated for the patient who has hypertension as well as heart failure. Preparations combining an ACE inhibitor and a thiazide diuretic are available (see Table 41-3). The pharmacokinetics of ACE inhibitors is discussed in Chapter 38.

DRUG CLASS • Angiotensin II–Receptor Blockers

candesartan (Atacand)

eprosartan (Teveten)

irbesartan (Avapro)

⚠ losartan (Cozaar)

telmisartan (Micardis)

valsartan (Diovan)

MECHANISM OF ACTION

Angiotensin II blockers bind tightly but reversibly to the AT_1 subtype of AII receptors. These receptors seem to be responsible for most of the clinically important effects of angiotensin on the heart, blood vessels, kidneys, and adrenal glands. AII-receptor blockers are thought to be more effective than ACE inhibitors in reducing activation of AT_1 receptors. By blocking the effects of the peptide at this receptor, these drugs relax vascular smooth muscle, resulting in vasodilation and a reduction in blood pressure. They also reduce salt and water retention (by preventing AII-induced stimulation of aldosterone secretion) and so reduce plasma volume, which also contributes to the fall in blood pressure. Other, unknown effects of AT_1-receptor blockade may contribute to their therapeutic response. These drugs do not directly influence AT_2 receptors but may increase their stimulation by increasing circulating AII levels. The consequence of this effect is unknown at this time.

USES

Angiotensin II antagonists (sometimes known as angiotensin II–receptor blockers [ARBs]) represent the newest important class of antihypertensive drugs. They are at least as effective as ACE inhibitors in lowering arterial pressure and have a superior adverse effect profile (see below). Like the ACE inhibitors, AII-receptor blockers are less effective in African-American patients. Because of the usefulness of ACE inhibitors in the treatment of heart failure, much interest is now focused on the potential therapeutic effect of AT_1-receptor blockade in hypertensive patients with evidence of left ventricular hypertrophy (enlargement of the ventricular muscle mass). The Evaluation of Losartan in the Elderly (ELITE) study suggested that losartan was more effective than the ACE inhibitor captopril in reducing mortality in older hypertensive patients with heart failure. A large clinical trial, the Losartan Intervention for Endpoint (LIFE) Reduction Study, as well as studies examining the effect of losartan or other AT_1-receptor blockers in different patient populations with heart failure or hypertension or after an MI are currently underway. Several preparations combining one of the AII blockers and a thiazide diuretic drug are available (see Table 41-3).

PHARMACOKINETICS

Oral bioavailability of these drugs is generally poor (30% or less) except for telmisartan (50%) and irbesartan (60% to 80%), and all are highly protein bound (90% to 99%). Candesartan is administered as the prodrug candesartan cilexetil. Most of the effect of losartan is produced by a metabolite with much more activity than the parent drug. Plasma half-lives are in the range of 6 to 9 hours for all except irbesartan (11 to 15 hours) and telmisartan (24 hours). All are eliminated from the body primarily in the feces usually unchanged or after biliary conjugation.

ADVERSE REACTIONS AND CONTRAINDICATIONS

The AII-receptor blockers produce few adverse reactions in the vast majority of patients. Unlike ACE inhibitors, the AII-receptor blockers do not usually cause cough and are rarely associated with angioedema. The most common adverse effect is dizziness and hypotension. As with the ACE inhibitors, though, they may provoke significant increases in plasma potassium in susceptible patients and should be avoided during pregnancy, especially after the first trimester. Also as with the ACE inhibitors, AII blockers should not be used by patients with renal artery stenosis.

INTERACTIONS

The AII-receptor blockers are more likely to produce significant hypotension when combined with diuretics. When used with potassium-sparing drugs, clinically significant increases in plasma potassium levels are possible. Telmisartan has been reported to increase the steady-state plasma digoxin level.

DRUG CLASS • Calcium Channel Blockers

diltiazem (Cartia, Cardizem, Tiamate, Tiazac)

felodipine (Plendil)

isradipine (DynaCirc)

nicardipine (Cardene)

nifedipine (Adalat, Procardia)

nisoldipine (Sular)

⚠ verapamil (Calan, Verelan)

MECHANISM OF ACTION

Calcium channel blockers are an alternative to diuretics and beta blockers as first-line drug therapy for hypertension. Most of the calcium channel blockers currently available are indicated for this purpose, including diltiazem, felodipine, isradipine, nicardipine, nifedipine, nisoldipine, and verapamil. Calcium channel blockers decrease the entry of calcium into smooth muscle and thereby reduce vascular tone, an action that in turn reduces peripheral resistance and blood pressure. This reduction in blood pressure can produce a reflex increase in heart rate. Cardiac function may also be depressed because of reduced intracellular calcium. Each of the various calcium channel blockers differs in its relative effect on vascular and cardiac tissue. Calcium channel blockers are especially effective as monotherapy for decreasing blood pressure in older adult patients, those with angina, and those with low plasma renin activity. Older adults and African-American patients have a better response to calcium channel blockers as the first-line drug to treat hypertension than to other antihypertensive drugs used alone. In general, calcium channel blockers are safe for patients with asthma, hyperlipidemia, diabetes, and renal dysfunction, and they are well tolerated by various age and ethnic groups. Because they are more sensitive to the effects of these drugs, a hypotensive response is more likely in older adults. Unlike beta blockers, calcium channel blockers do not improve the chances of survival for hypertensive patients who have had an MI; therefore they are not the antihypertensive drug of choice in these individuals. In fact, concern has been raised that some calcium channel blockers may increase the rate of heart attack or death. Two calcium channel blockers, verapamil and diltiazem, are also used to block cardiac calcium channels in the treatment of certain forms of cardiac arrhythmia (see Chapter 40). A more detailed discussion of calcium channel blockers and their use in the treatment of angina appears in Chapter 39.

 DRUG CLASS • Alpha Blockers

Alpha$_1$ blocking drugs such as prazosin are occasionally used as the initial antihypertensive drug but more often as second- or third-line drugs. A diuretic is usually necessary because the alpha$_1$ blockers tend to cause fluid retention. Another limitation is the orthostatic hypotension characteristic of these drugs. A favorable adverse effect is a reduction in cholesterol and triglyceride levels. Moreover, reflex tachycardia is not common with selective alpha$_1$ blockers, in contrast with nonselective alpha blockers and other classes of direct vasodilators. The reason for this is not known. Alpha blockers are discussed in detail in Chapter 12.

 DRUG CLASS • Centrally Acting Antihypertensives

⚠ clonidine (Catapres)

guanabenz (Wytensin)

guanfacine (Tenex)

methyldopa (Aldomet)

MECHANISM OF ACTION

All of these drugs reduce blood pressure by acting in the CNS to reduce the activity of the sympathetic nervous system. Clonidine, guanabenz, and guanfacine stimulate alpha$_2$-adrenergic receptors in the region of the medulla responsible for blood pressure regulation. Methyldopa does not directly stimulate alpha$_2$ receptors. Instead, it is taken up by nerve endings in this region and is biotransformed to methylnorepinephrine. The methylnorepinephrine is then stored in the nerve endings and released from the neuron instead of the normal transmitter. Therefore methylnorepinephrine is called a false transmitter, and like the other drugs in this class, is thought to lower blood pressure by stimulating alpha$_2$ receptors.

USES

The alpha$_2$ agonists are occasionally used in the treatment of essential hypertension, but because of their central adverse effects (see below) they are not first-line drugs and have been replaced by others. Because fluid retention is common when these drugs are used alone, they are usually given in combination with a diuretic. Methyldopa is often used to treat hypertension during pregnancy because of its safety for the developing fetus. Several preparations combining methyldopa and a thiazide diuretic are available (see Table 41-3).

Orally administered clonidine may be used in urgent situations to lower a dangerously elevated blood pressure (e.g., 210/118 mm Hg). Clonidine has also been used, usually as an adjunct, in a variety of different settings, including the treatment of opioid and nicotine withdrawal, dysmenorrhea, menopause, and pain.

PHARMACOKINETICS

All of these drugs are effective when given orally, and clonidine can also be administered by a transdermal patch. They are also relatively well absorbed and are highly bioavailable (greater than 50%) with the exception of guanabenz, which is subject to extensive first-pass hepatic biotransformation. Guanabenz has a relatively short half-life (about 6 hours) and unlike the others is highly protein bound. Clonidine and guanfacine have plasma half-lives ranging from 12 to 16 hours, and about half an administered dose is excreted unchanged in the urine. Although methyldopa disappears from plasma quickly, its duration of action may be as long as 24 hours because of its unique mechanism (see above).

ADVERSE REACTIONS AND CONTRAINDICATIONS

The most common and troubling adverse effects of these drugs are excessive sedation, mental depression, dizziness, headache, dry mouth, and sexual dysfunc-

tion. Some patients may develop severe bradycardia or atrioventricular block. Significant salt and water retention are also commonly seen with these drugs except for guanabenz and may limit or antagonize their antihypertensive effect.

Sudden withdrawal from clonidine or guanfacine can be dangerous. After discontinuing therapeutic doses for 12 to 48 hours, many patients experience symptoms of a sympathetic rebound: restlessness, insomnia, tremors, increased salivation, and tachycardia. If the drug is not reinstated, headaches, abdominal pain, and nausea follow. The most severe reaction is a hypertensive crisis that is best treated in the hospital with a combination of alpha and beta blockers such as phentolamine and propranolol. To avoid these withdrawal problems, dosages of these drugs should be gradually reduced over a week or more.

Methyldopa may cause Parkinson-like movement problems. Oversecretion of prolactin is also possible and may result in growth of breast tissue (gynecomastia) in men and excessive stimulation of breast tissue (galactorrhea) in women. Methyldopa also may cause potentially fatal hepatotoxicity, severe hemolytic anemia, and lupuslike symptoms. Patients should be closely monitored for signs of these conditions in the first few months after beginning therapy with the drug.

INTERACTIONS

The sedation and CNS depression produced by any of these drugs is greatly increased when they are combined with other CNS depressants. Tricyclic antidepressants antagonize the antihypertensive effects of clonidine or methyldopa, and methyldopa can cause agitation, headache, and severe hypertension in patients taking an MAO inhibitor. Other drug interactions with any of the central antihypertensive drugs are rare.

DRUG CLASS • Adrenergic Neuron-Blocking Drugs

deserpidine (Harmonyl)

guanadrel (Hylorel)

⚠ **guanethidine (Ismelin)**

rauwolfia serpentina (Raudixin, Rauval, Rauverid)

⚠ **reserpine (Serpalan, Serpasil)**

MECHANISM OF ACTION

Adrenergic neuron-blocking drugs interfere with the storage and release of norepinephrine from sympathetic nerve endings. However, two different mechanisms are involved for the various drugs.

Guanethidine and guanadrel are taken into peripheral sympathetic nerve endings by the same mechanism responsible for the reuptake of norepinephrine. Once inside the neuron, these drugs enter the vesicles where norepinehrine is stored and interfere with this process, so that the neuron eventually runs out of this neurotransmitter. These drugs may also act directly to interfere with norepinephrine release. Both actions serve to reduce the amount of norepinephrine released from sympathetic nerve endings. As a result, both peripheral vascular resistance and cardiac output are decreased, resulting in a reduction in blood pressure.

Reserpine, deserpidine, and rauwolfia serpentina are a class of naturally occurring compounds that have been used medicinally for thousands of years. These drugs can enter any neurons that release catecholamines or serotonin and block the mechanism responsible for transporting these neurotransmitters from the cytoplasm into the storage vesicles from which transmitter release occurs (see Chapter 10). In peripheral sympathetic nerve endings, this effect is thought to reduce the amount of norepinephrine available for release, ultimately producing an effect similar to that of guanethidine. However, reserpine and its relatives also act in the CNS in the same way to reduce sympathetic nervous system activity, an effect that contributes to their ability to lower blood pressure.

USES

Because these drugs impair the entire sympathetic nervous system, they cause a wide variety of troublesome adverse effects (see below). Therefore they are no longer commonly used to treat hypertension today but may prove effective in cases refractory to the newer drugs. They are never used alone and are almost always used in combination with a thiazide diuretic to counter fluid retention. The combination of reserpine and a thiazide drug is well tolerated in many patients. In contrast, guanethidine and guanadrel are very potent antihypertensive drugs that, because of their many adverse effects, are restricted for use in controlling severe hypertension, usually when other drug therapy has failed. They are also occasionally used in the treatment of renal hypertension, including that caused by pyelonephritis, renal amyloidosis, and renal artery stenosis.

PHARMACOKINETICS

Absorption of guanethidine after oral administration is poor and highly variable, ranging from 3% to 30%. In contrast, absorption of guanadrel is rapid and complete. Both guanethidine and guanadrel disappear rapidly from plasma because they are accumulated by sympathetic nerve endings, where their action is more prolonged. Therefore 1 to 3 weeks may be required to reach the maximum therapeutic response to a given dosage regimen of guanethidine, and the effects of the drug may persist for 7 to 10 days after therapy is discontinued. Most of a dose of guanadrel (85%) is eliminated unchanged by the kidneys, and 50% to 75% of guanethidine is biotransformed in the liver.

Reserpine and related drugs are all readily absorbed after oral administration. Although these drugs disappear rapidly from plasma (i.e., they have a half-life of about 4 to 6 hours), peak effect on blood pressure is not seen until 24 hours after a single dose and 1 to 6 weeks after beginning oral antihypertensive therapy. Most of a given dose is eventually excreted unchanged in the feces.

ADVERSE REACTIONS AND CONTRAINDICATIONS

A number of uncomfortable adverse effects arise from the depletion of peripheral norepinephrine stores. Orthostatic hypotension is a particular problem. The tone of blood vessels is diminished by the drugs, and if the patient moves suddenly from a reclining to a standing position, blood flow to the brain cannot be maintained, resulting in fainting. Other adverse effects resulting from the depletion of norepinephrine include bradycardia and diarrhea. The diarrhea, which often occurs after meals, can be severe and even explosive. In men, failure of erection or ejaculation may result from the loss of vascular tone. Guanethidine also causes sodium retention.

Contraindications for guanethidine therapy include the presence of angina, cerebral insufficiency, or coronary artery disease (CAD) conditions further compromised by the loss of vascular tone. The adverse effects of guanadrel are similar to those of guanethidine but less severe. Retention of water and salt are commonly seen with both drugs, and patients may develop edema. These drugs should not be used by patients with severe heart failure, and they may actually provoke heart failure in susceptible individuals. In certain rare circumstances, these drugs may cause initial release of sufficient catecholamines to provoke sympathetic responses such as increases in blood pressure. For this reason, these drugs are never given to patients with pheochromocytoma or tumors of the adrenal medulla.

Like guanethidine and guanadrel, reserpine, deserpidine, and rauwolfia may cause adverse effects related to decreased sympathetic tone. An example is vasodilation that results in a flushed, warm feeling, nasal congestion, and dizziness. Some of the adverse effects of reserpine are related to the predominant parasympathetic tone when sympathetic tone is depressed: salivation, stomach cramps, and diarrhea. Because reserpine augments gastric acid secretion, it should not be used by patients with a peptic ulcer.

Unlike guanethidine and guanadrel, however, reserpine and related drugs produce effects in the CNS. Common reactions to these drugs include sedation and tranquilization. Also, patients often complain of a lethargic feeling, increased appetite, increased dreaming, and sometimes nightmares. The reported incidence rate of depression with reserpine has varied from 27% to 40%. Occasionally, patients who take reserpine will become severely depressed to the point of attempting suicide. For this reason, reserpine and related drugs should not be given to patients with a history of depression, and treatment should be stopped immediately if signs of depression appear.

INTERACTIONS

A number of drug interactions have been noted with guanethidine and guanadrel. Patients taking these drugs are hypersensitive to administered catecholamines. Patients become less responsive to guanethidine or guanadrel when an indirect-acting adrenergic drug (e.g., amphetamine, ephedrine) or a tricyclic antidepressant is taken. Tricyclic antidepressants block the uptake of these drugs into the neuron so that they are unable to reach their site of action.

Reserpine and related drugs may greatly enhance the depression caused by other CNS depressants, and they should not be given to patients taking MAO inhibitors.

DRUG CLASS • Direct-Acting Vasodilators

diazoxide (Hyperstat, Proglycem)

hydralazine (Apresoline)

nitroprusside (Nipride)

MECHANISM OF ACTION

Direct-acting vasodilators act on vascular smooth muscle to cause relaxation and thus a decrease in blood pressure. The drop in arterial blood pressure is great enough to be detected by the baroreceptors, provoking a reflex stimulation of the heart that increases cardiac output and partially compensates for the fall in blood pressure (reflex tachycardia). The cardiac stimulation is especially severe with hydralazine, making this a poor choice for treating patients with angina, CAD, or heart failure. These drugs also cause sodium and water retention and are therefore useful in treating hypertension only when combined with a diuretic to counteract the sodium retention. Hydralazine is available in combination with a thiazide diuretic (see Table 41-3). Vasodilators are also often combined with beta blockers to prevent the reflex stimulation of the heart. Minoxidil causes additional adverse effects, including ECG changes and excessive hair growth, and these limit use in the chronic treatment of hypertension. Vasodilators are discussed further in Chapter 39.

TREATMENT OF HYPERTENSIVE EMERGENCIES

A hypertensive emergency cannot be defined simply. The blood pressure may be severely elevated or only moderately elevated. The important feature is that there is impending end-organ damage, usually to the brain, heart, kidneys, or eyes. Unstable neurologic symptoms that suggest damage to the brain include headache, restlessness, confusion, and even convulsions. Hemorrhaging may be apparent in the eye. In such a case, immediate and marked reduction of blood pressure is required. Therefore drugs used to treat hypertensive emergencies must act rapidly and be suitable for parenteral injection, usually by the intravenous route.

Because of their ability to produce suitably rapid effects, a number of the direct-acting vasodilators are commonly used to treat hypertensive emergencies. These include diazoxide (Hyperstat), nitroglycerin (Nitro-Bid IV, Nitrostat IV, Tridil), and sodium nitroprusside (Nipride). The advantage of diazoxide treatment is that a bolus of the drug can be given intravenously over 30 seconds, will usually take effect in 5 minutes, and will remain effective for 2 to 12 hours. The patient rarely becomes excessively hypotensive; thus blood pressure does not need to be continuously monitored as it does with nitroglycerin or nitroprusside treatment. Diazoxide causes retention of sodium and water, which must be treated with a diuretic, and hyperglycemia. The advantage of nitroglycerin or nitroprusside is their immediate action, but both must be continuously infused to maintain the effect. Because nitroglycerin is absorbed by polyvinyl chloride (PVC) plastic, special non-PVC infusion sets are used. These drugs can provoke excessive hypotension, necessitating the constant monitoring of blood pressure during their administration. Other than this, there are no notable adverse effects with the short-term use of nitroglycerin or nitroprusside. Adverse effects do arise, however, from the use of nitroprusside for several days. Some of the drug is biotransformed into thiocyanate, which can produce ringing in the ears (tinnitus), blurred vision, and hypothyroidism. Nitroprusside is unstable in light, so it should not be used more than 4 hours after it is dissolved. An injectable preparation of hydralazine is often used in the treatment of preeclampsia or eclampsia. These drugs and other direct-acting vasodilators are discussed in detail in Chapter 39.

Another drug sometimes used in hypertensive emergencies is trimethaphan. As discussed in Chapter 11, trimethaphan blocks the receptors for acetylcholine in the ganglia. Trimethaphan is used in treating specific hypertensive emergencies, particularly in surgery for an aortic dissecting aneurysm. Because this drug has a short duration of action, it is administered by continuous intravenous drip. During this time, blood pressure must be monitored constantly because severe hypotension can result from the inhibition of sympathetic tone. In this case, the intravenous drip is discontinued until the blood pressure begins to rise again. Another disadvantage of trimethaphan therapy is that the loss of pupillary reflexes makes it difficult to monitor ongoing neurologic damage to the brain (when signs of neurologic damage were present in the set of symptoms). In addition, trimethaphan can be unpredictable in its effects; patients already taking antihypertensive drugs or those with a reduced blood volume may be unusually sensitive to it. Some patients do not respond readily to this drug, whereas others are initially responsive but later become unresponsive. Trimethaphan decreases venous return of blood and reduces cardiac output. These actions are helpful when the patient has a condition such as a dissecting aortic aneurysm, hypertensive encephalopathy, acute left ventricular failure, or cerebral hemorrhage, because the pressure is removed from the weakened tissue.

Fenoldopam, a highly selective D_1 (dopamine) agonist, is another drug used in the management of severe hypertension in a hospital setting. D_1 receptors are found in vascular smooth muscle primarily in blood vessels in the kidneys, heart, and gut. Fenoldopam stimulates these receptors to produce selective vasodilation in these tissues. Thus fenoldopam lowers peripheral resistance and is especially useful when it is important to increase or maintain renal blood flow. This drug must be administered intravenously. Fenoldopam is discussed further in Chapter 39. Drugs used in the treatment of hypertensive emergencies are listed in Table 41-4.

TABLE 41-4	
Drugs Used in the Treatment of Hypertensive Emergencies	
Generic Drug	*Brand Name*
diazoxide	Hyperstat
hydralazine	Apresoline
fenoldopam	Corlopam
labetalol	Normodyne
methyldopa	Aldomet
nitroglycerin	Nitro-Bid IV, Nitrostat IV, Tridil
nitroprusside	Nipride
trimethaphan	Arfonad

APPLICATION TO PRACTICE

ASSESSMENT
History of Present Illness

Evaluation of patients with hypertension is directed at uncovering correctable secondary causes and establishing a pretreatment baseline in patients who have no end-organ damage. When symptoms do bring patients to seek health care, the symptoms often relate to the elevated pressure itself, vascular disease, or the underlying disease process of secondary hypertension.

Essential hypertension usually remains asymptomatic until the patient experiences severe blood pressure elevations (e.g., 220/110 mm Hg). Ask the patient about complaints associated with hypertension such as fatigue, an early morning occipital and pulsating headache that goes away as the day progresses, lightheadedness, flushing, epistaxis (nose bleeds), chest pains, visual and speech disturbances, and dyspnea. Tactfully ask the male patient if he has had problems with impotence.

Patients with disorders associated with secondary hypertension may have additional symptoms. For example,

intermittent claudication from lower extremity ischemia may be related to coarctation of the aorta. Other complaints may include hirsutism and easy bruising (seen in Cushing's syndrome), excessive diaphoresis, sustained or intermittent hypertension, paroxysmal headaches, palpitations, anxiety attacks, nausea and vomiting (seen with pheochromocytoma), hypokalemia, muscle weakness, cramps, polyuria, paralysis, nocturia (seen with primary hyperaldosteronism), and flank pain (seen with renal or renovascular disease).

Ask about lifestyle factors that may contribute to hypertension. Diet, levels of physical activity and stress, type of work, financial security, and education level should be included in the interview. Elicit information about factors that may affect treatment, such as the patient's feeling of well-being or illness, family support and acknowledgment of illness, concerns about potential adverse effects, and the requirement of lifelong treatment. A sexual history helps to document pretreatment level of sexual functioning should the patient have complaints after treatment is started.

Health History

The health history, which includes information about childhood illnesses, accidents, injuries, hospitalizations, operations, obstetric history (if applicable), immunizations, and allergies will give potential clues for secondary causes of hypertension.

A drug history including all current prescription and nonprescription drugs as well as any herbs or nontraditional interventions is necessary to decrease any chance of additive effects of antihypertensive drugs that may be prescribed. Older adults often take multiple drugs obtained from several different health care providers. Eye drops might not be mentioned when patients are asked to list drugs taken, yet ocular drugs (e.g., beta blockers) may cause significant systemic effects. Information related to alcohol and illicit street drug use is also important to elicit from all patients.

When asked, patients with essential hypertension may report a strong family history of hypertension along with documentation of or reports of intermittent elevations of blood pressure. Smoking history, comorbid conditions such as diabetes mellitus, lipid disorders, and a strong family history of early death from cardiovascular disease should be noted in the health history. This information is used in part to determine the patient's risk factors for hypertension or the risk of end-organ damage, or both.

Lifespan Considerations

Perinatal. Hypertension is a serious complication of pregnancy. The risk to both mother and fetus can be reduced by appropriate assessment, treatment, and evaluation. Hypertension may be an indication of an underlying maternal disease aggravated by pregnancy. It may also be the first sign of preeclampsia. The incidence rate of chronic hypertension in pregnant women ranges from 1% to 5%. The rates are higher in pregnant women who are older, obese, or African American.

During normal pregnancy, systolic pressure changes very little. Diastolic pressure decreases by 10 mm Hg in early pregnancy and rises to the prepregnancy level in the third trimester. The initial fall results from general vasodilation that occurs with pregnancy. An increase in renin and aldosterone levels occurs in normal pregnancy.

Preeclampsia most often develops after the twentieth week of gestation in susceptible women, although it can occur earlier in the pregnancy. An onset of preeclampsia during the second trimester is associated with increased risk of maternal and fetal harm. The disorder occurs during first and subsequent pregnancies, but blood pressure returns to normal between pregnancies.

Chronic hypertension during pregnancy may be mild or severe. Diagnostic criteria for hypertension in pregnancy include a rise in blood pressure of 20 to 30 mm Hg from the prepregnancy or first trimester value or an absolute level of blood pressure greater than 140/90 mm Hg at any stage of pregnancy. Severe hypertension is present when blood pressure readings are greater than 170/110 mm Hg.

Fetal death or intrauterine growth retardation may result from uteroplacental insufficiency caused by hypertension. Control of moderate and severe hypertension results in lower rates of perinatal morbidity and mortality.

Pediatric. The prevalence of hypertension in children varies from 0% to 13%. Criteria used for categorizing hypertension in adults are not applicable to children, although children are at higher risk for hypertension if both parents have the disorder. Blood pressure normally increases in children at a rate of 1.5 mm Hg systolic and 1 mm Hg diastolic values per year, leveling off between 18 and 20 years of age. There is a striking increase in sustained new hypertension in adolescents and young adults between the ages of 15 and 25 years. However, it is not clear if hypertensive adolescents continue to be hypertensive as adults. Premature labeling of an adolescent as hypertensive may interfere with some career choices and the ability to obtain life insurance later.

Frequent causes of persistent hypertension in children are renal hypertension and coarctation of the aorta. Children and adolescents whose blood pressure is consistently above the 95th percentile for height, weight, and age should be closely evaluated and treated.

Compliance with treatment regimens can be a major problem with adolescents who are asymptomatic. They often do not want to differ from peers in regard to diet and lifestyle.

Older Adults. The prevalence of hypertension among older adults is extremely common. Approximately two thirds of the U.S. population aged 65 years or older has hypertension. Elevated blood pressure occurs in about 60% of whites, 71% of African Americans, and 61% of Hispanic Americans aged 60 and over. Systolic blood pressure is a more accurate predictor of adverse events (i.e., CAD, heart failure, stroke, and end-stage renal disease) than is diastolic blood pressure, especially among older adults. Primary hypertension is the most common form of hypertension in older adults (see Evidence-Based Practice box).

Blood pressure must be measured with special care in older adults because some persons have pseudohypertension, a falsely high blood pressure reading, due to excessive vascular stiffness. In addition, older persons with hypertension and excessive variability in systolic blood pressure values may have white-coat hypertension (see Box 41-1). Additionally, older adults are more likely

EVIDENCE-BASED PRACTICE
Pharmacotherapy of Hypertension in Older Adults

Setting

Fifty million people in the United States have essential hypertension, with the onset usually occurring in adults 20 to 40 years old. Isolated systolic hypertension is more common in older adults. Complications associated with hypertension include heart failure, myocardial infarction, cerebrovascular accident (stroke), hypertensive heart disease, and renal failure. Beta blockers and diuretics have the most documented benefits and are thought to reduce the risk profiles of older adults on long-term antihypertensive therapy.

Objective of Literature Review

To characterize comorbid risk profiles of older adults on long-term antihypertensive therapy.

The search was carried out using electronic searches of WHO-ISH Collaboration Registry, The Cochrane Library, MEDLINE, and two Japanese databases. In addition, reference lists from the articles were reviewed, and the retrieved studies searched for additional potentially relevant citations. Experts in the field were also contacted.

Criteria for Inclusion of Studies in Review of Literature

Investigators included randomized, controlled studies that lasted at least 1 year, in which morbidity and mortality data were assessed in older adults (at least 60 years old) who had hypertension.

Data Extraction and Analysis

Two independent reviewers extracted the characteristics from the study as well as morbidity and mortality data. The data from three of the studies were restricted to that of older adults who had isolated systolic hypertension. Most studies were conducted in Western, industrialized countries and evaluated beta blocker and diuretic antihypertensive therapies. Available outcome data addressed the following:

1. Total mortality and morbidity from coronary heart disease
2. Combined mortality and morbidity data from coronary heart disease
3. Cerebrovascular mortality
4. Combined mortality and morbidity data from cerebrovascular disease
5. Cardiovascular mortality
6. Combined mortality and morbidity from cardiovascular disease

Results of Review

Fifteen studies ($N = 21,908$) were reviewed. Morbidity and mortality from cardiovascular disease were reduced from 17.7% to 12.6%; cardiovascular mortality from 6.9% to 0.5%, and total mortality from 12.9% to 11.1%. Older adults with isolated systolic hypertension benefited significantly from antihypertensive therapy, with a reduction in mortality and morbidity over 5 years from 157 events to 104 events. Disparities in treatment effects based on risk factors, preexisting cardiovascular disease, and competing comorbidities could not be established from available data.

Investigators' Conclusions

Event rates per 1000 participants over 5 years suggest that low-dose beta blockers or diuretics are clearly beneficial for adults 60 to 80 years old who have either diastolic or systolic hypertension. The average prevalence of cardiovascular risk factors, cardiovascular disease, and competing comorbid diseases was lower among study subjects than in the general population of older adults 60 to 80 years old who have hypertension.

Mulrow C, Lau J, Cornell J et al: *Pharmacotherapy for hypertension in the elderly* (Cochrane Review). In *The Cochrane Library*, Issue 2, Oxford, 2002, Update Software.

to experience orthostatic changes in blood pressure than younger patients. Thus blood pressure readings should always be measured with the patient standing as well as in the seated or supine positions.

The older adult is at increased risk for adverse drug reactions because of the physiologic changes associated with aging. These changes can affect the concentration and distribution of drugs (see Chapter 4). The effects of drugs at their sites of action may also be altered. Renal blood flow decreases with age, which affects the dosing of drugs eliminated by the kidneys.

Lean muscle mass decreases, whereas the proportion of fat in the body increases. This factor may extend the effects of fat-soluble drugs.

Cultural/Social Considerations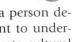

Cultural values and beliefs influence how a person defines health and health care. It is important to understand these cultural beliefs and to incorporate cultural sensitivity into delivery of care.

Patients cope differently when diagnosed with hypertension. Acceptance, denial, and retreat are some common reactions. It is important to allow patients to express fears and feelings in a nonjudgmental, empathetic atmosphere. Changes in attitudes and beliefs about self, illness, treatment, and relationships with family and health care providers are important to note. Identifying present life stressors that may be affecting the patient is helpful.

Furthermore, patients may not comply with their treatment regimen for a variety of reasons. For some patients, it is difficult to realize that treatment now, when they feel well, will prevent future complications. For others, the drugs interfere with their quality of life. The idea of life-long treatment is a difficult adaptation for some people. The cost of drugs may also be an issue for patients who have to pay for their drugs out of their pocket (see the Case Study: Hypertension).

Physical Examination

Elevated blood pressure readings should be verified at two subsequent office visits before confirming a diagnosis of hypertension (see Table 41-1). Blood pressure and apical pulse should be measured in both arms with the patient supine, seated, and standing. Verification of elevated blood pressure values should also be made in different settings (e.g., at home and at the workplace).

Postural blood pressure changes can occur in patients who have pheochromocytoma or diabetic nephropathy, in patients with hypertension who are taking tricyclic antidepressants, and in older adults. A rise in diastolic pressure when the patient moves from supine to a standing position is consistent with essential hypertension. A fall in blood pressure in the absence of antihypertensive drugs suggests secondary causes for the hypertension.

The initial physical examination of the patient with hypertension includes an assessment of end-organ damage and identification of signs suggesting a specific secondary cause. Signs of end-organ ophthalmic damage include arteriolar narrowing, arteriovenous compression, hemorrhages, exudates, or papilledema on funduscopic examination. A cardiac examination that finds carotid bruits and distended jugular veins, a loud aortic second sound, precordial heave, arrhythmia, or early systolic click may suggest cardiovascular end-organ damage. Diminished or absent peripheral arterial pulses, peripheral edema, abdominal bruit, and an abnormal neurologic assessment may also be noted with this damage.

Signs suggestive of secondary causes of hypertension include abdominal or flank masses (with polycystic kidneys), absence of femoral pulses (with coarctation of aorta), tachycardia, diaphoresis, orthostatic hypotension (with pheochromocytoma), abdominal bruits (with renovascular disease), truncal obesity, ecchymoses, pig-

mented striae (with Cushing's syndrome), and enlarged or nodular thyroid gland (with hyperthyroidism).

Laboratory Testing

Laboratory testing is important to assess for end-organ damage, to identify patients at high risk for cardiovascular complications, to determine if other cardiovascular complications exist, and to screen for possible secondary causes of hypertension. Routine tests for all patients with a new diagnosis of hypertension include hemoglobin and hematocrit, chemistry panel (i.e., potassium, creatinine, fasting glucose, calcium, and uric acid), fasting lipid panels, urinalysis, and ECG.

When specific secondary causes of hypertension are suspected, a chest x-ray study, dexamethasone suppression test (for Cushing's syndrome), urinary metanephrine and vanillylmandelic acid levels (for pheochromocytoma), intravenous pyelogram, renal scan, angiography (for renal vascular disease), or plasma renin activity levels (for primary aldosteronism or renovascular disease) may be ordered. By obtaining these laboratory tests, the patient's cardiovascular risk and potential for complications associated with antihypertensive therapy can be assessed.

GOALS OF THERAPY

The short-term goals of antihypertensive therapy are to reduce arterial pressure, minimize end-organ damage, and prolong life. These goals can be met by achieving and maintaining a systolic pressure below 135 mm Hg and a diastolic pressure under 85 mm Hg as well as controlling modifiable risk factors for cardiovascular disease. Treatment interventions that maintain blood pressure at or below 140/90 mm Hg may prevent stroke, preserve renal function, and prevent or slow progression of heart failure. Drug therapy used appropriately can enhance the patient's quality of life.

INTERVENTION

Treatment of hypertension has become more aggressive in the last several years. Dietary and lifestyle modifications are important components of this treatment. However, drug therapy is now recommended for patients whose blood pressure is in the high-normal range (130/85 to 139/89 mm Hg) if they also have diabetes, cardiovascular disease, target organ damage, or more than one major risk factor. Accumulated evidence shows that even high-normal hypertension is associated with an increased incidence of cardiovascular disease and stroke, especially when risk factors are present.

The Joint National Committee on Detection, Evaluation, and Treatment of High Blood Pressure (JNC-VI) recommends that initial therapy of hypertensive patients be customized based on a risk stratification for cardiovascular disease. Having one or more of the six major risk factors identified for hypertension is one component of the risk stratification. The six risk factors are cigarette smoking, high blood cholesterol or triglyceride levels, diabetes, age older than 60 years, being a man or a postmenopausal woman, and having a history of cardiovascular disease. The risk stratification also factors in whether the patient has clinical cardiovascular disease (left ventricular hypertrophy, heart failure, angina or prior myocardial infarction, or coronary revascularization) and whether there is target organ damage (stroke or transient ischemic attack, nephropathy, peripheral arterial disease, or retinopathy).

Risk Group A

Individuals in risk group A are those with no risk factors and no clinical cardiovascular disease or organ damage. These patients should be treated initially with counseling and follow-up for lifestyle changes. Risk group A patients need drug therapy if they fall into stage 2 or 3 hypertension or if they are in stage 1 and have not responded to lifestyle modifications after 1 year.

Risk Group B

Risk group B is comprised of those patients who have one or more major risk factors but who do not have diabetes, clinical cardiovascular disease, or end-organ damage. Most hypertensive patients are in this risk group. These patients are advised to adopt lifestyle changes, but patients with stage 2 or 3 hypertension are also started on drug therapy. Patients with stage 1 hypertension (140/90 to 159/99 mm Hg) are started on drug therapy if their blood pressure does not fall into normal ranges with lifestyle modifications.

Risk Group C

Risk group C includes patients with diabetes, clinical cardiovascular disease, or end-organ damage. Drug therapy is begun immediately for these patients. However, they are also counseled on lifestyle changes because such changes may reduce the dosage of drugs needed and thereby reduce adverse effects of drug therapy.

Drug therapy is generally advised for patients who have stage 1 or 2 hypertension, especially those with risk factors and with a blood pressure remaining at or above 140/90 mm Hg for 12 months despite attempts to change lifestyle factors. In general, drug therapy for hypertension is standard, but therapy is changing as more is learned about this disorder and as new drugs become available. Current drug therapy is based on a treatment algorithm (Figure 41-1) in which drug classes are substituted or added until blood pressure is brought under control.

Administration

Drug treatment of primary hypertension is usually lifelong. Thus it is important to use a flexible approach to drug therapy. Patients respond differently to individual drugs or combinations of drugs. Furthermore, simplified drug regimens make life easier for patients and increase compliance with treatment plans. Monotherapy with once- or twice-daily dosing is likely to achieve adequate blood pressure control in the compliant patient. However, effective dosages of antihypertensive drugs are often lower than the manufacturer's recommendations. For example, drug therapy in the older adult should begin at half the normal starting dose. Titration dosages should be small and spaced at longer intervals than those used for a younger patient.

Abruptly stopping antihypertensive drugs may result in a withdrawal syndrome characterized by sweating, palpitations, headache, tremor, and rebound hypertension. Withdrawal syndrome may precipitate heart failure and MI in patients with cardiac disease, a thyroid storm in patients with thyrotoxicosis, and peripheral ischemia in patients with peripheral vascular disease. Hypoglycemia may occur in patients with previously controlled diabetes.

Education

It is important to develop and implement an individualized teaching plan for each patient. Teaching the patient how to monitor blood pressure at home enables him or her to become a more active participant in care, reinforces treatment goals, and improves compliance. Advise the patient to check his or her blood pressure weekly and report significant changes to the health care provider. Reinforce the notion that hypertension may not produce symptoms but is a chronic disease that requires lifelong interventions. Patient beliefs about personal susceptibility to complications of hypertension, treatment effectiveness, and consequences of nontreatment should be discussed. Patients should be helped to understand that drug therapy controls, but does not cure, this disorder.

Patients are likely to comply with treatment regimens when they understand the plan and the plan is consistent with their own beliefs. Adequate information enables the patient to make informed choices about lifestyle changes.

Lifestyle changes are not an option if the patient does not want increased symptoms or possible end-organ damage. They are extremely important aspects of the management plan, particularly for patients with hyperlipidemia or diabetes. Lifestyle changes have been shown to prevent hypertension, are effective in lowering blood pressure, and can reduce cardiovascular risk factors with little cost and minimal risk. Even if changes in lifestyle are not sufficient to reduce blood pressure, the changes may reduce the need for multidrug therapy.

Exercise. A long-term regular exercise program can help control abnormally elevated arterial blood pressure. Blood pressure will increase if the patient returns to a sedentary lifestyle after as little as 3 months of exercise. However, subsequent blood pressure readings will still be lower than pre-exercise levels. Aerobic exercises (e.g., jogging or walking) reduce blood pressure by 30% to 50%. Isometric exercises (e.g., weightlifting) may raise arterial pressure. Exercise lowers blood pressure in African Americans more dramatically than in whites. In older adults, low-intensity training has resulted in a 20–mm Hg decrease in systolic pressure and a 12–mm Hg fall in diastolic pressure. An individualized exercise plan should be developed with the patient, and continuing encouragement should be provided. Regular aerobic activity enhances weight loss and functional health status, reduces cardiovascular risk factors, and other causes of morbidity and mortality.

Weight Reduction. A weight reduction of even 10 pounds reduces blood pressure in a large proportion of overweight patients. Furthermore, weight loss augments the effects of antihypertensive drugs and significantly reduces the patient's cardiovascular risk factors.

Sodium Restriction. Sodium restriction continues to be controversial. Patients with hypertension or diabetes, older adults, and African Americans are more sensitive to changes in sodium intake than persons in the general population. Sodium intake greater than 2360 mg daily plays a role in elevating blood pressure in some patients with essential hypertension. Thus mild sodium restriction is a practical approach in treatment. Teaching the patient to eliminate or at least restrict the use of frozen, canned, or processed foods can reduce sodium intake considerably (see Appendix A).

Calcium and Magnesium. There is some evidence that increased intake of calcium and magnesium may protect against hypertension and may actually improve blood pressure control in some patients as well as re-

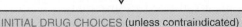

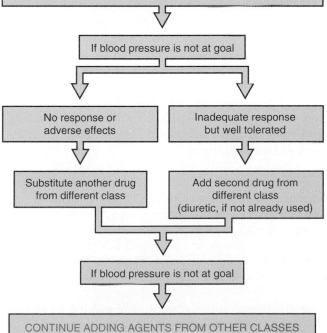

FIGURE 41-1 An algorithm for antihypertensive therapy replaces the stepwise approach to therapy used previously. The algorithm includes compelling indications for use of certain drug groups for specific patients. (Adapted from the Joint National Committee on Prevention, Detection, Evaluation and Treatment of High Blood Pressure: The sixth report of the Joint National Committee on Prevention, Detection, Evaluation and Treatment of High Blood Pressure, *Arch Intern Med* 157(21): 2430, 1997.)

duce the risk of osteoporosis. Supplemental potassium intake may be required, particularly for patients who are receiving a potassium-losing diuretic. Potassium supplementation, however, is contraindicated for patients taking ACE inhibitors or AII blockers as well as for those with renal dysfunction.

Dietary Fats. Diets that vary in total fat and in the proportion of saturated to unsaturated fats have had little, if any, direct effect on blood pressure. In some patients, a large intake of omega-3 fatty acids may lower blood pressure. However, some patients experience abdominal discomfort with a large intake of these fatty acids.

Caffeine. Some health care providers advise hypertensive patients to avoid caffeine intake. Although caffeine may raise blood pressure acutely, tolerance to the pressor effects of caffeine develops quickly. There has been no direct relationship found between caffeine intake and hypertension.

Tobacco. Hypertensive patients should avoid tobacco use in any form. Patients who continue to smoke while on antihypertensive therapy will not receive the full benefit of therapy. The cardiovascular benefits of discontinuing tobacco use can be seen in all age groups within a year of stopping. Smokers should be repeatedly and adamantly advised to stop smoking, but interventions directed at minimizing weight gain after stopping smoking may be required.

Alcohol. Excessive alcohol intake causes resistance to antihypertensive drugs and is a risk factor for stroke. Advise patients to limit their daily alcohol intake to no more than 1 ounce daily (e.g., 8 ounces of beer, 4 ounces of wine). A daily intake of $1/2$ ounce or less of alcohol is advised for women and lighter-weight persons. However, it should also be noted that significant hypertension can develop in patients with a heavy alcohol intake who abruptly stop consumption, with or without antihypertensive drug therapy.

Stress. Patients should be taught stress management techniques because these methods have been shown to decrease catecholamine release, oxygen consumption, respiratory rate, heart rate, and acute blood pressure elevation. A combination of biofeedback and stress management techniques has been shown to be more effective than either technique alone.

Drug Therapy. Patient education about the treatment regimen should be written and include identification of prescribed drugs by generic and trade names, the mechanism or mechanisms of action, and adverse effects. The patient should know the dosing frequency and what to do if a dose is forgotten. He or she should be encouraged to contact the health care provider before using OTC cold remedies, because many of these products contain adrenergic ingredients. Instruct the patient to continue taking the prescribed drug even if he or she is feeling well, because abrupt withdrawal can cause rebound hypertension. Also, advise the patient to inform other health care providers and dentists of the diagnosis of hypertension and its treatment regimen before any other treatment or surgery.

Although education has a substantial effect on the patient's knowledge and a positive effect on compliance, the effect of knowledge tends to diminish over time. Periodic dialogue between the health care provider and the patient tends to reinforce treatment goals and positive behaviors.

EVALUATION

Evaluation of the patient with hypertension is based on whether blood pressure has been reduced and end-organ damage prevented or minimized. A patient whose diastolic blood pressure when first diagnosed exceeds 115 mm Hg should be reevaluated after 48 hours of therapy to ensure that at least a 5- to 10-mm Hg drop in pressure has occurred. A patient whose diastolic pressure falls below this number may be followed up in 1 to 2 weeks. Blood pressure should be rechecked every 4 weeks, after each dosage or drug change, or until it is controlled. Once the blood pressure is controlled, the patient is ordinarily monitored two to four times yearly. If blood pressure remains controlled and there are no comorbid conditions, a serum creatinine, blood glucose, lipid values, and urinalysis should be checked a minimum of every 5 years.

The patient should be reassessed if the blood pressure has not decreased after 4 to 8 weeks of therapy. The present drug should be stopped and treatment restarted with a different drug at low dosage. If the blood pressure has decreased but not to the level desired, and if the patient has no adverse drug effects, the initial drug can be continued, and a second drug added at a low dosage titrated according to patient response. If, however, the patient's pressure has been reduced but not to the desired level and he or she is experiencing adverse effects, or if he or she cannot tolerate the treatment regimen, the drug should be discontinued and another started. Another option for the patient who is responding to drug therapy but is experiencing adverse effects is to decrease the dosage to a tolerable level of adverse effects. If this is not possible, the drug should be stopped and the patient changed to another drug.

Step-down therapy should be considered for patients whose blood pressure has been well controlled during the previous few visits. Fifty percent of patients remain stable. The drug dosage for a stable patient can be reduced by 50% and the patient reevaluated in 2 weeks. If the patient remains stable, the dosage may be decreased another 50% and the patient evaluated again in 2 weeks. If the patient is stable at this point, the drug may be discontinued and the patient once again evaluated in 2 weeks. Patients who may successfully withdraw from antihypertensive therapy include the following:

- Those whose blood pressure has been well controlled over the last few visits with the health care provider
- Those with a pretreatment diastolic blood pressure less than 100 mm Hg
- Those with no evidence of end-organ disease
- Those who have been on monotherapy only
- Those who have lost weight, are following a sodium-restricted diet, have decreased their alcohol intake, and have increased their exercise regimen

---

CASE STUDY  *Hypertension*

ASSESSMENT

HISTORY OF PRESENT ILLNESS

MD is a 57-year-old postmenopausal white woman who has come for a routine employment physical examination. Her last physical and eye examinations were 2 years ago. She is anticipating a midlife career change.

HEALTH HISTORY

MD has no known allergies. She was diagnosed with type 2 diabetes 10 years ago. She denies previous personal or family history of cardiovascular, renal, or hepatic disorders. Medical records indicate she is not always compliant with recommended treatment plans regardless of state of health. No regular exercise program. No other drugs currently taken.

LIFESPAN CONSIDERATIONS

MD lives with her husband, who is a traveling architect. Their three adult children have recently moved into apartments of their own. Husband and wife feel like their "nest is empty."

CULTURAL/SOCIAL CONSIDERATIONS

MD had a 40 pack/year smoking history, but quit 7 years ago because it exacerbated her asthma. She gained 50 lbs over this time. She denies alcohol use. MD's preferred health care provider is a naturopath. She would prefer to receive all health care from this individual because "he will be able to meet all of my health care needs with naturopathy." MD is covered for prescriptions under her current health plan. Copayments range from $5 to $10 per drug. MD is an accountant and does not rely on her husband for income.

PHYSICAL EXAMINATION

MD is 5'5" tall and weighs 182 lbs. Blood pressure is 210/118 mm Hg for right arm sitting and 206/114 mm Hg for left arm sitting; apical pulse 100 and regular. Previous three readings ranged from 152/88 mm Hg to 194/96 mm Hg; previous apical pulse readings 72 to 82 and regular. PMI not palpable. No lifts, heaves, thrills, murmurs, or extra heart sounds noted. No carotid, abdominal, or renal bruits noted. Breath sounds clear to auscultation bilaterally. Pulses 2+ for all four extremities, no peripheral edema. Brief neurologic examination nonfocal. Funduscopic examination unremarkable.

LABORATORY TESTING

Chest x-ray unchanged from 5 years ago. Urinalysis shows glycosuria, no protein. CBC count within normal limits; serum calcium 9.0 mg/dL; chloride 102 mg/dL; blood glucose 180 mg/dL; HgbA$_{1c}$ 8%; BUN 14 mg/dL; creatinine 1.0 mg/dL; uric acid 4.8 mg/dL; ALT 28 units/L; AST 34 units/L; total cholesterol 228 mg/dL; HDL 46 mg/dL; LDL 147 mg/dL; triglycerides 150 mg/dL. ECG normal sinus rhythm.

PATIENT PROBLEM(S)

Elevated blood pressure on three separate occasions and in different environments; history of poor adherence to treatment plan.

GOALS OF THERAPY

Patient's blood pressure will be within normal limits. Patient will not demonstrate signs or symptoms of end-organ damage. Patient will verbalize and demonstrate adherence to drug therapy and lifestyle modifications.

CRITICAL THINKING QUESTIONS

1. Given the patient's present blood pressure readings, describe three immediate interventions.
2. The health care provider orders clonidine 0.1 mg po one time STAT; losartan 50 mg po qd at bedtime. What are the mechanisms of action of clonidine and losartan?
3. What nursing actions are needed when clonidine is administered?
4. What are the treatment considerations when using losartan rather than an ACE inhibitor for MD?
5. Design a treatment plan to include lifestyle modifications related to diet, exercise, and stress reduction.
6. How will you respond to MD's request to use naturopathic interventions for her hypertension?

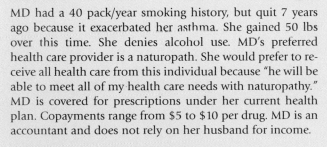

Bibliography

Aminoff UB, Kjellgren KI: The nurse—a resource in hypertension care, *J Adv Nurs* 35(4):582-589, 2001.

Arbour R: Aggressive management of intracranial dynamics, *Crit Care Nurse* 18(3):30-42, 1998.

Capriotti T: Nursing pharmacology. New recommendations: intensify control of patient blood pressure, *Medsurg Nurs* 8(3):207-213, 1999.

Davies N: When to use antihypertensives, *Nurs Times* 97(28):41-42, 2001.

Glaser V: ACE inhibitors: first-line therapy in diabetes, *Pat Care Nurse Pract* 4(4):28, 31, 36 passim, 2001.

Jacobson EJ: Hypertension: update on use of angiotensin II receptor blockers, *Geriatrics* 56(2):20-21, 25-28, 2001.

Joint National Committee on Detection, Evaluation, and Treatment of High Blood Pressure: The sixth report of the Joint National Committee on Prevention, Detection, Evaluation, and Treatment of High Blood Pressure, *Arch Intern Med* 157:2414-2446, 1997.

Mead M: Combination therapy, *Pract Nurse* 22(6):30, 32-33, 2001.

Reeder SJ, Hoffmann RL: Beta-blocker therapy for hypertension, *Dimens Crit Care Nurs* 20(2):2-12, 2001.

Smith A: The treatment of hypertension in patients with diabetes, *Nurs Clin North Am* 36(2):273-289, 2001.

Weir MR: Appropriate use of calcium antagonists in hypertension, *Hosp Pract* 36(9):47-48, 53-55, 2001.

Internet Resources

http://www.aafp.org/afp/20000515/3049.html.

http://www.ehendrick.org/healthy/00037930.html.

http://www.pharmj.com/Editorial/19990904/education/hypertension2.html.

http://www.ti.ubc.ca/pages/letter7.html.

http://www.ti.ubc.ca/pages/letter8.html.

http://www.who.int/ncd/cvd/PracticeGuidelinesSlideset2/sld068.htm.

CHAPTER

42

Antilipemic Drugs

LYNN ROGER WILLIS • KATHLEEN GUTIERREZ

 Visit **http://evolve.elsevier.com/Gutierrez/** for additional information.

KEY TERMS

Apoproteins, p. 678

Cholesterol, p. 678

Endogenous pathway, p. 678

Exogenous pathway, p. 678

Hyperlipidemia, p. 678

Hyperlipoproteinemia, p. 678

Myositis, p. 685

Rhabdomyolysis, p. 685

Xanthomas, p. 688

Xanthelasma, p. 688

OBJECTIVES

- Understand the various forms of hyperlipidemias.
- Explain the consequences of hyperlipidemias.
- Describe the mechanisms by which drugs may control hyperlipidemias.
- Discuss the benefits of drug therapy for hyperlipidemias.
- Construct a nursing plan for a patient receiving a drug for hyperlipidemia.

PATHOPHYSIOLOGY • Hyperlipoproteinemia

Diseases of the heart and blood vessels are the principal cause of death in the industrialized countries of the world. In the United States, more people die from heart and blood vessel disease than any other illness, including cancer. More than 75% of deaths resulting from cardiovascular disease can be attributed to hyperlipoproteinemia and resultant atherosclerosis (Figure 42-1). Effective treatment for hyperlipoproteinemia must be directed at causative factors and prevention rather than reversal, because it is a slowly developing disorder. Clinical investigation has shown that vigorous drug therapy slows progression, and in some cases produces regression, of atherosclerotic lesions that lead to coronary artery disease.

Hyperlipidemia is a general term for elevated concentrations of any or all of the lipids contained in plasma. **Hyperlipoproteinemia** is an excess of the lipoproteins in the blood and is caused by a disorder of lipoprotein metabolism. It may be acquired or hereditary. The acquired form occurs secondary to another disorder or as a result of environmental factors (e.g., diet, smoking). The hereditary form has been classified into five phenotypes on the basis of clinical features, enzymatic abnormalities, and serum lipoprotein patterns.

Cholesterol is a waxy, fatlike substance found in all animal fats and oils. Cholesterol can enter the body as dietary fat, and it is also manufactured by the liver from saturated fats. Cholesterol is an important component of cell membranes, bile acids, myelin sheath, and other body components as well as a precursor of steroid hormones and vitamin D. The liver produces about 1000 mg of cholesterol per day, enough for the body to maintain its required functions. Triglyceride is a different form of lipid that serves as an energy source for muscle and is stored in adipose tissue.

The production of atherogenic lipoproteins and atheromatous plaque involves both an exogenous and an endogenous pathway (Figure 42-2). The **exogenous pathway** follows absorption of dietary fat from the intestine to the tissue and back to the liver. Essentially no feedback mechanism exists within the exogenous pathway. The **endogenous pathway**, however, can exert feedback inhibition through receptors on cell surfaces. The endogenous pathway follows the formation of lipoproteins within the liver through metabolism in other parts of the body and returns to the liver.

Fats are not water soluble. To facilitate the transportation of lipids from the liver through the bloodstream to other tissues, cholesterol and triglycerides are bound to specialized proteins called **apoproteins.** The resultant lipoproteins move through the plasma, distributing and picking up the lipid components. Lipoproteins are classified according to their density: chylomicrons (lowest density), very low–density lipoprotein, intermediate-density lipoprotein, low-density lipoprotein, and high-density lipoprotein (Figure 42-3).

The four major classes of apoproteins are A (apos A-I, A-II, A-III, A-IV), B (apos B-48, B-100), C (apos C-I, C-II, C-III), and E (Table 42-1). Apoproteins are responsible for metabolic interactions and sometimes act as catalysts for enzymatic reactions (e.g., lipoprotein lipase) that allow the transfer of lipids to and from cells. Other apoproteins serve as cellular receptors for the metabolism of lipoproteins.

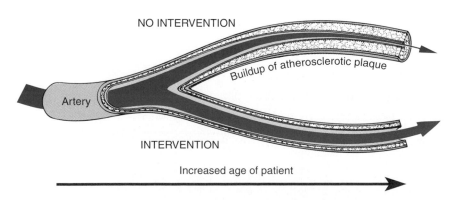

NO INTERVENTION

Buildup of atherosclerotic plaque

Artery

INTERVENTION

Increased age of patient

FIGURE 42-1 Diagram of increasing blockage of artery caused by atherosclerotic plaque. The buildup of plaque is shown as a time-dependent phenomenon. Intervention, through diet, exercise, or drugs, can slow buildup. Recent studies have shown that some interventions can reverse atherosclerosis.

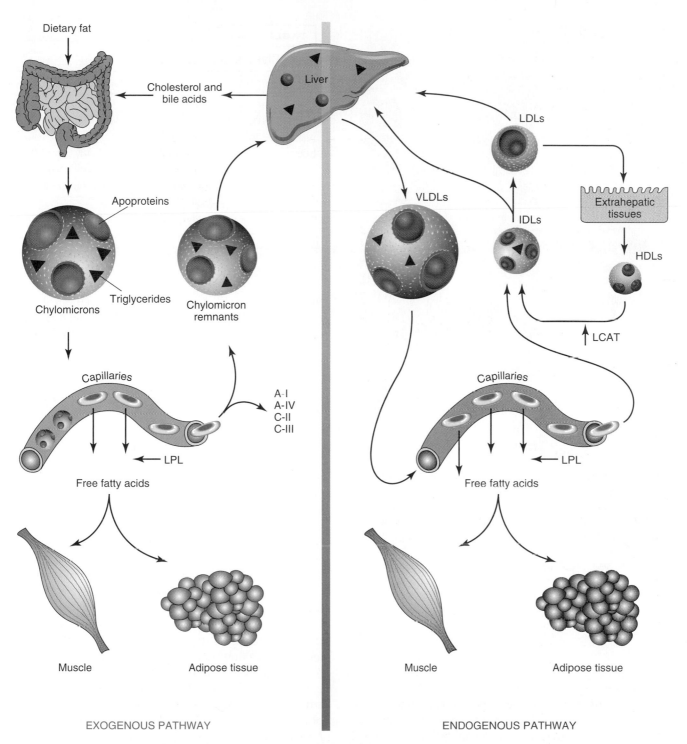

FIGURE 42-2 Metabolic pathways for lipoproteins. This diagram shows the exogenous and endogenous pathways that allow the transportation of lipids, in the form of plasma-soluble lipoproteins, from the intestine and liver to body tissues and back to the liver. Apoproteins, which bind with cholesterol and triglycerides to form lipoproteins, sometimes act as catalysts for enzymatic reactions. Apoproteins A-I, A-IV, C-II, and C-III activate lipolytic enzymes to remove lipids from lipoproteins; lecithin-cholesterol acyltransferase (LCAT) converts high-density lipoprotein (HDL) to intermediate-density lipoprotein (IDL) and low-density lipoprotein (LDL) for return to the liver. *LPL,* lipoprotein lipase; *VLDL,* very low–density lipoprotein.

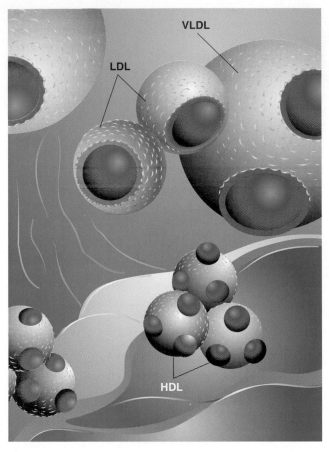

FIGURE 42-3 Density and function of lipoproteins. Lipoproteins are classified according to density, which reflects protein and lipid content: very low–density (VLDL), low density (LDL), and high density (HDL). Lipids are transported in plasma as components of these particles. The larger VLDL particles contain a higher percentage of lipid and are less dense, whereas the smaller HDL particles have less lipid and a higher percentage of protein, and are more dense. VLDLs and LDLs transport cholesterol and triglycerides away from the liver to organs and tissues. HDL particles move cholesterol toward the liver and away from tissues.

TABLE 42-1		
Major Classes of Lipoproteins		
Lipoprotein Class	*Major Lipid*	*Major Apoproteins*
Chylomicrons and remnants	Dietary triglycerides	A-I, A-II, B-48, C-1, C-II, C-III, E
VLDL	Endogenous triglycerides	B-48, C-I, C-II, C-III, E
IDL	Cholesterol esters, triglycerides	B-100, C-III, E
LDL	Cholesterol esters	B-100
HDL	Cholesterol esters	A-I, A-II

for the inverse relationship between HDL cholesterol and VLDLs. When the triglycerides have been removed from the VLDLs, the leftover remnants, which then contain about 45% cholesterol, are the intermediate-density lipoproteins.

Intermediate-Density Lipoproteins. Intermediate-density lipoproteins (IDLs) form when VLDLs lose their triglycerides. The remnant IDLs are either taken up by the liver through apo-E receptors or are converted to low-density lipoproteins by an intravascular process that removes much of the remaining triglycerides. IDLs are about 70% cholesterol. In normally healthy individuals, IDLs are not found in a significant amount.

Low-Density Lipoproteins. Low-density lipoproteins (LDLs) supply cholesterol to the tissues and carry proportionally more cholesterol than other lipoproteins. High levels of LDL, the "bad" cholesterol, have been implicated in atherogenesis. The core of LDL is composed of cholesterol esters (50%) and a relatively small amount of triglyceride (7% to 10%). The surface coat of LDL contains only one apoprotein, B-100. Although most LDL receptors are found in the liver, extrahepatic tissues (e.g., endothelial cells, lymphoid cells, smooth muscle cells, adrenal glands) use the receptor-dependent pathways to obtain the cholesterol needed for the synthesis of cell membranes and hormones. Serum LDL levels are increased in persons who consume large amounts of saturated fats or cholesterol, have defects in either their LDL receptors or in the structure of LDL apoprotein apo B, or have a familial form of increased LDL. The association of high levels of serum cholesterol with coronary artery disease (CAD) is predominantly a reflection of LDL levels.

Many of the mechanisms by which LDL contributes to atherosclerosis occur beneath the arterial wall. After traversing the tunica intima, LDL is oxidized by endothelial and smooth muscle cells. Oxidation of LDLs

Chylomicrons. The primary role of chylomicrons is to carry large quantities of triglycerides throughout the body. Triglycerides are synthesized primarily from carbohydrates in the liver and make up 85% to 95% of each chylomicron. Cholesterol esters make up 3% to 5% of the chylomicron. Triglycerides are removed from chylomicrons by the enzyme lipoprotein lipase.

Very Low–Density Lipoproteins. Very low–density lipoproteins (VLDLs) contain about 75% triglycerides and 25% cholesterol. The VLDLs transport triglycerides from the liver and intestines to capillary beds that service adipose and muscle cells. VLDLs also act as acceptors of cholesterol transferred from HDLs, possibly accounting

---

TABLE 42-2

Classification of Hyperlipoproteinemias

Type	Common Name	Chol*	VLDL	LDL	HDL	TriG	CAD Risk	Cause
I	Exogenous hypertriglyceridemia	N	NC	↓	↓	↑↑	Not known	Dietary fat not cleared from plasma
IIA	Familial hypercholesterolemia	↑	NC	↑	↓	N	Yes	Autosomal dominant
IIB	Combined hyperlipidemia	↑	↑	↑	NC	↑	Yes	Autosomal dominant
III	Familial dysbetahyperlipoproteinemia	↑	↑	↑†	NC	↑	Yes	Autosomal recessive
IV	Endogenous hypertriglyceridemia	N or ↑	↑	NC	NC or ↓	↑	Unclear	Excessive carbohydrate intake
V	Mixed hypertriglyceridemia	↑	↑	NC	NC or ↓	↑↑	Unclear	Possible metabolic defect

↑, ↓, Magnitude of change; *NC*, no change; *N*, normal.
*Most cases of elevated cholesterol values are multifactorial: genetics, nutrition, and metabolic disease.
†Beta VLDL particles.

results in an accumulation of monocytes, which take up the modified LDLs via alternative scavenger receptors. The monocytes become lipid-filled macrophages that further oxidize LDLs. Continued oxidation of LDLs appears to inhibit macrophage motility, and the first visible lesion of atherosclerosis (the "fatty streak") appears.

High-Density Lipoproteins. High-density lipoproteins (HDLs), the "good" cholesterol, are synthesized in the liver. HDLs contain relatively little lipid and much protein, and thus are the smallest and most dense of the lipoproteins. There are two subfractions of HDL: HDL_2 and HDL_3. The concentration of HDL_2 is the single most powerful indicator of risk for CAD. The HDLs probably

function in peripheral tissues as acceptors of free cholesterol. The cholesterol (17% to 20%) is esterified and stored in the central core of the HDL.

TYPES OF HYPERLIPOPROTEINEMIA

The Frederickson-Levy classification identifies five major types of hyperlipoproteinemia (Table 42-2). They are organized according to underlying cause and characteristic lipid and lipoprotein values. Type IIA, IIB, and III hyperlipoproteinemias have a positive correlation with CAD. The risk for CAD from Type IV and V hyperlipoproteinemias is unclear at this time. There is no known increase in the incidence of CAD with Type I hyperlipoproteinemia.

ANTILIPEMIC DRUGS

The most effective drugs for the treatment of hyperlipidemia are bile acid resins, fibric acid derivatives, HMG CoA (3-hydroxy-3-methylglutaryl coenzyme A) reductase inhibitors, and nicotinic acid. All of these drugs

reduce total cholesterol and LDL levels with varying effects on HDL and triglyceride levels (Table 42-3). They have additive effects when used in combination.

TABLE 42-3

Effects of Lipid Lowering Drugs

Drug Class	Total Cholesterol (%)	LDL (%)	HDL (%)	TriG (%)
Bile acid resins	↓ 15-20	↓ 15-30*	↑ or ↓ 3-5	↑ 3-10
Fibric acid derivatives	↓ 2-10†	↓ 15-20	↓ 15-20	↓ 20-50
HMG-CoA reductase inhibitors	↓ 20-45	↓ 18-55	↑ 5-15	↓ 7-30
Nicotinic acid	↓ 15-20	↓ 5-25	↑ 15-35	↓ 20-50

↑, ↓, Magnitude of change; *NC*, no change. Values in table represent percent of change in total cholesterol, LDL, HDL, or triglycerides; direction of change is indicated by the arrows.
*Fibric acid derivatives may increase LDL in patients with high triglyceride levels.
†Gemfibrozil does not reduce LDL levels.

DRUG CLASS • Bile Acid Resins

cholestyramine (Questran, Questran Light, Cholybar)

colestipol (Colestid)

MECHANISM OF ACTION

Cholestyramine and colestipol are quaternary ammonium anion-exchange resins that act indirectly to reduce LDL levels by binding bile salts in exchange for chloride ions. These drugs form an insoluble complex with the bile acids in the intestine, which prevents reabsorption of the bile acids from the gut and increases their elimination in feces. As compensation for the loss of bile salts, the liver increases the rate of bile acid synthesis. To increase bile acid synthesis, the liver requires an increase in the supply of cholesterol and increases the number of hepatic LDL receptors to increase the hepatic uptake of LDL. Increasing the hepatic uptake of LDL increases the hepatic supply of cholesterol. The increased hepatic uptake of LDL reduces the plasma concentration of LDL.

USES

Bile acid resins used in conjunction with a low-cholesterol diet can reduce LDL levels by 15% to 20% (see Table 42-3). They are useful for patients who have a low risk for CAD but in whom diet therapy alone has failed to reduce LDL. Bile acid resins are approved for use in the treatment of Type II hypercholesterolemia.

PHARMACOKINETICS

Bile acid resins are not absorbed in the GI tract. The onset of hypocholesterolemic effects occurs in 24 to 48 hours (Table 42-4). Peak action is achieved in 1 to 3 weeks, with a duration of action of 2 to 4 weeks for cholestyramine, and 4 weeks for colestipol. Once bound to the bile acids, the drugs are eliminated in the feces. The dose-response curves for bile acid resins are not linear, and when given in doses above the maximum recommended dosage, these drugs produce little additional cholesterol-lowering effect.

TABLE 42-4

Pharmacokinetics of Selected Antilipemic Drugs

Drug	Route	Onset	Peak	Duration	PB (%)	$t_{1/2}$	BioA (%)
Bile Acid Resins							
cholestyramine	po	24-48 hr	1-3 wk	2-4 wk	NA	UK	0
colestipol	po	24-48 hr	4 wk	4 wk	NA	UK	0
Fibric Acid Derivatives							
gemfibrozil	po	2-5 days*	4 wk*	Mo	95	1.3-1.5 hr	UA
fenofibrate	po	Varies	3-6 hr	Wk	UA	15 hr	UA
HMG-COA Reductase Inhibitors							
atorvastatin	po	Rapid	1-2 hr	UA	95	20 hr	30
fluvastatin	po	Slow	UA	4-6 wk	95	UK	30
lovastatin	po	3 days	2-4 hr, 4-6 wk†	UA	95	1–2 hr	30
pravastatin	po	1 hr	1-1.5 hr, wk‡	48 hr	50	77 hr	34
simvastatin	po	1 hr	1.3-2.4 hr	UA	95	UA	85
nicotinic acid	po	Hours-days	UK§	UK	UK	1 hr	UA

NA, Not applicable; *UA*, unavailable; *UK*, unknown.
*Time for gemfibrozil's onset and reduction of triglyceride–VLDL levels, respectively.
†The biphasic peaks of lovastatin and pravastatin, respectively.
‡Clinical effects of pravastatin take 4 to 6 weeks.
§Peak drug levels of niacin are reached in 1 hour; however, its peak effects on lipids is unknown.

ADVERSE REACTIONS AND CONTRAINDICATIONS

Because the bile acid–binding resins are not absorbed from the GI tract, they do not directly cause systemic adverse effects. However, the use of bile acid resins is not without problems. Resins are insoluble powders with the consistency of fine sand. They must be mixed with fluids to be ingested, and tend to cause bloating, nausea, indigestion, flatulence, and constipation. Because of the exchange of chloride ions for bile acids, greater chloride absorption can result in a hyperchloremic metabolic acidosis. Bile acid resins are contraindicated in patients with complete or partial biliary obstruction.

They should be used cautiously in patients with steatorrhea or preexisting constipation. These drugs can be used to treat hypercholesterolemia in children and pregnant women, although clear-cut data are not available as to the safety of their long-term use in children or their use during pregnancy and lactation.

INTERACTIONS

Bile acid resins diminish the absorption of many orally administered drugs (Table 42-5). The resulting decrease in absorption of antibiotics, cardiac glycosides, folic acid, and warfarin reduces their effects. The effect of bile acid resins on many other drugs has not been well studied.

TABLE 42-5

Drug Interactions of Selected Antilipemic Drugs

Drug	Interactive Drugs	Interaction
Bile Acid Resins		
cholestyramine, colestipol	Acetaminophen, antiinflammatory drugs, antibiotics, cardiac glycosides, corticosteroids, fat-soluble vitamins, folic acid, iron preparations, methotrexate, phenobarbital, propranolol, thiazide diuretics, thyroxine, warfarin	Decreased absorption of interactive drug
Fibric Acid Derivatives		
gemfibrozil	warfarin, lovastatin	Increased effects of interactive drug
	lovastatin	Increased risk of myositis, myalgia
fenofibrate	Anticoagulants, insulins, sulfonylureas	Increased effects of interactive drug
	probenecid	Increased toxicity of fenofibrate
	rifampin	Decreased effects of fenofibrate
HMG-COA Reductase Inhibitors		
atorvastatin, fluvastatin, lovastatin, pravastatin	cholestyramine, colestipol	Additive cholesterol-lowering effects
simvastatin	Azole antifungal drugs, cyclosporine, erythromycin, gemfibrozil, nicotinic acid	Increased risk of myopathy, rhabdomyolysis
	digoxin, warfarin	Increased serum drug levels of interactive drug
fluvastatin	cimetidine, omeprazole, ranitidine	Increased fluvastatin levels
Nicotinic Acid		
nicotinic acid	lovastatin	Increased risk of myopathy, rhabomyolysis
	guanethidine, guanadrel	Additive hypotension
	probenecid, sulfinpyrazone	Large doses may decrease uricosuric effects of interactive drugs

DRUG CLASS • Fibric Acid Derivatives

fenofibrate

gemfibrozil (Lopid)

MECHANISM OF ACTION

Gemfibrozil alters the rate of synthesis of specific lipoproteins (i.e., C-II, C-III) with activation of extrahepatic lipoprotein lipase. Synthesis of apoproteins (i.e., A-I, A-II) and, thus, formation of HDL increases. There is no explanation for how gemfibrozil raises HDL levels. However, because triglycerides make up the primary core of VLDLs, there is some speculation that the ability of gemfibrozil to reduce triglyceride production may be the mechanism by which this drug lowers LDL levels.

Fenofibrate inhibits the biosynthesis of LDL and VLDL, which are responsible for triglyceride development in the liver. It helps mobilize triglycerides from tissues and increases the elimination of neutral sterols. It also has antiplatelet effects.

USES

Gemfibrozil is used to treat Types III, IV, and V hyperlipoproteinemia and currently is approved by the FDA for patients with triglyceride concentrations exceeding 750 mg/dL. High triglyceride levels pose a risk not only for atherogenesis but more often for the development of pancreatitis. Gemfibrozil decreases serum triglyceride levels by 20% to 50% and VLDL levels by 40%, with variable reductions in total cholesterol (see Table 42-3). It increases HDL levels by 15% to 20%. Gemfibrozil does not reduce LDL levels.

Fenofibrate was recently approved by the FDA for patients with Types IV and V hypertriglyceridemia. It is used as adjunctive therapy in patients at risk for pancreatitis and whose very high triglyceride elevations do not respond adequately to determined efforts at dietary control.

PHARMACOKINETICS

The onset of triglyceride–VLDL reduction from gemfibrozil takes 2 to 5 days, although the drug reaches peak blood levels in 1 to 2 hours. It is 95% protein bound with a half-life of 1.5 hours (see Table 42-4). Biotransformation takes place in the liver with elimination in the urine.

Fenofibrate is well absorbed when taken by mouth, with varying times of onset. Its serum levels peak in 3 to 6 hours, and its duration of action is measured in weeks. It has a half-life of 15 hours and is eliminated in the urine.

ADVERSE EFFECTS AND CONTRAINDICATIONS

Gemfibrozil is generally well tolerated. Its most common adverse effect is GI disturbance, followed by fatigue, eczema, rash, vertigo, and headache. Head, neck, or extremity pain, anemia, leukopenia, and hyperglycemia (particularly in patients receiving insulin or oral antihyperglycemic drugs) are uncommon. Cholecystitis, cholelithiasis, acute appendicitis, pancreatitis, and malignancy rarely occur.

The most common adverse effects of fenofibrate are nausea, vomiting, dyspepsia, stomatitis, gastritis, increased risk of cholelithiasis, and weight gain. Impotence, decreased libido, dysuria, proteinuria, and oliguria have been noted. Skin rashes, urticaria, pruritus, dry hair and skin, and alopecia are possible. Flulike symptoms, including myalgias and arthralgias, are also common. Hematuria, pulmonary emboli, leukopenia, and eosinophilia have been documented and are the most life-threatening adverse effects.

Contraindications to the use of fibric acid derivatives are hepatic or renal disease and primary biliary cirrhosis. The drugs should be used cautiously in patients with a history of peptic ulcer disease.

INTERACTIONS

As with other antilipemic drugs, there are drug interactions for fibric acid derivatives (see Table 42-5). The action of warfarin is enhanced in the presence of gemfibrozil; thus, it is wise to monitor liver function, prothrombin times (PT), and international normalized ratios (INR) periodically when the two drugs are used concurrently. Increased bleeding tendencies have been noted when oral anticoagulants are given with fenofibrate. A dosage reduction of as much as 50% is often required.

DRUG CLASS • HMG-CoA Reductase Inhibitors

⚠ atorvastatin (Lipitor)

   fluvastatin (Lescol)

   lovastatin (Mevacor)

   pravastatin (Pravachol)

   simvastatin (Zocor)

MECHANISM OF ACTION

HMG-CoA reductase inhibitors lower total cholesterol, LDL, and apo B lipoprotein levels by inhibiting cholesterol synthesis in the liver. The inhibitors are selective for this enzyme. The decrease in cholesterol synthesis caused by the drugs is met by an up-regulation of cellular LDL receptors. As greater catabolism of LDL occurs, plasma concentrations of LDL fall.

USES

HMG-CoA reductase inhibitors are effective for most patients with hypercholesterolemia, decreasing total plasma cholesterol levels by 20% to 45% and LDL levels by 18% to 55%. There is emerging evidence of their ability to affect plaque progression, even when used alone. The HDL levels increase 5% to 15% in response to these drugs.

PHARMACOKINETICS

HMG-CoA reductase inhibitors differ in their bioavailability and in the effect of food on their absorption (see Table 42-4). Food reduces the bioavailability of these drugs (except lovastatin and simvastatin) but not their efficacy. All of these drugs are subject to significant first-pass biotransformation by the liver.

Maximum plasma levels for most HMG-CoA reductase inhibitors occur in approximately 1 to 2 hours, although their cholesterol-lowering effects may take several weeks. Plasma concentrations are lower with evening than with morning drug administration; however, LDL reduction is the same regardless of the time of day the drug is taken.

Some metabolites of these drugs are also active HMG-CoA reductase inhibitors. The drugs and their metabolites are primarily eliminated in the bile, following hepatic and extrahepatic biotransformation. Small amounts (less than 20%) of the unchanged drugs are eliminated in the urine.

ADVERSE EFFECTS AND CONTRAINDICATIONS

Headache is the most common adverse effect of HMG-CoA reductase inhibitors. Additionally, up to 10% of patients have GI symptoms consisting of diarrhea, constipation, dyspepsia, flatulence, abdominal pain or cramps, and nausea.

Myalgias have been reported in a small but significant percentage of patients who have taken HMG-CoA reductase inhibitors. Approximately 30% of immunosuppressed patients who received lovastatin developed **myositis** (inflammation of the muscles) within 1 year of starting the drug, but myositis has occurred as well in otherwise normal patients. If the HMG-CoA reductase inhibitor is not withdrawn, the myositis can progress to **rhabdomyolysis,** a disintegration of striated muscle fibers, possibly associated with acute renal failure.

Hepatotoxicity has been reported in a small percentage of patients taking HMG-CoA reductase inhibitors, although jaundice and other clinical signs were absent. Cautious use of these drugs is warranted in patients with liver disease and in those who consume alcohol to excess.

HMG-CoA reductase inhibitors are contraindicated in patients who are hypersensitive, because patients may develop cross-sensitivity among drugs. They are also contraindicated in patients with active liver disease. There is no compelling reason to use these drugs during pregnancy. Women of child-bearing age should be advised about the potential for fetal harm and warned against becoming pregnant while taking these drugs. HMG-CoA reductase inhibitors are also contraindicated during lactation.

INTERACTIONS

Niacin, erythromycin, gemfibrozil, cyclosporin, and azole antifungal drugs interact with HMG-CoA reductase inhibitors to increase the risk of myopathy and rhabdomyolysis (see Table 42-5). Warfarin and digoxin doses may need to be adjusted because of their increased serum drug levels. When an HMG-CoA reductase inhibitor is given with an antacid, the plasma concentration of the inhibitor is reduced but not its ability to reduce LDL levels.

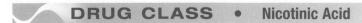

DRUG CLASS • Nicotinic Acid

niacin (Nia-Bid, Niacor, Nico-400, Nicobid, Nicolar, Nicotinex, Slo-Niacin)

MECHANISM OF ACTION

Nicotinic acid (niacin) is a water-soluble vitamin of the B complex, but the lipid-lowering action is independent of its vitamin activity. Indeed, the lipid-lowering effect of nicotinic acid requires substantially higher dosages than are needed to produce vitamin-related actions (i.e., in excess of 1000 mg per day to lower lipid levels versus 15 mg per day as a vitamin). Lipid-lowering doses of nicotinic acid also produce peripheral vasodilation, which causes facial flushing (discussed below).

The mechanism by which nicotinic acid lowers cholesterol levels is unclear, but the net result is a reduction of LDL and VLDL, with elevation of HDL.

USES

Nicotinic acid lowers both LDL and VLDL, and is the drug of choice for patients at risk for pancreatitis and for those with concurrent elevations of LDL and VLDL. Nicotinic acid reduces plasma triglyceride levels by 20% to 50% and total cholesterol levels by 15% to 20%. Levels of LDL may be reduced by 5% to 25% or more. A significant rise in HDL (approximately 15% to 35%) has also been reported.

PHARMACOKINETICS

Niacin is well absorbed in the intestine when given orally (see Table 42-4), and it is widely distributed throughout the body. When it is taken by mouth, peak drug concentrations are reached within 1 hour, but the time to peak effects on lipid levels is unknown. The half-life of nicotinic acid in plasma is approximately 1 hour. Large doses of nicotinic acid are eliminated unchanged in the urine. A small amount of niacin is converted to niacinamide for use as a B vitamin.

ADVERSE REACTIONS AND CONTRAINDICATIONS

The adverse effects of nicotinic acid include intense flushing and pruritus of the trunk, face, and arms. The flushing is mediated by the release of prostaglandin E_1, which can be partially inhibited by the ingestion of 325 mg of aspirin 30 to 60 minutes before administration of the nicotinic acid. The flushing usually decreases with prolonged administration, but this tolerance may not occur in warm climates.

The adverse reactions to nicotinic acid include dyspepsia, vomiting, and diarrhea. Activation of peptic ulcer disease has been documented. The GI problems are due, at least in part, to the increases in GI motility and gastric acid secretion stimulated by the released histamine. Less common adverse effects are acanthosis nigricans, vascular-type headaches, orthostatic hypotension (especially in older adults), and reversible blurred vision that results from macular edema. Nicotinic acid inhibits the tubular elimination of uric acid, thus predisposing the patient to hyperuricemia and gout. There also appears to be a higher incidence of arrhythmias, including, but not limited to, atrial fibrillation. Anaphylaxis is more likely with intravenous use of nicotinic acid.

Elevations in plasma glucose levels, attributed to a rebound in fatty acid concentrations, may occur after each dose of nicotinic acid in susceptible individuals. The larger amounts of free fatty acids may compete with the use of glucose by peripheral tissues.

Hepatotoxicity caused by nicotinic acid may manifest as cholestatic jaundice with marked elevations of serum transaminases (i.e., AST, ALT). Doses in excess of 2 g of nicotinic acid per day have been associated with hepatotoxicity.

Nicotinic acid is contraindicated in patients with known hypersensitivity, hepatic dysfunction, or active peptic ulcer disease. Some formulations may contain tartrazine (FD&C yellow dye #5) and should be avoided in patients with aspirin allergy. Nicotinic acid should be used cautiously in patients with arterial bleeding, gout, glaucoma, and diabetes mellitus.

INTERACTIONS

Large doses of nicotinic acid may decrease the uricosuric effects of probenecid or sulfinpyrazone and produce an increase in uric acid levels (see Table 42-5). There is a higher risk of myopathy with concurrent use of lovastatin. Additive hypotension is associated with the concurrent use of adrenergic neuronal blocking drugs (guanethidine, guanadrel).

APPLICATION TO PRACTICE

ASSESSMENT

History of Present Illness

Identify patient risk factors for hyperlipoproteinemia (Table 42-6). For example, a 45-year-old (1 risk factor) man who smokes (2) and has diabetes (3), hypertension (4), and a low HDL level (5) will have a 32-fold increase (i.e., five risk factors: $2 \times 2 \times 2 \times 2 \times 2 = 32$) in risk for CAD compared with a woman with no risk factors. Some health care providers "subtract" one risk factor in persons with an HDL level exceeding 60 mg/dL, and two risk factors for patients with an HDL level exceeding 70 mg/dL.

A diet history should be obtained from the patient, especially in regard to fat consumption. Saturated fat intake raises LDL levels. Polyunsaturated fats lower LDL and HDL values. Monounsaturated fat lowers LDL but does not affect HDL levels.

Health History

The patient should be asked about a history of constipation, peptic ulcer disease, gallstones or biliary obstruction, steatorrhea, iodism, impaired renal function, and bleeding disorders. Information on previously diagnosed heart disease in the patient or a first-degree family member is also significant.

A drug history is important, because of the possible drug-drug interactions that can occur with the use of antilipemic drugs. Particular attention should be paid to drugs that may increase lipid levels (e.g., hydrochlorothiazide, chlorthalidone). A history of allergy to fungal by-products should be specifically noted for patients who are candidates for HMG-CoA reductase inhibitors, which are derived from fungi.

Lifespan Considerations

Perinatal. Metabolic changes associated with pregnancy elevate cholesterol, lipoproteins, and triglycerides. The cholesterol level can increase by as much as 40% to 60%. The higher lipid levels are used to form new cells and synthesize new substances, and are also burned as fuel for energy.

During pregnancy, the use of glucose accelerates because of rapid fetal cell and organ growth. In addition, maternal sensitivity to insulin is diminished. As a result, pregnancy is said to produce a diabetes-like state. This diabetes-like state may contribute to the upset in lipid values, at least during the pregnancy. Although most pregnant women are young, healthy individuals, they remain at risk of developing lipid disorders, especially those that are genetically determined.

TABLE 42-6

Risk Factors for Coronary Artery Disease Other Than High LDL Levels

Risk Factors*	Comments
Age over 45 years for men	Men have higher total cholesterol levels than women until age 50.
Age over 55 years for women	Postmenopausal women without estrogen replacement have a drop in estrogen levels that triggers a rise in cholesterol levels.
Family history of CAD, definitive MI, or sudden death in first-degree male relative before age 55 or in first-degree female relative before age 65	Familial hypercholesterolemia affects 5% of general population.
Current cigarette smoking (particularly if more than 10/day)	HDL cholesterol levels are reduced.
HDL under 40 mg/dL	Low HDL levels are proven to contribute to CAD. An HDL level over 60 mg/dL is proven to be protective against CAD.
Treated or untreated systolic blood pressure over 135 mm Hg or diastolic blood pressure over 85	Other components all contribute to development of hypertension and thus increase the risk for CAD related to hyperlipidemia.
Diet high in saturated fats	Total cholesterol and LDL levels are raised.
Treated or untreated diabetes mellitus	Triglycerides, LDL, and total cholesterol levels are elevated with this condition.

Adapted from the Summary of the Third Report of the National Cholesterol Education Program Adult Treatment Panel (2001).
CAD, Coronary heart disease; *HDL,* high-density lipoprotein; *LDL,* low-density lipoprotein.
*Net risk for CAD is determined by adding the number of positive risk factors and then subtracting one risk factor if HDL level exceeds 60 mg/dL. Obesity is not listed as a separate risk factor because it operates through a variety of other mechanisms that include hypertension, low HDL levels, and diabetes. Obesity (i.e., 130% above ideal body weight) elevates triglyceride levels more than cholesterol levels and decreases HDL levels.

Pediatric. Childhood cholesterol levels appear to be a major population predictor for adult cholesterol levels. Current evidence indicates that a presymptomatic phase of atherosclerosis begins during childhood (in some cases as early as age 10 years). The more seriously affected children are customarily those for whom dietary and drug management is warranted.

Older Adults. Cholesterol levels have been reported to gradually increase with age in men and women. Women have higher levels of HDL in all age groups. Postmenopausal women have a drop in estrogen that triggers a rise in cholesterol levels. With changes in lipid metabolism, cholesterol levels rise to a maximum at 65 years and then decrease, but never as low as that in young adults. The LDL and HDL levels in combination with systolic blood pressure are significant in predicting coronary risk in older adults. Triglyceride values also rise with age. The increase in triglyceride levels is greater in females than males at age 50.

Older adults often have diabetes, impaired liver function, or other conditions that also raise blood lipid levels. They are also likely to have cardiovascular and other disorders for which they are taking drugs. For example, diuretics such as hydrochlorothiazide and chlorthalidone may be taken for hypertension or heart failure, but they can increase cholesterol levels by 10%. Beta blockers, such as propranolol, and estrogens can increase triglyceride levels by 25% to 50%.

Cultural/Social Considerations

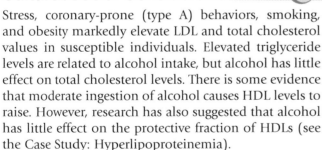

Stress, coronary-prone (type A) behaviors, smoking, and obesity markedly elevate LDL and total cholesterol values in susceptible individuals. Elevated triglyceride levels are related to alcohol intake, but alcohol has little effect on total cholesterol levels. There is some evidence that moderate ingestion of alcohol causes HDL levels to raise. However, research has also suggested that alcohol has little effect on the protective fraction of HDLs (see the Case Study: Hyperlipoproteinemia).

Physical Examination

Assessment of typical changes related to decreased oxygen supply, such as pallor around the lips and nail beds, rubor of the skin, thickened or clubbed nails, dry skin, or loss of hair on the extremities, should be noted. Arterial obstruction secondary to the build-up of atheromatous plaques contributes to these signs.

Most lipid disorders are detected through laboratory determinations rather than physical examination. Although uncommon, patients with extremely high triglyceride levels (over 1000 mg/dL) may complain of eruptive xanthomas and xanthelasma, which are deposits of cholesterol and other lipids, especially over the

buttocks, Achilles and patellar tendons, and on the backs of the hands. The presence of xanthomas usually indicates genetically based hyperlipoproteinemia. In patients with triglyceride levels over 2000 mg/dL, the appearance of cream-colored blood vessels in the fundus of the eye (lipemia retinalis) and retinal arteriovenous crossing changes may be seen.

Laboratory Testing

A lipid profile should be performed for any patient who is symptomatic or asymptomatic and has risk factors for CAD. Obtaining a lipid panel permits a reasonable estimate of CAD risk (see Table 42-6).

The ratio of total cholesterol to HDL cholesterol should be calculated. A ratio lower than 4.5 is desirable. As a rule of thumb, for every 10-mg/dL rise in total cholesterol levels, there is a 10% increase in risk for CAD. Although not routinely measured, apo B is a major component of LDL and is a more sensitive indicator of CAD in men than standard cholesterol measures. Apo A, a major component of HDL, is a much more sensitive predictor of CAD in women.

GOALS OF THERAPY

The ultimate goal in the treatment of hyperlipoproteinemia is to prevent the progression of coronary atherosclerosis and reduce the risk of CAD and other vascular disorders. Effective reduction in CAD risk requires identifying and aggressively treating all CAD risk factors responsive to intervention, including smoking, hypertension, diabetes, and obesity. The approach to treatment is guided by a total assessment of CAD risk, not just the lipid abnormality. For a given degree of LDL elevation, the threshold for initiation of therapy decreases and the intensity of therapy increases as CAD risk rises. Dietary modification, complemented by weight reduction and exercise, is the core of lipid management, with drug therapy reserved for patients at highest risk.

Target levels for LDL depends on the patient's risk for CAD. The goal for a patient with two or more risk factors for CAD is an LDL level under 100 mg/dL. The LDL for patients with zero to one risk factor is 130 mg/dL.

INTERVENTION
Dietary Modifications

Dietary modifications remain the cornerstone of treatment, effective for both treatment and prevention of lipid disorders. Decreases in the intake of cholesterol and saturated fat in controlled settings reduced total cholesterol and LDL levels by up to 30%. The reductions average about 10%, however, when a similar intensive treatment regimen is prescribed for outpatient use. The argument for dietary therapy as the initial step in treatment is based on the following considerations:

(1) diet is the most physiologic approach, (2) the change in lifestyle should be life-long, (3) no drugs are without known or potential adverse effects, and (4) in most cases, drug therapy is expensive.

It is recommended that all Americans adopt the Step I dietary plan published by the American Heart Association (Table 42-7). Step I dietary modifications do not require a dramatic alteration in eating habits and can be readily adopted by most persons. However, Step II dietary modifications require more effort, because they go beyond eliminating obvious sources of fat and cholesterol. Step II dietary modifications are indicated for patients who are already utilizing a Step I diet at the time of diagnosis, who do not achieve adequate results with Step I dietary management, or who have established CAD. If these limitations fail to reduce lipid levels to the desired range, an even more restrictive dietary regimen may be required.

Exercise and Weight Loss

Renewed emphases on exercise and weight reduction, as complements to dietary therapy, are essential components of a nondrug treatment program. They are helpful not only in correcting lipid abnormalities but also in reducing CAD risk factors. For example, regular exercise reduces LDL and raises HDL thus reducing the risk of CAD.

Dietary Supplements

Nonprescription dietary supplements are no substitute for dietary modification. There is some evidence to suggest that omega-3 fatty acids, available in fish oils, may be useful. Antioxidant vitamins such as vitamin C, vitamin E, and beta-carotene do not lower cholesterol levels. However, they may increase LDL resistance to oxidative change and, thus, reduce the risk of injury to vasculature. Additional study is needed, but daily doses of 400 IU of vitamin E, 0.5 to 1 g of vitamin C, and 25 mg of beta-carotene appear safe and, perhaps, may prove beneficial. Garlic supplements (Box 42-1) can reduce serum cholesterol levels by 5% to 10%.

Psyllium (found in Metamucil and other products) has been shown to lower LDL and total cholesterol levels an average of 5% to 10% in some patients (see Chapter 49). It is a logical drug of choice to treat moderately elevated LDL levels (130 to 159 mg/dL) when HDL levels are above 45 mg/dL, especially in older adults.

Drug Therapy

The range of available drugs is extensive, and they vary greatly in cost, effect on cholesterol fractions, efficacy, and adverse effects. No drugs currently available are effective in lowering all types of hyperlipoproteinemia, and all have adverse effects. Drug therapy is started when diet therapy and exercise for 3 to 6 months have been ineffective. Conditions known to increase serum lipid levels (i.e., diabetes, hypothyroidism, liver disease, long-term corticosteroid use) may impose the need for drug therapy. One effective treatment strategy includes administering two or more of the drugs in combination. This strategy enhances the net lipid-lowering effects of the drugs while reducing the incidence of adverse effects, since dosages of individual drugs in the combination can be reduced.

Administration

The bile acid resins are formulated as powders for suspension. Always mix the drug with liquids, food or fruit with a high fluid content such as applesauce or crushed pineapple, thin soups, or milk in hot or regular breakfast cereals. Fill a glass with 2 ounces of the chosen liquid. Put the correct dose on top of the liquid and mix thoroughly. Add an additional 2 to 4 ounces of the chosen liquid and mix again thoroughly. Instruct the patient to drink the mixture while the drug is still suspended. The drug will not dissolve in the liquid. Add a little more of the selected liquid to rinse the glass, and have the patient drink this also. If a carbonated beverage is chosen, use a large glass to prevent spillover because the mixture will foam up. Have the patient drink the mixture slowly to

---

TABLE 42-7			
Dietary Modifications			
Dietary Component	*Average Intake*	*Step I Diet*	*Step II Diet*
Dietary cholesterol	500 mg	<300 mg	200-250 mg
Total fat (as % of calories)	40%-45%	<30%	<30%
Saturated fat	17%	8%-10%	<7%
Monounsaturated fats	18%	<15%	<15%
Polyunsaturated fats	7%	<10%	<10%
Carbohydrates (as % of total calories)	40%-45%	55% or more	55% or more
Protein (as % of total calories)	15%-20%	Approximately 15%	Approximately 15%

BOX 42-1	Alternative Therapies: Antilipemics

Garlic

Garlic consists of the dried or fresh bulbs of *Allium sativum* of the lily family (Liliaceae). Although some advocates still recommend garlic for everything from cancer and tuberculosis to hemorrhoids and athlete's foot, the most frequent use of garlic in recent times has been in treating atherosclerosis and high blood pressure.

The main component of the volatile oil in garlic is an odorless, sulfur-containing amino acid derivative known as alliin (*S*-allyl-L-cysteine sulfoxide), which is considered to be the most important active ingredient. When the garlic bulb is in the ground, alliin comes in contact with the enzyme alliinase, which converts it to allicin. Unfortunately, allicin is extremely odoriferous, the carrier of the typical garlic odor.

The ability of garlic to provide some protection against atherosclerosis, coronary thrombosis, and stroke is believed to be directly related to its ability to inhibit aggregation of platelets. This activity is the result of a compound known as ajoene, a self-condensation product of allicin. To convert alliin to allicin, and, ultimately, to ajoene, requires the action of the enzyme alliinase. As an antithrombotic agent, ajoene is at least as potent as aspirin, and two breakdown products, which are also mildly antithrombotic, enhance its activity.

The daily dose of 4 g is equivalent to 5 to 20 average-sized cloves of fresh garlic, 400 to 1200 mg of dried garlic powder, which is equivalent to 2 to 5 mg of allicin. At these doses, garlic may cause discomfort. Garlic rarely causes allergic reactions or changes in the GI flora. It should be avoided if the patient is taking large amounts of aspirin or is on anticoagulants.

Omega-3 Fatty Acids

The clinical utility of omega-3 fatty acids is greater in patients with elevated triglyceride levels (i.e., Types II-B, III, IV, and V). Omega-3 fatty acids, contained in fish oils, produce a sustained reduction in plasma triglyceride levels by inhibiting VLDL and apo B-100 synthesis and decreasing postprandial lipemia. The effects on LDL or apo B and HDL levels are not as clear, but the effect on LDL appears to be dose dependent. Higher doses produce greater effects on lipid levels.

Omega-3 fatty acids affect many steps in atherogenesis, most notably as precursors of the prostaglandins that interfere with blood clotting. Ingestion of large quantities of omega-3 fatty acids can cause prolonged bleeding time because they inhibit platelet activity. This inhibition has led to concern about spontaneous or excessive bleeding in some patients. A prolonged bleeding time is common to Eskimo populations, who ordinarily have high dietary intake of omega-3 fatty acids and a low incidence of CAD. Other risks associated with the use of omega-3 fatty acids are vitamin A and D toxicity from fish oil contained in cod liver oil, and increased weight gain from the 9 calories per gram of fish oil.

---

prevent swallowing air. Other drugs should be administered 1 hour before or 4 to 6 hours after a bile acid resin. Because these drugs interfere with the absorption of fat-soluble vitamins, supplemental vitamin intake may be necessary.

The fibric acid derivative fenofibrate should be taken with meals to lessen gastric irritation. Nausea may diminish with continued use of the drug. Gemfibrozil should be taken 30 minutes before breakfast and the evening meal.

The highest rates of cholesterol synthesis are between midnight and 5 AM. For pravastatin and simvastatin, the drugs are given in the evening or at bedtime. For lovastatin, the drug is taken with the evening meal if ordered once daily, or with a meal or snack if ordered more than once daily.

Nicotinic acid formulations should be administered with meals or milk to minimize GI irritation. Timed-release formulations of nicotinic acid should be swallowed whole, without crushing, breaking, or chewing.

Contents of capsules may be poured into a small amount of food and swallowed but should not be chewed. Scored tablets may be broken in half.

Education

Patient education and discussion with family members are vital to foster an understanding of the importance of long-term commitment to antilipidemic therapy. Explanations of the lipid disorder, consequences, treatment regimens, and required lifestyle modifications are important. The patient should be advised that antilipemic drugs are used in conjunction with dietary restrictions of fat, cholesterol, calories, and alcohol. The importance of exercise, smoking cessation, weight reduction, and control of comorbid diseases should be included in the teaching.

It is important to work with the members of the patient's household who cook and shop for groceries, so that they understand how to select and prepare "heart-healthy" meals. Less pork and beef should be eaten, and more fish, chicken, turkey, and nonfat or low-fat milk. Minimal amounts of other whole-milk dairy products, such as cheese, butter, ice cream, and sour cream, are acceptable. Margarines and cooking oils that contain polyunsaturated oil products (e.g., safflower, corn, soybean) or monounsaturated oil products (e.g., olive oil) should be used. Oat bran, consumed as cereal or muffins, helps reduce total cholesterol and LDL levels an average of 5% to 10%. Refer the patient to a dietitian as needed.

As with all drugs, the patient should be instructed to take the prescribed antilipemic drug exactly as instructed and not to skip doses or to double up on missed doses. If a dose is missed, it should be taken as soon as remembered. Teach the patients that these drugs must be taken for weeks to months before their full benefit is known. If the drugs prove to be beneficial, they may then be prescribed on a long-term basis. Because antilipemic drugs may interfere with the absorption of other drugs, remind the patient to keep all health care providers informed of all drugs taken. Remind the patient not to stop using the drug without consulting with the health care provider. Discontinuing antilipemic drugs can result in incorrect dosages of other drugs being taken. The importance of regular follow-up visits and laboratory evaluations should be stressed.

Patients taking fibric acid derivatives should have liver function tests done every 3 to 6 months after the start of therapy or dosage change. Patients taking nicotinic acid should have liver function tests done every 6 to 12 weeks during the first year of therapy and every 6 months thereafter.

Liver function tests should be done 12 weeks after the start of therapy or a change in dosage and then every 6 months for patients taking the HMG-CoA reductase inhibitors atorvastatin, fluvastatin, and pravastatin. Liver function tests are done every 6 months or after a dosage increase for patients taking simvastatin. In dosages exceeding 80 mg/day, the liver function tests should be done at 3, 6, and 12-month intervals. For patients on lovastatin, liver function tests are done at 6 and 12 weeks after the start of therapy or a dosage increase and then every 6 months.

Constipation is possible with bile resins and other antilipemic drugs. Thus, explaining the importance of fluids and bulk in the diet as well as exercise, stool softeners, and laxatives (if necessary) is vital. The patient should be told to contact the health care provider if constipation, nausea, flatulence, and heartburn are persistent, or if the stools become frothy and foul smelling. The patient should also be told to report unusual bleeding or bruising, petechiae, or black, tarry stools. Treatment with vitamin K may be necessary. Advise the patient taking HMG-CoA reductase inhibitors to notify the health care provider immediately if they experience muscle aches or pains.

Correct preparation of the patient for evaluation of lipids is important. The patient should be advised to abstain from alcohol and smoking for 48 hours before testing. A 12-hour fast before testing is required, although water may be taken. These activities help to minimize transient increases in lipid levels that occur following a heavy meal or alcohol ingestion.

EVALUATION

The prognosis for patients with lipid disorders can be greatly improved by lasting lifestyle changes and, in many cases, long-term drug therapy. Reevaluate the patient's dietary intake, exercise regimen, and other lifestyle changes at each visit. The patient should exhibit weight loss, a consistently improved exercise regimen, and improvement in dietary intake of fats. Dietary changes continue throughout life.

Drug therapy for hyperlipidemia can continue for many years, and possibly a lifetime. Thus, the health care provider should consider reducing or stopping drug therapy if the desired LDL cholesterol level is maintained for a period of 2 years, in order to reestablish the diagnosis and check the efficacy of nondrug measures. For patients taking antilipemic drugs, baseline monitoring of liver function tests is done at the start of therapy, and then periodically thereafter, based on the drug used for treatment.

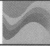

CASE STUDY *Hyperlipoproteinemia*

PATIENT HISTORY

HISTORY OF PRESENT ILLNESS

MM, a 66-year-old African-American man, comes to the clinic for a follow-up assessment of his hyperlipoproteinemia. His last visit was 6 months ago, at which time dietary interventions and an exercise regimen were prescribed. He reports feeling "a little sluggish" recently but attributes it to stress in the workplace, the need for a part-time second job, and perhaps an elevation in his blood pressure. His work requires him to travel three to four times a month, and he admits to noncompliance with diet and exercise regimen.

HEALTH HISTORY

MM has a positive family history for heart disease and hypertension. His father died at 53 of an MI, but his mother is alive and well. His brother has diabetes mellitus and a history of alcoholism. Except for the hyperlipoproteinemia, MM has an otherwise unremarkable health history. He has a 60 pack/year smoking history and has consumed 3 to 4 oz of alcohol daily for the past 5 to 6 months. Current drugs: none.

LIFESPAN CONSIDERATIONS

MM is attempting to support his family, including two sons in their early 20s and his aging mother, who is trying to remain independent at home.

CULTURAL/SOCIAL CONSIDERATIONS

MM admits he is a type A personality with a strong drive (i.e., need) to be the breadwinner in the family. His wife died 10 years ago in a motor vehicle accident. MM has health insurance and pharmacy coverage for his sons but does not carry his own insurance because of the expense. He is concerned about his health care needs but feels unable to obtain personal health insurance at this time, so he has been paying cash for visits to the health care provider and hopes hospitalization will not be necessary.

PHYSICAL EXAMINATION

Blood pressure is 158/88 mm Hg, pulse 100, respirations 24; temperature 98.6° F. MM is 5'11" tall and weighs 288 lb (up 25 lb from previous visit). Remainder of examination unremarkable.

LABORATORY TESTING

CBC count, electrolytes, BUN, creatinine, and thyroid tests are within normal limits. Total cholesterol 390 mg/dL; LDL 169 mg/dL; HDL 34 mg/dL; triglycerides 289 mg/dL.

PATIENT PROBLEM(S)

Type II hyperlipoproteinemia.

GOALS OF THERAPY

Prevent progression of coronary atherosclerosis; reduce LDL cholesterol levels while keeping treatment regimen affordable; improve adherence to diet and exercise regimen.

CRITICAL THINKING QUESTIONS

1. After reviewing MM's records, the health care provider orders nicotinic acid 250 mg po tid for 1 week; then 500 mg po tid for 1 week; then increase dosage at weekly intervals to 1500 mg po qd; one adult aspirin 30 minutes before the daily morning dose of nicotinic acid; atorvastatin 20 mg po qd. Why are both nicotinic acid and atorvastatin ordered?
2. Why was the nicotinic acid ordered to be titrated and what is the relationship of nicotinic acid with the daily aspirin?
3. What risk factors in MM's background place him at risk for coronary artery disease and stroke?
4. MM should be taught to watch for which adverse reactions?
5. What serious adverse reaction is possible with the concurrent use of nicotinic acid and atorvastatin?
6. What teaching is necessary for MM in regard to his diagnosis?

Bibliography

Best JD, Jenkins AJ: Novel agents for managing dyslipidaemia, *Expert Opin Investig Drugs* 10(11):1901-1911, 2001.

Chong PH, Seeger JD, Franklin C: Clinically relevant differences between the statins: implications for therapeutic selection, *Am J Med* 111(5):390-400, 2001.

Packard C: Lipid-lowering drug therapies: the evidence, *Proc Nutr Soc* 59(3):423-424, 2000.

Shek A, Ferrill MJ: Statin-fibrate combination therapy, *Ann Pharmacother* 35(7-8):908-917, 2001.

Internet Resources

This site supported by the National Institutes of Health contains various information relating to the National Cholesterol Education Program. Available online at http://hin.nhlbi.nih.gov/ncep.htm.

This site supported by the National Library of Medicine discusses acquired lipid disorders, as well as treatment for them. Available online at http://www.nlm.nih.gov/medlineplus/ency/article/000403.htm.

CHAPTER

43

Anticoagulant and Antiplatelet Drugs

LYNN ROGER WILLIS • SUSAN SCIACCA

 Visit http://evolve.elsevier.com/Gutierrez/ for additional information.

KEY TERMS

Anticoagulant drugs, p. 694
Antiplatelet drugs, p. 701
Antithrombotic drugs, p. 701
Coagulation, p. 694
Embolus, p. 694
Thrombin, p. 694
Thrombus, p. 694

OBJECTIVES

- Identify the various diseases/disorders for which anticoagulant drug therapy is an appropriate treatment.
- Identify the various diseases/disorders for which antiplatelet drug therapy is an appropriate treatment.
- Discuss the groups of drugs used in anticoagulation.
- Describe the mechanism of action of anticoagulant and antiplatelet drugs.
- Differentiate between the laboratory tests used in drug dosage monitoring.
- Identify the interventions and drug antidotes used for management of overdose.
- Identify patient outcomes that indicate successful therapy with anticoagulant and antiplatelet drugs.

PATHOPHYSIOLOGY • Coagulation

Steps in Coagulation

Coagulation, the complex process required to form a blood clot, is diagrammed in Figure 43-1. The process may begin in the intrinsic pathway with the activation of the blood component factor XII (the Hageman factor) by contact with exposed collagen or with an event in the extrinsic pathway (e.g., the release of tissue factor by damaged tissue). Either pathway results in the activation of factor X. Factor Xa (activated factor X) forms a complex with platelet phospholipids, calcium, and factor V. This complex, which is sometimes called thromboplastin, catalyzes the conversion of prothrombin (factor II) to thrombin. The enzyme thrombin then catalyzes the conversion of fibrinogen to fibrin. After cross-linking of fibrin by factor XIIIa, fibrin becomes insoluble, forming a mesh that is the blood clot, also called a thrombus.

Blood clots in the arterial system are initially composed largely of platelets with a fibrin mesh (white thrombi). Blood clots in the venous system have only a few platelet aggregates and are composed largely of fibrin with trapped red blood cells (red thrombi). A thrombus in the arterial or venous system may dislodge and be carried downstream as an embolus by the flow of blood. Venous emboli often lodge in the small arteries of the pulmonary circulation, thereby markedly impeding the oxygenating capability of the lungs and increasing the blood pressure in the pulmonary system, both of which may be life threatening. Thrombi form in veins in which blood flow is low, favoring the accumulation of activated clotting factors. Patients at risk for experiencing venous thrombosis include those immobilized as a result of trauma or surgery and those with a history of thromboembolism.

Role of Calcium in Blood Coagulation

Calcium is a cofactor for each of the steps in the coagulation cascade through the activation of prothrombin. The removal of calcium prevents coagulation. Citrate and ethylenediamine tetraacetic acid (EDTA) form complexes with calcium, making calcium unavailable for coagulation. When blood is drawn for testing or storage, citrate or EDTA may be used to keep the blood from clotting in the container. Because calcium is essential for many biochemical events, anticoagulants that complex calcium (i.e., that make calcium unavailable) can be used only in storage containers *(in vitro)*, not in a patient *(in vivo)*.

DRUG CLASS • Anticoagulant Drugs

Anticoagulant drugs prevent clot formation by interfering with many of the steps leading to the formation of fibrin (see Figure 43-1). Blood coagulation is often referred to as a cascade because the process becomes magnified at every step. Each activated factor is a catalyst leading to the formation of many molecules of the next activated factor.

Anticoagulant drugs prevent clot formation, but they do not affect existing clots (see Chapter 44 for a discussion of thrombolysis and thrombolytic drugs). The currently available anticoagulant drugs may be classified as acting either directly or indirectly on the coagulation cascade.

DRUG CLASS • Direct-Acting Anticoagulants

High Molecular Weight Heparin

 heparin (Calciparine, Liquaemin, Hep-Lock, Hep-Flush, Hepalean,✳ Heparin Leo✳)

Low Molecular Weight Heparins

   ardeparin (Normiflo)

   dalteparin (Fragmin)

   danaparoid (Orgaran)

   enoxaparin (Lovenox)

Recombinant Hirudin

   lepirudin (Refludan)

MECHANISM OF ACTION

Heparin is a heterogeneous mixture of sulfated, highly polar mucopolysaccharides that, when bound to antithrombin III, greatly accelerates the binding of antithrombin III to the clotting factors, thrombin, and factor Xa. When bound to antithrombin III, those clotting factors become less able to promote coagulation, and the clotting time for the blood increases. Once the bond between antithrombin III and the clotting factors has been formed, the heparin is released to facilitate formation of another such bond.

High molecular weight (HMW) fractions of heparin (MW 5000 to 30,000) markedly inhibit coagulation

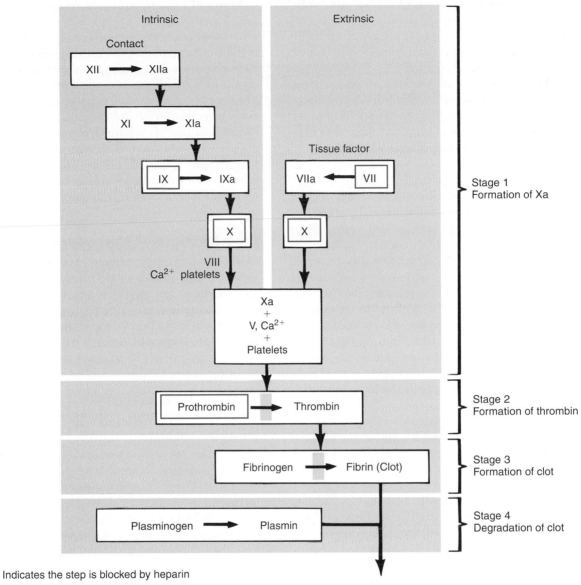

Indicates the step is blocked by heparin

Indicates a clotting factor that is not synthesized when oral anticoagulants are present

Fibrin degradation products

FIGURE 43-1 The four stages of blood coagulation: *Stage 1,* Antiplatelet drugs inhibit platelet aggregation in intrinsic pathway. Citrate and EDTA, which chelate calcium, prevent formation of factor Xa. Oral anticoagulants prevent synthesis of factors VII, IX and X, which are necessary for stage 1. Local hemostatic agents provide contact to activate intrinsic pathway. Not shown is the native inhibitor of anticoagulation, antithrombin III, which acts in stage 1 to inhibit the activity of factor Xa and in stage 2 to inhibit the conversion of prothrombin to thrombin. Heparin and LMW heparin drugs enhance the activity of antithrombin III by directly binding with it. In stage 1, the heparin/antithrombin III complex inhibits factor Xa. *Stage 2,* Oral anticoagulants prevent synthesis of prothrombin. *Stage 3,* The heparin/antithrombin III complex blocks thrombin (Factor IIa) activity. LMW heparin drugs are relatively ineffective at activating antithrombin III to block thrombin. *Stage 4,* Aminocaproic acid inhibits activation of plasminogen and thus inhibits clot degradation. Aprotinin inhibits plasmin. By contrast, alteplase, anistreplase, streptokinase, and urokinase activate plasminogen to promote clot digestion.

through their inhibition of factor Xa and thrombin. Low molecular weight (LMW) fractions, made by depolymerizing heparin, have less effect on coagulation than HMW heparin because they exert little effect on thrombin, even though they inhibit Xa.

Danaparoid sodium is a partially depolymerized mixture of heparin sulfate, dermatan sulfate, and chondroitin sulfate derived from porcine intestinal mucosa. This drug causes even less inhibition of thrombin than LMW heparin, but effectively inhibits factor Xa.

USES

The clinical uses of heparin differ on the basis of dose and route of administration. High-dose heparin is given to patients in the hospital to prevent the formation of venous thrombi. Large doses (35 to 100 units/kg) must be administered intravenously to achieve this degree of anticoagulation.

Heparin may also be given subcutaneously in relatively low doses to achieve slow, continuous absorption over 8 to 12 hours. Low-dose heparin is used in patients more than 40 years old undergoing thoracoabdominal surgery who are at increased risk for thrombosis. Heparin is not used in patients undergoing brain, spinal cord, or eye surgery, in which even minor hemorrhage could be catastrophic. A treatment regimen that involves preoperative and postoperative administration of heparin reduces the incidence of deep vein thrombosis by 50% in thoracoabdominal surgical patients without significantly affecting their bleeding or clotting times.

Heparin also prevents coagulation after blood has left the body. Tubing used in dialysis to transfer blood through the machine can be pretreated with heparin to prevent clotting. Heparin may also be added to containers used for blood collection to prevent coagulation.

The FDA has approved LMW heparin drugs and danaparoid for the prevention of deep vein thrombosis after abdominal and orthopedic surgery.

PHARMACOKINETICS
High Molecular Weight Heparin

The desired level of anticoagulation with HMW heparin occurs immediately on entry of the drug into the blood. Because heparin is highly charged even at the pH of the stomach, very little absorption takes place after oral administration, and therefore the drug is given only by intravenous or subcutaneous injection. Heparin is not given intramuscularly because subsequent bleeding may cause a large and painful hematoma. Absorption of heparin after subcutaneous injection can be erratic, probably because of the large size and electrical charge of the molecules.

Doses of heparin sufficient to cause anticoagulation are cleared from the blood at a constant rate by the reticuloendothelial system. That is, the concentration of heparin needed to produce anticoagulation will saturate the heparin-clearing mechanism, which runs at a constant rate; accordingly, the time required to reduce the plasma concentration of heparin by 50% depends on the concentration of the drug originally in the blood. Heparin administered intravenously in doses of 100, 400, or 800 units/kg has an elimination half-life of approximately 1, 2.5, and 5 hours, respectively. A small fraction of injected heparin is excreted in the urine. The pharmacokinetics of anticoagulant drugs is summarized in Table 43-1.

Low Molecular Weight Heparin

LMW heparin can be administered by subcutaneous injection, which provides good bioavailability. Peak plasma concentrations are usually reached in 3 to 5 hours, with the anticoagulant effect persisting for about 24 hours. LMW heparin is eliminated in the urine. Patients with renal impairment will need to have the dosage interval modified to prevent accumulation of the anticoagulant and subsequent toxicity.

ADVERSE REACTIONS AND CONTRAINDICATIONS
High Molecular Weight Heparin

Heparin is a natural compound, extracted from animal lungs or intestines, and some patients may become allergic to it. The usual symptoms of this allergy are chills, fever, and urticaria, but other allergic reactions such as rhinitis, asthma, and anaphylaxis have been reported. In some patients heparin has caused thrombocytopenia; thus the platelet count should be monitored regularly once therapy has begun.

Low Molecular Weight Heparin

LMW heparin causes pain at the injection site and nausea. Because these anticoagulants have only a small effect, routine coagulation tests cannot be used to monitor their anticoagulant activity. Coadministration of oral anticoagulants or inhibitors of platelet aggregation (see below) will increase the risk of bleeding with these drugs.

LMW heparin is not suitable for patients with blood dyscrasias, stroke, or ulcers, or those who are undergoing brain, spinal, or eye surgery. Patients sensitive to heparin, pork products, or sulfites may have an allergic response to these drugs. The risk for epidural or spinal hematomas with concurrent use of LMW heparin and spinal or epidural anesthesia or spinal puncture is increased by the use of indwelling epidural catheters; the concurrent use of nonsteroidal antiinflammatory drugs (NSAIDs),

TABLE 43-1

Pharmacokinetics of Selected Anticoagulant and Antiplatelet Drugs

Drugs	Route	Onset	Peak	Duration	PB (%)	$t_{1/2}$	BioA (%)
Anticoagulant Drugs							
ardeparin	SC	20-60 min	3-5 hr	12 hr	High	UA	92
dalteparin	SC	20-60 min	3-5 hr	12 hr	High	UA	92
enoxaparin	SC	20-60 min	3-5 hr	12 hr	High	4.5 hr	92
heparin	SC	20-60 min	2-4 hr	8-12 hr	High	1-2 hr*	100
	IV	Immediate	5-10 min	2-6 hr	High	1-2 hr*	100
warfarin	po	Slow	0.5-3 days	2-5 days	95%-97%	0.5-3 days	85-99
Antiplatelet Drugs							
abciximab	IV	NA	NA	48 hr	NA	30 min	NA
aspirin	po	5-30 min	15 min-2 hr	3-6 hr	Varies	2-3 hr; 15-30 hr†	Varies
clopidogrel	po	2 hr	1 hr	5 days	98	8 hr	50
dipyridamole	po	Varies	75 min	3-4 hr	95	10 hr	30-60
	IV	Immediate	6.5 min	30 min	UA	10 hr	100
eptifibatide	IV	Immediate	NA	NA	25	2.5 hrs	NA
pentoxifylline	po	2-4 wks	8 wks	UK	UA	25-50 min	UA
ticlodipine	po	48 hr	7 days	14 days	98	12.6; 4-5 days§	80
tirofibran	IV	Immediate	30 min	NA	low	2 hrs	NA
Anticoagulant Antagonists							
protamine sulfate	IV	30-60 sec	UK	2 hr‖	UA	UK	100
phytonadione	po	6-12 hr	UK	UK	UA	UA	UA
	SC/IM	1-2 hr	3-6 hr¶	12-24 hr	UA	UA	100

BioA, Bioavailability; *N/A,* not applicable; *PB,* Protein binding; $t_{1/2}$, elimination half-life; *UA,* unavailable; *UK,* unknown.
*Half-life of heparin increases with increasing dosage.
†Half-life of aspirin with low dosage and large dosage respectively.
‡Half-life of parahydroxysulfinpyrazone is 1 hour; 10 to 13 hours for sulfide metabolite.
§Half life of a single dose of ticlopidine is 12.6 hours; with multiple doses, 4-5 days.
‖Duration of action of protamine sulfate depends on body temperature.
¶Peak action of phytonadione for control of hemorrhage when given SC/IM; duration of drug action of phytonadione to achieve normal PT value.

platelet inhibitors, or other anticoagulants; or by repeated epidural or spinal puncture. These hematomas may cause neurologic injury, including paralysis.

The major adverse effect of heparin is bleeding; because the duration of action for heparin is short; discontinuing heparin therapy is usually sufficient to reverse a bleeding episode. If the bleeding must be stopped immediately, protamine sulfate may be given by slow intravenous infusion (Box 43-1).

Heparin causes thrombocytopenia in 25% or more of patients, presumably because the drug promotes platelet aggregation. In most cases the reduced platelet count is only temporary, but some patients may develop an allergic type of thrombocytopenia that may progress to thrombosis. Lepirudin, a recombinant form of hirudin, the anticoagulant produced by leeches, or danaparoid may be used as an alternative to heparin when heparin-induced thromboembolism threatens or when thrombocytopenia is detected.

INTERACTION

The number of potentially dangerous drug interactions with heparin is high. Table 43-2 lists a number of these interactions.

BOX **43-1** | **Patient Problem: Heparin Overdose**

The Problem

Heparin overdosage can lead to severe bleeding and may be life threatening.

The Solution

The highly charged protamine molecule forms a complex with the oppositely charged heparin molecule, thereby displacing the heparin from its binding site on antithrombin III and immediately terminating the anticoagulant action. However, protamine sulfate is an anticoagulant in its own right and should be given in doses that are just sufficient to reverse the effects of heparin. Otherwise, bleeding may persist under the influence of the protamine once the heparin has been cleared from the blood. Transfusion with whole blood or plasma may also be ordered for cases of severe overdose (the transfusion dilutes the heparin in the patient's body but does not neutralize it).

The dose of protamine sulfate is based on the amount of heparin or LMW heparin administered during the preceding 3 to 4 hour period. One milligram of protamine sulfate neutralizes 100 units of heparin.

Protamine sulfate may be given intravenously in undiluted form. Administer intravenously at a rate of 5 mg or less over 1 minute. Do not exceed 50 mg in 10 minutes. The solution may be diluted for infusion with 5% dextrose in water (D_5W) or 0.09% saline. Protamine sulfate is rarely used outside of a hospital setting.

Monitor the patient's vital signs; protamine sulfate may cause hypotension. Warn the patient that flushing and a feeling of warmth may occur. Patients receiving protamine zinc insulin may be sensitized to protamine and experience a severe reaction. Keep available appropriate emergency drugs and equipment to treat anaphylactic shock.

Continue to assess the patient and monitor blood laboratory values because the effects of heparin or LMW heparin may persist longer than the protamine, necessitating additional doses of protamine. Monitor the PTT/aPTT, activated clotting time (ACT), and thrombin time (TT). These tests may not be useful with overdose of a LMW heparin.

TABLE **43-2**

Drug-Drug Interactions of Selected Anticoagulant and Antiplatelet Drugs

Drug	*Interactive Drugs*		*Interaction*
Anticoagulants			
warfarin	acetaminophen	amiodarone	Increased effects of anticoagulant
	Androgens	aspirin	
	bumetanide	Cephalosporins	
	chloral hydrate	clofibrate	
	chloramphenicol	cimetidine	
	co-trimoxazole	danazol	
	disulfiram	erythromycin	
	ethacrynic acid	famotidine	
	furosemide	glucagon	
	meclofenamate	mefenamic acid	
	metronidazole	nalidixic acid	
	nizatidine	oxyphenbutazone	
	phenylbutazone	quinidine	
	quinine	ranitidine	
	aminoglutethimide	Barbiturates	Decreased effects of anticoagulants
	carbamazepine	colestyramine	
	ethchlorvynol	glutethimide	
	griseofulvin	rifampin	
	Oral contraceptives	vitamin E	
	vitamin K		
	phenytoin		Increased effects of interactive drug
	methimazole	propylthiouracil	Altered effects of warfarin

TABLE 43-2			
Drug-Drug Interactions of Selected Anticoagulant and Antiplatelet Drugs—cont'd			
Drug	*Interactive Drugs*		*Interaction*
Anticoagulants—cont'd			
heparin	Antiplatelet drugs	Cephalosporins	Increased effects of heparin
NSAIDs	Penicillins		
probenecid	Salicylates		
	nitroglycerin		Decreased effects of heparin
ardeparin	Oral anticoagulants	Cephalosporins	Increased effects of anticoagulant
enoxaparin	penicillins	Salicylates	
dalteparin			
Antiplatelet Drugs			
Aspirin	Oral anticoagulants	heparin	Increased effect of interactive drugs
	Insulin	methotrexate	
	Sulfonylureas	valproic acid	
	Beta blockers	captopril	Decreased effect of interactive drugs
	furosemide	probenecid	
	spironolactone	sulfinpyrazone	
	alcohol	Corticosteroids	Increased risk of GI ulceration
	NSAIDs	phenylbutazone	
	ammonium chloride	ascorbic acid	Increased serum salicylate levels
	furosemide	methionine	
	acetazolamide	Antacids	Decreased serum salicylate levels
	Alkalinizers	Corticosteroids	
	methazolamide		
dipyridamole	theophylline		Decreased coronary vasodilation effects
pentoxifylline	cimetidine		Increased effects of pentoxifylline
ticlopidine	digoxin		Decreased effects of interacting drug
clopidogrel	aspirin	theophylline	Increased effects of interacting drug
	cimetidine		Increased effects of ticlopidine
	Antacids		Decreased effects of ticlopidine
abciximab	Antiplatelet drugs	dextran	Increased risk of bleeding
eptifibratide	Oral anticoagulants		
tirofiban	Thrombolytic drugs		

 DRUG CLASS • **Oral Anticoagulants**

acenocoumarol (Sintrom✱)

anisindione (Miradon)

dicumarol (generic)

⚕ warfarin (Coumadin, Warfilone✱)

In the early 1920s, cattle fed spoiled, sweet clover silage developed a strange hemorrhagic disease, which led to the discovery of the coumarin class of anticoagulants. The disease, and the coumarin drugs, reduce clotting time by causing a deficiency of prothrombin. These drugs, unlike heparin, are effective when given orally.

Accordingly, their introduction in medicine revolutionized such practices as heart valve replacement.

MECHANISM OF ACTION

Clotting factors II (prothrombin), VII, IX, and X are synthesized in the liver, with vitamin K as a necessary cofactor. If vitamin K is deficient, the clotting factors synthesized are functionally inactive, thus impairing blood coagulation. Coumarin and indandione drugs interfere with the regeneration of active vitamin K in the liver and thereby produce vitamin K deficiency. Because the drugs interfere with the synthesis of functional clotting factors, and not the activity of the factors, the anticoagulant effect does not appear until the vitamin K–dependent factors are depleted by normal degradation, which usually takes several days. Factor II, prothrombin, is the longest lived of these clotting factors, and it usually takes 24 hours for the existing supply of prothrombin to be reduced by 50%.

USES

The major indications for oral anticoagulants are the same as for heparin: prophylaxis or treatment of thrombosis or thromboembolism.

PHARMACOKINETICS

Warfarin is the most widely used coumarin drug. Warfarin is well absorbed when given orally. Its peak effect occurs 36 to 72 hours after administration, and the duration of action is 4 to 5 days.

Dicumarol is longer acting than warfarin. The peak of action is 3 to 5 days after administration, and the duration of action is up to 10 days. However, dicumarol is not well absorbed and may cause flatulence and diarrhea.

Anisindione is well absorbed when given orally. The onset of action is 2 to 3 days, and duration of action after discontinuing therapy is 1 to 3 days.

Protein binding is important to the pharmacokinetics of coumarin drugs. These drugs stay in the body a long time because they are bound tightly to plasma albumin. As a result, only a small amount of the total drug in the body is free to diffuse to the site of action in the liver. The liver degrades coumarin to inactive forms that are then excreted in the urine, so only a small amount of the total coumarin is available for degradation of vitamin K–dependent factors. Other drugs can displace coumarin from albumin, thereby increasing the effective concentration of coumarin. For example, if only 1% of the total coumarin is not bound and displacement causes another 1% to be freed, the concentration of free (active) drug has doubled. The albumin-bound coumarin acts as a reservoir for the drug. After administration is discontinued, several days are required for the drug to dissociate from albumin and be degraded by the liver.

ADVERSE REACTIONS AND CONTRAINDICATIONS

The principal adverse effect of oral anticoagulant therapy is bleeding, commonly first seen as bleeding of the gingiva. Other signs of overdosage include blood in the urine or stools. The drug can be discontinued temporarily when minor bleeding occurs. When bleeding is severe, fresh or frozen plasma may be transfused to immediately replace clotting factors. Vitamin K_1 phytonadione can be used to treat less severe bleeding. The additional vitamin K in the blood overcomes the competitive inhibition of synthesis caused by coumarin and brings the prothrombin time (PT) to normal in about 24 hours. Adverse effects other than bleeding are rare with coumarin drugs.

Anisindione more commonly causes other adverse reactions, including rashes, depression of bone marrow functions, hepatitis, and renal damage.

INTERACTIONS

Drug interactions are not prominent with anisindione. However, drug interactions are especially numerous with dicumarol and warfarin. No drug should be added to or deleted from a therapeutic regimen that includes a coumarin without first considering the possible drug interactions and appropriately modifying the dosages.

Drugs that decrease platelet adhesion (e.g., aspirin, clofibrate, dextran, dipyridamole, hydroxychloroquine, ibuprofen, indomethacin, and phenylbutazone) enhance the anticoagulant action of both heparin and coumarin drugs. The anticoagulant action of coumarin is enhanced by drugs that inhibit coumarin degradation, such as clofibrate, disulfiram, metronidazole, oxyphenbutazone, phenylbutazone, and trimethoprim; drugs that displace bound anticoagulant, such as chloral hydrate, oxyphenbutazone, and phenylbutazone; and drugs that interact by unknown mechanisms, such as anabolic steroids, cimetidine, D-thyroxine, glucagon, quinidine, and sulfinpyrazone.

The anticoagulant action of coumarin is diminished by drugs that accelerate its degradation, such as barbiturates, ethchlorvynol, glutethimide, griseofulvin, and rifampin; drugs that decrease gastrointestinal (GI) tract absorption of coumarin, such as cholestyramine or psyllium products; and drugs that interact by unknown mechanisms, such as 6-mercaptopurine. Dicumarol enhances the action of phenytoin. This list summarizes the major drug interactions but is not comprehensive (see Table 43-2).

DRUG CLASS • Antiplatelet Drugs

Inhibitors of Cyclooxygenase

aspirin

Inhibitors of Phosphodiesterase

dipyridamole (Persantine, Apo-Dipyridamole✹)

pentoxifylline (Trental)

Inhibitors of Adenosine 5′ -Diphosphate (ADP) Binding

clopidogrel (Plavix)

ticlopidine (Ticlid)

Antagonists of Glycoprotein IIb/IIIa Receptors

abciximab (ReoPro)

eptifibatide (Integrilin)

tirofiban (Aggrastat)

MECHANISM OF ACTION

Platelets (thrombocytes) are the small cell fragments in blood derived from giant bone marrow cells called megakaryocytes. Ordinarily, platelets do not adhere to each other or to the endothelial lining of the blood vessels. However, when a break in the endothelial lining occurs, platelets readily attach to the collagen in the exposed tissue and to each other in the locality of the injury. This attachment causes the platelets to aggregate, rapidly forming a plug that stops the bleeding and aids in the formation of a thrombus. Platelet aggregation is the initial step in the normal repair system for blood vessels. Drugs that interfere with this process are termed **antiplatelet** or **antithrombotic drugs** (see Evidence-Based Practice box and Table 43-1). Several mechanisms are possible.

Inhibitors of Cyclooxygenase

Aspirin, which produces several pharmacologic effects by inhibiting prostaglandin synthesis (see Chapter 14), also prevents thrombus formation by preventing the production of thromboxane A (TXA_2), a prostaglandin that causes platelets to aggregate (clump together). Aspirin irreversibly inhibits (by acetylation) cyclooxygenase, which synthesizes TXA_2 in the platelet. Because platelets cannot synthesize more cyclooxygenase, aspirin effectively eliminates the platelet's ability to produce and release TXA_2 for the life of the platelet. Other salicylates and NSAIDs, such as ibuprofen (see Chapter 14), likewise inhibit cyclooxygenase in platelets and elsewhere in the body, but the inhibition is reversible (not involving acetylation), and the activity of the enzyme returns as the concentration of the drug in the platelet declines. Ac-

cordingly, aspirin is the only effective inhibitor of platelet aggregation in the NSAID class of drugs.

Inhibitors of Phosphodiesterase

Dipyridamole inhibits platelet function by increasing the cellular concentration of cyclic adenosine monophosphate (cAMP) either by inhibiting phosphodiesterase, which degrades cAMP or by increasing the cellular uptake of adenosine, which is converted to cAMP.

Pentoxifylline also inhibits phosphodiesterase and reduces platelet aggregation. In addition, this drug reduces the circulating levels of fibrinogen and improves red blood cell flexibility. These effects converge to improve the overall viscosity of the blood and reduce the risk of thromboembolism.

Inhibitors of Adenosine 5′ Diphosphate Binding

Clopidogrel and ticlopidine irreversibly inhibit the binding of adenosine diphosphate (ADP) to its receptor in platelets. This action prevents platelet-platelet aggregation and platelet-fibrinogen binding.

Antagonists of Glycoprotein IIb/IIIa Receptors

The glycoprotein IIb/IIIa complex serves as a receptor on platelets for fibrinogen, vitronectin, fibronectin, and von Willebrand factor. Activation of this complex promotes platelet aggregation. Eptifibatide and tirofiban prevent platelet aggregation by occupying this receptor. Abciximab is a humanized monoclonal antibody directed against the glycoprotein IIb/IIIa complex.

USES

The principal use of antiplatelet drugs is to prevent arterial thrombus formation. Aspirin has been shown to reduce the risk for recurrent transient ischemic attacks (TIAs) or stroke in men with a history of TIA. Aspirin also reduces the risk of death or nonfatal myocardial infarction (MI) in patients with a history of infarction or unstable angina pectoris.

Dipyridamole is used only in patients with prosthetic heart valves for prevention of thromboemboli, and only in combination with warfarin.

Pentoxifylline inhibits platelet aggregation but is currently approved by the FDA only for treatment of intermittent claudication.

Clopidogrel and ticlopidine are both used to reduce the risk of myocardial infarction, stroke, and vascular death in patients with documented atherosclerosis. Because ticlopidine has been shown to cause serious ad-

Setting

Atrial fibrillation is a chronic or paroxysmal arrhythmia characterized by chaotic atrial electrical activity. Atrial fibrillation thus increases the risk of cerebrovascular accident (stroke). The prevalence of atrial fibrillation increases with age, with approximately 2 to 3 cases per 1000 in patients 25 to 35 years old, 30 to 40 cases per 1000 in patients 55 to 64 years old, and 50 to 90 cases per 1000 in patients more than 64 years old. Antiplatelet drugs are proven effective for stroke prevention in other settings.

Objective of Literature Review

To determine the efficacy and safety of antiplatelet therapy for prevention of stroke in subjects with chronic non-valvular atrial fibrillation.

Investigators searched the electronic databases of the Cochrane Stroke Group Specialized Register of Trials, MEDLINE, and the database of the Antithrombotic Trialists Collaboration, as well as reference lists of relevant articles.

Criteria for Inclusion of Studies in Review of Literature

Investigators included all randomized trials that compared antiplatelet drugs to placebo in patients who had non-valvular atrial fibrillation and no history of transient ischemic attack or stroke.

Data Extraction and Analysis

Studies included in the review were independently selected by two investigators who extracted each outcome and double-checked the data. A special method was used for combining odds ratios. All analyses were, as far as possible, "intention-to-treat." Because the results of two trials included 3% to 8% of subjects who had a history of stroke or ischemic attack, unpublished results excluding these subjects were obtained from the Atrial Fibrillation Investigators.

Results of Review

In two trials, 1680 subjects who had no history of stroke or transient ischemic attack were randomized to aspirin or placebo. In these studies, aspirin was associated with nonsignificantly lower risks of ischemic stroke, all strokes, all disabling or fatal strokes, and the constellation of stroke, myocardial infarction, or vascular death. Taking into account all randomized subjects, including those who had a history of stroke or transient ischemic attack, reductions in these events by aspirin were consistently smaller and marginally statistically significant. No increase in major hemorrhage was seen, but the number of hemorrhagic events was small.

Investigator's Conclusion

Given all available randomized data, it appears that aspirin modestly (by about 20%) reduces stroke and major vascular events in patients with non-valvular atrial fibrillation. Aspirin used for primary prevention in subjects with atrial fibrillation reduces the average rate of stroke by 4.5% per year, or about 1 stroke per year for every 1000 subjects.

Benavente O, Hart R, Koudstaal P et al: Antiplatelet therapy for preventing stroke in patients with non-valvular atrial fibrillation and no previous history of stroke or transient ischemic attacks. In *The Cochrane Library*, Issue 2, Oxford, 2002, Update Software.

verse effects (see below), its use is recommended only for patients in whom aspirin is not tolerated or is ineffective.

Abciximab, eptifibatide, and tirofiban are each indicated for use with heparin or warfarin for prevention of acute cardiac ischemic complications associated with percutaneous coronary intervention and in patients not responding to conventional treatment for unstable angina.

PHARMACOKINETICS

The pharmacokinetics of aspirin are discussed in Chapter 14. The oral absorption and bioavailability of dipyridamole are variable. Enzymes in the liver convert the drug primarily to the glucuronide conjugate, which is secreted into bile. As much as 20% of the drug may be released from the glucuronide to be absorbed back into the blood via enterohepatic recirculation.

Pentoxifylline is well absorbed following oral administration. Food in the stomach delays but does not limit absorption. The drug binds to membranes of erythrocytes where the initial biotransformation of the drug occurs. Subsequent biotransformation to active and inactive metabolites occurs in the liver. The final pathway for elimination of metabolites is principally renal.

Clopidogrel is rapidly absorbed, with a bioavailability of about 50%. Food in the stomach does not appear to affect its bioavailability. Hepatic hydrolysis produces a carboxylic acid derivative, which accounts for 65% of the circulating drug-related compounds.

Neither this derivative nor the parent molecule inhibits platelet aggregation, therefore another unknown metabolite must be responsible for that action. Elimination of clopidogrel is primarily renal (50%) and fecal (46%). The long duration of action reflects the irreversible drug-platelet interaction and correlates with replacement of platelets.

Over 80% of ticlopidine is absorbed following oral administration. The drug is extensively biotransformed by the liver to numerous metabolites; the drug has only weak antiplatelet activity, but no active metabolites have yet been identified. Elimination is primarily renal (60%) and hepatic (23%) and involves mostly metabolites; very little of the parent drug is eliminated unchanged. The long duration of antiplatelet action of ticlopidine reflects the time required for replacement of platelets.

ADVERSE REACTIONS AND CONTRAINDICATIONS

The antiplatelet dose of aspirin is well below the dosage required for analgesia, antipyresis, and relief of inflammation. Adverse reactions are all but absent at that dosage, save for the potential for allergic and idiosyncratic reactions, which are not dose-related. See Chapter 14 for a detailed discussion of the adverse reactions and contraindications associated with aspirin.

Few adverse reactions are associated with dipyridamole. Hypotension may occur; GI disturbances, flushing, or pruritus of the skin, headache, and dizziness may develop but are rare. These symptoms, however, subside when the drug is discontinued. Fatal and nonfatal MIs, ventricular fibrillation, and bronchospasm have been documented with dipyridamole.

The most common adverse reactions to pentoxifylline are dizziness, headache, nervousness, nausea, dyspepsia, vomiting, and hand tremors. Thrombocytopenia and pancytopenia have also been noted.

The adverse effects most commonly associated with ticlopidine include nausea, dyspepsia, and diarrhea. Several serious, potentially fatal hematologic disorders may develop within the first 3 months of therapy with ticlopidine. These include neutropenia or agranulocytosis, thrombotic thrombocytopenic purpura and thrombocytopenia. Ticlopidine is contraindicated when there is a history of any of these reactions. Skin rash and bleeding complications may also occur with ticlopidine.

The adverse effect profile for clopidogrel is better than that for ticlopidine, but the possibility of serious hematologic reactions as described for ticlopidine still exists. The more common adverse effects of clopidogrel include chest pain, purpura, atrial arrhythmias, edema, and GI hemorrhage. Bleeding disorders are contraindications to the use of clopidogrel.

Adverse effects most commonly associated with the glycoprotein IIb/IIIa receptor blockers abciximab, eptifibatide, and tirofiban include bleeding, especially that occurring at the site of percutaneous access for arterial catheterization, hypotension, and thrombocytopenia. Preexisting bleeding disorders are contraindications to the use of these drugs.

INTERACTIONS

The number of potentially dangerous drug-drug interactions with antiplatelet drugs is high. See Table 43-2 for a list of a number of these interactions.

APPLICATION TO PRACTICE

ASSESSMENT
History of Present Illness

The symptoms exhibited by the patient typically depend on the location of the thrombus in the body. The patient with a deep vein thrombosis (DVT) usually complains of pain in the thigh or pain in the calf muscle that worsens during exercise.

Patients with the sudden onset of any of the following symptoms: dyspnea, substernal chest pain, hemoptysis, palpitations, pleuritic pain, and apprehension should be assessed for a suspected pulmonary embolism (PE). As with DVT, risk factors should also be elicited.

Patients having an MI most frequently complain of chest pain unrelieved by nitroglycerin (see Chapter 39). The patient's perception of the pain, its location and radiation to other sites, the quality of the pain, its onset and duration, and factors that alleviate or aggravate the pain should be explored. Determine if the patient has any feelings of uneasiness or impending doom, fear of death and the possibility of denial or depression, and the presence of associated symptoms such as dyspnea, nausea, diaphoresis, dizziness, and sleep disturbances.

Subjective data to be elicited from the patient with a suspected stroke include the presence, nature, and location of a headache or sensory deficits, presence of diplopia or blurred vision, weakness or partial paralysis of one side of the body, and complaints of an inability to think clearly. The patient's perception of what is happening is also important to note.

- Abdominal and pelvic surgery, surgery on long bones
- Advanced age (particularly patients more than 40 years old)
- Surgery lasting more than 30 minutes with general, spinal, or epidural anesthesia
- Bed rest, prolonged travel with limited mobility
- Cardiovascular disease (atrial fibrillation, heart failure, MI, hypertension, stroke)
- Cigarette smoking
- Dehydration or malnutrition
- Diabetes mellitus
- Estrogen therapy or use of oral contraceptives
- Excessive intake of vitamin E
- Fractured hip
- Intravenous therapy, venous catheterization
- Joint arthroplasty
- Neoplasms, especially hepatic and pancreatic
- Obesity
- Pregnancy, particularly the postpartum period
- Previous history of thrombophlebitis, varicose veins
- Selected blood dyscrasias (e.g., polycythemia vera)
- Sepsis

Health History

The health history provides information regarding existing disorders that can predispose the patient to the development of thrombosis. In addition, the patient's family history may provide information helpful in identifying individuals who may be more likely to develop thrombosis. The patient's history should note any risk factors associated with thrombophlebitis and thromboembolism (Box 43-2). A thorough drug history is vital.

Lifespan Considerations

Perinatal. The risk of thromboembolic disease in pregnancy is approximately 6 times greater than the nonpregnant state, with 3 to 12 occurrences per 1000 pregnancies. The true incidence may be significantly higher in the postpartum period. Risk factors for thromboembolic disease during pregnancy, in addition to those previously identified, include:

- Advanced maternal age (older than 40 years)
- Collagen-vascular disease
- Grand multiparity (more than four previous term pregnancies)
- Homocystinuria (predisposition to arterial and venous thrombosis)
- Nephrotic syndrome
- Cesarean section or instrumented delivery

Pregnancy-related alterations in the coagulation system may also predispose the patient to thrombus and related complications. Treatment for DVT and PE in pregnancy centers on anticoagulation. The incidence of TIA and stroke are relatively rare in pregnancy.

Pediatric. Infants and children lack mature body systems, which are required for drug absorption, distribution, biotransformation, and elimination. Thus there is a potential for drug accumulation and toxicity in this patient population.

Older Adults. Older adults frequently require anticoagulant and antiplatelet drugs, but normal changes of aging requires that their effectiveness must be monitored. Drug therapy used to treat other diseases common in this population increase the risk of drug interactions.

Cultural/Social Considerations

Anticoagulant and antiplatelet drugs themselves are relatively inexpensive, with the exception of some of the LMW heparin drugs. The inpatient treatment that may be initially required, however, is expensive. Furthermore, older adults are likely to require preventive treatment for thrombus formation. If cost is a concern, the patient should be referred to social services for assistance.

Physical Examination

Signs and symptoms of thrombosis vary according to the size and location of the thrombus and the adequacy of collateral circulation. The patient with superficial thrombophlebitis may have a palpable, firm, subcutaneous cordlike vein. The area surrounding the vein may be tender to the touch, reddened, and warm. A mild systemic fever and leukocytosis may be present. The most common sign of DVT is asymmetry and unilateral edema in a lower extremity. Occasionally the extremity feels warm to the touch or the patient has a fever greater than 100.4° F (38° C).

The patient should be examined with attention to risk factors for thrombus formation, such as hypertension, atrial fibrillation, heart murmurs, or infectious diseases of the heart. The peripheral pulses are noted and the extremities examined for temperature, pallor, and mottling.

Pulmonary embolism may cause tachypnea and tachycardia. Chest auscultation may reveal crackles, wheezes, pleural friction rubs, and increased S_2 heart sounds. Unilateral leg edema and pain may signal thrombophlebitis, which may be the origin of a PE.

Physical examination findings of the patient with an MI may include crackles or audible wheezes and a rapid pulse that may be barely perceptible. The skin is often cool and clammy with a pale or cyanotic appearance. The blood pressure usually falls and the patient may collapse. S_1 and S_2 heart sounds are often faint. An S_4 and sometimes an S_3 heart sound, which indicates left ventricular failure, can often be heard. A soft systolic murmur may be heard at the apex.

Objective data to be collected for the patient with a suspected stroke include motor strength, paresis, paralysis, any change in the level of consciousness, signs of increased intracranial pressure, and the presence or absence of aphasia. The patient's respiratory rate and depth should also be noted.

Laboratory Testing

Noninvasive compression/Doppler flow studies are effective for identifying proximal DVT but often fail to detect distal DVT. When the compression/Doppler flow studies are inconclusive, contrast venography allows for a definitive diagnosis of DVT. However, this invasive test is costly, requires injection of contrast dye, and may cause chemical phlebitis.

Diagnostic testing used to identify PE includes ventilation-perfusion scanning, spiral CT scanning, or pulmonary arteriography. Although a ventilation-perfusion scan rarely gives false positives, it often does not register small emboli. Pulmonary arteriography has been essentially replaced by spiral CT scanning as the gold standard for diagnosing PE, and is often used when a ventilation-perfusion scan is inconclusive or not tolerated by the patient who is short of breath.

Diagnostic testing for the patient with a suspected MI can be divided into three categories: nonspecific indicators of tissue necrosis and inflammation, electrocardiogram, and serum enzymes. Nonspecific indicators of MI include leukocytosis and an elevated erythrocyte sedimentation rate (ESR). An electrocardiogram (ECG) may indicate characteristic changes, depending on the location of the MI, as well as changes related to PE. It should be noted that the ECG does not always provide definitive evidence of an ischemic process. Troponin and serum enzymes such as creatine kinase (CK), serum glutamic-oxaloacetic transaminase (AST), and lactic acid dehydrogenase (LDH) are valuable diagnostic indicators of MI. It should be noted, however, that enzyme elevations are not solely specific to myocardial damage.

A CT scan may show the occurrence of a stroke but often not until several days after the onset. A lumbar puncture may reveal elevated spinal fluid pressure. If blood is noted in the spinal fluid, hemorrhage has occurred. CT scanning may be performed before a lumbar puncture if the patient is in a coma and the severity of increased intracranial pressure is unknown. After a TIA, a cerebral angiogram or digital subtraction angiogram may be obtained to look for blocked or occluded vessels.

Before initiating anticoagulant therapy, a complete blood cell count, platelet count, hemoglobin, and hematocrit should be obtained, as well as a baseline PT, partial thromboplastin time (PTT), or activated partial thromboplastin time (aPTT). Antiplatelet therapy with a glycoprotein receptor antagonist drug requires a baseline platelet count before treatment is instituted. Because many of the anticoagulant and antiplatelet drugs cause an elevation in liver function tests, it is important to establish a baseline for those values as well.

GOALS OF THERAPY

Treatment goals for the patient at risk for thrombus formation are directed toward prevention or slowing progression of thromboembolic disease, regardless of the site or sequelae. In addition, treatment is directed toward the speedy resolution of pain, inflammation, patient discomfort, and in reducing morbidity and mortality. The specific drug used depends on the location of the thrombus and the administration route most likely to be tolerated by the patient. The occurrence and recurrence of thromboembolic disease can be reduced to less than 5% if adequate anticoagulation is maintained (see the Case Study: Deep Vein Thrombosis).

INTERVENTION
Administration

It is recommended that patients with a history of allergies or asthma receive a test dose of heparin before receiving a full dose. Read medication labels carefully. Several strengths of heparin are available. Place an identification band on the patient's wrist or post a note above the patient's bed (or whatever is customary in the particular institution) stating that the patient is receiving anticoagulant therapy, so that laboratory personnel and other health care providers will use caution to avoid bleeding or bruising when caring for the patient or when performing venipuncture.

Parenteral anticoagulant solutions should be colorless to slightly yellow. Do not use solutions that contain particulate matter. Because there are numerous possible drug interactions with heparin, the health care provider should check for Y-site and additive compatibilities and incompatibilities before administration.

When heparin is given intravenously, loading doses usually precede a continuous infusion. An infusion pump is used thereafter to ensure dosage accuracy; however, remember that infusion pumps deliver milliliters/minute and the health care provider may order the heparin dose in units/hour, thus mathematical calculations may be required. Check calculations carefully and have the dose double-checked with a second professional health care provider before administration. The intravenous site should be checked for patency and evidence of inflammation according to hospital policy. Heparin blood levels will be erratic if the heparin infusion is interrupted frequently or for long periods.

Any subcutaneous site may be used for intermittent anticoagulation therapy, but the lower abdomen is preferred (avoiding the navel) because it contains few muscles and bruising is less of a cosmetic problem. Subcutaneous injections are given at a 45° to 90° angle using a 25- to 28-gauge, $3/8''$ to $5/8''$ needle. Do not aspirate the needle before injecting the drug or rub the area after injection. Aspiration or massage of the injection site may cause unnecessary bruising. Hematoma formation is possible with intramuscular injections, and this route should therefore be avoided. When venipuncture and injections are unavoidable, pressure should be applied to the site for a full 5 minutes to minimize bleeding. Keep a record of the sites used and rotate sites, even if the abdomen is used for all doses; avoid the arms.

To avoid bleeding complications, anticoagulant therapy must be individualized for each patient. Blood is drawn 20 to 30 minutes before heparin administration to establish baseline PTT/aPTT levels and then 4 to 6 hours after the start of the infusion or dosage change. The dosage of high molecular weight heparin is adjusted based on results of PTT or aPTT. The therapeutic range is typically a PTT or an aPTT value of 1 to 2 times baseline values. Notify the health care provider immediately if the PTT/aPTT exceeds the desired range. There will be little or no change in coagulation laboratory values when low-dose heparin is used. Monitor platelet count and hematocrit as well.

Blood for a PTT/aPTT should never be drawn from the intravenous tubing of the heparin infusion or from the infused vein because a falsely elevated PTT will result. A notice should be placed above the patient's bed to alert hospital personnel to apply pressure dressings after drawing blood from a patient on anticoagulants.

In recent years the World Health Organization instituted a standardized system based on the International Normalized Ratio (INR), which is used to determine the dosage for oral anticoagulants. Therapeutic dosages of oral anticoagulants increase the PT by 2 to 3.5 times the baseline values, depending on the purpose for use (Table 43-3). However, some patients require an INR value of up to 4.5 for adequate anticoagulation. A PT value of 1.3 to 1.5 times the control value is equivalent to INR values that are 2 to 3 times the control value; PT values of 1.5 to 2 times the control value are equivalent to INR values that are 3 to 4.5 times the control value. Notify the health care provider immediately if the PT value exceeds the desired range. If the patient is receiving both an oral and parenteral anticoagulant, monitor the appropriate laboratory work for both drugs.

INR laboratory testing typically requires a baseline value and then weekly monitoring initially, with some patients requiring daily monitoring. However, once a therapeutic INR is obtained, the frequency of monitoring may be reduced to every 4 to 6 weeks. Additional monitoring is recommended when adding drugs that interact with coumarin and indandione drugs or when changing the dosage. Patients receiving antiplatelet therapy with a glycoprotein receptor antagonist may require laboratory monitoring of platelet count 2 to 6 hours after a bolus dose and daily during therapy.

Handle the patient carefully to avoid bruising and avoid the use of restraints when possible. Inspect the pa-

---

TABLE 43-3

Therapeutic Goals for Oral Anticoagulation

Indication	*INR**	*Duration of Therapy*
Prophylaxis of DVT after high-risk surgery	2-3	7-10 days for total hip/knee replacement; clinical judgment otherwise
Treatment of DVT	2-3	3-12 months or indefinitely, depending on specific patient factors
Treatment of pulmonary embolism	2-3	First episode 3-6 months; indefinite if high risk for reoccurrence
Valvular heart disease	2-3	Indefinite
Atrial fibrillation	2-3	Weeks to indefinite, depending on specific patient factors
Prosthetic mechanical heart valves	2-3.5	Indefinite, depending on specific type of mechanical valve
Bioprosthetic heart valves	2-3	3-12 months, depending on specific patient factors

INR, International normalized ratio; *DVT,* deep venous thrombus.
*The goal is an INR in the middle of the range (e.g., 2.5 for a range of 2-3 and 3 for a range of 2.5-3.5).

tient's skin twice daily for evidence of bruising and bleeding. If necessary to use restraints, pad the extremities well and remove the restraints frequently to inspect the area.

Potential bleeding sites, including catheter insertion sites, arterial and venous puncture sites, needle puncture, sites, and cutdown sites should be inspected regularly for evidence of bleeding. Be alert for GI, genitourinary, retroperitoneal, or intracranial bleeding. Check the patient's stool for occult blood.

Monitor vital signs at regular intervals. A decrease in blood pressure may indicate hemorrhage. Assess the patient for signs of bleeding (petechiae, nosebleeds, bleeding gums, bruises on arms or legs, black tarry stools, hematuria, hematemesis) during anticoagulant therapy. For mild heparin overdosage, the health care provider may simply discontinue the heparin until the laboratory values return to the therapeutic range. Protamine sulfate may be used to treat a more severe case of overdose (see Box 43-1).

Education

Provide the patient and family with written as well as oral instructions about every drug being given, including the name, prescribed dose, reasons for receiving, and adverse reactions. They should also be instructed to avoid alcoholic beverages and OTC drugs, especially those containing aspirin, ibuprofen, or other NSAIDs without first consulting the health care provider or pharmacist, and not to significantly change their diet (Box 43-3).

Caution the patient taking anticoagulants or antiplatelet drugs to avoid alcoholic beverages, intramuscular injections, contact sports, and other activities that may lead to injury. Advise the patient not to walk barefoot, and to shave with an electric shaver and to use a soft toothbrush, but not to floss during anticoagulant therapy. Also, advise the patient to notify dentists or other health care providers of the anticoagulation therapy. Outpatients who are on anticoagulant therapy should be advised to carry medical alert identification at all times.

Tell the patient not to take any drugs (except those prescribed) without checking with the health care provider. This precaution applies especially to aspirin and OTC drugs that may contain aspirin.

If a LMW heparin is prescribed for home use, instruct the patient in the necessary techniques involved for subcutaneous administration and safe disposal of syringes. Provide positive reinforcement and encouragement. Supervise return demonstrations. If necessary, refer the patient to a community-based home health care agency.

Instruct the patient to take a missed dose of oral anticoagulant as soon as it is remembered, unless it is within 4 hours of the next dose, in which case the missed dose should be omitted and the regular dosing schedule resumed. Do not double up for missed doses. The health care provider should be notified of any missed doses at the time of check-up or laboratory testing.

Advise the patient to notify the health care provider if signs of bleeding or bruising occur, including nosebleeds; bleeding gums; blood in the urine, stool, or emesis; black tarry stools; unexplained or severe bruising, excessively heavy menstrual flow; severe headache; or stiff neck.

Other adverse reactions to anticoagulant therapy that require immediate notification of the health care provider include fast or irregular breathing, shortness of breath, tightness of the chest, skin rash, hives, itching, frequent or persistent erection, or fever. Other adverse effects include alopecia, a burning sensation of the feet, myalgia, and bone pain.

Inform the patient taking anisindione that it may turn alkaline urine orange, which may be mistaken for blood in the urine. If in doubt, the patient should consult with the health care provider.

Dietary Considerations for ANTICOAGULANT THERAPY

Anticoagulant drugs act by creating a vitamin K deficiency (see text). Instruct patients not to change their diet significantly while taking an oral anticoagulant, since large variances alter anticoagulant effects. They should not begin a weight-reduction diet or begin nutritional or vitamin supplements without consulting with the health care provider. Foods that should be avoided because they are high in vitamin K include the following:

- Asparagus spears
- Avocado
- Bean pods (raw)
- Broccoli (raw and cooked)
- Brussels sprouts
- Canola, salad, or soybean oil
- Coleslaw
- Collard greens
- Cucumber peel
- Dill pickles
- Dry soybeans
- Endive
- Green cooked peas
- Green scallion
- Leeks, kale
- Lettuce: head, Bibb, and red leaf
- Liver
- Margarine
- Mayonnaise and olive oil
- Red cabbage (raw)
- Sauerkraut

Patients taking aspirin for antiplatelet therapy should be advised that one OTC aspirin preparation is usually as good as another. They need not pay a high price to get the desired effects. Most oral antiplatelet drugs as well as warfarin should be taken with food or after meals to avoid GI upset. If postural hypotension occurs, as is sometimes the case with dipyridamole, the patient should be instructed to change positions slowly or to lie down for a short time after taking the drug to reduce the risk of falling. Patients should also be informed that worsening of gout or renal stones might occur with con-current use of sulfinpyrazone; but consuming plenty of fluids (2 to 3 L/day) should minimize this problem.

EVALUATION

Clinical response to parenteral and oral anticoagulants and antiplatelet therapy is considered successful if the patient experiences no further signs and symptoms of the disorder and negative sequelae have been avoided. The prevention and control of thromboembolic disease and its associated complications are evidence of overall treatment success.

CASE STUDY — *Deep Vein Thrombosis*

ASSESSMENT

HISTORY OF PRESENT ILLNESS

GR is a 65-year-old white man who had his left hip replaced 48 hours ago.

HEALTH HISTORY

GR has no known allergies. He has been treated for athero-sclerosis and mild hypertension for the past 2 years. He also smokes a pack of cigarettes per day. He states that he has had pain in his left hip and leg for the past several months and that it limits his mobility. Current drugs: furosemide 20 mg po qd; K-Lor 20 mEq po qd.

LIFESPAN CONSIDERATIONS

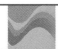

GR has changes of hepatic and renal function related to aging.

CULTURAL/SOCIAL CONSIDERATIONS

GR lives alone and is on Social Security income. He is un-able to drive because of his poor eyesight. He has four adult children who live in another state. He relies on friends for transportation.

PHYSICAL EXAMINATION

GR's vital signs are stable; his left dorsalis pedis and poste-rior tibial pulses are weak. He has restricted range of motion of his left hip. Deep tendon reflexes (DTRs) are intact; Homan's sign is negative.

LABORATORY TESTING

Preoperative PT, INR, and PTT are within normal limits. CBC and platelet counts, UA, BUN, and creatinine levels are within normal limits.

PATIENT PROBLEM(S)

Risk of developing deep vein thrombosis or pulmonary embolism during postoperative period related to surgical procedure and immobility.

GOALS OF THERAPY

GR will not develop deep vein thrombosis while recovering from hip replacement surgery.

CRITICAL THINKING QUESTIONS

1. The following drugs are ordered: enoxaparin 30 mg SC bid × 14 days or until GR is discharged and warfarin po qd dose titrated to PT and INR values to continue for 3 months postoperatively. What is the mechanism of ac-tion of enoxaparin? What is the mechanism of action of warfarin?
2. PT and INR are abbreviations for what tests? What pur-pose do these laboratory values serve during warfarin therapy?
3. What adverse effects should the nurse look for during enoxaparin therapy? What adverse effects should the nurse look for during warfarin therapy?
4. Why is it necessary to educate the patient taking warfarin about eating foods high in vitamin K?
5. When administering enoxaparin by the subcutaneous route, unlike other injections, aspiration does not pre-cede drug injection. Why is this?

Bibliography

Aquila A: Deep venous thrombosis, *J Cardiovasc Nurs* 15(4):25-29, 2001.

Boneu B, de Moerloose P: How and when to monitor a patient treated with low molecular weight heparin, *Semin Thromb & Hemost* 27(5):519-522, 2001.

Church V: Staying on guard of DVT and PE, *Nursing* 30(2), 2000.

Gibbar-Clements, S: The challenge of warfarin therapy, *Am J Nurs*, 100(3):38-41, 2000.

Gresele P, Agnelli G: Novel approaches to the treatment of thrombosis, *Trends Pharmacol Sci* 23(1):25-32, 2002.

Gylys K: Pharmacology department: low-molecular weight heparins, *J Cardiovasc Nurs* 15(4):91-98, 2001.

Lassiter T: Medications used to prevent adhesion and clotting, *Primary Care Practice: A Peer-Reviewed Series* 4(6), 2000.

Majid A, Delanty N, Kantor J: Antiplatelet agents for secondary prevention of ischemic stroke, *Ann Pharmacother* 35(10):1241-1247, 2001.

New Drugs of 2000, *J Am Pharm Assoc* 41(2):229-272, 2001.

Regensteiner JG, Hiatt WR: Current medical therapies for patients with peripheral arterial disease: a critical review, *Am J Med* 112(1):49-57, 2002.

Schainfeld RM: Management of peripheral arterial disease and intermittent claudication, *J Am Board Fam Pract* 14(6):443-450, 2001.

Shepard R: Pharmacology: antiplatelet and antithrombin therapy in acute coronary syndromes, *J Cardiovasc Nurs* 15(1):54-61, 2000.

Weinberger J: Stroke and TIA. Prevention and management of cerebrovascular events in primary care, *Geriatrics* 57(1):38-44, 2002.

Internet Resources

The American Academy of Family Physicians website contains information on warfarin use. Available online at http://www.aafp.org/afp/990201ap/635.html.

The FDA website contains information on various drugs, as well as specific alerts. Available online at http://www.fda.gov/bbs/topics/ANSWERS/ANS00839.html.

Medline plus Health Information. Available online at http://www.nlm.nih.gov/medlineplus/druginfo/medmaster/a682277.html.

The RxList for warfarin contains both specific information on the drug and general information about anticoagulants. Available online at http://www.rxlist.com/cgi/generic/warfarin.htm.

CHAPTER

44

Thrombolytic and Sclerosing Drugs

LYNN ROGER WILLIS • SUSAN SCIACCA

 Visit http://evolve.elsevier.com/Gutierrez/ for additional information.

KEY TERMS

Emboli, p. 713

Esophageal varices, p. 720

Myocardial infarction (MI), p. 712

Plasmin, p. 712

Plasminogen, p. 712

Plasminogen activator, p. 712

Pulmonary embolism (PE), p. 713

Sclerosing drugs, p. 720

Sclerosis, p. 720

Thrombolytic drugs, p. 713

Varicose veins, p. 720

OBJECTIVES

- Identify the various diseases and disorders for which thrombolytic drug therapy is an appropriate treatment.
- Identify the various disorders treated with sclerosing drugs.
- Discuss the rationale behind thrombolytic, hemostatic, and sclerotic therapy.
- Describe the mechanism of action of thrombolytic and sclerosing drugs.
- Describe the most common adverse effects of thrombolytic drug therapy and the management of potential hemorrhage.
- Describe the most common adverse effects of therapy with sclerosing drugs.
- Develop a nursing care plan, including a teaching plan, for a patient receiving thrombolytic or sclerosing therapy.
- Identify patient outcomes that indicate successful therapy with thrombolytic and sclerosing drugs.

PATHOPHYSIOLOGY • Thromboembolytic Diseases

Plasma contains the enzyme plasmin, which degrades the fibrin network of a clot into small, soluble fragments (see Chapter 43, Figure 43-1). Plasmin normally exists in an inactive form (i.e., plasminogen). Plasminogen is activated to plasmin by various factors in the plasma, primarily tissue plasminogen activator (tPA), which originates in the blood vessel wall. Plasminogen and tPA bind to fibrin, and tPA converts plasminogen to plasmin, which digests the fibrin. Degradation products of fibrin act as anticoagulants, thereby limiting further clot formation. These mechanisms normally protect the body from unnecessary clot formation, but there are conditions in which clot formation leads to serious medical consequences.

The heart muscle receives its blood supply through two major vessels located on the surface of the heart (i.e., the right and left coronary arteries) (Figure 44-1). An obstruction in any one of these vessels impedes the flow of blood carrying oxygen and nutrients to that area of the myocardium. In patients with coronary artery dis-

ease (CAD), atherosclerotic plaque builds up slowly over time. Because plaque has a rough surface, platelets adhere to it, fibrin is deposited, and blood cells become trapped. A clot forms that eventually occludes the vessel. In some cases, the clot breaks away and travels to a smaller vessel, where it will cause an occlusion.

Immediately after an acute coronary vessel occlusion, blood flow ceases to the area beyond the occlusion. Small amounts of collateral blood flow are available from surrounding vessels, but in areas with no oxygen available to the affected tissues, cells die.

Myocardial infarction (MI) is an occlusion of the arteries that provide blood, oxygen, and nutrients to the myocardium. Infarction is a dynamic process that occurs over several hours. Obvious physical changes do not begin in the heart muscle until approximately 6 hours after the infarct. The infarcted area appears blue and swollen. Approximately 48 hours later, neutrophils invade to remove necrotic cells and the area turns gray with yellow streaks. Granulation tissue forms at the edges 8 to 10 days

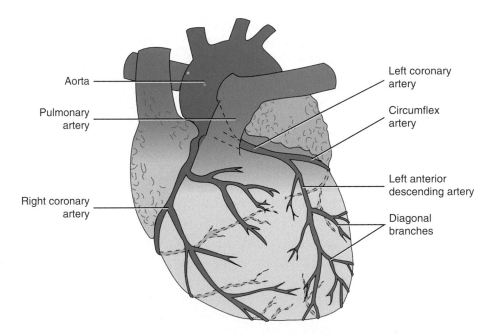

FIGURE 44-1 Major coronary arteries. The right and left coronary arteries originate from the aorta and divide into smaller arterioles that penetrate the heart muscle. The left coronary artery is divided into two parts. The left anterior descending artery supplies blood to the anterior surface of the left ventricle, and the left circumflex artery supplies blood to the lateral wall of the left ventricle. The right coronary artery supplies the inferior aspect of the left ventricle and the right ventricle. The right coronary artery also supplies the posterior aspect of the right and left ventricles. (From Black JM, Matassarin-Jacobs E: *Medical-surgical nursing: clinical management for continuity of care*, ed 5, Philadelphia, 1997, WB Saunders, p 1194. Used with permission.)

after the infarct. Over the next 2 to 3 months, the necrotic area is reduced to a shrunken, thin, firm scar. The presence of scar tissue permanently changes the structure and the function of the ventricle, which, in turn, increases morbidity and mortality.

Stasis of blood flow, damage to the endothelial lining of the vessel, and changes in the mechanics of coagulation (Virchow's triad) are the three primary causes of deep venous thrombosis. Once a clot has formed in a vessel, blood flow past the clot is likely to break it loose. Free-flowing clots are called **emboli.** When the embolus is dislodged, it may be transported to the right ventricle and then to the pulmonary arterial system, where it becomes lodged and obstructs circulation, causing a **pulmonary embolism (PE).** Platelets accumulate behind the embolus, triggering the release of serotonin and thromboxane A_2 (TXA_2), which in turn cause vasoconstriction. Circulation decreases further, causing some areas of the lung to be ventilated but not perfused, resulting in hypoxemia. Pulmonary vascular resistance increases because the size of the pulmonary vascular bed decreases, resulting in greater pulmonary arterial pressure. Accordingly, an increase in the workload of the right ventricule is needed to maintain pulmonary blood flow. When myocardial workload requirements exceed capacity, right ventricular failure occurs, which lowers cardiac output and may cause shock.

Arterial occlusions may occur in other sites, such as the lower extremity, brain, mesentery, and kidneys. Arterial emboli most often develop in the chambers of the heart as a result of atrial fibrillation or atrial flutter. Inadequate emptying of the atrium allows blood flow to stagnate and predisposes it to clotting. If a clot detaches, it is propelled from the heart into the arterial system and becomes lodged when it reaches an area smaller in diameter than the embolus. The result is the immediate cessation of blood flow below the area of occlusion. Clots typically lodge at arterial bifurcations and in narrowed vessels. Secondary vasospasm occurs, contributing to the ischemia. Thrombosis with emboli formation may also develop in an artery with advanced atherosclerosis because of roughening of the atheromatous plaque. A third site for stasis of blood with eventual clot formation is an arterial aneurysm, which is a ballooning of the vessel caused by a weakness in the intima of an artery. The force of the arterial pressure can propel the clot from the aneurysm into arterial circulation.

A cerebrovascular occlusion (also known as stroke or cerebrovascular accident [CVA]) is a sudden loss of brain function resulting from a disruption in the blood supply to a part of the brain. There are three major causes of strokes. Ischemic strokes are divided into those caused by a *thrombus* and those that are caused by *emboli*. Embolic strokes are more common in patients with a history of valvular disease, prosthetic valve replacements, atrial fibrillation, ischemic heart disease, or rheumatic heart disease. A *hemorrhagic stroke* produces bleeding into the brain. It generally results from a ruptured saccular aneurysm, rupture of an arteriovenous malformation, or more commonly, hypertension. Embolic strokes show an abrupt onset of symptoms, with steady worsening thereafter. The embolus tends to lodge in the middle cerebral artery or one of its branches. As it occludes the vessel, ischemia occurs in brain tissue supplied by the affected artery. Ischemia leads to hypoxia or anoxia and hypoglycemia, and brain dysfunction results. These processes can cause death of the neurons, glia, and vasculature in the involved areas.

Although the steps in coagulation occur very rapidly, the dissolution of a blood clot normally takes several days. **Thrombolytic drugs** speed the dissolution of blood clots and are widely used to treat conditions associated with the embolization of clots. For example, thrombolytic drugs are administered as quickly as possible after an acute MI to prevent the myocardial ischemia that leads to tissue death. Thrombolytic therapy is also used in patients with acute pulmonary embolism, deep vein thrombosis (DVT), and peripheral arterial occlusion. Thrombolytic drugs are also used to help clear blood clots from arteriovenous (AV) shunts in patients undergoing long-term renal dialysis.

DRUG CLASS • Thromboembolytic Drugs

First Generation

△ streptokinase (Streptase, Kabbikinase)

urokinase (Abbokinase)

Second Generation

alteplase (tissue plasminogen activator [tPA], Activase)

anistreplase (anisoylated plasminogen–streptokinase activator complex [Apsac], Eminase)

Third Generation

reteplase recombinant (Retavase)

tenecteplase recombinant (TNKase)

MECHANISM OF ACTION

Unlike anticoagulants, which prevent the formation or extension of thrombi (blood clots), thrombolytic drugs dissolve thrombi after they form. The drugs convert plasminogen to plasmin, which in turn degrades the fibrin networks present in the clots. Streptokinase combines with plasminogen to form activator complexes that then convert plasminogen to plasmin. Urokinase, which was initially isolated from human urine, activates plasminogen directly.

Alteplase, which is produced by recombinant DNA technology, is fibrin specific. Once it is injected into the circulation, it binds to fibrin in a thrombus and converts the trapped plasminogen to plasmin. There is less effect on circulating plasminogen.

Anistreplase is an active complex of streptokinase and plasminogen. Like alteplase, anistreplase was developed initially as a clot-specific (i.e., fibrin-specific) drug; however, it seems to work equally well on systemic plasminogen conversion. Anistreplase is an inactive derivative of a fibrinolytic enzyme in which the center of the activator complex is blocked temporarily by an anisoyl group. In solution, the anisoyl group is removed, and the enzymatically active lys-plasminogen streptokinase complex is activated.

Reteplase is a recombinant protein derived from tissue plasminogen activator. It, too, catalyzes the conversion of plasminogen to plasmin, with the activation stimulated by the presence of fibrin. Plasmin then degrades the fibrin matrix of the thrombus. Reteplase has a lower affinity for fibrin, which may result in better clot penetration.

Tenecteplase, the newest thrombolytic drug, is also a recombinant, fibrin-specific protein that catalyzes the conversion of plasminogen to plasmin. The fibrin specificity minimizes the systemic activation of plasminogen and reduces the degradation of circulating fibrinogen.

USES

Thrombolytic therapy is used to treat acute MI, pulmonary embolism, DVT, CVA, and arterial occlusions. Thrombolytics are also used to restore patency to occluded central venous catheters. Different drugs have been found to be more beneficial in some conditions than in others.

With prompt use of thrombolytic drugs and reperfusion following an MI there is a reduction in the size of the infarct, improvement in left ventricular function, and reduction of mortality. A thrombolytic drug usually is indicated for the patient who has chest pain consistent with an MI for at least 30 minutes but not longer than 6 hours.

Thrombolytic therapy has been indicated in the treatment of acute massive pulmonary embolism. Rapid dissolution of the clot helps normalize the patient's hemodynamic status. It is also indicated in the treatment of DVT. The Food and Drug Administration has approved alteplase for use in ischemic CVA confirmed by computed tomography (CT).

Streptokinase, the prototype thrombolytic, was the first drug widely available for clinical use. Streptokinase can be used to restore patency to occluded arteriovenous cannulae. Urokinase has been used successfully to restore patency to occluded central venous catheters when the occlusion is the result of a fibrous clot.

Alteplase is the drug of choice for patients who have previously received streptokinase, who have been given anisoylated plasminogen streptokinase activator complex, or who have been treated for a streptococcal infection within the previous year. These patients develop streptococcal antibodies that neutralize the streptokinase, causing severe allergic reactions.

PHARMACOKINETICS

Information on the pharmacokinetics of thrombolytic drugs is available but incomplete (Table 44-1). Streptokinase has an immediate action, with peak activity reached in 30 to 60 minutes. The duration of action is 4 to 12 hours, and the drug is cleared from the circulation by antibodies. The half-life of streptokinase is 23 minutes. This drug does not cross placental membranes, but the antibodies produced in response to it do cross over to the fetus.

Urokinase has an immediate onset, peaking by the end of the infusion. It crosses the placental membranes and may pass into breast milk. It has a duration of action of up to 12 hours. Urokinase is biotransformed and eliminated primarily by the liver; however, small amounts are eliminated in the urine. The half-life is 20 minutes or less but is prolonged if the patient has liver impairment.

TABLE 44-1

Pharmacokinetics of Thrombolytic Drugs

Drug	Route	Onset	Peak	Duration	Half-Life
alteplase	IV	Immediate	5-10 min	2.5-3 hr	5 min
anistreplase	IV	Immediate	45 min	4-6 hr*	70-120 min
reteplase	IV	Immediate	5-10 min	UA	13-16 min
streptokinase	IV	Immediate	30-60 min†	4-12 hr	23 min
tenecteplase	IV	Immediate	UA	UA	90-130 min

UA, unavailable.
*Systemic hyperfibrinolytic state may persist for 48 hours with the use of anistreplase.
†Clearance and thrombolytic activity of streptokinase appears to decline with continuous infusion.

Alteplase is rapidly absorbed intravenously with an immediate onset of action. This drug crosses the placental barrier and may pass into breast milk. It peaks in 5 to 10 minutes, with a duration of action of 2.5 to 3 hours. Biotransformation takes place in the liver, with small amounts eliminated in the urine.

Anistreplase's onset of action is immediate, reaching peak effect in 45 minutes. Like alteplase, anistreplase crosses the placenta and may pass into breast milk. Its duration of action is 4 to 6 hours. Biotransformation occurs in the plasma; inactivation is caused by binding to plasmin inactivators. The half-life is 70 to 120 minutes.

The half-life of reteplase is approximately 13 to 16 minutes. It is biotransformed in the liver and eliminated in the urine. It is not known whether it is excreted in human milk. The safety and efficacy of its use in children has not been established.

Tenecteplase, which distributes in a volume approximating the plasma volume, is cleared primarily by the liver and it has an elimination half-life of about 2 hours.

ADVERSE REACTIONS AND CONTRAINDICATIONS

Overall, bleeding represents the most common complication of thrombolytic therapy, occurring in 8% to 16% of patients. The bleeding occurs because plasminogen inactivates clotting factors in the plasma in addition to digesting fibrin. The inactivation of clotting factors confers a degree of anticoagulation on the blood. Avoidance or minimizing this effect forms the rationale for the development of tissue- or fibrin-selective activators of plasminogen (alteplase, anistreplase, and reteplase). Although valid in theory and to some extent in practice, even those tissue-selective drugs will inactivate systemic clotting factors and cause unwanted bleeding.

Bleeding as an adverse effect of thrombolytic therapy is more common in women than in men. Major bleeding severe enough to require a blood transfusion occurs in 12% to 15% of patients. Hemorrhagic CVA, which occurs in 0.5% to 1% of patients, is the single most dreaded complication associated with thrombolytic therapy. The risk of intracranial hemorrhage is higher in patients receiving thrombolytic drugs for the treatment of CVA than those receiving them for the treatment of MI. Drug-induced hypotension occurs infrequently but is reported more often with streptokinase and anistreplase.

Other adverse reactions to thrombolytic drugs include reperfusion arrhythmia, nausea and vomiting, and hypersensitivity reactions. Hypersensitivity reactions most commonly occur with streptokinase, with symptoms ranging in severity from minor breathing difficulty to bronchospasm, periorbital swelling, or angioedema. Other, milder allergic effects such as urticaria, itching, flushing, nausea, headache, and musculoskeletal pain have been observed. Anaphylaxis is rare. Approximately 33% of patients experience an increase in temperature.

Cross-sensitivity of anistreplase with streptokinase may occur. Streptokinase is a bacterial protein that can be antigenic. It can cause a hypersensitivity response in any patient who has been treated for streptococcal infection during the previous year. These patients develop streptococcal antibodies that neutralize the streptokinase, causing severe allergic reactions. Because urokinase is not a derivative of streptococci, there is a less frequent incidence of allergic reaction than with streptokinase.

Thrombolytic drug therapy carries serious risks, therefore it is contraindicated in patients who are at high risk for complications and those in whom the risks outweigh the benefits that they would receive. Such therapy might severely compromise the patient with surgery or organ biopsy within 10 days of administration, serious GI bleeding within 3 months, uncontrolled hypertension, an active bleeding or hemorrhagic disorder, history of cerebrovascular bleeding or neoplasm, or presence of an aneurysm.

Thrombolytic therapy is generally contraindicated during pregnancy. Urokinase has been classified as a pregnancy category B drug. The other thrombolytics are category C drugs.

INTERACTIONS

The concurrent administration of antiplatelet drugs, anticoagulants, dipyridamole, indomethacin, and phenylbutazone increases the risk of bleeding. The use of low-dose aspirin with thrombolytics reduces the incidence rates of reinfarction and CVA. The addition of aspirin seems to produce a slight increase in the incidence rate of minor bleeding but not in major bleeding.

APPLICATION TO PRACTICE

ASSESSMENT
History of Present Illness

A thorough and timely assessment of the patient is critical for the prompt treatment of disorders requiring thrombolytic therapy. The patient with an acute MI ordinarily complains of chest pain or pressure that usually radiates to the left arm, neck, or jaw that is unrelieved by nitroglycerin. The pain is often accompanied by other symptoms such as nausea, shortness of breath, diaphoresis, or a feeling of impending doom. The onset and duration of the pain and the patient's perception of the quality of the pain should be determined.

Thrombolytic drugs decrease the mortality rate associated with PE, but they must be administered within a few hours of the onset of symptoms to produce the beneficial effect. Therefore prompt recognition of the patient with a PE is essential. The patient with a PE usually presents with a history of chest pain and a sudden onset of shortness of breath. Ask if there is a history of known DVT or risk factors associated with this problem, which in turn increase the risk of a PE. The patient with a DVT usually complains of pain in the calf muscle that worsens during exercise. The patient may also complain of pain in the thigh.

Patients with a CVA have a variety of symptoms, depending on the location of the infarction. The most common symptoms are changes in mental status, weakness, or partial paralysis of one side of the body, diplopia, blurred vision, and slurred speech or aphasia.

Health History

The health history determines if the patient is a proper candidate for thrombolytic therapy. It is imperative to note whether the patient has any contraindications to thrombolytic therapy (Boxes 44-1 and 44-2). In addition, determine whether or not the patient has had a streptococcus infection in the past, as well as any previous administration of streptokinase or anistreplase. Identify allergies to any other drugs. It is important to know whether or not the patient is also taking anticoagulants, antiplatelet drugs, or indomethacin, because these drugs may cause an increased risk for bleeding if

thrombolytic drugs are used concurrently. The patient's and family histories should include information regarding past MI, PE, DVT, or stroke as well as any risk factors associated with thrombolytic disease.

Lifespan Considerations

The safety and efficacy of thrombolytic drugs have not been established for perinatal, lactating, or pediatric pa-

---

BOX 44-1 Contraindications to Thrombolytic Therapy

Absolute Contraindications

- Active internal bleeding
- Aneurysm
- Arteriovenous malformation
- Cerebral surgery, spinal surgery, or trauma in the previous 2 months
- History of CVA
- Intracranial neoplasm
- Known bleeding diathesis
- Severe, uncontrolled hypertension

Relative Contraindications

- Severe uncontrolled hypertension
- Acute pericarditis
- Age over 75 years
- Cerebrovascular disease
- Chronic renal failure
- Diabetic hemorrhagic retinopathy
- Hemorrhagic ophthalmic conditions
- Hypertension
- Liver dysfunction
- Mitral stenosis with atrial fibrillation
- Occluded A-V cannula at an infected intravenous site
- Patients taking anticoagulants
- Pregnancy or recent delivery
- Prolonged cardiopulmonary resuscitation
- Recent GI or urogenital bleeding
- Septic thrombophlebitis
- Subacute bacterial endocarditis

tients. Furthermore, patients 75 years of age or older are at higher risk for bleeding because of cerebrovascular disease. The older adult population is also at a higher risk for the disease processes that are typically treated with thrombolytic therapy.

Cultural/Social Considerations

MI, PE, and CVA are generally considered urgent to emergent conditions that may warrant treatment with thrombolytic drugs. It is a frightening experience not only for the patient but also for the family. Emotional support is essential at these times. Because health care providers become so focused on the medical status of a situation, the psychosocial aspects are often overlooked. Extra care should be taken to address these needs.

Physical Examination

Symptoms found during the physical examination are often the first indicators that a potentially lethal incident has occurred. Detections of subtle changes in the patient are the most important keys to early diagnosis and lead to rapid treatment decisions.

BOX 44-2 | **Contraindications to Thrombolytic Therapy for Acute Ischemic Stroke**

Absolute Contraindications

- Evidence of intracranial hemorrhage on pretreatment evaluation
- Suspicion of subarachnoid hemorrhage or history of intracranial hemorrhage
- Intracranial surgery within the previous 14 days
- Serious head trauma or CVA within previous 3 months
- Uncontrolled hypertension (e.g., systolic blood pressure over 185 mm Hg or diastolic over 110 mm Hg)
- Blood glucose value under 50 or over 400 mg/dL
- Seizure at onset of CVA
- Active internal bleeding
- GI or urinary bleeding within the past 21 days
- Intracranial neoplasm, A-V malformation, or aneurysm
- Known bleeding diathesis including but not limited to current use of anticoagulant with a prothrombin time exceeding 15 seconds; administration of heparin within 48 hours preceding onset of CVA; or an elevated aPTT upon arrival at health care facility
- Platelet counts less than 100,000/mm³
- Recent MI

Ablative Contraindications

- Patients with severe neurologic deficit (over 22 on National Institute of Health scale)
- Patients with early infarct signs on CT scan (e.g., substantial edema, mass effect, or midline shift)

The patient who is having an acute MI appears to be in obvious distress. The skin may be cool and clammy. The skin color may be pale or cyanotic. The blood pressure may be decreased, and the pulse and respiratory rate may be increased.

Pain in the affected extremity is a manifestation of DVT. The affected extremity is usually warm to the touch and may be reddened. Homan's sign may be present, although it is absent in about 50% of patients with this disorder. The affected extremity may be measurably larger than the unaffected one. Signs and symptoms exhibited by the patient with peripheral arterial occlusive disease are pain, absence of pulse, pallor, paresthesia, and paralysis of the affected extremity. These are the classic five Ps of arterial obstruction.

The patient with a PE exhibits signs and symptoms that include a sudden, marked shortness of breath, tachycardia, chest pain, and hemoptysis. A feeling of anxiety so intense that it may cause panic and a fear of impending death is also common.

Stroke should be considered in any patient whose level of consciousness suddenly deteriorates or who has focal neurologic deficits. Symptoms of acute ischemic stroke and hemorrhagic stroke often overlap, so clinical presentation cannot be relied on for treatment decisions. Further diagnostic testing must be performed.

Laboratory Testing

An elevated creatine kinase (CK) level with a myocardial band (MB) isoenzyme greater than 10% of the total is diagnostic of an acute MI. However, CK isoenzymes are not available immediately and the decision to treat with thrombolytic drugs must be made before the enzyme results return. Electrocardiographic (ECG) changes along with unrelieved chest pain are used as the definitive criteria for administration of thrombolytic therapy. Criteria for therapy are ECGs that exhibit ST segment elevation of 1-mm duration in two contiguous leads.

A newer test, thrombus precursor protein (TPP), is able to detect the formation of a blood clot. Earlier detection permits earlier diagnosis and treatment with thrombolytic drugs.

Patients with suspected PE should be diagnosed with a spiral CT scan or a ventilation-perfusion lung scan to obtain a correct diagnosis. There are diagnostic tests available for DVT, but because of the classic signs and symptoms, physical examination findings are usually enough to make a diagnosis.

When a patient presents with a CVA, it is impossible to differentiate an embolic stroke from a hemorrhagic stroke without the use of CT scanning or magnetic resonance imaging (MRI). A follow-up examination with a lumbar puncture or cerebral angiography may be performed if any doubt remains after obtaining the CT scan.

Very little change is seen on a CT scan in the early stages of an embolic event. If the scan shows massive edema, midline shift, or a mass, this may be an indication that the time interval has been longer than first thought or that the CVA is massive. These findings would put the patient at higher risk for intracranial hemorrhage.

GOALS OF THERAPY

Treatment goals for the patient receiving a thrombolytic drug include opening the occluded artery as soon as possible and maintaining patency after blood flow is reestablished. Preventing ischemia-related arrhythmia and minimizing the loss of tissues are also treatment objectives.

The patient must be screened carefully for contraindications to thrombolytic therapy. When a patient falls into the category of having relative contraindications, the risks must be weighed carefully against the benefits before a treatment decision is made. Careful consideration must be given to the time that has elapsed from the onset of symptoms to the beginning of treatment, especially in the patient with an acute MI or an acute ischemic CVA. Once tissue death has occurred, even though patency of the vessel is restored, there is little that can be done to improve the function of affected tissues. Therefore, the risks associated with late use of thrombolytic therapy heavily outweigh the possible benefits.

INTERVENTION
Administration

A baseline physical assessment should be conducted. Assess the patient's mental status, level of consciousness and orientation, heart rate and rhythm, and respiratory status before beginning therapy. Physical examination findings may also help identify the patient at risk for complications. Baseline vital signs should be obtained before drug administration for comparison during treatment. An increase in heart rate and a decrease in blood pressure may be an indication of bleeding. Assess for abdominal and back pain, which may indicate internal bleeding. Note changes in the color of urine and stool. Assess for neurologic changes indicative of intracranial bleeding. Document the patient's hematocrit and hemoglobin before administering the thrombolytic drug. Type and cross-match the patient for possible blood replacement.

There is a correlation between the amount of time that elapses before therapy and the risk for cardiac rupture. Initiation of thrombolytic therapy for acute MI often begins in the emergency department or in a prehospital setting. The window of time for successful treatment of an acute MI is 6 hours from the onset of chest pain. The earlier therapy is started after onset of symptoms, the better the chance of preserving myocardial tissue.

Patients who receive thrombolytics for the treatment of MI are usually maintained on heparin and nitroglyc-erin drips following treatment. Later the patient is started on aspirin to decrease platelet aggregation at the site.

Health care facilities that administer thrombolytic drugs must have access to cardiac catheterization laboratories. Institutions that do not have catheterization laboratories begin treatment for patients who fit the established protocol and then transfer the patient to a facility that can provide coronary angiography and angioplasty.

Initiation of thrombolytic therapy for the treatment of acute ischemic CVA cannot begin until the possibility of a hemorrhagic CVA has been ruled out. Facilities that do not have the ability to perform CT scanning usually transfer the patient to a facility that does before treatment can be begun. The optimal time to treat acute ischemic CVA is within 3 hours from the onset of symptoms.

Administration of thrombolytic drugs in the treatment of PE should begin as soon as possible after the onset of symptoms. Therapy may be started up to 7 days after the thrombotic event.

Observe the patient for signs and symptoms of allergic reactions (rash, dyspnea, fever, changes in facial color, swelling around the eyes, and wheezing). Allergic reactions are more common in the patient who is receiving streptokinase or anistreplase. If severe allergic manifestations occur, the drug is discontinued and the patient is treated with epinephrine, antihistamines, and steroids.

The possibility of bleeding exists up to 24 hours after thrombolytic therapy has been discontinued. Any unnecessary venipunctures or injections should be avoided during that time. When they are necessary, pressure should be applied manually for 10 minutes at venous sites and 30 minutes at arterial sites. Pressure dressings are then applied. Avoid venipunctures in noncompressible sites such as subclavian or internal jugular sites.

Careful monitoring and management of blood pressure are necessary, especially for the patient with an acute CVA. An elevated blood pressure is likely to contribute to the development of intracranial bleeding and can worsen ischemia. Frequent monitoring of the patient's neurologic status is imperative. If there is a sudden decrease in the level of consciousness, cerebral hemorrhage should be suspected. If the thrombolytic drug is being used to treat a PE, the patient should be monitored for indications that the clot has been lysed. If used for the treatment of DVT, monitor closely for symptoms of PE.

Education

Explain thrombolytic therapy and possible complications to the patient and family before starting treatment. Instruct the patient to report any adverse reactions, such as lightheadedness, dizziness, palpitations, or nausea. Explain the probability that bruising will occur as a result of the therapy and that bed rest and minimal handling of the patient are therefore required. The patient should be instructed to notify the health care provider if pain develops or intensifies.

Community education regarding the signs and symptoms of a heart attack and stroke and the importance of seeking help immediately should be a high priority for health care providers. It is common for patients having an MI to put off getting help as they work through their denial of what is happening. However, the sooner they seek help, the greater benefit thrombolytic therapy will provide.

Risk factors and preventive measures for MI, PE, and DVT should also be taught to the community because most of these disease processes can be prevented or lessened. Risk factors linked to the occurrence of CAD include advancing age, male gender, family history of heart disease, diabetes mellitus, smoking, elevated blood pressure, elevated serum cholesterol, excess weight, excess alcohol intake, sedentary lifestyle, and left ventricular hypertrophy. All risk factors, with the exception of age, gender, and family history of heart disease, can be modified somewhat to reduce the risk of cardiovascular disease and decrease the associated mortality. The risk factors of CAD are the same factors that are linked with peripheral artery occlusive disease. Essentially, it is the same disease process, only in different vessels.

EVALUATION

Evaluate the patient receiving thrombolytic therapy for drug effectiveness. In general, treatment has been effective if the patency of the vessel is restored, circulation to the area beyond the occlusion is restored, and the viability of tissues is maintained.

Indications of effective treatment in the patient with an acute MI include cessation of chest pain, onset of reperfusion arrhythmia, resolution of ST segment elevation, and a peak in the CK value at 12 hours. The patient who is treated for a PE should experience resolution of the chest pain and a return of pulmonary hemodynamics to a normal range. Patients with occluded arteries or veins should note a cessation of the accompanying symptoms. The desired outcome for the patient with a CVA is minimal or no disability at 3 months.

CASE STUDY *Acute Myocardial Infarction*

ASSESSMENT

HISTORY OF PRESENT ILLNESS

JH is a 40-year-old obese white man who has been admitted with complaints of substernal chest pain radiating to the left arm. The pain began approximately 1 hour ago. The ambulance crew administered three nitroglycerin tablets without relief.

HEALTH HISTORY

JH smokes two packs of cigarettes per day. He has a history of adult-onset diabetes mellitus and is on glyburide. His last cholesterol measurement was 465. He has no known allergies and no previous hospital admissions. However, he thinks that he has had strep throat infections on several occasions in the past year.

LIFESPAN CONSIDERATIONS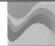

JH is a middle-aged adult completing the tasks of generativity versus stagnation. An MI will have an impact on role relationships, his earning capacity, and social relationships.

CULTURAL/SOCIAL CONSIDERATIONS

JH is an accountant for a very successful firm. He usually works 50 to 60 hours per week.

PHYSICAL EXAMINATION

JH's skin is moist; respirations 28 and slightly labored; lungs are clear. His blood pressure is 100/70 mm Hg; apical pulse 96 and irregular. Monitor shows sinus rhythm with PVCs.

LABORATORY TESTING

CK isoenzymes have been drawn; the ECG shows aVF and ST segment elevation in leads II, III, and aVF.

PATIENT PROBLEM(S)

Acute myocardial infarction with preexistant adult-onset diabetes mellitus and hypercholesterolemia; history of strep throat infections.

GOALS OF THERAPY

To restore the patency of the occluded vessel, prevent myocardial damage, and preserve myocardial function.

CRITICAL THINKING QUESTIONS

1. The health care provider orders alteplase 100 mg administered as intravenous bolus, followed by 50 mg over the next 30 minutes, and then 35 mg over the next hour. What is the mechanism of action of this drug?
2. What adverse effects should the nurse look for during therapy with alteplase?
3. JH has a history of strep throat infections. Why would consideration of this information in JH's health history be an important factor in the choice of thrombolytic drug ordered?
4. The earlier therapy is started to treat an acute MI, the better the chance of preserving myocardial tissue. What is the optimal time for treatment of an acute MI after the onset of symptoms?

PATHOPHYSIOLOGY • Varicosities

Varicose veins are varicosities most frequently found in the saphenous veins in the lower extremities. It is estimated that varicose veins affect one in five persons worldwide. They are most prevalent in women and in persons whose occupations require prolonged standing or sitting. There are two major types of varicose veins—primary and secondary. Primary varicosities are those in which the superficial veins are dilated. The valves in varicose veins may or may not be incompetent. Primary varicosities tend to be familial and probably are caused by a congenital weakness of the veins. Secondary varicosities are usually the result of a previous injury such as thrombophlebitis of a deep femoral vein with subsequent valvular incompetence. Secondary varicosities may also occur in the esophagus, in the anorectal area (hemorrhoids), and as abnormal arteriovenous connections.

Varicosities develop most often as a result of increased hydrostatic pressure resulting from obstruction of venous blood flow. Elevated venous pressure weakens venous walls and prevents the valves from closing completely. As pressure elevation continues, valves are damaged and the veins become tortuous and enlarged. Elevated venous pressure also increases capillary pressure, reduces capillary perfusion, and leads to pain and edema in the region. If stasis develops, ulcers may form and gangrene may set in.

Esophageal varices are dilated tortuous veins occurring in the submucosa of the lower esophagus; however, they may develop more proximally or extend into the stomach. Esophageal varices develop as a complication of hepatic cirrhosis and are one of the major causes of death from cirrhosis. The mortality rate resulting from an initial episode of esophageal bleeding is 45% to 50%.

Esophageal varices are almost always related to portal hypertension, which obstructs venous outflow and raises the hydrostatic pressure in the portal veins. The affected blood vessels become tortuous and brittle. Esophageal varices usually produce no symptoms until the pressure behind the obstruction suddenly increases, ruptures a weakened vessel, and causes massive hemorrhage.

Factors that may raise portal vein pressure and cause hemorrhage include straining, coughing, sneezing, heavy lifting, vomiting, poorly chewed foods, or irritating foods or fluids. Salicylates and any drugs that erode esophageal mucosa may also increase the risk of bleeding (see Chapter 14).

DRUG CLASS • Sclerosing Drugs

ethanolamine oleate (Ethamolin)

hypertonic saline (18% to 30%)

morrhuate sodium (Scleromate)

MECHANISM OF ACTION

Sclerosing drugs traumatize the endothelial lining of distended veins, causing thrombosis within the vessel and eventual **sclerosis** (a hardening of the vein). Some of the drugs act as detergents, producing vascular injury by altering the surface tension around endothelial cells. Drugs acting as detergents include ethanolamine oleate and morrhuate sodium. Other sclerosing drugs (such as hypertonic saline) act as osmotic agents and injure the endothelial cells by dehydrating them. The injury to the cells causes inflammation, which results in local fibrosis of the affected vessels. Eventually, the affected veins slough and disappear.

USES

Intravenous injection of sclerosing drugs is indicated in the treatment of superficial varicose veins of the lower extremities. Other possible uses for sclerosing drugs include treatment of internal hemorrhoids, closure of hernial rings, and the removal of condylomata acuminata. Sclerosing of varicose veins is an adjunct to, rather than a primary treatment for, varicosities. There have been some cases in which sclerosing drugs were used in place of surgery for varicose veins; however, the risk-to-benefit ratio must be heavily weighed.

Endoscopic sclerotherapy is used to treat both acute and chronic cases of esophageal varices. Prophylactic sclerotherapy may be performed on distended nonbleeding veins.

Morrhuate sodium is used in both the treatment of varicose veins and esophageal varices. Ethanolamine oleate is not recommended for the treatment of varicose veins.

PHARMACOKINETICS

Sclerosing drugs are injected directly into the varicose veins with small (31- to 33-gauge) needles. Sclerosing drugs are usually cleared from the circulation within minutes via the portal vein. Complete obliteration of the treated veins may not occur for several months after treatment.

ADVERSE REACTIONS AND CONTRAINDICATIONS

A common adverse effect of sclerosing drugs for treatment of varicose veins is burning or cramping at the injection site. Sloughing of tissue occurs if the drug is allowed to extravasate. Mild systemic responses include headache, dizziness, nausea, and vomiting. Significant adverse effects include urticaria, tissue sloughing and necrosis, and anaphylaxis. Allergic reactions may occur within a few minutes of the injection. Allergic reactions are more common when therapy is reinstituted after an interval of several weeks.

After endoscopic sclerotherapy the patient may experience chest pain for up to 72 hours. The pain is not cardiac in nature but is related to the procedure. Pleural effusion or infiltrate is a complication associated with the use of sclerosing drugs. Esophageal perforation, ulceration, and strictures have also been noted. Overdosage or overtreatment of esophageal varices may result in severe necrosis of the esophagus. Local reactions include esophagitis, tearing of the esophagus, and sloughing of the mucosa.

Sclerosing drugs are contraindicated in patients with a known hypersensitivity to the drug, acute superficial thrombophlebitis, valvular or deep vein incompetency, and large superficial veins that communicate freely with deep veins. Embolism can occur as late as 4 weeks after an injection. Sclerosing drugs are also contraindicated in patients with underlying arterial disease; varicosities caused by abdominal and pelvic tumors, uncontrolled diabetes mellitus, thyrotoxicosis, tuberculosis, a neoplasm, asthma, sepsis, blood dyscrasias, or acute respiratory or skin disease; and in bedridden patients. Continued use of the drug is contraindicated when a local reaction occurs. The sclerosing drugs are classified as pregnancy category C. It is not known whether they are excreted in human breast milk.

INTERACTIONS

There are few documented drug interactions with sclerosing drugs. Heparin is incompatible and therefore should not be mixed in the syringe with a sclerosing drug.

 DRUG CLASS • Antihemorrhagic Drugs

octreotide (Sandostatin)

MECHANISM OF ACTION

The mechanism of action of octreotide is unknown, but it may involve suppression of vasoactive GI hormones and vasoconstriction within the splenic circulation.

USES

Octreotide is used to control bleeding associated with esophageal varices, acromegaly, and GI endocrine tumors (carcinoid tumors and tumors secreting vasoactive intestinal polypeptide) (see Chapter 49). For esophageal varices, the drug is usually administered in conjunction with a sclerosing drug. Octreotide has been shown to improve the 5-day survival rate in patients with esophageal varices.

PHARMACOKINETICS

Octreotide is usually given by subcutaneous injection but may also be injected intravenously. Systemic absorption after subcutaneous injection is rapid and complete. The drug has a long duration of action (about 12 hours) and an elimination half-life in plasma of 1.7 hours. Elimination is renal.

ADVERSE REACTIONS AND CONTRAINDICATIONS

Arrhythmia, hyperglycemia, and pancreatitis may occur. Long-term therapy may result in GI pain, alopecia, dizziness, edema of the lower limbs, and fatigue.

TOXICITY

Symptoms of toxicity to octreotide include abdominal cramps, bradycardia, diarrhea, and facial flushing.

INTERACTIONS

The potential exists for interactions to occur between octreotide and oral hypoglycemic drugs, diazoxide, glucagon, growth hormone, or insulin.

 APPLICATION TO PRACTICE

ASSESSMENT
History of Present Illness

The patient with varicose veins may present with a history of pain, muscle weakness, and edema if there has been valvular damage. Esophageal varices appear much like upper GI bleeding with abdominal pain, nausea, and vomiting. Because bleeding from esophageal varices is an emergency situation, time should not be wasted trying to differentiate between the two disorders.

Health History

Factors associated with the onset of varicose veins include pregnancy, obesity, abdominal tumors, and standing for long periods. The patient should also be questioned about a family history of varicose veins because there is a genetic tendency toward primary varicosities. A history of cirrhosis or known alcoholism should immediately suggest the origin of esophageal varices. Patients often maintain secrecy regarding the extent of alcohol use; screening for abuse requires a nonthreatening approach, where compassion and respect for the patient is maintained.

A previous history of sclerosing drug injections, vein stripping, or phlebitis is an important assessment parameter because obliteration of too many vessels can occlude venous circulation. Other information to be noted in the health history is that of recurrent DVT.

Lifespan Considerations

Perinatal. The normal changes associated with pregnancy may predispose the woman to varicosities in the lower extremity. These varicosities usually do not require sclerotherapy.

Pediatric. The disease processes for which sclerosing drugs are indicated are not ordinarily found in children.

Older Adults. Both esophageal varices and peripheral varicosities are typically progressive states that occur when the primary problem has been present over a prolonged period of time. Hence the older population may be at increased risk given the associated risk factors for the disorders.

Cultural/Social Considerations

The psychosocial considerations related to peripheral varicosities may be significant. The disease can be exacerbated in patients whose employment requires long periods of standing or sitting. If the patient is unable to work because of the discomfort or because the varicosities are unsightly, feelings of powerlessness and changes in self-image may have an impact on their state of wellness.

Esophageal varices are often a complication of cirrhosis of the liver, which in turn may be the result of chronic alcohol use. These patients have often not admitted to themselves or others just how extensive their drinking problem is until they are diagnosed with cirrhosis. The efficacy of sclerotherapy for patients with habitual alcohol use is less than would otherwise be desired. Another important aspect to be considered is the high mortality rate associated with bleeding and the fear and anxiety experienced by these patients.

Physical Examination

The patient with varicose veins has tortuous veins in the lower extremity. If there has been valvular damage, there may also be swelling and pain in the extremity. Secondary varicosities may occur in areas other than the legs (e.g., hemorrhoids).

The Trendelenburg test is used to help diagnose varicose veins. The patient is placed in a supine position with the legs elevated. A tourniquet is placed above the knee after the legs have been elevated. As the patient sits

up, normal veins will fill from the distal end. However, if varicosities are present, the veins fill from the proximal end. A venogram and phlebogram may be performed to assess for adequate circulation before performing a sclerosing procedure.

Dilated abdominal veins, ascites, and hemorrhoids may indicate portal hypertension with esophageal varices. The patient will be in acute distress and shock, with acute bleeding from esophageal varices. Diagnosis of esophageal varices is made by endoscopic examination. During an acute bleeding episode, diagnosis is made by history and physical examination because there is no time for an endoscopy.

Laboratory Testing

No laboratory test can be used to monitor the effectiveness or possible adverse effects of sclerosing drugs. Because there is a significant risk for DVT and PE with the administration of sclerosing drugs, the degree of valvular incompetency should be evaluated by angiography or Doppler venous examination before injection.

GOALS OF THERAPY

The objective of treatment of varicose veins is directed toward improving circulation, relieving discomfort and swelling, and avoiding complications. The objective of sclerotherapy for esophageal varices is to control the bleeding and avoid hemorrhage. It does not eliminate the possibility that the varicosities will recur.

INTERVENTION
Administration

Sclerosing drugs are administered directly into the affected veins. Care must be taken to avoid extravasation because of the possibility of necrosis of the surrounding tissues. The minimal effective volume is used at each injection site. It is recommended that a small test dose be given first and the patient observed for hypersensitivity before the full dose is administered. Written consent is usually required for the procedure.

Sclerosing drugs are introduced via endoscopy for the treatment of bleeding esophageal varices. Before the therapy is performed, baseline vital signs and informed consent should be obtained. Vital signs are monitored throughout the procedure. A sedative is usually administered before the procedure.

The patient may be taken to the GI laboratory, or if the patient's condition is critical, the procedure can be performed at the bedside. The patient's throat is sprayed with a topical anesthetic. A dose of the sclerosing drug is injected through a flexible injector into the varicosity. The procedure usually takes about an hour. After treatment, the patient is observed for bleeding from perforation of the esophagus, aspiration pneumonia, and esophageal stricture. Because bleeding can occur for up to 24 hours after treatment is completed, patients must be closely monitored.

Education

As with all types of intervention, patient education is vital to the success of the treatment. The patient should be told what to expect during the procedure and what unusual sensations or adverse effects may occur. They should also be advised of the behaviors and or activities that should be avoided after therapy and when to return for follow-up care.

Prevention is a key factor related to varicose veins. The patient who is predisposed to varicose veins should be taught to avoid occupations that require prolonged periods of standing or sitting. They should also avoid wearing tight girdles or garters and not cross the legs at the knee. Any activity that increases venous stasis or increases pressure in the venous system in the lower extremities can lead to the formation of varicose veins. Patients who are obese have a higher incidence of varicose veins; dietary teaching about weight loss for these patients is warranted.

The patient with esophageal varices should be taught to avoid alcoholic beverages, nonsteroidal antiinflammatory drugs, and irritating foods. These substances can irritate varices and cause bleeding. After sclerotherapy for esophageal varices, achiness and feelings of chest stiffness develop and may persist for 48 hours. Varices have a tendency to recur, so the need for follow-up endoscopy must be stressed. Assistance in finding support groups for patients who abuse alcohol should be offered.

EVALUATION

During the first 24 hours after treatment for varicose veins, the vein will remain hard and tender to the touch. The surrounding skin is typically a light bronze color, which is a temporary condition. However, there may be a permanent but barely discernible discoloration that remains along the path of the sclerosed vein.

When sclerosing drugs are administered for esophageal varices, bleeding should stop within 2 minutes after the introduction of the drug. If bleeding continues, a second injection attempt is made below the bleeding site. The health care provider should conduct a follow-up examination to determine whether or not assistance with alcohol abuse has been obtained.

Bibliography

Bottiger B, Bode C, Kern S, et al: Efficacy and safety of thrombolytic therapy after initially unsuccessful cardiopulmonary resuscitation: a prospective clinical trial, *Lancet* 357(9268): 1583-1585, 2001.

Hiele M, Rutgeerts P: Combination therapies for the endoscopic treatment of gastrointestinal bleeding, *Best Pract Res Clin Gastroenterol* 14(3):459-466, 2000.

Henderson-Martin B: No more surprises: screening patients for alcohol abuse, *Am J Nurs* 100(9):26-32, 2000.

Herrine S: Portal hypertension/variceal bleeding: an update, American Association for the Study of Liver Diseases 51st Annual Meeting, 2000.

Hoffmeister HM, Szabo S, Helber U, et al: The thrombolytic paradox, *Thromb Res* 103(Suppl)1:S51-S55, 2001.

Rijken DC, Sakharov DV: Basic principles in thrombolysis: regulatory role of plasminogen, *Thromb Res* 103(Suppl)1:S41-S49, 2001.

Ross AM: Combination therapies to enhance reperfusion in acute myocardial infarction, *Thrombo Res* 103(Suppl)1:S81-S90, 2001.

Sadick N, Li C: Small-vessel sclerotherapy, *Dermatol Clin* 19(3):475-481, 2001.

Sinnaeve P, Van de Werf F: Thrombolytic therapy: state of the art, *Thromb Res* 103(Suppl)1:S71-S79, 2001.

Spinler S, Inverso S: Update on strategies to improve thrombolysis for acute myocardial infarction, *Pharmacotherapy* 21(6):691-716, 2001.

Strauss-McErlean E: Thrombolytic therapy versus primary angioplasty in the treatment of acute myocardial infarction, *J Cardiovasc Nurs* 13(3):46-48, 1999.

Tsikouris J, Tsikouris A: A review of available fibrin-specific thrombolytic agents used in acute myocardial infarction *Pharmacotherapy*, 21(2), 207-217, 2000.

Internet Resources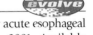

Ioannou C, Doust J, Rockey D: Terlipressin for acute esophageal variceal hemorrhage, *The Cochrane Library* 2, 2001. Available online at http://www.cochranelibrary.com/enter/.

Wardlaw J, del Zoppo G, Yamaguchi T: Thrombolysis for ischaemic stroke, *The Cochrane Library* 2, 2001. Available online at http://www.cochranelibrary.com/enter/.

CHAPTER

45

Blood and Blood Products

KATHLEEN GUTIERREZ

 Visit http://evolve.elsevier.com/Gutierrez/ for additional information.

KEY TERMS

ABO typing, p. 726

Autologous transfusion, p. 727

Hematopoiesis, p. 726

Hemolytic disease of the newborn, p. 727

Hemophilia, p. 737

Homologous transfusion, p. 727

Hypovolemia, p. 728

Packed red blood cells (PRBCs), p. 731

Rh factor, p. 726

Transfusion reaction, p. 726

von Willebrand's factor, p. 735

Whole blood, p. 727

OBJECTIVES

- Identify the various diseases/disorders for which administration of blood or blood products is appropriate.

- Distinguish among the different blood groups and blood types.

- Explain the nursing responsibilities for proper administration of blood and blood products.

- Describe the most common adverse reactions of administration of blood and blood products.

- Develop a nursing care plan, including a teaching plan, for a patient receiving blood or blood products.

- Identify patient outcomes that indicate successful therapy after administration of blood or blood products.

In the mid-seventeenth century, Denis, a physician in the court of Louis XIV, performed the first blood transfusion when he successfully administered lamb's blood to a 15-year-old boy using a quill and an animal's bladder. The French physician's subsequent attempts at animal-to-human transfusion and the efforts of other physicians were not successful and, in fact, resulted in a number of fatalities. These failures and the demonstrated risk of mortality led the French Parliament, with the backing of the Church, to ban further animal-to-human transfusions. Knowledge associated with blood transfusions remained stagnant until 1818, when an

725

English physician, Blundell, using human blood, successfully transfused women who had childbirth-related hemorrhages.

Early in the twentieth century, the efforts of Landsteiner, Ottenberg, and Epstein led to the development of the **ABO typing** and matching system, thus decreasing the number of incompatible transfusions. In 1940, Landsteiner and Weiner pinpointed the anti-Rh antigen as the cause of hemolytic disease of the newborn as a result of alloimmunization during gestation. Thus, **Rh factor** determination joined the ABO matching system in defining donor and recipient compatibility. By the late 1940s, the medical community had discovered how to preserve blood for future use with the addition of sodium citrate as an anticoagulant. This discovery set the stage for the development of blood banks.

BASIC PRINCIPLES OF IMMUNOHEMATOLOGY

Blood defends the body against foreign material, supplies oxygen, and transports nutrients, waste, and hormonal messengers to each of the 60 billion cells in the body. Each cubic millimeter of blood contains 4.5 to 5.5 million red blood cells (RBCs) and an average total of 7500 white blood cells (WBCs). Because both RBCs and WBCs are continually being destroyed, the body must continue to produce new ones by a process called **hematopoiesis.** Hematopoiesis takes place primarily in the red bone marrow of axial skeletal bones and the proximal heads of the femur and humerus. Most cells mature in the bone marrow, but some mature in the thymus, spleen, lymph nodes, and tonsils.

Immunohematology deals with the body of knowledge associated with the antigens and antibodies of the blood. Because the transfusion of incompatible blood triggers life-threatening reactions in the body, it is important to understand the basics of blood antigens and antibodies.

Antigens

An antigen stimulates the formation of an antibody (see Chapter 35). Some antigens occur naturally whereas others are acquired. Antigens in the ABO typing system (agglutinogens) are hereditary ones located on the surface of the RBC. Agglutinogens are also components of WBCs and are present in plasma.

The two most important antigens are antigen A and antigen B. The presence or absence of these two antigens determines an individual's blood type. People with an A antigen have blood type A, and those with a B antigen have blood type B. Individuals with both an A and B antigen on their red cells have blood type AB. Those with neither an A nor a B antigen on their red cells have blood type O.

Other antigens important in the understanding of immunohematology include the Rhesus, or Rh system, antigens. The Rh system consists of almost 50 different RBC antigens. The most important of these antigens is antigen D. The presence or absence of the D antigen on the RBC helps determine if a person is Rh positive or Rh negative.

Human leukocyte antigens (HLA) are on the surface of lymphocytes and other nucleated cells. HLAs determine the degree of compatibility between donors and transplant recipients. A transfusion of blood or blood products is essentially a transplant. Some patients may reject their transfusions because of the presence of incompatible HLAs on the surface of white cells present in the blood product.

Antibodies

Antibodies are proteins (immunoglobulins) that float freely in the plasma (see Chapter 35) and develop in response to stimulation by an antigen. The body recognizes the antigen as foreign, and the immune system responds by producing an antibody.

In the ABO system, antibodies A and B are naturally occurring. Their names derive from the antigens with which they react. Anti-A and anti-B antibodies react with A and B antigens, respectively. RBC antigens and their corresponding antibodies do not exist naturally in the same person. For example, an individual with an A antigen on his or her RBCs does not normally have anti-A antibody in the plasma.

The Rh antigen is very immunogenic (i.e., capable of initiating the body's immune responses) and, therefore, is likely to stimulate antibody formation. For example, an individual with Rh-negative blood who is transfused with Rh-positive blood will develop anti-Rh antibodies after the exposure to the Rh D antigen or the D^u subantigen. Individuals with the D antigen are Rh-positive donors and Rh-positive and Rh-negative recipients. Individuals with the subantigen D^u are Rh-positive donors but Rh-negative recipients.

The reaction generally does not occur with the initial exposure because the Rh antibodies develop slowly. Once sensitized, the individual will likely experience a **transfusion reaction** and associated hemolysis of the RBCs with the next exposure.

Transfusion is not the only way for an Rh-negative individual to be exposed to Rh-positive antigens. For example, an Rh-negative pregnant woman who has an Rh-positive fetus is exposed to the Rh antigen during her pregnancy. Until 30 years ago, a subsequent pregnancy with an Rh-positive fetus produced anti-Rh antibodies that in turn attacked fetal RBCs. This phenomenon became known as **hemolytic disease of the newborn.** Giving human immune globulin (RhoGAM) to the mother within 72 hours of delivery, miscarriage, or abortion prevents the formation of anti-Rh antibodies and prevents the disorder. The intramuscular injection of RhoGAM reduces the formation of anti-Rh antibodies to 1% to 2%. Anti-Rh antibodies can be decreased to 0.1% by administering one dose of the immunoglobulin at 28 weeks' gestation and the other 72 hours after delivery. Although this drug was developed to prevent hemolytic disease of the newborn, it is now also given after transfusion of an Rh-positive blood product to an Rh-negative recipient.

Blood and Blood Products

Blood and blood products (e.g., red blood cells, leukocyte-poor red blood cells, plasma, platelets, granulocytes, cryoprecipitate AHF) are living tissues. With an **autologous transfusion** the individual donates a unit of blood, which is then given back during medical or surgical procedures. The risk of disease transmission with this type of transfusion is little to none. In contrast, a **homologous transfusion** is the transfer of living tissue from one person to another. All homologous blood products carry the risk of disease transfusion and transfusion reactions. Although the development of sensitivity screening has reduced the incidence of transfusion-related diseases, it has not eliminated transmission.

Blood banks screen donors carefully and test blood to ensure safe, compatible transfusions. Current donor screening protocols used by the American Red Cross include an extensive, confidential, and private interview with the donors. Donors may complete a confidential exclusion process, which notes that any blood collected should not be used for transfusion for reasons the donor found too sensitive to disclose during the interview portion of the screening process. In addition to identifying the donor's ABO group and Rh type, the American Association of Blood Banks (AABB) requires that blood banks test each unit of blood for antibodies to the human immunodeficiency virus (anti-HIV), hepatitis B surface antigen, hepatitis B core antigen, hepatitis C virus, the type 1 human T cell lymphotropic virus, and syphilis. Despite the extensive screening process, the risk of transmitting infectious diseases is always present. It is because of this ever-present potential that the American Red Cross and the AABB, in conjunction with the Food and Drug Administration, strongly recommend that blood products be used only in patient conditions that cannot be remedied by other methods.

Since 1985, all donated blood is tested for antibodies to HIV by enzyme-linked immunosorbent assay (ELISA), a procedure that is over 99% accurate in detecting potentially infectious units of blood. In the United States, these efforts translate to a 1 in 400,000 chance of acquiring HIV per unit of blood or blood product transfused. HIV transmission via transfusion remains a major problem in developing countries because of lack of donor screening.

For over 40 years hepatitis has been a common hazard for patients receiving transfusions. Hepatitis may be transmitted by whole blood, RBCs, platelets, fresh frozen plasma (FFP), cryoprecipitate AHF, clotting factors, and RhO (D) immune globulin. Before 1980, the risk for hepatitis C (non-A, non-B hepatitis) transmission among those receiving multiple transfusions was 7% to 10%. Although the incidence of hepatitis has dramatically decreased since the advent of specific tests for hepatitis B and C, hepatitis remains the most common transfusion-related infection. Currently, the risk is estimated to be 1 in 65,000 per unit of blood product transfused.

BLOOD PRODUCT • Whole Blood

Whole blood consists of 45% cells and 55% plasma combined with an anticoagulant or preservative. The cellular components include erythrocytes (RBCs), leukocytes (WBCs), and platelets. Plasma consists of 90% water and 10% solutes. Solutes present in plasma include crystalloids (e.g., ions or glucose) and colloids (e.g., proteins of all types). Proteins make up the largest quantity of all solutes present in plasma. Other solutes include food substances, such as amino acids and lipids; products of biotransformation, such as urea, uric acid, creatinine, and lactic acid; respiratory gases such as oxygen and carbon dioxide; and regulatory substances, such as hormones and enzymes.

MECHANISM OF ACTION

Whole blood immediately provides the recipient with the oxygen-carrying capability of RBCs. It is an intravascular volume expander and a source of proteins with oncotic properties and stabile coagulation factors. A unit of whole blood contains enough hemoglobin to raise an anemic adult's hematocrit by about 3%. Only when the donor and recipient are ABO identical should whole blood be used (Table 45-1).

A unit of whole blood contains approximately 500 mL of which 240 to 275 mL is plasma, and 62 mL is anticoagulant. The hematocrit of whole blood is about 35% to 40%. The label of the blood unit lists the volume of the unit (+/− 10%) and the anticoagulant solution used.

USES

Whole blood is used to treat acute, massive blood loss requiring the oxygen-carrying capacity of RBCs along with the volume expansion provided by plasma. Patients with symptomatic anemia and **hypovolemia** or shock (a loss of 25% to 30% or more of circulating blood volume) are candidates for transfusion with whole blood. When the patient does not exhibit signs of hypovolemia, a transfusion with RBCs only is the treatment of choice (see below).

Neonates, infants, or adults who require exchange transfusions receive whole blood that is less than 7 days old to ensure that any cellular breakdown associated with the age of the unit of blood will not cause potentially dangerous electrolyte imbalances in the recipient. Whole blood should not be considered a source of viable platelets, WBCs, or the labile coagulation factors V and VIII. Factors V and VIII begin to break down 24 hours after collection. Patients requiring these components are better managed with the actual clotting factors.

The number of units or volume of the transfusion depends on the patient's condition. Unless the patient's condition dictates otherwise, the infusion should begin at a rate not to exceed 5 mL/minute for the first 15 minutes of the transfusion. During this initial period, the patient requires close observation because life-threatening

---

TABLE 45-1

ABO-Rh Compatibility of Whole Blood

Recipient Blood Type	Donor Blood Type					
	A	B	O	AB	Rh₁	Rh₂
A	X		X			
B		X	X			
O			X			
AB		X	X			
Rh₁					X	
Rh₂						X

X, compatibility.

---

reactions may occur after only a small volume of incompatible blood has been infused. After the first 15 minutes, the remainder of the transfusion should be infused as quickly as necessary. Patients who do not tolerate a rapid administration rate should be considered candidates for treatment with RBCs rather than with whole blood. Follow agency guidelines for administering blood and blood products to children.

ADVERSE REACTIONS AND CONTRAINDICATIONS

Hypothermia, circulatory overload, hypocalcemia, hyperkalemia, coagulopathies, and febrile, nonhemolytic reactions are primarily associated with whole blood and RBC transfusions. Table 45-2 provides an overview of other immunologic reactions to blood products.

Febrile Nonhemolytic Reactions

Febrile nonhemolytic reaction, the most common adverse effect of blood and blood products, manifests as facial flushing, chills and fever, headache, low back pain, rash, red urine, shock, and a burning sensation along the vein where the transfusion is given.

Circulatory Overload

Patients with cardiopulmonary disorders may experience circulatory overload in the form of heart failure. Additionally, each unit of whole blood contains about 56 mEq of sodium that contributes to fluid retention. Older adult patients, those of small stature, or patients with chronic severe anemia are at particular risk when the RBC mass is decreased and the plasma volume is increased. Patients with cardiopulmonary disorders who require multiple transfusions are also at risk for pulmonary edema. Another difficulty that may be encountered when blood is administered under pressure is that of air embolism.

Hypocalcemia

Patients requiring massive transfusions, especially those with liver disease, are at risk for hypocalcemia. The citrate anticoagulant binds with calcium ions in the recipient's blood, removing them from circulation and thereby reducing the calcium level below that essential for normal coagulation. Although a rare occurrence, the citrate-induced hypocalcemia is characterized by intestinal cramping, muscle twitching, tingling of the fingertips, decreased urine output, and possible renal failure. If the condition is left untreated, the patient may experience seizures, arrhythmias, or cardiac arrest. Metabolic alkalosis may also develop as citrate is converted to pyruvate and bicarbonate.

For the patient with mild symptoms of hypocalcemia, treatment consists of slowing or discontinuing

TABLE 45-2

Immunologic Reactions to Blood Transfusion

Cause	*Characteristic*	*Manifestations*	*Implications*
Immediate Reactions			
Intravascular hemolytic reaction	Incompatibility between recipient plasma and donor RBCs	Chills, fever, low back pain, flushing, tachycardia, tachypnea, hypotension, vascular collapse, hemoglobinuria, hemoglobinemia, bleeding, acute renal failure, shock, cardiac arrest, death.	Treat shock. Draw blood for serologic testing. Maintain BP with intravenous colloid solutions. Give diuretics to maintain urine flow. Measure urinary output.
Extravascular hemolytic reaction	Sensitization to an incompatible antigen through previous transfusion or pregnancy.	Fever, hemoglobinuria, hyperbilirubinemia. Continued fall in hemoglobin 4 to 14 days after the transfusion or continued anemia.	Rarely preventable. A complete and accurate transfusion history given to the blood bank may assist in identifying patients at risk.
Febrile, nonhemolytic reaction (most common)	Antigen-antibody response of HLA antigens on donor leukocytes reacting with patient antibodies.	Sudden chills, fever (rise in temperature greater than 2° F), headache, flushing, anxiety, muscle pain.	Do not restart transfusion. Give antipyretics as prescribed. Do not give aspirin to thrombocytopenic patients. Leukocyte-poor products or leukocyte-depleting filters are used for patients with a recurrent history of reaction.
Transfusion-related acute lung injury	Anti-HLA antibodies in donor plasma react with antigens on recipient's WBCs or platelets.	Fever (to 104° F), chills possible, cyanosis. Pulmonary edema in severe cases.	Symptom relief. Give antipyretics as prescribed. Oxygen and intravenous steroids if needed. Symptoms usually abate in 48 hours. Use leukocyte-poor products or leukocyte-depleting filters to prevent recurrence.
Allergic reactions (mild to anaphylaxis)	Sensitivity to donor's IgA antibody.	Urticaria, itching, flushing. Chills and fever at times. Bronchospasm, dyspnea, pulmonary edema if severe.	Antihistamines if reaction is mild. Epinephrine and corticosteroids if severe reaction. Donors with allergies should be eliminated from the donor pool. Frozen or washed RBCs and IgA-deficient plasma required for future transfusions require frozen or washed red blood cells and IgA-deficient plasma for future transfusion.

Continued

TABLE 45-2			
Immunologic Reactions to Blood Transfusion—cont'd			
Cause	*Characteristic*	*Manifestations*	*Implications*
Immediate Reactions—cont'd			
Acute nonimmune-mediated hemolytic reaction	Giving hypotonic fluid with blood product, bacterial infection, or contamination of donor's blood, acute hemolytic anemia from any cause, improper handling by the blood bank.	Fever, chills, hemoglobinuria. DIC and renal failure in severe cases.	Treat shock. Draw blood samples for serologic testing. Maintain BP with intravenous colloid solutions. Give diuretics to maintain urine flow. Measure urinary output.
Transfusion-related bacterial sepsis	Contamination of blood or blood product with bacteria.	Rigors, fever, nausea, vomiting, diarrhea, chest or back pain, hypotension, tachycardia, dyspnea, and cyanosis. May progress to respiratory failure, DIC.	Peripheral blood smears positive for hemolysis, a positive Gram's stain of a sample from the suspected blood unit, and an elevated WBC count differentiates bacterial sepsis from acute hemolytic reactions. Antibiotic therapy warranted.
Delayed Reactions			
Graft-versus-host disease	Immunodeficient person receives lymphocytes. These lymphocytes reject donor cells 4 to 30 days after transfusion.	High fever, skin rash, diarrhea and jaundice possible. Death.	Symptomatic, supportive care. Irradiation of RBCs or removal of all plasma from the blood product may prove beneficial.
Delayed hemolytic reaction	Sensitization to RBC antigen, not ABO system. Anamnestic immune response occurs 7 to 14 days after transfusion.	Fever, chills, back pain, jaundice, anemia, hemoglobinuria.	Give antipyretics as prescribed. Monitor adequacy of urinary output. Do more specific type and cross-match when giving blood.

DIC, disseminated intravascular coagulation.

the transfusion. The hypocalcemia will eventually correct itself without further intervention. For the patient with severe symptoms, a slow infusion of calcium chloride may be ordered.

Hyperkalemia

Another possible complication, particularly in patients with cardiac or renal disease is hyperkalemia, an excess of potassium in the blood. If the condition is not corrected, a flaccid paralysis develops, affecting the muscles of respiration and eventually the heart muscle, which can lead to bradycardia and cardiac arrest. High levels of potassium in donor blood are likely to occur when the blood is several days old. It is estimated that the breakdown of RBCs in the stored blood increases the level of potassium at the rate of 1 mEq/L/day. After 3 weeks of storage, potassium levels in donor plasma may reach 18 to 30 mEq/L. This is normally not a problem for patients receiving 1 or 2 units of blood because the serum potassium level is ordinarily self-correcting. However, when large quantities of RBCs are given, signs and symptoms of hyperkalemia can appear. Laboratory data will show high serum potassium levels and the ECG will show high, peaked T waves and wide QRS complexes.

To decrease potassium levels, the health care provider may order sodium polystyrene sulfonate. This cation-exchange resin may be administered orally or as a retention enema (see Chapter 51). When the patient is expected to receive large quantities of blood, requesting that the blood bank use the freshest blood available decreases the potential for hyperkalemia.

Coagulopathies

Some patients may hemorrhage as a result of platelet loss and deficiency of coagulation factors V and VIII in stored whole blood. Factors V and VIII begin to degrade 24 hours after collection. These coagulopathies can usually be prevented by administering platelets and FFP or by only using fresh units (less than 24 hours old) of unaltered whole blood.

Hypothermia

Hypothermia occurs when patients receive large quantities of cold blood, particularly through a central intravenous line. The patient exhibits shaking chills, hypotension, and cardiac arrhythmias. If the condition is left untreated, the patient's condition may proceed to arrhythmias and cardiac arrest. Treatment includes stopping the transfusion, warming the patient with blankets, and if tolerated, encouraging warm liquids. Warming the blood to 37° C with automatic blood warmers prevents hypothermia.

Patients with anemias who can be managed with drugs such as iron, vitamin B_{12}, recombinant erythropoietin, or folic acid, and whose condition permits sufficient time for these measures to promote erythropoiesis are not candidates for blood transfusions. Whole blood is not considered first-line treatment to expand circulating volume because of the risks of complications. Crystalline solutions, such as 0.9% sodium chloride solution or lactated Ringer's, and colloids such as albumin or plasma protein fraction are the treatments of choice for hypovolemia. In coagulation deficiencies, the appropriate coagulation products and derivatives are superior to whole blood.

◢ BLOOD PRODUCT • Packed Red Blood Cells

Blood banks prepare a unit of **packed red blood cells (PRBCs)** by removing plasma from a unit of whole blood. The red blood cell concentrate has the same RBC mass as a unit of whole blood, but only 20% to 30% of the plasma and a much smaller quantity of leukocytes and platelets.

Leukocyte-poor preparations of PRBCs are units in which the number of WBCs has been reduced to less than 5×10^8. Washing RBCs with saline solution removes 80% to 95% of the WBCs, 99% of the plasma, and 100% of the platelets from a unit. At least 80% of the RBCs remain.

MECHANISM OF ACTION

Unlike whole blood, PRBC transfusions must be ABO compatible but not ABO identical, because most of the plasma, and therefore, the ABO antibodies have been removed (Table 45-3). A unit of PRBCs has a volume of about 300 mL, with a hematocrit of 65% to 80%. PRBC units may be divided by the laboratory into several smaller bags with less volume.

PRBCs with additive solution (AS) contain red cells with 90% of the plasma removed and 100 mL of a special solution containing the necessary preservative to increase the shelf life (42 days) and decrease viscosity. PRBCs with CPDA-1 solution have a shelf life of 35 days. Because of the presence of additional preservative solution, the AS units have a higher volume and lower hematocrit than do PRBCs containing CPDA-1 solution.

USES

Patients who are not hypovolemic but who have heart failure, older adults, and debilitated patients as well as patients with normal or expanded plasma volumes who cannot tolerate rapid shifts of blood volume receive PRBCs. In some cases, RBCs may be used for exchange transfusions, but as with whole blood, these cells must be less than 7 days old to avoid potential electrolyte imbalances.

Leukocyte-poor PRBCs are used to prevent recurrence of febrile, nonhemolytic transfusion reactions caused by donor WBC antigens reacting with recipient

---

TABLE 45-3

ABO-Rh Compatibility with Packed Red Blood Cells

Recipient Blood Type	Donor Blood Type					
	A	B	O	AB	Rh_1	Rh_2
A	X		X			
B		X	X			
O			X			
AB	X	X	X	X		
Rh_1					X	X
Rh_2						X

X, compatibility.

WBC antibodies. Leukocyte-poor PRBCs are preferred for patients who require multiple transfusions (e.g., patients with leukemia or aplastic anemia) and as a result have become HLA alloimmunized. Washed or frozen deglycerolized PRBCs may be used to reduce the incidence of urticarial and anaphylactic reactions. Washed PRBCs may be indicated for patients with paroxysmal nocturnal hemoglobinuria or other conditions that require the transfusion of RBCs containing minimal amounts of plasma.

Irradiated blood products are used to prevent post-transfusion graft-versus-host disease (GVHD) in patients with Hodgkin's or non-Hodgkin's lymphoma, acute leukemia, congenital immunodeficiency syndromes, low-birth-weight neonates, intrauterine transfusions, and bone marrow transplants. Irradiated blood products have been exposed to a measured amount of radiation, thereby rendering the donor lymphocytes incapable of replication. The product carries no radiation risk to the health care provider or the recipient.

The number of units to be transfused depends on the patient's condition. The rate of administration and clinical interventions are the same as for whole blood, beginning at 5 mL/minute for the first 15 minutes and then proceeding as rapidly as the patient tolerates the infusion and as clinically indicated. One unit of PRBCs is usually infused over a period of 2 to 3 hours. Follow agency protocol for pediatric infusion rates.

ADVERSE REACTIONS AND CONTRAINDICATIONS

Simply put, RBCs should not be given to recipients with matching antibodies in their plasma, and plasma should not be given to recipients with matching antigens on their RBCs. In general, the adverse reactions associated with whole blood transfusions are found with PRBCs, but there is a reduced risk of febrile, nonhemolytic reactions and circulatory overload. However, hypovolemia without significant deficit in red blood cell mass is best treated with other volume expanders and not PRBCs. PRBCs should not be used for volume expansion, in place of a hematinic drug, to enhance wound healing, or to improve the general well-being of the patient.

BLOOD PRODUCT • Plasma

Plasma is the clear portion of blood. It may be in the form of plasma, liquid plasma, or fresh frozen plasma (FFP). Plasma and liquid plasma are the clear portions of the blood that have been separated from the cells with anticoagulant added. Plasma is stored frozen, whereas liquid plasma is refrigerated. Plasma and liquid plasma contain stable coagulation factors but not the labile coagulation factors VI and VIII.

FFP is separated from a fresh unit of whole blood (less than 6 hours old) and frozen. It is 91% water, 7% protein (i.e., albumin, globulins, antibodies, clotting factors), and 2% carbohydrate. When FFP is frozen within 6 hours of collection, it can be stored for up to 1 year without loss of labile or nonlabile coagulation factors.

MECHANISM OF ACTION

Plasma and liquid plasma provide the patient with stable clotting factors such as fibrinogen and factor IX. Cross-matching is not required before transfusing plasma or liquid plasma, but the transfusion must be compatible with the patient's donor or recipient ABO status (Table 45-4). Rh compatibility is not an issue because blood cells are not part of the transfusion, and consequently, the Rh D antigen and subantigen D^u are not present.

A cross-match between donor and recipient is not required to use FFP, but the plasma must be ABO compatible with the recipient's blood cells. One unit of plasma or liquid plasma contains between 180 and 300 mL of anticoagulated plasma. One unit of FFP contains about 250 mg of fibrinogen, although there is great variability from one donor unit to another. One unit of FFP contains 2 to 4 mg of fibrinogen and raises the recipient's plasma fibrinogen level about 10 mg/dL.

TABLE 45-4

ABO-Rh Compatibility of Fresh Frozen Plasma

Recipient Blood Type	Donor Blood Type					
	A	B	O	AB	Rh_1	Rh_2
A	X		X			
B		X		X		
O	X	X	X	X		
AB				X		
Rh_1					X	X
Rh_2					X	X

X, compatibility.

USES

Plasma is used for the treatment of stable clotting factor deficiencies for which no concentrates are available. In some cases, even when clotting factor concentrates are available, plasma is the product of choice. Plasma keeps patient exposure to multiple-donor products to a minimum.

FFP is used to control bleeding in patients who have a demonstrated deficiency that requires labile plasma coagulation factors and blood volume expansion. It is essential in the management of idiopathic thrombocytopenic purpura (ITP).

The individual patient's clinical situation determines the volume of the treatment. Knowledge of the patient's size and laboratory assays of coagulation function assists in determining the dosage. FFP should be used within 24 hours after thawing if the therapeutic objective is to provide labile coagulation factors. The rate of administration is 200 mL/hour, or more slowly if circulatory overload is a potential problem.

The infusion rate for pediatric patients who are hemorrhaging is dictated by the clinical situation. When FFP is used for pediatric clotting deficiency, the infusion rate is 1 to 2 mL/minute.

ADVERSE REACTIONS AND CONTRAINDICATIONS

Plasma and liquid plasma can produce the same adverse reactions as those of whole blood. FFP is an isotonic volume expander, so the patient receiving more than 1 unit is at risk for circulatory overload.

Plasma carries the same risk of disease transmission (except for cytomegalovirus [CMV]) as whole blood. Plasma or liquid plasma is contraindicated when volume can be safely replaced with other methods such as 0.9% sodium chloride, Ringer's lactate, albumin, and plasma protein fraction. FFP should not be used for volume expansion, as a nutritional supplement, prophylactically with a massive blood transfusion, or in patients following cardiopulmonary bypass.

BLOOD PRODUCT • Platelets

Normal hemostasis requires the plasma component platelets. Platelet masses act as a patch to physically occlude breaks in small blood vessels. Platelets are also a source of phospholipids required for blood coagulation. Each unit of platelets contains approximately 5.5×10^{10} platelets suspended in 20 to 70 mL of plasma.

Single-donor platelets are concentrates harvested using a procedure known as hemipheresis. Units of hemipheresed platelets contain at least 3×10^{11} platelets (equivalent to about 5 to 6 units of pooled donor units) suspended in 200 to 500 mL of plasma. This product contains varying numbers of lymphocytes, depending on the type of blood cell separator that is used.

In some cases, the patient may require HLA-matched platelets. Platelets for these patients are obtained from a donor who is an HLA-match to the recipient. HLAs, which are located on all nucleated cells of the body and most of the circulating body cells, play a vital role in tissue transplantation.

MECHANISM OF ACTION

Factors V and VIII are bound to platelets and may contribute to hemostasis in patients receiving multiple transfusions, in those with disseminated intravascular coagulopathy (DIC), or in patients who have a factor V deficiency. Each unit of platelets raises the platelet count of a nonbleeding 70 kg adult by 5000 to 10,000/mL. A bag of pheresed platelets is equivalent to five to eight bags of platelets.

USES

Platelet transfusions are used for patients who are actively bleeding and who have a platelet count less than 50,000/mm³ or a qualitative defect. Patients requiring surgery whose platelet counts are less than 50,000/mm³ (less than 90,000/mm³ if the surgery is on the central nervous system or the eye) receive platelets. Patients undergoing antineoplastic therapy or who have leukemia require multiple, repeated platelet infusions. The multiple infusions place the patients at risk for alloimmunization to the donors' leukocytes and platelets. It is thought that with increased exposure to multiple donors, the recipient's risk of alloimmunization increases and the recipient can become refractory to the transfusions. In these patients, the use of single-donor hemipheresed platelets reduces the patient's exposure to foreign leukocyte antigens from 6 to 1.

Patients who are unresponsive to single-donor and pooled platelets may respond to HLA-matched platelets (but only if the HLA antibodies are the primary cause of platelet destruction). A family member such as a sibling is the most likely suitable match for HLA-matched platelets, but this matching should be avoided if the family member plans to donate bone marrow for use by the patient.

Patients with a history of febrile, nonhemolytic reactions may require leukocyte-poor platelets. Filters specifically designed for administration of leukocyte-poor platelets should be used. Removal of leukocytes reduces the risk of alloimmunization and risk of CMV transmission.

Platelets from Rh-negative donors should be used for Rh-negative women of childbearing age. If that is not possible, administration of RhoGAM should be considered if Rh-positive platelets must be transfused.

The patient's clinical state determines the number of platelet concentrate units to be administered. The usual amount given to a bleeding adult patient with a platelet count below $20 \times 10^9/L$ is six to eight bags. The patient may require a repeat dose in 1 to 3 days because transfused platelets have a life span of only 3 to 4 days. Another acceptable dosage calculation is to infuse 1 unit of platelets per 10 kg of patient body weight. The average pediatric dose of platelet concentrates is 1 unit for every 7 to 10 kg of body weight. Platelet infusions may be administered as rapidly as tolerated but should be completed within 4 hours.

ADVERSE REACTIONS AND CONTRAINDICATIONS

Patients who require multiple or frequent platelet infusions may become refractory to treatment. When the pa-

tient becomes refractory, platelet counts no longer respond to the infusion. Instead, previously acquired HLA antibodies destroy the infused platelets.

Immunization to RBC antigens may occur as a result of the presence of red blood cells in pheresed platelet concentrates. Platelets incompatible with recipient RBCs may cause low-grade hemolysis caused by isoagglutinins in the plasma.

Platelet concentrates contain few RBCs. Hence, ABO compatibility is not required. However, ABO red blood cell compatibility enhances platelet recovery and survival. Rh compatibility should be considered, particularly in Rh-negative women of childbearing age. If it is impossible to use platelets from Rh-negative donors, consideration should be given to immunizing the recipient with RhoGAM.

Platelets should not be transfused to patients with ITP (unless there is life-threatening bleeding). Platelets also should not be given prophylactically with a massive blood transfusion, nor given to patients following cardiopulmonary bypass.

 BLOOD PRODUCT • Granulocytes

Granulocytes are phagocytes that migrate toward and kill bacteria. This cellular product is obtained from a single donor and contains other leukocytes, platelets, and 20 to 50 mL of RBCs. The cells are suspended in 200 to 300 mL of anticoagulant and plasma. Granulocyte infusions contain at least 20 to 30×10^9 granulocytes.

MECHANISM OF ACTION

Because the granulocyte product contains a considerable number of RBCs and plasma, cross-matching of donor to recipient is necessary. Pretransfusion testing for granulocyte transfusions is ordinarily the same as for RBC transfusion (Table 45–5).

An infusion of granulocytes does not cause the patient's granulocyte count to increase. This may be because of prior immunization to leukocyte antigens and subsequent sequestration of the granulocytes by the body. It may also be to the result of consumption of the granulocytes as they fight the infection.

USES

Granulocyte infusions are indicated as supportive therapy for patients with acquired neutropenia (usually less than $0.5 \times 10^9/L$) or in patients who have WBC dysfunction from a documented gram-negative infection that is unresponsive to antibiotics or other treatments. These

patients are very ill and may not have the bone marrow capacity to generate granulocytes on their own. The clinical course of those who will not recover bone marrow function is generally not altered with the use of granulocyte infusions. Only CMV-seronegative granulocytes should be given to profoundly immunosuppressed CMV-seronegative recipients (e.g., bone marrow transplant recipients). The long-term benefits of granulocyte infusions remain questionable and continue to be evaluated.

TABLE 45-5

ABO-Rh Compatibility for Granulocyte Transfusions

Recipient Blood Type	Donor Blood Type					
	A	B	O	AB	Rh_1	Rh_2
A	X		X			
B		X	X			
O			X			
AB	X	X	X	X		
Rh_1					X	X
Rh_2						X

X, compatibility.

When the decision is made that granulocyte infusion is appropriate, the patient should receive daily infusions until the infection is cured, the patient's fever abates, or the absolute granulocyte count returns to at least 0.5×10^9/L. Ideally, granulocytes are administered within 24 hours of harvesting. The recommended dosage is 3×10^8 cells/kg per infusion. The unit is administered over 4 hours (based on a 200-mL volume) through a standard infusion set. Depth-type microaggregate or leukocyte reduction filters remove granulocytes and are not appropriate for use with this blood product.

ADVERSE REACTIONS AND CONTRAINDICATIONS

It is not unusual for patients receiving granulocyte infusions to exhibit febrile, nonhemolytic reactions. Chills, fevers, and pulmonary insufficiency may be avoided with slow administration and pretreatment (meperidine, acetaminophen, or antihistamines); however, patients may experience these adverse reactions in spite of interventions. The same types of reactions and hazards associated with the administration of whole blood may occur with granulocyte infusions.

Granulocyte infusions are contraindicated in the treatment of infections responsive to antibiotics. Only patients whose conditions have not responded to broad-spectrum antibiotics are candidates for treatment with granulocytes.

The systemic antifungal drug amphotericin B should not be administered within 4 hours of granulocyte infusion because of the risk of pulmonary insufficiency.

BLOOD PRODUCT • Cryoprecipitate AHF

Cryoprecipitate AHF is prepared by thawing FFP and recovering the precipitate. On the average, each bag contains 80 to 120 units of factor VIII (antihemolytic factor [AHF]), 250 mg of fibrinogen, and 20% to 30% of factor XIII present in the original unit.

MECHANISM OF ACTION

Cryoprecipitate AHF contains a small volume of plasma and no RBCs. Cross-matching and Rh determination is preferred but not required (Table 45-6).

USES

Cryoprecipitated AHF assists in controlling bleeding in patients with coagulopathies associated with deficits of factors VIII, XIII, fibrinogen, and **von Willebrand's factor** by replacing selected clotting factors. It is used to control bleeding caused by deficiency of factor VIII (i.e., hemophilia A), von Willebrand's factor (AHF-VWF), factor XIII, and fibrinogen. It is occasionally used to control bleeding in patients with uremia. Cryoprecipitate AHF is also indicated in the treatment of hypofibrinogenemia. This deficiency may be caused by an inherited coagulopathy or DIC. Cryoprecipitate AHF is the only source of concentrated fibrinogen available.

The dosage of cryoprecipitate is based on plasma volume. Eight to ten bags supply 2 g of fibrinogen (a hemostatic dose).

When treating bleeding patients with hemophilia, a rapid infusion of 10 mL/min of factor VIII as a loading dose yields the desired effect; this infusion is followed by a smaller maintenance dose every 8 to 12 hours. After surgery, a 10-day or more regimen of therapy may be needed. Patients with circulating antibodies to factor VIII require larger doses. Managing and monitoring cryoprecipitated AHF responses in factor VIII–deficient patients requires periodic plasma factor VIII:C assays. Smaller doses of cryoprecipitated AHF usually control the bleeding time of patients with von Willebrand's disease. Fibrinogen assays are necessary to monitor patients with hypofibrinogenemia.

ADVERSE REACTIONS AND CONTRAINDICATIONS

Adverse reactions of cryoprecipitate are similar to those described for whole blood and may include allergic reactions, transmission of infectious diseases, and bacterial contamination.

TABLE 45-6

ABO-Rh Compatibility for Cryoprecipitate AHF

Recipient Blood Type	Donor Blood Type					
	A	B	O	AB	Rh₁	Rh₂
A	X			X		
B		X		X		
O	X	X	X	X		
AB				X		
Rh₁					X	X
Rh₂					X	X

X, compatibility.

APPLICATION TO PRACTICE

ASSESSMENT
History of Present Illness

The symptoms and complaints of the patient with blood loss depend on the rapidity with which the loss occurred, the volume of loss, and the ability of the patient's compensatory mechanisms to maintain homeostasis.

Patients with bleeding disorders may have a history of bleeding following minor surgical procedures, dental procedures, childbirth, or other trauma, and they may also have a family history of bleeding. The patient may note that bleeding has occurred from multiple sites without a history of trauma.

The examiner should determine whether the patient has had a recent viral or bacterial infection, particularly involving the upper respiratory tract. Autoimmune ITP frequently follows upper respiratory infections or other viral infections.

Health History

A history of jaundice, blood loss, coagulopathy, alcohol abuse, diarrhea, or chronic diseases may assist in determining the cause of the patient's symptoms. Attempt to get a thorough drug history because many drugs contribute to or exacerbate bleeding (Box 45-1). Allergy and transfusion history, as well as any history of coagulopathies, provide the health care provider with information about the potential risks should a blood or blood product infusion become necessary. The patient presenting with acute blood loss secondary to major trauma will likely be unable to assist with a history, and

---

BOX 45-1 **Drugs Contributing to Bleeding Disorders**

acetylsalicylic acid
Alcohol
Barbiturates
Cephalosporins
chlorpromazine
dipyridamole
heparin
isoniazid (INH)
methyldopa
Nonsteroidal antiinflammatory drugs
phenytoin
quinidine
rifampin (RIF)
Semisynthetic penicillins
Sulfonamides
Thiazides
warfarin

---

all initial efforts when dealing with the patient in this condition are directed at maintaining the patient's airway, breathing, and circulation.

Lifespan Considerations

Perinatal. In pregnancy, fibrinogen, platelet adhesiveness, and factor VIII levels are increased but antithrombin III and the activators of plasminogen are decreased. Plasminogen itself is increased. Therefore, the equilibrium of coagulation and fibrinolysis is skewed toward coagulation.

Disseminated intravascular coagulation (DIC) is a secondary disorder that may occur in the pregnant woman (as well as in patients with surgical, infectious, hemolytic, and neoplastic disorders) as a result of an abruptio placentae, intrauterine fetal death (especially if the products of conception are retained longer than 5 weeks), preeclampsia and eclampsia, postpartum hemorrhagic sepsis, a rapid traumatic labor and delivery, or amniotic fluid embolism. These disorders cause infusion of tissue extract from injured tissues, severe injury to endothelial cells, red blood cell or platelet injury, build up of bacterial debris or endotoxins, immune reactions, and thrombocytopenia. All of these factors activate the intrinsic coagulation sequence in some way. Paradoxically, the intravascular clotting ultimately produces hemorrhage because of rapid consumption of fibrinogen, platelets, prothrombin, and clotting factors V, VIII, and X.

The tendency toward excessive bleeding can appear suddenly and, with little warning, rapidly progress to severe or even fatal hemorrhage. Signs of DIC include continued bleeding from a venipuncture site, occult and internal bleeding, and in some cases, profuse bleeding from all orifices. Other less obvious and more easily missed signs of bleeding are generalized sweating, cold and mottled fingers and toes (due to capillary thrombi and hypoxia), and petechiae.

Pediatric. The causes of bleeding disorders in children are similar to those of adults, although there are some disorders that are seen more often in children. For example, von Willebrand's disease is a hereditary bleeding disorder characterized by a factor VIII deficiency and low levels of factor VIII–related antigen. In addition, the functional component of factor VIII that is required for platelet adhesion to vascular subendothelium is reduced. This factor results in prolonged bleeding time because the platelets fail to adhere to the walls of ruptured vessels.

The patient with von Willebrand's disease has an increased tendency to bleed from mucous membranes. The most common symptom is frequent nosebleeds, followed by gingival bleeding, easy bruising, and menorrhagia in female patients. Von Willebrand's disease can be mild, moderate, or severe. Unlike hemophilia, it affects both males and females because it is an autosomal dominant disorder.

Hemophilia is an X-linked recessive disorder that can be mild, moderate, or severe. It is most often transmitted via an unaffected male and a trait-carrier female. Hemophilia A, or classic hemophilia makes up about 75% of the cases. Factor IX deficiency (hemophilia B, or Christmas disease) makes up the remainder of cases.

The risk of bleeding in hemophilia is variable, depending on the level of clotting factor deficiency. Approximately 60% of children with hemophilia A or B are severely affected and may have spontaneous bleeding without recognized trauma. Soft tissue bleeding from the neck, lower face, and tongue may cause grave consequences if it is not treated. Hematuria and GI bleeding are likely. Hemarthrosis (bleeding into the joints) can lead to painful stiffening and permanent disability. The leading cause of death, however, is intracranial bleeding. Hemorrhagic complications can be avoided or minimized with early and adequate factor replacement therapy.

Older Adults. The older adult who presents with bruising requires the health care provider to differentiate between a bleeding disorder and senile purpura, the bleeding under the skin associated with increased capillary fragility as a result of the aging process.

Cultural/Social Considerations

Culture and religious beliefs influence patients' explanations of the cause of illness, perception of its severity, and the choice of health care providers. In times of crisis, religion may influence the course of action believed to be appropriate. For example, blood and blood products are generally acceptable to Hindus, Mennonites, Seventh-Day Adventists, Unitarians, and followers of Islam. Catholicism, according to the Roman Rite, permits the use of blood and blood products as long as they are used for the good of the whole person. There is a prohibition in Judaism against ingesting blood (e.g., blood sausage, raw meat). However, this does not apply to receiving blood transfusions. Blood and blood products are not ordinarily used by members of the Church of Christ (Christian Scientists).

Jehovah's Witnesses must refuse blood in any form and products in which blood is an ingredient. Blood volume expanders are acceptable if they are not derivatives of blood. Mechanical devices for circulating the blood are acceptable as long as they are not primed with blood initially. Courts of justice have often upheld the principle that each person has a right to bodily integrity.

Yet, some health care providers and hospital administrators have turned to the courts for legal authorization to use blood as an intervention for an individual whose religious convictions prohibit the use of blood. In some cases, children have been made wards of the court so that they could receive blood when a life-threatening medical condition occurred.

Other patients may refuse blood or blood products because of their fear of contracting infectious diseases. In all cases, health care providers should explain to patients in terms that they can understand the potential outcomes related to their decisions and support these patients in their informed decisions.

Physical Examination

Vital signs reflect the patient's volume status. But before there are discernible changes in vital signs, the patient with hypovolemia displays restlessness, thirst, and generalized anxiety, much as that seen in dehydration. Urinary output is reduced. Patients with blood loss via the GI tract may complain of black, tarry stools. Blood in the GI tract functions as an effective cathartic, and the patient may have diarrhea. The stool may first appear as black and tarry, proceed to maroon-colored loose stools, and then become liquid, frank blood.

A loss of at least 10% of circulating volume is usually necessary before there is a decrease in systolic blood pressure. In advanced blood loss, as the patient's blood pressure and cardiac output fall, the heart rate increases as the body attempts to compensate for the fall in cardiac output. The patient may have postural changes in blood pressure. Mucous membranes and extremities become pale and cool because of vasoconstriction as the body shunts blood away from the periphery to vital organs. There may also be peripheral edema and systolic ejection murmurs.

Patients with platelet defects generally experience bleeding immediately after trauma. Bleeding may be evident on the skin in the form of petechiae (less than 3 mm) or ecchymoses (greater than 3 mm). Other common areas of bleeding in platelet disorders are the mucous membranes, nose, and GI or urinary tracts. Patients with platelet disorders may have hepatosplenomegaly as a result of increased platelet destruction. A rectal examination determines the presence of blood in the GI tract.

Laboratory Testing

Laboratory testing includes a complete blood cell (CBC) count with differential, platelet count, and reticulocyte count. Additionally, prothrombin (PT), activated partial thromboplastin (aPTT), and bleeding times assist in determining the cause of symptoms. If it becomes necessary, blood for type and cross-match or for type and hold are drawn and sent to the laboratory to prepare for transfusion.

Initially, the patient's hemoglobin and hematocrit may be falsely high because the compensatory vasoconstriction caused by hypovolemia initially prevents the extravascular fluids from replacing the intravascular fluid loss. Eventually, the hemoglobin and hematocrit fall. Reticulocyte counts in acute blood loss are elevated because the bone marrow is trying to replace lost cells.

Laboratory tests done for patients with platelet-associated bleeding disorders include a CBC and platelet counts. Platelet counts of less than $100,000/mm^3$ are associated with mildly prolonged bleeding times. Platelet counts of less than $50,000/mm^3$ result in easy bruising. Patients whose platelet counts are less than $20,000/mm^3$ are at increased risk for spontaneous bleeding. A PT evaluates the function of the extrinsic coagulation system whereas the PTT or aPTT evaluates the function of the intrinsic coagulation system. The clotting cascade is discussed in Chapter 43.

Determination of bleeding time is used when diagnosing patients with bleeding disorders. Patients with bleeding times over 9 minutes in the presence of normal platelet counts have a qualitative platelet defect. In the patient with thrombocytopenia, a bone marrow biopsy is helpful in determining whether the patient has bone marrow aplasia caused by malignancy or fibrosis. If the bone marrow biopsy reveals an increase in megakaryocytes, ITP is the likely diagnosis.

GOALS OF THERAPY

Treatment goals for patients with fluid volume deficits are to reverse hypovolemia, restore fluid volume, and prevent ischemic complications. To accomplish these goals, treatment modalities may include the use of blood and/or blood products, other colloids or crystalloid solutions. The guiding principle used in clinical decision-making is to use the least extreme measure to safely accomplish treatment goals. Blood and blood products are always considered extreme measures.

INTERVENTION
Administration

Obtain informed consent from the patient for the administration of the blood or blood product and take the patient's vital signs before starting the transfusion. The transfusion should begin within 30 minutes of obtaining the blood or blood product from the laboratory. Strict adherence to verification before blood or blood product administration greatly reduces the risk of transfusing the wrong blood type. With another registered nurse at the bedside, verify the blood product and the

patient's identity by comparing the laboratory blood record with the following:
- Patient's name and identification number, both verbally and against the patient's wristband
- The unit number on the blood bag label
- Blood group and Rh type on the blood bag label
- Type of blood component with the health care provider's order
- Expiration date noted on the blood bag label

An 18- or 19-gauge cannula, which facilitates transfusion flow and prevents hemolysis of RBCs, must be used. Restart the intravenous unit if necessary. A 0.9% sodium chloride solution used as a priming solution should be infused into the primary line with the blood piggybacked to the primary solution. Because blood and blood products are fragile, handle the bag carefully. Under no circumstances should any drugs be mixed with the blood product.

For routine administration of whole blood, a standard blood filter with a minimum pore size of 170 microns is recommended. If the patient requires three or more units of blood or if the blood product is over 5 days old, microaggregate blood filters with pore sizes of 30 to 40 microns are effective in removing any tiny clots or debris that may have developed during storage.

Unless the patient's condition dictates otherwise, the infusion of whole blood or RBCs begins at a rate of 5 mL/minute for the first 15 minutes of the infusion. After this initial period, the transfusion should proceed as quickly as possible. During the first hour of the transfusion, vital signs should be taken every 15 minutes or according to agency policy. During the remaining time of the transfusion, observe the patient very closely while monitoring for signs of a transfusion reaction. Should the patient exhibit signs of a transfusion reaction, stop the transfusion, maintain the intravenous line with 0.9% sodium chloride solution, and notify the health care provider immediately. No single unit of blood product should infuse for more than 4 hours, and platelets should be infused as rapidly as possible.

Although such cases are rare, transfusions can result in fatal reactions. Approximately 30 people in the United States die each year as a direct result of blood product transfusion. Each year, 10% to 15% of patients receiving transfusions experience adverse reactions, with 1% experiencing serious adverse reactions. By law, when complications from the transfusion of blood or blood components result in death, the blood bank must notify the FDA by phone within 24 hours and file a written report of the investigation of the reaction with the FDA within 7 days.

Patients with a history of severe febrile transfusion reactions may benefit from leukocyte-depleting filters. The use of leukocyte-depleting filters will decrease the patient's risk of alloimmunization to HLA. If the situation is such that the patient will likely require multiple platelet transfusions over a period of time, it is prudent to use a leukocyte-reduction filter with the patient's first platelet infusion.

When a rapid transfusion of multiple units of blood is needed or if there is a patient history of cold agglutinins (antibodies that agglutinate RBCs at temperatures below 37° C), a blood warmer should be used. Be aware before administration of blood products where emergency drugs and equipment are kept.

Education

Explain the transfusion procedure to the patient. Instruct the patient to report signs and symptoms that may suggest adverse reactions. Frequently, it is the patient who will report a problem before the health care provider is able to discern it by physical examination. Instruct the patient to report low back pain, chest pain, headache, fever, chills, tachycardia, tachypnea, dizziness, urticaria, itching, anxiety, pain at the intravenous site, or nausea. Any of these signs and symptoms should alert the health care provider to potential problems with the patient's transfusion.

EVALUATION

Patients who have received whole blood or PRBCs will likely have resolution of symptoms of hypovolemic shock and anemia. If a patient is actively bleeding, the hematocrit and hemoglobin may fluctuate because of rapid fluid shifts. In a nonbleeding adult, one unit of whole blood should increase the hematocrit by 3% and the hemoglobin by 1 g/dL.

Treatment effectiveness of plasma infusions is assessed by monitoring coagulation function, which is measured by the PT, international normalized ratio (INR), aPTT, or by specific factor assays.

A transfusion of platelets to a bleeding patient yields a cessation of bleeding, correction of prolonged bleeding times, and an increase in the patient's platelet count. One unit of platelets raises the platelet count of a 70-kg adult by 5000 to 10,000/mL and an 18-kg child by 20,000/mm^3 if the underlying cause of thrombocytopenia is resolved or controlled. To assess therapeutic effects, a platelet count should be performed within 1 hour of the transfusion.

The expected outcome of granulocyte infusion is improvement in or resolution of the infection and is the only measure of treatment effectiveness. No increase in peripheral WBC count is usually seen following granulocyte infusion in adults; however, an increase may be seen in children.

Bibliography

Gabrilone J: Overview: erythropoiesis, anemia, and erythropoietin, *Semin Hematol* 37(4 suppl 6):1-3, 2000.

Goodnough L: Universal leukoreduction of cellular blood components in 2001? *Am J of Clin Pathol* 115(5):674-677, 2001.

Horrell C, Rothman J: Establishing the etiology of thrombocytopenia, *Nurse Pract* 25(6):68-77, 2000.

Lipson S, Shepp D, Match M, et al: Cytomegalovirus infectivity in whole blood following leukocyte reduction by filtration, *Am J Clin Pathol* 116(1):52-55, 2001.

Mantovani L, Lentini G, Hentschel B, et al: Treatment of anemia in myelodysplastic syndromes, *Br J Haematol* 109(2): 367-375, 2000.

Nichols W, Boeckh M: Pathogen inactivated blood products and granulocyte transfusions, 42nd Annual Meeting of the American Society of Hematology, 2000.

Piron M, Leo M, Gothot A, et al: Secondary anemia after intensive treatment with erythropoietin, *Blood* 97:442-448, 2000.

Internet Resources

Meremikwu M, Smith H: Blood transfusion for treating malarial anaemia, *The Cochrane Library*, ed 2, Oxford, 2001, Update Software. Available online at http://www.cochranelibrary.com/enter/.

CHAPTER

46

Diuretics

LYNN ROGER WILLIS • ELIZABETH KISSELL

 Visit **http://evolve.elsevier.com/Gutierrez/** for additional information.

KEY TERMS

Aldosterone, p. 743

Carbonic anhydrase, p. 743

Diuretics, p. 741

Homeostasis, p. 742

Hyperkalemia, p. 751

Loop diuretics, p. 744

Metabolic alkalosis, p. 744

Nephrons, p. 741

Osmotic diuretics, p. 753

Potassium-sparing diuretics, p. 751

Thiazides, p. 745

OBJECTIVES

- Explain why increasing sodium excretion is a desirable action of diuretics.
- Identify the class of diuretics with the highest efficacy.
- Name the loop and potassium-sparing diuretics.
- List conditions for which loop and thiazide diuretics are used.
- Create a nursing care plan for the patient receiving a diuretic.

 PHYSIOLOGY • **Renal Function**

The kidneys regulate water and electrolyte balance in the body so that the extracellular fluid volume may be held constant, a function that can influence blood pressure and the actions of several organs. Diuretics act at various renal sites to modify salt and water excretion. The mechanisms by which these drugs act can be understood by first recalling normal renal function and then considering how diuretics alter the normal processes.

MAINTENANCE OF EXTRACELLULAR FLUID VOLUME

Urine is produced by the thousands of nephrons that comprise the kidneys (Figure 46-1), and glomerular filtration is the first step in forming urine. Blood flowing through the kidneys contacts a filtering surface in the glomerulus, where water and small molecules pass freely into the tubule, leaving behind most proteins and the molecules bound to proteins. The filtered fluid then travels down the tubular portion of the nephron where specialized transport systems reabsorb most (more than 99%) of the filtered electrolytes and water, leaving on average less than 1% of the filtered water and electrolytes for excretion in the urine.

The quantities of water, sodium, chloride, potassium and other constituents of the glomerular filtrate that finally end up in the urine each day ordinarily reflect a person's daily dietary intake of these substances. That is, the kidneys normally excrete only that fraction of the filtered water and electrolytes in excess of what is needed to maintain the desired volume and concentration of extracellular fluid. This process and others like it for maintaining physiologic stability are called **homeostasis.** Homeostasis amounts to maintaining a balance between those con-

stituents of the extracellular fluid volume obtained each day in the diet and those excreted each day in the urine. Conditions that upset this balance (e.g., heart, liver, or kidney failure) cause retention of electrolytes and water by reducing the production of urine. The fluid retention expands the extracellular fluid volume compartment. If not stopped, fluid retention leads ultimately to the formation of edema, which can be life threatening (the so-called congestion in heart failure results from the accumulation of edema fluid in a pathologically significant amount). Diuretics are used to increase the kidneys' ability to excrete the excess salt and water that caused the edema to form.

To understand how diuretics intervene in diseases and conditions in which fluid and electrolyte balance is

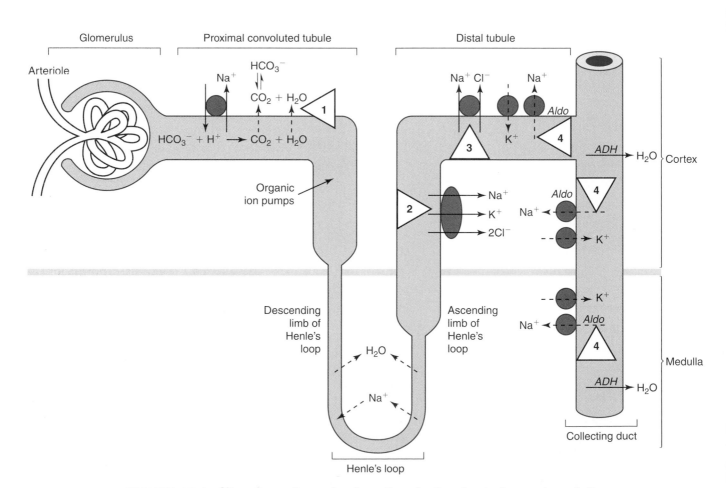

FIGURE 46-1 Sites of secretion and reabsorption of salt and water in a nephron. Active (energy-requiring) processes are designated by solid arrows; passive transport is designated by broken arrows. Symporters, antiporters, and channels are shown as circles or ovals. The sites of major classes of diuretic agents are shown by the numbered triangles. *1,* carbonic anhydrase inhibitors; *2,* loop diuretics acting on the Na^+-K^+-Cl^- symporter; *3,* thiazide and thiazide-like drugs acting on the Na^+-Cl^- symporter; *4,* potassium-sparing diuretics acting on aldosterone-regulated sodium channels.

upset, several elements of normal renal physiology must be considered.

Renal Transport Mechanisms

Membranes are composed of lipids, which water and water-soluble materials such as ions do not easily cross. Several specific renal transporters facilitate and regulate the passage of selected ions and other molecules across renal membranes. These transporters have been given names based on their function. Symporters move two or three ions all in the same direction in a process called cotransport. For example, a chloride ion might be cotransported with a sodium ion. Antiporters are exchangers, which move two ions in opposite directions. For example, a sodium ion might be taken into a cell in exchange for a hydrogen ion, which then leaves the cell. Such transporters may be either active (requiring the expenditure of metabolic energy) or passive (no direct expenditure of energy required). Active transporters (e.g., Na^+-K^+-ATPase) move ions from regions of low to high concentration, that is, against a concentration gradient. Passive transporters move ions down a concentration gradient, from regions of higher to lower concentration. Several of the symporters and antiporters affected by diuretics are passive. The energy needed for them to function comes from the energy expended to operate the Na^+-K^+-ATPase antiporter.

Sodium Ion Transport. Sodium ions freely enter tubular fluid from the glomerulus, so fluid entering the proximal convoluted tubule has the same sodium ion concentration as blood. The proximal convoluted tubule removes from the tubular fluid two thirds of the sodium ions presented to it. The transporters at this site include sodium symporters of glucose, amino acids, or phosphate, and antiporters of sodium exchanged with hydrogen ions. In the ascending limb of Henle's loop, sodium ions are removed from tubular fluid by the symporter of Na^+, K^+, and Cl^- (see Figure 46-1). In the distal tubule, sodium is removed by a symporter of Na^+ and Cl^- as well as an antiporter of Na^+ and H^+. When tubular fluid reaches the end of the distal tubule, nearly 99% of the sodium that entered the tubular fluid from the glomerulus has been reabsorbed. Final adjustments to regulate sodium excretion occur in the collecting duct, where the adrenal steroid **aldosterone** promotes sodium reabsorption.

Chloride Ion Transport. Chloride reabsorption occurs at all tubular sites where sodium ions are reabsorbed (see Figure 46-1).

Potassium Ion Transport. Potassium is not the only ion involved in the action of any diuretic except those drugs classified as potassium sparing. The major diuretics are

designed to relieve edematous conditions by reducing the tubular reabsorption of sodium, chloride, and water, which are the principal constituents of edema fluid. Potassium ions do not play a significant role in edema formation. Even so, diuretics also affect the renal excretion of potassium, which has potentially detrimental consequences for patients if serum potassium concentration is not properly monitored during treatment.

Most of the filtered potassium is reabsorbed in the proximal tubule and ascending limb of the loop of Henle such that potassium that appears in the urine will have been added to tubular fluid by secretion from distal tubule and collecting ducts (see Figure 46-1). Indeed, the effects of diuretics to decrease or increase the tubular reabsorption of potassium are entirely linked to the secretion of potassium in the distal portion of the nephron, not to potassium reabsorption. The secretion of potassium in the distal segments of the nephron is directly linked to the reabsorption of sodium at those same sites (see below).

Water Reabsorption. Water may be reabsorbed from the proximal convoluted tubule, the descending limb of the loop of Henle, and the collecting ducts. The ascending limb of the loop of Henle is relatively impermeable to water. In the proximal tubule, water flows into the interstitium and then into the blood by following the osmotic gradient created by the transport of sodium, chloride, and other ions into the interstitium. Final urine concentration is achieved primarily in the collecting duct. Removal of water at this site is regulated by antidiuretic hormone (ADH), which increases permeability of the tissue to water. The water then moves from the tubule to the hypertonic medullary interstitium.

Bicarbonate Reabsorption. Bicarbonate, the main buffer in blood, freely enters tubular fluid from glomeruli and must be reabsorbed for the body to maintain proper acid-base balance. This reabsorption occurs in the proximal convoluted tubule and depends on the enzyme **carbonic anhydrase.** Carbonic anhydrase converts carbonic acid in tubular fluid to carbon dioxide and water. The carbonic acid forms when a bicarbonate ion in the filtrate combines with a hydrogen ion. The carbon dioxide, being electrically uncharged and lipid soluble, then passes freely across the membranes of cells lining the tubules. Once inside the cell, carbonic acid catalyzes the conversion of carbon dioxide and water back into carbonic acid, which immediately dissociates into bicarbonate ions and hydrogen ions. The bicarbonate ions are then transported back to blood by a symporter of sodium and bicarbonate. This symporter exists only in the membrane on the blood side of the tubular cell, thus necessitating the enzymatic conversion of bicar-

TABLE 46-1

Diuretic Effects on Tubular Transport of Ions

Drug	Excretion Increased				Excretion Reduced			
Loop diuretics	Na^+	K^+	Ca^{++}	Cl^-	Uric acid	$(Li^+)*$		
Thiazides and related drugs	Na^+	K^+		Cl^-	Uric acid	$(Li^+)*$	$(Ca^{++})*$	
Potassium-sparing diuretics	Na^+		Ca^{++}		Uric acid	$(Li^+)*$	K^+, H^+	
Carbonic anhydrase inhibitors	Na^+	K^+	Ca^{++}		Uric acid			Cl^-
Osmotic diuretics	$(Na^+)†$	$(K^+)†$		$(Cl^-)*$				

Ca^{++}, calcium ion; Cl^-, chloride ion; H^+, hydrogen ion; K^+, potassium ion; Li^+, lithium ion; Na^+, sodium ion.
NOTE: The effects on ion transport shown are those commonly observed in humans during long-term therapy with normal clinical doses. With prolonged therapy, ions whose excretion is increased may become depleted from the body, whereas those whose excretion is blocked may accumulate. Lithium ion accumulation is clinically important only for those patients receiving lithium carbonate therapy for bipolar disorder. Uric acid accumulation is usually important only for those patients predisposed to gout.
*Excretion reduced because diuretic-induced volume depletion causes compensatory increases in reabsorption.
†In large doses.

bonate in tubular fluid to carbon dioxide to facilitate the net reabsorption of bicarbonate.

Organic Ion Transport.   The kidneys rapidly secrete complex organic ions such as amino acids and other natural compounds. This secretion occurs in late portions of the proximal tubule. Many drugs, including several diuretics, are themselves organic ions and enter tubular fluid by this transport mechanism. Because some diuretics work only from within the tubule, the action of the drug depends at least in part on the proper function of this transporter.

Mechanism of Diuretic Action

The diuretics discussed in this chapter achieve their effects mainly by increasing sodium chloride excretion. Because osmotic forces cause water to follow these ions as they are moved across renal membranes, water is also excreted when sodium and chloride are excreted; hence the diuresis. The sites of action of the classes of diuretics are shown in Figure 46-1. Specific patterns of ion excretion produced by these drugs are summarized in Table 46-1, and mechanisms are discussed in detail in the following sections.

DRUG CLASS • Loop Diuretics

bumetanide (Bumex)

ethacrynic acid (Edecrin)

 furosemide (Lasix, Apo-Furosemide,✶ Novosemide✶)

torsemide (Demadex)

MECHANISM OF ACTION

Bumetanide, ethacrynic acid, furosemide, and torsemide (see Table 46-1) are called **loop diuretics** because the primary site of their diuretic action is in the loop of Henle. These drugs inhibit the powerful symporters of Na^+, K^+, and Cl^- in the ascending limb of the loop of Henle (see Figure 46-1). Therefore increased amounts of sodium chloride stay in tubular fluid and are excreted in urine with the osmotic equivalent of water. The higher than normal delivery of sodium ions to the dis-

tal tubule and collecting duct promotes the exchange of sodium for potassium and hydrogen ions, increasing the urinary excretion of both ions. This exchange contributes nothing to the diuretic action of the drugs but may produce serious depletion of potassium and hydrogen ions, leading in time to hypokalemia and **metabolic alkalosis**. Calcium excretion also increases in response to these drugs (see Table 46-1).

Although all loop diuretics are similar in their mechanism of action and maximum diuretic efficacy, bumetanide is much more potent than other loop diuretics. For example, 1 mg of bumetanide given orally is as effective as approximately 40 mg of furosemide.

USES

Because loop diuretics promote the loss of excess salt and water, they can relieve edematous conditions such

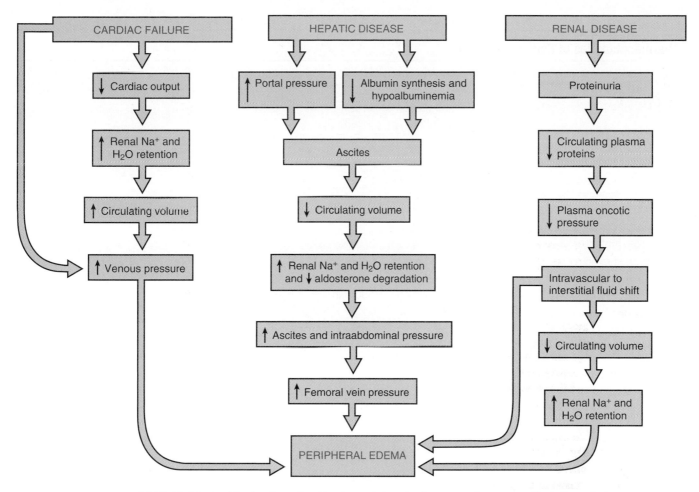

FIGURE 46-2 Mechanisms leading to peripheral edema, a primary manifestation of alteration in capillary dynamics as well as sodium and water balance caused by cardiac failure, hepatic disease, and renal disease.

as those occurring in heart failure, renal disease, and hepatic cirrhosis (Figure 46-2). In fact, the loop diuretics are by far the most effective drugs in this class for mobilizing edema fluid, causing the elimination of up to 30% of the filtered salt and water. Loop diuretics are also effective antihypertensive drugs, although the **thiazides** are the diuretics of choice for this application (see following drug class). Because loop diuretics also increase urinary calcium excretion, they are used to treat hypercalcemia.

PHARMACOKINETICS

Loop diuretics are well absorbed from the GI tract and generally increase urine flow within 1 hour of administration. With intravenous doses, diuresis occurs within 5 to 10 minutes (see Table 46-2).

Ethacrynic acid should not be given by intramuscular or subcutaneous injection, because the drug can cause severe pain and irritation at the injection site. Torsemide is also only used intravenously. Other loop diuretics can be given intramuscularly, but the intravenous route is preferred for parenteral administration.

Loop diuretics are extensively bound to plasma proteins and are not readily available for glomerular filtration. However, because the organic ion transporter in the proximal tubule readily secretes the drugs, they have ready access to their binding site on the Na^+-Cl^- transporter in the thick ascending limb of the loop of Henle. Were it not for tubular secretion, these drugs would not be effective diuretics.

The elimination of loop diuretics is primarily renal, because of their rapid and efficient secretion in the proximal tubule, but some biotransformation to active and inactive products occurs. In moderate renal failure the elimination half-life of torsemide is unchanged, but a relatively inactive metabolite accumulates.

```
TABLE 46-2
```

Pharmacokinetics of Selected Diuretics

Drug	Route	Onset	Peak	Duration	PB (%)	$t_{1/2}$	BioA (%)
Loop Diuretics							
bumetanide	po	30-60 min	1-2 hr	4-6 hr	95	1-1.5 hr	100
	IV	minutes	15-30 min	0.5-1 hr	95		100
ethacrynic acid	po	30 min	2 hr	6-8 hr	95	30-70 min	UA
	IV	5 min	15-20 min	2 hr	95		100
furosemide	po	60 min	1-2 hr	6-9 hr	95	2 hr	60
	IV	5 min	30 min	2 hr	95		100
torsemide	po	60 min	1-2 hr	6-8 hr	98	2-4 hr	80
	IV	10 min	1 hr				
Thiazides							
bendroflumethiazide	po	1-2 hr	6-12 hr	6-12 hr	UA	3-3.9 hr	UA
chlorothiazide	po	2 hr	4 hr	6-12 hr	95	1-2 hr	10
	IV	15 min	30 min	6-12 hr	UA		100
cyclothiazide	po	6 hr	7-12 hr	18-24 hr	UA	UA	UA
hydrochlorothiazide	po	2 hr	4 hr	6-12 hr	65	1-2 hr	UA
hydroflumethiazide	po	1-2 hr	3-4 hr	18-24 hr	UA	17 hr	UA
methyclothiazide	po	2 hr	6 hr	24 hr	UA	UA	UA
polythiazide	po	2 hr	6 hr	24-48 hr	UA	25 hr	UA
trichlormethiazide	po	2 hr	6 hr	24 hr	UA	2-7 hr	UA
Nonthiazide Diuretics							
chlorthalidone	po	2 hr	4-6 hr	24-72 hr	UA	40 hr*	UA
metolazone	po	1 hr	2 hr	12-24 hr	33	8 hr	UA
quinethazone	po	2 hr	6 hr	18-24 hr	UA	UA	UA
Potassium-Sparing Diuretics							
amiloride	po	2 hr	6 hr	24 hr	40	6-9 hr	20
spironolactone	po	8 hr	2-4 hr	48 hr	90	17-22 hr	UA
triamterene	po	2-4 hr	2-4 hr	72 hr	60	2-4 hr	UA
Carbonic Anhydrase Inhibitors							
acetazolamide	po	1 hr	2-4 hr	6-12 hr	90	13 hr	UA
	SR	2 hr	8-12 hr	18-24 hr			UA
dichlorphenamide	po	1 hr	2-4 hr	6-12 hr	UA	UA	UA
methazolamide	po	2-4 hr	6-8 hr	10-18 hr	Moderate	14 hr	UA
Osmotic Diuretics							
mannitol	IV	30-60 min	IOP: 30-60 min Diuresis: 6-12 hr	4-8 hr	UA	15 min-1.5 hr	UA
urea	IV	15 min	IOP: 1-2 hr Diuresis: 6-12 hr	5-6 hr	UA	3-4 hr	UA

BioA, bioavailability; *IOP*, intraocular pressure; *PB*, protein binding; *SR*, sustained release; $t_{1/2}$, elimination half-life; *UA*, unavailable.
*Chlorthalidone is sequestered in red blood cells; the $t_{1/2}$ is longer if blood rather than plasma is analyzed.

ADVERSE REACTIONS AND CONTRAINDICATIONS

Electrolyte depletion, marked by weakness or lethargy, dizziness, leg cramps, anorexia, vomiting, and possibly mental confusion, may occur gradually during treatment with loop diuretics. GI disturbances common with loop diuretics include diarrhea, loss of appetite, and stomach pain or cramping. Ethacrynic acid causes GI disturbances more often than other loop diuretics, especially in patients receiving the drug continually for several months. A sudden, severe, watery diarrhea indicates that the drug should be withdrawn.

Orthostatic hypotension is a common reaction with these powerful diuretics because of the large fluid losses (with accompanying reduction of blood volume) they cause. Patients who tend to rise quickly from a sitting or lying position must learn to move slowly to accommodate the shift in blood pressure. The most serious danger to such patients comes from the risk of injury from falls.

Loop diuretics increase the loss of potassium and calcium ions as well as sodium and chloride ions (see Table 46-1). Excessive potassium loss impairs proper functioning of the heart, skeletal muscle, kidneys, and other organs. Many health care providers routinely prescribe potassium replacement for patients receiving loop diuretics for prolonged periods. Dietary sources of extra potassium sometimes are sufficient for preventing excessive urinary losses of potassium, but potassium supplements may be required (see Appendix A).

Calcium losses associated with loop diuretics are rarely severe enough to produce tetany. In fact, most patients do not even require calcium replacement, but serum calcium levels should be monitored periodically. Uric acid excretion is partially blocked by loop diuretics. In susceptible patients gout may develop in association with the accumulation of uric acid, but for most patients the increase in serum uric acid produces no symptoms.

Loop diuretics affect ion transport in several organs other than the kidneys. Altered sodium and potassium transport may be associated with toxicity to certain cells in the inner ear. Transient or permanent deafness has been observed in patients receiving loop diuretics, especially those who receive high doses or who have reduced renal function. The drug may accumulate to toxic concentrations in such patients. Ototoxicity is more likely with ethacrynic acid than with other loop diuretics.

These diuretics impair glucose tolerance in some patients and may, albeit rarely, precipitate diabetes mellitus. Some patients experience sensitivity to sunlight while taking furosemide. Ethacrynic acid and furosemide may activate lupus erythematosus. Large doses of bumetanide may cause severe muscle pain (myalgia), chest pain, and premature ejaculation.

TOXICITY

Loop diuretics are the most effective diuretics in use today. Their rapid, powerful action must be carefully monitored to avoid profound dehydration and salt depletion. Dehydration with reduction in blood volume can precipitate circulatory collapse. Vascular thromboses and emboli may be generated, especially in older adults.

INTERACTIONS

There are many drug interactions with loop diuretics (Table 46-3). The potassium-depleting effect of these drugs makes them dangerous for patients receiving cardiac glycosides. Reduced potassium content in cardiac tissue predisposes the heart to toxicity from cardiac glycosides, the effects of which may include fatal arrhythmia. Corticosteroids also deplete potassium and may add to the danger of electrolyte imbalance when given with these diuretics.

Loop diuretics may inhibit the renal clearance of lithium, a drug used to control manic cycles in manic-depressive psychosis (see Chapter 18). Accordingly, lithium may accumulate in the blood and severe toxicity may occur. Patients undergoing lithium treatment should not take loop diuretics.

The ototoxic effect of loop diuretics may be potentiated by aminoglycoside antibiotics, which are also ototoxic (see Chapter 29). This combination should be avoided because permanent deafness may result.

When given with loop diuretics, amphotericin B has the potential for increasing the risk of nephrotoxicity, ototoxicity, and hypokalemia.

Finally, loop diuretics may displace other drugs from their binding sites on plasma proteins. This action increases the concentration of the free, active form of the displaced drug. The anticoagulant warfarin is displaced in this way by these drugs. Higher concentrations of unbound warfarin produce increased anticoagulant effects and may produce toxicity.

TABLE 46-3

Drug-Drug Interactions of Selected Diuretics

Drugs	Interactive Drugs	Interactions
Carbonic anhydrase inhibitors	Thyroid drugs	Decreased uptake of thyroidal iodine
	methenamine	Alkalinization of urine, interferes with action of interactive drug
	Salicylates	Severe metabolic acidosis and salicylate toxicity
	quinidine, amphetamines, ephedrine, pseudoephedrine, flecainide	Alkalinization of the urine, promotes reabsorption of interactive drug
Loop diuretics	Oral hypoglycemic drugs	Increased potential for hyperglycemia
	Aminoglycosides, cisplatin	Increased potential for ototoxicity
	lithium carbonate, salicylates	Decreased elimination of lithium and salicylates; lithium or salicylate toxicity
	digoxin	Increased potential for digoxin toxicity related to potassium loss
	NSAIDs	Decreased antihypertensive and diuretic effect of diuretic
	Neuromuscular blockers	Increased effects of neuromuscular blockers
	phenytoin	Decreased absorption and effectiveness of furosemide
	Theophyllines	Increased diuresis from furosemide
Thiazide and thiazide-like drugs	Antihypertensive drugs	Increased action of antihypertensive
	digoxin	Increased potential for digoxin toxicity due to potassium loss
	Oral hypoglycemics, insulin	May cause hyperglycemia and hyponatremia, resulting in thiazide resistance
	Corticosteroids, ACTH	Increased loss of potassium
	probenecid	Decreased uric acid elimination; may precipitate gout
	lithium carbonate, salicylates	Decreased elimination of lithium or salicylates; lithium or salicylate toxicity
	NSAIDs	Decreased antihypertensive effect of thiazide
	Depolarizing skeletal muscle relaxants	Increased responsiveness to skeletal muscle relaxants
	methenamine	Neutralized effect of methenamine because of alkaline urine from thiazides
	Cation exchange resins	Decreased absorption of thiazides if taken concurrently
Potassium-sparing diuretics	Other potassium-sparing diuretics, potassium supplements, ACE inhibitors	Increased risk of hyperkalemia
	digoxin	Decreased elimination of digoxin; digoxin toxicity
	Salicylates	Decreased effectiveness of spironolactone
	Antihypertensives	Increased effectiveness of antihypertensive drug
	norepinephrine	Decreased vascular response to norepinephrine
Osmotic diuretics	lithium	Decreased effectiveness of lithium in presence of mannitol

ACE, Angiotensin-converting enzyme; *ACTH,* adrenocorticotropic hormone; *NSAIDs,* nonsteroidal antiinflammatory drugs.

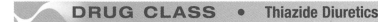

DRUG CLASS • Thiazide Diuretics

bendroflumethiazide (Naturetin)

⚠ chlorothiazide (Diuril)

hydrochlorothiazide (Esidrix, HydroDIURIL)

hydroflumethiazide (Diucardin, Saluron)

methyclothiazide (Aquatensen, Enduron)

polythiazide (Renese)

trichlormethiazide (Metahydrin, Naqua)

MECHANISM OF ACTION

Thiazide diuretics block sodium and chloride ion reabsorption in the distal tubule by inhibiting the Na^+-Cl^- symporter (see Figure 46-1). Because this transporter affects only about 10% of the filtered sodium, the maximal diuretic effect possible with these drugs is substantially less than that for the loop diuretics. Accordingly, the risk of dangerous depletion of extracellular fluid volume occurring with these drugs is relatively low, although it is not negligible.

USES

Because thiazide diuretics are less effective than loop diuretics, they are generally considered safer for use by outpatients. These drugs control edema associated with heart or renal disease as well as that caused by corticosteroid or estrogen therapy. The use of thiazide diuretics for the treatment of hypertension is discussed in Chapter 41. Hydrochlorothiazide is one of the most widely used drugs in this class.

PHARMACOKINETICS

Thiazide diuretics are well absorbed from the GI tract and take action in the kidneys within 1 hour of ingestion. Peak diuretic action occurs within 2 to 6 hours after an oral dose, depending on which thiazide and dosage form are used. Formulations differ in timing and duration of diuretic effects (see Table 46-2).

Thiazides are secreted into renal tubules by the organic anion pump. Most of an administered dose leaves the body by this route, but the liver, which secretes these drugs into bile, eliminates some of the drug.

Many drugs are available in this class of diuretics. They differ primarily in potency and duration of action. Several drugs in this class, the so-called nonthiazide diuretics, are structurally unrelated to the thiazides but behave in the body in similar fashion. The single effect that distinguishes this group from the true thiazide diuretics is their longer duration of action.

ADVERSE REACTIONS AND CONTRAINDICATIONS

Long-term use of thiazide diuretics can cause fluid and electrolyte imbalance characterized by thirst, weakness, lethargy, restlessness, muscle cramps, and fatigue. These effects are not unique to the thiazide diuretics but are caused by loop diuretics as well. The electrolyte imbalance most likely to occur results from excessive urinary losses of potassium and chloride ions. The loss of potassium leads to hypokalemia, and the loss of chloride leads to metabolic alkalosis. Potassium supplements may be required.

Thiazide diuretics initially increase urinary calcium excretion, but if the ensuing urinary losses of salt and water are large enough to cause a deficit of extracellular fluid volume, the reabsorption of glomerular filtrate, including calcium, will undergo a compensatory increase in the proximal tubule, leading to reduced calcium excretion and net calcium retention. The treatment of edematous conditions with a thiazide diuretic does not usually require depletion of the extracellular fluid volume; rather, the rationale for the treatment is merely to eliminate the edema. The rationale for using a thiazide diuretic to promote calcium retention applies to pathologic conditions of hypocalcemia, which normally are not edematous.

Thiazide diuretics often inhibit uric acid excretion, which increases the blood level of urate and may precipitate an attack of gout in susceptible individuals.

Thiazide diuretics irritate the gastrointestinal tract and may cause adverse effects ranging from simple nausea and vomiting to constipation, jaundice, and pancreatitis.

Thiazides are usually not to be given to patients with severe impairment of renal function or anuria, because the drugs are less likely to be effective in these patients.

TOXICITY

Thiazides may cause CNS symptoms such as dizziness, headache, and paresthesia. At high concentrations, such as those found in drug overdose, mental lethargy may progress to coma, although heart function and respiration are not markedly depressed. Overdose requires stomach evacuation as well as monitoring of electrolyte balance and renal function.

INTERACTIONS (see Table 46-3)

The hypotensive effect of thiazide diuretics adds to the action of other antihypertensive drugs. Accordingly, several drug manufacturers provide formulations consisting

---

TABLE 46-4

Drug Combinations Including Thiazide or Thiazide-like Diuretics

Thiazide or Thiazide-like Diuretics in Combination with	
ACE inhibitors	captopril with hydrochlorothiazide (Capozide) enalapril maleate with hydrochlorothiazide (Vaseretic) lisinopril with hydrochlorothiazide (Zestoretic, Prinzide) quinapril with hydrochlorothiazide (Accuretic)
Alpha blockers	prazosin with polythiazide (Minizide)
Beta blockers	atenolol with chlorthalidone (Tenoretic) bendroflumethazide with nadolol (Corzide) labetalol HCL with hydrochlorothiazide (Normozide) metoprolol with hydrochlorothiazide (Lopressor HCT) nadolol with bendroflumethiazide (Corzide) pindolol with hydrochlorothiazide (Viskazide✳) propranolol with hydrochlorothiazide (Inderide LA) pimolol with hydrochlorothiazide (Timolide)
Centrally acting antihypertensives	clonidine with chlorthalidone (Combipres) guanethidine with hydrochlorothiazide (Esimil) methyldopa with chlorothiazide (Aldoclor) methyldopa with hydrochlorothiazide (Aldoril)
Angiotensin II blockers	gandesartan with hydrochlorothiazide (Atacand HCT) irbesartan with hydrochlorothiazide (Avalide) losartan with hydrochlorothiazide (Hyzaar) telmisartan with hydrochlorothiazide (Micardis HCT) valsartan with hydrochlorothiazide (Diovan HCT)
Potassium-sparing diuretics	amiloride with hydrochlorothiazide (Moduretic, Moduret✳) spironolactone with hydrochlorothiazide (Aldactazide) triamterene with hydrochlorothiazide (Dyazide, Maxzide)

ACE, Angiotensin-converting enzyme.
✳ Available only in Canada.

---

of a thiazide diuretic and another antihypertensive drug, such as captopril, in the same tablet. Such formulations are commonly referred to as fixed-dose combinations because it is not possible to adjust the dose of one drug, such as by breaking a tablet in half, without altering the dose of the second drug. Some physicians consider the fixed, unalterable dosage of these products to be a shortcoming, but many patients view the convenience of taking one tablet instead of two as an advantage. A list of the most widely prescribed thiazide-antihypertensive combinations is provided in Table 46-4. The pharmacology of antihypertensive drugs is covered in Chapter 41.

Thiazide-induced excretion of potassium may be enhanced when thiazide diuretics are given with corticosteroids or adrenocorticotropic hormone (ACTH). Regardless of the cause, hypokalemia may make patients more sensitive to digoxin toxicity.

Thiazide diuretics often alter the requirement for insulin or other hypoglycemic drugs. A patient with diabetes who must receive one of the thiazides should be carefully observed during the first few days of thiazide therapy to prevent loss of diabetes control.

Thiazides reduce lithium excretion. The increased danger of lithium toxicity prevents the safe concurrent use of these two drugs.

Cholestyramine and colestipol are solid resins used orally to treat hyperlipidemias (see Chapter 42). These drugs can reduce absorption of thiazide diuretics.

DRUG CLASS • Potassium-Sparing Diuretics

amiloride (Midamor)

spironolactone (Aldactone)

triamterene (Dyrenium)

Potassium-sparing diuretics (see Table 46-2) are rather weak diuretics that reduce the urinary loss of potassium. These drugs are often used in combination with loop or thiazide diuretics to counteract the tendency of those drugs to enhance urinary potassium losses.

MECHANISM OF ACTION

Amiloride and triamterene inhibit sodium channels found in the distal tubule and collecting duct. The movement of sodium ions through these channels normally provokes excretion of potassium by an exchange mechanism (see Figure 46-1). Inhibition of the sodium channels by amiloride and triamterene inhibits the exchange, thereby reducing urinary losses of potassium.

Spironolactone competitively inhibits binding of the mineralocorticoid hormone aldosterone to its intracellular receptor. Aldosterone bound to its receptor normally induces proteins in the nucleus of the cell to activate sodium channels in the late distal tubule and collecting duct, thereby promoting sodium reabsorption. Movement of sodium ions through these channels evokes excretion of potassium ions by the exchange mechanism discussed above. By binding to the aldosterone receptor, spironolactone reduces sodium reabsorption and urinary losses of potassium. Aldosterone is present in greater than normal amounts in edematous states resulting from heart failure, nephrotic syndrome, and hepatic cirrhosis. Spironolactone is most effective when aldosterone levels are high.

USES

Amiloride, spironolactone, and triamterene can be used to control edema in heart failure, cirrhosis of the liver, and nephrotic syndrome. Spironolactone may lessen the effects of excessive aldosterone levels in patients with the endocrine disorder hyperaldosteronism. It may also be useful in treating hypertension and reversing potassium loss. Amiloride is also used for hypertension.

PHARMACOKINETICS

Spironolactone, a steroid derivative, is not highly water soluble but is formulated using very fine particles to improve absorption from the GI tract. Peak therapeutic effects with this drug are observed several days after treatment begins (see Table 46-2). This delay is related to the mechanism of action of the drug and is not a result of delay in absorption or other pharmacokinetic properties of the drug. Spironolactone is extensively biotrans-

formed, much the same as the natural mineralocorticoids it chemically resembles. Metabolites of spironolactone appear in urine and in lesser quantities in bile.

Triamterene, although not a steroid like spironolactone, is also relatively insoluble in water. Intestinal absorption is somewhat variable but usually satisfactory. Elimination is by hepatic and renal mechanisms. The peak effect of triamterene is usually observed within a day.

Amiloride is more water soluble than either triamterene or spironolactone and is excreted primarily by the kidneys. About 50% of an oral dose is recovered unchanged in urine within 48 hours of administration.

Spironolactone is highly protein bound in the blood, whereas triamterene is only moderately bound, and amiloride exists primarily as free drug.

ADVERSE REACTIONS AND CONTRAINDICATIONS

The potassium retention caused by spironolactone, triamterene, and amiloride may cause dangerous increases in serum potassium concentration. Patients with impaired renal function or high potassium intake are especially at risk. The earliest sign of **hyperkalemia** (high levels of potassium in the blood) may be an irregular heartbeat. Fatal arrhythmia can occur.

Spironolactone can cause various endocrine alterations, because the drug chemically resembles not only mineralocorticoids but also androgens and progestins. Women may observe menstrual irregularities, hirsutism, and deepening of the voice. Men may observe gynecomastia and have difficulty in achieving or maintaining erection. Symptoms in both sexes are usually reversed when the drug is discontinued.

Spironolactone produces tumors in rodents exposed to the drug for long periods; carcinomas have been reported in breasts of both men and women taking this drug, but controlled trials have not been performed to prove cause and effect. Nevertheless, the use of spironolactone should be restricted to cases in which the benefit clearly outweighs this risk. Spironolactone should not be used to control edema in pregnancy. If lactating women use the drug, breast-feeding should be discontinued because its metabolites appear in breast milk.

Triamterene and amiloride may produce a reversible azotemia revealed by an increased BUN level. Triamterene has also been linked to blood dyscrasias and to photosensitivity. Skin rashes, GI disturbances (especially with spironolactone), dizziness, and fever have been observed in patients receiving potassium-sparing diuretics.

All potassium-sparing diuretics are contraindicated for patients with hyperkalemia or those who may be prone to develop hyperkalemia. Examples of the latter include hypertensive patients being treated with ACE inhibitors (e.g., captopril) or AII blockers (e.g., losartan).

TOXICITY

Patients who overdose on potassium-sparing diuretics should have their stomachs evacuated. Electrolyte balance and renal function should be carefully monitored.

INTERACTIONS (see Table 46-3)

Two potassium-sparing diuretics should not be administered concurrently, nor should these drugs be administered to a patient receiving potassium supplements or ingesting a diet high in potassium.

Use of potassium-sparing diuretics with antihypertensives may require reduction in doses of the latter because spironolactone, triamterene, and amiloride may have additive antihypertensive effects. When spironolactone is combined with other diuretics, dosages may require reduction. Spironolactone can prevent distal tubular reabsorption of sodium, making diuretics that act upstream of this site in the nephron even more effective. Amiloride is less effective than spironolactone or triamterene when given in combination with hydrochlorothiazide.

Anticoagulant drugs are more potent when given with potassium-sparing diuretics, which may result in excessive anticoagulation and the risk of bleeding.

Potassium-sparing diuretics may promote lithium retention and toxicity and should not be used in patients who are being treated with lithium. Spironolactone increases the half-life of digoxin, leading to accumulation of that substance. Careful monitoring and dosage adjustment is required to keep the level of digoxin in the blood in a safe range.

 DRUG CLASS • **Carbonic Anhydrase Inhibitors**

acetazolamide (Diamox, Acetazolam❋)

dichlorphenamide (Daranide)

methazolamide (Neptazane)

MECHANISM OF ACTION

Bicarbonate ions are freely filtered at the glomerulus, but, by a quirk of nature, cannot be reabsorbed back into the blood as bicarbonate ions. Instead, the bicarbonate must be converted to a form that *can* be reabsorbed. The process begins after the bicarbonate ions have been filtered into proximal tubular fluid. There they form carbonic acid by combining with hydrogen ions secreted from the tubular cells. The enzyme carbonic anhydrase, located in the membranes of the tubular cells, then catalyzes the conversion of carbonic acid to carbon dioxide and water. The resulting carbon dioxide, which is uncharged and freely diffusable across cell membranes, then moves down its concentration gradient into the tubular cells, where the enzyme catalyzes its conversion with water back into carbonic acid. Being a weak acid, carbonic acid spontaneously dissociates into bicarbonate and hydrogen ions. The hydrogen ions cycle back into the tubular fluid to combine with more bicarbonate ions to keep the cycle going, and the bicarbonate ion formed within the cell is then transported from the cell back into the bloodstream.

Inhibition of carbonic anhydrase by one of the drugs in this class interrupts this efficient cycle for reabsorbing bicarbonate and forces elimination of the ion in the urine (with sodium and water). The urine thus produced is alkaline by virtue of its high concentration of bicarbonate.

The diuresis caused by carbonic anhydrase inhibitors normally lasts only a few days because plasma bicarbonate concentration eventually declines to a level at which the spontaneous conversion of bicarbonate to carbon dioxide prevents further urinary losses of bicarbonate. By this time, mild metabolic acidosis will have developed, which along with the excretion of alkaline urine, constitute the hallmarks of carbonic anhydrase inhibition.

USES

Carbonic anhydrase inhibitors are not used to treat edematous conditions, because the drugs cause the excretion mainly of sodium bicarbonate and not sodium chloride. Edema fluid will not be mobilized unless sodium ions are excreted with chloride ions.

The most common clinical use for carbonic anhydrase inhibitors is in the treatment of glaucoma, which is characterized by high intraocular pressure (see Chapter 65). Carbonic anhydrase is believed to be involved in the production of intraocular fluid, and inhibition of the enzyme slows the rate at which intraocular fluid is produced, thereby reducing pressure within the eyes.

Acetazolamide is used for treatment of a variety of convulsive disorders and for prevention and treatment of altitude sickness. It is believed, but not proven, that the drug's effectiveness against convulsive disorders may involve some retardation of neuronal conduction associated with elevated carbon dioxide tension in the CNS. The effectiveness of acetazolamide against altitude sickness may be related to the metabolic acidosis induced by the drug, but this mechanism is not yet understood.

PHARMACOKINETICS

Carbonic anhydrase inhibitors are well absorbed from the GI tract. The most widely used drug of this class, acetazolamide, is concentrated in the kidneys, where tissue levels may be two to three times the plasma concentration within 30 minutes to 2 hours of an oral dose. Acetazolamide enters tubules by the organic anion pump. The drug also inhibits carbonic anhydrase in other tissues.

Acetazolamide is sometimes given on alternate days rather than continuously. This regimen is designed to prevent the kidneys from becoming resistant to the action of the drug (e.g., to prevent bicarbonate depletion and the resulting metabolic acidosis). During the day without the drug, acetazolamide is cleared from the body, and bicarbonate levels in the blood are replenished. When the drug is readministered on the following day, it is as effective as when first given.

ADVERSE REACTIONS AND CONTRAINDICATIONS

Reactions to carbonic anhydrase inhibitors are uncommon, especially when they are used in intermittent or short-term therapy.

Carbonic anhydrase inhibitors are sulfonamide derivatives. Patients who are sensitive to thiazide diuretics, antibacterial sulfonamides, or other sulfonamide-related diuretics (e.g., furosemide) may have a cross-allergenicity to these drugs.

Carbonic anhydrase inhibitors act directly on the CNS, causing paresthesia, nervousness, sedation, lassitude, depression, headache, vertigo, and other symptoms. Patients may complain of unusual fatigue or weakness. The conditions of patients already experiencing respiratory acidosis may worsen from these drugs, which tend to produce metabolic acidosis.

Carbonic anhydrase inhibitors cause a range of GI symptoms, including diarrhea, loss of appetite, nausea, vomiting, metallic taste, and weight loss.

Carbonic anhydrase inhibitors are usually not given to patients at risk for electrolyte disturbances (e.g., those with adrenocortical insufficiency, hypokalemia, acidosis, hepatic disease, or renal failure).

TOXICITY

Renal function and acid-base balance must be carefully monitored in patients who have excessively high blood levels of carbonic anhydrase inhibitors.

INTERACTIONS (see Table 46-3)

Carbonic anhydrase inhibitors produce more marked excretion of potassium than sodium. Potassium depletion is therefore likely to occur. This possibility is made even more likely by combining carbonic anhydrase inhibitors with corticosteroids or ACTH. Digoxin toxicity is increased in the presence of low serum potassium levels.

Excretion of amphetamines, anticholinergics, mecamylamine, and quinidine is slowed because carbonic anhydrase inhibitors alkalinize urine. Alkaline urine also blocks the effects of the urinary antiseptic methenamine, which requires an acidic environment to be converted to formaldehyde, the active metabolite.

DRUG CLASS • Osmotic Diuretics

mannitol (Osmitrol)

urea (Ureaphil, Urevert)

MECHANISM OF ACTION

Osmotic diuretics are nonelectrolytes that are filtered by the glomerulus but are not significantly reabsorbed or metabolized. The high osmolality in tubules caused by the presence of these drugs reduces reabsorption of water, which increases the production of urine. With a high urine output, sodium excretion is somewhat increased, accompanied by smaller increases in potassium, calcium, chloride, and bicarbonate excretion.

USES

Osmotic diuretics are used clinically to prevent permanent renal damage during acute renal failure. The usefulness of osmotic diuresis in these cases often depends on maintaining adequate urine volume without altering electrolyte balance. Osmotic diuretics also increase the osmolality of plasma, which allows reduction of osmotic pressure inside the eye and in the CSF.

PHARMACOKINETICS

The drugs currently used as osmotic diuretics, mannitol and urea, are usually administered intravenously. Mannitol is the preferred drug. Mannitol and urea are rapidly distributed when administered intravenously. They are filtered by the glomeruli and eliminated unchanged in the urine. The elimination rate is reduced in patients with renal insufficiency (see Table 46-2).

ADVERSE REACTIONS AND CONTRAINDICATIONS

Pulmonary congestion, acidosis, thirst, blurred vision, seizures, nausea and vomiting, diarrhea, tachycardia, fever, and angina-like pain may be noted occasionally. Local irritation of the intravenous site with thrombophlebitis can also occur. Urea should not be used in patients with liver failure, because high levels of urea may place additional demands on liver function. Other contraindications to osmotic diuretics include active intracranial bleeding and marked dehydration. Safe use of the drugs during pregnancy and lactation as well as in children has not been established.

TOXICITY

Toxicity produced by these drugs depends on how much drug is administered and how much the drug affects fluid balance. These drugs are retained within the extracellular space and can cause an acute expansion of extracellular fluid volume during intravenous administration. This volume expansion may be hazardous to a patient with reduced cardiac reserve.

Fluid and electrolyte imbalances may develop, especially if a degree of renal impairment exists. Under these circumstances the diuretics tend to accumulate in the blood and may cause dangerous shifts in salt and water balance.

APPLICATION TO PRACTICE

ASSESSMENT
History of Present Illness

The patient who reports symptoms related to fluid volume excess should be asked the following questions:

- Has there been a change in the amount, color, or odor of the urine?
- Has there been dysuria, frequency, urgency, hesitation, or incontinence?
- Do you awake from sleep to void?
- Has there been unusual swelling around the eyes or in the hands or feet?
- Has there been an unexplainable change in your weight?
- Are rings, a wristwatch, or shoes too tight?
- Do you have leg swelling that increases during the day and decreases at night?
- Do your legs feel more swollen after you have been up during the day?

Furthermore, patients with fluid volume excess often report headache, anorexia, nausea, vomiting, and abdominal pain. Changes in mental status may include mood and personality changes, restlessness, confusion, and anxiety. Some patients may report shortness of breath or shallow respirations.

When evaluating symptoms, determine when they began. Does the patient consider them to be mild, moderate, or severe in nature? Is there something that aggravates or provokes the symptoms, and does the patient have methods for lessening or alleviating the symptoms?

Health History

The medical history may reveal a preexisting condition that contraindicates the use of certain diuretics or that requires special caution. A thorough history includes any known electrolyte imbalance, hypertension, cardiac disease, hepatic or renal dysfunction, diabetes, pregnancy and lactation, and allergies.

Patients with a history of diabetes, hypertension, heart failure, or liver or renal disease likely have a history of diuretic therapy, or the patient may be taking a drug that interacts with the diuretic that may be prescribed. Any prescription or OTC drugs as well as herbal supplements the patient is taking need to be documented.

Lifespan Considerations

Perinatal. Diuretics are not commonly used in pregnancy. Water retained during pregnancy increases blood volume and aids in providing nutrients to the fetus. There is no evidence supporting the notion that diuretics prevent the development of hypertension in pregnancy. In general, before diuretics are used, the effects of the drug must be weighed against the potential risk to the fetus. Furthermore, many diuretics are contraindicated for lactating patients because the diuretic passes into breast milk, exposing the infant to the drug.

Pediatric. In infants and children, the most common causes of heart failure are congenital heart disorders and rheumatic fever. These two conditions result in decreased renal blood flow and urinary insufficiency. Pediatric dosage considerations include the age and size of the child, with attention directed toward the reasons for administering the diuretic. Dosage should be calculated as 1 mg/kg of body weight.

Older Adults. Because of altered physiology and underlying diseases, older adults are more sensitive to diuretics and tend to experience more adverse effects than younger people. The renal function of older adults is diminished because of the normal changes of aging; thus they may be unable to handle shifts in electrolyte balance. For this reason, serum electrolyte levels (especially that of potassium) should be checked at least every 3 to 4 months.

Compliance with a drug regimen implies a few economic considerations. Older adults are generally taking several drugs at any given time and may not be able to afford all of them because of fixed incomes or Medicare restrictions. These patients sometimes exhibit poor nutritional status or a change in condition because they are using financial resources for drugs rather than for food. Furthermore, many of the lower-cost food choices are high in sodium. Failure to restrict sodium intake increases the potential for fluid volume excess and electrolyte imbalance.

Cultural/Social Considerations

In some instances, diuretics have been abused by those seeking quick weight loss. The abuse of diuretics has been observed in some obese individuals and in athletes who must meet a weight limit. (The diuretic is used before weigh-in, and the athlete later attempts to rehydrate before competition.) The use of diuretics for weight control is not justified in the absence of edematous conditions. Some patients, however, receive diuretics from more than one health care provider or from an authorized source (see the Case Study: Fluid Volume Excess).

Physical Examination

Physical assessment of the patient who requires a diuretic includes a baseline assessment of neurologic, cardiovascular, respiratory, renal, skin, and nutritional systems. Each system is assessed to detect real and potential problems that may compromise diuretic therapy.

Assessment of the patient's neurologic status includes orientation, mental status, cranial nerve testing, deep tendon reflexes, muscle strength, and hearing. Neurologic deficits may be attributed to other medical conditions such as uncontrolled diabetes or encephalopathy related to hepatic disease rather than to the diuretic.

Assessment of the patient's cardiovascular status includes, at minimum, blood pressure (lying, sitting, and standing), heart rate and rhythm, heart sounds, and peripheral pulses. Capillary refill should be noted, as well as the skin color, temperature, and turgor. A baseline ECG may also be appropriate. Changes in cardiovascular status indicative of fluid overload include an increased heart rate, the presence of an S_3 heart sound, blood pressure changes, jugular venous distention, and an increase in central venous pressure and pulmonary artery wedge pressure.

The respiratory assessment includes rate, depth, and pattern. The presence of adventitious breath sounds (e.g., crackles, wheezes, rales, rubs), if any, should be noted. Assessment of renal status includes measurements of fluid intake and output as well as any changes in weight.

Skin assessment factors to address include temperature, color, and turgor, as well as the presence and degree of edema. Edema is first seen in the submalleolar spaces in the ambulatory patient, and overlying the sacrum, flanks, and lateral thighs of a bedridden patient. When pressure is applied with a finger to an edematous area, the small depression that is left usually disappears within 30 seconds. This so-called pitting edema can be quantified further by measuring the depth of the depression in millimeters. Extremity circumference should be measured bilaterally. Comparisons made from side to side assist in determining and documenting the extent of the edema.

Local swelling that is firm and nonpitting is the major sign of capillary edema. The swelling results from the increased protein content of the edematous fluid. A severe form of such swelling is common in patients with lymphedema and is usually unilateral rather than bilateral.

Laboratory Testing

Much of the laboratory testing for the patient receiving diuretics is performed to monitor therapy and to watch for complications such as hypokalemia or hyperuricemia. Elevated BUN and creatinine levels suggest alterations in renal function. Elevated uric acid levels have been identified in 65% to 70% of patients treated with diuretics. However, signs and symptoms of gout rarely occur, and when they do, then only in susceptible individuals. Cholesterol and triglyceride levels should be monitored for elevation, particularly with prolonged use of diuretics. Blood gas values may be done for patients who are in respiratory distress caused by pulmonary edema.

A urinalysis is a helpful parameter. The volume of urine should be documented, as well as specific gravity, osmolality, and electrolytes before and after administration of a diuretic. A random sample may be obtained for a quick analysis, or a 24-hour collection may be required to evaluate therapy.

An ECG is important for some patients because of the risk of hypokalemia. This disorder manifests as flattened T waves.

GOALS OF THERAPY

Treatment goals for the patient with fluid volume excess or edema are to decrease that excess or edema, to improve hemodynamics, to bring intake and output volumes closer to equal, to increase the patient's ability to participate in activities of daily living and verbalize an understanding of the effects of medications, and to maintain or increase quality of life.

INTERVENTION
Administration

Determine the desired daily fluid balance with the health care provider. Read the package insert of the prescribed drug for precautions and intravenous administration rates, and question the patient about allergies to sulfonamides, thiazide diuretics, or other drugs before administering the first dose of a diuretic.

Administer intravenous diuretics slowly, following the manufacturer's recommendations. Discolored (yellow) injectable solutions should not be used. A slow administration rate decreases the risk of adverse effects. Be sure to check the intravenous site for extravasation because some drugs (e.g., chlorothiazide) are extremely alkaline. Furosemide is light sensitive and must be stored in light-resistant containers. In rare instances, a diuretic drug is administered by intramuscular injection. Furosemide given intramuscularly causes transient pain at the injection site. Be sure to warn the patient of the discomfort before administration.

Monitor the patient's blood pressure regularly while he or she is standing, sitting, and lying down. Compare the measurements from each arm. Although all patients receiving diuretics would be expected to have an initial drop in blood pressure, older adults, those receiving intravenous diuretics, and those also taking antihypertensive drugs may experience a more precipitous fall in blood pressure and in rare instances go into shock.

Weigh the patient who is in an acute care setting daily under standard conditions (i.e., at the same time every day [usually in the morning, after the patient has voided or the catheter bag emptied, but before breakfast]). Use the same scale each time and have the patient wear the same amount of clothing. Continuous weight gain should always be evaluated.

The bedpan or urinal must be readily available for the patient on bed rest. For some patients a urinary catheter may be needed initially for a short time. For the ambulatory patient, bathroom facilities should be readily available. Carefully measure and record fluid intake and output. Report unexpected findings to the health care provider. For example, oliguria or anuria are unexpected after an increase in the dose of a diuretic. Patients at home are not usually required to measure intake and output except in the case of severe kidney or heart disease, but encourage the patient to report abnormal output.

The patient should be evaluated for fluid volume deficit as well as for drug resistance. In the face of a shrunken intravascular volume, the part of the tubular system not affected by the diuretic reacts by reabsorbing more sodium. For this reason, it is important to obtain answers to the following questions.

- Is the patient compliant with sodium restriction requirements?
- Are the optimal drug and dosage being used?
- Are there electrolyte imbalances that should be corrected?
- Is the patient's general cardiovascular status optimal?
- Are inotropic drugs being used judiciously?

Signs of fluid volume deficit should also be evaluated, particularly if the patient has overresponded to the diuretic therapy. Changes in blood pressure or vital signs may be the first indication that the patient is experiencing excessive diuresis. Orthostatic hypotension may be a problem, putting the patient at a greater risk for falls.

Monitor serum electrolytes, glucose, uric acid, creatinine, and lipid levels. Observe for evidence of dehydration, including thirst, decreased skin turgor, nausea, light-headedness, weakness, increased pulse, oliguria, decreased blood pressure, and elevated hemoglobin, hematocrit, and BUN levels. Dehydration and hypovolemia can contribute to thromboembolic disorders. Assess the patient for pain in the chest, calves, and pelvis that may indicate thromboembolism. In addition, assess the patient for signs or symptoms of hyponatremia, hypokalemia, hypocalcemia, and metabolic (hypochloremic) alkalosis (see Table 64-1).

To monitor for fluid retention, measure the patient's abdominal girth or the circumference of one or both legs. To ensure accurate measurement, mark the patient's skin with small ink marks to indicate the correct placement of the tape measure from day to day. Check dependent areas daily for the presence of or changes in the amount of edema. In pitting edema, an indentation or depressed area made by the examiner's finger remains visible in the skin for seconds to minutes after the pressure has been released. Dependent areas where this is more likely to appear include the sacral area as well as the feet and legs.

Education

To reach the goals of diuretic therapy effectively, patient cooperation is most important. Compliance is best encouraged by teaching the patient about the disease process and the drugs used to treat the problem. Family members or significant others should be included in this teaching. Information to be included in the teaching plan includes the name of the drug, the dose, the reason for prescribing the drug, and the expected effects of taking the drug. The patient also needs to be aware of any special precautions and adverse reactions.

Teach the patient to take the diuretic as ordered; once-daily diuretics are taken in the morning. Twice-daily diuretics are taken in the morning and again before 6 PM to avoid interrupting sleep to urinate. For some patients, intermittent therapy (e.g., every other day or Monday-Wednesday-Friday) will achieve the desired effects with fewer adverse effects. Poor compliance may stem from patient annoyance caused by frequent or excessive urination. The patient should be advised to remain close to bathroom facilities the first few hours after taking the drug. Statistically, diuretics are associated with urinary incontinence, particularly in older adult women; thus patients may require information on how to manage the problem. A patient caught in an embarrassing situation is less likely to be compliant with drug therapy. At times, the peak period of drug activity interferes with work or leisure plans. Patients should be helped to adjust their schedule so as not to be caught in an embarrassing situation.

Instruct the patient to take oral doses of the diuretic with food to minimize gastric irritation. If a dose is missed, it should be taken as soon as remembered unless within a few hours of the next dose (this varies with the frequency of the dosing schedule), in which case it should be omitted and the regular dosing schedule resumed. Advise the patient not to double up for missed doses. Patients taking the oral liquid form of a diuretic should measure their dose with the calibrated dropper provided with the drug or to use a specially marked measuring spoon or medication cup to measure the dose.

Teach patients the importance of taking potassium supplements if prescribed, and work with them to find a formulation they are willing to take. Many effervescent formulations are unpalatable. Enteric-coated tablets have been implicated in small bowel ulceration. Oral solutions are the preferred formulation, but they often taste unpleasant. Dilute these solutions in juice or milk to reduce the risk of gastric irritation and to make the taste tolerable. Instruct patients to take potassium with meals to reduce gastric irritation. Encourage patients with hypokalemia to increase their dietary intake of potassium-rich foods (see Appendix A). A dietitian may assist with the teaching in some cases.

Caution the patient taking diuretics not to use salt substitutes without first consulting with the health care provider. Salt substitutes contain a variety of electrolyte salts, and the exact proportions may vary from product to product. A patient may inadvertently contribute to electrolyte abnormalities by using a salt substitute. For example, a patient taking a potassium-sparing diuretic may develop hyperkalemia if a salt substitute containing a high portion of potassium salts is used.

The patient should be taught to identify and avoid foods high in sodium content (see Appendix A). Fast foods, canned foods, and prepackaged foods are often high in sodium and sugar. Many of the foods that are beneficial for the patient to prepare and consume, however, require more time and effort in preparation and are more costly.

If appropriate to their ability and resources, teach patients who are at home how to keep daily or weekly weight records. Instruct patients to report to the health care provider weight gains or losses greater than 2 pounds per day or 5 pounds per week unless otherwise instructed.

Postural hypotension can occur in patients taking diuretics. It is important that the patient sit up a few minutes before standing to minimize these effects. Another adverse reaction is photosensitivity. Advise patients to wear appropriate sunscreen, a hat, and protective clothing on arms and legs, as well as to report any episodes of delayed sunburn or the development of a rash.

If the diuretic is prescribed for hypertension, emphasize the importance of taking all drugs prescribed, even if the patient has no symptoms of hypertension. Explain to the patient that drug therapy for hypertension may be required for life. Emphasize the importance of continuing all other therapies (i.e., weight loss, sodium restriction, stopping smoking, regular exercise, and antihypertensive drugs).

Explain to the patient that diuretics are not to be used for weight loss purposes (Box 46-1).

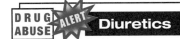

DRUG ABUSE ALERT   **Diuretics**

Background
Patients obsessed with weight loss may abuse diuretics. The acute weight loss produced by these drugs has been exploited by some diet clinics that may initiate the program with a diuretic so that dramatic weight loss will occur early; however, this weight loss is short-lived and related only to water loss. The lost weight returns as soon as the person rehydrates. Such acute weight loss is also occasionally exploited in high school and college wrestling programs—the drugs enable a wrestler to meet a weight limit at weigh-in, and the athlete usually attempts to rehydrate before wrestling. Patients who are obsessed with excretory functions and use the drugs to achieve large volumes of urine excretion may also abuse diuretics. Such patients may also abuse cathartics.

Pharmacology
Diuretics promote an acute loss of body water and therefore cause an immediate drop in body weight. The amount of diuresis is related to the dose and strength of the drug used and also to the patient's water balance.

Health Hazards
The use of diuretics over several days or longer can cause severe electrolyte imbalances, especially if patients are not receiving careful counseling on dietary practices. If patients are receiving diuretic or other drugs from more than one physician or from unauthorized sources, follow-up care to monitor for the development of side effects may be lacking. The use of these drugs in weight control is unjustified, especially in healthy young athletes with no preexisting edema.

EVALUATION

Evaluation of the effectiveness of diuretic therapy is based on the pretreatment goals. In most cases, the optimum outcome includes an informed patient and family who understand the disease processes and the treatment regimen, a reduction in symptoms as a result of compliance with the plan of care, dietary guidelines, and minimum adverse effects related to therapy. The decrease in uncomfortable symptoms such as swollen feet and legs, puffy hands, or dyspnea on exertion may be sufficient incentive to comply with the regimen.

With effective therapy, the patient's urine output increases, electrolyte balance is corrected or maintained, and edema is decreased. If these goals are not met, a review should be undertaken to develop realistic goals with the patient and family that take into consideration the limits of the patient's illness.

CASE STUDY

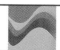

Fluid Volume Excess

ASSESSMENT

HISTORY OF PRESENT ILLNESS

JR is a 60-year-old white man in moderate distress who reports recurring dyspnea and increased edema in his lower extremities over the last 2 weeks. He has also noted a gradual increase in shortness of breath on exertion, orthopnea, nocturia, and edema in his lower extremities. He notes that he is compliant with his drug regimen but has problems staying on his sodium-restricted diet. He has no complaints of chest pain or diaphoresis.

HEALTH HISTORY

JR denies allergies to food or prescription drugs. He has a history of previous hospitalizations for cardiomyopathy, heart failure, and renal insufficiency, the last of which was 4 weeks ago. He has no known history of hypertension. He has a history of smoking but stopped 2 years ago. He denies alcohol use. Current drugs include enalapril 5 mg po qd; digoxin 0.25 mg po qd; furosemide 80 mg po bid. JR has a documented history of noncompliance with planned treatment regimens.

LIFESPAN CONSIDERATIONS

In older adults, relatively minor illnesses may precipitate decompensation that can rapidly progress to a severe state. Warning signs, such as those seen in patients with heart failure, and a history of prolonged weight gain of as little as 2 pounds per week warrant special attention.

CULTURAL/SOCIAL CONSIDERATIONS

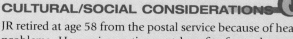

JR retired at age 58 from the postal service because of health problems. He receives retirement benefits from the postal service and for his military service. He visits his health care provider on a regular basis. He first began having health problems at age 52, before which he rarely sought medical care. He is married with two children and six grandchildren. He receives much emotional support from his family.

PHYSICAL EXAMINATION

JR is 5'11" tall and weighs 189 pounds (an increase of 20 pounds since discharge from hospital 2 weeks ago); his vital signs are: BP 148/82 mm Hg, respirations 24, apical heart rate 96 beats/min and regular. He has wet crackles at the bases of his lungs, distended jugular veins, and 4+ pitting edema bilaterally from his feet to his mid-thighs; S_3 heart sound is present.

LABORATORY TESTING

Laboratory findings unremarkable except for a BUN of 52 mg/dL and plasma creatinine of 2.2 mg/dL.

PATIENT PROBLEM(S)

Heart failure; cardiomyopathy; renal insufficiency.

GOALS OF THERAPY

Relieve symptoms of fluid volume excess; improve exercise tolerance and the quality of life; improve hemodynamics and prolong survival.

CRITICAL THINKING QUESTIONS

1. What questions would you ask to assess for compliance with present therapy regimen?
2. Describe the mechanism of action of furosemide.
3. Why would JR be susceptible to digitalis toxicity?
4. What signs and symptoms would you assess JR for or teach him to report to his health care provider related to digitalis toxicity or hypokalemia?
5. Which class of diuretics has the highest degree of efficacy?
6. A BUN of 52 mg/dL and creatinine of 2.2 mg/dL gives a BUN/creatinine ratio of 24:1 (normal range is 10:1 to 20:1). What might this elevated ratio lead the provider to suspect? Why is JR at risk?

Bibliography

Brater DC: Pharmacology of diuretics, *Am J Med Sci* 319(1):38-50, 2000.

Dumont L, Mardirosoff C, Tramer MR: Efficacy and harm of pharmacological prevention of acute mountain sickness: quantitative systematic review, *Br Med J* 321(7256):267-272, 2000.

Greenberg A: Diuretic complications, *Am J Med Sci* 319(1):10-24, 2000.

Hardman J, Limbird L, Gilman A, eds: *Goodman and Gilmans' The pharmacologic basis of therapeutics*, ed 10, New York, 2001, McGraw-Hill.

Moser M: Diuretics revisited—again, *J Clin Hypertens* 3(3):136-138, 2001.

Rasool A, Palevsky PM: Treatment of edematous disorders with diuretics, *Am J Med Sci* 319(1):25-37, 2000.

Internet Resources

The Altruis Biomedical Network d-Kidneys.net website summarizes function and drugs. Available online at http://www.e-kidneys.net/diuretics.html.

The National Library of Medicine and the National Institutes of Health sponsor Medline plus Health Information, with entries for all classes of diuretics. Available online at http://www.nlm.nih.gov/medlineplus/druginfo/uspdi/202208.html.

http://www.nlm.nih.gov/medlineplus/druginfo/uspdi/202205.html.

http://www.nlm.nih.gov/medlineplus/druginfo/uspdi/202206.html.

Drugs to Treat
Renal Dysfunction

LYNN ROGER WILLIS • KATHLEEN GUTIERREZ

 Visit http://evolve.elsevier.com/Gutierrez/ for additional information.

KEY TERMS

Acute renal failure (ARF), p. 762

Acute tubular necrosis (ATN), p. 762

Azotemia, p. 762

Chronic renal failure (CRF), p. 763

Intrarenal causes, p. 762

Postrenal obstruction, p. 763

Prerenal failure, p. 762

OBJECTIVES

- Relate the physiologic and pathophysiology changes that occur with renal dysfunction.

- Identify the treatment goals of drug therapy for the patient with renal dysfunction.

- Identify the principles of drug dosing for the patient with renal disease.

- Explain the patient and laboratory parameters that are available to support and monitor drug therapy.

- Recognize drug interactions that may be clinically significant for the patient with renal dysfunction.

- Create a nursing care plan for a patient with renal failure who is receiving drugs from multiple classes.

PATHOPHYSIOLOGY • Renal Failure

The kidneys receive 20% to 25% of the cardiac output every minute and are very sensitive to changes in blood supply. A number of prerenal and intrarenal events can cause a critical fall in renal perfusion pressure (supplied by the arterial pressure of the blood), which may reduce renal blood flow (RBF). When RBF is diminished, the nutrients and oxygen for basic renal cellular metabolism and tubular transport systems are also diminished. Further, when RBF decreases, the fundamental driving force for glomerular filtration, the arterial blood pressure, may also be reduced. A reduction in renal perfusion pressure may result in a further decline in RBF because vasoconstrictive hormones, including angiotensin, vasopressin, and catecholamines, will have been released in response to the fall in perfusion pressure. As a result, glomerular filtration may no longer be maintained. A failure of glomerular filtration reduces urine flow and causes blood urea nitrogen (BUN) and creatinine levels in the blood to rise. Correcting the factors that contribute to reduced RBF helps reestablish adequate circulation, thereby preventing ischemic injury.

ACUTE RENAL FAILURE

Acute renal failure (ARF) is defined as a sudden, rapid, partial or complete loss of renal function that occurs over a matter of hours or, at most, a few days. The failure may be oliguric (less than 500 mL of urine excreted per day) or nonoliguric (more than 800 mL of urine per day) and is usually accompanied by azotemia. **Azotemia** is a buildup of nitrogenous waste in the blood.

Acute renal failure can occur in seriously ill people of any age, sex, or community, and in any hospital unit or extended care facility. Numerous renal insults can cause acute renal failure, but the acute syndrome, unlike chronic renal failure, is usually reversible.

The causes of ARF are divided into three groups based on anatomic location: prerenal, intrarenal, and postrenal (Figure 47-1 and Table 47-1). **Prerenal failure** occurs when there is a loss or shift of circulating blood volume, decreased cardiac output, decreased peripheral vascular resistance, or renal vascular obstruction.

Acute tubular necrosis (ATN) is the most common cause of intrarenal azotemia and of ARF in general. Acute tubular necrosis is basically ARF caused by ischemia or toxins, or both. Urinary output in ATN is related to the number of injured nephrons and the location of the injury (i.e., cortex versus medulla). Approximately 50% of patients with ATN have oliguric renal failure. **Intrarenal causes** of ARF are the most serious, and have the greatest morbidity and mortality. Other intrarenal causes of ARF include trauma, infection, glomerulonephritis, and vascular lesions.

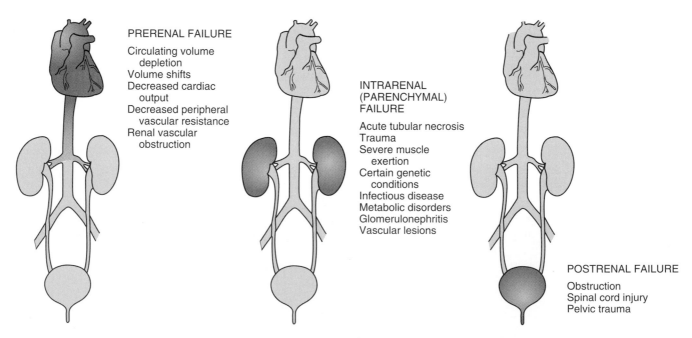

PRERENAL FAILURE

Circulating volume
    depletion
Volume shifts
Decreased cardiac
    output
Decreased peripheral
    vascular resistance
Renal vascular
    obstruction

INTRARENAL
(PARENCHYMAL)
FAILURE

Acute tubular necrosis
Trauma
Severe muscle
    exertion
Certain genetic
    conditions
Infectious disease
Metabolic disorders
Glomerulonephritis
Vascular lesions

POSTRENAL FAILURE

Obstruction
Spinal cord injury
Pelvic trauma

FIGURE 47-1 Anatomic location of prerenal, intrarenal, and postrenal failure. (From Black JM, Matassarin-Jacobs E: *Medical-surgical nursing: clinical management for continuity of care,* ed 6, Philadelphia, 2001, Saunders.)

Postrenal obstruction is the major cause of postrenal azotemia, accounting for 2% to 15% of all cases of ARF and the second most common cause of ARF in infants.

ARF is characterized by an initial oliguric phase, followed in 10 to 14 days to a few weeks by a diuretic phase. Problems seen during the oliguric phase include an inability to eliminate solute loads, regulate electrolytes, and eliminate metabolic waste. During the diuretic phase, large amounts of dilute urine (4 to 5 L/day) and electrolytes are lost. The recovery phase may take as long as 6 months to a year before renal function returns to normal.

CHRONIC RENAL FAILURE

Chronic renal failure (CRF) develops insidiously over several years. More than 100 different disease processes contribute to a progressive loss of renal function, but diabetes mellitus and hypertension account for over 60% of patients who develop end-stage renal disease (ESRD) in the United States. The third most common cause of CRF is glomerulonephritis, an inflammation of the glomeruli that frequently follows streptococcal infec-

tions of the upper respiratory tract. Acute glomerulonephritis can completely resolve or progress to chronic glomerulonephritis and eventual renal failure.

Chronic renal failure is characterized by histologic evidence of irreversible renal damage, which progresses in three stages. Initially, there is diminished renal reserve without accumulation of metabolic wastes. The unaffected kidney compensates for decreased function of the diseased kidney. The failure then moves from mild to severe renal insufficiency, involving the steady accumulation of metabolic waste products in the blood. Severe fluid and electrolyte imbalances develop. The patient ultimately enters ESRD, which ends with dialysis, transplant, or death.

As renal failure progresses, the progressive failure of multiple systems leads to anemia, uremia, disorders of calcium and phosphorus biotransformation, and acidosis. Anemia, an expected complication of advanced renal failure, primarily results from the inability of diseased kidneys to manufacture erythropoietin. However, it can be further aggravated by deficiencies of iron and certain vitamins. Although iron

---

TABLE 47-1

Causes of Renal Failure

Prerenal Factors	
Hypovolemia	Hemorrhage, burns, shock, excessive sweating, GI losses, peritonitis, nephrotic syndrome, diuretics, diabetes insipidus
Altered peripheral vascular resistance	Antihypertensive drugs, sepsis, drug overdose, anaphylaxis, neurogenic shock
Cardiac disorders	Heart failure, myocardial infarction, cardiac tamponade, arrhythmias
Renal artery disorders	Emboli, thrombi, stenosis, aneurysm, occlusion, trauma
Drug-induced hepatorenal syndrome	ACE inhibitors, NSAIDs
Intrarenal Factors	
Inflammatory processes	Bacterial, viral, preeclampsia
Immune processes	Autoimmunity, hypersensitivity, rejection
Trauma	Penetrating injury (e.g., knife, bullet), nonpenetrating injury (e.g., fall, crushing injury, motor vehicle accident, sports injury)
Obstruction	Neoplasm, stones, scar tissue
Systemic and vascular disorders	Diabetes mellitus, systemic lupus erythematosus (SLE), sickle cell disease, multiple myeloma, renal vein thrombosis
Drug induced	Anesthetics, antimicrobials, NSAIDs, antineoplastics, contrast media
Nephrotoxins	Tumor toxins, heme pigments (e.g., hemoglobin, myoglobin), pesticides, fungicides, organic solvents, heavy metals, mushrooms, snake venom
Postrenal Factors	
Obstruction	Congenital anomalies (e.g., ureteropelvic stricture), benign prostatic hypertrophy (BPH), pelvic cancer, trauma, surgical injury

ACE, Angiotensin-converting enzyme; *GI,* gastrointestinal; *NSAIDs,* nonsteroidal antiinflammatory drugs.

deficiency is not uncommon in renal failure alone, it is common in patients who are maintained on hemodialysis for long periods of time. The anemia is a consequence of continued blood sampling for diagnostic studies and losses associated with the dialysis. Because of recombinant DNA technology, the anemic state can now largely be prevented and cured with epoetin alfa (see Chapter 36).

The uremic state is associated with abnormal platelet function that manifests as prolonged bleeding times and a predisposition to bleeding. A number of abnormal mechanisms contribute to the potential for bleeding. Platelet factor III activity is decreased; there are decreased levels of thromboxane A_2, increased levels of the platelet inhibitor prostacyclin, and suboptimal activity of factor VIII (von Willebrand's factor). The defects in platelet function can be partially corrected by repeated dialysis. Desmopressin acetate (DDAVP), a synthetic analog of ADH, increases von Willebrand's factor concentrations and shortens bleeding times.

Disorders of calcium and phosphorus metabolism, including hypocalcemia, hyperphosphatemia, secondary hyperparathyroidism, bone disease, and metastatic calcification, are common findings in patients with advanced renal failure. These disturbances are largely a consequence of the kidneys' inability to eliminate phosphate, synthesize the active metabolite of vitamin D (calcitriol) (see Chapter 63), and eliminate hydrogen ions. Retention of phosphorus results in hyperphosphatemia, promoting soft tissue calcification and suppression of serum calcium levels. The hypocalcemia, in turn, causes secondary hyperparathyroidism and promotes bone disease. The hyperparathyroid state is further intensified by an inability of the diseased kidney to synthesize calcitriol, which normally exerts a suppressive effect on parathyroid hormone synthesis. Therapy is directed at normalizing serum phosphorus levels and suppressing the hyperparathyroid state. This goal can be accomplished by administering phosphate binding drugs and calcitriol, a vitamin D supplement.

Acidosis represents a compounding factor in the genesis of bone disease. The patient with CRF has a positive hydrogen ion balance as a result of the inability to eliminate diet-derived acids. The retained hydrogen ions are thought to be buffered by bone salts, resulting in the dissolution of bone. Sodium bicarbonate given orally effectively corrects the acidosis and prevents the dissolution of bone.

PHARMACOTHERAPEUTIC OPTIONS

The management of a patient with renal failure ordinarily includes multidrug therapy, diet therapy, and dialysis. Managing drug therapy in patients with renal disease is a complex endeavor because of the numerous drugs used. As the patient's renal function deteriorates, adjustments in dosages are repeatedly required.

Drug classes used in the management of renal failure include angiotensin-converting enzyme (ACE) inhibitors, antianemia drugs, iron supplements, antihemorrhagic drugs, phosphate binders, vitamin D supplements, heavy metal antagonists (chelating drugs), systemic antacids, loop diuretics, vasopressors, and cation-exchange resins.

DRUG CLASS • Angiotensin-Converting Enzyme (ACE) Inhibitors

captopril (Capoten)

Other ACE inhibitors (see Chapter 41)

MECHANISM OF ACTION

The conversion of angiotensin I to angiotensin II is blocked by ACE inhibitors. By blocking angiotensin II formation, efferent arteriolar vasoconstriction is reduced and the stimulus for secretion of the mineralocorticoid hormone, aldosterone, is diminished. Withdrawal of angiotensin II–induced constriction of efferent arterioles reduces filtration pressure, which when high, damages the glomerular basement membrane and increases the permeability of the membrane to proteins, resulting in proteinuria. Consequently, ACE inhibitors reduce proteinuria and help to restore normal glomerular filtration. Decreased aldosterone secretion reduces sodium retention caused by the hormone, promotes the excretion of excess salt and water, and normalizes arterial blood pressure. Overall, the ACE inhibitors slow the rate of renal deterioration in CRF.

USES

The major goal in the treatment of CRF is to slow the progression of renal failure to ESRD and alleviate the complications and consequences of advancing renal failure. Captopril and other ACE inhibitors are most useful in patients with type 1 diabetic nephropathy who have decreasing renal function, but the ACE inhibitors are also thought to exert similar effects in all types of proteinuric renal diseases.

PHARMACOKINETICS

The pharmacokinetic characteristics of captopril are summarized in Table 47-2. The pharmacokinetics of other ACE inhibitors are discussed in Chapter 41.

TABLE 47-2

Pharmacokinetics of Selected Drugs Used to Treat Renal Dysfunction*

Drug	Route	Onset	Peak	Duration	PB (%)	$t_{1/2}$	BioA (%)
ACE Inhibitors							
captopril	po	15-60 min	0.5-1.5 hrs	6-12 hr	25-36	1.5-2 hr	65
Antianemic Drugs							
epoetin alfa	IV/SC	7-14 days	2-6 wks†	2 wks	UA	4-13 hr	UA
Iron Supplements							
ferrous formulations	po	4 days	7-10 days‡	2-3 months	UA	UK	UA
Iron dextran	IM	Slow	1-2 wks	Months	UK	6 hr	UK
Antihemorrhagic Drug							
desmopressin acetate	IV/SC	Min	15-30 min	90-120 min	UA	75 min	100
	IN	1 hr	1-5 hrs	8-20 hr	UA	75 min	10-20
Phosphate-Binding Drugs							
aluminum hydroxide§	po	Hr to days	Days to wks	Days	UA	UK	UA
calcium salts	po	UK	UK	UK	45	UK	UK
	IV	Immed	Immed	0.5-2 hr	45	UK	100
Vitamin Supplement							
calcitriol	po	2-6 hr	2-6 hr	1-5 days	Variable	3-8 hr	UK
Heavy Metal Antagonist							
deferoxamine	IM/IV/SC	UK	UK	UK	UA	1 hr	UK
Loop Diuretic							
furosemide	po	30-60 min	1-2 hr	6-8 hr	95	30-60 min	60
	IV	5 min	30 min	2 hr	95	UA	100
Vasopressor							
dopamine	IV	1-2 min	10 min	Duration of infusion	UA	2 min	100
Systemic Antacids							
sodium bicarbonate	po	Immed	30 min	1-3 hr	UA	UK	UK
	IV	Immed	Rapid	UK	UA	UK	100
Cation-Exchange Resin							
kayexalate	po	2-12 hr	UK	6-24 hr	UA	UK	0
	PR	2-12 hr	UK	4-6 hr	UA	UK	0

BioA, bioavailability; *IM*, intramuscular; *IN*, intranasal; *IV*, intravenous; *PB*, protein binding; *SC*, subcutaneous; $t_{1/2}$, elimination half-life; *UA*, unavailable; *UK*, unknown.

*Therapeutic serum drug levels for these renal drugs are not routinely measured.

†Epoetin alfa: peak effect, which is the targeted hematocrit level, may be achieved in 8 weeks with adequate dosing. Elevation in red blood cell count lasts for approximately 2 weeks following discontinuation of the drug.

‡Peak levels and the amount of iron absorbed are approximately in linear relationship to dose ingested.

§Aluminum hydroxide has hypophosphatemic effects when given orally.

ADVERSE REACTIONS AND CONTRAINDICATIONS

Adverse reactions of ACE inhibitors include skin rash, hypotension, angioedema, and cough. A major adverse effect noted in patients with renal failure is hyperkalemia. Hyperkalemia results from reduced circulating aldosterone concentrations. A loss of taste perception may also occur, which may lessen after 2 to 3 months of therapy. ACE inhibitors are contraindicated in patients with hypersensitivity. These drugs are pregnancy category C for the first trimester, but are considered category D for the remainder of the pregnancy. They are avoided, if possible.

INTERACTIONS

There are several potentially adverse interactions between ACE inhibitors and other drugs used in the treatment of renal failure. The concurrent use of nonsteroidal antiinflammatory drugs (NSAIDs) may reduce the antihypertensive effect of captopril by inhibiting the synthesis of renal prostaglandin or causing sodium and water retention. Concurrent use of diuretics and some antihypertensive drugs with ACE inhibitors produces additive hypotensive effects. See Chapter 41 for additional discussion of drug interactions with ACE inhibitors.

 DRUG CLASS • Antianemia Drug

epoetin alfa (erythropoietin, EPO, Epogen, Procrit)

MECHANISM OF ACTION

Epoetin alfa induces erythropoiesis by stimulating the division and differentiation of erythroid progenitor cells (see Chapter 36). Newly formed reticulocytes are released from the bone marrow and mature to erythrocytes. Clinically significant increases in the reticulocyte count occur within 7 to 10 days of starting treatment with epoetin alfa, with a rise in hemoglobin and hematocrit occurring in 2 to 6 weeks.

USES

Anemia universally accompanies chronic renal disease. In fact, hematocrit values of 16% to 22% were common in the days before epoetin alfa was available. Epoetin alfa is now a well-accepted drug for the treatment of the anemia associated with CRF.

Epoetin alfa is not a substitute for blood transfusions and is not intended as an emergency treatment for severe anemia or blood loss. However, it has decreased the transfusion dependency of many patients with CRF. Patients treated with this drug have an increase in hematocrit, improved energy, and less fatigue. Other favorable outcomes include improvements in cardiovascular status and cognitive function, exercise tolerance, and quality of life.

Epoetin alfa is also indicated for the management of anemia secondary to zidovudine therapy in patients with human immunodeficiency virus. Patients with nonmyeloid malignancies who have anemia secondary to antineoplastic therapy may also be candidates for epoetin alfa.

PHARMACOKINETICS

Epoetin alfa is well absorbed following subcutaneous and intravenous administration; its distribution, bio-

transformation, and elimination are presumed to be the same as natural erythropoietin. An increase in reticulocyte count is observed in 7 to 14 days with peak activity noted in 2 to 6 weeks. The increase in RBC counts lasts for approximately 2 weeks following discontinuation of the drug. The half-life of epoetin alfa is 4 to 13 hours (see Table 47-2).

ADVERSE REACTIONS AND CONTRAINDICATIONS

Hypertension is the most common adverse effect of epoetin alfa. Headache, transient rashes, and thrombotic events (in patients on dialysis) are also possible. Female patients may have a resumption of menses and fertility may be restored; therefore, the risk of pregnancy should be evaluated.

Although they are rare, seizures are the most serious adverse effect, occurring in about 1.1% of the patients receiving epoetin alfa. If the hematocrit increases more than four points in a 2-week period, the likelihood of a hypertensive reaction and seizures increases.

Epoetin alfa is contraindicated in patients with hypersensitivity to albumin or mammalian cell–derived products or in those with uncontrolled hypertension. It is also contraindicated in patients with erythropoietin levels exceeding 200 mU/mL. The drug should be used cautiously in patients with a history of seizures. Safe use during pregnancy, lactation, or in children has not been established.

INTERACTIONS

There are few drug interactions with epoetin alfa. The drug may increase the requirement for heparin in patients on dialysis or interfere with drug control of blood pressure.

DRUG CLASS • Iron Supplements

ferrous fumarate (Femiron, Feostat, Fumasorb, Fumerin, Hemocyte, Ircon, Palafer✱)

ferrous gluconate (Apo-Ferrous Gluconate,✱ Fergon, Ferralet, Simron)

ferrous sulfate (Apo-Ferrous Sulfate,✱ Feosol, Ferospace, Fer-In-Sol, Fer-Iron, Fero-Grad,✱ Fero-Gradumet Filmtabs, Ferralyn, Ferra-TD, Mol-Iron, PMS-Ferrous Sulfate,✱ Slow Fe)

iron dextran (Imferon, InFeD)

MECHANISM OF ACTION

Iron is an essential mineral found in hemoglobin, myoglobin, and a number of enzymes, and it is necessary for effective erythropoiesis and for the transport and utilization of oxygen. Parenteral iron enters the bloodstream and organs of the reticuloendothelial system (i.e., liver, spleen, bone marrow), where it is separated from the dextran complex and becomes part of the body's iron stores.

USES

Patients on dialysis are prone to iron deficiency because of repeated blood testing, surgical interventions, and blood loss during hemodialysis. A minority of dialysis patients will have an increase in hematocrit and symptomatic improvement with correction of iron deficiency alone. However, iron is a necessary component of erythropoiesis. Therapy with epoetin alfa will be hindered if patients do not have adequate iron stores.

PHARMACOKINETICS

In general, only 5% to 10% of dietary iron is absorbed. In deficiency states, this may increase to 30%. Iron supplements are well absorbed following intramuscular administration. Iron remains in the body for many months (see Table 47-2), crosses the placenta, enters breast milk, and is over 90% protein bound. Iron supplements are mostly recycled, with small daily losses occurring through desquamation, sweat, urine, and bile.

ADVERSE REACTIONS AND CONTRAINDICATIONS

Oral iron preparations are usually well tolerated, although nausea, epigastric pain, constipation, diarrhea, abdominal cramping, GI bleeding, and black stools may result. Contact irritation of the throat may occur with oral formulations, particularly liquids. Hypotension is the most common adverse reaction of parenteral iron. Headache, dizziness, syncope, tachycardia, urticaria, flushing, arthralgias, and phlebitis have also been reported. Seizures and anaphylaxis are the most serious adverse reactions.

Iron supplements are contraindicated in patients with primary hemochromatosis, hemolytic anemias, and other anemias not associated with iron deficiency. They should be used with caution in patients with peptic ulcers, ulcerative colitis, or regional enteritis, whose conditions may be aggravated. Some products contain alcohol or tartrazine and should be avoided in patients with known intolerance or hypersensitivity. Indiscriminate use of iron supplements may lead to iron overload. Patients with autoimmune disorders and arthritis are more susceptible to allergic reactions. Extreme caution should be used when administering iron supplements to patients with severe liver impairment.

INTERACTIONS

Iron preparations may decrease the antimicrobial actions of fluoroquinolone antibiotics if they are taken concurrently. The absorption of iron is decreased when it is taken with antacids, and the effectiveness of levodopa is decreased. Serum iron levels may increase when iron preparations are taken with chloramphenicol. Because there are no physiologic means of removing toxic amounts of iron from the body, a heavy metal antagonist (e.g., deferoxamine) may be needed to chelate the iron.

 DRUG CLASS • Heavy Metal Antagonist

deferoxamine (Desferal)

MECHANISM OF ACTION

Deferoxamine has a strong affinity for trivalent iron and aluminum, forming soluble stable complexes (chelates) that are readily eliminated by the kidney or removed with dialysis. One hundred milligrams of deferoxamine binds 8.5 mg of ferric iron or 17 mg of aluminum.

USES

Deferoxamine alleviates bone pain, muscle weakness, and the anemia that results from iron and aluminum toxicities. It is also used in the management of secondary iron overload syndrome associated with multiple transfusion therapy. Musculoskeletal symptoms and anemia are ordinarily corrected in 2 or 3 months. Aluminum neurotoxicity is more resistant to treatment, with 6 months to 1 year of continuous therapy required before improvement is noted.

PHARMACOKINETICS

Deferoxamine is poorly absorbed by the GI system following oral administration; therefore, it must be given intramuscularly or subcutaneously. It is rapidly biotransformed by tissue and plasma enzymes, with a serum half-life of approximately 1 hour (see Table 47-2). The chelated complexes that are formed have an extended plasma half-life. Elimination is totally dependent on either renal function or removal by dialysis. Thirty-three percent of iron is removed through biliary elimination.

ADVERSE REACTIONS AND CONTRAINDICATIONS

The most common adverse reactions to deferoxamine are fever, tachycardia, diarrhea, and abdominal discomfort. A red coloration to the urine, anaphylactic reactions, auditory neurotoxicity, and ocular toxicity has been reported. Hypotension, shock, skin rash, hives, itching, and wheezing can result and are often caused by too-rapid infusion of deferoxamine. Because deferoxamine is a naturally occurring iron siderophore (a molecule facilitating iron uptake), it acts as a growth factor for *Yersinia* and *Rhizopus* (mucormycosis). In susceptible individuals, deferoxamine increases the proliferation and virulence of these organisms, resulting in severe, often fatal, infection.

INTERACTIONS

Ascorbic acid improves the chelation action for iron and increases the amount of iron eliminated. However, deferoxamine should be used judiciously because concurrent use enhances tissue iron toxicity, especially in the heart, causing cardiac decompensation.

 DRUG CLASS • **Antihemorrhagic Drug**

desmopressin acetate (DDAVP, Stimate)

MECHANISM OF ACTION

DDAVP is a synthetic polypeptide structurally related to the posterior pituitary hormone, antidiuretic hormone (ADH). The mechanism for antihemorrhagic action is unclear, but DDAVP is thought to increase factor VIII activity. DDAVP-induced vasoconstriction may also aid in reducing the tendency to bleed.

USES

DDAVP is effective in reversing the bleeding disorder present in uremia and is useful for preventing postrenal biopsy bleeding. It is also used in the management of diabetes insipidus caused by a deficiency of vasopressin and to control bleeding in certain types of hemophilia and von Willebrand's disease (factor VIII deficiency).

PHARMACOKINETICS

Ten to twenty percent of DDAVP is absorbed from the nasal mucosa when given intranasally, and it is 100% bioavailable when given intravenously (see Table 47-2). DDAVP is biotransformed by the kidney with a half-life of 75 minutes. The onset of drug effects when DDAVP is given intranasally is 1 hour, with peak activity noted in 1 to 5 hours. The intranasal form of DDAVP has a duration of action of 8 to 20 hours. The onset of drug action occurs within minutes of intravenous administration. Peak effects are noted in 15 to 30 minutes, with a duration of action of 3 hours.

ADVERSE REACTIONS AND CONTRAINDICATIONS

The major adverse reactions of DDAVP are mild hypertension (caused by constriction of vascular smooth muscle) and water retention (caused by increased permeability of the renal collecting ducts to water). Other adverse reactions include rhinitis, headache, nausea, and abdominal or stomach cramps. Large intravenous doses can cause tachycardia. Phlebitis at the intravenous injection site is possible. Water intoxication and hyponatremia are possible after long-term use.

Desmopressin is contraindicated in patients with hypersensitivity to DDAVP or hypersensitivity to chlorobutanol, and in patients with type IIB or platelet-type (pseudo) von Willebrand's disease. It should be used with caution in patients with angina pectoris or hypertension. Safe use during pregnancy and lactation has not been established.

INTERACTIONS

When used in the presence of chlorpropamide, clofibrate, or carbamazepine, DDAVP may elicit an enhanced diuretic response. Demeclocycline, lithium, or norepinephrine may diminish the antidiuretic response to desmopressin.

DRUG CLASS • Phosphate-Binding Drugs

aluminum hydroxide (AlternaGEL, Alu-Cap, Alu-Tab, Amphojel, Basaljel, Dialume, Nephrox)

calcium acetate (Phos-Ex, PhosLo)

calcium carbonate (Apo-Cal,✶ Calcite,✶ Calsan,✶ Caltrate, Maalox Antacid Caplets, Mylanta Lozenges,✶ Nephro-Calci, Nu-Cal,✶ Os-Cal, Rolaids Calcium Rich, Titrilac, Tums, others)

MECHANISM OF ACTION

Patients with renal failure often have a buildup of phosphate. Calcium salts prevent absorption of dietary phosphorus from the GI tract by combining with phosphorus to form the insoluble compound calcium phosphate. Aluminum hydroxide binds phosphate in the GI tract to lower serum phosphate levels.

USES

Phosphate-binding drugs are used in renal failure to normalize serum phosphorus levels and to decrease the severity of secondary hyperparathyroidism and the incidence and severity of bone disease. The major drugs in this class include calcium carbonate and calcium acetate. Aluminum hydroxide may be used as a phosphate binder in adults when calcium compounds prove ineffective. Overall, the use of aluminum hydroxide as a phosphate binder is discouraged because of the potential for aluminum-induced neurotoxicity.

PHARMACOKINETICS

Absorption of calcium salts from the GI tract requires the presence of vitamin D. Elimination is mostly through the feces, with only 20% eliminated by the kidneys (see Table 47-2). The half-life of calcium salts has not been determined.

Aluminum salts are absorbed poorly when given orally, but over time substantial amounts of aluminum may accumulate. Absorbed aluminum distributes widely in the body and concentrates in the central nervous system. Aluminum is mostly eliminated in the feces.

ADVERSE REACTIONS AND CONTRAINDICATIONS

The major adverse reactions of calcium salts are mild GI complaints such as diarrhea, gas, and constipation. Hypercalcemia may also occur, but it is unusual if the patient takes the calcium compounds with meals and they are not receiving vitamin D supplements. Arrhythmias have been noted with excess calcium intake. The phosphate depletion that results in bone disease can be induced with excessive use of calcium.

Calcium salts are contraindicated in patients with hypercalcemia, renal calculi, or ventricular fibrillation. They should be used cautiously in patients receiving cardiac glycosides, and in patients who have severe respiratory insufficiency, or renal or cardiac disease.

Aluminum is retained in patients who have uremia causing severe skeletal, hematopoietic, and neurologic toxicity. Children with renal failure should not receive aluminum-containing phosphate binding compounds because of the risk of aluminum toxicity.

Aluminum hydroxide is contraindicated in patients with severe abdominal pain of unknown cause. It should be used with caution in patients with hypercalcemia or hypophosphatemia. Use during pregnancy is generally considered safe, although chronic high-dose therapy should be avoided.

INTERACTIONS

Calcium compounds prevent the absorption of other elements (e.g., iron), antibiotics (i.e., tetracyclines, fluoroquinolones), and digoxin. Calcium acetate should not be given with other calcium supplements.

Aluminum hydroxide should not be taken concurrently with compounds containing citrate (i.e., sodium citrate, calcium citrate) because they markedly enhance the absorption of aluminum.

 DRUG CLASS • Vitamin D Supplement

calcitriol (Rocaltrol)

MECHANISM OF ACTION

Calcitriol is a synthetic steroid hormone identical to that synthesized by the renal proximal tubule cells. Calcitriol is the active form of vitamin D and binds to receptors in the small intestine to promote the production of a calcium-binding protein. The calcium-binding protein is essential for the absorption of dietary calcium and phosphorus.

USES

Calcitriol, a fat-soluble vitamin and a synthetic form of vitamin D_3, is well accepted in the treatment of CRF. It replaces a hormone that can no longer be synthesized by the diseased kidney. Calcitriol also suppresses parathyroid hormone production and improves bone disease resulting from secondary hyperparathyroidism. To achieve maximum suppression of parathyroid hormone levels and improve bone disease, a treatment regimen of a year or more may be needed.

PHARMACOKINETICS

Calcitriol is readily absorbed from the small intestine following oral administration (see Table 47-2). It is bound in the serum to alpha globulins. The onset of action occurs in 2 to 6 hours, with a duration of action of 1 to 2 days. Its plasma half-life of calcitriol is 3 to 8 hours, with biotransformation and degradation occurring partly in the kidneys. Elimination occurs primarily through biliary mechanisms.

ADVERSE REACTIONS AND CONTRAINDICATIONS

Hypercalcemia is the primary adverse effect associated with calcitriol. However, because of the relatively short duration of action of calcitriol, any hypercalcemia asso-

ciated with its administration is of brief duration and is usually associated with minimal symptoms. Manifestations of hypercalcemia include weakness, nausea, vomiting, and muscle and bone pain.

Calcitriol is contraindicated in patients with hypersensitivity, hypercalcemia, vitamin D toxicity, and during lactation (in large doses). It should be used with caution in patients with sarcoidosis and hyperparathyroidism, and in those receiving cardiac glycosides. Safe use of large doses during pregnancy has not been established.

INTERACTIONS

Barbiturates, primidone, and hydantoin may reduce the effect of calcitriol by accelerating its biotransformation. Calcitriol-induced hypercalcemia potentiates the effect of cardiac glycosides, causing arrhythmias. Aluminum hydroxide precipitates bile acids in the small intestine, decreasing absorption of calcitriol and other fat-soluble vitamins. Additionally, calcitriol promotes the absorption of phosphorus from dietary sources, resulting in hyperphosphatemia.

 DRUG CLASS • **Cation-Exchange Resin**

sodium polystyrene sulfonate (Kayexalate, SPS)

MECHANISM OF ACTION

Sodium polystyrene sulfonate is a cation-exchange resin used in the treatment of hyperkalemic states in both ARF and CRF. When administered as an enema, the resin exchanges sodium ions for potassium and, to a lesser extent, other cations (e.g., calcium and magnesium), which have higher affinities for binding to the resin than sodium and are then eliminated in the feces. After oral administration of the resin, sodium ions are exchanged for hydrogen ions in the stomach. The hydrogen ions are subsequently exchanged for potassium ions in the large intestine (see also Chapter 51).

USES

Sodium polystyrene sulfonate is used in uremic patients to remove potassium from blood and extracellular fluid because renal mechanisms for eliminating potassium have failed.

PHARMACOKINETICS

Sodium polystyrene sulfonate is nonabsorbable and is not biotransformed. The exchange efficiency is approximately 33%. One gram of resin has the capacity to exchange approximately 1 mEq of potassium for 1 mEq of sodium. Virtually 100% of administered doses, oral or rectal, are eliminated in the feces (see Table 47-2).

ADVERSE REACTIONS AND CONTRAINDICATIONS

Because sodium polystyrene sulfonate exchanges sodium for potassium, fluid retention caused by the added sodium may occur. Hypokalemia can occur.

INTERACTIONS

Concurrent use of antacids and laxatives that contain magnesium should be avoided because of the risk of metabolic alkalosis. This risk is decreased with rectal administration of the resin.

DRUG CLASS • Systemic Antacids

sodium bicarbonate (Citrocarbonate, Neut, Soda Mint)

sodium citrate (Bicitra, Oracit, Shohl's Modified Solution)

MECHANISM OF ACTION

Sodium bicarbonate is a systemic alkalizing drug used for the treatment of metabolic acidosis caused by renal failure. The logic for its use in the treatment of ARF also applies to the treatment in CRF. By increasing plasma bicarbonate levels, excess hydrogen ions are buffered and blood pH is raised, thus reversing the clinical manifestations of acidosis. The increase in serum pH results in translocation of potassium from the extracellular pool and a corresponding acute fall of plasma potassium levels.

USES

Correction of acidosis results in improvement of GI symptoms associated with uremia. In addition, by buffering the retained dietary acids, sodium bicarbonate saves bone buffers and retards the development of renal osteodystrophy. Chronic correction of acidosis in uremia is accomplished by the oral administration of either sodium bicarbonate or sodium citrate. Both are equally effective in correction of the acidotic state. However, because of citrate's ability to enhance the absorption of some toxic elements, namely aluminum, bicarbonate is the preferred drug.

PHARMACOKINETICS

Sodium bicarbonate is always administered intravenously for acute acidosis. Bicarbonate replacement is calculated based on the difference between actual plasma bicarbonate and the desired bicarbonate levels. With acute acidosis, the volume of distribution of bicarbonate is assumed to be 50% of body weight. In most cases, half of the calculated bicarbonate deficit is initially replaced. Replacement therapy is monitored by serial determinations of serum CO_2 content and arterial pH.

ADVERSE REACTIONS AND CONTRAINDICATIONS

Administration of sodium bicarbonate can result in modest sodium and fluid retention. The retention of sodium and fluids has the potential for aggravating a hypertensive state and edema formation.

INTERACTIONS

Interactions primarily result from altering pH in various compartments (Chapter 51).

 DRUG CLASS • Diuretics (see Chapter 46)

furosemide (Apo-Furosemide,✳ Furoside,✳ Lasix, Lasix Special,✳ Myrosemide, Novosemide✳)

mannitol (Osmitrol)

In patients with renal failure, diuretics are mostly used for the conversion of oliguric ATN to nonoliguric ATN. Loop diuretics (e.g., furosemide) and osmotic diuretics (e.g., mannitol) are most often used, although the efficacy of diuretics in renal failure varies. Because of failure-induced reduction in renal function, large doses of the diuretics are usually required. Diuretics should be administered only after vital signs are stabilized and extracellular fluid volume is optimized.

Loop diuretics are used in the early stages of renal insufficiency and in ARF caused by ATN. The non-oliguric form of ATN rarely requires dialysis and has a better prognosis than oliguric ATN. Osmotic diuretics are used for the prevention of radiocontrast media-induced ATN.

Although diuretics have some effect on renal blood flow, their major therapeutic efficacy is in improving tubule flow rate. The increased flow rate is thought to wash out debris, mostly tubule cells that were sloughed off as a result of the initial injury. Diuretics are seldom used in patients with end-stage renal disease after dialysis has been initiated. See Chapter 46 for more discussion of diuretic drugs.

DRUG CLASS • Renal Vasodilator

dopamine (Intropin)

Low-dose dopamine has been used to improve renal blood flow, glomerular filtration rate (GFR), and renal salt and water elimination. In hypotensive states associated with increased renal vasoconstriction, dopamine improves renal blood flow, thereby reducing oliguria and preventing the development of ARF. Additional uses of dopamine are discussed in Chapter 41.

Dopamine has two distinct actions. It stimulates adrenergic receptors to cause vasoconstriction and it acts on dopaminergic receptors to cause vasodilation. In addition, dopamine causes a decrease in sodium reabsorption and it also increases the rate of sodium elimination in the urine (a natriuretic effect). Low-dose dopamine (0.5 to 2 mcg/kg/minute intravenous infusion) causes renal vasodilation. In so doing, it increases renal blood flow, GFR, and sodium elimination, with minimal effect on the vasoconstrictive adrenergic receptors.

There are few adverse effects with low-dose dopamine. However, at doses of 2 to 10 mcg/kg/minute given intravenously, dopaminergic and beta receptors are stimulated, producing cardiac stimulation and greater renal vasodilation. Hypotension and arrhythmias are potentially problematic at higher doses.

APPLICATION TO PRACTICE

ASSESSMENT
History of Present Illness

The history of present illness should address each of the body systems that are commonly implicated in renal failure, including the genitourinary system; GI tract; and neurologic, cardiovascular, respiratory, and dermatologic systems. The symptoms associated with renal failure are often mistakenly interpreted by the patient as the flu or some other infection.

The frequency of voiding, urine quantity, the appearance, and any difficulty starting or controlling urination should be described. This information helps identify the stage of renal dysfunction, determine the cause of renal damage, and monitor treatment. Patients with chronic lower urinary tract obstructive disease (e.g., prostatic disease) may relate a long history of strangury, frequency, urgency, nocturia, incontinence, hesitancy, and decreased stream size. With more advanced renal disease, the patient experiences increasing symptoms of uremia.

Ask about a change in the taste of food, as well as nausea and vomiting that often accompanies renal failure. This change occurs as a result of azotemia and nervous system disruptions, drug therapies, and changes in diet and fluid intake. Excessive intake of high-protein foods and sodium contributes to electrolyte imbalance and accelerates the build up of metabolic wastes. Also ask about diarrhea and constipation, because they are common symptoms and the result of a buildup of metabolic and nitrogenous waste.

Ask the patient about neurologic disruptions such as excitement and insomnia alternating with weakness and lassitude with periods of extreme drowsiness. The patient may complain of a short attention span and peripheral neuropathies, with numb, weak extremities, particularly of the hands. Neurologic disruptions also generate complaints of headache and muscle twitching, which in severe cases can progress to seizures and coma.

Ask about fluid intake. Excessive fluid intake contributes to cardiovascular overload, eventually resulting in peripheral edema, pulmonary edema, and heart failure. Complaints of edema, dizziness, weakness, lethargy, and abnormal bleeding may be indications of worsening renal failure. Symptoms reported by the patient may also be related to the hypertension associated with certain types of ARF and are the result, in part, of altered function of the renin-angiotensin-aldosterone system. Anemia associated with renal failure may be evidenced in complaints of weakness, pallor, lethargy, shortness of breath, and dizziness.

Health History

Inquire about a history of renal calculi, difficulty voiding, or acute abdominal or flank pain secondary to a distended bladder or ureteral stone. A positive history of hypertension, diabetes mellitus, systemic lupus erythematosus, cancer, tuberculosis, and many other disorders can contribute to or worsen renal function. Frequently, there is a recent history of infection; severe trauma; a complicated surgical procedure; an episode of sepsis; or the administration of nephrotoxic drugs, such as contrast media, antimicrobials, or antineoplastic drugs.

Some OTC drugs can precipitate or aggravate renal failure; therefore, obtaining a thorough drug history is important. A history of analgesic abuse (most notably NSAIDs) is associated with both ARF and CRF. Occupational exposure to some trace elements such as cadmium and lead can also result in CRF. Furthermore, a history of intravenous drug abuse represents an additional risk factor.

Family history is also relevant in assessing the patient with renal disease. A patient with a family history of diabetic nephropathy and hypertension places the patient at additional risk for renal failure. Similarly, patients with a family history of hereditary renal disease (e.g., Alport's syndrome, polycystic kidney disease), and recessive or sex-linked diseases (e.g., Fabry's disease, tuberous sclerosis, medullary cystic disease, type I glycogen storage disease, cystinosis, oxalate nephropathy) frequently know of another family member with a similar condition.

Lifespan Considerations

Perinatal. Renal disease can be caused by a urinary tract infection before or during pregnancy, can be the result of other diseases such as diabetes, or can occur during pregnancy from complications such as preeclampsia, HELLP syndrome (*h*emolysis, *e*levated *l*iver enzymes, *l*ow *p*latelets), or abruptio placentae. Treatment of sudden ARF during pregnancy resembles that of the nonpregnant population. The goal is to retard the development of uremic symptoms, restore acid-base and electrolyte balance, and volume homeostasis.

In general, renal disease is not affected by pregnancy if it is mild and the patient is not hypertensive at the time of conception. However, in the presence of renal disease and hypertension, pregnancy is often complicated with worsening hypertension, a decline in renal function, or both.

Pediatric. Chronic renal disease affects children in many of the same ways it affects adults. However, because the child's body, character, and personality are still forming, the effects on maturation are even more pronounced. Furthermore, because childhood illness often results in stunted physical, psychologic, and educational development, it is generally true that the older the child is when he or she becomes ill, the better the chances are of having established a secure sense of self.

Growth failure is an important consequence of childhood renal disease. The growth rate may be somewhat improved with control of acidosis and calcitriol supplementation. Recombinant human growth hormone has been used in children with uremia and in those with transplants who subsequently experienced substantially increased growth rates. In addition, adequate peritoneal dialysis, especially continuous cycle-assisted peritoneal dialysis, is the therapy of choice for improved growth rate. However, none of the previously mentioned therapies produce catch-up growth.

The recurrent hospitalizations and lengthy treatment regimens often make a child's reintegration to school and social activities a challenge. The return to school and activities, however, helps minimize the depression, isolation, and low self-esteem associated with chronic illness. The child needs encouragement to assume as much responsibility for self-care as possible. The child's ability to cope with what may be a complex drug regimen can foster self-esteem and improve the outcomes of the treatment regimen. However, the age and maturity of the child will determine the degree to which they participate in their drug therapies.

Older Adults. The effects of normal aging result in a decrease in the size and function of the kidneys, and a subsequent decrease in GFR and tubular function. Because of the physiologic changes of aging, older adults are more susceptible to dehydration, hypotension, fever, and acute renal insufficiency. Advanced age also represents an additional risk factor for the development of ARF secondary to antimicrobial use (e.g., aminoglycosides) as well as radiocontrast drugs.

The incidence of ESRD increases dramatically with advanced age. Between the ages of 20 and 44, the incidence of ESRD is 91 per million population, compared with 680 per million population between the ages of 65 and 75 years. The cause of renal failure also changes with aging.

As a consequence of social, financial, psychologic, and comorbidity factors, older adults frequently do not cope well with chronic dialysis and drug therapies associated with renal failure. These factors result in chronic fatigue, depression, concerns regarding quality of life, and suicidal ideations. Over 40% of patients 65 years and older discontinue dialysis for these reasons.

Cultural/Social Considerations

In assessing cultural and social factors that influence the patient and family, ask about understanding of the diagnosis, implications, and treatment regimens (e.g., diet, drugs, dialysis). The coping mechanisms used by the patient and family members should also be noted because family relations, social activities, work patterns, body image, and sexual activities are altered by renal disease. Introducing a life-threatening illness such as ESRD to the already stressful demands placed on the contemporary family system taxes coping mechanisms.

Role changes are common in families with renal disease, such that spouses often take on the role responsibilities of the sick partner while maintaining their own role. This leads to reduced rest and leisure for the spouse and lowers physical reserve. Major changes in thinking and living must be made, and, at the same time, relationships must be maintained and nurtured.

The cultural and social support required is determined by the reversibility and severity of the underlying disease or condition responsible for producing renal failure. Further, complex drug regimens and any associated medical or surgical conditions determine whether the patient and the family are compliant with the plan of care.

Other factors to be considered when assessing the patient are the health beliefs about what is considered a healthy state, personal beliefs related to religious and cultural practices, and financial considerations. Compliance with drug therapy is impacted by the expense of the required drug regimens.

Physical Examination

The patient's height, weight, vital signs, intake, and output should be noted, with attention to fluid balance. Any recent, unintended weight gain or edema may suggest cardiovascular overload and fluid retention. Fluid overload is supported by the presence of shortness of breath, activity intolerance, increased jugular pulsations, crackles on pulmonary auscultation, and the presence of edema. In contrast, volume depletion is seen as orthostatic changes in blood pressure and pulse, poor skin turgor, and dry mucous membranes. A pericardial friction rub may also be present.

The normal flora of the mouth is altered in uremia. The ammonia generated from the hydrolysis of urea contributes to a breath odor that smells like urine. It also causes uremic stomatitis (mouth inflammation). With advanced uremia, the patient's skin develops a sallow appearance because of the presence of urochrome pigments. Skin excoriations are the result of severe pruritus, although the cause of the pruritus is unknown. In ARF, a dusting of urea crystals (uremic frost) from evaporated perspiration is sometimes seen on the face and eyebrows. Evidence of bleeding from the nose, gums, vaginal tract, GI tract, or skin surfaces may indicate decreased erythrocyte production, thrombocytopenia, and a resultant defect in platelet activity.

Assessment of other body systems should include neurologic evaluation because myoclonic jerks, asterixis, and hyperreflexia may also be noted with renal disease.

Laboratory Testing

Renal function is evaluated by measuring the GFR. Although an indirect measurement, creatinine clearance (CrCl) is the most commonly used clinical means of estimating GFR. It is classically measured with a blood test and a timed urine collection; however, this combination of tests may not always be possible. Alternatively, CrCl can be estimated from serum creatinine determination alone using the Crockcroft and Gault equation. The normal CrCl for men is 140 ± 27 mL/minute, and for women, it is 112 ± 20 mL/minute.

Like CrCl, BUN is a measure of renal function. However, unlike creatinine, the production rate of urea varies as a result of the ingestion of dietary protein, and the catabolic status of the patient. In addition, urea clearance depends on urine flow. Thus, urea clearance fluctuates, making it a less reliable marker of GFR.

Urinalysis can be of value in establishing and monitoring the patient with intrarenal disease. The majority of renal diseases, whether acute or chronic, will have abnormalities consisting of increased numbers of white blood cells or red blood cells, casts, and proteins. Chronic renal disease causes hematuria and proteinuria, and the urine may become cloudy with heavy sediment. In ESRD, the urine becomes more dilute and clear, which reflects the diminished GFR of a diseased kidney. Serum electrolytes, bicarbonate, and hemoglobin should also be evaluated.

Patients with uremia are frequently anemic, acidotic, and have electrolyte disturbances and alterations in calcium and phosphorus balance. Therefore, a complete blood cell count, serum bicarbonate, electrolytes, phosphate, and calcium levels should be serially evaluated. Owing to the proteinuria accompanying some CRF states, serum albumin may be low. Urinary protein should be measured and serum albumin determined.

GOALS OF THERAPY

The primary objective in the management of renal failure is prevention. The avoidance or removal of nephrotoxic drugs, along with rapid correction of cardiovascular alterations that lead to renal ischemia, will prevent or minimize progression of the disease. Once renal failure has developed, however, treatment goals are directed at supporting the patient and maintaining existing system functioning. Achieving and maintaining acceptable fluid and electrolyte balance, and minimizing the risk of complications from fluid and electrolyte imbalances are also relevant objectives. Maintenance of adequate nutritional status and compliance with the plan of care are also desirable outcomes.

One of the risk-reduction objectives listed in the Healthy People 2000 document of the United States Public Health Service and the Department of Health and Human Services is to reverse the increase in ESRD (requiring maintenance dialysis or transplantation) to attain an incidence of no more than 13 per 100,000 cases (baseline: 13.9/100,000 in 1987).

Financial Considerations

Recent studies strongly suggest that ACE inhibitors (e.g., captopril) are highly effective in decreasing the progression of diabetic nephropathy. Because over 30% of the patients with ESRD have diabetes mellitus there is a major impact on ESRD programs. In addition, there is reasonable evidence that other types of proteinuric renal disease may also benefit from the use of ACE inhibitors. Because the average cost of treating a patient with ESRD is over $50,000 annually, preventive therapy with ACE inhibitors at the recommended dosage would cost less than $1500 annually. Furthermore, it has been estimated that the use of captopril in patients with type 1 diabetic nephropathy could reduce national health costs by over 3 billion dollars over the next decade.

In contrast, recent advances in therapies directed at improving the quality of life of patients with ESRD have done little to improve rehabilitation but have markedly increased costs. For example, epoetin alfa, an antianemic drug, has increased the annual cost of treating a patient with ESRD by $5000 to $7000. It is also estimated that the cost of recombinant human growth hormone for treatment of growth failure in children with renal disease will be even more expensive than epoetin alfa.

INTERVENTION

Drug treatment regimens are initiated and modified based on the degree of the patient's functional impairment by using interval extension and dose reduction strategies. Using the interval extension method, the time between each dose is lengthened, but the dosage remains the same. The interval extension method is useful for drugs with wide therapeutic ranges and long plasma half-lives. With the dose reduction method, the size of the individual dose is reduced, but the interval between each dose remains unchanged. The dose reduction method is preferred when constant blood levels of a drug are required, and for drugs with narrow therapeutic ranges and rather short half-lives. At times, a combination of these two methods is employed to achieve maximum therapeutic benefits. Guidance regarding dose reduction and interval modification for most drugs can be found in a number of books, including *Drug Prescribing in Renal Failure*, published by the American College of Physicians.

Measurement of peak and trough serum drug levels is useful in documenting the effectiveness of the dosing schedule. The levels are indicators of drug elimination and reflect potential drug accumulation. Peak levels are most useful when obtained 30 minutes to 1 hour after the third dose of the drug. Trough levels are obtained immediately before the next dose. Reliable clinical assessment of changes in the patient's condition and knowledge of drug interactions must be used to aid in the interpretation of test results. Further, the following principles are used when the health care provider is adjusting the dosage:

- The loading dose given is usually the same as the initial dose given to a patient with normal renal function.

- The maintenance dose can be adjusted by using the interval extension or dose reduction method.
- In patients with substantial edema or ascites, the initial dose may be somewhat higher than that usually given to achieve desired blood levels.

The importance of consistency in obtaining peak and trough values cannot be overstated. Regardless of the sampling procedure used, it is important that the same time interval between sampling and dose administration be used consistently when comparing results from serial samples on the same patient.

Administration

Drugs that are to be taken on an empty stomach should be taken 1 hour before or 2 hours after meals to enhance absorption. Drug regimens should not be stopped without first checking with the health care provider. OTC drugs should be avoided, especially cough, cold, and allergy preparations containing ingredients that interact with the drugs used in the treatment regimens.

Iron Supplements. Iron preparations should be taken with meals if GI discomfort is severe, but milk, eggs, coffee, and tea should be avoided because they alter absorption of the iron. Liquid iron preparations should be mixed with water or juice to mask the taste and given through a straw to prevent staining of the teeth. The patient should be informed that iron turns the stool dark green or black. Periodic monitoring of hematocrit and hemoglobin levels should be done to monitor effectiveness and prevent possible toxicity.

Antihemorrhagic Drugs. Intranasal formulations of DDAVP should be administered by drawing the solution into the flexible calibrated tube that is supplied with the drug. The patient is instructed to insert one end of the tube into the nostril and to blow into the other end to deposit the solution deep into the nasal cavity. Inappropriate administration technique can lead to nasal ulcerations. Be sure to check the manufacturer's instructions for use. The nasal solution and injectable formulations should be stored in the refrigerator.

Phosphate-Binding Drugs. Phosphate-binding drugs should be taken 1 to 3 hours after meals and at bedtime, or as prescribed by the health care provider. Other drugs should not be taken within 1 to 2 hours of the phosphate binder. Encourage the patient to chew the phosphate-binding (e.g., calcium carbonate) tablets thoroughly before swallowing and follow with a glass of water or milk. Patients should be reminded to avoid magnesium-containing antacid preparations because of the possibility of magnesium toxicity. Serum calcium and phosphorus levels should be measured before beginning therapy with the vitamin D supplement and calcitriol, and at least weekly during therapy to monitor for hypercalcemia.

Heavy Metal Antagonist.   Deferoxamine is used most often in the acute care environment. When an intravenous route is required, the drug should be infused slowly, preferably using an infusion pump. Pain at the injection site with administration of subcutaneous or intramuscular forms is common.

Diuretics.   Furosemide should be taken with food or milk to prevent gastric upset. The dosage of the diuretic may be reduced with concurrent use of antihypertensives. It should be administered early in the day so increased urination will not disturb sleep. Intravenous use should be avoided if oral routes are at all possible. Oral solutions of furosemide should be refrigerated.

Vasopressors.   Extreme caution should be used when calculating and preparing dopamine for intravenous infusion. Small errors in dosage can cause serious adverse reactions. The drug should always be diluted before use, if it is not already diluted. The large veins of the antecubital fossa are preferred to veins in the hands or ankle. The initial dose should be reduced by 10% in patients who have been on monoamine oxidase inhibitors. Phentolamine, an alpha blocker, should be available in case extravasation occurs. If required, infiltration with 10 to 15 mL of saline containing 5 to 10 mg of phentolamine is effective in reducing tissue damage.

Cation Exchange Resin.   Sodium polystyrene sulfonate is a suspension that is mixed with either food or liquid to improve palatability. Liquid vehicles include warm water, 1% methylcellulose, or 5% to 10% dextrose in water. The osmotic cathartic effect of the ingredient sorbitol hastens elimination of potassium and prevents constipation and, more importantly, fecal impaction.

For rectal use, a cleansing enema precedes administration of the resin. The resin is mixed with an aqueous solution (i.e., 25% sorbitol, 1% methylcellulose, or 10% dextrose) and instilled at least 20 cm into the colon as a retention enema. Following instillation, the tubing is flushed with 100 to 200 mL of a non–sodium-containing solution to ensure complete instillation of the solution. The enema should be retained for at least 30 to 60 minutes and up to 4 to 10 hours, followed by a non–sodium-containing cleansing enema. The resin should not be administered as a thick paste because it is less effective in that form.

Rectal administration of sodium polystyrene sulfonate is recommended when the patient is receiving nothing by mouth or is vomiting, or if there is an upper GI tract disorder. However, the rectal route is less effective in reducing potassium levels than the oral method of administration. Further, constipation, fecal impaction, and colonic necrosis have been reported either as the result of the omission of cleansing enemas before or after the resin enema or because of failure to give sorbitol with the oral formulation.

Serum electrolytes, including calcium and magnesium levels, should be monitored when cation exchange resin therapy continues for more than one day. Serum potassium levels should be monitored at least daily to determine the effectiveness of therapy. Bicarbonate levels should be monitored at least weekly with chronic therapy, especially if the resin is prescribed concurrently with laxatives and antacids.

Systemic Antacids.   Serum potassium levels should be checked before the administration of sodium bicarbonate. The risk of metabolic acidosis is increased in states of hypokalemia, and the dosage of sodium bicarbonate may need to be reduced. Dosage is based on arterial blood gases and patient response. Complete correction of acid-base imbalance within the first 24 hours should be avoided because of the increased risk of metabolic alkalosis. In most cases, drug interactions with sodium bicarbonate may be avoided by not administering other oral drugs within 1 to 2 hours.

Education

The most important role of the health care provider for the patient with renal failure and his or her family is patient teaching. Most patients receive their care on an outpatient basis, so whenever possible the patient should be encouraged to take the major responsibility for compliance with the treatment plan. However, because of the changes in cognitive functioning of the patient with renal failure or the level of understanding from age limitations, it is important to involve family members in the teaching process.

Both the patient and family should have a thorough understanding of renal disease and its consequences to adjust to the numerous limitations imposed by the disease. An understanding of the reasons for dietary restrictions, drug regimens, and adherence to the dialysis schedule, when applicable, is necessary for acceptance and compliance with the treatment regimen.

All patients with decreased renal function must limit their protein consumption to some degree because the accumulation of nitrogenous waste products from protein metabolism is the primary cause of uremia. Protein restriction is based on the degree of renal insufficiency and the severity of the symptoms. The GFR, albumin, creatinine, and BUN levels are often used as a guide to safe levels of protein consumption.

Low-protein diets are usually deficient in vitamins, and water-soluble vitamins are removed from the blood during dialysis. In addition, anemia is a chronic problem because of the limited iron content of low-protein diets and decreased erythropoietin production by the kidneys. For these reasons, all patients with renal failure are given vitamin and mineral supplements. The patient should be taught to take them after dialysis rather than before because they will be dialyzed out of the body if taken before, and the patient would receive no benefit.

Phosphate-binding drugs, often referred to by the patient as antacids, are necessary because the metabolism of calcium and phosphorus is altered in renal failure. The patient should be taught the purpose of these drugs and the importance of avoiding preparations containing magnesium. The inability to get rid of magnesium predisposes the patient to dangerous levels of magnesium toxicity. Further, the patient should be taught to monitor for signs and symptoms of hypophosphatemia (muscle weakness, anorexia, malaise, tremors, and bone pain).

Diuretics are often used in the early stages of renal failure and should be taken early in the day to avoid disturbance of sleep. The diuresis produced is useful in treating fluid overload in patients who still have some urinary function. Teach the patient to keep careful intake and output records, because as kidney function deteriorates, these drugs become increasingly nephrotoxic. Diuretics are seldom used in patients with ESRD after dialysis has been initiated.

Many patients with renal failure also have diabetes mellitus, so patient teaching should include the need for close monitoring of blood glucose levels. As renal disease progresses, the patient with diabetes mellitus requires a decrease in insulin dosage because insulin is partially biotransformed by the kidneys (see Chapter 58). Urinary glucose measurements may be inaccurate because of the renal disease and, if possible, should not be used.

Patients with uremia are particularly sensitive to the respiratory depressant effects of opioid analgesics and should be taught to use them with caution (see Chapter 13). The effects of opioids last much longer in patients with renal failure than in persons with healthy kidneys. Because opioids are biotransformed by the liver and not the kidneys, dosage recommendations are often the same regardless of kidney function. The patient should also be taught to avoid aspirin because it is normally eliminated by the kidneys and may rapidly build to toxic levels and prolong bleeding time.

Infection related to altered immune, nutritional, and biochemical states represent an additional cause of morbidity and mortality in patients with renal failure.

Meticulous handwashing is essential, and the patient should be taught to avoid contact with people with known infections. It is important that patients understand aseptic technique and that it be used with all necessary invasive procedures. Additionally, invasive procedures by the health care provider should be avoided whenever possible, especially the use of indwelling catheters. Antibiotics are given prophylactically before any dental procedures to prevent pericarditis, which may result if oral bacteria enter the circulation. The patient should be taught to discuss the need for antibiotics and the preferred protocol because it varies with the patient's needs and the preference of the health care provider. Drug dosing with antibiotics is based on the degree of renal dysfunction.

Patients with little or no financial resources will have difficulty obtaining their drugs and, thus, complying with treatment plans. Federal, state, and local resources may provide assistance with the cost of therapy. The End-Stage Renal Disease Program, a part of Medicare, was initiated in 1972 to relieve kidney patients of the catastrophic costs of dialysis by covering 80% of the costs of service. It does not cover the cost of drugs.

Patients and their families should also be informed of other resources that are available. Home care nurses may monitor the patient's status and evaluate maintenance of the treatment regimen. Social service personnel are usually involved because of the complex process of paying for the required care and in applying for financial aid. Physical and occupational therapists often work with patients who have renal failure, depending on their needs. The patient and family may benefit from joining support groups or obtaining other services locally. Resources such as the National Kidney Foundation and the American Kidney Fund are good initial contacts.

EVALUATION

Successful achievement of treatment goals is indicated by a number of factors. The patient is free from peripheral edema, hypertension, respiratory distress, and other signs of fluid and electrolyte imbalance. There are no signs of infection, and the patient is feeling more rested and less fatigued. Blood pressure is maintained within an acceptable range. There are no signs of bleeding; anorexia, nausea, and pruritus are controlled; and there is no muscle cramping. The patient demonstrates mental clarity and an ability to perform activities of daily living independently and safely. Any comorbid illness, including heart failure, anemia, electrolyte imbalance, and dehydration, is controlled or resolved. Furthermore, the patient should be able to correctly describe the nature of his or her illness, treatment and drug regimens, and plans for follow-up care.

Bibliography

Holt SG, Moore KP: Pathogenesis and treatment of renal dysfunction in rhabdomyolysis, *Intensive Care Med* 27(5):803-811, 2001.

Horl MP, Horl WH: Hemodialysis-associated hypertension: pathophysiology and therapy, *Am J Kidney Dis* 39(2):227-244, 2002.

Mantel GD: Care of the critically ill parturient: oliguria and renal failure, *Best Pract Res Clin Obstet Gynaecol* 15(4):563-581, 2001.

Salem M: End-stage renal disease survival in blacks and whites, *Am J Med Sci* 323(2):100-101, 2002.

Internet Resources

www.merck.com/pubs/mmanual/section17/chapter222/222a.htm.

www.nlm.nih.gov/medlineplus/ency/article/000501.htm.

CHAPTER

48

Hyperacidity and Related Drugs

ALAN P. AGINS • KATHLEEN GUTIERREZ

 Visit http://evolve.elsevier.com/Gutierrez/ for additional information.

KEY TERMS

Acid reflux, p. 779

Gastroesophageal reflux disease (GERD), p. 779

H$_2$ antagonists, p. 783

Helicobacter pylori, p. 780

Hydrochloric acid, p. 780

Peptic ulcer, p. 780

Secretin, p.. 780

Ulcer, p. 799

OBJECTIVES

- Discuss the use of drugs to control gastrointestinal reflux disease.
- Discuss the use of antihistamines and proton pump inhibitors to treat ulcers.
- Explain the role of antibiotics in treating ulcers.
- Develop a nursing care plan for patients receiving one of the drugs in the classes discussed in this chapter.

PATHOPHYSIOLOGY • GERD and Ulcers

Acid reflux, or gastroesophageal reflux disease (GERD), occurs when stomach acid backs up into the esophagus. Unlike the lining of the stomach, the esophageal surface is much less protected by mucus. The result is heartburn or indigestion, a burning pain that begins in the pit of the stomach and moves upward toward the throat. Triggers of acid reflux include large meals and overeating; exercise or exertion immediately after a meal; and con-

sumption of caffeine, nicotine, fatty or fried foods, alcohol, chocolate, or peppermint.

Acid reflux generally occurs as a result of insufficient closure of the lower esophageal sphincter. Treatment, therefore, is aimed at either (1) decreasing the acidity of the stomach contents that come in contact with the esophagus or (2) increasing the lower esophageal tone. An ulcer is the loss of the mucosal tissue that provides the protective layer of cells normally surrounding an organ. A **peptic ulcer** can occur in the lower esophagus, stomach, or duodenum after the mucosal barrier is destroyed, exposing the underlying tissue to stomach acid; as a result, the anatomic structure of the stomach and the regulation of stomach secretions are affected. The common symptom is a gnawing or burning pain in the upper abdomen that usually occurs between meals and early in the morning and is often relieved by food or antacids. Ulcers can also cause nausea, vomiting, and loss of appetite and weight.

An esophageal ulcer occurs when there is reflux of stomach acid into the esophagus because of a defective esophageal sphincter. An ulcer in the duodenum results from overactive secretion of acid in the stomach so that stomach contents cannot be neutralized in the duodenum. The acidic contents then damage the duodenal mucosa. Stomach ulcers can be caused by the reflux of duodenal contents back into the stomach because of a faulty pyloric sphincter. The duodenal contents contain bile acids that disrupt the mucosal barrier normally protecting the stomach from acid and pepsin.

Control of Acid Secretion

Factors controlling the secretion of **hydrochloric acid** by the parietal cells of the stomach are diagrammed in Figure 48-1. The neurotransmitter acetylcholine (released from a branch of the vagus nerve), the hormone gastrin, and histamine stimulate the secretion of acid. Hydrochloric acid aids in the breakdown of connective tissue in food, activates pepsinogen to pepsin (which degrades protein), and kills any bacteria ingested in food. The acidic digest leaves the stomach and enters the duodenum. This movement of digested food lessens stomach distension and thereby removes a stimulus for the release of gastrin and for vagal activity. In response to acidity the duodenum releases **secretin**, a hormone that stimulates the release of bicarbonate and digestive enzymes from the pancreas. Secretin also depresses the release of hydrochloric acid by the parietal cells and depresses the motility of the stomach. The bicarbonate released by the pancreas neutralizes the acidity of the partially digested food entering the duodenum. This neutralization is also necessary for the digestive enzymes in the intestine to be active.

Risk Factors for Peptic Ulcer Disease

Bacteria. Recent attention has focused on a bacterial cause of ulcers. The bacterium *Helicobacter pylori* accounts for 70% to 90% of all stomach and duodenal ulcers. This bacterium attaches to the mucus-secreting gastric epithelial cells that line the stomach and survives by converting urea into bicarbonate, which, in turn, neu-

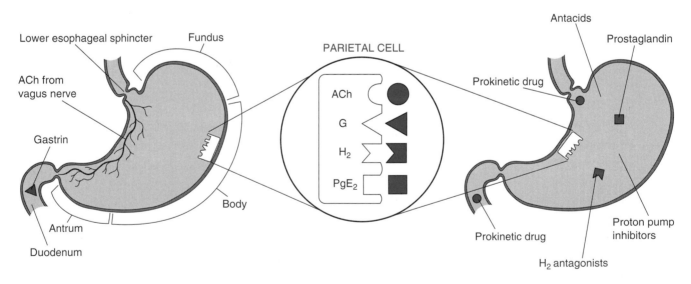

FIGURE 48-1 Various factors influence acid secretion in the stomach and sites of drug action. Secretion of acid by parietal cells of the stomach is controlled by the hormone gastrin *(G)* released from the duodenum, by the neurotransmitter acetylcholine *(ACh)* released from a vagus nerve branch from the parasympathetic nervous system, and by histamine. Histamine is the most effective stimulant of gastric acid secretion, acting through H_2 receptors. Acid secretion is discontinued when food reaches the duodenum, where hydrochloric acid inhibits gastrin release and stimulates secretin release, and where distension of the stomach is lessened, decreasing vagal stimulation. Prostaglandin E_2 *(PgE$_2$)* is a major inhibitor of stomach acid secretion.

tralizes the acid in its microenvironment. In time, the bacteria give rise to a local inflammatory state that leads to the loss of the mucus that protects the lining of the stomach and duodenum from acid. However, most persons infected with this organism do not develop an ulcer, so other risk factors also play a role. Evidence is accumulating that chronic *H. pylori* infection can also lead to acid hypersecretion and gastritis as well as stomach cancer and some B cell lymphomas.

Eradication of *H. pylori* can be achieved with a combination therapy that includes suppression of acid production and antibiotics. When eradication therapy is used, the recurrence rate for ulcers drops to 5%. Previous therapies had a recurrence rate of 60% to 80%.

NSAIDs. Nonsteroidal antiinflammatory drugs (NSAIDs) inhibit prostaglandin synthesis. Because prostaglandins play a critical role in maintaining the gastric mucosal cytoprotective system, the loss of prostaglandins with NSAID use is associated with upper gastrointestinal (GI) tract bleeding, and prolonged use can cause peptic ulcers. Older adults, or anyone on chronic high doses of NSAIDs, are especially sensitive to this effect. The newer COX-2 selective NSAIDs may help reduce this problem for some. Corticosteroids, because they also reduce prostaglandins and slow the growth of new gastric mucosal cells, also enhance the incidence of ulcer formation in patients, especially those also taking NSAIDs.

• • •

In the past, much attention was given to dietary and emotional factors. However, these are exacerbating factors and not causes for ulcers. Cigarette smoking is also an aggravating factor.

Until recently, the control of acid secretion was the goal of ulcer or reflux treatment. Now control of acid secretion is just part of the treatment. Drugs to treat acid secretion are listed in Table 48-1. The introduction of H_2 receptor antagonists and proton pump inhibitors in the past decade dramatically improved the ability to control acid secretion and allow ulcer healing. Mucosal protective agents also aid ulcer healing. Antacids and anticholinergic drugs, once a mainstay of ulcer therapy, now play a minor role. The recognition that a bacterial cause underlies many ulcers has led to therapies that include antibiotics for eradicating the causative agent, *H. pylori*.

TABLE 48-1
Drugs to Treat Acid Secretion and Reflux

Generic Name	Brand Name	Comments
H_2-Receptor Antagonists		
cimetidine	Tagamet, Apo-Cimetidine,✻ Novocimetidine,✻ Peptol✻	Administer with meals because food slows and prolongs action of cimetidine. Administer at least 1 hr after antacids or metoclopramide, which reduces absorption of cimetidine if taken concurrently. Available OTC.
cimetidine hydrochloride	Tagamet HCl	Switch to oral doses when ulcer bleeding stops.
famotidine	Pepcid, Ulcidine✻	Famotidine acts longer than cimetidine. Available OTC.
nizatidine	Axid	Nizatidine acts longer than cimetidine. Available OTC.
ranitidine HCl	Zantac, Apo-Ranitidine✻	Ranitidine HCl acts longer than cimetidine. Available OTC.
ranitidine bismuth citrate	Tritec	Bismuth salt formulated to eradicate *H. pylori*.
Proton Pump Inhibitors		
esomeprazole	Nexium	Esomeprazole is the S-isomer of omeprazole.
lansoprazole	Prevacid	Delayed-release capsules. Also used in combination with clarithromycin and/or metronidazole or amoxicillin to eradicate *H. pylori*.
omeprazole	Losec,✻ Prilosec	Delayed-release capsules/tablets. Also used in combination with clarithromycin and/or metronidazole or amoxicillin to eradicate *H. pylori*.
pantoprazole	Protonix, Pantoloc✻	Available in enteric-coated tablets; also only drug in this class available for intravenous use.
rabeprazole	AcipHex	Delayed release tablets.

✻ Available in Canada.

Continued

TABLE 48-1

Drugs to Treat Acid Secretion and Reflux—cont'd

Generic Name	Brand Name	Comments
Mucosal Protective Drugs		
aluminum hydroxide gel	AlternaGEL, Amphojel	OTC antacid. Aluminum hydroxide gel is constipating. Long-term use may cause hypophosphatemia. The drug complexes with tetracycline and can interfere with absorption of warfarin, digoxin, quinine, and quinidine.
aluminum carbonate gel	Basaljel	OTC antacid. See aluminum hydroxide gel.
bismuth subsalicylate	Pepto-Bismol, others	Used in combination therapy with antibiotics to eradicate *H. pylori*. Available OTC.
calcium carbonate	Dicarbosil, Titralac, Tums, others	OTC antacid. Calcium carbonate is constipating. It can be used hourly to keep acid neutralized, but some patients become hypercalcemic.
magnesium carbonate	Milk of Magnesia, others	OTC antacid. These magnesium salts are laxatives and must be taken with aluminum or calcium antacid to maintain normal stool consistency.
misoprostol	Cytotec	Misoprostol protects against ulcers from nonsteroidal antiinflammatory drugs used for arthritis. It is also effective for healing peptic ulcers.
sucralfate	Carafate, Sulcrate ❋	If antacids are prescribed for pain relief, they should not be taken 30 min before or after sucralfate.
Antimicrobials Effective against *H. pylori*		
amoxicillin	Amoxil, Trimox, others	Requires acid suppression with proton pump inhibitor or H_2 antagonist to be effective.
clarithromycin	Biaxin	Requires acid suppression with proton pump inhibitor or H_2 antagonist to be effective.
metronidazole	Flagyl, Prostat, Novonidazol, ❋ others	Resistance develops rapidly. Best if given with another antimicrobial, bismuth, and acid suppressor with proton pump inhibitor or H_2 antagonist.
tetracycline	Achromycin, Novotetra, ❋ Sumycin, others	Oxytetracycline may be substituted. Best if given with another antimicrobial, bismuth, and acid suppressor with proton pump inhibitor or H_2 antagonist.
bismuth subsalicylate with metronidazole and tetracycline HCl	Helidac	Fixed combination to eradicate *H. pylori*.
Prokinetic Drug		
metoclopramide	Reglan	Oral solution, tablet, or injectable.

DRUG CLASS • Histamine (H₂) Receptor Antagonists

cimetidine (Tagamet)

famotidine (Pepcid)

nizatidine (Axid)

ranitidine (Zantac)

ranitidine bismuth citrate (Tritec)

MECHANISM OF ACTION

The H_2 antagonists specifically block the H_2 receptors that control the basal and stimulated secretion of hydrochloric acid by the parietal cells (see Figure 48-1). H_1 receptors are blocked by antihistamines (see Chapter 53). Gastrin and acetylcholine are thought to act through histamine as a final common pathway to cause the release of hydrochloric acid. This hypothesis is supported by the fact that H_2 antagonists are so effective in decreasing acid secretion stimulated by pentagastrin (an active analog of gastrin) or bethanechol (an agonist of acetylcholine), as well as by food, insulin, and caffeine.

USES

H_2 antagonist drugs became available in 1995 as did OTC drugs for the prevention and relief of heartburn (or indigestion). Because H_2 antagonists dramatically decrease stomach acid, they alleviate many conditions in which stomach acid impedes therapy, including the following:

- *Duodenal and gastric ulcers*: H_2 antagonists are used in combination with other drugs in the treatment of ulcers.
- *Zollinger-Ellison syndrome*: A pancreatic tumor that secretes excessive gastrin, which stimulates excessive acid production. H_2 antagonists depress this acid production; however, much higher doses are needed than those used for the other listed conditions.
- *GI hemorrhage*: Stomach acid intensifies inflammation of the stomach, worsening the hemorrhaging.
- *Pancreatic insufficiency*: Digestive enzymes must be administered orally. Without H_2 antagonists, stomach acid inactivates most of the administered enzymes.
- *Gastroesophageal reflux disease (GERD)*: By decreasing acidity of the stomach, the contents that are refluxed into the lower esophagus are less irritating to the mucosal lining.

PHARMACOKINETICS

The H_2 antagonists are taken orally and absorbed rapidly. They are generally effective within an hour. Although they all have half-lives ranging from 2 to 4 hours, cimetidine has a duration of action of up to 6 hours, whereas other H_2 antagonists have a duration of up to 12 hours. They are partially biotransformed by the liver and excreted in the urine. Patients with diminished renal function, especially those with severe renal disease, should receive reduced doses.

ADVERSE REACTIONS AND CONTRAINDICATIONS

H_2 antagonists are remarkably well tolerated and typically free of general adverse effects. Central nervous system (CNS) effects include mental confusion, agitation, and hallucinations; these symptoms are usually mild and reversible when the drug is discontinued. CNS effects are more common in patients with liver or renal disease.

Cimetidine given in large doses over a long time may have an antiandrogen (feminizing) effect on men, producing gynecomastia, impotence, and loss of libido. These effects are not characteristic of the other H_2 antagonists.

There are no absolute contraindications for the H_2 antagonists other than hypersensitivity to that class of drugs. Caution should be exercised in patients with renal impairment. Patients should also be warned not to use H_2 antagonists chronically for undiagnosed conditions.

INTERACTIONS

Because H_2 antagonists decrease gastric acidity, they can also cause altered absorption of other drugs or nutrients. The absorption of ketoconazole and itraconazole in particular are reduced unless they are taken at least 2 hours before the H_2 antagonist. The absorption of two cephalosporin antibiotics, cefpodoxime and cefuroxime, may also be reduced by H_2 antagonists. Vitamin B_{12} absorption also depends to some degree on a relatively acidic environment and may be compromised by H_2 antagonists.

Another potential site for drug interactions with H_2 antagonists is in the kidney. It has been shown that these drugs can compete with other drugs for the renal tubular active transport system (cationic transporter). Such an action may decrease the elimination of drugs such as metformin and lead to potential toxicity from that drug.

Cimetidine inhibits the liver cytochrome P-450 system that biotransforms many drugs. Some of the drugs whose biotransformation is inhibited include warfarin, theophylline, and phenytoin. The dosages of these drugs should be reduced. Cimetidine also inhibits the gastric metabolism of alcohol. The other H_2 antagonists do not affect drug metabolism.

DRUG CLASS • Proton (Acid) Pump Inhibitors

esomeprazole (Nexium)

lansoprazole (Prevacid)

omeprazole (Prilosec)

pantoprazole (Protonix)

rabeprazole (AcipHex)

MECHANISM OF ACTION

Proton (acid) pump inhibitors block the enzyme that pumps hydrogen ion (or proton) into the luminal (or secretory) side of the parietal cells of the stomach. This enzyme blockade is more effective than histamine-receptor blockade at reducing stomach acid production. As a result, these drugs are often preferred over the H_2 antagonists.

USES

Proton pump inhibitors (PPIs) are more potent than the H_2 receptor antagonists but are used for the same indications. They are effective in treating severe erosive esophagitis that has not responded to therapy with H_2 receptor antagonists. They also are used in the short-term treatment of active peptic ulcer disease, especially when combined with an antibiotic to eradicate *H. pylori* (Box 48-1). Pathologic gastric hypersecretion disorders such as Zollinger-Ellison syndrome are treated with PPIs. All of the PPIs appear to be similar with respect to symptom relief and healing rates for gastric and duodenal ulcers and moderate to severe gastroesophageal reflux disease.

BOX 48-1 | **Examples of Combination Therapy for Eradication of *H. pylori****

1. Proton pump inhibitor twice daily, plus
   - clarithromycin twice daily, plus
   - metronidazole twice daily or amoxicillin twice daily.
2. Proton pump inhibitor once daily or H_2 antagonist at bedtime, plus
   - bismuth subsalicylate four times daily, plus
   - metronidazole four times daily, plus
   - tetracycline four times daily.
3. Proton pump inhibitor once daily or H_2 antagonist at bedtime, plus
   - amoxicillin three times daily, plus
   - clarithromycin three times daily, plus (optional)
   - bismuth subsalicylate four times daily.

*These are examples and not exhaustive of therapeutic combinations for eradication of *H. pylori*. Combination 1 is given for 7 days; combinations 2 and 3 for 7 to 14 days.

PHARMACOKINETICS

The onset of action for these drugs is fairly rapid, typically within 1 hour. Although the half-lives for all PPIs range from about 1 to 2 hours, the durations of action are longer and more varied. For example, the duration of action is approximately 24 hours for pantoprazole, more than 39 hours for lansoprazole, and 72 hours for omeprazole. All proton-pump inhibitors are biotransformed by the liver into inactive metabolites that are excreted in the feces. The elimination of these drugs may be slowed in patients with mild liver impairment or in older adults; however, dosage adjustments are not necessary.

ADVERSE REACTIONS AND CONTRAINDICATIONS

PPIs are generally well tolerated with few adverse effects. The most frequent adverse reactions during short-term therapy are headache, diarrhea, nausea and vomiting, and abdominal pain. The major concern for long-term therapy is the potential for overproduction of gastrin (hypergastrinemia), which has been shown to cause gastric carcinoid tumors in animals. At present this is a theoretical rather than an observed risk for humans, but more experience with these drugs will be needed to assess safety with long-term use.

INTERACTIONS

PPIs are extensively biotransformed in the liver, therefore careful monitoring is recommended when using these drugs along with others that are changed in the liver. Similarly, omeprazole and esomeprazole inhibit the hepatic biotransformation of oral anticoagulants, diazepam, and phenytoin, leading to high blood levels of these drugs.

PPIs change the pH of the stomach, thereby altering the bioavailability of drugs such as ketoconazole, iron salts, ampicillin, or digoxin, which depend on a specific gastric pH for absorption. Similarly, the absorption of vitamin B_{12} may be reduced.

ANTIMICROBIAL THERAPY FOR *H. PYLORI*

amoxicillin (Amoxil, Trimox)

clarithromycin (Biaxin)

metronidazole (Flagyl)

tetracycline

The identification of *H. pylori* as the major causative agent for peptic ulcers has added antimicrobials as the key to effective treatment of ulcers. *H. pylori* infection is endemic worldwide. The highest infection rates are associated with food and water contamination. For instance, the infection rate is lowest in Australia at 20% and highest in West Africa at 90%. Although infection occurs during childhood, the individual may remain asymptomatic throughout life. For individuals with symptoms of an ulcer, the presence of *H. pylori* can be confirmed by serologic testing or by the urease breath assay. A 2-week therapy with two appropriate antimicrobial drugs and acid suppression or bismuth leads to eradication of *H. pylori* in 80% of cases. In the future, a vaccine may be developed to prevent infection.

Amoxicillin is concentrated in gastric secretions and can therefore achieve effective antimicrobial concentrations in the lumen. Because amoxicillin is not very active in an acidic environment, suppression of acid secretion enhances antimicrobial activity. *H. pylori* does not become resistant to amoxicillin. Adverse effects of amoxicillin include diarrhea and yeast infections (see Chapter 25).

Clarithromycin can replace metronidazole in treatment therapies for *H. pylori*. Adverse reactions include diarrhea, nausea, headache, and a bad taste in the mouth. Resistance can develop to clarithromycin (see Chapter 26).

A two-drug combination therapy of clarithromycin (antimicrobial) and omeprazole (proton pump inhibitor) has been approved by the FDA for treatment of ulcers and *H. pylori* infection. The goal of two-drug combination therapies is to increase the patient compliance rate, which can be low with the more complicated triple and quadruple combination therapies.

Metronidazole is selective against bacteria that grow under low oxygen. It is secreted in gastric secretions and is not affected by acidic conditions. Although *H. pylori* is sensitive to metronidazole, resistance rapidly develops. Adverse reactions such as diarrhea, nausea, vomiting, and a metallic taste in the mouth are common. A disulfiram-like reaction can develop if the patient drinks an alcoholic beverage while taking metronidazole (see Chapter 30).

Tetracycline combined with bismuth and metronidazole is used to eradicate *H. pylori*. Similar to amoxicillin, tetracycline concentrates in the gastric mucosa, but it is also active in an acidic environment. To treat ulcers, tetracycline is taken with bismuth at meals to promote binding of the tetracycline to bismuth, a combination that promotes activity against *H. pylori*. Adverse effects of tetracycline include diarrhea and photosensitivity. Tetracycline is not recommended for pregnant women or children less than 8 years old (see Chapter 28).

Bismuth subsalicylate is used in combination with one or more antimicrobial drugs to treat ulcers. Bismuth is toxic to *H. pylori* and the organism does not develop resistance. Because of its short half-life, bismuth subsalicylate should be taken four times daily. Bismuth subsalicylate can turn the tongue and stools black. Caution should be exercised when treating children with fevers because of the salicylate content and the risk of Reye's syndrome.

Bismuth has been added to the H_2 antagonist ranitidine as ranitidine bismuth citrate. This combination of the bacteriocidal activity of bismuth with the suppression of acid secretion by ranitidine is approved for the treatment of ulcers.

DRUG CLASS • Antacids

Aluminum Compounds
  aluminum hydroxide (AlternaGel, Amphojel, Basajel)

  dihydroxyaluminum sodium carbonate (Rolaids)

Magnesium Compounds
  magaldrate (Riopan, Isopan✽)

  magnesium hydroxide (Milk of Magnesia)

  magnesium oxide (Uro-Mag)

Calcium Compounds
  calcium carbonate (Titralac)

Combination Compounds
  aluminum hydroxide and magnesium hydroxide (Maalox, Mylanta, Gelusil)

  aluminum hydroxide and magnesium trisilicate (Gaviscon)

MECHANISM OF ACTION

Antacids are weak bases that can be ingested to neutralize the hydrochloric acid secreted by the stomach. Although their mechanism for increasing the pH of the stomach differs and their effectiveness may be inferior to the drugs discussed earlier, the end result can be similar. The decrease in stomach acid can help to relieve the irritation of acid reflux in GERD as well as create an environment that is conducive for healing of peptic ulcers.

USES

These days, antacids are typically used to treat the symptoms of acid reflux or heartburn (indigestion). Although antacids were once the only available treatment for peptic ulcers, the more efficacious and convenient H_2 antagonists and PPIs have become the primary choices for that condition.

PHARMACOKINETICS

Antacids are not systemic drugs. For aluminum- or magnesium-containing products, very small amounts of aluminum and up to 10% of magnesium are absorbed from the GI tract. The remainder is excreted in the feces. In patients with significant renal impairment, the amount of magnesium absorbed may be significant enough to produce hypermagnesemia. Absorbed salts are then excreted in the urine. When calcium carbonate reacts with hydrochloric acid in the stomach, it mostly forms insoluble salts that are not well absorbed in the intestine. Small amounts of calcium and bicarbonate are absorbed, however, which can cause hypercalcemia.

ADVERSE REACTIONS AND CONTRAINDICATIONS

Aluminum and calcium salts tend to cause constipation, whereas magnesium salts tend to loosen the bowels. Therefore most antacids combine a magnesium salt or hydroxide and an aluminum or calcium salt or hydroxide. The most common adverse effect is diarrhea or constipation, even with a combination antacid. Calcium carbonate has a greater potential for allowing acid rebound and leading to the formation of kidney stones. As an adjunct to ulcer therapy, 1444 mEq of acid-neutralizing capacity taken 1 to 3 hours after meals and at bedtime gives adequate acid control and relieves the pain of ulcers (Table 48-2).

INTERACTIONS

Antacids impede the absorption of certain drugs by binding to them (chelation) and forming insoluble complexes. Drugs that may have decreased absorption because of chelation include antibiotics such as tetracyclines and fluoroquinolones and oral thyroid hormones. Antacids may also cause decreased absorption of digoxin, captopril, and acetaminophen. The absorption of drugs that require a strong acid environment for absorption, such as ketoconazole, itraconazole, and ampicillin, may be reduced.

Calcium containing antacids may alter urine pH (more alkaline), which reduces the clearance of drugs such as quinidine and enhances the urinary excretion of salicylates.

It should be remembered that enteric-coated drugs are designed to dissolve in more alkaline environments than the stomach. However, any drugs that increase the pH of the stomach may cause the enteric coating to be compromised.

TABLE 48-2

Neutralizing Capacity of Selected Antacids*

	Ingredient (mg/5 mL)					Neutralizing Capacity (mEq/5 mL)
	$Al(OH)_3$	$Mg(OH)_2$	$CaCO_3$	Simeth	Na Content	
Alternagel	600	0	0	—	<2.5	16
Aludrox	307	103	0	—	2.3	12
Amphojel	320	0	0	—	<2.3	10
Basaljel	400†	†	†	—	2.9	12
Di-Gel	200	200	0	20	<5	—
Gaviscon	31.7‡	‡	‡	—	4	13
Gelusil	200	200	0	25	0.7	12
Gelusil-M§	300	200	0	25	1.2	15
Maalox	225	200	0	0	1.4	13
Milk of Magnesia	0	390	0	0	0.12	14
Mylanta	200	200	0	20	0.7	13
Mylanta II	400	400	0	40	1.1	25
WinGel	180	160	0	0	—	10

Simeth, simethicone; *Na*, sodium content.

*Many of these antacid preparations are also available in solid dosage forms (i.e., tablets). Although the composition of these forms is often similar to that of suspensions, there are variations.

†Basaljel: $Al(OH)CO_3$ equivalent to 400 mg of $Al(OH)_3$.

‡Gaviscon: $Al(OH)_3$ plus 137 $MgCO^3$ plus sodium alginate.

§Therapeutic concentrate of Gelusil; *M*, medium strength.

DRUG CLASS • Prokinetic Drugs

metoclopramide (Reglan)

MECHANISM OF ACTION

Prokinetic drugs are those that enhance the contractile force of GI smooth muscle, including the lower esophageal sphincter, and accelerate luminal transit of contents in the GI tract. Metoclopramide is a peripherally (GI tract) and centrally acting dopaminergic antagonist that indirectly increases parasympathetic (cholinergic) activity in the gut. These actions lead to increased esophageal peristalsis, increased lower esophageal sphincter pressure, increased antral contractions, and relaxed pyloric sphincter and duodenal tone. The combined effect is to accelerate gastric emptying and intestinal transit from the duodenum to the ileocecal valve. Metoclopramide appears to have little effect on gastric acid secretion or motility of the colon.

USES

Prokinetic drugs are used for conditions such as GERD, diabetic gastroparesis and postsurgical GI stasis. In the treatment of GERD, metoclopramide may be as effective as H_2 antagonists for managing symptoms and acute healing but is inferior to therapy with PPIs.

PHARMACOKINETICS

Metoclopramide is administered orally and parenterally. It appears to undergo minimal biotransformation, but the elimination and half-life of metoclopramide is prolonged in patients with renal insufficiency. Metoclopramide is distributed into breast milk, and it crosses the blood-brain barrier and the placenta.

ADVERSE REACTIONS AND CONTRAINDICATIONS

Metoclopramide antagonizes dopamine receptors in the CNS. Central dopaminergic blockade may produce sedation and extrapyramidal (movement) adverse effects such as dystonic reactions, akathisia, and facial grimac-

ing. Inhibition of dopamine receptors by metoclopramide in the pituitary and hypothalamus increases prolactin secretion. Chronic treatment may cause gynecomastia in men, breast enlargement in women, and galactorrhea in both sexes. Impotence, resulting from hyperprolactinemia, may develop in men, whereas women may experience menstrual irregularity.

Metoclopramide should be used cautiously in patients with a known hypersensitivity to procainamide. It is contraindicated in patients with GI obstruction, perforation, or ileus. Metoclopramide should be administered cautiously, if at all, to patients with a preexisting seizure disorder or Parkinson's disease.

INTERACTIONS

Because it can increase gastric emptying, metoclopramide may affect the rate or extent of absorption of other drugs, such as acetaminophen, aspirin, diazepam, lithium, and tetracycline.

Drugs with significant anticholinergic activity (the antimuscarinics) block the therapeutic potential of metoclopramide on the GI tract. Diphenoxylate, loperamide, and opiate agonists antagonize GI motility, thus enhancing the effects of metoclopramide.

Because it blocks central dopamine receptors, metoclopramide cancels the actions of dopamine agonists used for treating Parkinson's disease. Conversely, if metoclopramide is used with drugs such as the antipsychotics chlorpromazine and haloperidol, which antagonize dopamine receptors, the extrapyramidal or dystonic effects may be additive.

DRUG CLASS • Miscellaneous Drugs

misoprostol (Cytotec)
sucralfate (Carafate)

Misoprostol is an ester of prostaglandin E_1, a chemical relative of the prostaglandins, and is normally synthesized in the stomach, where they (i.e., the prostaglandins) block gastric acid secretion. NSAIDs, including aspirin, inhibit the synthesis of naturally occurring prostaglandins when

they dissolve in the stomach. Therefore bleeding from gastric ulcers is a significant problem with long-term use of NSAIDs. Patients with arthritis who must take NSAIDs to relieve inflammation and pain are often prescribed misoprostol to replace the prostaglandins. Misoprostol blocks the secretion of excess acid and therefore protects the stomach mucosa. Misoprostol is also used to treat duodenal and peptic ulcers caused by NSAID use.

Minor adverse reactions such as diarrhea, mild nausea, abdominal discomfort, and dizziness are occasionally reported with misoprostol use. Serious adverse reactions include vaginal bleeding and abortion in pregnant women, an action expected of a prostaglandin E_1 analog. One study reported bleeding in 50% of pregnant women and a 7% incidence of abortion. Therefore misoprostol is contraindicated for pregnant women and should be used cautiously in women of childbearing age.

Sucralfate is a complex of sulfated sucrose and aluminum hydroxide that is changed by stomach acid into viscous material that binds to proteins in ulcerated tissue. This action protects the ulcer from the destructive action of the digestive enzyme pepsin. Sucralfate may be used in the initial treatment (first 1 to 2 months) of a duodenal ulcer. Sucralfate does not neutralize stomach acid or inhibit acid secretion.

Sucralfate should be given alone 30 to 60 minutes before meals so that it can be activated by stomach acid and coat the ulcer. Because sucralfate binds digoxin, tetracycline, warfarin, phenytoin, quinidine, and theophylline, these drugs should be taken at a different time. Sucralfate also decreases the bioavailability of ciprofloxacin and norfloxacin.

APPLICATION TO PRACTICE

ASSESSMENT
History of Present Illness

Patients with ulcers or gastroesophageal reflux may have a variety of complaints; thus the reason for the hospitalization or clinic visit should be determined. The patient's perception of the problem, its onset, recent stressors, lifestyle changes during the previous 2 years, and any other precipitating factors should be noted. Elicit information about recent fever, nausea, vomiting, heartburn or indigestion, tarry stools, changes in bowel patterns (constipation or diarrhea), abdominal cramping, or recent weight changes. Activities or factors that precipitate, exacerbate, or alleviate symptoms should be noted. For example, eating often alleviates epigastric pain for a short time.

It is common for patients with peptic ulcer disease (PUD) to have no pain or other symptoms because gastric and duodenal mucosa do not have pain sensory fibers. The pain of gastric ulcers is located high in the epigastrium and occurs spontaneously 1 to 2 hours after meals. It is often described as a burning, gaseous pain. The pain occurs when the stomach is empty and when food has been ingested. If the ulcer has eroded through the gastric mucosa, food tends to aggravate rather than alleviate the pain. Some patients do not experience pain until a perforation or hemorrhage has occurred.

The pain of duodenal ulcers usually occurs 2 to 4 hours after meals, when the stomach is empty, and is described as burning or cramplike. The pain is located in the mid-epigastrium, beneath the xiphoid process. The pain is relieved by antacids and sometimes by foods that neutralize and dilute gastric acid. Some patients claim their symptoms are worse in the spring and fall of the year, thus supporting the seasonal trend in occurrence. Ulcers located on the posterior aspect of the duodenum may manifest as back pain.

Lack of symptoms does not necessarily indicate the absence of an ulcer. Asymptomatic ulcers are common, especially in older adults and in patients who are on chronic NSAID therapy. It is estimated that 30% to 50% of peptic ulcer complications occur in asymptomatic patients.

Patients with GERD often complain of heartburn. Other signs and symptoms the patient may note include regurgitation, dysphagia or a sensation of "something stuck in the throat," angina-like chest pain, bronchospasm, laryngitis, and a chronic cough, particularly worse at nighttime. Twenty-four percent of these patients have had symptoms for over 10 years. Seventeen percent use indigestion aids at least once weekly, but only 24% of affected persons have seen their health care provider.

Health History

Information important in the assessment of a patient complaining of GI distress includes the patient's and family's health history, allergies, drug history, concomitant diseases or illnesses, and associated risk factors. The patient should also be questioned about respiratory or cardiovascular disease, current traumas, burns, and recent intake and output values.

If the patient reports having chronic allergies, ask about the type of allergies and symptoms, all drugs used in the treatment of allergies, and the patient's reactions to the drugs. H_2 blockers are frequently used in the management of allergies but have no effect on GI histamine receptors and the GI tract's ability to secrete gastric acid.

Specific drugs may produce GI discomfort; therefore, the drug history should include the patient's current and past drug use. It should include OTC drugs, alcohol, tobacco, prescription drugs including antineoplastic drugs, radiation, vitamin and mineral supplements, household items such as baking soda, laxatives and enemas as well as items ingested based on cultural beliefs such as paint chips, specific herbs, and other items. The use of aspirin, aspirin-containing products and other NSAIDs, corticosteroids, and anticoagulants place the patient at greater risk for bleeding episodes. Because many OTC drugs contain aspirin, it is not unusual for the patient to deny taking aspirin but self-treat with products such as Alka-Seltzer, Bufferin, or Excedrin. Therefore, a careful history of all commonly used drugs is necessary.

Lifespan Considerations

Perinatal. Nausea and vomiting during the first trimester is usually caused by the body's response to human chorionic gonadotrophin secreted by the implanted fetus and reactions to changes in carbohydrate metabolism (see Chapter 3). However, the perinatal patient's gastric contents become more acidic during pregnancy as a result of elevated gastrin levels produced by the placenta. During the second and third trimesters, several GI symptoms are attributable to the physical pressure from the growing uterus, as well as the smooth muscle relaxation triggered by elevated progesterone levels. Relaxation of the cardiac sphincter frequently causes heartburn as the gastric contents from the stomach move into the lower esophagus. Gastric emptying time and intestinal motility are also delayed, which lead to frequent complaints of constipation and bloating. Once delivery has taken place, the woman's pregnancy-related GI symptoms usually abate.

Pediatric. The exact cause of PUD in children is unknown, although infectious, genetic, and environmental factors are implicated. There is an increased familial incidence and an increased incidence in persons with blood group O. The ulcers may occur in the stomach or duodenum and are characterized as multiple and superficial. The signs and symptoms of PUD vary according to the age of the child and the location of the ulcer.

Chronic abdominal pain or weight loss may be the only signs of primary PUD. The abdominal pain may be nonspecific, but epigastric pain, especially if it penetrates to the back and is relieved temporarily by eating, points to the possibility of an ulcer. The presence of anemia or occult stool blood are further indications of possible PUD.

Approximately 1:300 to 1:1000 children have a significant problem with GERD. The condition may occur in infants who are premature; who have undergone tracheoesophageal or esophageal atresia repair; or who have bronchopulmonary dysphasia, neurologic disorders, scoliosis, asthma, cystic fibrosis, or cerebral palsy. Upper GI contrast studies are less effective if the child is unable to cooperate fully, thus making endoscopic ex-

aminations of infants and children more frequent. In most cases, the best treatment for hyperacidity and reflux in children is prevention. Children at risk should be treated prophylactically. Children with chronic ulcers often receive histamine antagonist drugs or PPIs.

Older Adults. Peptic ulcers and GERD occur at all ages, but the incidence is on the rise in older adults. An older adult experiencing a major body insult, whether medical or psychologic, is at risk for ulcer development, particularly if a preexisting gastritis is present. In addition to stress, diet, and genetic predisposition, other factors are believed to account for the increased incidence of ulcers in the aged. Longevity, more precise diagnostic evaluation, and the fact that ulcers can be a complication of chronic airway limitation disorders also increase the incidence.

Early symptoms commonly associated with peptic ulcers or GERD may not be as evident in the older adult. Epigastric pain is not a prominent feature. More frequently, the outstanding symptoms the older adult exhibits include poorly localized pain, decreased appetite, decreased general energy level, melena, weight loss, vomiting, and anemia. Even with a perforation, symptoms may be vague. Regardless of the cause, the consequences of GI bleeding are much more severe in the older adult.

Cultural/Social Considerations

A patient's diet has both a direct and indirect effect on the GI tract mucous membranes. Food choices, fluid, and fiber intake should be noted as well as any anorexia and weight loss. Poor nutrition contributes to the occurrence of PUD and GERD. It is helpful to assess the relationship that food and drink have to the patient. Does the patient eat alone? What percentage of income is spent on food? Is help required for meal preparation or transportation?

The stressor or stressors that exist in the patient's life and the coping mechanisms used to respond should be determined. The amount of stress needed to affect a patient's physiology is idiosyncratic. A person's perception of the stressor and methods of handling stress are, for a large part, a product of his or her environment.

The effectiveness of a patient's support network may be an indicator of the level of stress a patient may be experiencing. If the patient has an effective support network and uses the network, studies have shown that the patient experiences a lower level of overall stress than a patient without a support network.

A regular employment pattern is important because it relates to the ability of the patient to meet life's needs. An individual looks to employment to satisfy any number of needs, such as the need to be productive, to provide for individual and family financial needs, to meet social needs, and more. When an imbalance exists between the patient's needs and the job's ability to meet those needs, stress results. A patient's activity level is an additional factor in the overall data. It is important to evaluate the patient's employment and activity level from the patient's perspective and the effect on the patient's state of health.

The patient's educational level has an indirect effect on the patient's health as it relates to stress and seeking medical care. If a low level of education results in poverty, the consistent stress that is present has a chronic effect on hyperacidity, PUD, and GERD. Studies have shown that patients with lower educational levels are less informed regarding the benefits of medical care and are less likely to be compliant with follow-up care. In addition, fewer are covered by health insurance.

The patient's past experiences with the health care system should be evaluated because it affects patient care management. The point at which the patient sought medical care, the patient's level of trust in health care providers, the degree of compliance with the long-term and short-term plan of care, and the integration of lifestyle changes into the patient's life are all important. Awareness of the patient's past experiences may permit a more appropriate plan of care that will provide maximum benefit for the patient (see the Case Study: GERD with *H. pylori* Infection).

Physical Examination

Before starting the physical examination, it is important to have the patient identify the area or areas causing the most pain. The examiner should then avoid that area until the end of the examination. It is also necessary to assess any acute or chronic signs briefly that may dictate the need for urgent interventions.

The more acute the abdominal pain, the greater the likelihood of perforation. If the pain is acute, the response needs to be immediate, without a thorough history or assessment. If the patient complains of chills or is febrile, the situation is more acute in that sepsis may be present. The absence of liver dullness may indicate an air viscus from perforation.

The patient's vital signs rarely provide clues to the cause of chronic abdominal pain, but close monitoring helps identify early changes in condition. Inspection of the abdomen usually does not provide significant data regarding peptic ulcer and gastroesophageal reflux. However, note whether the patient has any scars that may indicate previous abdominal surgery and whether the patient is guarding the abdomen. Muscle spasms and altered bowel sounds are unusual. Listen for tympanic sounds over all four quadrants. Abdominal pain when coughing or rebound tenderness may be apparent when peritoneal irritation is present.

Laboratory Testing

Laboratory test results are normal in patients with uncomplicated PUD but tests may be ordered to rule out ulcer complications or confounding disease states. Anemia caused by acute blood loss from a bleeding ulcer or, less commonly, from chronic blood loss may be reflected in the CBC. Urine and stool are routinely tested for occult blood.

Vomiting may occur in response to excessive pain or may reflect intraabdominal irritation and should be tested for blood. A coffee-ground appearance to the emesis suggests that blood has been in the stomach long enough to interact with the hydrochloric acid. On the other hand, bright red blood indicates active bleeding of the esophagus lining or cardiac portion of the stomach.

Liver function tests may be done to help evaluate patient complaints. An elevated serum amylase level in a patient with severe epigastric pain suggests ulcer penetration into the pancreas. A fasting serum gastrin level to screen for Zollinger-Ellison syndrome is obtained in some patients.

Serologic tests may be helpful in the initial diagnosis of *H. pylori* but are not reliable in documenting eradication. The FDA-approved breath test, Meretek UBT, can be used to test for eradication but costs over $300. To use the test, the patient drinks a liquid containing carbon-13 (^{13}C, which is not radioactive) and breathes into a container, which is then sent to the laboratory. In the presence of *H. pylori*, bacterial urease hydrolyzes the urea, releasing $^{13}CO_2$, which can be detected by a mass spectrometer. This new test appears to be highly specific but can yield 5% to 10% false-negative results.

Given the importance of *H. pylori* in the pathogenesis of PUD, testing for this organism is ordinarily performed in all patients with suspected PUD. In patients for whom an ulcer is diagnosed by endoscopy, gastric mucosal biopsies may be obtained for both a rapid urease test and histology. The histology specimen is discarded if the urease test is positive.

A gastric analysis may also be used to determine the acidity of gastric secretions in a basal state (without stimulation) and the maximal secretory state (with stimulation of gastric secretions). Elevated levels of free hydrochloride may indicate either a duodenal or gastric ulcer or Zollinger-Ellison syndrome. It has been suggested that the reason for the low level of acid recovered by gastric analysis in patients with a gastric ulcer is an increase in the backward diffusion of gastric acid rather than lower production.

GOALS OF THERAPY

Until recently, the control of acid secretion was the goal of treatment for PUD and GERD. Now control of acid secretion is just part of the treatment. The introduction of H_2 receptors and PPIs in the past decade dramatically improved the ability to control acid secretion and allow ulcer healing. Antacids and anticholinergic drugs, once a mainstay of ulcer therapy, now play a minor role. Mucosal protective drugs also aid ulcer healing. The recognition that a bacterial cause underlies many ulcers has led to therapies that include antibiotics for eradicating of the causative agent, *H. pylori*. Now, the primary goal in the treatment of PUD and GERD is to ameliorate symptoms and promote healing while preventing complications.

INTERVENTION
Peptic Ulcer Disease

For persons at high risk for PUD, identification of contributory factors should be carried out. Once those factors have been identified, the person can take primary preventative action. Smoking, although not a primary cause of PUD or of hyperacidity, has an irritating effect on the mucosa, increases gastric motility, and delays mucosal healing. The combination of inadequate rest and smoking accelerates ulcer development.

Secondary prevention involves the detection and treatment of the disease early in its course. For example, the use of aspirin and NSAIDs should be discontinued when possible. Interventions are aimed at detecting problems early in their course so that prompt treatment can forestall the serious consequences of advanced disease. When irritating drugs must be continued, enteric-coated or highly buffered preparations are more suitable.

Tertiary prevention of PUD is time intensive. The healing and subsequent cure of PUD requires 8 to 12 weeks of therapy, depending on the ulcer size and the specific treatment regimen (see Box 48-1). Although the pain may be alleviated in less than a week, healing is much slower. For many patients, better-tolerated, shorter treatment regimens that require fewer pills per day may prove to be more effective than more complicated regimens with higher eradication rates. Recurrence of duodenal ulceration after healing can be as high as 80% within 1 year when elimination of *H. pylori* is not part of treatment. The recurrence rate is less than 5% when *H. pylori* is eradicated.

In general, duodenal ulcers are treated with nighttime acid suppression, whereas gastric ulcers and GERD usually require 24-hour acid suppression. With this principle in mind, available treatment options include the nonsystemic antacids, H_2 antagonists, PPIs, or a cytoprotective drug. A combination of these drugs may be used in some circumstances.

Gastroesophageal Reflux Disease

Otherwise healthy patients with a classic history of uncomplicated GERD can be treated empirically, employing step 1 and 2 measures (Box 48-2). In many cases, these measures will suffice. If the patient fails to respond or if the reflux is complicated by dysphagia, weight loss, anemia, or if the stool tests positive for occult bleeding, a more comprehensive diagnostic evaluation is indicated.

Administration

It is important that drugs be administered on time, for the full duration of therapy, and that other drugs be administered at other times.

In most cases, antacids decrease the absorption of other drugs taken concurrently. Therefore, it is recommended that the administration of other drugs be separated by at least 1 hour. To ensure healing, antacids, when used to treat PUD, should be continued for 4 to 8 weeks after all symptoms have disappeared. The healing period is variable, depending on the depth, number, and

---

BOX 48-2 | **Stepwise Treatment for GERD**

Step 1: Lifestyle Changes

- Avoid foods high in fat or carbohydrates (chocolate can be particularly problematic because it is high in both elements).
- If obese, lose weight.
- Avoid large meals within 2 hours of bedtime or before exercise.
- Take advantage of gravity. Sleep with the head of the bed elevated on 6-inch blocks under the bedposts (pillows are not sufficient for elevation).
- Avoid tight clothing around the waist.
- If possible, avoid drugs that decrease lower esophageal sphincter tone (e.g., theophylline, calcium channel blockers, meperidine, anticholinergics).
- If possible, avoid drugs that may injure esophageal mucosa (e.g., tetracycline, wax matrix potassium supplements, NSAIDs, steroids).
- Significantly reduce or eliminate tobacco use.
- Avoid the following foods: alcohol, caffeine-containing beverages (e.g., coffee, tea, soda), yellow onions, chocolate, mint in any form, grapefruit or grapefruit juice, oranges or orange juice, and tomatoes in any form (e.g., salsa, spaghetti sauce, pizza, ketchup).

Step 2: Drug Therapy

- Add an oral H_2 antagonist. If not effective after 6 to 8 weeks, add a proton pump inhibitor but limit therapy to no more than 3 to 6 months (drug of choice for erosive esophagitis).
- Add metoclopramide or bethanechol.

Step 3: Surgical Intervention

- Consider antireflux surgery (e.g., Nissen fundoplication, crural tightening) for incapacitating refractory disease.

location of ulcers. Some antacids contain large amounts of sodium and should be used cautiously in patients on sodium restriction.

Follow the manufacturer's recommendations when administering H₂ antagonists. Too rapid administration of ranitidine has been associated with bradycardia, tachycardia, and premature ventricular contractions (PVCs). Prefilled syringes of cimetidine are intended for intramuscular use or for diluting for intermittent infusion, not for direct intravenous injection. Check for compatibilities with intravenous H₂ antagonists. Cimetidine is not compatible with many other drugs for infusion.

The PPI pantoprazole, like rabeprazole, is available in tablets that can be crushed and given with liquid through feeding tubes that are placed distal to the stomach. The tube placement is critical to effective treatment because these drugs are inactivated by gastric acid.

Education

The successful management of PUD and reflux depends on the patient's compliance with diet, drugs, and postural measures. A thorough explanation of the mechanisms of ulcer disease or reflux and its aggravating factors help provide a rational basis for patient action. The patient and family members, as appropriate, should be taught the name of the drug, the dosage, purpose for taking the drug, benefits anticipated from therapy, and the time period over which drug therapy is expected.

Patients should be taught that no single measure will alleviate the discomfort of PUD or reflux, but when all of the interventions are performed together, relief is extremely likely. Nondrug measures, such as relaxation and stress management, help prevent or minimize symptoms and are often as effective as drugs when they are used concurrently.

Unlike GERD, diet therapy has little role in the prevention or treatment of PUD. Although many patients consider milk an alkali, it has little effect on the pH of gastric secretions. The calcium and protein content of dairy products stimulate gastric acid secretion. A treatment regimen that includes the frequent ingestion of dairy products may actually aggravate PUD. Smoking cessation, avoiding highly spiced foods, gas-forming foods, alcohol, and caffeine-containing beverages may help relieve symptoms and promote healing.

It is also critical that the patient be instructed to take the drug for the full duration of therapy. Halting therapy when symptoms improve is a major cause for exacerbation of symptoms. Instruct the patient to swallow capsules whole, not to break or chew them. Remind the patient to take missed doses as soon as remembered, unless it is almost time for the next dose, in which case the missed dose should be omitted and the regular dosing schedule resumed. Do not double up for missed doses.

Remind patients to chew antacid tablets thoroughly and then follow with a full glass of water. Instruct them to take a small amount of water after an antacid suspension to ensure that the dose is carried to the stomach. Antacids used in the treatment of PUD are often administered 1 hour and 3 hours after meals and at bedtime. Be sure to review the health care provider's orders with the patient.

Have the patient who is taking antacids increase the daily fluid intake to 3000 mL so as to reduce the risk of kidney stone formation. For patients bothered by diarrhea or constipation as a result of antacid use, suggesting the use of a combination antacid product may help. A high-fiber diet and consuming 2000 to 3000 mL of fluid daily also helps in preventing constipation.

Advise patients taking a once-daily H₂ antagonist to do so at bedtime; twice-daily doses in the morning and at bedtime, and more frequent doses with meals and at bedtime. If antacids or metoclopramide are also ordered, they should be taken 1 hour before or 2 hours after the dose of the H₂ antagonist. Teach patients taking ranitidine effervescent granules or tablets to dissolve the dose in 6 to 8 ounces of water before drinking. Warn patients taking nonprescription-strength H₂ antagonists to take doses no longer than 2 weeks on a regular basis unless approved by the health care provider.

Instruct the patient taking the PPIs lansoprazole and omeprazole capsules to do so immediately before a meal, preferably in the morning. Omeprazole tablets may be taken on an empty stomach, with food, or with antacids as ordered.

Encourage patients to comply with therapy and continue with follow-up care for at least 1 year. The patient and family should also be instructed that any change in symptoms or the appearance of blood, tarry stools, or coffee-ground emesis signals the need to contact the health care provider.

EVALUATION

As with all patient care, perceived susceptibility to disease and its seriousness influences treatment outcomes. The need for long-term drug regimens should raise questions regarding the patient's commitment to the plan of care. It is necessary to work with the patient and family members, as appropriate, to solicit support and cooperation from all parties. A plan that is relevant to the patient and family increases the level of compliance.

The primary determination of treatment effectiveness is in the healing of peptic ulcers and a reduction in acid reflux. In evaluating the patient's response to the regimen, the health care provider would expect to find fewer complaints of abdominal pain and discomfort, and few or no complaints of adverse drug effects.

CASE STUDY

GERD with Helicobacter pylori *Infection*

ASSESSMENT

HISTORY OF PRESENT ILLNESS

NJ, a 46-year-old woman reports to the medical clinic today with complaints of increasing gastric distress for the past 4 weeks. She has tried an occasional dose of Maalox with short-term relief from the epigastric pain. NJ also notes that she has had a cough that is particularly bad at night and it worsens when she eats before going to bed. Two weeks ago she had an abscessed tooth and has been taking a NSAID several times a day for the discomfort.

HEALTH HISTORY

Past history negative for peptic ulcer disease. She had a cholecystectomy 5 years ago. NJ reports she does not drink alcohol, nor does she take any drugs on a routine basis. She has a 15 pack/yr smoking history. The remainder of her past health history is unremarkable.

LIFESPAN CONSIDERATIONS

NJ is worried that she will be admitted to the hospital and not be available to help her husband on the family farm.

CULTURAL/SOCIAL CONSIDERATIONS

NJ is a housewife who lives on a farm with her husband of 27 years. Her 57-year-old husband was hospitalized 3 months ago with an MI. Although his condition has improved, NJ worries about him a great deal. NJ has two grown daughters who live nearby. NJ is active in community and church affairs. NJ and her husband are self-employed with the family farm. They carry only catastrophic health insurance and have no pharmacy coverage. NJ is concerned about the cost of treatment.

PHYSICAL EXAMINATION

NJ's vital signs are stable; she is 5'3" tall and weighs 145 lbs. Bowel sounds are present in all four quadrants. No palpable hepatosplenomegaly or masses. No abdominal bruits noted. Epigastric area is tender to light and deep palpation.

LABORATORY TESTING

CBC count, electrolytes, BUN, creatinine level, and sedimentation rate are within normal limits. *H. pylori* organisms present on analysis. Stool is negative for occult blood.

PATIENT PROBLEM(S)

Gastroesophageal reflux disease (GERD).

GOALS OF THERAPY

Ameliorate symptoms, promote healing, prevent complications, and prevent recurrence of reflux.

CRITICAL THINKING QUESTIONS

1. The health care provider orders Prevpac 1 dose bid for 14 days (a Prevpac contains 30 mg of lansoprazole, 1000 mg of amoxicillin, and 500 mg of clarithromycin). What is the mechanism of action of these drugs?
2. What are the common adverse effects that NJ should be made aware of during Prevpac therapy?
3. What factors in NJ's life may be contributing to her GERD?
4. What information does NJ need regarding dietary habits to help reduce her symptoms?
5. What can you tell NJ that will help her avoid the nighttime coughing episodes she is experiencing?
6. How did the health care provider know that NJ had an *H. pylori* infection?

Bibliography

Abramowicz M: Pantoprazole (Protonix), *The Medical Letter* 42(1083):65-66

Abramowicz M: Pantoprazole through feeding tubes: a clarification, *The Medical Letter* 42(1084):72.

Anonymous. Clinical upate. Preventing and treating NSAID-induced ulcers: ACG guidelines. *Crit Illness,* 14(2):73-74, 77, 1999.

Anonymous. Which drug class is best for GERD? *Pat Care* 34(17):26-28, 34-35, 39-40 passim, 2000.

Aronson BS: Applying clinical practice guidelines to a patient with complicated gastroesophageal reflux disease, *Gastroenterol Nurs*, 23(4).143-147, 2000.

Bailey MA, Katz PO: Gastroesophageal reflux disease in the elderly, *Clin Geriatr* 8(8):64-72, 2000.

Chiba N, DeGara CJ, Wilkinson JM, et al: Speed of healing and symptom relief in grade UU to IV gastroesophageal reflux disease: a metaanalysis, *Gastroenterology* 112:1798-1820, 1997.

DeVault KR: Guidelines for the diagnosis and treatment of gastroesophageal reflux disease, *Am J Man Care* 6(9 Suppl):S476-S479, S508-S511, 2000.

Humphries TJ: Safely treating acid-related diseases in the elderly, *Home Healthcare Consultant* 7(8):23-28, 2000.

Mead M: Duodenal ulcer, *Prac Nurse* 18(9):622-623, 1999.

Smith C: Pantoprazole: a new benzimidazole proton pump inhibitor for oral and IV administration, *Formulary* 35(1):28 30, 33-34, 37, 2000.

Webb DD: New therapeutic options in the treatment of GERD and other acid-peptic disorders, *Am J Man Care* 6(9 Suppl): S467-S475, S508-S511, 2000.

Laxatives and Antidiarrheal Drugs

LYNN ROGER WILLIS • KATHLEEN GUTIERREZ

 Visit http://evolve.elsevier.com/Gutierrez/ for additional information.

KEY TERMS

Bulk-forming laxatives, p. 799

Cathartics, p. 796

Constipation, p. 796

Diarrhea, p. 806

Hyperosmotic laxatives, p. 800

Laxatives, p. 796

Purgatives, p. 796

Stimulant laxatives, p. 797

Stool softeners, p. 799

OBJECTIVES

- Relate the physiologic and pathophysiologic changes that occur with constipation and diarrhea.
- Describe the factors that contribute to constipation and diarrhea.
- Identify the treatment goals for the patient with constipation and the patient with diarrhea.
- Recognize drug interactions that are clinically significant.
- Identify the patient and laboratory parameters available to support and monitor drug therapy for patients receiving laxatives and antidiarrheal drugs.

Normal physiologic functions of the lower gastrointestinal (GI) tract include motility, absorption, and secretion. Alterations in one or more of these functions result in constipation or diarrhea. Although various drugs can be used for symptomatic relief of constipation or diarrhea, drug therapy does not correct the underlying cause and in some cases may even worsen the problem. This chapter focuses on drugs used to prevent or alleviate constipation and diarrhea.

PATHOPHYSIOLOGY • Constipation

The primary function of the colon is to absorb water and dissolved minerals. By removing 90% of the fluid each day, the colon converts 1000 to 2000 mL of isotonic chyme from the ileum into about 150 g of semisolid stool. In general, the first remnants of a meal reach the hepatic flexure in 6 hours, the splenic flexure in 9 hours, and the pelvic colon in 12 hours. Transport is much slower from the pelvic colon to the anus; as much as 25% of the residue from a meal may still be in the rectum 72 hours later.

Constipation is defined as infrequent defecation, a hardening or reduced caliber of stool, a sensation of incomplete evacuation, and strained bowel movements. Defecation less than three times a week is a commonly accepted criterion for the diagnosis of constipation. In bowel-conscious America, the amount of misinformation and inordinate apprehension about constipation probably exceeds that of any other health concern. Approximately 4 million people in the United States have frequent constipation. This figure corresponds to a prevalence of 2%, which makes constipation the most frequent GI problem seen in ambulatory care settings. The prevalence is highest in the southern United States and is reported more often by patients over the age of 65. In this age group, the problem is often a result of physical inactivity rather than intrinsic bowel changes related to aging.

Constipation of recent onset is usually related to changes in lifestyle or health status. Inadequate fluids or dietary fiber is the most common cause of chronic constipation. Other culprits include dietary changes related to aging and restrictive weight-loss programs as well as poor dentition. In contrast, constipation of long duration indicates a functional cause (i.e., not responding to the urge to defecate) or chronic organic disease. Busy schedules with no established time for regular elimination also contribute to constipation. Disorders that may originally manifest as constipation include hypothyroidism, diabetes mellitus, hypokalemia, hypercalcemia, and neurologic disorders. In some instances, constipation may be drug induced (Box 49-1).

BOX 49-1	**Drugs Likely to Cause Constipation**

Analgesics (opioids and NSAIDs)
Aluminum-containing antacids
Anticholinergic drugs
Antidiarrheal drugs
Antiparkinson drugs
atropine
barium sulfate
Beta blockers
Calcium channel blockers
Cation exchange resins
cimetidine
clonidine
Diuretics
Ganglionic blocking drugs
Heavy metals (especially lead)
Iron supplements
MAO inhibitor antidepressants
Muscle relaxants
Phenothiazines
phenylephrine
pseudoephedrine
ranitidine
Saline laxatives (habitual use)
Stimulant laxatives (habitual use)
sucralfate
terbutaline
trazodone
Tricyclic antidepressants

Drugs used for the symptomatic relief of constipation are often classified as laxatives, cathartics, or purgatives. The terms are frequently used interchangeably, although not necessarily accurately. **Laxatives** loosen the bowel contents and encourage evacuation of soft stool. **Cathartics** and **purgatives** promote intense elimination activity and loss of water. The same drug can produce any of these effects, depending on the dosage and the patient's sensitivity to the drug (Figure 49-1).

DRUG CLASS • Stimulant Laxatives

bisacodyl (Dulcagen, Dulcolax, Fleet Laxative)

cascara sagrada

casanthranol

castor oil (Neoloid)

senna (Black-Draught, Fletcher's Castoria, Senexon, Senokot, Senolax)

MECHANISM OF ACTION

Stimulant laxatives act on the intestinal wall of the small bowel and colon to increase the amount of fluid and electrolytes within the intestinal lumen. Additionally, they cause the release of prostaglandins and produce an increase in cyclic adenosine monophosphate (cAMP) concentration, which in turn increases

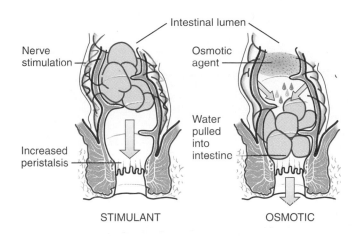

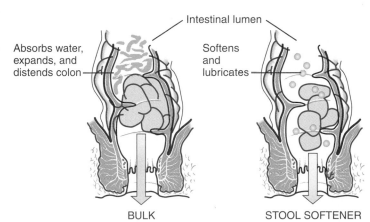

FIGURE 49-1 Mechanism of action of four types of laxatives. Stimulant laxatives act on the intestinal wall of the small bowel or colon to increase the amount of fluid and electrolytes within the intestinal lumen. Osmotic laxatives act by drawing water into the intestinal lumen and causing peristalsis. The greater the concentration of solutes, the greater the osmotic activity. Bulk-forming laxatives combine with water in the intestine to form an emollient gel or viscous solution. The result is an increase in peristalsis. Stool softeners produce an emollient action that reduces surface tension and thus facilitates penetration of water and lipids into the stool.

the secretion of electrolytes and contributes to the cathartic effect.

Specifically, bisacodyl, cascara, and senna stimulate the submucosal and mesenteric plexus to produce semi-soft or soft, formed stool. Cascara produces propulsive movements of the colon by direct chemical irritation.

USES

Stimulant laxatives are used to treat constipation associated with prolonged bed rest, constipating drugs, slowed transit times, and irritable bowel syndrome. They can also be used to evacuate the bowel before radiologic studies or surgery. Stimulants are included as part of a bowel regimen for patients with spinal cord injuries or neurologic disorders. Castor oil is obsolete and should not be used, because it causes serious toxicity.

PHARMACOKINETICS

The pharmacokinetics of stimulant laxatives are identified in Table 49-1. Their onset times vary from less than 15 minutes for bisacodyl suppositories to more than 24 hours for senna preparations. Bisacodyl is minimally absorbed (less than 5%) following oral administration. Small amounts of bisacodyl metabolites are found in

breast milk. Biotransformation takes place in the liver. The half-life of bisacodyl is unknown, although evacuation takes place in 6 to 12 hours.

ADVERSE REACTIONS AND CONTRAINDICATIONS

The most common adverse reactions of stimulant laxatives include mild cramping, nausea, vomiting, diarrhea, and even dehydration in susceptible individuals. Continued use of these laxatives produces diarrhea similar to that seen in irritable bowel syndrome and can be severe enough to cause fluid and electrolyte imbalances. Stimulant laxatives can cause proctitis in men. Hypokalemia, tetany, and protein-losing enteropathy also occur with long-term use of stimulant laxatives.

Stimulant laxatives are contraindicated for patients with hypersensitivity to these drugs, abdominal pain of unknown cause (especially when associated with fever), rectal fissures, and ulcerated hemorrhoids. The aromatic fluid extract formulation of cascara sagrada contains alcohol and should not be given to patients with known intolerance to alcohol. Excessive or prolonged use of stimulant laxatives may lead to dependence.

---| **TABLE 49-1** |---

Pharmacokinetics of Selected Laxatives

Drug	Route	Onset	Evacuation	Site	Stool Type
Stimulant Laxatives					
bisacodyl	po	6-10 hr	6-12 hr	C	SS
	pr	15-60 min	15-60 min	C	SS
castor oil	po	2-6 hr	2-3 hr	SB	W
cascara sagrada	po	6-10 hr	6-10 hr	C	SS
senna	po	6-24 hr	1-3 days	SB, C	SF
Stool Softeners					
docusate calcium	po	24 hr-5 days	3-5 days	SB, C	SF
docusate potassium	po	24-72 hr	3-5 days	SB, C	SF
docusate sodium	po	24-72 hr	3-5 days	SB, C	SF
	pr	2-15 min	Hours	C	SF
Bulk-Forming Laxatives					
methylcellulose	po	12 hr	2-3 days	SB, C	SF
polycarbophil	po	12 hr	2-3 days	SB, C	SF
psyllium	po	12 hr	2-3 days	SB, C	SF
Saline Laxatives					
magnesium sulfate	po	3-6 hr	3-6 hr	SB, C	W
magnesium hydroxide	po	0.5-3 hr	3-6 hr	SB, C	W
magnesium citrate	po	0.5-3 hr	3-6 hr	SB, C	W
sodium phosphate and	po	0.5-3 hr	3-6 hr	C	W
sodium biphosphate	pr	2-15 min	60 min	C	W
polystyrene glycol electrolyte solution	po	30-60 min	60 min	SB, C	W
Lubricant Laxatives					
mineral oil	po/pr	6-8 hr	6-8 hr	C	SS
Hyperosmotic Laxatives					
glycerine	pr	0.25-5 hr	15-30 min	C	SF
lactulose	po	24-48 hr	1-3 days	C	SF

C, Colon; *pr*, per rectum (i.e., suppository); *SB*, small bowel; *SF*, soft-formed stool in 1-3 days; *SS*, semisoft stool in 6-12 hr; *UK*, unknown; *W*, watery stool in 2-6 hr.

TOXICITY

Overdose with stimulant laxatives leads to sudden and severe symptoms (e.g., nausea, vomiting, cramping, or diarrhea) and may require prompt medical attention.

INTERACTIONS

Stimulant laxatives decrease the absorption of other orally administered drugs because of increased motility and decreased transit times.

Cascara is minimally absorbed when taken orally. It is converted to an active metabolite in the colon and circulates throughout the body to be eliminated in the bile, urine, saliva, colonic mucosa, and breast milk. Evacuation of the bowel occurs in 6 to 10 hours.

Senna is also minimally absorbed following oral administration. Its distribution, biotransformation, elimination, and half-life are unknown. It produces soft, formed stools in 1 to 3 days.

DRUG CLASS • Stool Softeners

docusate calcium (Pro-Cal-Sof, Surfak)

docusate potassium (Diocto-K)

docusate sodium (Colace, Correctol Extra
Gentle, Dialose, Modane, many others)

MECHANISM OF ACTION

Stool softeners incorporate water and lipids into the
stool, producing an emollient action that reduces surface tension. The drugs act primarily in the jejunum and
colon. By incorporating water into the stool, a softer fecal mass results.

USES

Orally administered stool softeners are used to prevent
constipation in patients who should avoid straining
(e.g., patients with an MI or those who have had rectal
surgery). When administered as an enema, they help
soften fecal impactions.

PHARMACOKINETICS

Small amounts of docusate may be absorbed from the
small bowel following oral administration. The extent
of absorption from the rectum is unknown. The onset
time of drug action varies from 2 to 15 minutes for the
rectal formulation to 24 to 72 hours for the orally administered tablets or capsules (see Table 49-1). It may
take 1 to 2 days or more before a softened fecal bolus
reaches the rectum and evacuation occurs.

ADVERSE REACTIONS AND CONTRAINDICATIONS

The adverse effects of orally administered stool softeners include throat irritation, mild cramps, and rashes.
Diarrhea may occur with excessive use.

Stool softeners are contraindicated for patients with
hypersensitivity, abdominal pain, nausea, or vomiting,
especially if the constipation is associated with fever or
other signs of an acute abdominal condition. Excessive or
prolonged use of stool softeners may lead to dependency.

INTERACTIONS

There are no significant drug interactions with docusate
laxatives.

DRUG CLASS • Bulk-Forming Laxatives

psyllium (Effer-Syllium, Metamucil, Modane
Bulk, Perdiem, many others)

polycarbophil (Fiberall, Fibercon, Fiber-Lax,
Mitrolan)

methylcellulose (Citrucel)

MECHANISM OF ACTION

Bulk-forming laxatives include natural and semisynthetic
polysaccharides as well as cellulose derivatives. They
combine with water in the intestine to form an emollient
gel or viscous solution. The result is an increase in peristalsis and reduced transit time. Bulk-forming laxatives
produce the same action as 6 to 10 g per day of dietary
fiber. Antidiarrheal activity occurs because the drug takes
on water within the intestinal lumen.

USES

Bulk-forming laxatives such as psyllium and methylcellulose may be safely used for the long-term management of simple, chronic constipation, particularly when
the disorder is related to a low-fiber diet. They are useful in situations in which straining should be avoided
(e.g., MI or rectal surgery) and are useful for managing
chronic watery diarrhea. Polycarbophil is used to manage constipation or diarrhea associated with diverticu-
losis or irritable bowel syndrome.

Bulk-forming laxatives are the least harmful of the
various types of laxatives. They do not hinder the absorption of nutrients and are less likely to be habit forming than other laxatives. Compared with stimulant laxatives, which act quickly and empty the entire bowel,
bulk-forming laxatives have a longer onset of action and
evacuate only the descending sigmoid colon and rectum.

PHARMACOKINETICS

Bulk-forming laxatives are indigestible and thus not absorbed in the GI tract. They attain their expanded bulk
in approximately 12 hours and produce a soft, formed
stool in 2 to 3 days (see Table 49-1).

ADVERSE REACTIONS AND CONTRAINDICATIONS

Bloating and flatulence are common, undesirable adverse
reactions of bulk-forming laxatives. Bowel obstruction
may occur if fluid intake is inadequate; accordingly, these
preparations should always be taken with copious quantities of water or juice. In addition, allergic reactions such

---

TABLE 49-2

Drug Interactions of Selected Laxatives and Antidiarrheal Drugs

Drug	*Interactive Drugs*	*Interaction*
Stimulant Laxatives		
bisacodyl, phenolphthalein, cascara	Antacids	Removes enteric coating
	disulfiram	Disulfiram-like reaction
Bulk-Forming Laxatives		
psyllium polycarbophil	Cardiac glycosides	May reduce absorption of interactive drug
	Salicylates, tetracycline	
	Warfarin	
Saline Laxatives		
magnesium salts	Neuromuscular blockers	Potentiates effects of interactive drug
	Fluoroquinolone antibiotics	May reduce absorption of interactive drug
Opioid Antidiarrheals		
diphenoxylate	alcohol	Additive CNS depression
	difenoxin	Antihistamines
	loperamide	Opioids
	Sedative-hypnotics	
	Anticholinergics, disopyramide	Additive anticholinergic properties
	Tricyclic antidepressants	
	MAO inhibitors	May result in hypertensive crisis
Absorbent Antidiarrheals		
attapulgite	aspirin	Potentiates salicylate toxicity
bismuth subsalicylate	tetracycline, enoxacin, heparin	Decreases absorption of interactive drug
	enoxacin, heparin, thrombolytics, warfarin	Large doses may increase risk of bleeding

CNS, Central nervous system; *MAO*, monoamine oxidase.

as urticaria, dermatitis, rhinitis, and bronchospasm can result from inhaling the powder. Esophageal obstruction has occurred in patients who have dysphagia or esophageal strictures. These laxatives are not recommended for patients with conditions that cause the esophageal or intestinal lumen to be narrowed.

INTERACTIONS

Bulk-forming laxatives decrease the absorption of warfarin, salicylates, and cardiac glycosides (Table 49-2). Polycarbophil may decrease the absorption of tetracycline when taken concurrently. There are no known direct drug interactions with methylcellulose.

DRUG CLASS • Hyperosmotic Laxatives

glycerin suppositories (Fleet Babylax, Sani-Supp)

lactulose (Cephulac, Cholac, Chronulac, Lactulax,✳ others)

magnesium sulfate (Epsom Salts)

magnesium hydroxide (Phillips' Milk of Magnesia [MOM])

magnesium citrate (Citrate of Magnesia, Citro-Mag✳)

polystyrene glycol electrolyte solution (Colovage, Colyte, GoLytely, Nulytely, OCL, Peglyte, Klean-Prep✳)

sodium phosphate/diphosphate (Phospho-Soda, Fleet Enema)

MECHANISM OF ACTION

Hyperosmotic laxatives produce their effects by drawing water into the intestinal lumen, where the increased volume stimulates peristalsis. With hyperosmotic laxatives, the higher the tonicity of the solutes, the greater the laxative action. Magnesium salts also cause an increase in the secretion of cholecystokinin from the duodenum. This activity is thought to increase the secretion and motility of the small bowel and colon, thus contributing to the cathartic effect.

Glycerin is applied directly into the rectum as a suppository where it draws water from the extravascular spaces, expands the contents of the rectum and stimulates evacuation. Glycerin suppositories contain sodium stearate, which irritates the mucous membranes of the rectum. The irritation may contribute to the laxative effect by promoting contraction of rectal muscle.

Lactulose, a semisynthetic disaccharide, is administered orally as a hyperosmotic solution. In the colon, lactulose is hydrolyzed mainly to lactic acid and, to a lesser extent, to formic acid and acetic acid. Hyperosmotic concentrations of the acids draw water from the extravascular space, expanding the colonic contents, and stimulating defecation.

USES

Hyperosmotic laxatives are often used to cleanse the entire intestinal tract for diagnostic purposes, to flush poisons, or to remove parasites. Glycerin is used in adults and infants for those conditions in which the rectum is filled with stool but the defecation reflex is not triggered or transit time is severely delayed.

In addition to its use as a laxative, lactulose is used to promote the elimination of ammonia in treatment of portal-systemic encephalopathy because the acids produced by the metabolism of lactulose convert intestinal ammonia to ammonium ions which, being charged, cannot be systemically absorbed (see Chapter 51).

PHARMACOKINETICS

The onset times for most hyperosmotic laxatives after oral administration vary from 30 minutes to 6 hours, depending on the preparation (see Table 49-1). Most hyperosmotic laxatives produce a watery stool in 3 to 6 hours.

Glycerin is poorly absorbed after rectal administration and usually produces a bowel movement within 30 minutes.

Lactulose is poorly absorbed after oral administration (less than 3%) and does not exert its effects until it reaches the colon; the onset of action may require 24 to 48 hours.

ADVERSE REACTIONS AND CONTRAINDICATIONS

The most serious adverse reaction of magnesium-containing laxatives derives from the systemic absorption of an average of 20% of the ingested magnesium. If renal function is normal, the magnesium will be quickly eliminated in the urine with no physiologic consequence. However, if renal function is impaired, or if the patient is a neonate or an older adult, magnesium toxicity may ensue with resultant depression of the CNS, hypotension, and respiratory depression.

All hyperosmotic laxatives are contraindicated for patients with nausea and vomiting of unknown origin, abdominal pain, impaction, intestinal obstruction, colostomies, or ileostomies. Magnesium salts are contraindicated for patients with renal disease.

Glycerin produces minimal adverse reactions. Irritation from the stearate content of glycerin suppositories elicits the most complaints. Chronic use or overuse may cause hypokalemia.

The most common adverse reactions to lactulose include cramps, distention, flatulence, belching, and diarrhea. Lactulose is contraindicated for patients with hypersensitivity and those on a low-galactose diet. Hyperglycemia has been noted in patients who have diabetes mellitus; therefore it should be used with caution in these patients, as well as in older adults or debilitated patients.

TOXICITY

Overdose with a magnesium-containing laxative can cause hypotension, muscle weakness, changes in the electrocardiogram, and CNS depression. An overdose of a laxative containing phosphate can lead to a coma resulting from hyperphosphatemia.

INTERACTIONS

Magnesium salts potentiate the action of neuromuscular-blocking drugs (see Table 49-2). The absorption of fluoroquinolone antibiotics is reduced in the presence of magnesium salts. Polystyrene glycol electrolyte solutions interfere with the absorption of orally administered drugs by decreasing the transit time through the bowel. Oral drugs should not be given within 1 hour of starting laxative therapy.

DRUG CLASS • Lubricant Laxatives

mineral oil (Agoral, Fleet Mineral Oil Enema, Kondremul,✷ Lansoÿl,✷ others)

MECHANISM OF ACTION

Mineral oil coats the surface of the stool and intestine with a film and retards water reabsorption to allow passage of the stool through the intestine. It does not stimulate intestinal peristalsis.

USES

Mineral oil is the only lubricant laxative in use today. It is used to soften impacted stool in the management of constipation.

PHARMACOKINETICS

Mineral oil is minimally absorbed following oral administration. Distribution is to the liver, spleen, mesenteric lymph nodes, and intestinal mucosa. It produces a semisoft stool in 6 to 8 hours (see Table 49-1).

ADVERSE REACTIONS AND CONTRAINDICATIONS

The adverse effects of mineral oil are few but potentially troublesome. They include anorexia, nausea, vomiting, and nutritional deficiencies. Anal irritation and leakage can occur. Aspiration pneumonia has been documented in cases where some of the oil flowed into the trachea. Repeated use of mineral oil decreases the absorption of fat-soluble vitamins (A, D, E, K), food, and bile salts.

Mineral oil is contraindicated for patients who are hypersensitive to it. The rectal route is contraindicated for children less than 2 years of age, and the oral route is contraindicated for children less than 6 years of age. Mineral oil should be used cautiously in older adults or debilitated patients because of the increased risk of aspiration pneumonia. It should also be used cautiously during pregnancy because it decreases the absorption of fat-soluble vitamins and can cause hypoprothrombinemia in the newborn.

INTERACTIONS

The absorption of fat-soluble vitamins is decreased in the presence of mineral oil (see Table 49-2). Similarly, concurrent use of mineral oil with stool softeners may increase the absorption of mineral oil.

APPLICATION TO PRACTICE

ASSESSMENT
History of Present Illness

A careful description of the patient's usual and current elimination patterns should be elicited during the health history, including information about the frequency, consistency, size, and color of stools (Box 49-2). Ask about any related symptoms such as abdominal pain, flatulence, or sensation of incomplete evacuation, as well as the onset and duration of the elimination problem and any precipitating, aggravating, or mitigating factors. It is also helpful to ask about the patient's perception of normal bowel patterns, because many patients describe themselves as constipated if they do not have a daily bowel movement.

Health History

Ask about the patient's health history. Does he or she have a history of colorectal disease, hemorrhoids, or rectal fissures that may be causing discomfort? Neurologic diseases and spinal cord lesions that disrupt colon and abdominal motor nerves may provide insight into the cause of constipation. When questioning the patient about drug use, it is important to include OTC drugs, especially laxatives and enemas. Chronic laxative or enema use can cause megacolon (dilation and hypertrophy of the colon). A history of intermittent or partially obstructing bowel lesions as well as metabolic disorders such as diabetes mellitus, hypothyroidism, hypokalemia, hypercalcemia, and uremia can contribute to constipation.

Lifespan Considerations

Perinatal. Constipation during pregnancy is not uncommon. The effect of progesterone on smooth muscle reduces gastric emptying time and intestinal motility, effects that contribute to constipation. This problem is also caused by mechanical compression of the bowel by the enlarging uterus and the effects of iron supplements. The increase in electrolyte and water absorption during pregnancy adds to the problem. Constipation may increase the likelihood of developing hemorrhoids.

Pediatric. Stool patterns of children vary widely. Normally, neonates pass more than four stools daily during

---

BOX **49-2** | **Patient Problem: Constipation**

The Problem

The patient is not having bowel movements as often as necessary.

Signs and Symptoms

Abdominal discomfort; feeling a need to defecate but inability to do so; dry, firm, hard stools when bowel movements do occur; infrequent defecation (the meaning of infrequent may vary with each patient).

Associated or Contributing Factors

Dehydration or inadequate fluid intake; constipating medications; misuse or overuse of antidiarrheal medications; improper use of cathartics (which causes the patient to move from constipation to diarrhea); immobility.

Measures to Help Eliminate Constipation

- Keep a record of bowel movements to help verify the problem, and note any associated factors.
- Increase daily fluid intake to 2500 to 3000 mL.
- Increase dietary intake of fruit and fruit juices.
- Increase dietary intake of fiber (see Dietary Considerations box in this chapter).
- Increase level of exercise.
- Examine the use of any drugs that cause diarrhea or constipation.
- Examine the use of foods that may contribute to constipation, especially cheese and sweets (such as cake, pastries, and pudding).

Additional Nursing Care Measures

- Keep a record of bowel movements for all hospitalized, immobilized, or institutionalized patients, because constipation is easier to prevent than to treat, and easier to treat if found early.
- Auscultate bowel sounds in patients complaining of constipation.

---

the first week of life. The frequency declines to one or two stools daily by the age of 4 years. Factors such as emotional distress, family conflict, dietary changes, febrile illness, or recent travel can alter the child's bowel habits.

A significant number of children have chronic functional constipation that often begins in infancy and tends to be self-perpetuating. Large, hard stools are retained because elimination is difficult. Chronic distention of the rectum and colon gradually decrease a child's awareness of the need to defecate. This problem results in more retention, more water reabsorption, and

hardening of the stool. As the rectum becomes dilated, liquid stool oozes around the hard mass, resulting in involuntary soiling.

Older Adults. Although intestinal motility decreases with age, constipation is not necessarily a problem in the older age group. Inactivity, poor appetite, tooth loss, and poor-fitting dentures contribute to the risk of constipation. Furthermore, many older adults habitually use laxatives to produce bowel movements. Chronic laxative use causes the mesenteric plexus to be less sensitive to stimulation.

Cultural/Social Considerations

Pertinent lifestyle factors to assess in the patient with constipation include their usual activities, occupation, type and frequency of exercise, dietary habits, and elimination patterns. Could the patient be depressed or socially isolated and thus less active? Some cultures and patients believe that autointoxication occurs if bowel movements do not occur on a regular basis (see the Case Study: Constipation).

Physical Examination

Signs of constipation found during the physical examination include abdominal masses with palpable tenderness. Silent or abnormal bowel sounds may be auscultated in the abdomen. A rectal examination may reveal painful areas indicating external hemorrhoids, strictures, anal tears, or abrasions. The presence of a rectal mass indicates impaction or an obstructing lesion. Anal sphincter tone is increased in patients with functional problems and strictures, but is decreased in cases of constipation caused by neurologic diseases. The diameter of the rectal ampulla is markedly increased in megacolon, and bowel sounds may be reduced. Abdominal radiographs may demonstrate stool in the colon. Guaiac-positive stools may help identify an underlying cause of the constipation.

Laboratory Testing

Diagnostic testing is not usually required in acute constipation. However, cases resistant to treatment may require some testing to establish the cause of the problem. Fecal occult blood testing provides information about ulcerative or cancerous lesions. Although it carries a 50% to 90% sensitivity rate, this procedure is an inexpensive method of screening for bleeding lesions that may be contributing to constipation. Occult testing is not indicated if the patient has hemorrhoids or fissures, because the lesions may cause misleading positive results.

Hypokalemia evidenced in the serum potassium level may manifest as constipation. Thyroid function testing may detect hypothyroidism as a possible cause of constipation. A serum calcium level test may eliminate hypercalcemia as a cause of constipation.

GOALS OF THERAPY

Prevention of constipation is the best overall treatment goal. However, when this is not possible, the goal is to reestablish a normal bowel pattern and to effect comfortable bowel movements. The goal includes using the least number of drugs in the lowest dosages for the shortest duration of time.

INTERVENTION

Treatment for constipation covers three main areas: correction of underlying conditions that may be causing the constipation, patient education, and nondrug therapies.

The initial drug of choice for constipation depends on the type and severity, the effect desired, and the underlying cause. In cases of drug-induced constipation, correction is accomplished by adjusting the drug dosage or by using alternative drugs before resorting to concurrent laxative use.

Administration

Keep a record of bowel movements on all institutionalized, immobilized, or incapacitated patients. Prevention, early detection, and treatment of constipation are much easier and less time-consuming than treatment of severe constipation or impaction. Assess bowel sounds before administering any drug to relieve constipation. If bowel sounds are absent, withhold the drug dose and notify the health care provider.

Read drug orders and labels carefully, because many drugs have similar names. Be alert to the action of each component drug in combination products. For example, Colace contains the stool softener docusate sodium, whereas Peri-Colace contains docusate and casanthranol, a mild stimulant laxative.

All laxatives should be taken with a full glass of water. Enteric-coated laxatives (e.g., bisacodyl, phenolphthalein) should not be chewed or taken within 1 hour of drinking milk or taking an antacid. Other laxatives (e.g., cascara sagrada, docusate) should not be taken by patients who abuse alcohol.

Castor oil does not mix with a water-based diluent. Adding a small amount of baking soda (less than ¼ teaspoon) immediately before administering causes the mixture to fizz, and the castor oil will be partially suspended in the juice for 1 or 2 minutes. Patients may find it easier to take castor oil this way. In an institution, routine use of baking soda for this purpose must be cleared by the pharmacy or health care provider.

Bulk-forming laxatives such as psyllium should be diluted at the bedside with 8 ounces of water, milk, or juice. The mixture should be taken immediately after mixing because it congeals in a few minutes. Psyllium granules should not be chewed, taken at bedtime, or given to patients who are unable to sit upright, because they may cause esophageal or intestinal obstruction. Additionally, some dosage forms of psyllium contain sugar, aspartame, or excessive sodium and should not be taken by patients on restricted diets. To promote absorption, bulk-forming laxatives should be taken 1 hour before or 2 hours after other drugs.

Mineral oil should not be given to bedridden patients or children because it can cause lipid pneumonia should the patient aspirate it. When use is necessary, the patient should remain in an upright position, and other drugs should be administered at least 2 hours before or 2 hours after the mineral oil.

Monitor the serum electrolyte levels of patients receiving lactulose, especially older adults.

Education

Instruct the patient that a daily bowel movement is not necessary for normal bowel function. Correct misconceptions about bowel function; autointoxication does not occur when bowel movements are less frequent.

Advise the patient that, although there are valid indications for the use of laxatives, constipation can generally be resolved by increasing fluid and fiber intake (Box 49-3) and exercise as well as appropriate bowel training. Drug therapy should be used in cases of constipation resistant to simple treatment measures.

To help keep a regular bowel schedule, advise the patient to increase daily fluid intake to 2500 to 3000 mL. If necessary, suggest that the patient drink a full (8-ounce) glass of water before and with each meal.

Instruct the patient to increase the daily dietary intake of fiber as found in bran cereals and other foods such as fruits, vegetables, and fruit juices as well as foods that are known to stimulate defecation (e.g., hot chocolate, coffee). Encourage the patient to exercise regularly to promote bowel regularity.

Remind patients that laxatives are temporary measures not intended for long-term use and to use them only as directed. Many laxatives are available without

---

 Dietary Considerations for FIBER

Adequate amounts of dietary fiber may help prevent constipation and colon diseases, maintain blood glucose levels, and lower blood cholesterol levels. Good sources of dietary fiber include fruits and vegetables (especially raw, unpeeled, or those with edible seeds) as well as whole grains and whole-grain products, such as bread, cereals, pastas, bran, oats, peas, beans, and lentils.

prescription and thus may be misused or abused by patients who do not understand that increasing dependence on these drugs can develop with regular use.

Advise the patient to take daily doses of stimulant laxatives (but not castor oil) at bedtime to promote regular defecation in the morning. It is essential to review the importance of following the prescribed regimen with patients taking laxatives in preparation for GI diagnostic procedures. The major reason that many studies of the GI tract are poor in quality or must be repeated is that the preparation of the colon is inadequate.

Inform patients that storing suppositories in the refrigerator will make them firmer and easier to insert. Encourage them to chill magnesium citrate before drinking to make it more palatable. Patients should drink the entire prescribed amount at once for best results. Instruct patients adhering to a sodium-restricted diet to avoid saline cathartics.

Patients should be warned that when mineral oil is used regularly there may be leakage of the oil or fecal material from the anus. Mineral oil stains clothing; suggest that patients wear a perianal pad or incontinence shield to protect clothing and sheets. Regular mineral oil use is associated with increased incidence of lipid pneumonia, especially in older adults. Encourage the patient to always sit upright or stand when taking this medication. For long-term treatment of constipation, drugs other than mineral oil are preferred. Instruct patients not

---

CASE STUDY *Constipation*

ASSESSMENT

HISTORY OF PRESENT ILLNESS

SB is a 26-year-old woman who reports to the OB clinic today with complaints of constipation. She states she is 32 weeks pregnant. Her last BM was 3 days ago, and it was hard and dry. She ordinarily has one soft, formed bowel movement a day. She acknowledges not drinking enough fluids and eating primarily carbohydrates, such as "fast-food stuff. It's quick and easy to fix." Her activity level has declined with gestation and since it started snowing. She reports she is afraid she will fall, so she has given up her daily walk. She thinks the iron in her vitamins is contributing to her constipation and adding to her hemorrhoidal discomfort.

HEALTH HISTORY

SB's past health history is unremarkable. She had an appendectomy at age 13 and an episode of mononucleosis at age 18. She has been faithful about taking her prenatal vitamin with iron but is taking no other drugs.

LIFESPAN CONSIDERATIONS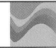

Constipation in SB is related to a combination of intestinal smooth muscle relaxation associated with progesterone secretion, mechanical compression of the bowel by an enlarging uterus, and the effects of iron supplements.

CULTURAL/SOCIAL CONSIDERATIONS

SB reports that her husband is excited about the pregnancy but is worried about her increasing constipation. She and her husband carry health insurance that covers perinatal care and pharmacy needs.

PHYSICAL EXAMINATION

SB's vital signs are within normal limits. Her skin is pink and warm; mucous membranes are dry. Abdominal examination reveals 32-week pregnancy. Rectal examination reveals several small, external hemorrhoids. Percussion is dull on the left with palpable stool in the colon.

LABORATORY TESTING

Stool guaiac is negative. Serum electrolytes, hemoglobin and hematocrit, and thyroid function tests are within normal limits.

PATIENT PROBLEM(S)

Constipation.

GOALS OF THERAPY

Reestablish regular, comfortable BMs that empty rectum, using the least number of drugs in the lowest dosage possible for the shortest duration of time.

CRITICAL THINKING QUESTIONS

1. The health care provider orders docusate calcium 240 mg po once daily for 3 to 10 days and psyllium hydrophilic muciloid 2 teaspoons in a full glass of water bid. What is the mechanism of action of these two drugs?
2. What teaching is required for SB to safely use psyllium hydrophilic muciloid?
3. SB asks why she cannot take castor oil as her mother used to when she was pregnant. What is the appropriate response?
4. What is the most common adverse effect of stool softeners such as docusate calcium?
5. SB develops a mild case of diarrhea after taking the two drugs for 1 week. She wishes to stop the psyllium hydrophilic muciloid and blames this drug for the diarrhea. What is the appropriate response?

to take doses of mineral oil within 2 hours of meals, because the mineral oil may interfere with absorption of fat-soluble vitamins and other nutrients. Do not give mineral oil to children less than 6 years of age.

Explain the action of stool softeners to the patient. Many patients misunderstand their function and expect defecation to occur a few hours after taking a single dose. Inform the patient that best results are achieved by using stool softeners daily as prescribed. The patient may take liquid forms in milk or fruit juice, if desired.

Encourage the patient taking saline cathartics or lactulose to follow doses with an additional glass of water, if possible, to facilitate laxative action. If the laxative leaves an unpleasant taste in the mouth, the patient should drink a glass of fruit juice or carbonated beverage after the dose rather than water.

Caution patients with diabetes to monitor blood glucose levels carefully when taking lactulose, because the drug contains high concentrations of lactose and galactose. Warn patients taking lactulose that flatulence and abdominal cramps are common initially but will subside with continued therapy.

Many laxatives change the color of urine; warn the patient about these changes. Anthraquinone laxatives (i.e., phenolphthalein) are eliminated in the urine. For this reason, the patient should be advised that the drug may tint acid urine a yellow-brown color and alkaline urine a pinkish-red color. Castor oil can turn alkaline urine pink as well.

Review with the patient how to administer suppositories or enemas if these routes of administration are prescribed. Suppositories containing mineral oil should not be lubricated before administration, because the lubricant interferes with the action of the suppository. Moisten the suppository with water.

Inform women who are pregnant or lactating that drugs to relieve constipation should be used only under the direction of the health care provider.

Inform patients that sudden or persistent changes in bowel habits should be thoroughly evaluated by a health care provider. Patients with abdominal pain, nausea, vomiting, or fever should be advised not to use laxatives without first consulting their health care provider.

EVALUATION

Normal bowel patterns are individually determined and may vary from three times a day to three times a week. Clinical response to treatment is demonstrated by the passage of a soft, formed bowel movement, usually within 12 to 24 hours. In some cases, 3 days of therapy may be required to produce results. Evidence suggests that 50% of patients who regularly use laxatives reestablish normal bowel habits once laxative administration is discontinued.

PATHOPHYSIOLOGY • Diarrhea

Diarrhea is not a disease but a symptom experienced by most people at some point in their lifetime. Diarrhea is characterized by an increase in the frequency of profuse, watery, loose stools during a limited time period. This condition is considered chronic if it persists for at least 2 weeks, produces over 300 g of stool daily, or subsides and returns more than 2 to 4 weeks after the initial episode.

In essence, diarrhea is caused by any factor that decreases fluid absorption in the small or large bowel, increases fluid secretion (e.g., deranged electrolyte transport), alters bowel motility, or is associated with mucosal injury. Diarrhea can be acute or chronic. Acute diarrhea is usually of bacterial or viral origin. It can be caused by bacterial overgrowth because of antimicrobial suppression of normal flora. It can also be an undesired, adverse response to drug therapy (Box 49-4).

Although avoiding laxatives in the presence of diarrhea seems all too obvious, concealed abuse of stimulant laxatives is a surprisingly frequent cause of chronic diarrhea of supposedly unknown origin. Other common causes of chronic diarrhea include malabsorption and irritable bowel disease, as well as surgical procedures that shorten the intestinal tract (i.e., short-gut syndrome) or cause rapid emptying of the stomach (i.e., dumping syndrome).

BOX 49-4 | **Drugs and Drug Classes Likely to Cause Diarrhea**

Antimicrobials
Antineoplastics
Bile acids
Cardiac glycosides
Cholinergic drugs
Cholinesterase inhibitors
guanethidine
Magnesium-containing antacids
methyldopa
Osmotic laxatives
quinidine
reserpine
Stimulant laxatives

DRUG CLASS • Opioids

camphorated tincture of opium (Paregoric)

difenoxin with atropine sulfate (Motofen)

diphenoxylate with atropine sulfate (Lomotil, Lofene, Logen, Lonox)

loperamide (Imodium, Imodium A-D, Kaopectate II Caplets, Maalox Anti-Diarrheal Caplets, Pepto Diarrhea Control)

opium tincture

MECHANISM OF ACTION

Opioids such as diphenoxylate, difenoxin, and opium (morphine is the main active constituent of the opium tinctures) act at the mu (μ) and possibly delta opioid receptors to decrease intestinal motility, thereby slowing transit time. The prolonged transit time facilitates absorption of fluid, electrolytes, and solutes throughout the intestinal tract. In addition, stimulation of the opioid receptors also decreases secretion of fluid into the small intestine. Rectal sphincter tone is also increased. As a result of these actions, the fluidity and volume of stools as well as the frequency of defecation are reduced.

Loperamide inhibits peristalsis and prolongs transit time through a direct effect on nerves in the intestinal muscle wall. It reduces fecal volume and increases viscosity and bulk while diminishing loss of fluid and electrolytes. Loperamide reduces the volume of discharge from an ileostomy and can be used in the treatment of traveler's diarrhea or chronic diarrhea associated with inflammatory bowel disease, and provides symptomatic relief of acute, nonspecific diarrhea.

USES

Opioids are the most effective antidiarrheal drugs. Although water/alcohol solutions of opium powder (e.g., camphorated tincture of opium, opium tincture) have long been used to treat diarrhea, synthetic opioids are now preferred. Atropine, an anticholinergic drug (see Chapter 11), is combined with diphenoxylate and difenoxin in subtherapeutic doses to discourage abuse of the preparation.

Opium tincture and camphorated tincture of opium are used less often today than in the past. However, camphorated tincture of opium has been especially useful in treating diarrhea associated with HIV. Opium tincture may be added to enteral feedings to help minimize the diarrhea typically caused by such feedings.

PHARMACOKINETICS

Diphenoxylate is well absorbed from the GI tract. Most of the drug is biotransformed in the liver; some converts to an active antidiarrheal metabolite difenoxin. Difenoxin, in turn, is biotransformed in the liver to an inactive metabolite. The half-life of difenoxin is about 12 hours (Table 49-3).

Loperamide is slowly and incompletely absorbed following oral administration. It apparently crosses the blood-brain barrier relatively slowly, because doses greatly in excess of those recommended for treatment of diarrhea produce only modest effects on the CNS. Loperamide is 97% protein bound, and is biotransformed in the liver. Thirty percent of the drug is eliminated in feces, and there is minimal elimination in the urine. The half-life of loperamide is 11 hours.

TABLE 49-3

Pharmacokinetics of Selected Antidiarrheal Drugs

Drug	Route	Onset	Peak	Duration	PB (%)	$t_{1/2}$	BioA (%)
Opioids							
diphenoxylate with atropine	po	45-60 min	2 hr	3-4 hr	UA	2.5 hr	UA
difenoxin with atropine	po	45-60 min	2 hr	3-4 hr	UA	UA	UA
Absorbents							
activated attapulgite	po	UK	UK	UK	UK	UK	UK
bismuth subsalicylate	po	24 hr	UK	UK	UA	2-3 hr; 15-30 hr	UA
Anticholinergic							
loperamide	po	60 min	2.5-5 hr	10 hr	97	10.8 hr	UA

BioA, Bioavailability; *NA*, not applicable; *PB*, protein binding; $t_{1/2}$ elimination half-life; *UA*, unavailable; *UK*, unknown.
*Half-life of salicylate component of bismuth subsalicylate for low doses; it is longer for higher doses.

ADVERSE REACTIONS AND CONTRAINDICATIONS

The adverse reactions of diphenoxylate are caused by both mu agonist activity and nonselective muscarinic antagonism. The most common of these includes constipation and dizziness. Blurred vision, dry mouth and eyes, tachycardia, epigastric distress, nausea and vomiting, ileus, drowsiness, headache, insomnia, nervousness, and confusion are also possible. Urinary retention and flushing may occur as well.

Although difenoxin and diphenoxylate are effective in the treatment of mild to moderate diarrhea, they should not be given to patients with chronic ulcerative colitis or acute bacillary or amebic dysentery. When the drugs are used in these patients, it appears that they potentiate ulcerating processes in the colon and provoke the development of toxic megacolon. Opioids are also contraindicated for patients with hypersensitivity, severe liver disease, infectious diarrhea (caused by *Escherichia coli, Salmonella,* or *Shigella*), and diarrhea associated with pseudomembranous colitis (*Clostridium difficile*). Diphenoxylate preparations should not be given to patients who are dehydrated, who cannot tolerate alcohol, or who have narrow angle glaucoma as well as children younger than 2 years of age.

The adverse reactions of loperamide are fewer than those of diphenoxylate with atropine. Drowsiness and constipation are the most common, but dizziness, nausea, and dry mouth also occur. Loperamide is contraindicated for patients who are hypersensitive to the drug, who must avoid constipation, who have abdominal pain of unknown cause (especially if associated with fever), or who cannot tolerate alcohol. Loperamide should be given with caution to patients who have liver disease, children younger than 2 years of age, and older adults as well as pregnant or lactating women.

Opioids should be given cautiously to patients with inflammatory bowel disease or prostatic hypertrophy, pregnant women, and children. Difenoxin is not recommended for children less than 12 years of age.

Large doses of the opium tinctures can cause dizziness, drowsiness, fainting, flushing, and CNS depression. Adverse effects are typically dose related and include nausea, vomiting, dysphoria, constipation, and increased biliary tract pressure. Anaphylaxis is rare.

Opium tincture and camphorated tincture of opium are contraindicated for patients with hypersensitivity and those who have pseudomembranous colitis or severe ulcerative colitis (toxic megacolon may develop). The drugs should be given with caution to patients with liver disease or severe prostatic hypertrophy, pregnant women, or patients who may be prone to opioid dependence.

Euphoria, analgesia, and dependence are unlikely with opium tincture or camphorated tincture of opium when using the recommended doses for short periods of time. Nevertheless, the tinctures have a demonstrated history of being abused and as a result are regulated as controlled substances. Opium tincture contains 10% opium by weight and is classified as a schedule II drug. Camphorated tincture of opium contains only 0.04% morphine (25 times less concentrated than opium tincture) together with camphor, anise oil, benzoic acid, and alcohol (45%). It is classified as a schedule III drug. See Chapter 7 for a discussion of the laws regulating controlled substances.

INTERACTIONS

Table 49-2 lists the drug interactions with opioid antidiarrheal drugs. The interactions are not unlike those found when the opioid is used for analgesia (see Chapter 13).

DRUG CLASS • Absorbents

activated attapulgite (Kaopectate, Parepectolin, Diar-Aid, Diasorb)

bismuth subsalicylate (Pepto-Bismol, Bismatrol, Pink Bismuth)

MECHANISM OF ACTION

Bismuth subsalicylate is a relatively insoluble compound with absorbent, demulcent, astringent, and weak antacid characteristics. Although the mechanism of action is poorly understood, it is thought that the antiinflammatory actions of salicylate are primarily involved, which decreases the synthesis of intestinal prostaglandins. Antibacterial actions of bismuth may also be involved, especially in the prevention of traveler's diarrhea.

Attapulgite is thought to act by absorbing bacteria and toxins as well as by decreasing water loss. The therapeutic effect is thus a decrease in number and water content of stools.

USES

Bismuth subsalicylate is used in the adjunctive treatment of diarrhea. It has also been used in the treatment of enterotoxigenic *E. coli* (traveler's diarrhea). Bismuth subsalicylate has also been added to the armamentarium in the treatment of gastritis and peptic ulcer disease associated with *Helicobacter pylori* and is sometimes used as a local skin protectant. The availability of this relatively inexpensive drug promotes its overuse and increases the potential for toxicity to both the salicylate and bismuth components.

Attapulgite is a nonspecific antidiarrheal drug. Although this absorbent clay produces stools with a more normal appearance, fluid loss may remain unchanged and electrolyte losses may actually increase. The claim that attapulgite facilitates removal of bacterial toxins has not been supported by research.

PHARMACOKINETICS

Bismuth is not absorbed; however, the salicylate is hydrolyzed from the parent compound and is 90% absorbed from the small bowel. The onset of action occurs within 24 hours (see Table 49-3). Salicylates are highly bound to plasma proteins with bismuth subsalicylate distributed to the placenta. It also enters breast milk. The salicylate component undergoes significant biotransformation. The half-life of the salicylate component is 2 to 3 hours for low doses and 15 to 30 hours for larger doses.

ADVERSE REACTIONS AND CONTRAINDICATIONS

The adverse effects of bismuth subsalicylate include constipation and impaction, as well as gray-black tongue and stools. It is contraindicated for older adults with impacted stool and patients hypersensitive to aspirin. The Centers for Disease Control and Prevention recommend that bismuth subsalicylate not be given to children or teenagers during or after recovery from chickenpox (varicella) or flu-like illnesses, because of the association of salicylate with Reye's syndrome. Cautious use is warranted for infants, older adults, and debilitated patients because impaction is possible.

Because bismuth is radiopaque, it is generally not given to patients who will be undergoing radiologic examination of the GI tract. Safe use during pregnancy and lactation has not been established. Cautious use is also warranted in patients who have diabetes mellitus or gout.

Attapulgite stays within the GI tract and causes few adverse effects. It may increase the fecal elimination of sodium and potassium, but the most common adverse effect is constipation.

INTERACTIONS

If bismuth subsalicylate is taken with aspirin, it may potentiate salicylate toxicity. It decreases the absorption of tetracycline antibiotics. Large doses may increase the risk of bleeding in the presence of thrombolytic drugs, warfarin, or heparin. For example, a 2-ounce dose of bismuth salts can produce the same salicylate blood level as one 5-grain tablet of aspirin. Large doses can also increase the risk of hypoglycemia from insulin or oral hypoglycemics and may decrease the effectiveness of probenecid. This drug has a cross-allergenicity with NSAIDs and oil of wintergreen.

Much like bismuth subsalicylate, attapulgite may decrease the GI absorption of concurrently administered drugs. Other drugs should be administered 2 to 3 hours before or 2 to 4 hours after taking attapulgite.

DRUG CLASS • Miscellaneous Antidiarrheal Drugs

belladonna alkaloids (Donnagel)

cholestyramine (Questran)

kaolin and pectin

Lactobacillus acidophilus (Lactinex, Bacid)

batreotide (Sandostatin)

BELLADONNA ALKALOIDS

Many traditional remedies have little or no value in the treatment of acute diarrhea. These remedies include kaolin and pectin, lactobacilli, and anticholinergic preparations (muscarinic antagonists). Belladonna alkaloids are classified as anticholinergic drugs and include atropine, hyoscine, and hyoscyamine. However, there is no conclusive evidence that drugs in this class are effective in the treatment of diarrhea. They do, however, prevent the spasms and cramping frequently associated with acute or chronic diarrhea when given in a sufficient dose.

CHOLESTYRAMINE

Cholestyramine, an antihyperlipidemic drug, has a direct affinity for acidic materials such as bile salts and the toxin produced by *C. difficile*. It is thought to relieve diarrhea caused by excessive bile salts and may be effective for antibiotic-induced pseudomembranous colitis, although it is not approved by the FDA for such use.

KAOLIN AND PECTIN

Kaolin is a natural aluminum silicate clay that has been used for hundreds of years to treat diarrhea. It is most often mixed with pectin, a purified carbohydrate obtained from the peel of citrus fruits or from apple pulp. When pectin is cooked with sugar at the proper pH, a gel forms.

The combination of the two drugs may add bulk to the stool but rarely reduce stool fluid or frequency. The FDA recognizes neither kaolin nor pectin as effective.

LACTOBACILLUS ACIDOPHILUS

Lactobacillus acidophilus and *Lactobacillus bulgaricus* are OTC preparations that are thought to promote the growth of normal intestinal flora, particularly *E. coli*. There is also the notion that increased dietary intake of products containing lactobacillus as well as lactose and dextrose (e.g., milk, buttermilk, and yogurt) are all equally effective in recolonizing the intestine. The effectiveness of this preparation is questionable.

OCTREOTIDE

Octreotide is identical to the natural hormone somatostatin (see Chapter 51) but also acts to increase absorption of fluid and electrolytes from the GI tract and in-crease the transit time. It has been used as an investigational drug to control severe, refractory diarrhea. Refractory diarrhea may occur with dumping syndrome, severe enterotoxic infections, short-gut syndrome, graft-versus-host disease, carcinoid and vasoactive intestinal peptic tumors (vipomas), and AIDS. It is described as a universal inhibitor of secretory cells.

Common adverse reactions to octreotide include transient nausea, diarrhea, abdominal cramping, and fat malabsorption. Headache, drowsiness, dizziness, fatigue, and weakness have also been reported. Palpitations and orthostatic hypotension is possible. Gallstones may form because octreotide decreases the emptying of the gallbladder. This drug also alters the secretion of insulin and glucagon, which leads to hyperglycemia or hypoglycemia. Because it is available only for subcutaneous or intravenous use, the patient may experience discomfort at the injection site.

APPLICATION TO PRACTICE

ASSESSMENT
History of Present Illness

Much like the patient with constipation, the patient with diarrhea should be asked about usual and current elimination patterns, including information about the frequency, consistency, size, and color of stools. Ask also about any related symptoms such as abdominal pain and flatulence, as well as onset and duration of the problem and any precipitating, aggravating, or mitigating factors. Determine whether there has been an increase in the consumption of laxative-like foods such as bran, lactose, sorbitol, fructose, brassica vegetables, coffee, or tea. Has the patient experienced an unexplained weight loss or been exposed to possible carriers of enteric infection? Has the patient consumed potentially contaminated food or water or traveled in foreign countries?

Ask the patient about his or her perception of normal defecation patterns. Some patients describe themselves as having diarrhea if they have more than one stool per day regardless of the consistency. Alternating periods of constipation and diarrhea are characteristic of irritable bowel syndrome.

Assess the patient with diarrhea for a history of recent travel, especially international travel; recent antibiotic use; recent antineoplastic therapy; and recent work with children in day-care centers or other settings where harmful microorganisms are easily spread.

Health History

A number of groups are at high risk for infectious diarrhea, particularly patients with a recent travel history (e.g., Peace Corps workers) and campers. Often there is a history of eating raw seafood or shellfish. Patients may also report having eaten in restaurants or fast-food restaurants, having recently attended a picnic or banquet, or having been in close contact with children or ill family members.

When questioning the patient about drug use, ask about the use of laxatives, magnesium-containing antacids, excess alcohol, caffeine-containing beverages, and herbal teas. Note whether the patient has recently taken antibiotics, digoxin, quinidine, loop diuretics, or antihypertensive drugs or ingested excessive amounts of sugar-free gums and mints that contain sorbitol.

Lifespan Considerations

Perinatal. Intestinal disorders during pregnancy mirror the range of GI diseases in the normal population. Common causes include antibiotic-induced diarrhea (related to overgrowth of *C. difficile* after antibiotic therapy), functional bowel disorders, infectious gastroenteritis (bacterial, parasitic, and viral), and inflammatory bowel disorders (regional enteritis and ulcerative colitis). Acute-onset diarrhea is usually associated with a viral or bacterial infection; although it is problematic, it is not usually voluminous in nature. Ordinarily, gastroenteritis in pregnancy does not pose significant risk to the fetus if maternal hydration is maintained. Most infections tend to be localized to the bowel mucosa and do not present a risk for infection of the fetus. Most cases of infectious diarrhea resolve without antibiotic therapy in several days, although antibiotic therapy should be considered for severe infections. The detrimental perinatal effects of GI diseases generally result from their impact on maternal nutrition.

Pediatric. Diarrhea occurs more often during infancy, is a lesser threat in early childhood, and usually constitutes only a minor problem in older children. Acute diarrhea is the leading cause of illness in children less than 5 years of age. The dehydration, electrolyte disturbances, and malnutrition caused by diarrhea are fatal for approximately 400 children a year in the United States. As a general rule, the younger the child, the greater the susceptibility and the more severe the diarrhea. Malnourished or debilitated children are more susceptible and tend to have more severe diarrhea.

The frequency of diarrhea in infancy is closely related to the ingestion of contaminated milk. There is a lower incidence rate of diarrhea in breast-fed infants. Diarrhea occurs more often when there is overcrowding, substandard sanitation, inadequate facilities for preparation and refrigeration of food, and generally inadequate health care education.

Most cases of diarrhea in children are caused by bacterial, viral, and parasitic pathogens. Metabolic acidosis may be present with severe diarrhea and dehydration. Malnutrition may contribute to the severity of the condition and may be a consequence of diarrheal disease because of reduced dietary intake, malabsorption, and the catabolic response to infection. Because a child's metabolic rate is higher than that of an adult, the child is predisposed to a more rapid depletion of nutritional reserves.

Fluid replacement is important when diarrhea develops in infants and toddlers, because it can lead to life-threatening dehydration. However, antidiarrheal drugs have limited value in this age group, and there is a concern about possible toxicity. Although pediatric dosages are identified for diphenoxylate with atropine and loperamide, the World Health Organization does not recommend giving either of these drugs to children. The Centers for Disease Control and Prevention and the American Academy of Pediatrics recommend the use of oral fluid and electrolyte replacement therapy as the treatment of choice for most cases of dehydration caused by diarrhea.

Older Adults. The causes of diarrhea in the older adult are not unlike those of others. In the older adult, 15% of diarrhea cases are related to an infectious source; 19% of those cases are caused by bacterial infection, 68% by viral infections, and 3% by parasitic infections. Fecal impaction can be mistaken for diarrhea because liquid stool comes around the impaction and is eliminated frequently. Fecal impaction accounts for 16% of diarrhea cases; other mistaken accounts include antibiotic use (11%), laxative abuse (6%), and inflammatory bowel disease (4%). Dietary indiscretions (e.g., too much fruit, especially bananas), hyperosmolar tube feedings, protein-calorie malnutrition, and anxiety are also culprits. Diarrhea can be a serious problem contributing to mortality that increases dramatically in patients older than 74 years of age.

Cultural/Social Considerations

American culture is very bathroom oriented. Status—even the assessed value of a home—is determined by the number of bathrooms in a house. However, persons from foreign countries may have totally different experiences with bathroom facilities. Toileting is a private activity for most people and takes place behind closed doors. During illness or hospitalization, this formerly private activity suddenly may be exposed for all to discuss and possibly view (and perhaps even worse, for others to smell).

Pertinent lifestyle factors to assess include usual activities, occupation, type and frequency of exercise, dietary patterns, and elimination habits. What is the patient's stress level? Could the stress be manifesting in part as diarrhea? In addition, a sexual history is important when the patient complains of diarrhea, because it may be a manifestation of gay bowel syndrome.

GOALS OF THERAPY

The excessive loss of fluid and electrolytes, as well as stool that characterizes diarrhea, is an important aspect of many infectious and noninfectious GI disorders. Although acute-onset diarrhea is most often of infectious origin, it is usually self-limiting and specific drug therapy is seldom warranted (unless there is evidence of GI erosion or systemic disease). Therefore treatment goals include the maintenance of adequate hydration and skin integrity as well as the limited use of select antidiarrheal drugs.

Treatment goals for the patient with chronic diarrhea include reestablishing bowel habits to a pattern that is normal for the patient. To do so, treating the underlying cause of the diarrhea is important.

Although an otherwise healthy adult may not be harmed by dietary abstinence during an episode of mild to moderate diarrhea, the ingestion of soft, easily digested foods and noncarbonated beverages is suggested (Box 49-5). The oral administration of solutions containing electrolytes, glucose, and amino acids usually suffices. However, parenteral fluids may be warranted in some cases to help the patient achieve adequate hydration.

BOX 49-5 | **Patient Problem: Diarrhea**

The Problem
The patient is experiencing diarrhea: frequent loose or unformed stools.

Signs and Symptoms
Frequent urge to defecate; abdominal cramping or discomfort; dizziness; symptoms of dehydration (e.g., weight loss, poor skin turgor, confusion, dry mucous membranes); anal tenderness and irritation (severity will vary with the patient and the cause).

Associated or Contributing Factors
Misuse or overuse of drugs to treat constipation; antibiotics or other drugs that may cause diarrhea; concurrent gastrointestinal pathologic condition; excessive intake of food items that are irritating to that individual; gastrointestinal infection; exposure to contaminated water.

Measures to Help Treat Diarrhea
- Initially, switch to a clear liquid diet; gelatin or carbonated drinks add glucose and carbonate. Avoid diet and caffeine-containing carbonated drinks.
- Adding broths and clear soups, Gatorade, Pedialyte, Lytren, or other commercially available replacement will add sodium and chloride to the patient's diet.
- Avoid alcohol, caffeine, acidic fruit or juices, fried foods, milk and milk products, and raw fruits. Slowly add bland foods such as crackers, bread, and cooked cereals.

- Clean the rectal area carefully after each bowel movement: wash with mild soap or just water, or use a cleansing wipe, and pat thoroughly dry. Consider sitz baths three or four times a day. For irritated skin, apply a thin layer of petroleum jelly, zinc oxide, or Desitin around the anus.
- Wash hands thoroughly with soap and water after each bowel movement or after changing an infant's diaper. If it is suspected that the diarrhea may be infectious, have patient use bathroom facilities separate from others in the family. Dispose of contaminated diapers in closed container, away from kitchen and food preparation areas, or put into closed hamper. In the home, wash contaminated linens promptly; in the hospital, use infection control guidelines.
- Wash the dishes and eating utensils of the person with diarrhea thoroughly with soap and hot water, or put them into a dishwasher. Do not let others in the family share dishes with the patient if the diarrhea might be infectious.

Additional Nursing Care Measures
- Monitor weight and blood pressure.
- Take diet history, if indicated.
- If contaminated well water is a possible source of microorganisms, have water tested.

INTERVENTION
Administration
The frequency and consistency of stools and bowel sounds should be assessed before and periodically throughout the course of therapy. Monitor intake and output, daily weight, skin turgor, level of consciousness, blood pressure, pulse, and serum electrolyte levels.

Opioid antidiarrheal drugs may be administered with food if GI upset occurs. The tablets may be crushed and administered with the patient's choice of food or fluids. If a liquid formulation is required, a calibrated measuring device should be used. Dilute opium tincture in 15 to 30 mL of water to ensure that the patient receives the entire dose.

Dependency on diphenoxylate or difenoxin is theoretically possible. Overdose with this drug resembles an overdose of an opioid analgesic and is treated similarly (see Chapter 13). The risk of dependence on opioid antidiarrheal drugs increases with high-dose, long-term use. As discussed previously, subtherapeutic doses of atropine has been added to these drugs to discourage abuse. A single dose of these preparations causes few adverse effects

from the atropine, but the accumulated dose after 1 or 2 days of treatment might cause problems. Review the adverse effects of and contraindications to atropine use (see Chapter 11). The patient can minimize the dry mouth associated with the atropine component of opioid antidiarrheal drugs by frequent mouth rinses, good oral hygiene, and the use of sugarless gum or candy.

Health care providers also sometimes prescribe bulk-forming drugs to treat diarrhea, especially diarrhea associated with tube feedings. If the drug is to be given through a feeding tube, dilute the solution with sufficient fluid to prevent clogging of the tube and flush the tube with water after administration. Large-bore tubes are better suited to administer these drugs.

Education
Because most acute diarrhea is self-limiting, the patient with no evidence of serious underlying disorders can be reassured and advised to concentrate on maintaining hydration. Instruct the patient to consult the physician if any of the following occur: diarrhea persists longer than 3 to 5 days, the prescribed antidiarrheal drugs do

not afford relief, stools are particularly foul smelling or contain flecks of blood or large amounts of mucus, or the patient is unable to take in sufficient replacement fluids. Review with the patient the symptoms of hypokalemia (muscle weakness, fatigue, anorexia, vomiting, drowsiness, irritability, and eventually coma and death) and hypochloremia (hypertonic muscles, tetany, and depressed respiration).

Sugar and electrolyte preparations are easy to take and should be encouraged. Many people think that taking fluids will worsen their diarrhea and therefore request opiates. The proper role of these drugs should be discussed. In addition, the patient should be instructed as to the role of antibiotics and the emergence of resistant bacterial strains, potential complications of antibiotic use, and efficacy of antidiarrheal preparations.

Patients using opioid antidiarrheal drugs should be cautioned to take the drug exactly as directed and to avoid consuming alcohol or taking other CNS depressants concurrently with these drugs. Patients should not take more than the prescribed amount because of the habit-forming potential and the risk of overdose in children. If the patient is on a scheduled dosing regimen, missed doses should be taken as soon as possible unless it is almost time for the next dose. Double doses should not be taken. Patients should be advised to avoid driving or other activities that require alertness until their response to the drug is known.

Caution the patient to avoid giving bismuth salts to infants or children who are recovering from the flu or chicken pox. If nausea and vomiting are present, the patient should check with the health care provider because these symptoms may indicate Reye's syndrome.

Instruct patients taking bismuth subsalicylate to read the labels of other drugs they may be taking and to avoid other salicylate-containing drugs. Large amounts of bismuth salts may also interfere with urine glucose tests. Instruct patients with diabetes to be alert to this possibility.

Much can be done to relieve the perianal discomfort associated with diarrhea. It may help to wash the area with warm water on absorbent cotton after each stool in lieu of using toilet paper, which can be irritating. Avoiding soap is important to prevent perianal irritation. A short course of treatment with hydrocortisone cream may be useful when there is considerable perianal irritation. Some patients report that cleansing gently with cotton pads soaked in witch hazel (Tucks) provides considerable relief. The patient should be advised that ointments containing topical anesthetics should be avoided because they can cause irritation themselves.

Once the diarrhea is relieved, it is usually best to have the patient avoid milk and dairy products for another 7 to 10 days, because mild lactose intolerance commonly accompanies many cases of diarrhea. The best foods to consume are those that are easily digested, such as high-carbohydrate substances (including rice, baked potato, toast, and applesauce). Continued fluid replacement is important. Furthermore, once the underlying cause of the diarrhea has been identified, the patient should be advised to avoid the causative activity.

EVALUATION

The therapeutic outcome of antidiarrheal treatment is relief of diarrhea. Treatment effectiveness is noted by the absence of abdominal cramping, flatulence, and other discomforts associated with diarrhea. However, if symptoms of acute diarrhea continue, fever persists, or blood or mucus appears in the stool, antidiarrheal drugs should be discontinued and the patient reevaluated. Patients who are unable to maintain oral hydration and who become significantly volume depleted (as evidenced by postural hypotension) require serious consideration for hospital admission and parenteral fluid replacement.

Bibliography

Castiglia PT: Constipation in children, *J Pediatr Health Care* 15(4):200-202, 2001.

Ramzan NN: Traveler's diarrhea, *Gastroenterol Clin North Am* 30(3):665-678, viii, 2001.

Scheidler MD, Giannella RA: Practical management of acute diarrhea, *Hosp Pract* 36(7):49-56, 2001.

Schiller LR: Review article: the therapy of constipation, *Aliment Pharmacol Ther* 15(6):749-763, 2001.

Wingate D, Phillips SF, Lewis SJ, et al: Guidelines for adults on self-medication for the treatment of acute diarrhoea, *Aliment Pharmacol Ther* 15(6):773-782, 2001.

Xing JH, Soffer EE: Adverse effects of laxatives, *Dis Colon Rectum* 44(8):1201-1209, 2001.

Internet Resources

The Centers for Disease Control and Prevention website features information on diarrhea with infectious causes, as well as information on how to avoid infectious diarrhea. Available online at http://www.cdc.gov/ncidod/dpd/parasiticpathways/diarrhea.htm and http://www.cdc.gov/travel/foodwatr.htm.

The Medical Letter: advice for travelers. Available online at http://www.medicalletter.com/#1128.

The National Institutes of Health website includes background information and information about specific drugs for many conditions, including constipation and diarrhea. Available online at http://www.niddk.nih.gov/health/digest/pubs/const/const.htm and http://www.niddk.nih.gov/health/digest/summary/conchild/ and http://www.niddk.nih.gov/health/digest/pubs/diarrhea/diarrhea/htm.

The National Library of Medicine has overviews and information about constipation and diarrhea, as well as information about clinical trials. Available online at http://www.nlm.nih.gov/medlineplus/constipation.html and http://www.nlm.nih.gov/medlineplus/diarrhea.html.

CHAPTER

50

Antiemetic Drugs

MICHAEL R. VASKO • KATHLEEN GUTIERREZ

 Visit http://evolve.elsevier.com/Gutierrez/ for additional information.

KEY TERMS

Antiemetic drugs, p. 816

Chemoreceptor trigger zone (CTZ), p. 816

Emesis, p. 816

Emesis center, p. 816

Hyperemesis gravidarum, p. 824

Nausea, p. 816

Regurgitation, p. 823

OBJECTIVES

- Discuss the physiology of emesis.
- Identify the uses, pharmacokinetics, adverse effects, and contraindications for antiemetic drugs.
- Identify the treatment goals of drug therapy for the patient with nausea and vomiting.
- Develop a nursing care plan for patients receiving one of the various antiemetic drugs.

PATHOPHYSIOLOGY • Emesis

Nausea and vomiting are most commonly associated with overindulgence in rich and abundant food; with drugs, toxins, inflammation, and infection; and with vestibular disorders, motion sickness, anesthesia, radiation therapy, and antineoplastic therapy (Table 50-1). Vomiting is an involuntary act of emptying the stomach (**emesis**). Under normal conditions, vomiting provides a way for the body to rid itself of potentially toxic substances. Under stressful conditions or with drug therapy, vomiting is not desired and not only can make the patient uncomfortable, but can cause electrolyte imbalances, dehydration, and malnutrition. Nausea is the unpleasant sensation that usually precedes vomiting.

Vomiting is a reflex under CNS control. It occurs when the **emesis center** located in the lateral reticular formation of the brainstem near the **chemoreceptor trigger zone (CTZ)** is stimulated by various inputs (Figure 50-1). The CTZ lacks an intact blood-brain barrier. As a result, neurons in this region are sensitive to stimulation by circulating drugs and toxins and can relay excitatory inputs to the emesis center. Another input to the emetic center is from the cerebral cortex and is usually associated with vomiting because of emotion, pain, or anticipation of sickness. Additional inputs arise from peripheral stimuli activating sensory afferent neurons. Irritation of the mucosa of the GI tract or bowel or biliary distension stimulates the vomiting center by way of the vagus nerve or splanchic nerves through the nucleus tractus solitarius (NTS). Vestibular dysfunction sends impulses to the emesis center by way of vestibular nerve connections and causes vomiting resulting from disequilibrium or motion sickness.

When stimulated, the emesis center initiates efferent impulses that cause a sequence of events including alterations in respiration, salivation, autonomic responses, and motor activity in the GI tract. The glottis closes and the diaphragm and abdominal muscles contract. The gastroesophageal sphincter relaxes, and reverse peristalsis moves stomach contents upward toward the mouth for expulsion.

There are a number of neurotransmitters that mediate the stimulatory inputs to the emesis center. The CTZ has high levels of dopamine, opioid, and $5-HT_3$ receptors and receives input from dopamine, opioids, and serotonin. The NTS has opioid, $5-HT_3$, dopamine, histamine (H_1), and muscarinic receptors, whereas vestibular input involves activation of histamine (H_1) and muscarinic receptors. Given the transmitters involved in inducing vomiting, a variety of **antiemetic drugs** (drugs to treat vomiting with different mechanisms of action) are effective against selected causes of nausea and vomiting (Table 50-2, and below). Antiemetics include serotonin receptor antagonists, antihistamines,

---

TABLE 50-1

Examples of Disorders Associated with Nausea and Vomiting

Category	*Disorders*
GI tract inflammation or infection	Appendicitis; cholecystitis; cholelithiasis; hepatitis; pancreatitis; peptic ulcer disease; postgastrectomy states; pyelonephritis; Reye's syndrome
Motility disorders	Gastroduodenal motor dysfunction; gastroparesis (autonomic neuropathy); postvagotomy states
GI obstruction	Achalasia; gastric outlet obstruction; incarcerated hernia; small bowel obstruction; volvulus
Vestibular disorders	Labyrinthitis; Meniere's disease; motion sickness
Increased intracranial pressure	Meningitis; space-occupying lesions
Metabolic derangements	Adrenal insufficiency; diabetic ketoacidosis; electrolyte imbalances; thyrotoxicosis; uremia
Psychogenic vomiting	Eating disorders; physical or sexual abuse; posttraumatic stress disorder; pain; stress; unpleasant sights, sounds
Toxins	Staphylococcal enterotoxin
Drugs	Aspirin, NSAIDs; bromocriptine; cisplatin; cyclophosphamide; carboplatin; dacarbazine; digoxin; doxorubicin; erythromycin; ifosfamide; levodopa; lithium; nitrofurantoin; opioids; phenytoin; quinidine; tetracycline; theophylline

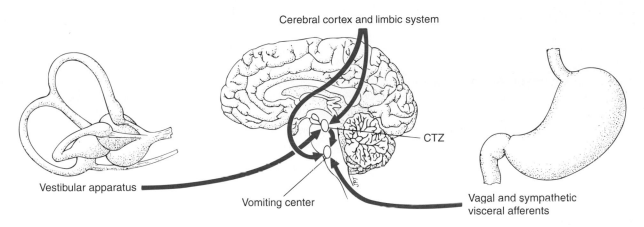

FIGURE 50-1 Vomiting action. Once stimulated, emesis center acts on cranial nerves, spinal nerves to diaphragm, and abdominal muscles, which results in autonomic response of vomiting. *CTZ,* Chemoreceptor trigger zone. (From Beare PG, Myers JL: *Adult health nursing,* ed 3, St Louis, 1998, Mosby.)

anticholinergic drugs, dopamine receptor antagonists, cannabinoids, and a variety of miscellaneous drugs. The choice of an antiemetic is determined by the cause of the nausea and vomiting. Benzodiazepines are also used to reduce the anxiety and anticipation of nausea and vomiting (see Chapter 17) and glucocorticoids are used as adjuncts in patients with cancer (see Chapter 57).

Many drugs (e.g., levodopa and opioids) cause nausea and vomiting because they act directly on the CTZ. The effective treatment is to lower the dosage of the offending drug or to increase the dosage slowly. Drugs (e.g., aspirin) irritate the gastric mucosa, thus causing a reflex stimulation of nausea and vomiting. To dilute the drug, patients should take it with a large volume of liquid or with a meal.

TABLE 50-2

Antiemetic Drugs

Generic Name	Brand Name	Comments
Serotonergic Receptor Antagonists		
dolasetron	Anzemet	Effective in controlling nausea and vomiting associated with emetogenic antineoplastic drugs including cisplatin. Intravenous administration can be given over 30 seconds or diluted up to 50 mL and infused over up to 15 minutes.
granisetron	Kytril	Effective in controlling nausea and vomiting associated with emetogenic antineoplastic drugs including cisplatin. Also used to control emesis associated with cancer radiation therapy.
ondansetron	Zofran	Effective in controlling nausea and vomiting associated with emetogenic antineoplastic drugs including cisplatin. Also used to control emesis associated with cancer radiation therapy.
Dopamine Receptor Antagonists (See Chapter 19 for further discussion.)		
chlorpromazine hydrochloride	Largactil,✽ Novo-Chlorpromazine✽ Sonazine Thorazine	Effective for postoperative nausea and vomiting and that caused by toxins, radiation therapy, and antineoplastic drugs. Watch for orthostatic hypotension with initial injection. Drug may cause considerable drowsiness.

✽ Available only in Canada.

Continued

TABLE 50-2

Antiemetic Drugs—cont'd

Generic Name	Brand Name	Comments
Dopamine Receptor Antagonists—cont'd		
perphenazine	Trilafon	Effective for postoperative nausea and vomiting and that caused by toxins, radiation therapy, and antineoplastic drugs.
prochlorperazine	Compazine, Prorazin✸	Same as perphenazine.
thiethylperazine	Norzine, Torecon	Same as perphenazine.
triflupromazine	Vesprin	Same as perphenazine.
trimethobenzamide	Tigan	Relieves nausea and vomiting of radiation therapy in immediate postoperative period and in gastroenteritis.
Cannabinoids		
dronabinol	Marinol	Chemical name is delta-9-tetrahydrocannabinol, the major active ingredient in marijuana. It is a particularly effective antiemetic when combined with phenothiazine. It is a schedule II drug in the United States and schedule N in Canada.
nabilone	Cesamet✸	Especially effective antiemetic for cisplatin chemotherapy. It is a controlled substance in Canada.
Muscarinic Receptor Antagonists		
scopolamine	Bucospan,✸ Pamine, Transderm-Scop, Transderm-V✸	Sustained release protects most patients from motion sickness while greatly reducing anticholinergic adverse effects (blurred vision, sensitivity to light, dry mouth, and drowsiness).
Histamine Receptor Antagonists		
dimenhydrinate	Dramamine, Gravol,✸ others	Effective for preventing vertigo, motion sickness, and nausea and vomiting of pregnancy. It also causes drowsiness.
diphenhydramine	Benadryl, others	Causes sedation. It is effective for preventing vertigo, motion sickness, and nausea and vomiting of pregnancy.
hydroxyzine	Atarax, Vistaril	Antianxiety drug effective for preventing motion sickness and postoperative nausea and vomiting.
meclizine	Antivert, others	Effective for preventing motion sickness, vertigo, and nausea and vomiting of radiation therapy. It acts longer than most antihistamines.
promethazine	Prometh Plain, Phenergan, others	Effective for preventing motion sickness, vertigo, and postoperative nausea and vomiting.
Miscellaneous Antiemetics		
benzquinamide	Emete-Con	Used for preventing and treating nausea associated with anesthesia. May be administered prophylactically at least 15 minutes before emergence.
dexamethasone	Decadron, others	Effective against moderately emetogenic chemotherapy; enhances overall antiemetic effect of other drugs.
diphenidol	Vontrol	Acts on vestibular apparatus to prevent vertigo after surgery on middle ear. It is effective for postoperative nausea and vomiting as well as that caused by toxins, radiation therapy, or chemotherapy.
metoclopramide	Apo-Metoclop,✸ PMS-metoclopramide Reglan	Acts centrally to block stimulation of CTZ and peripherally to enhance GI tone. High-dose therapy is effective in reducing nausea and vomiting caused by cisplatin therapy; or used in low doses with corticosteroid.

DRUG CLASS • Serotonin Receptor Antagonists

dolasetron (Anzemet)

granisetron (Kytril)

ondansetron (Zofran)

MECHANISM OF ACTION

Serotonin is the major neurotransmitter for emesis. A specific subtype of serotonin receptor, the 5-HT$_3$ receptor, is located in the CTZ and the NTS as well as on vagal nerve terminals in the stomach and small intestine. Serotonin antagonists block the action of serotonin at the 5-HT$_3$ receptors, preventing initiation of the signal for nausea and vomiting.

USES

The serotonin antagonists are effective in preventing nausea and vomiting after radiation therapy for cancer or bone marrow transplantation. They also are effective in treating postoperative vomiting. Antineoplastic drugs that are destructive to cells release serotonin from the enterochromaffin cells in the GI tract, which sets off a severe emetic response. The serotonin antagonists block the action of serotonin at the 5-HT$_3$ receptors in the GI tract, the CTZ, and the NTS. Studies have demonstrated an efficacy of 60% to 90% in preventing significant nausea or vomiting following antineoplastic therapy. For the severely emetic antineoplastic drugs (e.g., cisplatin), the serotonin receptor antagonists are the most effective antiemetic drugs, especially when combined with the glucocorticoid dexamethasone.

PHARMACOKINETICS

Serotonin antagonists are available in oral and intravenous formulations. They often are administered for prophylaxis before chemotherapy or surgery. They are well absorbed after oral administration. Bioavailabilities are approximately 60% to 80%, depending on the drug administered. The onset of drug action is rapid when taken orally or intravenously, with onset times of 30 to 60 minutes. Peak drug actions are reached in 15 to 60 minutes; the duration of drug action ranges from 4 to 24 hours. Dolasetron and ondansetron are 70% to 80% bound to plasma proteins, whereas granisetron binds at 65%. The half-lives of these drugs range from 3 to 4 hours for ondansetron to 5 to 9 hours for dolasetron and granisetron. These drugs are biotransformed by the cytochrome P-450 enzyme system, with dolasetron biotransformed to hydrodolasetron, an active metabolite. Large portions of the metabolites are excreted in the urine, and a smaller portion is eliminated in the bile.

ADVERSE REACTIONS AND CONTRAINDICATIONS

Serotonin antagonists have few adverse effects other than headaches, constipation, or diarrhea. Dolasetron can cause alterations in blood pressure, changes in heart rate, chest pain, and paranoia. This drug also can widen the QRS interval in a dose-related but reversible manner. Granisetron can produce fever, arrhythmia, and chest pain. Ondansetron's adverse effects also include chest pain and bronchospasm.

The major contraindication for these drugs is a history of an allergic reaction, because they can produce anaphylaxis. Dolasetron is contraindicated in patients with a history of substance abuse.

INTERACTIONS

No significant drug interactions have been reported. Because these drugs are acted on by the P-450 mixed function oxidases, their biotransformation may be augmented by drugs that induce the P-450 enzymes (e.g. phenobarbital, rifampin) or inhibited by drugs like cimetidine.

DRUG CLASS • Dopamine Receptor Antagonists

chlorpromazine (Thorazine, Largactil,✲ Novo-Chlorpromazine,✲ Sonazine)

perphenazine (Trilafon)

prochlorperazine (Compazine, Prorazin)

thiethylperazine (Norzine, Torecan)

triflupromazine (Vesprin)

trimethobenzamide (Tigan)

MECHANISM OF ACTION

These drugs suppress nausea and vomiting by blocking dopamine receptors in the CTZ. To varying degrees, these drugs also produce blockade of acetylcholine (muscarinic), histamine, and norepinephrine receptors. Most of these dopamine receptor antagonists are used as antipsychotic drugs, and their actions are discussed in detail in Chapter 19.

USES

Dopamine receptor antagonists are effective in reducing vomiting from antineoplastic and radiation therapy of cancer. They also control postoperative vomiting, although they do not prevent motion sickness. Chlorpromazine and prochlorperazine are used to prevent nausea and vomiting associated with use of mildly emetic antineoplastic drugs. Perphenazine is effective in treating nausea and vomiting associated with surgery, opioid use, and radiation. Thiethylperazine and triflupromazine are considered very effective in preventing postoperative nausea and vomiting. Thiethylperazine also is effective in treating nausea and vomiting caused by the use of mildly emetogenic antineoplastic drugs, radiation, and toxins.

ADVERSE REACTIONS AND CONTRAINDICATIONS

Phenothiazines produce a variety of serious adverse effects (see Chapter 19), including extrapyramidal reactions such as pseudoparkinsonism, dystonia, akathisia, and tardive dyskinesia. Other adverse effects include those related to anticholinergic actions, hypotension, and sedation. Chlorpromazine causes considerable sedation and orthostatic hypotension, actions that limit its use. Prochlorperazine does not produce the profound sedation associated with chlorpromazine. The drugs also can produce photosensitivity and agranulocytosis. Liver function abnormalities may warrant discontinuation of therapy.

PHARMACOKINETICS

In addition to oral administration, most of these drugs are available for intramuscular or intravenous injection. In the majority of cases, onset occurs in 30 minutes to 1 hour when the drugs are taken by mouth; more rapid action is noted when taken by other routes. In general, the drug is biotransformed by the liver and excreted in the urine. The pharmacokinetics of these drugs are discussed in detail in Chapter 19.

INTERACTIONS

The major drug interaction of these antiemetics is a synergistic depression with drugs depressing the CNS, particularly when respiratory depression is involved. For instance, vomiting related to alcohol intoxication or ingestion of narcotic analgesics can be relieved with dopamine receptor antagonists, but the resultant respiratory depression makes this treatment undesirable. Interactions with other drugs are numerous and are discussed in Chapter 19.

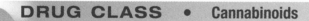

DRUG CLASS • Cannabinoids

dronabinol (Marinol)
nabilone (Cesamet✳)

MECHANISM OF ACTION

The mechanism by which cannabinoids suppress nausea and vomiting is unknown. It is thought, however, that they inhibit the emesis center in the brainstem by an action at the CB_1 cannabinoid receptor.

USES

Dronabinol and nabilone are used for nausea and vomiting associated with antineoplastic therapy. Dronabinol (delta-9-tetrahydrocannabinol, THC) is the primary active ingredient in marijuana. It is also used to treat anorexia in patients with AIDS, since it stimulates the appetite. Nabilone is an active cannabinoid-like dronabinol that appears to be especially effective for relieving the nausea from low-dose cisplatin therapy. It is available in Canada but not in the United States. The use of these drugs has declined somewhat since ondansetron became available.

PHARMACOKINETICS

The cannabinoids are well absorbed after oral administration, but the bioavailability of dronabinol is only 10% to 20%, because of an extensive first-pass effect. The time to peak plasma concentration is 2 to 4 hours, with a duration of action of 4 to 6 hours, although the appetite stimulant actions of dronabinol last up to a day. Dronabinol is 97% bound to plasma proteins, but the cannabinoids are highly lipid soluble and enter breast milk in high concentrations. They are extensively biotransformed: 50% of the metabolites are eliminated through biliary routes and 50% through the kidneys.

ADVERSE REACTIONS AND CONTRAINDICATIONS

Cannabinoids produce subjective effects similar to those evoked by marijuana (see Chapter 9). Patients experience euphoria or dysphoria, detachment, and depersonalization. In addition to the subjective effects, cannabinoids cause tachycardia and hypotension and therefore must be used cautiously in patients with cardiovascular disease. Because of their CNS effects, cannabinoids are contraindicated in patients with psychiatric disorders. They are also contraindicated in patients with hypersensitivities to cannabinoids. Dronabinol and nabilone are schedule II drugs. Chronic use may lead to drug dependence (see Chapter 9).

INTERACTIONS

Cannabinoids produce additive CNS depression if they are used concurrently with alcohol, antihistamines, opioids, tricyclic antidepressants, and sedative-hypnotics. They cause an increased risk of tachycardia when combined with amphetamines, cocaine, sympathomimetics, anticholinergics, antihistamines, and tricyclic antidepressants.

 DRUG CLASS • **Muscarinic Receptor Antagonist**

scopolamine (Pamine, Transderm-Scop, Transderm-V,＊ Bucospan＊)

MECHANISM OF ACTION

Scopolamine is a reversible inhibitor of the actions of acetylcholine at muscarinic receptors. Thus it prevents the actions of acetylcholine in the vestibular system. This drug and other muscarinic antagonists are discussed in detail in Chapter 11.

USES

Scopolamine is considered the most effective drug available for prophylaxis and treatment of motion sickness and vertigo. It has some antiemetic action for patients with postoperative vomiting. Scopolamine is also administered as a preanesthetic agent to depress respiratory secretions and salivation.

PHARMACOKINETICS

Scopolamine is well absorbed and readily crosses the blood-brain barrier. When administered orally, scopolamine causes significant anticholinergic effects. For preventing motion sickness, a transdermal patch is preferred to decrease adverse effects. The patch is applied at least 4 hours in advance of travel and delivers scopolamine over 3 days. Because of their sensitivity to the anticholinergic effects, children should not use the patch. Administered orally, scopolamine is effective in 30 minutes and has a duration of action of 4 to 6 hours. It is biotransformed by the liver and excreted in the urine.

ADVERSE REACTIONS AND CONTRAINDICATIONS

Anticholinergic effects of scopolamine include dry mouth, blurred vision, decreased sweating, urinary retention, and constipation (see Chapter 11). Drowsiness, amnesia, and fatigue may also be experienced. Because vagal tone is depressed, patients with cardiac disease may experience an undesirable increase in heart rate. Children and older adults are more sensitive to the effects of urinary retention, constipation, and disorientation. Men with prostatic hypertrophy are also likely to have difficulty with urination.

Scopolamine is contraindicated for patients who are hypersensitive to this drug or to bromides (injection formulation only) and those who have narrow-angle glaucoma or tachycardia resulting from cardiac insufficiency or thyrotoxicosis. This drug should be used cautiously in patients with suspected intestinal obstruction, prostatic hyperplasia, and chronic cardiac disease.

INTERACTIONS

Scopolamine causes additive anticholinergic effects with other drugs having this activity. In particular, antiparkinsonian drugs, phenothiazines, tricyclic antidepressants, and some antihistamines have significant anticholinergic activity (see Chapter 11).

DRUG CLASS • Histamine Receptor Antagonists

dimenhydrinate (Dramamine, Gravol, others)

diphenhydramine (Benadryl)

hydroxyzine (Atarax, Vistaril)

meclizine (Antivert, others, Bonamine,✦ Antivert✦)

promethazine (Prometh Plain, Phenergan, others)

MECHANISM OF ACTION

Selected antihistamines have been developed that help prevent motion sickness and vertigo, although their exact mechanism remains unknown. Stimulation of receptors in the labyrinth of the ear from which signals governing the sense of equilibrium arise is suppressed. A central anticholinergic action depresses the CTZ. Not all antihistamines are effective as antiemetics, however, and there is no correlation between their ability to prevent motion sickness and their potency as antihistamines or anticholinergics. Antihistamines are discussed in detail in Chapter 53.

USES

Antihistamines are primarily effective for treating motion sickness and vertigo. Therapy is most effective when given prophylactically, 30 minutes before travel. Dimenhydrinate and hydroxyzine are effective for motion sickness and vertigo. Promethazine is the most effective drug for motion sickness prophylaxis. Unfortunately, the sedating effect of the drug limits its usefulness. Given intramuscularly, hydroxyzine also reduces postsurgical nausea and vomiting. Meclizine is especially useful in treating the nausea of vestibular disorders such as labyrinthitis and Meniere's disease.

Diphenhydramine is effective in treating dystonic reactions caused by antipsychotic drugs. The use of antihistamines for symptom relief associated with allergies, including rhinitis, urticaria, and angioedema, is discussed in Chapter 53.

PHARMACOKINETICS

For antiemesis, most antihistamines are taken orally 30 minutes before travel and every 4 to 6 hours as needed. Dimenhydrinate can be administered intramuscularly, intravenously, orally, or rectally. The antihistamines are well absorbed when taken orally and distributed throughout body fluids and tissues. Peak activity occurs in 1 to 4 hours and lasts 3 to 8 hours. The half-lives vary from 2 to 7 hours. Meclizine has a slower onset (60 minutes) and longer duration (24 hours) than other antihistamines. These drugs are biotransformed in the liver and eliminated in the urine (see Chapter 53).

ADVERSE REACTIONS AND CONTRAINDICATIONS

The most common adverse reactions are drowsiness and dry mouth. Headache and jitters may also occur. Older adults tend to be more sensitive to the anticholinergic effects of antihistamines, including dry mouth, urinary retention, sedation, and confusion.

Antihistamines are contraindicated for patients with hypersensitivity or narrow-angle glaucoma as well as premature or newborn infants. These drugs should also be used cautiously in patients with pyloric obstruction, prostatic hypertrophy, hyperthyroidism, cardiovascular disease, or severe liver disease.

INTERACTIONS

Antihistamines cause additive depression with concurrent use of CNS depressants including alcohol, antidepressants, opioid analgesics, and sedative-hypnotics. Anticholinergic effects are enhanced with concurrent administration of other drugs that have anticholinergic activity. Thus therapy for glaucoma may require alteration.

DRUG CLASS • Miscellaneous Drugs

benzquinamide (Emete-Con)

diphenidol (Vontrol)

metoclopramide (Apo-Metoclop,✦ PMS-Metoclopramide, Reglan, Maxeran✦)

MECHANISM OF ACTION

Benzquinamide acts by depressing the CTZ in the brain stem, whereas diphenidol acts on the aural vestibular apparatus to inhibit function and at the CTZ to inhibit nausea and vomiting. Metoclopramide blocks dopaminergic (specifically, D_2) receptors at the CTZ to reduce afferent input. It also is a blocker at serotonergic (HT_3) receptors. In the GI tract, it enhances motility of smooth muscle from the esophagus through the proximal small bowel, and accelerates gastric emptying and the transit of intestinal contents, which counteracts the loss of tone in vomiting.

USES

Benzquinamide is used for the prevention and treatment of nausea associated with anesthesia and surgery. Diphenidol prevents nausea associated with Meniere's disease and surgery on the middle and inner ear. It is also effective in treating postoperative nausea and vomiting as well as emesis associated with radiation therapy and some antineoplastic drugs. Metoclopramide is effective in preventing severe antineoplastic drug–induced vomiting, especially when combined with dexamethasone.

PHARMACOKINETICS

Benzquinamide is administered parenterally, preferably by the intramuscular route, because of the risk of arrhythmia resulting from intravenous administration. Onset occurs within 15 minutes by either route; the duration of action is 3 to 4 hours. Diphenidol is well absorbed after oral administration and has a time to peak of 1 to 3 hours. It has a half-life of approximately 4 hours and is largely eliminated unchanged in the urine.

Metoclopramide is well absorbed from the GI tract, from rectal mucosa, and from intramuscular tissue sites. It is widely distributed to body tissues and fluids crossing the blood-brain barrier and placenta. The onset of drug action varies from minutes for the intravenous formulation to 30 to 60 minutes for the oral form. The duration of action is 1 to 2 hours, and the half-life is 2.5 to 5 hours. Metoclopramide is partially biotransformed in the liver, but 85% of the drug is eliminated unchanged in the urine.

ADVERSE REACTIONS AND CONTRAINDICATIONS

The most common adverse effects of benzquinamide are drowsiness, although insomnia, restlessness, tremors, hypotension, and hypertension also occur. This drug should be used cautiously in patients with a history of cardiovascular disease. Older adults or debilitated patients are prone to the adverse CNS effects of this drug and thus require lower dosages.

Diphenidol produces adverse reactions such as drowsiness, confusion, insomnia and sleep disturbances, visual hallucinations, headache, and restlessness. It is contraindicated for patients with hypersensitivity, psychosis, or anuria. Cautious use is warranted in children and older adults as well as in patients with prostatic hyperplasia, glaucoma, or pyloric or duodenal stenosis.

Sedation and diarrhea are common with high doses of metoclopramide. Although metoclopramide does not have useful antipsychotic effects, it can cause significant extrapyramidal symptoms, especially at high doses and in children. Because of its ability to increase GI motility, metoclopramide is contraindicated in the presence of obstruction, hemorrhage, and perforation of the GI tract.

INTERACTIONS

Additive toxicity can occur when benzquinamide is taken concurrently with other CNS depressants. Hypertension can develop in patients concurrently receiving vasopressors or epinephrine. Although metoclopramide can accelerate the absorption of many drugs, the decreased transit time may decrease the bioavailability of others, most notably digoxin. In addition, the delivery of food to the intestine may be altered to such an extent in patients with diabetes that an insulin dosage adjustment may be required.

APPLICATION TO PRACTICE

ASSESSMENT
History of Present Illness

The patient should be interviewed about the frequency, duration, and precipitating causes of nausea and vomiting. Accompanying symptoms and any measures that relieve the episode of nausea and vomiting should be elicited. A patient's previous experiences with nausea and vomiting may help explain the severity of the present episode. A distinction should be made between vomiting and regurgitation. **Regurgitation** is the passage of food into the esophagus and frequently into the mouth as well, without nausea or vomiting.

Elicit information from the patient about nausea and vomiting that does not have a clear relationship to meals. The timing of this type of nausea and vomiting can result from any cause but is most likely related to metabolic or vestibular disorders, drugs, or toxins. Nausea and vomiting occurring more than 2 hours after eating (especially if recurrent and not associated with significant abdominal pain) suggests gastric outlet syndrome, especially if the emesis contains food material that was eaten several hours earlier. Vomiting within 2 hours after eating may also occur with motility disorders (gastroparesis associated with diabetic autonomic neuropathy and postvagotomy states), or esophageal disorders such as Zenker's diverticulum and achalasia, in which the emesis is typically undigested food. Gastroparesis is characterized by bloating, early satiety, and intractable nausea and vomiting.

Repetitive vomiting during or soon after a meal suggests different causes in children versus adults. In children, a feeding disorder associated with overfeeding or too-rapid feeding is possible. In adults, the problem is psychoneurotic, especially when there is no history of dysphagia and vomiting can be suppressed long enough to make it to the toilet.

Acute-onset nausea and vomiting lasting less than 72 hours in a previously healthy person is usually caused by viral gastroenteritis or toxin exposure. Ask about such exposures. Nausea and vomiting lasting over 24 hours (especially if associated with weight loss and impaired nutrition) is most often caused by GI obstruction or motility dysfunction (e.g., diarrhea). In addition, nausea and vomiting are early manifestations of toxicity of antineoplastic therapy.

Vomiting in the early morning before eating is characteristic in the first 12 to 14 weeks of a normal pregnancy. Early morning vomiting also occurs frequently in patients with increased intracranial pressure (e.g., meningitis and space-occupying lesions of the CNS).

Health History

The patient should be questioned about his or her previous history of nausea and vomiting. A number of conditions and states have been associated with nausea and vomiting (see Table 50-1).

Lifespan Considerations

Perinatal. Nausea and vomiting is common during the first trimester of pregnancy. It usually is self-limited and intermittent, beginning at about the sixth week and disappearing by about the twelfth week of gestation. It is commonly worse in the morning. If it is severe (**hyperemesis gravidarum**), acid-base and electrolyte imbalances, dehydration, or starvation may occur.

Pediatric. Vomiting in infants and children may be associated with acute gastroenteritis or an acute illness (e.g., urinary tract infection, otitis media, or asthma), feeding disorders, hypertrophic pyloric stenosis, or intussusception. If there is no fever, no weight loss, and no abdominal distension and the child does not appear sick, the cause may be a feeding disorder.

Older Adults. Older adults are at risk for fluid volume depletion and electrolyte disturbances with vomiting as well as a potential for injury related to drowsiness. Changes of aging may contribute to the potential for

nausea and vomiting. Esophageal motility is decreased, and the distal end becomes slightly dilated. Esophageal emptying is slower, and gastric motility and emptying is reduced.

Cultural/Social Considerations

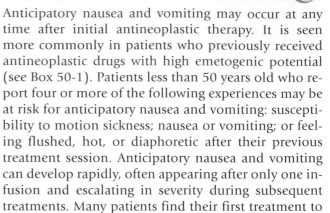

Anticipatory nausea and vomiting may occur at any time after initial antineoplastic therapy. It is seen more commonly in patients who previously received antineoplastic drugs with high emetogenic potential (see Box 50-1). Patients less than 50 years old who report four or more of the following experiences may be at risk for anticipatory nausea and vomiting: susceptibility to motion sickness; nausea or vomiting; or feeling flushed, hot, or diaphoretic after their previous treatment session. Anticipatory nausea and vomiting can develop rapidly, often appearing after only one infusion and escalating in severity during subsequent treatments. Many patients find their first treatment to be much easier than they expected. However, as treatment continues, patients begin to notice the anticipatory adverse effects. With repeated treatments, the problem becomes worse.

Psychogenic vomiting can be associated with a physical syndrome, sexual abuse, post-traumatic stress, and eating disorders. Formal psychiatric assessment and psychologic testing (e.g., the Minnesota Multiphasic Personality Inventory [MMPI]) may be helpful for patients in whom psychogenic vomiting is suspected (see the Case Study: Motion Sickness).

Physical Examination

The physical examination is unremarkable in many cases of nausea and vomiting stemming from some of the more common causes or from motility disorders, metabolic disorders, drugs, or toxins. However, physical examination findings associated with recurrent episodes of nausea and vomiting can include an unexplained increase in tooth decay and gum disease as well as evidence of dehydration or fluid and electrolyte imbalances. The physical examination in patients with gastroparesis or gastric outlet obstruction may reveal a succession splash. Patients with either acute or chronic symptoms should undergo a neurologic examination.

Laboratory Testing

Laboratory testing should be directed by the history and physical examination. Many of the causes of nausea and vomiting have nonspecific physical findings. In patients with acute vomiting, flat and upright abdominal x-ray studies are obtained. Testing may include serum electrolytes to evaluate for hydration, derangements, and evidence of metabolic disorders. Blood urea nitrogen (BUN) and creatinine level tests can be useful in identifying renal

BOX 50-1	Emetogenic Potential of Selected Antineoplastic Drugs

Almost Certain (90%) Risk of Nausea and Vomiting

Drugs that Directly Attack DNA
cisplatin
cyclophosphamide
dacarbazine
mechlorethamine
Drug that Blocks DNA Synthesis
cytarabine

High (60% to 90%) Risk of Nausea and Vomiting

Drugs that Directly Attack DNA
carboplatin
carmustine
lomustine
streptozocin
Drugs that Block RNA or Protein Synthesis
dactinomycin
daunorubicin
doxorubicin

Moderate (30% to 60%) Risk of Nausea and Vomiting

Drugs that Attack DNA
altretamine
etoposide
ifosfamide
procarbazine
topotecan
Antimetabolite
pentostatin

Drugs that Block RNA or Protein Synthesis
idarubicin
L-asparaginase
mitomycin
plicamycin
Drug that Blocks DNA Synthesis
mitoxantrone

Low (0% to 30%) Risk of Nausea and Vomiting

Drugs that Directly Attack DNA
bleomycin
busulfan
chlorambucil
melphalan
thiotepa
Drugs that Block DNA Synthesis
cytarabine
floxuridine
fludarabine
fluorouracil
hydroxyurea
mercaptopurine
methotrexate
thioguanine
Mitotic Inhibitors
paclitaxel
vinblastine
vincristine
vindesine
vinorelbine

toxicity resulting from drugs. Complete blood cell counts may provide evidence of infection or blood loss. Liver function tests can be used to evaluate the possibility of hepatitis, pancreaticobiliary disease, or Reye's syndrome.

For patients with acute vomiting, flat and upright abdominal x-ray studies may be necessary. Gastroparesis is confirmed by nuclear scintigraphic studies, which show delayed gastric emptying. Endoscopy or barium upper GI studies may reflect obstruction. Disorders of the CNS suspected of causing nausea and vomiting should be investigated by brain scan or MRI.

GOALS OF THERAPY

Treatment goals include preventing or relieving the distressing symptoms associated with nausea and vomiting. The potentially life-threatening complications such as electrolyte imbalances, dehydration, and malnutri-

tion should also be avoided. Additionally, treatment goals for the patient with relentless nausea and vomiting related to antineoplastic therapy include preventing or reducing the nausea and vomiting, thus allowing completion of effective antineoplastic regimens.

INTERVENTION

The treatment of vomiting should be directed primarily at finding and correcting the underlying cause. Most causes of acute vomiting are self-limited and require no special treatment. Patients should take clear liquids (e.g., broths, tea, soups, carbonated beverages) and small quantities of dry foods (e.g., soda crackers). Hospitalization may be required for more acute vomiting. Because of the inability to eat and the loss of gastric fluids, patients can become dehydrated and develop hypokalemia and metabolic alkalosis. Intravenous fluids and nasogastric suctioning may be needed to maintain hydration and to allow for gastric decompression.

The choice of an antiemetic is usually directed at symptomatic relief, but it depends primarily on the cause of the nausea and vomiting. Combinations of drugs from different classes may provide better symptom control with less toxicity in some patients. Combination strategies take advantage of the synergistic mechanisms afforded to each drug. This makes possible more complete and extended prophylaxis, use of lower doses of individual drugs, and thus fewer adverse effects. For example, treatment of a patient with anticipatory, acute, or delayed forms of emesis might include a benzodiazepine (e.g., lorazepam), a serotonin antagonist (e.g., ondansetron), and a corticosteroid (e.g., dexamethasone). The decision to use a specific drug is thus based, in part, on potential adverse effects, because no one drug has proved to be more effective than any other drug.

Administration

Most antiemetics are available in oral, parenteral, and rectal dosage forms. Be sure to read the manufacturer's instructions before administration. As a general rule, oral dosage forms are preferred for prophylaxis. Administration should be planned so that peak drug effects correspond to the time of anticipated nausea. For example, antiemetics used in the prevention of motion sickness are usually administered at least 30 minutes (preferably 4 hours) before travel. This allows time for drug dissolution and absorption. Some preparations can then be used every 3 to 4 hours as needed thereafter. Box 50-2 provides examples of combination antiemetic regimens that may be used for nausea and vomiting in cancer patients.

Rectal or parenteral antiemetics are preferred for therapeutic use. Parenteral antiemetics should not be mixed in a syringe with other drugs. An exception is promethazine, which may be mixed with meperidine and atropine sulfate for preanesthetic use. Intramuscular injections should be given deeply into a large muscle mass to decrease tissue irritation.

Use antiemetics with caution in children who may have Reye's syndrome, which is characterized by an abrupt onset of persistent severe vomiting, lethargy, irrational behavior, progressing to encephalopathy, seizures, coma, and death. Avoid giving intramuscular trimethobenzamide to children. Dolasetron may be administered orally, diluted in apple or grape juice, and administered 1 hour before antineoplastic therapy is begun.

Excessive sedation may occur with usual therapeutic doses of antiemetics and is more likely to occur with high doses. Avoiding high doses when possible and assessing the patient for responsiveness before each dose can sometimes reduce sedation. Notify the health care provider if the patient appears excessively drowsy or is hypotensive.

The patient's blood pressure should be checked before administration of the antiemetic. Hypotension, including orthostatic hypotension, and anticholinergic effects may occur with any of the drugs but is most likely to occur with phenothiazines and droperidol. When cannabinoids are used, the patient should be observed for alterations in mood, cognition, and perception of reality. According to the manufacturer, these adverse effects are well tolerated, particularly by young individuals. If necessary, tachycardia associated with the use of cannabinoids can be prevented with a beta-blocking drug such as propranolol.

Education

To help minimize nausea and vomiting, bland foods should be eaten and very sweet, fatty, salty, and spicy foods avoided. Patients are advised to sip clear liquids slowly and take foods served cool or at room temperature. Some patients receiving antineoplastic therapy are unable to tolerate plain water or red meat.

Visual, auditory, and olfactory stimulation should be minimized, and noxious stimuli should be removed from the environment. Avoid or decrease activity during episodes of nausea. The patient should be advised to change positions slowly to minimize orthostatic hypotension.

BOX 50-2 | **Examples of Combination Antiemetic Regimens**

For Drugs with Low to Moderate Emetogenic Potential

Oral prochlorperazine every 6 hours, starting 24 hours before treatment (continue combination until 24 hours after last treatment) + oral dronabinol every 6 hours, starting 24 hours before treatment.

For Drugs with Moderate Emetogenic Potential

Intravenous metoclopramide 20 minutes before and 90 minutes after treatment + intravenous dexamethasone 20 minutes before treatment + intravenous diphenhydramine 30 minutes before treatment.

For Drugs with High Emetogenic Potential

Intravenous ondansetron and dexamethasone 30 minutes before treatment + oral prochlorperazine SR, oral lorazepam, and oral diphenhydramine at bedtime.

Antiemetic Drugs CHAPTER 50 **827**

Good oral hygiene and frequent rinsing of the mouth with water helps relieve the bad taste and corrosion of tooth enamel caused by gastric acid. To relieve mouth dryness caused by the anticholinergic effects of some antiemetics, frequent rinsing and sugarless gum or candy may be used. A cool wet washcloth to the face and neck may help the patient feel more comfortable. Because pain may cause nausea and vomiting with some individuals, administration of analgesics before the event can help.

Patients should be informed that drowsiness may occur with antiemetics and that driving and other activities requiring alertness should be avoided until response to the drug is known. Advise the patient who has motion sickness to ride in the front seat of the car if possible, facing forward. If dry eyes are a problem, suggest that the patient regularly use artificial tears.

Review the adverse effects of antiemetics with the patient. Warn the patient to use these drugs only as prescribed and not to self-treat with leftover doses. The use of these drugs is contraindicated for pregnant women unless the benefit outweighs the risks. Patients should also be taught to take the drug as ordered and cautioned to avoid concurrent use of alcohol or other CNS depressants (e.g., tranquilizers, sleeping pills, and opioid analgesics) without first checking with the health care provider.

CASE STUDY   *Motion Sickness*

ASSESSMENT

HISTORY OF PRESENT ILLNESS

CM is a 52-year-old man who reports to the medical office today for a required annual employment physical examination. He is also requesting a prescription for motion sickness. He will once again be crossing "the treacherous Drake Passage by ship" on his way to Antarctica and is worried he will not be able to perform his job as an engineer should he experience motion sickness. The Drake Passage takes 3 days to cross. He has made the trip three times previously and reports having persistent nausea and vomiting while aboard ship. He states that he has tried OTC Benadryl and other "motion sickness pills" but found them to be less than effective.

HEALTH HISTORY

CM's medical history is unremarkable except for hay fever and an early benign prostatic hypertrophy that causes occasional urinary hesitancy. He had an intramedullary rod inserted in his right femur without sequelae after a motor vehicle accident (MVA) at age 25. He reports taking no OTC or prescription drugs.

LIFESPAN CONSIDERATIONS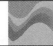

CM is unmarried and feels he must remain so because of the extended periods of time he is away from his home in the United States.

CULTURAL/SOCIAL CONSIDERATIONS

CM reports no history of psychiatric disorders. He denies use of tobacco or alcohol since the MVA at age 25. He enjoys basketball and playing cards with fellow employees as well as occasionally dating a fellow employee. His employer covers the cost of an annual physical examination and prescriptions when a formulary drug is used. Preauthorization is needed from the insurance company if a nonformulary drug is prescribed.

PHYSICAL EXAMINATION

CM's physical examination is unremarkable. Heart rhythm and rate are regular (RRR); breath sounds are clear bilaterally; cranial nerves II to XII are intact. Strength of bilateral upper and lower extremities are equal; bowel sounds are present in all four quadrants; prostate is enlarged on palpation; hernia examination is negative.

LABORATORY TESTING

Laboratory test results reveal CBC count, electrolytes, urinalysis, and ECG within normal limits. Drug screen is negative.

PATIENT PROBLEM(S)

Motion sickness.

GOALS OF THERAPY

Prevent or relieve distressing symptoms associated with nausea and vomiting; prevent complications such as electrolyte imbalances, dehydration, and malnutrition.

CRITICAL THINKING QUESTIONS

1. What are the three major pathways that stimulate vomiting?
2. The health care provider considers prescribing scopolamine (Transderm-Scop) patches and meclizine for CM. What are the mechanisms of action for these drugs?
3. CM should be aware of which adverse effects of scopolamine?
4. How and when should CM use the scopolamine patch?
5. What other actions can CM take to help prevent or minimize his motion sickness?

For the patient using sustained release transdermal formulations, emphasize the importance of reading the manufacturer's instructions. Instruct the patient to wash hands before and after applying the device. The patch is usually applied behind the ear, in front of the hairline. The patient should avoid cut or denuded skin and replace the patch every 3 days or as directed by the health care provider. If the patch falls off, the patient should apply a new one. Instruct the patient to apply the patch at least 30 minutes before travel and preferably 4 hours before the trip (for Transderm-Scop) or 12 hours ahead of the trip for the Canadian brand (Transderm-V).

Because of its tendency to cause mood changes, advise patients taking a cannabinoid to use the drug only when supervised by a responsible adult. Other drugs should not be taken without the knowledge and consent of the health care provider.

EVALUATION

Therapeutic effects of antiemetics can be observed through verbal reports of decreased nausea and a decreased frequency or complete absence of vomiting. Note the patient's ability to maintain adequate intake of food and fluids, comparing current weight with a baseline weight. Determine whether the dosage and administration times of the antiemetic drugs are the most effective for the individual patient.

Bibliography

Anastasia PJ: Effectiveness of oral 5-HT$_3$ receptor antagonists for emetogenic chemotherapy, *Oncol Nurs Forum* 27(3):483-493, 2000.

Cox F: Systematic review of ondansetron for the prevention and treatment of postoperative nausea and vomiting in adults, *Br J Theatre Nurs* 9(12):556-563, 1999.

Doherty KM: Closing the gap in prophylactic antiemetic therapy: patient factors in calculating the emetogenic potential of chemotherapy, *Clin J Oncol Nurs* 3(3):113-119, 1999.

Eckert RM: Understanding anticipatory nausea, *Oncol Nurs Forum* 28(10):1553-1560, 2001.

Eremita D: Dolasetron for chemo nausea, *RN* 64(3):38-40, 2001.

Ouellette SM: Newer trends in the prevention or treatment of postoperative nausea and vomiting, *CRNA* 10(1):24-33, 1999.

Thompson HJ: The management of post-operative nausea and vomiting, *J Adv Nurs* 29(5):1130-1136, 1999.

Zeidenstein L: Alternative therapies for nausea and vomiting of pregnancy, *J Nurse Midwifery* 43(5):392-393, 1998.

Internet Resources

www.nlm.nih.gov/medlineplus/ency/article/003117.htm.
www.nlm.nih.gov/medlineplus/nauseaandvomiting.html.

CHAPTER

51

Drugs to Treat Liver, Gallbladder, and Pancreatic Diseases

SHERRY F. QUEENER • KATHLEEN GUTIERREZ

 Visit http://evolve.elsevier.com/Gutierrez/ for additional information.

KEY TERMS

Amylase, p. 833

Bile, p. 830

Cholecystitis, p. 831

Cholecystectomy, p. 831

Cholelithiasis, p. 831

Cirrhosis, p. 836

Fetor hepaticus, p. 840

Hepatic coma, p. 836

Hepatic encephalopathy, p. 836

Lipase, p. 833

Proteases, p. 833

Steatorrhea, p. 834

OBJECTIVES

- Explain the mechanism of drugs used to dissolve gallstones.
- Explain the role of the pancreas in digestion.
- Discuss the drugs used for pancreatic enzyme replacement.
- Discuss the causes of liver disease and options for treatment.
- Develop a nursing care plan for patients receiving one of the drugs discussed in this chapter.

The liver, gallbladder, and pancreas all function in maintaining effective digestion of food. In addition, the liver has a role in the biotransformation of drugs (see Chapter 1). The relationship of the pancreas to diabetes mellitus is discussed in Chapter 58.

 ## PATHOPHYSIOLOGY • Gallbladder Disease

The gallbladder is a small organ located beneath the right side of the liver (Figure 51-1). The liver produces **bile**, a yellow-brown, watery fluid consisting of cholesterol, lipids, bile salts, and bilirubin. As much as 600 to 800 mL are produced daily, and up to 250 mL of concentrated bile is stored by the gallbladder. A duct connects the gallbladder with the small intestine. As food leaves the stomach and enters the small intestine, the gallbladder contracts and propels stored bile into the small intestine, where it disperses the fat in

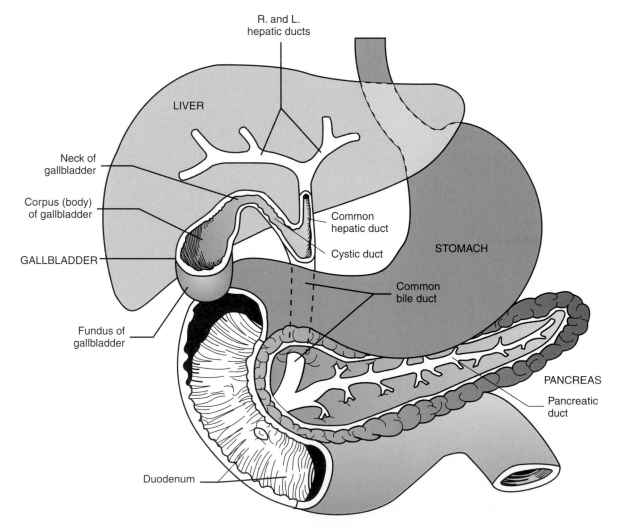

FIGURE 51-1 Bile is secreted by the liver and stored in the gallbladder. As food passes into the small intestine, the gallbladder contracts and sends stored bile into the cystic duct, which connects to the common bile duct. Bile salts enter the intestine, where they aid in digestion by dispersing lipids. Symptomatic gallstones usually become lodged in the cystic duct and less often in the common bile duct. The pancreas is a major source of digestive enzymes: amylase to digest carbohydrates; trypsin, chymotrypsin, and carboxypeptidase to digest proteins; and lipase to digest lipids. Bicarbonate is also released to neutralize stomach acid. Pancreatic secretions enter the intestine at the lower end of the common bile duct. *R*, right, *L*, left. (Courtesy Donald O'Conner.)

food. Therefore it is important for the digestion of lipids in the small intestine. Normally, most of the bile is reabsorbed by the small intestine and returned to the liver.

Cholelithiasis refers to the presence of gallstones, which are usually small (less than 2 cm in diameter). Most gallstones are composed almost entirely of cholesterol and are believed to result when crystals form in bile that is supersaturated with cholesterol. In about 20% of cases, the gallstone is composed of pigment. Poor motility of the gallbladder contributes to the development of gallstones.

A gallstone attack usually gives rise to a steady, severe pain in the upper abdomen that lasts from 20 or 30 minutes to several hours. The pain may also be felt in the back between the shoulder blades or in the right shoulder. Nausea and vomiting may also occur. Attacks may not happen often. A common complication of gallstones is that they lodge in the cystic duct, the channel connecting the gallbladder with the common bile duct, and cause **cholecystitis**, an inflammation of the gallbladder. A more serious problem is blockage of the common bile duct, obstruction of the flow of bile from the liver, or even blockage of the flow of digestive fluids from the pancreas. Blockage of any of the ducts can cause severe damage to the gallbladder, liver, or pancreas.

About 1 in every 12 adults in the United States has gallstones, and more than 1 million people are newly diagnosed each year. Risk factors for gallstones include age, female gender (especially with multiple pregnancies), obesity, and rapid weight loss (Box 51-1). Most people with gallstones have no symptoms. Gallstones are most commonly detected by an abdominal x-ray study, a computed tomography (CT) scan, or an abdominal ultrasound scan taken for an unrelated prob-

lem. Complications arising from gallbladder disease appear most commonly in patients who develop manifestations of biliary colic. The younger the age at initial diagnosis, the more likely the development of complications.

Removal of the gallbladder, **cholecystectomy**, is the most common method for treating gallstones. More than 500,000 patients undergo this surgery each year in the United States. Laparoscopic surgery has made cholecystectomy a relatively simple procedure with a recovery period of a few days. Although surgery is the treatment of choice for symptomatic gallstones, pharmacologic treatment is available for small stones that consist mostly of cholesterol. Because the gallbladder is left in place in all interventions except a cholecystectomy, recurrence of stones is likely.

BOX 51-1	Risk Factors for Gallstones

Partly because gallstones are so common, it has been possible to identify many risk factors:
- Age more than 60 years old
- Obesity
- Ethnicity (Native Americans have the highest prevalence of gallstones in the United States, followed by Hispanic Americans)
- Use of birth control pills or estrogen replacement therapy
- Rapid weight loss
- Female gender (women between the ages of 20 and 60 years are twice as likely as men to develop gallstones)

DRUG CLASS • Anticholelithic Drugs

 ursodiol, or ursodeoxycholic acid (Actigall, Urso, Ursofalk✦)

MECHANISM OF ACTION

Ursodiol is concentrated in bile and decreases biliary cholesterol saturation by suppressing hepatic synthesis and secretion of cholesterol. This mechanism is effective only for gallstones composed of cholesterol. Ursodiol also increases bile flow. The drug is related to natural bile acids.

USES

Ursodiol is used to treat uncomplicated gallstone disease (i.e., in which stones are less than 2 cm in diameter) in patients with a functioning gallbladder. Gallstones that are radiolucent are predominantly composed of cholesterol. Patients with complications from gallstones are

usually treated surgically because of the long response time to therapy with ursodiol.

Ursodiol is also used to treat some chronic liver diseases because of its ability to increase bile flow and to reduce the detergent properties of bile salts. Ursodiol appears to protect liver cells from the damaging activity of toxic bile salts, which increase in chronic liver disease (see discussion that follows).

PHARMACOKINETICS

Ursodiol is usually given orally three times a day with meals. It is well absorbed from the intestine and is biotransformed in the liver into several forms, including another bile acid called chenodiol. Ursodiol is also converted to taurine and glycine conjugates that are excreted into the bile.

ADVERSE REACTIONS AND CONTRAINDICATIONS

Ursodiol has few adverse reactions. Those taking it occasionally experience diarrhea. The drug does not have adverse effects on the fetus in animal studies and is not contraindicated during pregnancy.

INTERACTIONS

Cholestyramine, antacids, and colestipol may bind ursodiol and prevent its absorption. Clofibrate, estrogens, progestins, and neomycin counteract the action of ursodiol because they tend to increase the concentration of cholesterol in bile.

 APPLICATION TO PRACTICE

ASSESSMENT
History of Present Illness

Less than half of the population with gallstones report any distress, because gallstones cause no manifestations unless complications develop. However, ask patients with gallbladder disease if they have had any pain, particularly steady, severe pain in the upper abdomen. Does the pain radiate? Often the pain radiates around to the back and right shoulder blade. Ask how long the pain lasts and when it occurs (e.g., before meals or after meals). Is the pain worse when eating fatty foods? Contraction of an inflamed gallbladder to release bile precipitates pain. Ask about the pain severity (on a scale of 1 to 10). Ask also where the pain is located, because discomfort may also be felt not only in the upper right quadrant but also in the back between the shoulder blades or in the right shoulder. Determine if the patient has had any nausea, vomiting, or if the stool has changed to a light, chalky color.

Health History

There are many risk factors for gallbladder disease. Ask the patient about a history of diabetes mellitus, multiple pregnancies, vagotomy, regional enteritis, ileal disease or resection (which results in bile salt depletion). Long-term parenteral nutrition (which decreases gallbladder motility), cirrhosis, chronic hemolytic disorders (resulting in increased bile pigments), obesity, and calorie restriction with certain diets are also risk factors to be identified. Be sure to obtain a thorough drug history that includes the use of clofibrate or cholestyramine.

Lifespan Considerations

Perinatal. Gallbladder disease during the perinatal period is not uncommon, because the gallbladder is influenced by estrogen and becomes hypotonic. This causes an increased concentration of bile and an increased risk of gallstone formation.

Pediatric. Ask whether the patient has a history of sickle cell anemia. Although uncommon, children with sickle cell anemia may be found to have anorexia, jaundiced sclera, and gallstones.

Older Adults. The incidence of gallstones increases with age and affects women more frequently than men. With advancing age, the liver becomes smaller and consequently has less storage capacity. Less efficient cholesterol stabilization and absorption predispose the individual to develop gallstones.

Cultural/Social Considerations

Genetics seem to play some role in gallstone formation, as evidenced by its prevalence in Pima and Chippewa Native Americans, followed by Hispanic Americans. African Americans who have a history of sickle cell anemia are also at higher risk for developing gallstones.

Physical Examination

The patient with acute gallbladder disease is often restless, changing positions frequently to relieve the intensity of the pain. In addition to the basic physical examination, a thorough abdominal examination is required. Ask the patient to take a deep breath. Murphy's sign is noted if the patient experiences tenderness and stops breathing on inspiration while the examiner is palpating the right upper quadrant. If a gallstone lodges in the common bile duct, the condition may be complicated by cholangitis (inflammation of the bile ducts) and pancreatitis. Jaundice appears only when the common bile duct is obstructed. If the stone is blocking the cystic duct, the patient may show signs of acute cholecystitis (fever, leukocytosis, and worsening abdominal pain). Nausea and vomiting are caused by distension of the bile ducts, which sends impulses to the emesis center in the brain.

Laboratory Testing

Patients with gallbladder disease often have fever and leukocytosis, which are responses to inflammation. Leukocyte count is elevated in 85% of patients, with the exception of the older adult and those on glucocorticoid therapy. Aminotransferase (ALT, AST), alkaline phosphatase, and bromosulfaphthalein values may be slightly abnormal. Cholelithiasis and cholecystitis both cause increased serum bilirubin levels. The serum amylase value is measured to determine the presence of secondary pancreatitis.

Ultrasound of the gallbladder may reflect cholelithiasis, thickening of the gallbladder wall (greater than 3 mm), and distension of the lumen of the gallbladder (greater than 5 mm). In 15% of cases, gallstones contain enough calcium to be visible on an abdominal x-ray study.

GOALS OF THERAPY

The treatment goals for the patient taking ursodiol for the treatment of gallstones are to dissolve the stone(s), relieve pain, maintain adequate hydration, and prevent complications.

INTERVENTION
Administration

Administer ursodiol with food or milk. Do not administer within 2 hours of aluminum-based antacids, clofibrate, or cholestyramine. Monitor the patient's bowel function, because the drug can cause diarrhea.

Education

Emphasize the importance of concomitant therapies such as dietary restrictions and weight loss. Maintaining ideal or low body weight and eating a high-fiber diet may help prevent and treat gallstones.

Teach the importance of taking the drug as ordered for the full course of therapy. Dissolution of gallstones with ursodiol generally requires many months and may take 2 years of daily therapy. Response is monitored with oral cholecystograms or ultrasonograms performed every 6 to 9 months. If no response is seen in 18 months, therapy is discontinued. If a response is seen, therapy is continued until dissolution has been confirmed by two successive ultrasonograms. In most cases, ursodiol will need to be taken for 1 to 3 months after the stone is dissolved.

Remind the patient of the importance of returning for regular follow-up visits to monitor treatment effectiveness, even if the patient feels better. Frequent blood work will be necessary to follow drug effects. Instruct the patient to notify the health care provider if severe or persistent diarrhea, nausea, and vomiting, severe abdominal pain, or right upper quadrant pain develops.

EVALUATION

Ursodiol treatment is effective if the gallstones dissolve, the patient is more comfortable, and surgery and its associated complications have been avoided.

PATHOPHYSIOLOGY • Pancreatic Diseases

Like the gallbladder, the pancreas secretes agents to aid in digestion in the small intestine. Pancreatic secretions enter the small intestine through the common bile duct via the pancreatic duct (see Figure 51-1). The pancreas secretes the enzymes **lipase** and **amylase** as well as **proteases** such as trypsin and chymotrypsin, which are important in the digestion of fats, carbohydrates, and proteins. Bicarbonate is also secreted to neutralize stomach acid. These functions are lost when drugs or diseases such as chronic pancreatitis or cystic fibrosis damage the pancreas. Protein malnutrition is a major cause of this disease in developing countries of the world. Obstruction of the pancreatic duct may also result from tumors or other injuries; removal of the pancreas may be required. Patients who have undergone this surgical intervention require replacement therapy with the products of the pancreas.

Characteristically, chronic pancreatitis is characterized by progressive loss of the *exocrine* functions, that is, the production of pancreatic enzymes essential for normal digestion. There is relative preservation of the organ's *endocrine* functions until late in the disease. The specific cause of chronic pancreatitis can rarely be identified, but most of the factors associated with the acute form of the disease are also associated with the chronic form. In the United States and other industrial countries, alcoholism is considered by many to be one of the primary causes of the disease since prompt diagnosis and treatment of biliary obstruction have reduced the incidence of pancreatitis resulting from obstruction.

Chronic pancreatitis can progress to pancreatic insufficiency as acinar tissue becomes replaced with fibrous tissue. Because the acini secrete pancreatic enzymes necessary for the digestion of proteins, carbohydrates, and fats, dysfunction of acinar tissue results in malabsorption of nutrients from the small intestine.

The extent of GI involvement in children with cystic fibrosis varies. In the pancreas of many patients, the thick secretions block the ducts, leading to cystic dilations of the acini, which then undergo degeneration and progressive diffuse fibrosis. This even prevents pancreatic enzymes from reaching the duodenum, which causes marked impairment in the digestion and absorption of nutrients, particularly fats, proteins, and to a lesser degree, carbohydrates. The disturbed absorption is reflected as excessive fat in the stool. The endocrine function of the pancreas in children with cystic fibrosis remains unchanged. The islets of Langerhans are normal but may decrease in number as pancreatic fibrosis progresses.

Children with cystic fibrosis demonstrate decreased pancreatic secretion of bicarbonate and chloride. The secondary degeneration of the pancreas leads to malabsorption syndrome.

 DRUG CLASS • Pancreatic Enzymes

 pancrelipase (Cotazym, Creon, Pancrease, Ultrase, Viokase, others)

MECHANISM OF ACTION

Pancrelipase is derived from hog pancreata. The preparation is adjusted to contain 8000 USP units of lipase to aid in digestion of lipids, 30,000 USP units of protease to aid in digestion of proteins, and 30,000 USP units of amylase to assist in digestion of carbohydrates.

USES

Pancrelipase is used as replacement therapy in symptomatic treatment of malabsorption syndrome resulting from conditions that cause pancreatic insufficiency such as chronic pancreatitis, benign or malignant pancreatic tumors, cystic fibrosis, and pancreatectomy. There is no rationale for replacement therapy as a digestive aid. However, the drug is occasionally used to open occluded feeding tubes.

PHARMACOKINETICS

Pancrelipase is available in capsules, enteric-coated microspheres, microtablets, delayed release formulations, powders, and tablets to be taken orally before or with meals. If the capsule dissolves completely in the presence of high acidity in the stomach, the activity of the enzymes may be impaired. Best results occur when the enzymes reach the more pH-neutral regions of the small intestine.

ADVERSE REACTIONS AND CONTRAINDICATIONS

The major complications of replacement therapy include diarrhea, nausea, abdominal cramps, and pain, especially when the preparation is taken in large doses. Occasionally, individuals may be allergic to the animal protein in these preparations. Safe use during pregnancy or lactation has not been established.

INTERACTIONS

Drugs that lower gastric pH may be used with pancrelipase to prevent premature destruction of the enzymes in the stomach. Blockers of H_2 receptors or antacids may play a role, but if antacids are used, care should be taken to avoid those that contain calcium carbonate or magnesium hydroxide, because these compounds impair the actions of pancrelipase. Pancrelipase may decrease the absorption of concurrently administered iron preparations.

APPLICATION TO PRACTICE

ASSESSMENT
History of Present Illness

The classic manifestation of chronic pancreatitis is abdominal pain, weight loss, diabetes, and steatorrhea (high fat content in the stool). Ask the patient with pancreatic insufficiency about problems with bulky, fatty, foul-smelling stools, weight loss, fever, malaise, and nausea and vomiting.

Because of the negative nitrogen balance resulting from wasting of muscles and malabsorption of fat-soluble vitamins, there may be bruising and bleeding from even a mild injury. Ask about these and any pain the patient is having. Dull pain will often alternate with severe pain, vomiting, fever, and jaundice. Note if the patient's pain is relieved by sitting in bed with the knees flexed and pressing a pillow to the abdomen. The patient may note more pain when supine.

Health History

Ask the patient about a history of hyperparathyroidism, congenital anomalies, and pancreatic trauma. Patients with pancreatitis often have a history of abusing opioid analgesics in an effort to control pain. The pain and steatorrhea often motivates the patient to seek help.

Ask about food consumption. Because eating often aggravates the pain, the patient usually reduces consumption, resulting in weight loss. Because of involvement of islet cell tissues, the patient develops hyperglycemia with manifestations of diabetes mellitus. Ask about polyuria, polyphagia, and polydipsia.

Lifespan Considerations

Perinatal. Gallbladder disease is common during and shortly after pregnancy. If stones obstruct the common bile duct, the pancreas could be affected. Perinatal women who complain of upper abdominal pain should be evaluated for gallstones and any related pancreatic involvement.

Pediatric. Cystic fibrosis is an autosomal recessive trait; that is, the affected child must inherit the defective gene from both parents. It is estimated that 3.3% of whites in the United States are symptom-free carriers of cystic fibrosis. The chronic nature of the disease affects the growth and development of children and young adults.

Older Adults. The pancreas of the older adult produces normal amounts of bicarbonate, amylase, and trypsin, but there is a decrease in lipase, resulting in subclinical abnormalities in fat absorption. Reduced fat absorption reduces in turn the absorption of fat-soluble vitamins as well as vitamins B_1 and B_{12}, calcium, and iron. Pancreatitis and pancreatic insufficiency is no more common in older adults than in middle-aged adults.

Cultural/Social Considerations

Although more than 95% of documented cases of cystic fibrosis affect whites, the disease is also present in Hispanic Americans, African Americans, and Asian Americans. It is estimated that in the 1990s patients with cystic fibrosis could be expected to survive into their forties.

Physical Examination

Dull pain may alternate with severe pain, vomiting, fever, and jaundice. Monitor the patient's stools for steatorrhea. Stools will be foul smelling and frothy.

Laboratory Testing

Because of a reduced amount of functional tissue in chronic pancreatitis, pancreatic enzyme analysis may be normal. Blood tests may reveal a mild leukocytosis, mild hyperglycemia, and an elevated sedimentation rate. Serum amylose and urinary amylase test results are also elevated in pancreatic disease. The patient may also have hypocalcemia resulting from saponification of calcium by fatty acids in areas of fat necrosis as well as hyperlipidemia resulting from the release of free fatty acids by lipase. Alkaline phosphatase and serum bilirubin levels may also be elevated.

X-ray studies may show reduced GI motility, calcification, and adhesions. Both ultrasound and pancreatic CT scans may provide useful data. Cholangiography and cholecystography show biliary alterations, which may be either a cause or a consequence of the pancreatic disorder.

GOALS OF THERAPY

The treatment goal for the patient with pancreatic insufficiency is chiefly substitutive and palliative: to improve nutritional status and normalize stools. Symptomatic relief from pain can make the patient more comfortable. Substitutive therapy with pancreatic enzymes can help maintain adequate nutrition and strengthen the patient's resources so that the activities of daily living can be carried out.

INTERVENTION

Pain relief is not easily accomplished but should begin with nonopioid analgesics and progress to opioid analgesics such as codeine, morphine, or meperidine if necessary (see Chapter 13). Some patients experience less pain when they assume positions that flex the trunk and draw the knees up to the abdomen. A side-lying position with the head elevated 45 degrees decreases tension on the abdomen and may help ease the pain. It is important to control pain and restlessness because they increase body metabolism and subsequent stimulation of pancreatic secretions. Control of pain is the sole indication for surgical intervention.

Control of diet may reduce the painful stimulation of pancreas enzyme secretion. A nasogastric tube or NPO status is helpful in reducing GI stress.

Administration

The actual dosage of pancrelipase depends on the severity of the insufficiency, the digestive requirements of the patient, and the philosophy of the health care provider. Usually 300 mg of pancrelipase is necessary to digest 17 g of dietary fat. Observe the patient's stools for evidence of steatorrhea to help determine the effectiveness of the enzymes. In children, the dosage is adjusted to achieve normal growth and a decrease in the number of stools to two or three per day.

Administer pancrelipase immediately before or with meals and snacks. The patient should take the drug while in an upright position. Eating immediately after taking the drug helps to further ensure that the drug is swallowed and does not remain in contact with the mouth and esophagus for extended periods. Be aware, however, that alkaline foods destroy the coating on enteric-coated formulations.

Capsules filled with enteric-coated beads should not be chewed; capsules may be opened and sprinkled on soft foods that can be swallowed without chewing, such as applesauce or flavored gelatin. If a dose is missed, it should be omitted and not doubled up.

Assess the patient's nutritional status (height, weight, skinfold thickness, arm muscle circumference, and laboratory values) before and periodically throughout therapy. Monitor the serum and urine uric acid concentrations as well because pancrelipase can cause these to be elevated.

Education

Emphasize the importance of taking the drug as ordered and not to change brands of pancrelipase without checking first with the health care provider. Advise the patient not to chew tablets and to swallow them quickly with plenty of liquid to prevent mouth and throat irritation. Advise the patient to avoid sniffing the powdered contents of capsules, because the nose and throat may become sensitized (nasal stuffiness or respiratory distress). Instruct the patient to store the drug at room temperature in a tightly sealed container. If antacids or iron are also prescribed, advise the patient to avoid concurrent administration of these products.

Advise the patient to avoid alcoholic beverages. If the patient has developed dependence on alcohol or opioids, referral to other agencies or resources may be advised.

Encourage the patient to return for regular follow-up visits to monitor drug effectiveness and adverse effects, even if he or she feels better. Emphasize the importance of concomitant therapies including dietary restrictions. Have the patient notify the health care provider if joint pain, swelling of legs, gastric distress, abdominal pain, cramping, blood or the urine, or a rash develops.

EVALUATION

The effectiveness of therapy for pancreatic insufficiency is demonstrated by improved nutritional status. Patients with steatorrhea should have a normalization of stools.

The prognosis for chronic pancreatitis is good if acute attacks decrease in frequency. Enzyme replacement therapy permits a fairly normal life. However, if the patient continues to drink alcohol, the prognosis is poor. Repeated attacks eventually cause death from shock or renal failure.

PATHOPHYSIOLOGY • Liver Disease

Liver disease may range from transient minor impairment of function to profound and irreversible organ failure. Several factors are known to contribute to liver dysfunction. For example, hepatitis A, B, and C all cause disease, but the forms differ. Hepatitis A mostly occurs as an acute illness lasting less than 6 months, and the immune system ultimately eliminates the virus. Hepatitis B infections in most people also clear without treatment, although up to 10% of infections become chronic and lead to long-lasting or progressive health problems. Hepatitis C is a more serious infection for most people. About 85% of cases of this form of hepatitis progress to chronic forms that lead to cirrhosis, liver cancer, or liver failure. In the United States, hepatitis C is now the leading cause of liver failure that requires transplantation. Treatment of the viral infections before they produce these serious outcomes is covered in Chapter 31. Unfortunately for many patients, they acquired hepatitis C years ago through blood transfusion or other intravenous injections in which blood exchange can occur, and liver damage progressed silently until symptoms appeared.

Liver disease may be caused by drugs or alcohol as well as by viral infection. Abuse of ethyl alcohol has long been known to cause **cirrhosis** of the liver (Laënnec's cirrhosis), a condition in which scar tissue replaces normal liver cells. More recently it has become clear that drugs are also significant causes of serious liver failure. The most common cause among OTC drugs is acetaminophen. This drug has a limited capacity for detoxification in the liver through sulfation and glucuronida-

tion. With excessive doses of the drug or with normal doses in patients whose metabolic capacity is damaged by preexisting liver disease, toxic metabolites may accumulate and cause centrilobular necrosis of the liver. Drugs and vitamins known to cause liver injury are listed in Table 51-1.

Advanced liver failure can lead to **hepatic encephalopathy,** a state of disordered CNS function, and ultimately to **hepatic coma,** in which the patient loses consciousness (Box 51-2). Hepatic encephalopathy or coma results from failure of the liver to detoxify nitrogen-containing substances of GI origin because of hepatocellular dysfunction or portal-systemic shunting. Ammonia is the most readily identified toxin but is not solely responsible for the patient's disturbed mental status.

Ammonia is formed in the body in several ways: by the liver during deamination of amino acids, by epithelial cells of the proximal and distal tubules and the collecting duct of the nephron as part of the regulation of hydrogen ions, and by bacteria of the GI tract acting on dietary protein. A normally functioning liver converts the absorbed ammonia to urea, a less toxic substance. Urea is then eliminated in urine.

Damage to the liver or shunting of blood flow around the liver inhibits conversion of ammonia to urea. The elevated serum ammonia level that results leads to hepatic encephalopathy with a decreasing level of consciousness, impaired neuromuscular functioning, and in some cases, death. Serious GI bleeding decreases perfusion to the liver, brain, and kidneys but also contributes 15 to

TABLE 51-1

Drugs and Vitamins Associated with Liver Failure*

Drug	Primary Use	Comments
acetaminophen	Analgesic (Chapter 14)	Dose-dependent toxicity
amiodarone	Antiarrhythmic (Chapter 40)	May cause fatty liver or cirrhosis
cyclophosphamide	Antineoplastic (Chapter 37)	Damages endothelial cells in liver
diclofenac	NSAID (Chapter 14)	Idiosyncratic reaction
isoniazid	Tuberculosis (Chapter 33)	Risk increases with age
valproic acid	Anticonvulsant (Chapter 22)	May cause fatty liver or cirrhosis
Vitamin A	Food supplement (Chapter 63)	Cirrhosis may be slow to develop

*This list is not exhaustive. Reference material should be consulted to ascertain specific risk for any other individual drug.

BOX 51-2   **Stages of Hepatic Encephalopathy**

Stage 1: Prodromal Period

- Changes in sleep patterns
- Slowed responses
- Shortened attention span
- Depressed or euphoric mood
- Irritability
- Tremors
- Incoordination
- Impaired ability to write

Step 2: Impending Encephalopathy

- Disorientation to time
- Lethargy
- Impaired calculation ability
- Decreased inhibition
- Anxiety or apathy
- Inappropriate behavior
- Slurred speech
- Decreased reflexes
- Ataxia and asterixis

Stage 3: Stupor

- Disorientation to place
- Confusion, somnolence
- Stupor but still with capacity to be aroused
- Anger, rage, paranoia
- Hyperreflexia
- Clonus
- Presence of Babinski's sign
- Asterixis

Stage 4: Coma

- No intellectual functioning
- Lack of consciousness
- Loss of deep tendon reflexes
- Responsiveness only to deep pain
- Hyperventilation
- Fetor hepaticus
- Increased body temperature
- Increased pulse rate

---

20 g of protein per 100 mL as ammonia substrate when absorbed from the bowel.

Acid-base balance and electrolyte shifts also contribute to ammonia toxicity. Alkalosis leads to diffusion of unionized ammonia across the blood-brain barrier. Hypokalemia may also contribute to this form of toxicity, because as serum levels decrease, potassium moves from intracellular compartments in exchange for sodium and hydrogen. The shift of hydrogen ions into the intracellular compartment increases the relative amount of base in the extracellular compartment. This extracellular alkalosis liberates hydrogen from ammonium (NH_4^+) ions, thus creating ammonia (NH_3). Ammonia readily crosses into cells, where it accumulates and exerts toxic effects.

Constipation also allows for increased production and absorption of ammonia because of the longer contact time for bacteria and substrates. Constipation may also provoke Valsalva's maneuver during bowel movements and thus precipitate bleeding from esophageal varices or hemorrhoids.

DRUG CLASS • **Ammonia-Detoxifying Drugs**

lactulose (Cephulac, Cholac, Chronulac,
  Constilac, Constulose, Enulose, Evalose,
  Generlac, Heptalac, Laxilose,✸ Ratio-
  Lactulose✸)
neomycin (Mycifradin)

MECHANISM OF ACTION

Lactulose is a semisynthetic disaccharide that decreases blood ammonia concentration. The mechanism of action is not completely known, but the decrease in ammonia level appears to be associated with metabolism of the sugar in the bowel. The breakdown of lactulose to organic acids causes a drop in the pH of colon contents from 7 to 5. It also inhibits the diffusion of ammonia from the colon into the blood. In addition, because the contents of the colon are more acidic than blood, ammonia is converted to ammonium ions, thereby preventing its absorption. The cathartic action of lactulose is probably caused by the osmotic effect of the drug's organic acid metabolites. The metabolites expel trapped ammonium ions and other nitrogenous substances from the colon. The osmotic effect of the metabolites causes an increase in the water content of the stool and subsequent softening.

Neomycin is an aminoglycoside antibiotic (see Chapter 29) that is unabsorbed when given orally. Because the drug is bactericidal, it eliminates many of the bacteria that produce nitrogenous wastes in the bowel and thus reduces the buildup of ammonia.

USES

Lactulose is used as an adjunct to protein restriction and supportive therapy for the prevention and treatment of hepatic encephalopathy. This drug has been useful in the management of hepatic encephalopathy resulting from surgical portacaval shunts or from chronic hepatic diseases such as cirrhosis. Lactulose reduces blood ammonia concentration, improving the mental state of the patient. This drug is not useful in the management of drug-induced encephalopathy or for encephalopathy caused by inborn errors of metabolism and electrolyte disturbances. It is not effective in the treatment of coma associated with hepatitis or with other acute liver disorders. Lactulose is also used as a laxative (see Chapter 49).

Neomycin is used like lactulose in the management of hepatic encephalopathy. It is also sometimes used in conjunction with erythromycin, a low-residue diet, and a laxative or enema for preoperative bowel preparation. Neomycin is also found in topical preparations as an antibiotic (see Chapter 67).

PHARMACODYNAMICS

Neither lactulose nor neomycin is absorbed in appreciable amounts from the bowel when given orally. When lactulose reaches the colon, it is transformed by bacteria to lactic acid and small amounts of acetic and formic acids, both of which contribute to the osmotic effect of the drug. The cathartic effect of lactulose may not be seen for 24 to 48 hours after administration. The reduction of ammonia production may take several days to fully develop with both drugs.

ADVERSE REACTIONS AND CONTRAINDICATIONS

The adverse reactions of lactulose primarily affect the GI tract. During the first few days of therapy, anorexia, nausea, vomiting, and abdominal cramping are common. These effects usually subside with continued therapy, although dosage reduction may be required in some cases. Diarrhea, flatulence, distension, and belching have been noted. Lactulose is contraindicated for patients on a low-galactose diet. It should be used with caution by patients with diabetes mellitus or by women who are pregnant.

The adverse effects of neomycin are ototoxicity and nephrotoxicity, but the risks are low unless the drug is used parenterally or absorption is abnormally high because of bowel disease. Neomycin is contraindicated for patients with preexisting ototoxicity, nephrotoxicity, or renal impairment.

INTERACTIONS

Theoretically, the effects of lactulose are decreased in the presence of neomycin and other oral antimicrobial drugs. The antibiotics may eliminate colonic bacteria necessary to transform lactulose and thereby prevent acidification of colon contents.

Neomycin, like other aminoglycosides, may interact with a number of drugs (see Chapter 29). Most of the potential interactions, such as the increased risk of ototoxicity with loop diuretics and nephrotoxicity with nephrotoxic drugs, are unlikely because most patients absorb so little neomycin from the bowel.

APPLICATION TO PRACTICE

ASSESSMENT
History of Present Illness

Ask the patient or family about the presence of anorexia, nausea, vomiting, indigestion, flatulence, constipation, fatigue, restlessness, irritability, or sleep pattern reversal (see Box 51-1). Reports of vague, dull, mild, or steady wavelike abdominal pain may be noted. The pain is usually in the right upper quadrant. As the disease progresses, family members may note diminished short-term memory, personality changes, and activity intolerance.

Health History

The patient usually has a past history of Laënnec's cirrhosis; therefore ask about the frequency and quantity of alcohol consumed. Cirrhosis can also result from viral hepatitis, biliary tract obstruction, right-sided heart failure, and metabolic derangement. Therefore a history of these disorders warrants attention because as much as 75% of the liver can be destroyed before physiologic function is altered. Ask about the use of high-protein diets or GI bleeding since these processes increase protein in the intestine, causing elevated blood ammonia levels and manifestations of encephalopathy.

A thorough drug history is important because diuretics and drugs containing aluminum or amino compounds can cause or precipitate an episode of hepatic encephalopathy. Ask too about the use of herbal remedies, since many of these can contribute to liver failure (Box 51-3).

Herbal Interactions
Contributing to Hepatotoxicity

Several herbal preparations are known to carry the risk of hepatotoxicity (Chapter 8). When these herbal preparations are taken with hepatotoxic drugs such as those mentioned in Table 51-1, the result can be additional hepatic damage or even liver failure and death. Patients who have preexisting liver damage or who are taking hepatotoxic drugs should not take the following herbal supplements:

- Comfrey
- Chaparral
- Germander
- Ma huang
- Mistletoe
- Pennyroyal
- Sassafras
- Senna
- Skullcap
- Valerian

Lifespan Considerations

Perinatal. A woman with a history of alcohol abuse has a reduced chance of conceiving. However, when pregnancy does occur, alcohol use places both the mother and the fetus at risk. Maternal complications of alcohol use during pregnancy include increased risk of spontaneous abortion, stillbirth, and abruptio placentae.

In the United States approximately 7% to 10% of childbearing women are heavy drinkers, consuming five to six drinks on occasion and at least 45 drinks per month, and 65% of fetuses are exposed to alcohol. Alcohol use during pregnancy interferes with the absorption of many nutrients as well as overall fetal cell growth and division, causes abnormal migration of neural and nonneural brain cells, inhibits DNA synthesis, interferes with amino acid availability to the fetus, and directly suppresses fetal breathing. The teratogenic manifestations of alcohol abuse can range from no effect to fetal alcohol syndrome, depending on factors such as genetic sensitivity, time of exposure, and dose size.

Pediatric. Common causes of cirrhosis and potential hepatic encephalopathy in infancy, childhood, and adolescence include hepatitis, cystic fibrosis, alpha$_1$ antitrypsin deficiency, and biliary atresia. The adolescent population is at particular risk for cirrhosis because hepatitis B is more widespread among teenagers who are parenteral drug abusers. The prognosis depends on the cause of the liver disease and the severity of the hepatic damage.

Older Adults. Cirrhosis or other liver disease superimposed on the physical changes of an aging hepatic system increases the risk of hepatic encephalopathy. Approximately 8% to 10% of Americans over 65 years old abuse alcohol. Although older adults consume less alcohol overall than their younger counterparts, the physical changes of aging cause it to be metabolized more slowly.

Also compounding cirrhosis is the potential for fluid and electrolyte imbalance resulting from comorbid diseases the patient may have. Additionally, only about 3% of older adults meet 100% of the recommended daily allowances for protein, vitamins A and C, thiamine, riboflavin, and iron. Differentiation between the mental status changes caused by fluid and electrolyte imbalances or nutritional deficiencies and the signs and symptoms of hepatic encephalopathy can be difficult to discern. Therefore a thorough patient history is vital.

Cultural/Social Considerations

The patient with hepatic encephalopathy resulting from cirrhosis or other liver diseases may experience changes in body appearance and in role relationships. Assessment of the patient's self-esteem, body image, and role relationships is important to successful treatment outcomes. If the patient is not helped to reestablish or maintain positive self-esteem, it can add to the problem of alcohol abuse and its complications (see the Case Study: Hepatic Encephalopathy).

Physical Examination

Manifestations of hepatic encephalopathy vary and may occur rapidly or gradually over the course of a few days. Assessment findings reflect alterations in the level of consciousness; intellectual function, behavior, and personality; and neuromuscular function (see Box 51-2). Asterixis may be present. Evaluate the patient's handwriting and speech patterns for significant changes. Weight loss masked by water retention can also be seen. The presence of methylmercaptan causes a characteristic odor on the breath called **fetor hepaticus**. Assess respiratory status, since some patients with hepatic encephalopathy develop hyperventilation and respiratory alkalosis because high ammonia levels stimulate the respiratory center.

Laboratory Testing

Patients with hepatic encephalopathy have a number of abnormal laboratory tests including increased levels of total, unconjugated, and conjugated bilirubin; urine bilirubin and urobilinogen; and ALT, AST, LDH, and alkaline phosphatase. Increased prothrombin time, decreased platelets, decreased leukocyte count, decreased red blood cell count, decreased serum albumin and serum glucose levels, and hypokalemia and hyponatremia may also be noted.

GOALS OF THERAPY

The treatment goals for hepatic encephalopathy are directed toward control or reduction of further degenerative processes, correction or prevention of factors that may precipitate or aggravate encephalopathy, and preservation of remaining physiologic functioning. In a practical sense, the goal is to increase the patient's overall cognitive ability from baseline status, and if the patient was comatose, a return to consciousness.

INTERVENTION

Several principles guide intervention in hepatic encephalopathy: (1) reducing protein in the diet to reduce protein in the intestine (if no other precipitating factors are present, this alone may eliminate manifestations of encephalopathy); (2) preventing GI bleed-

ing, or, if present, quickly removing the blood from the intestinal lumen with the use of lactulose enemas (GI bleeding transports a protein load through the GI tract); (3) reducing bacterial production of ammonia through the use of neomycin or lactulose; (4) maintaining safety and function in the unconscious patient who lacks reflexes and thus is vulnerable to the complications of immobility; (5) eliminating or correcting fluid and electrolyte imbalances, hypoxia, infection, and sedation; (6) preventing infections that lead to increased tissue catabolism and increased protein load; and (7) avoiding the use of drugs or herbal remedies that are hepatotoxic.

Administration

Lactulose should be administered with 8 ounces of fruit juice, water, or milk to increase its palatability. Rapid results are achieved when lactulose is given on an empty stomach. Fluid intake should be increased to 2 L daily. Dilute the lactulose in water, usually 60 to 120 mL, before administration through a gastric or feeding tube. When lactulose is administered as an enema, a rectal balloon catheter should be used and the drug retained for 30 to 60 minutes. If inadvertent evacuation occurs, the enema may be repeated.

Instruct the patient to take neomycin as directed for the full course of therapy. This drug can be taken without regard to meals, but caution the patient that neomycin can cause nausea, vomiting, or diarrhea. The patient should be well hydrated during therapy.

A good clinical response to lactulose is achieved in 75% to 85% of patients and is defined as two to three soft stools daily. Because lactulose is relatively nontoxic, it is a valuable alternative to neomycin, especially when prolonged therapy is required, or when neomycin is contraindicated. Patients who previously failed to respond to neomycin and dietary protein restriction may respond to lactulose, and vice versa. Some health care providers recommend neomycin for acute episodes of hepatic encephalopathy and lactulose for long-term management of chronic disease.

Education

Dietary protein may be reduced for the patient with hepatic encephalopathy. Teach the patient the common sources of protein and help them develop a low-protein dietary regimen. The usual protein restriction is 20 to 40 g daily. The patient with chronic hepatic encephalopathy may need to adjust to a long-term low-protein diet (50 to 60 g daily), which can be difficult. Inform patients that they may tolerate vegetable and dairy proteins better than meat protein. Vegetable and dairy proteins contain fewer amino acids that form ammonia than do meat protein. A diet high in vegetables and dairy products also helps prevent constipation, which further reduces ammonia production.

Teach the patient taking lactulose to dilute it to counteract the sweet taste and to take it on an empty stomach, thereby promoting drug action. It should be stored in a cool environment but not where the drug may freeze. The patient should report any change in bowel habits, particularly diarrhea, because diarrhea may indicate an overdose. The importance of consistent use and titration to the number of stools should be emphasized.

Instruct the patient taking neomycin to report any signs of hypersensitivity, tinnitus, vertigo, rash, dizziness, or difficulty urinating. Remind the patient of the importance of drinking plenty of fluids.

EVALUATION

A clearing of confusion, lethargy, restlessness, and irritability demonstrates effective treatment of hepatic encephalopathy with lactulose. Improvement may occur within 2 hours following rectal administration

---

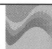

CASE STUDY   *Hepatic Encephalopathy*

ASSESSMENT

HISTORY OF PRESENT ILLNESS

MM, a 59-year-old man, comes to this appointment accompanied by his wife. He has a 3-day history of increasing confusion, lethargy, restlessness, and irritability. She also notes that his writing has been impaired; he has involuntary muscle tremors, especially in the hands; his speech is slurred; and he has "bad breath—like a diaper pail." She reports a consumption history of a pint of whiskey a day for 15 years. She reports he has not eaten much for the last 3 days but she generally sees that he follows a high-calorie, low-protein diet. His last drink was 3 days ago.

HEALTH HISTORY

MM has a history of Laënnec's cirrhosis with three previous hospitalizations for GI bleeding. His last episode of bleeding was 1 year ago. He is taking no other drugs at this time but has a history of noncompliance with treatment regimens.

LIFESPAN CONSIDERATIONS

No specific age-related changes; however, because of history of cirrhosis he has loss of liver function. His ability to progress through ages and stages of growth and development are impaired by his alcohol intake.

CULTURAL/SOCIAL CONSIDERATIONS

MM has been a confectionery worker at a national bakery for 24 years. He was recently relieved of his duties. He has been married 37 years to the same woman, who oversees his health care needs and drug regimens. MM's wife reports he has consistently lost time from work because of his alcohol consumption and hospitalizations. He has attempted several times to participate in the corporation-sponsored rehabilitation program but with little success. He acknowledges that the alcohol abuse started when he began accompanying fellow employees to the local saloon after work.

PHYSICAL EXAMINATION

MM is 5'9" tall and weighs 167 pounds (up 9 pounds from previous visit); BP 139/88 mm Hg, and his vital signs are stable. Spider angiomas are noted over MM's nose and cheeks, and dilated vessels are seen over upper body and lower extremities. Multiple ecchymotic areas are noted over his extremities with 2+ edema of lower extremities. Bowel sounds are diminished in all four quadrants; liver is not palpable. General body odor of urine.

LABORATORY TESTING

Electrolyte level is low normal. Urine bilirubin and urobilinogen, total and conjugated bilirubin, ALT, AST, LDH, and alkaline phosphatase levels are elevated. Serum ammonia level is elevated.

PATIENT PROBLEM(S)

Hepatic encephalopathy.

GOALS OF THERAPY

Decrease blood ammonia levels by 25% to 50%; facilitate overall increase in cognitive ability from baseline status.

CRITICAL THINKING QUESTIONS

1. The health care provider orders neomycin 500 mg po qid until symptoms improve and then to discontinue and start lactulose 30 to 45 mL po tid–qid titrated to two to three stools daily. What are the mechanisms of action of these two drugs?
2. Of what adverse effects should MM and his family be made aware?
3. What laboratory testing is required for MM during drug treatment?
4. How is the dosage of lactulose determined?
5. What is the usual protein restriction for the patient with pancreatitis?

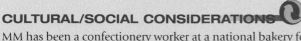

and 24 to 48 hours following oral administration of lactulose. Passage of soft, formed stool usually occurs within 24 to 48 hours. Improved neurologic status should be noted with effective neomycin therapy.

Bibliography

Aithal PG, Day CP: The natural history of histologically proved drug-induced liver disease, *Gut* 44:731-735, 1999.

Beckingham IJ: ABC of diseases of liver, pancreas, and biliary system: gallstone disease, *BMJ* 322(7278):91-94, 2001.

Field AE, Coakley EH, Must A, et al: Impact of overweight on the risk of developing common chronic diseases during a 10-year period, *Arch Intern Med* 161(13):1581-1586, 1683-1684, 2001.

Schuppan D, Jia JD, Brinkhaus B, et al: Herbal products for liver diseases: a therapeutic challenge for the new millennium, *Hepatology* 30:1099-1104, 1999.

Simon JA, Hunninghake DB, Agarwal SK, et al: Effect of estrogen plus progestin on risk for biliary tract surgery in postmenopausal women with coronary artery disease: The Heart and Estrogen/progestin Replacement Study, *Ann Intern Med* 135(7):493-501, I24, 2001.

Internet Resources

The National Institute of Diabetes and Digestive and Kidney Diseases website's information about gallstones. Available at www.niddk.nih.gov/health/digest/pubs/gallstns/gallstns.htm and www.niddk.nih.gov/health/nutrit/pubs/dietgall.htm.

CHAPTER

52

Drugs to Treat Asthma and Other Pulmonary Diseases

ALAN P. AGINS • LYNN ROGER WILLIS • KATHLEEN GUTIERREZ

 Visit http://evolve.elsevier.com/Gutierrez/ for additional information.

KEY TERMS

OBJECTIVES

- Discuss the role of inhaled corticosteroids, nonselective and selective beta agonist bronchodilators, xanthines, cromolyn, and ipratropium in treating asthma.

- Describe the action and the resulting central nervous system effects of sympathomimetic bronchodilators on the alpha, $beta_1$, and $beta_2$ adrenergic receptors.

- Discuss the role of $alpha_1$-proteinase inhibitor in the treatment of chronic obstructive pulmonary disease.

- Explain the role of surfactant in infants with respiratory distress syndrome.

- Develop a nursing care plan for patients receiving one or more of the groups of drugs discussed in this chapter.

PATHOPHYSIOLOGY • Asthma

Asthma was once regarded as a disease of airway smooth muscle but is now known to be a chronic inflammatory disease characterized by an increased reactivity of the trachea and bronchi to various stimuli and by narrowing of the airways. An asthma attack typically includes the following three processes: (1) constriction of the bronchioles, (2) edema or swelling of the bronchial mucosa, and (3) excessive secretion and accumulation of mucus. These three early-phase actions combine to restrict the caliber of the airway (Figure 52-1). Thus symptoms

of asthma include shortness of breath, coughing, and wheezing.

Late-phase responses clearly demonstrate the inflammatory nature of asthma. Even patients with mild asymptomatic asthma have obvious, though microscopic, inflammatory changes in their airways. These changes are distinguished by infiltration of the mucosa and epithelium by activated T cells, mast cells, and eosinophils. T cells and mast cells secrete an array of chemicals in asthmatic individuals, some of which direct eosinophil

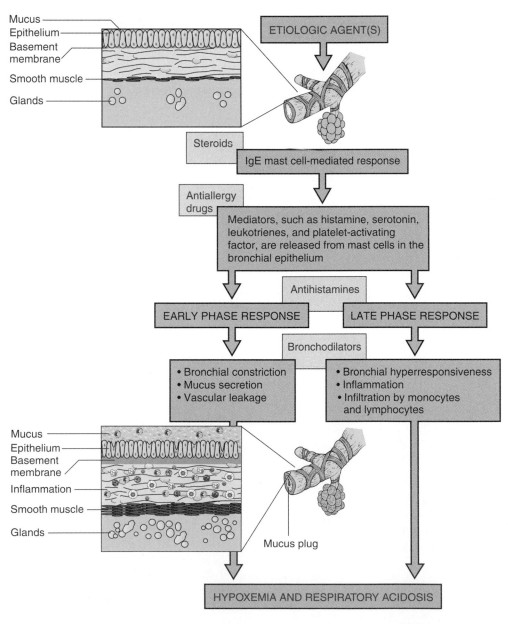

FIGURE 52-1 Pathophysiology of bronchial inflammation and airway hyperresponsiveness.

growth and maturation, providing an explanation for the inflammatory response of asthma. The aftermath of this response is increased capillary permeability, stimulation of local and central neural reflexes, epithelial disruption and stimulation of mucus-secreting glands, smooth muscle hypertrophy, and airway wall remodeling.

Extrinsic asthma results if an allergic response is the primary stimulus for bronchial constriction (Box 52-1). When no such trigger or stimulus can be identified, the condition is classified as **intrinsic asthma.** Bronchial constriction induced by allergens or antiimmunoglobulin E (IgE) is entirely mediated by a specific group of leukotrienes (LTs) together with a minor histamine-dependent component. In the lung, mast cells are primarily located in the epithelial layer and exposed to the surface. Immunoglobulin E antibodies bind to mast cells; when an antigen appears, it binds to IgE. The formation of the antigen-antibody complex causes mast cells to degranulate, releasing several substances, including histamine and leukotrienes C and D. The LTs are more potent mediators that cause long-term contraction of bronchial smooth muscle (Figure 52-2).

The LT family includes metabolites of arachidonic acid, an essential fatty acid that cannot be synthesized by animal tissues. Arachidonic acid is also the precursor of prostaglandins (see Chapter 14). Specific LTs are produced by the activity of 5-lipoxygenase. Arachidonic acid is presented to the 5-lipoxygenase enzyme by 5-lipoxygenase–activating protein, a cofactor present in the nuclear membrane. The interaction leads to the formation of LTA_4, an unstable intermediate LT (Figure 52-3). Depending on the cell type, further conversion of LTA_4 may occur by the actions of enzymes that are widespread in the tissues and circulation. Leukotrienes induce numerous biologic effects, including augmentation of neutrophil and eosinophil migration, monocyte aggregation, leukocyte adhesion, increased capillary permeability, and smooth muscle contraction. These effects contribute to inflammation, edema, mucus secretion, and bronchoconstriction of the airways.

Recently, drugs that block the actions of LTs have been approved for the treatment of asthma. Although histamine induces both bronchoconstriction and vasodilation, which can lead to the mucosal edema characteristic of asthma, antihistamines have not been widely used for the treatment of asthma. This restriction has been in place because the anticholinergic adverse effects of many antihistamines cause drying or thickening of mucus in the lungs, which can be harmful to a patient with asthma. In recent years, however, some of the newer, second-generation antihistamines have been shown to have less drying effects and may be useful in treating mild cases specifically caused by seasonal allergic triggers (see Chapter 53).

BOX 52-1 **Conditions that Commonly Trigger Asthma Attacks**

Environmental Factors
- Allergens such as pollens, spores, mold, dust, feathers, animal dander, dust mites, and cockroaches
- Air pollutants such as aerosol sprays, cigarette smoke, exhaust fumes, oxidants, perfumes, and sulfur dioxide

Occupational Exposure
- Industrial chemicals, plastics, and metal salts
- Pharmaceuticals
- Airborne particulates

Foods and Food Additives
- Sulfites, bisulfites, and metasulfites
- Monosodium glutamate (MSG)
- Nuts
- Milk or other dairy products

Drugs
- Antibiotics
- Nonsteroidal antiinflammatory drugs (e.g., aspirin, indomethacin)

- Beta blockers (e.g., propranolol)
- Drugs containing tartrazine
- Angiotensin-converting enzyme (ACE) inhibitors

Diseases/Conditions
- Respiratory conditions such as colds, flu, sore throats, bronchitis, sinusitis, and nasal polyps
- Gastroesophageal reflux or tracheoesophageal fistula
- Hormone shifts in women (resulting from menses or pregnancy)
- Thyroid disease

Other Triggers
- Very cold or windy weather or sudden changes in weather
- Sudden excessive exertion
- Emotional stress such as excessive fear or excitement, anger
- Environmental change (e.g., moving to new house, starting a new school)

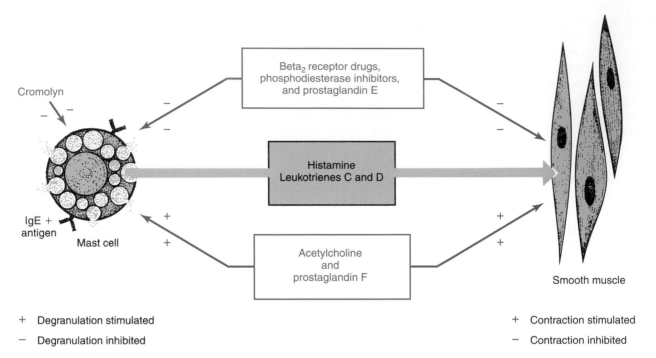

FIGURE 52-2 Histamine and leukotrienes C and D released from mast cells stimulate smooth muscle contraction to produce bronchoconstriction. Mast cell degranulation and smooth muscle contraction are stimulated by acetylcholine and prostaglandin F. Smooth muscle relaxation and inhibition of mast cell degranulation are promoted by beta$_2$ receptor agonists, phosphodiesterase inhibitors, and prostaglandin E.

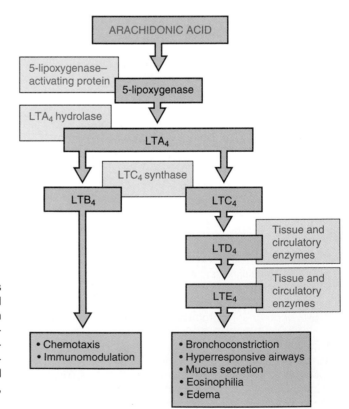

FIGURE 52-3 Leukotriene synthesis and activity. Five types of leukotrienes (LTA$_4$, LTB$_4$, LTC$_4$, LTD$_4$, and LTE$_4$) are generated from arachidonic acid released from mast cell membranes by an intracellular phospholipase that acts on membrane phospholipids. Leukotrienes are acidic, sulfur-containing lipids that produce effects similar to those of histamine. LTB$_4$ is a chemotactic agent that causes aggregation of leukocytes. LTC$_4$, LTD$_4$, and LTE$_4$ all cause contraction of smooth muscle, bronchospasm, and increased vascular permeability.

Acetylcholine, the neurotransmitter of the parasympathetic nervous system, stimulates muscarinic receptors to cause bronchoconstriction through the second intracellular messenger, cyclic guanosine monophosphate (cGMP). Mast cell degranulation is also promoted by drugs that stimulate the formation of cGMP. Intrinsic asthma may arise from direct stimulation of the enzyme guanylate cyclase, which synthesizes cGMP. Irritants such as noxious gases can also stimulate guanylate cyclase. Asthmatic individuals develop bronchospasm with low inhaled dosages of a cholinergic agonist such as methacholine, but high dosages are required to induce bronchospasm in nonasthmatic individuals. Intrinsic asthma may therefore involve a parasympathetic response, mediated by cGMP, to inhaled bronchial irritants. Blocking the muscarinic receptor with atropine or scopolamine causes bronchodilation. However, since atropine also causes mucus to dry out and inhibits the sweeping motion of bronchial tract cilia, it is not given to patients with asthma. Instead, the atropine-like drug ipratropium, which has less drying action than atropine, is used for bronchodilation.

Asthma is a common disease, affecting upwards of 12 million people in the United States. Morbidity associated with asthma is dramatic, affecting physical activity, school or work attendance, occupational choices, and many other aspects of daily living. The prevalence of asthma has increased more than 60% in the last 10 to 12 years, and the mortality rate from asthma has doubled since the late 1970s. These disturbing trends have led to a renewed focus of research on the disease, resulting in a better understanding of the disease process as well as the development and marketing of new drug therapies. Antiasthmatic drugs covered in this chapter include drugs to control bronchospasm as well as drugs to control the release or action of the various inflammatory mediators that have been discovered to contribute to the disease process in asthma (Table 52-1).

TABLE 52-1

Drugs for Asthma Maintenance

Generic Name	Brand Name	Comments
Corticosteroids		
beclomethasone dipropionate	Beclovent, Vanceril	Corticosteroid used by metered inhaler. Patients changing from oral corticosteroids to beclomethasone must be carefully monitored because adrenal function is impaired and may require months to begin functioning adequately.
budesonide	Pulmicort, ✸ Nebuamp ✸	Inhalation suspension not available in the United States.
flunisolide	AeroBid, Bronalide ✸	Inhaled corticosteroid. See comments for beclomethasone.
fluticasone propionate	Flovent	Inhaled corticosteroid. See comments for beclomethasone.
flucatisone + salmeterol	Advair	Inhaled corticosteroid combined with bronchodilator (see Table 52-3).
triamcinolone	Azmacort	Inhaled corticosteroid. See comments for beclomethasone.
Inhaled Nonsteroidal Antiallergy Drugs		
cromolyn sodium	Intal	Prophylactic drug used to inhibit mast cell degranulation. Cough or bronchospasm is occasionally experienced after dosing.
nedocromil	Tilade	Inhaled prophylactic drug used to inhibit mast cell degranulation.
Leukotriene Modifiers		
montelukast	Singulair	Blocks receptor for LTs. Prophylaxis for asthma.
zafirlukast	Accolate	Blocks receptor for LTs.
zileuton	Zyflo	Selective inhibitor of enzyme-synthesizing LTs. Prophylaxis for asthma.
Other Drugs		
ipratropium	Atrovent	Anticholinergic bronchodilator.
ketotifen	Zaditor	Prophylaxis for asthma in children.

✸ Available only in Canada.

DRUG CLASS • Beta Agonist Bronchodilators

Selective Beta₂ Agonists

⚠ albuterol (Ventolin, Proventil, Gen-Salbutamol, ✱ Novo-Salmol✱)

bitolterol (Tornalate)

formoterol (Foradil)

isoetharine (Bronkometer)

levalbuterol (Xopenex)

metaproterenol (Alupent, Metaprel)

pirbuterol (Maxair, Maxair Autohaler)

salmeterol (Serevent)

salmeterol + fluticasone (Advair Diskus)*

terbutaline (Brethine, Bricanyl)

Nonselective Beta Agonists

epinephrine inhalation (OTC, generic)

epinephrine systemic (Adrenalin)

isoproterenol (Medihaler-Iso)

ephedrine (generic✱)

MECHANISM OF ACTION

Beta agonists (see Chapter 12) relax smooth muscle in the bronchioles by activating adenylate cyclase and increasing intracellular concentrations of cyclic adenosine monophosphate (cAMP). This action produces a functional antagonism of bronchoconstriction. In addition to increasing cAMP, beta agonists inhibit release of mast cell mediators, decrease vascular permeability, and increase mucociliary clearance. They inhibit neither the late-phase inflammatory response nor the bronchial hyperresponsiveness that subsequently develop.

The beta₂ receptor mediates the bronchodilating action of the beta agonists. The first drugs to be used as beta agonists for the treatment of asthma were ephedrine and epinephrine, which stimulated beta₂ receptors well enough but also stimulated beta₁ and alpha₁ receptors. As a result, unwanted and potentially unsafe elevations of heart rate (from beta₁ stimulation) and arterial blood pressure (from alpha₁ stimulation) occurred. The so-called pure beta agonist, isoproterenol—which was introduced some years later—eliminated the risk of alpha₁-mediated increases in arterial blood pressure but not the risk of cardioacceleration, since the drug stimulated both beta₁ and beta₂ receptors.

The subsequent introduction of the selective beta₂ agonists brought several improvements to the treatment

---

*A combination of corticosteroid and bronchodilator.

of sudden attacks of asthma. The marked selectivity of these drugs for beta₂ receptors minimizes for most patients the hazards associated with stimulation of cardiac beta₁ receptors. Moreover, the drugs are effective both by inhalation and by oral administration, and they have long durations of action.

Another strategy is the use of purified isomers of active drugs. For example, albuterol is a racemic drug, which means it contains two isomers that are exact chemical twins but mirror images of one another. Only one isomer (the R isomer) is effective in stimulating beta₂ receptors. The inactive isomer (the S isomer) may actually compete with and decrease the effectiveness of the active form of albuterol. Levalbuterol is, in fact, the R-isomer of albuterol. Since it is a more purified form of active drug, reduced doses can be used, which in turn reduces the potential for adverse effects.

USES

Beta agonists are categorized as both quick-relief drugs and long-term controllers. A number of beta agonists have been developed to treat asthma. Most are available in metered-dose inhalers (aerosol canisters) that deliver the drug in a spray taken by inhalation. They are also available in nebulizer solutions. With the exception of salmeterol and formoterol, these drugs are used to relieve acute episodes of asthma. Oral and parenteral forms are available for some beta agonists when the inhalation route is not possible. Salmeterol and the newer formoterol are long-acting beta agonists used only prophylactically and considered long-term controllers.

Beta agonists may also be used prophylactically for exercise-induced asthma or when exposure to antigens is anticipated, for instance, during contact with animals or periods when pollen counts are high.

PHARMACOKINETICS

The onset of action for short-acting beta agonists occurs in 5 to 30 minutes, depending on the drug and the route of administration (Table 52-2). Peak effects are reached in 30 minutes to 2 hours; the duration of action is 3 to 8 hours for most drugs. Compared with short-acting beta agonists, salmeterol has a slower onset of action (15 to 30 minutes) but a longer duration of action (8 to 12 hours). Terbutaline rapidly undergoes first-pass biotransformation when taken by mouth but has minimal absorption following inhalation. Distribution of inhaled drugs is essentially limited to the respiratory tract, although most drugs have a minimal systemic uptake and may appear in breast milk in small amounts.

TABLE 52-2

Pharmacokinetics of Selected Antiasthmatic and Bronchodilator Drugs

Drugs	Route	Onset	Peak	Duration	PB (%)	$t_{1/2}$	BioA (%)
Inhaled Corticosteroids							
beclomethasone	INH/po	Rapid	Up to 4 wk	3.25 days	91	3-15 hr	20
budesonide	INH	24 hr	3-7 days	UK	91	2 hr	11
flunisolide	INH	Rapid	UA	UA	91	1-2 hr	20
fluticasone	INH	Few days	1-2 weeks	UK	91	UA	1
triamcinolone	INH	Few days	3-4 days	UK	91	4 hr	10.6
Antiallergy Drugs (Mast Cell Stabilizers)							
cromolyn	INH	15 min	2-4 weeks	4-6 hr	UA	80 min	2½-3
nedocromil	INH	2 weeks	20-40 min	4-6 hr	89	1.5-2.3 hr	2½-3
Beta Agonists							
albuterol	po	30 min	2-2½ hr	4-8 hr	UK	2-4 hr	UA
	INH	5 min	1½-2 hr	3-8 hr			
bitolterol	INH	3-4 min	½-2 hr	5-8 hr	UK	3 hr	UA
metaproterenol	po	15-30 min	1 hr	4 hr	UK	UK	UA
	INH	1-4 min	1 hr	3-4 hr			
pirbuterol	INH	5 min	1-5 hr	6-8 hr	UK	2 hr	UA
salmeterol	INH	10-25 min	3-4 hr	8-12 hr	UK	UK	UA
terbutaline	po	1-2 hr	2-3 hr	4-8 hr	UK	UK	30-50
	INH	5-30 min	1-2 hr	3-6 hr			
Leukotriene Antagonists							
montelukast	po	UA	3-4 hr	UA	99	2.7-5.5 hr	63-73
zafirlukast	po	UA	3 hr	UA	UA	10 hr	40
zileuton	po	1.7 hr	2 hr	UA	93	1.5 hr	UA
Xanthine Derivatives							
aminophylline	po	1-6 hr*	4-6 hr	6-8 hr	UA	3-15 hr	UA
	IV	Immediate	30 min	4-8 hr			100
dyphylline	po	1 hr*	1 hr	6 hr	UA	1.8-2.1 hr	75
	IM	30-45 min	UK				
oxtriphylline	po	15 min-1 hr*	5 hr	6-8 hr	UA	3-15 hr	UA
	po/ER	UK	4-7 hr	12 hr			
theophylline	po	Varies	1-2 hr	6 hr	60; 36; 35†	4-5 hr; 3-15 hr‡	UA
	po/ER	Delayed	4-8 hr	8-24 hr		3-13 hr	UA
	IV	Rapid	End of inf	6-8 hr			100
Anticholinergic							
ipratropium	INH	5-15 min	1-2 hr	3-6 hr	UA	2 hr	

*Provided a loading dose of methylxanthine drug has been given and steady/state serum levels exist.
†Protein binding of theophylline in healthy adults, neonates, and patients with cirrhosis, respectively.
‡Half-life of theophylline in smokers and nonsmokers, respectively.
BioA, Bioavailability; *ER*, extended-release formulation; *INH*, inhalation; *IV*, intravenous; *PB*, protein binding; $t_{1/2}$, serum half-life; *UA*, unavailable; *UK*, unknown.

Biotransformation and elimination of beta agonists vary with the drug. Albuterol and metaproterenol are extensively biotransformed by the liver and other tissues. Bitolterol is converted in the lungs to colterol, the active compound. Pirbuterol and terbutaline are biotransformed by the liver and eliminated through the kidneys. The half-life of the drugs generally varies from 2 to 4 hours.

The inhalation route of **bronchodilators** is particularly advantageous, since it delivers the drug rapidly and in its highest concentration directly to the site of action, the bronchioles. The inhalation route also helps to limit the potential for rapid degradation by systemic biotransforming enzymes. Bronchodilators available for inhalation include albuterol, bitolterol, epinephrine, fenoterol, isoetharine, isoproterenol, and metaproterenol.

Albuterol, ephedrine, fenoterol, isoproterenol, metaproterenol, and terbutaline are available in oral forms. Although oral administration is convenient, especially for children, the patient is exposed to more adverse effects than with aerosol administration. Albuterol, ephedrine, epinephrine, ethylnorepinephrine, isoproterenol, and terbutaline are available in parenteral formulations. These are generally reserved for relieving severe bronchospasm or conditions in which inhalation or oral administration is not possible.

ADVERSE REACTIONS AND CONTRAINDICATIONS

The older beta-adrenergic bronchodilators—ephedrine, epinephrine, and isoproterenol—are not selective for the beta$_2$-adrenergic receptor and thus have a range of adverse effects resulting from their nonselective action. These effects are generally related to stimulation of the heart and include palpitations, tachycardia, and arrhythmia. Stimulation of the CNS can cause tremors, headache, nervousness, and hypotension. Beta$_1$-adrenergic activity promotes the breakdown of glycogen to glucose, which impairs glucose control in patients with diabetes mellitus. Isoproterenol may cause saliva to turn pinkish to red; this effect is harmless.

The newer beta-adrenergic bronchodilators are relatively selective for the beta$_2$ receptor. In most patients using low to moderate doses, the drug is more likely to bind to and stimulate beta$_2$ receptors while having a minimal effect on beta$_1$ receptors. However, in those patients who require higher doses or greater frequency of the beta$_2$-selective agonists to control their asthma, there can be significant crossover stimulatory effects at beta$_1$ receptors, increasing the risk of tachycardia and irregular cardiac rhythm. Patients with preexisting cardiovascular disease, especially older adults, are more likely to experience adverse cardiovascular effects with inhaled adrenergic drugs.

Other adverse effects of the beta agonists include headache, tachycardia, hypokalemia, hyperglycemia, skeletal muscle tremors, and increased lactic acid. In general, the inhaled route causes few systemic adverse effects except when high doses are administered.

TOXICITY

Overdose with beta agonists can cause chest discomfort and pain with an irregular heartbeat and irregular blood pressure. Chills, fever, light-headedness, and dizziness may be experienced. Other symptoms of overdose include nervousness, restlessness, unusual anxiety, and trembling.

INTERACTIONS

The additive effects of beta agonists when used concurrently with other adrenergic drugs or monoamine oxidase inhibitors may lead to hypertensive crisis. When they are used with beta-blocking drugs, the therapeutic effects of the beta agonist may be lost.

 DRUG CLASS • Leukotriene Modifiers

montelukast (Singulair)

zafirlukast (Accolate)

zileuton (Zyflo)

MECHANISM OF ACTION

The newest class of drugs for control of persistent asthma are the leukotriene (LT) modifiers. Arachidonic acid is converted to inflammatory mediators that include prostaglandins, thromboxanes, and LTs. Zileuton selectively inhibits the path to LTs by blocking the enzyme 5-lipoxygenase (Figure 52-3). Montelukast and zafirlukast block cysteinyl LT$_1$ receptors for LTs. The result is that the bronchoconstrictive and inflammatory action of LTs are prevented; thus these drugs are not direct-acting bronchodilators.

USES

Zafirlukast and zileuton are indicated for the prophylaxis and chronic treatment of asthma in adults and as alternatives to low doses of inhaled corticosteroids or antiallergy drugs in mild, persistent asthma in patients more than 12 years old. Zafirlukast and zileuton therapy can be continued during acute exacerbations of asthma but are not indicated for acute episodes. Montelukast is indicated for the prophylaxis and chronic treatment of asthma in adults and pediatric patients 6 years of age and older. These drugs are not appropriate for acute asthma attacks, including status asthmaticus, because they are not bronchodilators.

PHARMACOKINETICS

Zileuton is well absorbed following oral administration; it has a mean peak plasma level of 1.7 hours (see Table 52-2). The absolute bioavailability of zileuton is unknown. Plasma concentrations are proportional to dose, and steady-state levels are predictable from single-dose pharmacokinetics. Zileuton is highly bound to plasma albumin and has minor binding to alpha$_1$ glycoprotein. Elimination of zileuton is predominantly via the liver; the drug has a half-life of 2.5 hours. It is eliminated through the urine and feces.

Zafirlukast is rapidly absorbed from the GI tract, reaching its peak serum concentration in about 3 hours. Taking the drug with food reduces its bioavailability by 40%. Zafirlukast is biotransformed in the liver and eliminated primarily in the feces; it has a half-life of about 10 hours. However, the half-life may be twice as long in older adults.

Montelukast is rapidly absorbed following oral administration; peak activity is noted in 3 to 4 hours. The mean oral bioavailability is 64% to 73%. It is highly bound (99%) to plasma proteins and extensively biotransformed in the liver. Elimination takes place exclusively through the bile. The mean plasma half-life of montelukast is 2.7 to 5.5 hours in healthy young adults. With once-daily dosing, there is little accumulation of the parent drug.

ADVERSE REACTIONS AND CONTRAINDICATIONS

The main adverse reactions to LT antagonists to date include headache, dry mouth, and somnolence. Unspecified pain, abdominal pain, dyspepsia, nausea, asthenia, and myalgias have also occurred. Less common adverse effects include arthralgia, chest pain, conjunctivitis, constipation, dizziness, fever, flatulence, hypertonia, insomnia, lymphadenopathy, malaise, neck pain and rigidity, nervousness, pruritus, urinary tract infection, vaginitis, and vomiting.

Leukotriene antagonists are contraindicated for patients with hypersensitivity to these drugs. Additionally, zileuton is contraindicated for patients with active liver disease and should be given with caution to patients who consume substantial quantities of alcohol or who have a past history of liver disease.

INTERACTIONS

Zafirlukast and zileuton inhibit the activity of common drug-biotransforming enzymes such as CYP2C9 or CYP3A4 in vitro, but clinical data regarding interactions with these drugs are limited. Therefore zafirlukast and zileuton should be given very cautiously to patients taking drugs biotransformed by either the CYP2C9 or CYP3A4 isoforms. Examples of interacting drugs include celecoxib, diclofenac, ibuprofen, imipramine, phenytoin, alprazolam, carbamazepine, citalopram, some corticosteroids, cyclosporine, diazepam, calcium channel blockers, lovastatin, midazolam, quinidine, simvastatin, tolterodine, triazolam, and zonisamide.

Erythromycin (and perhaps clarithromycin) can decrease the bioavailability of zafirlukast by roughly 40% and hence reduce the effectiveness of the LT antagonist.

Montelukast is relatively free from drug interactions. Drugs such as carbamazepine, phenytoin, and rifampin, which induce cytochrome P-450, may decrease the effectiveness of this drug.

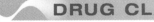 **DRUG CLASS** • **Inhaled Corticosteroids**

beclomethasone (Beclovent, Beconase, QVAR, Vancenase, Vanceril)

budesonide (Pulmicort, Rhinocort)

flunisolide (AeroBid, Bronalide, ✱ Nasalide, Nasarel)

fluticasone (Flonase, Flovent)

fluticasone + salmeterol (Advair)*

triamcinolone (Azmacort, Nasacort)

MECHANISM OF ACTION

Corticosteroids are potent antiinflammatory drugs that, among other actions, inhibit the production or release of inflammatory mediators including leukotrienes, prostaglandins, cytokines, histamine, and others from lymphocytes, macrophages, mast cells, fibroblasts, and eosinophils (see Chapter 57). Because they affect multiple mediators of inflammation, these drugs are highly effective antiasthmatic drugs.

USES

Aerosolized corticosteroids are the mainstay of therapy to prevent asthma attacks in patients with persistent asthma,

---

*A combination of corticosteroid and bronchodilator.

especially in adults. Corticosteroids do not relieve acute bronchospasm or bronchitis not caused by asthma. Asthma specialists now advocate the use of aerosol glucocorticoids over theophylline or beta-adrenergic agonists in the daily management of persistent asthma. Aerosolized, oral, or intravenous corticosteroids may also be used to treat patients with chronic obstructive pulmonary disease (COPD) who have some reversibility to their symptoms (see later sections in this chapter).

PHARMACOKINETICS

Aerosol corticosteroids have been developed that can be used daily with reduced risk for producing adrenal suppression or Cushing's syndrome. The aerosol cannot be used during an episode of acute bronchospasm because the powder causes further irritation and the bronchospasm prevents adequate inhalation. An oral glucocorticoid is indicated instead.

Beclomethasone is biotransformed in the lungs to an active metabolite. The other corticosteroids are unchanged. The portion of the drug that reaches the plasma is rapidly degraded in the liver to inactive metabolites. Maximum improvement in pulmonary function may take up to 4 weeks. Reduction in airway responsiveness occurs over weeks to months. If patients discontinue these drugs when they begin to feel better, the benefits may be lost.

ADVERSE REACTIONS AND CONTRAINDICATIONS

Some individuals may experience bronchospasm or cough following use of an inhaled corticosteroid. Systemic adverse effects are uncommon with inhaled corticosteroids. However, children may be at risk for retarded growth and depressed adrenal function when high dosages are used. It is recommended that growth rates be monitored in children receiving inhaled corticosteroid therapy.

Patients using corticosteroid inhalers over long periods of time may develop a *Candida* infection in the mouth or throat.

INTERACTIONS

There is little risk for significant drug interactions when using normal doses of inhaled corticosteroids.

 DRUG CLASS • **Inhaled Nonsteroidal Antiallergy Drugs**

cromolyn (Intal, Nalcrom,* Rynacrom,* Vistacrom*)
nedocromil (Tilade)

MECHANISM OF ACTION

Cromolyn and nedocromil work at the surface of the mast cell to inhibit its degranulation, which in turn prevents the release of histamine and other inflammatory mediators. Cromolyn may also reduce the release of LTs and other factors that recruit inflammatory cells into the airways (chemotaxis). It has been proposed that cromolyn produces these effects by inhibiting calcium influx, but its exact mechanism of action is still unclear. These drugs do not treat an ongoing asthma attack or prevent asthma attacks brought on by vagal reflexes rather than by mast cell degranulation. Cromolyn and nedocromil do not have bronchodilator or antiinflammatory activity.

USES

These drugs, sometimes referred to as mast cell stabilizers, are controller drugs for persistent asthma. Cromolyn and nedocromil are used prophylactically, especially in children, to treat asthma. No tolerance develops to these drugs. They are used in place of glucocorticoids or to allow the gradual reduction in the dose of glucocorticoids. These drugs are more effective in treating children than adults for asthma. They may be effective for adults as well when taken before exercise or exposure to allergens.

PHARMACOKINETICS

Cromolyn is available as a metered-dose inhalation (MDI) aerosol. In addition, this drug is formulated for nasal administration (Nasalcrom and Rynacrom) as prophylaxis for allergic rhinitis, for ophthalmic administration (Opticrom and Vistacrom) in cases of allergic conjunctivitis, and for oral administration in cases of food allergies. Cromolyn is rapidly excreted unchanged in the urine such that the blood level is negligible.

Nedocromil is available as a MDI aerosol. It is effective when administered 30 minutes before exposure to an allergen or chemical or before exercise. The drug is rapidly excreted unchanged in bile and the urine.

ADVERSE REACTIONS AND CONTRAINDICATIONS

Because cromolyn and nedocromil are rapidly excreted unchanged, they are practically nontoxic. The major adverse effect that limits their use is bronchospasm caused by the dry powder form of the drug in sensitive individuals. Some individuals become allergic to cromolyn or nedocromil.

INTERACTIONS

Few interactions occur with these drugs.

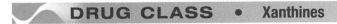

DRUG CLASS • Xanthines

aminophylline (Amoline, others)

♠ theophylline (Slo-Bid, Slo-Phyllin, Theobid, Theo-Dur, others)

MECHANISM OF ACTION

Similar to beta agonists, theophylline probably increases cellular concentrations of cAMP, which relaxes bronchial smooth muscle and inhibits mast cell degranulation. Theophylline and the other xanthines are believed to accomplish this, in part, by inhibiting the degradation of cAMP by the enzyme phosphodiesterase. In addition to inhibiting cAMP-phosphodiesterase it is believed that theophylline also blocks adenosine receptors in bronchial smooth muscle, thereby preventing the bronchoconstriction caused by adenosine. The action of theophylline complements that of the beta agonists; the drugs may be combined in therapy when the effect of either drug alone is insufficient to control bronchospasm.

USES

Theophylline and related drugs are used for the prophylaxis and treatment of asthma, bronchospasm, maintenance therapy in COPD, and the apnea of premature neonates. Short-acting forms are used to treat acute asthma. Although theophylline may be used as a prophylactic drug for asthma, inhaled steroids are now preferred as prophylaxis for persistent asthma because of the adverse effects associated with theophylline. However, long-acting formulations of the drug are effective and are considerably less expensive than other drugs. Theophylline is also used to treat Cheyne-Stokes respiration, in which the medullary sensitivity to hypoxia is decreased. Theophylline stimulates respiration in newborns who do not breathe well.

PHARMACOKINETICS

Theophylline can be used intravenously (as aminophylline) to control acute bronchospasm in status asthmaticus or orally to control the bronchospasm of mild, moderate, or severe asthma. Aminophylline, the most common soluble form of theophylline, is the only form that can be administered intravenously.

Theophylline is not highly water soluble, and there are many formulations to improve the solubility; dosage is determined by the theophylline content. The drug is also available in slow- and fast-release preparations, alcoholic or aqueous solutions, and suppositories. Only the suppository is erratically absorbed and therefore unreliable. Rectal solutions are well absorbed. Studies have shown that theophylline tablets are well absorbed: more than 96% of the drug appears in the plasma within 2 hours. Intramuscular injections of theophylline are not used, because they are painful. Theophylline is not effective when administered by inhalation.

Theophylline is combined with ephedrine and a sedative in several combination products for treating asthma. Most clinicians prefer to individualize doses of each ingredient to minimize adverse effects while maximizing therapeutic effects and therefore do not favor combination drugs.

Theophylline is biotransformed by the liver into inactive compounds excreted in the urine. There is a wide variability among individuals in the plasma half-life of theophylline. In normal, nonsmoking adults the plasma half-life is about 6 hours but can vary from 3 to 12 hours. In smokers and children the plasma half-life is shorter, whereas in older adult patients, premature infants, and patients with liver disease or heart failure with pulmonary edema, the plasma half-life is prolonged.

ADVERSE REACTIONS AND CONTRAINDICATIONS

Theophylline has a narrow therapeutic index. The most common adverse effects of this drug after oral administration are nausea and epigastric pain. Headache, dizziness, and nervousness are also common. The effectiveness of theophylline is determined by its plasma concentration. Its traditional therapeutic range has been 10 to 20 mcg/mL, but there is a recent trend to lower the target range to 5 to 15 mcg/mL. Agitation, exaggerated reflexes, and mild muscle tremors (fasciculation) are often seen when the plasma level reaches 20 to 30 mg/mL. Seizures and arrhythmia may occur when the plasma level exceeds 20 mg/mL; the risk is very high above 30 mg/mL.

Other adverse reactions of theophylline seen in the therapeutic dose range are dilation of blood vessels and mild diuresis resulting from the increased renal blood flow and glomerular filtration. Stomach acid secretion is increased, which may be a problem for a patient with an ulcer.

INTERACTIONS

Drugs such as phenytoin, carbamazepine, rifampin, and phenobarbital increase the biotransformation of theophylline so that larger doses of theophylline are required. Similarly, cigarette or marijuana smoking induces hepatic biotransformation of theophylline. Smokers may require a 50% to 100% increase in the dose of theophylline. Serum concentration of theophylline is increased by cimetidine, erythromycin, or the influenza virus vaccine. Adrenergic agonist drugs enhance CNS stimulation caused by theophylline. This drug itself decreases the effects of phenytoin, lithium, nondepolarizing muscle relaxants, and beta blockers.

DRUG CLASS • Anticholinergic Drugs

ipratropium bromide (Atrovent)

MECHANISM OF ACTION

Airway diameter is predominantly controlled by the parasympathetic nervous system. The effects of acetylcholine, the neurohormone, are increased mucus secretion and smooth muscle contraction, resulting in bronchoconstriction. Anticholinergic drugs (i.e., ipratropium) inhibit only the component of bronchoconstriction mediated by the parasympathetic nervous system. Cholinergic receptor activity in bronchial smooth muscle is inhibited, resulting in decreased concentrations of cyclic guanosine monophosphate (cGMP). Decreased levels of cGMP produce local bronchodilation. The end result is bronchodilation without systemic anticholinergic adverse effects. Anticholinergic drugs are discussed in more depth in Chapter 11.

USES

The anticholinergic ipratropium is used as a bronchodilator in maintenance therapy of reversible airway obstruction caused by asthma. It is not designed for use in acute bronchospasm. A combination of ipratropium with albuterol is used in other pulmonarydiseases (see later section on obstructive pulmonary diseases).

PHARMACOKINETICS

The onset of action of ipratropium occurs 5 to 15 minutes after inhalation, reaching a peak in 1 to 2 hours. Effects may last as long as 6 hours. There is minimal systemic absorption. Small amounts are biotransformed in the liver. The half-life of this drug is about 2 hours (see Table 52-2).

ADVERSE REACTIONS AND CONTRAINDICATIONS

Systemic adverse effects of ipratropium are uncommon because it is poorly absorbed. Possible adverse effects include nervousness, dizziness, and headache. Ipratropium is contraindicated for hypersensitive patients and those allergic to atropine, belladonna alkaloids, bromide, or fluorocarbons. Its use should be avoided during acute bronchospasm. Ipratropium should be given with caution to patients who have bladder-neck obstruction, glaucoma, or urinary retention. Safe use during pregnancy, lactation, or with children has not been established.

INTERACTIONS

Because ipratropium is an anticholinergic drug, it may cause additive anticholinergic effects with other drugs of this class. In practice this risk is low because ipratropium is poorly absorbed systemically.

PATHOPHYSIOLOGY • Other Airflow-Obstructive Lung Diseases

Obstruction of airflow is a component of other pulmonary diseases as well. Chronic bronchitis and emphysema are referred to as **chronic obstructive pulmonary diseases (COPD)**. Chronic **bronchitis** is characterized by inflammation of the bronchi. In contrast to acute bronchitis, the clinical manifestations of chronic bronchitis continue for at least 3 months of the year for 2 consecutive years. These patients have an increase in the size and number of submucous glands in the large bronchi, which increases mucus production; an increased number of goblet cells, which also secrete mucus; and impaired ciliary function, which reduces mucus clearance. Thus the lungs' mucociliary defenses are impaired, and there is increased susceptibility to infection. When infection develops, mucus production increases, and the bronchial walls become inflamed and thickened. The thick mucus and inflamed bronchi obstruct airways, which leads to reduced alveolar ventilation.

Patients with **emphysema** can get air in but not out, because the alveolar walls are weakened, causing a permanent overdistension of the airspaces and difficult expiration. Air passages are obstructed as a result of these changes, rather than from mucus production. Difficult expiration is the result of destruction of the walls between alveoli, partial airway collapse, and loss of elastic recoil. As the alveoli and septa collapse, pockets of air form between the alveolar spaces and within the lung parenchyma. This process leads to increased ventilatory dead space, areas that do not participate in gas or blood exchange. The work of breathing increases because there is less functional lung tissue to exchange oxygen and carbon dioxide.

Although the precise cause of emphysema is unknown, research has shown that protease enzymes such as elastase can attack and destroy the connective tissue of the lungs. Emphysema may result from a breakdown of the lungs' normal defense mechanism, alpha$_1$-antitrypsin.

About 60,000 to 70,000 premature infants in the United States develop **respiratory distress syndrome** each year, and 6000 to 10,000 of these infants die. Despite the growth of knowledge and technology, respiratory failure remains the leading cause of infant morbidity and mortality in neonatal intensive care units. In addition, about half of the 150,000 adult Americans who develop respiratory distress syndrome as a result of injuries or blood infections die.

Respiratory distress syndrome, also called hyaline membrane disease, in preterm infants is caused by several factors. Anatomic and functional development in the fetus occurs in stages; the final stage occurs in the third trimester. The final stage includes lung growth, development of ventilatory muscle strength, development of alveoli, and maturation of the surfactant system. Surfactant is a lipoprotein material coating the air sacs in mature lungs; it lowers the surface tension and thereby allows ready inflation of the lungs. Without sufficient surfactant the preterm infant exhibits clinical signs of cyanosis, tachypnea, or apnea. Nasal flaring, chest wall retraction, or an audible expiratory grunt is generally present as an early sign of the disorder.

DRUG CLASS • Drugs for Chronic Obstructive Pulmonary Disease

alpha$_1$-proteinase inhibitor (Prolastin)

beractant (Survanta)

colfosceril palmitate, cetyl alcohol, and tyloxapol (Exosurf)

ipratropium with albuterol (Combivent)

methylprednisolone (Medrol, Solu-Medrol)

MECHANISM OF ACTION

Lung damage in COPD results from the destruction of elastin, a major structural protein of the lung. Elastin is destroyed when there is an imbalance between the lung proteinase, elastase, which breaks down elastin, and alpha$_1$-proteinase inhibitor (also called alpha$_1$ antitrypsin), a protein that inhibits elastase. Smoking depresses alpha$_1$-proteinase inhibitor, which accounts for the high association between smoking and COPD. Some people have a genetic defect that results in a low level of alpha$_1$-proteinase inhibitor.

Surfactants supply the function missing in premature infants whose lungs have not sufficiently matured before birth. The combination of colfosceril palmitate, cetyl alcohol, and tyloxapol is a synthetic surfactant mixture. The colfosceril palmitate is the lipid and active ingredient. Cetyl alcohol is a spreading agent, and tyloxapol is a nonionic detergent that serves as a dispersing agent. Beractant is derived from cows' lungs. Both synthetic and natural surfactants improve gas exchange across the air-alveolus interface in the lung.

Ipratropium bromide is the first anticholinergic drug available to treat asthma and conditions such as chronic bronchitis and emphysema, in which bronchoconstriction is present. Ipratropium opens narrowed breathing passages by blocking vagal nerve impulses that tighten the muscles in the walls of the bronchial tubes. Mucus secretion is also reduced. Ipratropium tends to offer greater advantage in COPD and other so-called lower airway diseases, since the lower airways have a high density of cholinergic receptors. When using ipratropium, there may be a significant advantage in combining it with a beta agonist. The latter opens the upper airways, which allows for greater deposition of the former into the lower airways. A product that combines ipratropium and albuterol in a single metered-dose inhaler is available (Combivent).

Oral glucocorticoids (corticosteroids) are general inhibitors of inflammatory processes and may be effective in high doses for short periods, especially when used with bronchodilating drugs. This class of drugs is covered in detail in Chapter 57.

USES

Alpha$_1$-proteinase inhibitor is available for replacement therapy for patients with a congenital deficiency of the inhibitor. Surfactant preparations (beractant; the combination of colfosceril palmitate, cetyl alcohol, and tyloxapol) are used for respiratory distress in newborns. Ipratropium with albuterol is indicated for patients with COPD.

Oral glucocorticoids are often used to treat patients with asthma or COPD who have severe symptoms not controllable by bronchodilator therapy alone. Initially, large doses of a glucocorticoid drug may be administered for as long as 5 days to bring a severe attack under control when intravenous aminophylline and adrenergic agonists have proven inadequate.

PHARMACOKINETICS

Alpha$_1$-proteinase inhibitor is currently purified from human plasma and administered intravenously.

Surfactant preparations reduce the mortality rate from respiratory distress syndrome in infants, but it is not clear whether it is preferable to give surfactant for prophylaxis as well or as treatment only. All doses are calculated based on the infant's weight and are administered directly into the trachea.

Ipratropium is administered by inhalation. The onset of action is 5 to 15 minutes, and the duration of action is 3 to 6 hours. The drug is primarily excreted unchanged in the feces. It has negligible cardiovascular effects. Atropine-like adverse effects are rare with inhalation administration.

ADVERSE REACTIONS AND CONTRAINDICATIONS

Alpha$_1$-proteinase inhibitor may cause allergic reactions. Surfactants may be associated with pulmonary hemorrhage or tachycardia. Ipratroprium rarely causes skin rashes, bronchospasm, or other signs of allergies.

High dosages of glucocorticoids can be tolerated for short periods but cause many severe adverse effects when used on a long-term basis. To minimize these long-term toxic effects, glucocorticoids are administered in small doses every other day. This schedule minimizes suppression of adrenal function and also avoids excessive use, which could cause Cushing's syndrome (characteristic of excessive glucocorticoid administration; see Chapter 57).

INTERACTIONS

Used properly, these drugs rarely cause significant interactions.

APPLICATION TO PRACTICE

ASSESSMENT
History of Present Illness

Patient history is the most important component in the evaluation of a patient with a respiratory disorder. The patient should be asked if he or she has had sudden and severe or recurrent episodes of coughing, wheezing, or shortness of breath in the last 12 months. Does the coughing, wheezing, or shortness of breath occur during a particular season or time of the year? Does it occur in certain places or when the patient is exposed to certain things (e.g., animals, tobacco smoke, perfumes)? Have the symptoms occurred during the night, early morning, or after moderate exercise, running, or other physical activity? Has the patient had colds that settle in the chest or take more than 10 days to resolve?

Determine the frequency and severity of attacks, as well as precipitating and alleviating factors. Ask if the patient uses any drugs that help him or her to breathe better and how often the drugs are used. Ask if the drugs are taken regularly or occasionally. Ask what the highest and lowest peak flow reading has been since the patient's last visit and what was done with the information.

A careful search of environmental factors should be conducted. The patient should be questioned in detail about the home environment: location, type of heating (e.g., wood-burning stove or fireplace), type and quality of construction, type of insulation, humidity level, nature of furnishings, presence of plants, draperies and bedding, pets and their habits, housecleaning methods, cigarette smoking, and so on. Variations in symptoms with seasons and with changes in location should be carefully recorded. Ask about the work environment, any exposure to chemical irritants or sensitizers, physical demands, and job stressors. Does the patient cough or wheeze during the week but not on weekends when away from the workplace? Do the patient's eyes and nasal passages get irritated soon after arriving at work? The patient's clothing and dietary history should not be overlooked, especially with children, because fabrics and foods are potential allergens.

Be sure to obtain a smoking history, since the major risk factor for COPD is cigarette smoking. Smokers have a higher death rate from chronic bronchitis and emphysema; they also have a higher prevalence of lung function abnormalities, respiratory symptoms, and all forms of COPD. Cigarette smokers also have a greater annual rate of decline in forced expiratory volume (FEV_1). Other factors that increase the likelihood of developing or worsening COPD include passive smoking, ambient air pollution, and hyperresponsive airways. Even controlling for smoking, there is a higher prevalence of respiratory symptoms in men.

Health History

When interviewing the patient, the health care provider should take pains to identify any previous allergic problems in the patient and also any allergies in close family members. This information is particularly helpful in providing support for the diagnosis of an atopic disease. The onset of symptoms in childhood is typical of allergic disease, but the onset of symptoms during adulthood does not rule out atopy. Apart from homozygous alpha$_1$-antitrypsin deficiency, COPD may aggregate in families.

A drug history is important, especially any prescription or OTC drug used to treat present or past symptoms. Determine what drugs the patient is taking, how much, and how often. Ask the type and how many puffs of an inhaler the patient is using daily. How many inhalers has the patient used in the last month? For some patients, ask them to demonstrate the technique for using the inhaler. Information regarding the use of inhaled cocaine or nasal decongestants and antihistamines should be carefully noted.

Lifespan Considerations

Perinatal. A number of changes take place in the respiratory tract during pregnancy that are mediated by the mechanical effects of an enlarging uterus, increased oxygen demands, and the respiratory stimulant effect of progesterone. Estrogen causes hyperemia of nasopharyngeal mucosa with edema and increased production of mucus. This leads to a feeling of stuffiness and an increased tendency for epistaxis. Pregnant women should be warned of this normal change and advised against using OTC drugs and nasal sprays to alleviate the symptoms. A normal saline spray may be helpful in reducing some of the discomfort and should be encouraged for women who find the stuffy feeling uncomfortable.

Although studies show that about 4% of pregnancies are complicated by asthma, the true prevalence may be much higher. Asthma may occur at any time during pregnancy. If it is diagnosed before pregnancy, it may be worsened by the pregnancy. About 33% of pregnant women with asthma are adversely affected, 33% remain the same, and 33% improve. Women with asthma usually have a return to their prepregnancy level of the disease by about 3 months postpartum.

Maternal and fetal morbidity and mortality rates are increased if asthma is not controlled during pregnancy. Maternal complications include preeclampsia, gestational hypertension, hyperemesis gravidarum, vaginal hemorrhage, and complications of labor. Fetal complications include increased risk of perinatal mortality, intrauterine growth retardation, preterm birth, low birth weight, and neonatal hypoxia. If asthma is controlled, the woman can maintain a normal pregnancy with little or no increased risk to herself or the fetus.

Pediatric. A strong relationship exists between viral infections and the development of asthma in infants. Allergens play a less important role in this age group because it takes time for allergic sensitivity to develop. In children, however, allergy influences the persistence and severity of the disease (see Box 52-1).

Assessment of symptoms in the child is much like that of the adult but also includes a feeding history for a very young child, with attention to cow's milk, eggs, and wheat consumption. The stability of family members' relationships and stress level in the home should not be overlooked. Information about the child's toys, bedroom, and other rooms of the house where the child spends waking hours should be noted. The presence or absence of symptoms in all of these areas should be noted. The source of present and past health information (often the parents) is important because valid recall of times and events associated with symptoms is critical in providing clues to the causal antigen. Poorly controlled asthma may delay growth in children. In general, children with asthma tend to have longer periods of reduced growth rates before puberty, boys more so than girls.

Older Adults. Commonly, older adults who develop asthma late in life have intrinsic asthma, which does not have allergic or environmental triggers. Common estimates of the incidence of new-onset asthma after age 65 vary from 1% to 3%. Some health care providers indicate, however, that asthma develops in almost half of the patient population older than 65. The chronic bronchitis of COPD is not a genetic disorder, although some studies have hinted at a predisposition for development of this condition. It affects 10% to 20% of adults and is the fourth most common cause of death in the United States. Fourteen million people have chronic bronchitis and 2 million have emphysema. The predominant age of people with these diseases is over 40 years, and men are affected more often than women.

Neither IgE nor skin testing is useful in the older adult, probably because of the decrease in allergic response associated with aging. Unfortunately, treatable airway disorders in older adults often go undiagnosed, perhaps because of the high prevalence of other forms of respiratory disease and heart failure that may have similar clinical presentations. Some older adults may not be able to perform spirometry testing reliably. Additional tests, such as symptom scores and distance walked without dyspnea and wheezing, can be used to evaluate the patient.

Cultural/Social Considerations

Many of the drugs used in the treatment of allergies, asthma, and COPD are purchased by consumers over the counter. They are easily accessible to almost all persons, easy to use, and in many cases are generally effective. For these reasons, many patients with asthma and COPD have not been diagnosed or adequately treated. Family and societal health care beliefs and norms may keep the patient from seeking help (see the Case Study: Moderate Persistent Asthma).

Mortality rates for COPD are higher in whites than in nonwhites, but the difference is decreasing in men. Morbidity and mortality rates are inversely related to socioeconomic status and are higher in blue-collar than in white-collar workers.

Physical Examination

A general respiratory examination includes assessment of the rate and character of respirations and skin color. Percussion of the chest may reveal hyperresonance. On auscultation, breath sounds are coarse and loud with sonorous crackles throughout the lung fields. The ratio of inspiration to expiration is abnormal (i.e., expiration is prolonged in patients with asthma). In asthma, coarse rhonchi may be heard along with generalized inspiratory and expiratory wheezing. The wheezing becomes high-pitched as obstruction progresses. If the lungs sound clear, auscultate during forced expiration, which may bring out asthmatic wheezing.

Abnormal breathing patterns (e.g., rate below 12 or above 24, dyspnea, cough, orthopnea, wheezing, and stridor) suggest respiratory distress. Severe respiratory distress is characterized by tachypnea, dyspnea, use of accessory muscles of respiration, and hypoxia. Early signs of hypoxia include restlessness, confusion, anxiety, increased blood pressure, and tachycardia. Late signs of hypoxia include cyanosis as well as decreased blood pressure and pulse. Hypoxemia is confirmed when the pulse oximetry (SaO_2) and arterial blood gas analyses reflect decreased partial pressure of oxygen (PaO_2).

The nose is often overlooked or given only a cursory inspection during a physical examination. The nasal mucosa should be inspected for erythema, pallor, atrophy, edema, crusting, and discharge. The presence of polyps (not to be confused with turbinates), erosions, and septal perforations or deviations should be noted. A pale, boggy appearance to the mucosa is allegedly a classic sign of allergic disease, but erythema sometimes occurs in allergy and a boggy appearance certainly does not rule out sinusitis, which may also be present at the time of the examination. Mucopurulent discharge from the nares or seen in the posterior pharynx raises the possibility of this condition.

A child with atopy may have dark circles under the eyes (allergic shiners) and have a transverse crease above the tip of the nose from frequent upward nose rubbing (allergic salute). Erythematous conjunctiva, tearing, photophobia, and papillary edema of the eyelids provide supportive evidence of an allergic mechanism. Transillumination and palpation of the sinuses, a pharyngeal examination for erythema and discharge, checking the ears for evidence of otitis, and cervical node examination for adenopathy are included in the examination.

Laboratory Testing

Few general laboratory procedures are appropriate for the patient with a respiratory disorder. Pulmonary function tests provide an objective and reproducible means of evaluating the presence and severity of lung disease as well as the response to therapy. A key measurement is peak expiratory flow rate (PEFR), or the greatest flow velocity that can be obtained during a forced expiration. PEFRs place the disease into physiologic categories: red, yellow, and green zones (Figure 52-4). In general, spirometry testing can be reliably performed by adults as well as children by the age of 5 or 6 years. In addition, skin testing is specifically recommended for patients with persistent asthma who are exposed to perennial indoor allergens.

GOALS OF THERAPY

Active partnership with patients remains the cornerstone of management of respiratory diseases because there are many goals of therapy, all of which are important in managing the disease effectively. The goals include the following:

- Preventing chronic, troublesome symptoms (e.g., coughing or shortness of breath at night, in the early morning, or after exercise)
- Providing optimal drug therapy (i.e., inducing bronchodilation, decreasing the inflammatory reaction, and facilitating expectoration) with minimal or no adverse effects
- Maintaining normal or near-normal pulmonary function
- Maintaining exercise and other physical activities
- Preventing recurrent exacerbations and minimizing the need for acute-care interventions
- Meeting patient and family expectations of satisfaction with care

Respiratory diseases are clearly not treatable with one drug. Thus multidrug therapy is generally the rule rather than the exception.

INTERVENTION

As shown in Table 52-3, a stepwise approach is recommended with the type and amount of drug dictated by the severity of the respiratory disorder. Drug therapy is divided into quick-relief drugs and (long-term) con-

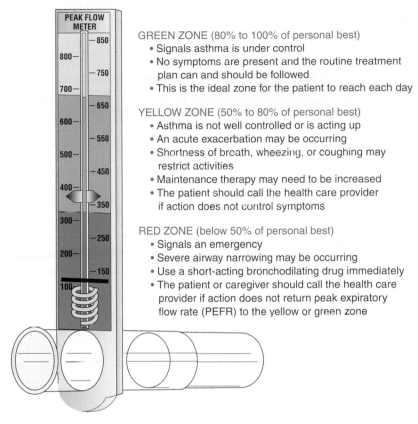

PEAK FLOW METER

GREEN ZONE (80% to 100% of personal best)
- Signals asthma is under control
- No symptoms are present and the routine treatment plan can and should be followed
- This is the ideal zone for the patient to reach each day

YELLOW ZONE (50% to 80% of personal best)
- Asthma is not well controlled or is acting up
- An acute exacerbation may be occurring
- Shortness of breath, wheezing, or coughing may restrict activities
- Maintenance therapy may need to be increased
- The patient should call the health care provider if action does not control symptoms

RED ZONE (below 50% of personal best)
- Signals an emergency
- Severe airway narrowing may be occurring
- Use a short-acting bronchodilating drug immediately
- The patient or caregiver should call the health care provider if action does not return peak expiratory flow rate (PEFR) to the yellow or green zone

FIGURE 52-4   Interpreting peak expiratory flow rates. A baseline reading is required for accurate interpretation of the expiratory flow rate zones, because expiration measurements are based on the patient's personal best effort rather than set levels.

troller drugs. This reflects a shift in treatment guidelines, which previously emphasized symptomatic relief with bronchodilators.

Three documents set the standards for the diagnosis and treatment of asthma and COPD: the *Guidelines for the Diagnosis and Treatment of Asthma* (1991, 1997), *International Consensus Report on Diagnosis and Treatment of Asthma* (1992), and the American Thoracic Society's *Standards for the Diagnosis and Care of Patients with Chronic Obstructive Pulmonary Disease* (1995). According to these documents, therapy should be started when avoidance of bronchospasm-triggering factors does not control symptoms or when beta agonists are required more than twice daily for 1 week. Short-acting beta agonists and anticholinergic drugs are used for acute attacks. Corticosteroids, antiallergy drugs, LT antagonists, long-acting beta agonists, and xanthine derivatives are used for long-term control.

Prophylaxis should be instituted before exercise for all patients with demonstrated exercise-induced or seasonal asthma (in the latter case, ideally before the season for the known allergen).

Administration

Patients with acute respiratory distress may require admission to the intensive care unit. Characteristics of acute asthma attack include poor air exchange, diminished breath sounds, marked retraction of accessory muscles of respiration, dulled thinking processes, cyanosis, confusion, signs of exhaustion, and an FEV_1 less than 1 L.

Anxiety, insomnia, fear, and other emotional responses may aggravate bronchospasm and air hunger. Maintain a calm but efficient attitude in caring for the patients. Do not leave the patient unattended for long periods. Keep the call bell within easy reach of the patient. Hyperglycemia may appear in diabetic patients receiving bronchodilators. Be sure to monitor blood sugar level as well as intake and output.

Check pulse oximetry and obtain arterial blood gases if indicated. Establish an intravenous line to provide access for drugs and to keep the patient hydrated. Auscultate for breath sounds. Monitor the patient's pulse, blood pressure, and respiratory rate. The frequency of monitoring varies with the patient's condition, drug,

TABLE 52-3

Drug Therapy for Asthma

Characteristics	*Controller Drugs*	*Reliever Drugs*
Mild Intermittent Asthma Episodes of wheezing, coughing, or chest tightness twice a week or less. Nighttime problems with breathing less than twice a month. Often associated with exercise. Few severe attacks.	No daily drug treatment needed	Short-acting inhaled bronchodilator, usually a beta$_2$ agonist; inhaled beta$_2$ agonist or cromolyn before exercise or exposure to antigen; alternatively, ipratropium
Mild Persistent Asthma Episodes of wheezing, coughing, or chest tightness more than twice a week but less than daily (especially effective for children). Nighttime problems with breathing more than twice a month. Severe attacks that affect activity.	Low daily dosage of inhaled corticosteroids or mast cell inhibitor, sustained-release theophylline or LT modifier (for patients 12 years and older)	Short-acting inhaled bronchodilator, usually a beta$_2$ agonist; alternatively, an oral beta$_2$ agonist as needed up to 4 times daily, ipratropium, or an oral short-acting theophylline
Moderate Persistent Asthma Daily episodes of wheezing, coughing, or chest tightness. Nighttime problems with breathing more than once a week. Severe attacks that affect activity two or more times weekly.	Medium daily dosage of inhaled corticosteroids or small daily dosage of inhaled corticosteroid combined with long-acting drug such as salmeterol or sustained-release theophylline	Short-acting inhaled bronchodilator, usually beta$_2$ agonist; alternatively, an oral beta$_2$ agonist as needed up to 4 times daily (for children) or ipratropium if excessive tachycardia develops with beta$_2$ agonist
Severe Persistent Asthma Continual wheezing, coughing, or chest tightness and frequent nighttime breathing problems. Limited physical activity because of breathing problems. Frequent serious attacks.	High daily dosages of inhaled corticosteroid combined with long-acting drugs such as salmeterol or sustained-release theophylline and oral doses of corticosteroid	Short-acting inhaled bronchodilator, usually a beta$_2$ agonist; alternatively, an oral beta$_2$ agonist as needed up to 4 times daily (for children)

dosage, and route of administration. During intravenous drug administration, monitor vital signs every 5 to 15 minutes until stable. With subcutaneous or inhalation administration, monitor every 15 minutes.

With subcutaneous or intramuscular injections, perform aspiration before administering the drug to avoid inadvertent intravenous administration. For continuous intravenous infusion, use an infusion control device and (usually) a microdrip tubing.

Sublingual tablets should be allowed to dissolve under the tongue. Instruct the patient not to swallow saliva until the tablet is completely dissolved. Oral doses should be taken with meals or snacks to lessen gastric irritation.

Inhalation Devices. There are several aerosol delivery devices: metered-dose inhalers (MDIs), breath-actuated MDIs, dry-powder inhalers, and nebulizers. Each has advantages and disadvantages. The decision for a particular delivery device is matched to patient needs and the likelihood of compliance. The advantages and disadvantages of each are outlined in Table 52-4.

The administration technique varies with the specific aerosol delivery device and whether or not a spacer or holding-chamber device is used. The drug dose contained in an MDI is expressed as the actuator dose, the amount of drug leaving the actuator and delivered to the patient. This is a labeling requirement in the United States. The actuator dose is different from the dosage expressed, because the valve dose, the amount of drug leaving the valve, is not completely available to the patient. The valve dose is commonly used in many European countries and in some scientific literature. The dosages of dry-powder inhalers are expressed as the amount of drug in the inhaler following activation.

Peak expiratory flow rate (PEFR) measurements should be performed when symptoms appear, when there has been a change in therapy, and every 1 to 2 years thereafter. PEFRs are usually measured on waking, before bedtime, and before and after administration of a

TABLE 52-4

Comparison of Aerosol Delivery Devices

Advantage(s)	Disadvantage(s)
Metered-Dose Inhaler (MDI) (Actuated during slow,* deep inhalation, followed by 10-second held breath)	
Mouth rinsing may reduce systemic absorption.	Slow inhalation is difficult for some patients. Patients may have difficulty coordinating actuation with inhalation. Patients may incorrectly stop inhalation at actuation. 80% of drug is deposited in the oropharynx.
Breath-Actuated MDI (slow, deep inhalation, followed by 10-second held breath)	
Helpful for patients unable to coordinate actuation with inhalation.	Slow inhalation is difficult for some patients. Patients may incorrectly stop inhalation at actuation. This form requires more rapid inspiration to activate than is optimal for deposition. It cannot be used with the currently available spacer.
Dry-Powder Inhaler (DPI) (rapid, deep inhalation with mouth closed tightly around mouthpiece)	
Dose delivery is greater than MDI depending on device and technique. Can be used in children less than 4 years old. Similar delivery efficacy as MDI with or without spacer. Mouth rinsing effectively reduces systemic absorption.	Dose is lost if patient exhales through device. Some devices deliver greater doses of drug than that of an MDI.
Nebulizer (slow, tidal breathing with occasional deep breaths, requiring a tightly fitting face mask if patient is unable to use mouthpiece)	
This form is less dependent on patient coordination or cooperation. It is the delivery method of choice for cromolyn in children. It is the delivery method of choice for high-dose beta$_2$ agonists and anticholinergics in moderate to severe exacerbations in all patients.	It is expensive and time-consuming. It is bulky, and output is device dependent. There are significant differences in the output of devices.
Spacer or Holding Device (slow inhalation or tidal breathing immediately after actuation; one actuation into device per inhalation. If face mask is used, three to five inhalations per actuation)	
This form is easier to use than MDI alone. With a face mask, it allows MDI to be used with small children. Large volume devices (>600 mL) increase lung delivery over MDI alone for patients with poor MDI technique. It decreases deposition of drug in the oropharynx, reducing the potential for systemic absorption of inhaled corticosteroids that have higher oral bioavailability. It is recommended for patients on medium to high doses of inhaled corticosteroids. It is effective as a nebulizer in delivering high doses of beta$_2$ agonists during severe exacerbations.	It does not eliminate need for coordinating actuation with inhalation. It is bulky, and output may be reduced in some devices after cleaning. Output from an MDI with a spacer is dependent on both the MDI and the spacer.

Adapted from the National Institutes of Health, National Heart, Lung, and Blood Institute: *Highlights of the expert panel report 2: guidelines for the diagnosis and management of asthma,* Pub. No. 97-4051A, Bethesda, Md., 1997, U.S. Department of Health and Human Services.
*Slow inhalation means 30 L/minute for a period of 3 to 5 seconds. Rapid inhalation means 60 L/minute for a period of 1 to 2 seconds.

beta agonist; that is, a minimum of twice daily and the best of three measurements on each occasion. Patients are often instructed to double the dose of inhaled corticosteroid if their PEFR is less than 75% of the best value, start a short course of oral corticosteroids if the PEFR is less than 50% of the best value, and call the health care provider if the PEFR is less than 25% of personal best.

Surfactant Formulations. Protocols for administration of these drugs are being developed and refined. Check hospital protocol for guidelines, because administration may be restricted to the health care provider.

Reconstitute colfosceril palmitate, cetyl alcohol, and tyloxapol with diluent provided by manufacturer. See manufacturer's instructions for preferred method. Reconstitute

---

| BOX 52-2 | **Patient Problem: Using an MDI Correctly*** |

The Problem

Many patients are unable to coordinate activation with inhalation or activate an MDI in the mouth while breathing through their nose. Some patients do not have adequate strength to activate an MDI or are unable to hold their breath for the required length of time after use. Some patients inhale more than one puff with each inspiration or do not wait a sufficient amount of time between each puff (1 to 5 minutes is recommended). Not shaking the MDI before use or holding it upside down or sideways contributes to ineffective use. Not tilting the head back and opening the mouth causes the drug to bounce off the teeth, tongue, or palate, thus limiting the amount of the drug that reaches the airways. Furthermore, recent studies indicate that overuse of inhalers (more than one incident per month) may be associated with increased morbidity and mortality.

The Solution

Review the manufacturer's instruction sheet. The following technique maximizes the drug's benefit:

1. Use the drug only as prescribed.
2. Have the patient assemble the inhaler and shake the canister.
3. Exhale deeply while holding the device upright.
4. Put the mouthpiece into the mouth with the head tilted back and the opening of the device mouthpiece directed to the back of the throat. Grasp the mouthpiece with the teeth and lips.
5. Inhale deeply for 5 to 10 seconds while depressing the aerosol container or activating the spray mechanism, then hold breath as long as possible before exhaling.
6. Wait several minutes before taking a second dose (if prescribed). When two drugs are ordered via inhalation device, use the bronchodilating drug first, wait at least 1 minute, then take the corticosteroid drug. Remember to shake the canister again before administering the second dose. Also, by waiting, the potential toxicity from inhaled chlorofluorocarbon propellants is reduced. Some of the newer aerosols (e.g., Proventil HFA) are formulated using hydrofluoroalkane rather than chlorofluorocarbons. Even though chlorofluorocarbons are safe for human use, they damage the ozone layer of the atmosphere.
7. For children, it may be necessary to hold the nose closed. Special devices can help children use inhalation drugs if they are having trouble using the MDI, including the Inhal-Aid and InspirEase devices. Consult with the pharmacist.
8. Wash and dry the mouthpiece after use.

*The nurse should periodically watch the patient use the inhalation device or MDI to verify that the patient is using it correctly.

---

immediately before use because the product does not contain antibacterial preservatives.

Beractant suspension should be warmed before administration. Let it stand at room temperature for 20 minutes, or warm it in the hand for at least 8 minutes. Do not use artificial warming methods. For prophylactic doses, begin warming the drug before infant's birth. Rotate vial to suspend or resuspend drug in diluent. Use each vial for a single dose, discarding any unused suspension.

Aspirate an infant's lungs before administration of surfactant; avoid suctioning if possible for at least 2 hours after administration of the drug and for as long as 6 hours, if tolerated by the infant. Dosage is based on weight. Inject the drug into the trachea via an endotracheal tube. The manufacturer of Exosurf provides an endotracheal tube adapter to permit injection. To distribute the drug throughout the lungs, it may be necessary to rotate the infant's body gently from side to side.

Monitor the infant's clinical appearance, pulse oximetry, partial pressure of oxygen, carbon dioxide partial pressure, arterial blood gases, lung sounds, and cardiac status. Keep the parents and family members informed of the infant's condition.

Education

Patient and family education begins at the time of diagnosis and should be integrated into each step of care. Education about self-management should be tailored to the needs of each patient, maintaining a sensitivity to cultural beliefs and practices. Begin patient teaching after the acute respiratory distress episode is over. The patient should be advised to stop smoking. Provide the patient with information about local resources available.

The patient should be able to describe or demonstrate the correct way to take ordered drugs, including frequency, route of administration, and use of inhalation devices; the patient should also know under what circumstances to return to the health care provider or emergency room if the drugs are ineffective.

Caution the patient to use the drugs only as prescribed and not to increase the dosage or frequency unless directed to do so by the health care provider. Many bronchodilators are dispensed with patient information leaflets; review the leaflets with the patient. When two drugs are ordered via inhalation, the patient should be instructed to use the bronchodilating drug first, then use the second inhaler. If tachycardia is a problem, suggest that the patient limit caffeine intake.

Patients with asthma should be advised to avoid sulfite-containing foods such as acidic juices, dried fruits, instant potatoes, and shrimp (see Appendix A). Additionally, some drugs used to treat respiratory disorders contain sulfites. If the patient is allergic to sulfites, instruct him or her to read carefully all literature provided with the prescription. The occurrence and severity of sulfite reactions depend on the nature of the food or drug, the level of residual sulfite, the sensitivity of the individual, and perhaps the form of residual sulfite and the mechanism of the reaction. Work with the pharmacist to obtain sulfite-free brands.

In some patients, bronchospasm is triggered by exercise. Strategies that may be helpful for exercise-induced bronchospasm include extending the warm-up period before exercise, choosing a less strenuous sport, avoiding exercise during periods of high air pollution, and using a bronchodilating or antiallergy drug approximately 20 to 30 minutes before exercise. Use of these drugs before exercise is better than avoiding exercise altogether, especially for children.

Decrease exposure to common irritants. Teach the patient to vacuum the home often, encase mattresses and pillows with plastic, use an air conditioner if possible, use high-energy particulate air (HEPA) filters for the heating and air conditioning systems, and keep the windows closed. Routine use of chemicals to kill dust mites and denature the antigen is no longer recommended as a control measure.

Teach the patient and family how to check the supply of drugs on hand to avoid running out at inopportune times. To check the amount of drug in the inhaler canister, drop the canister into a container of water (without the mouthpiece). Full containers sink to the bottom, whereas half-full containers float with part of the container out of the water. An empty container floats on its side, half submerged. Unlike other drugs administered via inhalation, neither the cromolyn nor the nedocromil canister can be floated to estimate the number of doses remaining. Consult the manufacturer's instructions for additional information.

Patients should be encouraged to have an influenza vaccine annually and an inoculation of a pneumococcal vaccine every 5 to 7 years if they have chronic lung disease or other chronic conditions. Adult patients with severe persistent asthma, nasal polyps, and a history of sensitivity to aspirin or nonsteroidal antiinflammatory drugs should be counseled regarding the risk of severe and even fatal exacerbations from using these drugs.

Instruct patients to notify the health care provider if they experience unusual stressors such as surgery or illness, have an asthma attack that does not respond to usual treatment, develop an infection of the mouth or throat, or if their general condition deteriorates. Patients should also be encouraged to seek treatment for rhinitis, sinusitis, and gastroesophageal reflux, if present.

Glucocorticoids. For best effect, glucocorticoids should be used at evenly spaced intervals throughout the day. Several weeks of therapy may be required before full benefits of therapy are seen. Glucocorticoids for inhalation are dispensed with an inhaler and a patient instruction booklet, which should be reviewed with the patient. Glucocorticoids are also available as powder or capsules containing powder. These forms require a special device that punctures the capsule or blister containing the powder and releases it into the inhaler. Review the manufacturer's instructions with the patient. These patients should also be instructed to carry medical alert identification indicating that they are using glucocorticoid drugs.

Instruct the patient to gargle and rinse the mouth (but not to swallow the gargle liquid) after each use of the glucocorticoid inhaler to help reduce the risk of oral fungal infections. The inhalation device should be washed at least daily in warm running water. Patients should be taught to observe for hoarseness, cough, throat irritation, and fungal infection of the mouth and throat. When present, candidiasis responds well to antifungal drugs such as nystatin mouthwash or clotrimazole troches.

Antiallergy Drugs. Unlike other drugs administered via inhalation, neither the cromolyn nor the nedocromil canister can be floated to estimate the number of doses remaining. Teach patients using this form to keep a record of doses used. There are either about 112 or about 200 inhalations per canister of cromolyn, depending on the size of canister prescribed. Cromolyn capsules for inhalation are used with the Spinhaler or Halermatic devices only. The cromolyn capsule is placed in the turbohaler, which punctures the capsule. When the turbohaler is placed in the mouth and the patient inhales, the capsule spins and vibrates, causing the micronized powder to be released. The solution formulation is used with a power-operated nebulizer. Hand-operated nebulizers are unsuitable for administration of these drugs.

A canister of nedocromil holds either about 56 or about 122 inhalations, depending on the size prescribed. Nedocromil is available only in aerosol canisters.

For missed doses, instruct the patient to take dose as soon as remembered, then space remaining doses for that day evenly throughout the day.

Leukotriene Modifiers. Teach patients that these drugs are used to *prevent* attacks of asthma, not to *treat* acute attacks. For best effect, they need to be used regularly as prescribed, even if the patient is feeling better. It may require several weeks of therapy for the full effect to be realized.

For missed doses, instruct the patient to take the dose as soon as remembered, unless it is almost time for the next dose; in this case, omit the missed dose and resume the usual schedule. Do not double up for missed doses. Do not discontinue other asthma drugs while taking an LT modifier without first consulting with the health care provider.

Beta-Adrenergic Bronchodilators. Review the general guidelines for these drugs. The first dose from an MDI may contain an inadequate amount of drug. When the canister is new or when it has not been used in a while, especially if stored in an upright position, the patient should activate the canister at least once into the air before using it again to administer a dose. Avoid spraying the priming mist into the eyes.

Caution the patient to contact the health care provider if the usual doses of drug are not controlling his or her asthma and not to increase doses without medical advice. The need for an increased amount of a given drug may signal a worsening of the condition, in which case, the health care provider needs to be consulted.

Instruct patients to keep a record of inhalations from each canister. Floating the canister in water provides only a rough estimate of the amount of drug remaining. Consult the pharmacist or the manufacturer's literature for information about the number of doses per canister prescribed, or consult the manufacturer's literature.

Beta agonists are available in a variety of dosage forms: oral solution, oral syrup, tablets, extended-release tablets, capsules, and forms for injection, as well as aerosol, solution, and powder for inhalation. Review the patient's drug formulation to verify that the patient is taking the prescribed formulation correctly.

Xanthines. Instruct the patient to read drug prescriptions and labels carefully. Many xanthines are available in regular and sustained-release formulations; they cannot be interchanged on the same dosing schedule. In addition, various brands are not interchangeable. Inform the patient not to switch brands or dosage forms without checking with the health care provider.

Instruct the patient to take oral doses of a xanthine on an empty stomach with a full glass (8 ounces) of water, 1 hour before or 2 hours after meals. Doses can also be taken with meals or a snack to lessen gastric irritation. Inform patients who have difficulty swallowing extended-release capsules that the contents may be sprinkled on a small amount of food such as jam, jelly, or applesauce and swallowed without chewing. Instruct the patient to limit or avoid coffee, tea, chocolate, and other xanthines because they may affect xanthine biotransformation. Inform the patient taking once-daily doses to take the dose after fasting through the night and 1 hour before eating or in the evening with or without food, depending on the product. Whichever way the patient takes the drug, it should be taken the same way each day to minimize fluctuations in the serum level.

Instruct the patient to avoid smoking cigarettes or marijuana, which may also alter the serum drug level. The patient should be told not to start or stop smoking without talking with the health care provider, because the dose of xanthine may need to be adjusted.

Instruct the patient to notify the health care provider if fever, diarrhea, or symptoms of the flu develop. Warn the patient to avoid driving or operating hazardous equipment if dizziness, light-headedness, or vertigo develops; if any of these symptoms occur, tell the patient to notify the health care provider. Encourage the patient to return for follow-up visits so that blood work can be performed to monitor serum drug levels.

Alpha$_1$-Proteinase Inhibitor. This drug is administered intravenously. If used by the patient for self-administration, teach the patient how to store the drug; prepare doses; manage infusion; and dispose of contaminated needles, tubing, and equipment. Advise the patient to be immunized against hepatitis B because this drug is prepared from pooled human plasma.

Advise the patient not to discontinue any prescribed drugs without first consulting with the health care provider. Remind the patient to keep these and all drugs out of the reach of children.

EVALUATION

New emphasis has been placed on evaluating treatment outcomes in terms of patient perception of improvement, quality of life, and the ability to engage in activities of daily living. Clinical improvement is demonstrated by an increase in the distance the patient can walk, decreases in the use of rescue drugs, and fewer reports of shortness of breath, chest tightness, coughing, and wheezing.

Chronic asthma symptoms are relieved with corticosteroids or antiallergy drugs. Effectiveness of beta agonists is demonstrated by prevention or relief of bronchospasm and a reduction in the frequency of acute asthma attacks. Exercise-induced bronchospasm is prevented or reduced. Patients with COPD should strive for normal exercise tolerance, and sleep should not be interrupted by coughing or wheezing.

Although the health care provider manages a wide range of respiratory disorders, when conservative methods fail to control symptoms, one must consider referral to an appropriate allergist or respiratory specialist.

The FEV_1 should be assessed once to determine the reversibility of bronchoconstriction. Reversibility is indicated by an increase of 15% to 20% in FEV_1 after administration of a bronchodilator. Measure arterial blood gases if the patient's PEFR is less than 40% of predicted, the FEV_1 is less than 1.2 L, or the patient is not responding to treatment. Hospitalization is considered for patients with acute respiratory distress who manifest any one of the following:

- Subjective report of severe difficulty breathing
- Failure to respond fully and promptly to inhaled beta agonist therapy that was followed promptly by full doses of prednisone

- Use of accessory muscles of respiration
- A pulsus paradoxus in excess of 10 mm Hg
- An FEV_1 less than 1 L per second
- An arterial $PaCO_2$ inappropriately high for respiratory rate
- Presence of an underlying cardiac condition
- Inadequate home situation or a history of poor compliance with therapy

CASE STUDY *Acute Asthma Attack*

ASSESSMENT

HISTORY OF PRESENT ILLNESS

RL is a 25-year-old Native American woman who has had asthma since age 7, resulting in recurrent episodes of acute attacks. She has been treated in the emergency room or hospitalized for asthma attacks once a month for the last 10 months. Today's attack began when she awoke this morning, although she reports wheezing during the night and having a headache. Symptoms of an upper respiratory tract infection had been present for the past 48 hours. She reports a 10 pack/year history of cigarette smoking. Her wheezing this morning was not relieved by her metaproterenol MDI. She reports using up two, 14-g MDI canisters this month alone trying to control her asthma.

HEALTH HISTORY

RL was hospitalized at age 17 for severe respiratory distress and since then has used intermittent steroid therapy to maintain control. Her family history reveals that both parents and three of her five siblings have diabetes mellitus. Her mother has a 40-year history of asthma and eczema. RL's current drugs include cromolyn sodium four times daily and metaproterenol MDI prn.

LIFESPAN CONSIDERATIONS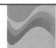

RL is in Erikson's stage of intimacy versus isolation. She is attempting to establish intimate bonds of love and friendship, although her attempts have been hindered by her asthma.

CULTURAL/SOCIAL CONSIDERATIONS

RL was married at age 20, divorced a year later, and has one child, a daughter now age 4. RL is presently in college full-time and living with her parents until she completes her education. She tries to participate in social activities at the local Native American center. She has no income of her own. Her parents are supporting her and their grandchild while RL is in school. Health care needs are covered through her parents' insurance coverage.

PHYSICAL EXAMINATION

RL is 5'2" tall and weighs 190 pounds. Her blood pressure is 120/80 mm Hg, temperature 97.2° F, pulse 90 and regular, and respirations 24. Audible wheezes on inspiration and expiration over bilateral lung fields. Altered ratio of inspiration to expiration. Heart sounds not audible because of the wheezes. Her skin is pink and diaphoretic.

LABORATORY TESTING

Spirometry reveals an FEV_1 74% of predicted with a variable PEFR that exceeds 30%.

PATIENT PROBLEM(S)

Acute asthma attack.

GOALS OF THERAPY

Prevent chronic, troublesome symptoms (e.g., coughing or shortness of breath at night, in the early morning, or after exercise). Maintain near-normal pulmonary function exercise and other physical activities.

CRITICAL THINKING QUESTIONS

1. The health care provider initially orders an aminophylline drip for RL. What is the mechanism of action of this drug?
2. What benefit should RL have received from her metoproterenol inhaler?
3. RL insists on keeping her metoproterenol inhaler at the bedside. What are the adverse effects that the nurse needs to warn her about if this request is granted?
4. The health care provider stops RL's cromolyn for the time being. Why?
5. Which nursing measures are necessary to monitor RL's bronchodilation therapy?
6. On discharge RL will be using a triamcinolone inhaler in addition to her beta agonist. What patient teaching is needed for RL to use these inhalers correctly?

Bibliography

Barnes PJ: The role of inflammation and anti-inflammatory medication in asthma, *Respir Med* 96(suppl A):S9-S15, 2002.

Blaiss MS: Efficacy, safety, and patient preference of inhaled nasal corticosteroids: a review of pertinent published data, *Allergy Asthma Proc* 22(6 suppl 1):S5-S10, 2001.

Jain N, Puranik M, Lodha R, et al: Long-term management of asthma, *Indian J Pediatr* 68(Suppl 4):S31-S41, 2001.

Kabra SK, Pandey RM, Singh R, et al: Ketotifen for asthma in children aged 5 to 15 years: a randomized placebo-controlled trial, *Ann Allergy Asthma Immunol* 85(1):46-52, 2000.

Kips JC, Tournoy KG, Pauwels RA: New anti-asthma therapies: suppression of the effect of interleukin (IL)-4 and IL-5, *Eur Respir J* 17(3):499-506, 2001.

Kowalski AF: Reducing asthma morbidity and mortality: cost containment strategies, *AAOHN J* 48(9):418-422, 2000.

MacDonald P: Managing asthma in adolescence, *Nurs Times* 97(38):40-41, 2001.

McAllister J: PN plus. Treatment options for asthma. *Pract Nurse* 22(3):43i-46iv, 50v-52vii, 54viii-55ix, 2001.

Miller AL: The etiologies, pathophysiology, and alternative/complementary treatment of asthma, *Altern Med Rev* 6(1):20-47, 2001.

National Institutes of Health, National Heart, Lung, and Blood Institute: National Asthma Education and Prevention Program expert panel report 2: *guidelines for the diagnosis and management of asthma*, NIH Publication No. 97-4051, Bethesda, MD, 1997, U.S. Department of Health and Human Services.

Papiris S, Kotanidou A, Malagari K, et al: Clinical review: severe asthma, *Crit Care* 6(1):30-44, 2002.

Quarton J: On demand use of beta₂-agonists led to better asthma control than regular use in moderate to severe asthma: a randomized controlled trial. Commentary on Richter B, Bender R, Berger M: Effects of on-demand beta₂-agonist inhalation in moderate-to-severe asthma: a randomized controlled trial, from *J Intern Med* 247:657-666, 2000; in *Evid Based Nurs* 4(1):14, 2001.

Reicin A, White R, Weinstein SF, et al: Montelukast, a leukotriene receptor antagonist, in combination with loratadine, a histamine receptor antagonist, in the treatment of chronic asthma, *Arch Intern Med* 160(16):2481-2488, 2551, 2000.

Slawson DC: Can patients with asthma well controlled on low doses of inhaled corticosteroids be switched to salmeterol monotherapy? Commentary on Lazarus SC, Boushey HA, Fahy JV, et al: Long-acting B₂-agonist monotherapy vs continued therapy with inhaled corticosteroids in patients with persistent asthma: a randomized controlled trial, from *JAMA* 285:2583-2593, 2001; in *Evid Based Pract* 4(8):9, insert 2p, 2001.

Somerville LL: Theophylline revisited, *Allergy Asthma Proc* 22(6):347-351, 2001.

Thoonen B, van Weel C: Self management in asthma care: professionals must rethink their role if they are to guide patients successfully, *BMJ* 321(7275):1482-1483, 2000.

Wales S, Harrod ME, Crisp J: The nurse's role in the child and family's adherence to asthma treatment, *Aust Nurs J* 9(1):suppl 1-4, 2001.

Internet Resources

American Lung Association. Available online at http://www.lungusa.org/asthma/.

Asthma and Allergy Foundation of America. Available online at http://www.aafa.org/.

National Heart Lung and Blood Institute. Available online at http://www.nhlbi.nih.gov/index.htm.

Sestini P, Renzoni E, Robinson S, et al: Short-acting beta₂ agonists for stable chronic obstructive pulmonary disease. In *The Cochrane Library*, Issue 2, Oxford, 2002, Update Software. Available online at http://www.cochranelibrary.com/enter/.

CHAPTER

53

Antihistamines

SHERRY F. QUEENER • KATHLEEN GUTIERREZ

 Visit **http://evolve.elsevier.com/Gutierrez/** for additional information.

KEY TERMS

Allergen, p. 869
Allergy, p. 869
Anaphylaxis, p. 868
Angioedema, p. 868
Antibodies, p. 869
Antigens, p. 870
Antihistamine, p. 872
Complement, p. 870
Eczema, p. 868
Histamine, p. 868
Purpura, p. 868
Rhinitis, p. 868
Urticaria, p. 868

OBJECTIVES

- Describe the localized and generalized allergic responses.
- Discuss the role of histamine in allergic responses.
- Describe the common adverse effects of antihistamines, including the anticholinergic effects.
- Describe the differences between first- and second-generation antihistamines.
- Develop a nursing care plan for a patient taking an antihistamine.

PATHOPHYSIOLOGY • Allergies

Histamine is a naturally occurring amine formed from the amino acid histidine. Histamine is found in mast cells, which are numerous in the lung and skin, and basophils, the counterparts of mast cells in the blood. The histamine released from mast cells causes many of the symptoms associated with allergic reactions. It is also found in the gastrointestinal (GI) tract, where histamine is a potent stimulant for the secretion of acid in the stomach. Histamine is also found in parts of the brain, where it is believed to function as a neurotransmitter. At present, the role of histamine in the brain is speculative but may involve regulating the level of arousal, biologic rhythms, and thermoregulation.

Histamine in mast cells and basophils is stored in granules as a complex with heparin and is released in response to antigens in anaphylactoid or atopic (Type I) reactions (see Physiology: Allergic Reactions below). The released histamine and other compounds alter capillary permeability and attract phagocytes (Figure 53-1).

Degranulation of mast cells and basophils is induced not only by antigens but also by many chemicals and venoms, including drugs and dyes that carry a positive charge, large molecules that occur in animal sera and dextran solutions, and venoms and enzymes that damage tissue. Once histamine is released, it is rapidly biotransformed into inactive compounds, but the effects may persist. Local and systemic allergic responses involving histamine include:

- **Anaphylaxis:** Systemic; onset usually indicated by a generalized itching and tingling sensation and a feeling of apprehension; profound hypotension leading to shock may follow; bronchioles become constricted, causing a choking sensation.
- **Angioedema:** Swelling caused by plasma leakage and blood vessel dilation in the skin or mucous membranes (giant hives).
- **Asthma:** Spasm of the bronchial smooth muscle (see Chapter 52).
- **Eczema:** Inflamed areas of skin.
- **Purpura:** Red spots on the skin caused by the leakage of blood from small vessels.
- **Rhinitis:** Inflammation of the nasal mucous membranes that allows fluid to escape.
- **Urticaria:** Hives, which are large wheals caused by leakage of plasma and are accompanied by severe itching.

Histamine released systemically causes anaphylaxis as a result of fluid loss from the vascular system, vasodilation, and severe constriction of the bronchioles. Local effects of histamine are also pronounced, as histamine exerts these same physiologic effects. Initially, a red spot reflects the dilation of the small blood vessels; as fluid leaks into the extravascular space, the bump, representing local edema, appears. Histamine also stimulates the contraction of smooth muscle, particularly the bronchial smooth muscle. When mast cells are degranulated in the lung, as in asthma, the airway is narrowed and patients have difficulty breathing.

The symptoms for which patients seek antihistamines tend to involve asthma, rhinitis, urticaria, and other skin reactions. These symptoms affect the 15% to 20% of the population that suffer from chronic or recurrent allergies. Asthma was discussed in Chapter 52.

There are several types of rhinitis, which is an acute or chronic inflammation of the mucous membranes of the nose. Rhinitis is found in 8% to 10% of the population younger than 20 years of age. Its cause involves interplay of allergens, viruses, and bacteria. Allergic rhinitis (i.e., hay fever) is most common. It occurs most often in families with atopy, a hereditary predisposition for allergy. The interaction of an antigen-IgE complex on the surface of mast cells produces the symptoms associated with allergic rhinitis. Fluid rapidly moves into the tissues of the nose, causing edema of nasal mucosa. In certain indi-

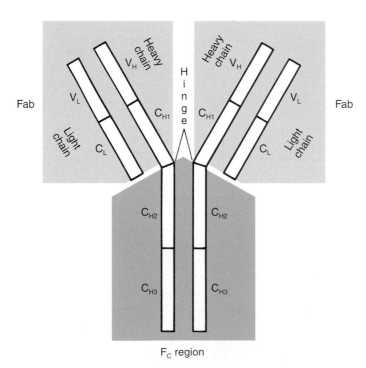

FIGURE 53-1 Schematic diagram of antibody molecule. Heavy and light chains composed of variable *(V$_H$, V$_L$)* regions and constant *(C$_H$, C$_L$)* regions. The *Fab* portions of the molecule are responsible for antigen binding, and the *F$_c$* portion mediates biologic activity.

viduals, antihistamines can help prevent the edematous reaction if the drug is taken before antigen exposure.

Acute episodes of allergic rhinitis tend to be seasonal, occurring for a few weeks at the same time each year. In North America, seasonal allergies are triggered by tree pollens in the spring; grasses in midsummer; and weeds in the fall, a period that typically lasts from August 15 until the first frost.

Chronic or perennial allergic rhinitis presents intermittently or continuously when the patient is exposed to allergens such as animal dander, wool, or certain foods. Exposure to dust mites and mold in upholstered furniture, mattresses, and pillows causes symptoms that may be worse in the morning. Perennial allergic rhinitis occurs half as often as seasonal rhinitis.

Nonallergic rhinitis produces symptoms similar to those of perennial allergic rhinitis. Allergy skin testing is not diagnostic for these patients and antihistamines are ineffective.

Urticaria is a vascular reaction of the skin marked by transient appearance of wheals that are redder or paler than the surrounding skin. It is often accompanied by itching. Twenty percent of the population has experienced acute urticaria at least once. However, at any given time, the prevalence is little more than one in 1000. Of these patients, about 66% have chronic urticaria. The majority of cases are acute and self-limited. Cases that persist for longer than 6 weeks are referred to as chronic urticaria. By far the most common causes of urticaria are drug reactions, stinging insect venoms, and allergenic extracts used in immunotherapy. Only persons with atopic allergy who are extremely sensitive are likely to react to ingested foods or contact with allergens through unbroken skin. Urticaria caused by an inhaled allergen is extremely rare.

Drug allergies characterized by urticaria can develop in susceptible individuals who have shown no previous adverse response to the first dose of a drug. However, a second or subsequent exposure to even a small amount of the drug elicits an exaggerated antigen-IgE response either locally or systemically. In some patients, even limited contact with the allergen can produce fatal systemic anaphylaxis. Drugs known for producing allergic responses include aspirin, chloramphenicol, penicillin, streptomycin, and sulfonamides. Contact urticaria can be a toxic effect of formaldehyde or dimethyl sulfoxide (DMSO), a penetrating solvent used to hasten absorption of drugs through the skin. Shellfish and certain foods (e.g., strawberries) may produce urticaria. Coffee and alcohol can aggravate urticaria although they do not cause it directly.

Histamine binds to three classes of receptors in the body: H_1, H_2, and H_3. The histamine that binds to H_2 receptors in the stomach stimulates acid production. The role of histamine in the stomach is discussed in Chapter 48. H_3 receptors are found in presynaptic sites in histamine-containing neurons in the brain and other sites. Antagonists or agonists for the H_3 receptor have not yet been developed as drugs, but studies of this receptor have clarified the role of histamine in the level of alertness. Histamine binding to H_1 receptors is responsible for increased capillary permeability, vasodilation, urticaria, bronchial constriction with wheezing and coughing, and increased muscle contraction in the gut. This chapter focuses on the role of antihistamines in relieving allergic reactions mediated through the H_1 receptor.

PHYSIOLOGY • Allergic Reactions

The role of the immune system is to recognize and inactivate foreign substances. However, after an individual develops an immune response to a substance, the reactivity may be altered so that there is a pathologic reaction when reexposed to the substance. Hypersensitivity, or **allergy,** refers to this pathologic, exaggerated reaction to a foreign substance. The chemical that sets off the reaction is called an **allergen.** Drugs as well as other chemicals can be allergens. Contrary to popular belief, allergic reactions do not occur with the first exposure to an allergen. An allergic reaction occurs only after a second or subsequent exposure.

Antibodies, the soluble mediators of humoral immunity, are specialized proteins called immunoglobulins. The immunoglobulin molecule is comprised of two light chains and two heavy chains (see Figure 53-1).

The light chain is made up of a variable region *(V)* and a constant region *(C)*. Heavy chains contain three or four constant regions and the variable region. Each variable portion of the immunoglobulin molecule includes three hypervariable regions, which vary widely in amino acid composition. The combination of these hypervariable regions makes up the antibody-combining site of the immunoglobulin molecule. This portion of the molecule binds the antigen against which the antibody was generated. Each antibody molecule has two combining sites. There are five classes of immunoglobulins: IgA, IgD, IgE, IgG, and IgM. Five different constant regions define these major immunoglobulin classes, which are discussed in more detail in Chapter 35. IgD, IgE, and IgG are monomeric, each composed of one antibody molecule. IgA is composed of two antibody mol-

---

TABLE 53-1		

Major Classes of Immunoglobulins

Class	Distribution	Biologic Properties
IgA	Intravascular and secretions	Most common antibody in secretions, where it protects mucous membranes; bactericidal in presence of lysozyme; efficient antiviral antibody.
IgD	On surface of B lymphocytes; trace in serum	Serves as antigen-specific receptor on B cells; may be involved in differentiation of B lymphocytes.
IgE	On basophils and mast cells; in saliva and nasal secretions	Mediates hypersensitivity and allergic reactions; protects against parasite infections.
IgG	Intravascular and extravascular	Responsible for most responses to antigens, including activation of complement, sensitization of target cells for destruction by killer cells, neutralization of toxins and viruses, and immobilization of bacteria. Can pass through placenta.
IgM	Mostly intravascular	First type of antibody produced during primary immune response; activates complement as well; efficient agglutinating antibodies; natural isohemagglutinins.

ecules, and IgM is composed of five. A protein called the J chain joins the five basic molecules that make up the IgM molecule. A secretory component, synthesized by epithelial cells, connects the two IgA molecules that compose the dimer. Table 53-1 summarizes the immunoglobulin classes and their functions.

Antigens are large molecules, usually proteins that trigger the formation of an antibody and bind specifically to that antibody. Because drugs and other allergens are ordinarily not proteins, they do not act directly as antigens, but they can combine with endogenous proteins to form potent antigens.

The **complement** system is a group of enzymes found in serum that work together to "complement" the action of antibodies in destroying antigens. The major functions of the complement system include mediating inflammatory responses and opsonization, or coating, of antigenic particles (including microorganisms). The result is damage to the membrane of the microorganism, which in turn often results in lysis. The complement system is a classic enzyme cascade in which a small stimulus can be amplified to activate large amounts of complement.

The classic and the alternate pathway can activate complement. The pathways share many components but differ in the ways they become activated. Antigen-antibody complexes activate the classic pathway. The alternate pathway is activated by suitable surfaces or molecules, including cell walls of some bacteria, cell walls of yeast, endotoxin derived from cell walls of gram-negative bacteria, and aggregated IgA. Several steps in the complement cascade result in the release of a fragment of some of the proteins of the complement system. Some

of these small molecules act as chemotaxins or anaphylatoxins. *Chemotaxins* cause phagocytic cells to migrate from an area where there is less chemotaxin to an area of higher concentration. *Anaphylatoxins* cause mast cell degranulation, smooth muscle contraction, and increased capillary permeability. The end result of complement action is to activate the lytic pathway, leading to the formation of the membrane attack complex, a series of proteins with detergent properties that produce "holes" in the target cell membrane, resulting in lysis of the target cell.

Allergens, antigens, antibodies, complement, and various immune cells interact to cause a variety of allergic reactions. Allergic reactions may be classified as anaphylactoid or atopic (type I), cytotoxic (type II), autoimmune (type III), and cell-mediated (type IV); these types of reaction were first introduced in Chapter 1 (see Table 1-2). This classification system is based on which parts of the immune system are involved in producing the reaction. The first three of these classes are referred to as immediate hypersensitivity reactions because the allergic responses occur within minutes to hours. These responses are initiated by interaction of an antibody and an antigen.

Type I hypersensitivity refers to the release of histamine from basophils or tissue mast cells. The antibody is IgE bound to the surface of the basophil or tissue mast cell, and the antigen induces cross-linking of the IgE molecules, a process that leads to the release of histamine and other proinflammatory chemical mediators (Figure 53-2). Type I hypersensitivity is characteristic of asthma, hay fever, and hives. The most extreme reaction is classic systemic anaphylaxis, a generalized release of

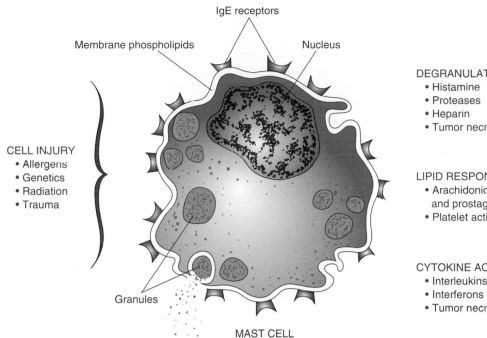

FIGURE 53-2 Immunologic mechanism underlying release of histamine from mast cells. Antibodies of immunoglobulin E (IgE) class are bound to surface of mast cells. Binding of antigen to IgE triggers degranulation of mast cell, releasing histamine and other mediators. Histamine is responsible for many allergy and asthma symptoms.

histamine leading to a profound fall in blood pressure and shock, as well as a constriction of the airways, which can be fatal if not treated immediately. Drugs that can cause type I reactions include penicillins, cephalosporins, aspirin, and iodides. Other common causes of type I hypersensitivity include insect stings and antitoxins prepared from animal serum.

Type II hypersensitivity arises from an antigen on a cell surface that is complexed by IgG or IgM antibody. This complex may lead to tissue destruction through cell lysis by complement or phagocytosis. Examples are hemolytic responses during blood transfusions and the hemolytic response of an Rh-positive fetus to an Rh-negative mother. In these cases an antibody against a foreign red blood cell membrane antigen binds to the red blood cell and initiates complement-mediated destruction of the red blood cell. Some complexes lead to altered cell function without cell destruction such as in Graves' disease, where the end result is hyperthyroidism. External chemicals including drugs can also bind to a red blood cell or other tissue membrane and act as an antigen, leading to type II hypersensitivity. Such drug reactions include hemolytic anemia induced by methyldopa and thrombocytopenic purpura induced by quinidine. Examples of autoimmune diseases

involving type II hypersensitivity include autoimmune hemolytic anemia, autoimmune thrombocytopenia, Goodpasture's syndrome, pemphigus, pernicious anemia, myasthenia gravis, and Graves' disease.

Type III hypersensitivity, or immune complex disease, is characterized antigen-antibody complexes that become deposited in tissues such as the kidney, skin, and serous membranes and activate complement, leading to cell destruction. The reaction leads to increased vascular permeability and the recruitment of neutrophils. Depending on the location, the result can be skin rashes, glomerulonephritis, or arthritis. Normally, immune complexes are cleared by macrophages in the spleen and elsewhere. Serum sickness is a generalized immune complex reaction. Examples of immune complex diseases include systemic lupus erythematosus, polyarteritis nodosa, and poststreptococcal glomerulonephritis. Stevens-Johnson syndrome is a life-threatening form of serum sickness involving many organ systems. One of the most common triggers of this response is a sulfonamide antibacterial drug.

In contrast to the immediate hypersensitivity reactions, type IV reactions are delayed; T cells, rather than antibodies mediate type IV reactions. The reaction is seen 2 or 3 days after reexposure to the antigen, not minutes to hours. The classic delayed hypersensitivity reaction is the tuberculin test in which the test antigen is applied to the skin and the reaction read after 2 to 3 days. In delayed hypersensitivity the sensitized T cells release cytokines that recruit macrophages and neutrophils, which ultimately produce widespread tissue damage. Delayed hypersensitivity is a reaction to infections caused by intracellular pathogens such as *Mycobacterium tuberculosis* or Leishmania species. Contact dermatitis is a common delayed hypersensitivity response to a variety of compounds, including such agents as poison ivy.

Any of the undesirable immunologic responses described above are possible with drugs. In practice, drug allergy is a term that is often used imprecisely to describe unusual responses or toxicity to a drug arising from genetic variations in the patient or from unknown causes (idiosyncratic reactions). Documented allergic reactions account for as few as 10% of all adverse reactions to drugs.

DRUG CLASS • Antihistamines (Histamine H₁ Receptor Antagonists)

First-Generation Antihistamine

⚠ **diphenhydramine (Benadryl, others)**

Second-Generation Antihistamine

⚠ **fexofenadine (Allegra)**

For other members of this class, see Table 53-2.

MECHANISM OF ACTION

The term **antihistamine** refers to drugs that block any histamine receptor. In this chapter, the term antihistamine refers to drugs that specifically block the H_1 receptors. Drugs that block H_2 receptors are covered in Chapter 48.

TABLE 53-2

Selected H₁ Receptor Antagonists

Class or Generic Name	Brand Name	Route/ Availability	Indications Primary	Indications Other	Duration of Action
Alkylamines					
First Generation					
brompheniramine	Veltane	po/Rx	Allergies	—	4-6 hr
	Bromanate, Dimetane-DX	po/Rx	Allergies*	Colds*	4-6 hr
	Dimetapp, Drixoral	po/OTC	Allergies*	Colds*	4-6 hr
chlorpheniramine	generic	po/Rx	Allergies	—	4-8 hr
	Tussionex	po/Rx	Allergies*	Colds*	Extended release†
	Chlor-trimeton	po/OTC	Allergies	—	Extended release†
	Contac, Demazin	po/OTC	Allergies*	Colds*	Extended release†
dexbrompheniramine	Disophrol, Drixoral	po/OTC	Allergies*	Colds*	Extended release†
dexchlorpheniramine	Mylaramine, Polaramine	po/Rx	Allergies	—	4-8 hr
pheniramine	Naphcon-A, Visine-A	Eye/OTC	Allergies*	—	4-6 hr
triprolidine	Corphed, Triacin-C	po/Rx	Allergies*	Colds*	—
Second Generation					
acrivastine	Semprex-D	po/Rx	Allergies*	Colds*	4-6 hr
Ethanolamines					
First Generation					
clemastine	Tavist	po/Rx, OTC	Allergies	—	12 hr
	Tavist Allergy Sinus	po/OTC	Allergies*	Colds*	12 hr
bromodiphenhydramine	Ambenyl, Bromanyl	po/Rx	Allergies*	Colds*	4-6 hr
diphenhydramine	generic	po/Rx	Allergies	Antidyskinetic; sedative/ hypnotic	4-8 hr

*In combinations with decongestants, analgesics, and/or cough suppressants.
†Extended-release preparations have longer duration of action.

TABLE 53-2

Selected H₁ Receptor Antagonists—cont'd

Class or Generic Name	Brand Name	Route/ Availability	Indications Primary	Indications Other	Duration of Action
Ethanolamines—cont'd *First Generation—cont'd*					
	Benadryl	Injection/Rx	Allergies	Antiemetic; antivertigo	4-8 hr
dimenhydrinate	generic	Injection/Rx	Antivertigo	Antiemetic	4-6 hr
	Dramamine	po/OTC	Antivertigo	Antiemetic	4-6 hr
doxylamine	Unisom	po/OTC	Sedative/ hypnotic	Allergies	6-8 hr
Ethylenediamines *First Generation*					
antazoline	Vasocon-A	Eye/OTC	Allergies*	—	4-6 hr
pyrilamine	generic	po/Rx	Allergies	—	—
	Prefrin-A	Eye/Rx	Allergies	—	—
tripelennamine	PBZ	po/Rx	Allergies	—	4-6 hr
	PBZ-SR	po/Rx	Allergies	—	Extended release†
Phenothiazines *First Generation*					
promethazine	Phenergan	po/Rx	Allergies	Antivertigo	4-6 hr
	Phenergan	Injection/Rx	Sedation	Analgesia adjunct	4-6 hr
	Promethacon	Rectal	Sedation	Antiemetic	4-6 hr
Phthalazinones *Second Generation*					
azelastine	Astelin	Nasal/Rx	Allergies	—	12-24 hr
	Optivar	Eye/Rx	Allergies	—	12 hr
Piperidines *First Generation*					
azatadine	Optimine	po/Rx	Allergies	—	8-12 hr
	Trinalin	po/Rx	Allergies*	Cold*	Extended release†
cyproheptadine	Periactin	po/Rx	Allergies	Appetite stimulant; vascular headaches	8 hr
Second Generation					
desloratadine	Clarinex	po/Rx	Allergies	—	24 hr
fexofenadine	Allegra	po/Rx	Allergies	Antiasthmatic	12 hr
	Allegra-D	po/Rx	Allergies*	—	Extended release†
loratadine	Claritin	po/Rx	Allergies	Antiasthmatic	24 hr
	Claritin-D	po/Rx	Allergies*	—	Extended release†
Piperazines *First Generation*					
hydroxyzine	Atarax, Vistaril	po/Rx	Allergies	Antianxiety; antiemetic; sedative-hypnotic	4-6 hr
meclizine	Antivert	po/Rx	Antivertigo	Antiemetic	12-24 hr
	Bonine	po/OTC	Antivertigo	Antiemetic	24 hr
Second Generation					
cetirizine	Zyrtec	po/Rx	Allergies	Antiasthmatic	12-24 hr
	Zyrtec-D	po/Rx	Allergies*	—	12-24 hr

Antihistamines prevent the action of histamine at several key sites in the body and thus block allergic reactions. These drugs block H_1 receptors in nerve endings and in capillaries; as a result, fluid does not escape from the capillaries, edema does not develop, and redness and itching are prevented. Although antihistamines do inhibit the constrictor effects of histamine on smooth muscle, these drugs are not sufficient alone to control bronchoconstriction induced by allergic mechanisms because leukotrienes and other mediators are also involved (see Chapter 52).

First-generation antihistamines may have dual actions in the CNS, but the most common effect is sedation. The ethanolamine class of antihistamines is actually used clinically for their sedative/hypnotic effects (see Table 53-2), but for other first-generation drugs this action is usually an unwanted adverse reaction.

The first-generation of H_1 receptor antagonist drugs are characterized by actions not only on H_1 receptors but also on muscarinic receptors. The so-called anticholinergic effects of these drugs produce many of the common adverse reactions of the class (i.e., dry mouth, reduced fluidity of mucus, and urinary retention). Anticholinergic effects in the CNS may account for the antiemetic actions of certain antihistamines, because the antiemetic action seems to correlate with the strength of the anticholinergic effect of the drug. For example, promethazine is one of the best antiemetic antihistamines and also has the strongest anticholinergic actions.

Four second-generation antihistamines are now available for use to systemically control allergies: loratadine, fexofenadine, cetirizine, and desloratadine. These drugs block H_1 receptors the same as the traditional antihistamines, but are less likely to produce the major adverse reaction of sedation. This difference is because the second-generation drugs do not cross the blood-brain barrier in sufficient concentrations to affect histamine receptors in the brain. In addition to reducing the likelihood of sedation, these drugs have fewer anticholinergic effects. In addition to these drugs, azelastine is a second-generation H_1 antagonist that also inhibits mast cell histamine release (see Table 53-2). Azelastine is used intranasally or in the eyes.

USES
Antihistamines for Allergies

Antihistamines are primarily effective in decreasing the discomfort of acute allergic reactions that involve the upper respiratory system (e.g., hay fever) or the skin (e.g., hives). Hay fever is most successfully treated when therapy is begun while the pollen count is still low. Sneezing, runny nose, and swollen eyes are reduced in more than 70% of patients. Antihistamines reduce the swelling and itching (pruritus) of urticaria and related

conditions. Many of the older antihistamines are available over the counter, but the newer generation drugs are available by prescription.

Antihistamines do not prevent or treat colds, although they are often combined with a decongestant or other ingredients in many OTC and prescription cold remedies (see Table 53-2). Because most antihistamines have anticholinergic actions, they can dry up a runny nose and appear to relieve the symptoms of a cold. However, the drying action may be counterproductive to the body's own mechanisms for ridding itself of the damage produced by the cold virus. The drying caused by many antihistamines can make mucus more viscous and hence more difficult to clear from the sinuses and lungs.

Antihistamines have traditionally not been used to treat asthma because substances other than histamine are responsible for the prolonged bronchiole constriction characteristic of asthma. In addition, the potential for antihistamines to dry out and thicken mucus can be detrimental to the patient with asthma. However, because antihistamines may prevent or reduce asthma symptoms triggered by allergic rhinitis, there is an increasing trend to use antihistamines in certain patients with asthma. In that regard, the second-generation, nonsedating antihistamines (cetirizine, fexofenadine and loratadine) are the preferred option for most people because they have minimal or no anticholinergic effects.

Antihistamines as Sedatives

Sedation is a common adverse effect of antihistamines. Many OTC sleeping aids use a first-generation antihistamine as the active ingredient. The antihistamines approved as sleep-aid ingredients are doxylamine succinate and diphenhydramine. Hydroxyzine is an antihistamine often used as an antianxiety agent (see Chapter 17).

Antihistamines as Antiemetics and Antiparkinsonism Agents. Selected antihistamines have other uses. Some antihistamines prevent nausea and vomiting, particularly from motion sickness and vertigo. These antihistamines are discussed in Chapter 50. Antihistamines that suppress the tremors of parkinsonism are discussed in Chapter 23.

PHARMACOKINETICS

Antihistamines are generally well absorbed orally. Their onset of action is typically observed in 15 to 30 minutes and lasts for 4 to 6 hours. Timed-release preparations are active for 8 to 12 hours. The second-generation antihistamines have slightly slower onsets of action but have longer durations (see Table 53-2).

Antihistamines are distributed well throughout the body, but the older drugs have not been as well studied as some of the newer ones. For example, it is not known how these drugs distribute to the skin or how long they persist at tissue sites. Nevertheless, it is known that for many patients, control of skin reactions persists well beyond the time when drug can be measured in plasma. First-generation antihistamines are biotransformed into inactive compounds by the liver and kidneys. These drugs also induce liver metabolic enzymes, which create the potential for strong drug interactions.

Second-generation antihistamines do not distribute to the brain as readily as first-generation drugs and the newer drugs have a more variable biotransformation. Loratadine is biotransformed by the liver and excreted in urine and feces, mostly as metabolites. Cetirizine relies more on renal excretion than other antihistamines, with over half of the drug being excreted in an active form in urine.

ADVERSE REACTIONS AND CONTRAINDICATIONS

Although the antihistamines are so named because they specifically compete with histamine for the H₁ receptors, they have other pharmacologic properties. Antihistamines also act as muscarinic antagonists. The main secondary action of these drugs is, therefore, an anticholinergic (antimuscarinic) or atropine-like action. This action is the origin of adverse effects such as inhibition of secretions, blurred vision, urinary retention, fast heart rate (tachycardia), and constipation. Because of their atropine-like effects, antihistamines should be used with caution in patients with glaucoma, hyperthyroidism, cardiovascular disease, or hypertension. In the CNS the anticholinergic effect can cause insomnia, tremors, nervousness, and irritability. These effects are particularly predominant in children. Sedation and drowsiness, the central antihistaminic

effects, are more common in adults. Tolerance to the sedative effects usually develops after several days of treatment. The spectrum of antihistaminic and anticholinergic properties depends on the drug and the dosage as well as the individual. These adverse effects are more likely with first-generation antihistamines.

In addition to the adverse effects common to most antihistamines, azelastine nasal spray can also leave a bitter taste (dysgeusia).

Antihistamines are contraindicated for nursing mothers because the drugs are secreted in milk. Antihistamines taken by young children can cause paradoxical excitement, whereas older adult patients tend to be more sensitive to the sedative actions.

TOXICITY

Antihistamine overdose can cause CNS depression or stimulation, the latter being more common in adults receiving very high doses of the drugs or in children. CNS stimulation produces nervousness, insomnia, restless behavior, or, on rare occasions, convulsions. Atropine-like symptoms (flushed skin and fixed, dilated pupils) are also prominent in overdose with first-generation drugs.

INTERACTIONS

The main drug interaction associated with antihistamines is the additive depression of the CNS when taken with alcohol, hypnotics, sedatives, antipsychotics, anxiolytic drugs, or opioid analgesics. Additive anticholinergic effects may be observed with tricyclic antidepressants, antipsychotics, atropine and other antimuscarinic drugs. Most manufacturers recommend that H₁ antagonists not be used within 2 weeks of therapy with a MAOI (monoamine oxidase inhibitor).

APPLICATION TO PRACTICE

ASSESSMENT
History of Present Illness

Patient history is the most important component in the evaluation of a patient with a suspected or confirmed allergy. Ask about the frequency and severity of attacks, precipitating or alleviating factors, drugs used, and whether they are taken regularly or intermittently. Elicit known sources of allergies, the patient's status between attacks, and any restrictions in the activities of daily living.

Patients with seasonal allergic rhinitis complain of sneezing, nasal or ocular pruritus, bilateral clear watery or mucoid nasal secretions, and nasal congestion. Patients may also complain of pruritus of the upper palate and ears, and dry, scratchy, erythematous conjunctiva. These symptoms are related to elevations of specific

pollen counts. Symptoms of dust and mold allergies are less distinct in that the nasal congestion and clear drainage frequently occur without sneezing or pruritus but vary significantly throughout the year.

A careful search of environmental factors should be conducted. The patient should be questioned in detail about the home environment, including its location, type of heating, type and quality of construction, type of insulation, and humidity. The nature of furnishings (e.g., upholstered furniture), the presence of plants, carpeting, draperies and bedding, pets and their habits, housecleaning methods, and cigarette smoking should also be noted. Variations in symptoms with changes in seasons and with changes in location should be carefully recorded. Ask also about the work environment and note exposure to chemical irritants or sensitizers, physical demands, and job stressors. Information about the type of clothing worn and dietary history should not be overlooked. Clothing and food are potential antigens, particularly in children. Smokers have increased nasal congestion and thick postnasal drainage, and may be predisposed to sinusitis.

A history of pruritic wheals lasting several hours is typical of urticaria. A history of a swollen tongue or lips and epigastric discomfort may indicate GI involvement. The presence of wheezing or pharyngeal swelling suggests an anaphylactoid reaction.

Health History

Take time to identify previous allergic problems the patient has had and any allergies in close family members. This information is particularly helpful in providing support for the diagnosis of an atopic disease. The onset of symptoms in childhood is typical of allergic disease. The onset of symptoms during adulthood, however, does not rule out atopy.

Record the patient's drug history, especially any prescription, OTC drugs, or herbs used to treat present or past symptoms. Information regarding the use of inhaled cocaine or nasal decongestants should be carefully noted. These drugs have been associated with allergy as well as rhinitis medicamentosa.

Lifespan Considerations

Perinatal. A number of changes take place in the respiratory tract during pregnancy. The changes are mediated by the enlarging uterus, increased oxygen demands, and the respiratory stimulant effect of progesterone. There is also an estrogen-induced hyperemia of the nasopharynx mucosa with concurrent edema and increased production of mucus. These changes lead to a feeling of stuffiness and an increased tendency for epistaxis (nosebleeds). Pregnant women should be warned of this normal change and advised against using OTC nasal sprays to alleviate the symptoms. However, normal saline nasal spray may be helpful in reducing some of the discomfort.

Pediatric. Assessment of symptoms in the child is much like that in the adult but also includes a feeding history for a very young child, with attention to the intake of cow's milk, eggs, and wheat. The stability of family relationships and the stress level in the home should not be overlooked. Information about the child's toys, bedroom, and other rooms where the child spends waking hours should be noted. The child's exposure level to baby-sitters, relatives, day care, and school environments is included. The presence or absence of symptoms in all of these areas should be noted.

Older Adults. It is difficult to determine whether losses in somesthetic sensitivity can be attributed to changes of aging itself or to disease states that occur with greater frequency in older adults. Local sinus and respiratory tract factors and comorbid diseases probably play a larger role in the allergic response than age-related changes in immunity. Clinically, older adults are more susceptible to respiratory tract and other infections and are also likely to purchase OTC drugs for self-treatment.

Cultural/Social Considerations

Consumers purchase many of the drugs used in the treatment of allergies and asthma over the counter. They are easily accessible to almost all persons, easy to use, and in many cases generally effective. By using OTC drugs to treat allergies, patients save a trip to the health care provider and the associated costs of a visit (see the Case Study: Seasonal Rhinitis with Secondary Rhinitis Medicamentosa).

Physical Examination

Examine the conjunctiva for erythema and the eyes for tearing and photophobia. Edema of the lids provides supportive evidence of an allergic mechanism. Transillumination and palpation of the sinuses, a pharyngeal examination for erythema and discharge, the ears for evidence of otitis, and palpitation of cervical nodes for adenopathy is included in the exam.

The nose is often overlooked or is given only a cursory examination. Nasal mucosa should be inspected for evidence of erythema, pallor, atrophy, edema, crusting, and discharge. The presence of polyps (not to be confused with the turbinates), erosions, and septal perforations or deviations should be noted. A pale, boggy appearance to the mucosa is allegedly a classic sign of allergic disease, but erythema sometimes occurs in allergy, and its presence certainly does not rule out sinusitis. Sinusitis may be present at the time of the examination. Mucopurulent discharge from the nares or seen in the posterior pharynx raises the possibility of sinusitis. Tenderness of the maxillary, ethmoid, or frontal sinus regions on palpation helps support a diagnosis of sinusitis.

A general respiratory examination includes assessment of the rate and character of respirations and skin color. The lungs should be examined during forced expiration, which may bring out asthmatic wheezing. Abnormal breathing patterns (e.g., rate below 12 or above 24, dyspnea, cough, orthopnea, wheezing, stridor) indicate respiratory distress. Severe respiratory distress is characterized by tachypnea, dyspnea, use of accessory muscles, and hypoxia. Early signs of hypoxia include restlessness, confusion, anxiety, increased blood pressure, and pulse. Late signs include cyanosis and decreased blood pressure and pulse. Hypoxemia is confirmed when arterial blood gas analyses demonstrate decreased partial pressure of oxygen (PaO_2).

A description and location of any skin lesions should be recorded. Urticarial lesions range in size from 0.5-cm papules to 20-cm plaques. The lesions can be circular, annular, or serpiginous in shape. Central clearing is common, and any area of the body can be involved.

A child with atopy may have dark circles under the eyes (allergic shiners) and have a transverse crease above the tip of the nose from frequent upward nose rubbing (allergic salute).

Laboratory Testing

Few general laboratory tests are appropriate for the patient with an allergic disorder. A nasal or sputum smear may be examined for the presence of eosinophils. Blood eosinophilia is helpful if it is present, but its absence does not exclude allergic disease. The measurement of total serum IgE is costly and generally of limited value. In some cases, patients with acute respiratory illness may have arterial blood gases drawn, a pulse oximetry, and pulmonary function testing.

Allergy testing can be helpful in patients who have significant symptoms. RAST (radioallergosorbent test) is a serum test that determines the amount of IgG immunoglobulin present against a specific allergen or allergen group. Prick or scratch testing measures clinical response but is not diagnostic.

Skin testing is selective based on clues provided by the patient's history. In adults, testing is limited to pollens, house dust, feathers, animal danders, and mold spores. If the patient's history warrants, skin tests to some foods may also be performed. Food testing is more useful in young children than in adults.

GOALS OF THERAPY

Treatment goals for the patient with an allergy centers on relief of symptoms. Minimizing exposure to external trigger factors and ensuring compliance with treatment plans are also important objectives.

INTERVENTION

Approaches to cost containment in the treatment of rhinitis consists of a first-generation antihistamine and switching to a nonsedating preparation only if daytime sedation becomes a problem. (Daytime sedation occurs in 10% to 25% of patients.) Tolerance to sedative effects is common. Substituting an inexpensive, sedating drug for the nighttime dose of a twice-daily preparation may help. Some degree of psychomotor impairment may occur with daytime use of a first-generation drug, even without noticeable sedation. Second-generation antihistamines (except for azatadine) are 15 to 30 times more expensive than many first-generation preparations (al-

though not all first-generation drugs are inexpensive). Inhaled cromolyn and aerosol solutions are generally more expensive than nedocromil (see Chapter 52). Corticosteroids, whether for nasal use or inhalation, are generally consistent in price with antiallergy drugs.

Identifying factors that cause allergic symptoms and strategies for elimination or avoidance of those factors provides the most satisfactory treatment regimen.

Administration

Anaphylaxis requires immediate diagnosis and treatment, usually with 1:1000 epinephrine injected subcutaneously or intramuscularly (see Chapter 12) followed by parenteral antihistamines. Supportive care is symptomatic and based on rapid assessment of the cardiovascular and respiratory response.

Management of the less acute allergic response is not an emergency and not all patients respond to drugs in the same fashion. If one drug is not effective in relieving symptoms or if excessive sedation or GI distress results, another drug from a different class may be tried. Table 53-3 provides a comparison of the various antihistamines effects.

Antihistamines prevent nasal congestion but do not relieve existing congestion. Thus, they are more effective if they are taken before symptoms occur. Sensitive patients should use antihistamines regularly just before and during the seasonal exposures, even when symptoms are absent. Furthermore, because these drugs may thicken respiratory tract secretions, making them more difficult to expel, the patient should be encouraged to drink 2000 to 3000 mL of fluids daily (if it is not contraindicated).

Oral antihistamines are given with meals to minimize GI distress. Read drug labels carefully. Some antihistamines are for intramuscular use only and should not be used for intravenous administration. Use a large muscle mass for an intramuscular injection of an antihistamine. Record and rotate injection sites. Aspirate before injecting the drug to prevent inadvertent intravenous administration. Warn the patient that intramuscular injection of antihistamine may burn as the drug is injected.

Patients taking first-generation antihistamines should be monitored for excessive drowsiness during the first few days of therapy. Concurrent use of sedating antihistamines with other CNS depressant drugs should be avoided. If a drug with a long half-life is used, administering the entire daily dose at bedtime can minimize daytime sedation.

Management of antihistamine overdose includes maintaining the airway and treating hypotension. In children a high temperature is common, which can be reversed with ice packs and sponge baths. If the antihistamine is not a phenothiazine, vomiting is induced, gastric lavage is carried out, and cathartics are used to empty the

TABLE 53-3

Comparison of Antihistamine Drug Effects

Class or Drug Name	H_1 Receptor Specificity	Anticholinergic Effects	Performance Impairment	Relieves Sneezing and Rhinorrhea	Relieves Nasal Congestion	Relieves Ocular Symptoms and Provides Rapid Allergy Relief
Single-Entity First-Generation Antihistamines						
alkylamines	Effective	Moderate	Mild	Yes	No	Yes
ethanolamines	Moderate	Significant	Marked			
ethylenediamines	Effective	Variable–mild	Variable			
phenothiazines	Potent	Marked	Marked			
piperidines	Effective	Moderate	Slight			
Single-Entity Second-Generation Antihistamines						
cetirizine	Moderate	Little or none	Little or none			
fexofenadine	Moderate to high	Little or none	Little or none			
loratadine	Moderate to high	Little or none	Little or none			
Combination Antihistamine and Decongestant						
First generation	Moderate to potent	Mild to marked	Yes	Yes	Yes	Yes
Second generation	Moderate to high	Mild to marked	Yes	Yes	Yes	Yes
Related Drugs						
Antiallergy drugs	Moderate	NA	No	No	No	No
Topical nasal corticosteroids	No antihistamine action	No	No	Yes	Yes	No

GI tract of remaining drug. Vomiting should not be induced with phenothiazines because they can cause uncoordinated movements of the head and neck, which could cause aspiration of vomitus. Antihistamines that are phenothiazine derivatives are identified in Table 53-1.

Education

The most important aspect of allergy care is patient education. Patients must understand the nature of their disease and how to prevent and treat symptoms. Avoiding allergens has important clinical significance in limiting the severity of the disease. Teach the patient to wipe the face with a cool cloth frequently throughout the day to remove dust and pollen from around facial features. Brush the hair thoroughly before going to bed to remove the day's dust and pollen, and wash the hands frequently and thoroughly. Patients should be told to stop smoking and to avoid other irritants or precipitating factors. This aspect is often overlooked when teaching patients who have mild allergies.

Appropriate avoidance procedures relate to the responsible allergens and differ for seasonal and perennial disease. For seasonal allergic rhinitis, patients should be advised to refrain from long walks in the woods during pollination periods. Remaining indoors with the windows closed when symptoms are severe and the pollen count is high (e.g., hot, windy, sunny days) helps reduce exposure to allergens. Some patients find air conditioners helpful, but the filter does little to remove pollen from the air. Air conditioning only makes staying indoors with the windows closed on a hot day more tolerable. The outside air intake on the conditioner should be kept closed to avoid bringing in more pollinated air. If ragweed is a problem, daisies, dahlias, and chrysanthemums should not be kept indoors because these flowers are cousins to ragweed. Minimizing dust accumulation in the bedroom and avoiding irritants such as tobacco smoke, chemical vapors, and strong perfumes lessens symptoms.

Control of perennial allergic rhinitis demands specific attention to allergens in the home. Housecleaning with a damp mop two to three times a week reduces dust. Dacron or polyester pillows should replace feather pillows. Mattresses should be covered. Areas where mold can collect (e.g., damp basements and furniture) should be cleaned thoroughly. Furnishings made of synthetic fabrics minimize dust collection and are preferable to cotton and wool. Humidification reduces dust. Patients with allergies to mold should not keep African violets or geraniums indoors. In some cases pets may need to be removed from the home if allergic symptoms become disabling. Merely keeping the pet out of the home does not sufficiently reduce dander in the air.

Instruct patients to take antihistamines only as prescribed or as instructed on the patient package insert contained in OTC preparations. Have the patient take oral doses with meals or a light snack to decrease gastric irritation. Advise the patient to swallow sustained-release formulations whole without crushing or chewing. Scored tablets may be broken before swallowing. Capsules may be opened and contents poured into soft food for ease in taking. The patient should chew gum formulations for 15 minutes or longer (see manufacturer's literature). Review administration technique for patients using suppository formulations. Instruct the patient about the correct technique for using antihistamine nasal sprays and inhalers (see Chapter 52). Teach the patient correct intramuscular administration technique if this route is prescribed for self-administration.

Teach the patient that aerosolized drug canisters should be stored with the valve pointed downward and to replace the canister every 3 months, even if it is not completely empty. Patients keep inhalers in their purse or jacket pockets for extended periods, many times long after the drug has expired. By replacing the inhaler every 3 months, the patient is assured that active drug will be available when it is needed. Additionally, the delivery device of inhaled formulations should be cleaned after its use to minimize unnecessary repeated exposure to bacteria that may collect in the device. Proper cleaning also helps maintain patency of the device.

Advise patients to avoid driving or operating machinery until the sedative effects of antihistamines are known or the period of drowsiness has worn off. Alcohol and other drugs should not be used without first contacting the health care provider because the combined CNS depressant effects can cause excessive respiratory depression and death. As with all drugs, antihistamines should be stored out of the reach of small children to avoid accidental ingestion.

The anticholinergic properties of some antihistamines limit their use in patients with prostatic hypertrophy, those with a predisposition to urinary retention, or those who have narrow-angle glaucoma. Individuals with these disorders should be told to contact their health care provider before using an antihistamine.

Teach the patient to consume 2000 to 3000 mL of fluids daily to help thin secretions and make them easier to remove. They should also be advised to maintain dental hygiene by brushing and flossing. The diminished salivary flow that results from the anticholinergic effects of many antihistamines contributes to dental caries and gum disease. Regular dental check-ups should be advised. Using ice, sugarless gum, or hard candy can minimize mouth dryness.

Warn patients that an antihistamine is often included in prescription and OTC combination products for the common cold. However, they do not relieve cold symptoms any better than a placebo. Moreover, their use exposes the patient to adverse effects without therapeutic advantage.

Patients who are using a corticosteroid (see Chapter 52) or an antihistamine nasal spray concurrently with a decongestant nasal spray (see Chapter 54) should be taught to use the decongestant 5 to 15 minutes before the other drug. Using the decongestant first causes shrinkage of mucous membranes, whereby the other drugs can better reach deeper nasal passages. The patient should be taught to blow the nose in advance of nasal drug administration so as to not place the drug on the surface of secretions. The patient should also be advised to contact the health care provider if allergic symptoms do not improve within 1 month or if nasal discharge becomes purulent.

EVALUATION

The principal outcomes of antihistaminic therapy are based on the reason the drugs were used. Treatment effectiveness is demonstrated most often through patients' verbal statements. If the antihistamine was used for seasonal or perennial allergic symptoms, symptoms are relieved. If it was specifically used for its sedative characteristics, drowsiness or sleep resulted.

When conservative methods fail to control allergic symptoms the patient should be referred to an allergist. An allergist may be of help when an allergic cause cannot be distinguished from vasomotor rhinitis and when the antigen or antigens must be identified for management purposes.

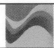

CASE STUDY

Seasonal Rhinitis with Secondary Rhinitis Medicamentosa

ASSESSMENT

HISTORY OF PRESENT ILLNESS

AR is a 54-year-old woman who presents to the outpatient clinic with complaints of headache, nasal stuffiness and sneezing, puffy, red eyes, scratchy throat, and a dry cough over the past 6 weeks. She has self-treated with saline nasal irrigations that "helped a little," aspirin for the headache, and cold compresses over her eyes but with no real relief. She has also been using OTC oxymetazoline nasal spray, but the "congestion continues to get worse."

HEALTH HISTORY

AR has a family history of atopy, with two sisters and a brother who have hay fever. All three have asthma of varying severity. AR denies a history of asthma or other respiratory disorders, hypertension, heart disease, or difficulty urinating. Except for hay fever she is otherwise healthy. Except for the oxymetazoline nasal spray, she uses no other OTC drugs and has no known food or drug allergy. She has two longhair cats that sleep on her bed at night.

LIFESPAN CONSIDERATIONS

AR is a third grade elementary schoolteacher who is continuously exposed to sick children.

CULTURAL/SOCIAL CONSIDERATIONS

AR is a single parent with four teenage sons at home. She acknowledges that she is on a very tight budget and has limited resources. AR has health insurance but no pharmacy coverage.

PHYSICAL EXAMINATION

AR's blood pressure is 124/72 mm Hg, temperature 99.4° F, pulse 76, respirations 20. TMs are clean; nasal mucosa is pale and boggy; no palpable sinus tenderness. Oropharynx is without redness or exudate. Breath sounds are clear to auscultation bilaterally.

LABORATORY TESTING

No diagnostic testing indicated for AR at this time.

PATIENT PROBLEM(S)

Seasonal rhinitis with secondary rhinitis medicamentosa.

GOALS OF THERAPY

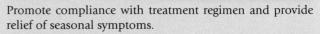

Promote compliance with treatment regimen and provide relief of seasonal symptoms.

CRITICAL THINKING QUESTIONS

1. The health care provider left the following orders: stop oxymetazoline nasal spray now; start fexofenadine 180 mg, $\frac{1}{2}$ to 1 tablet po daily and pseudoephedrine 60 mg po bid for 3 days only. Why did the health care provider stop the oxymetazoline nasal spray when AR is complaining of nasal stuffiness?
2. What is the mechanism of action for fexofenadine?
3. Pseudoephedrine has no antihistaminic activity. Why would the drug be ordered for AR?
4. Of what adverse effects of fexofenadine should AR be aware?
5. In addition to teaching AR how and when to take the fexofenadine and pseudoephedrine, what else should the nurse teach her about self-care during allergy season?

Bibliography

Banov CH, Lieberman P: Efficacy of azelastine nasal spray in the treatment of vasomotor (perennial nonallergic) rhinitis, *Ann Allergy Asthma Immunol* 86(1):28-35, 2001.

Blankenship CR: Nursing notes. Adverse reactions related to phenergan, *Gastroenterol Nurs* 24(3):149-150, 2001.

Crystal-Peters J, Crown WH, Goetzel RZ, et al: The cost of productivity losses associated with allergic rhinitis, *Am J Manag Care* 6(3):373-378, 2000.

Diphenhydramine and cognitive decline, *Nurses Drug Alert* 25(11):84, 2001.

Graft DF, Bernstein DI, Goldsobel A, et al: Safety of fexofenadine in children treated for seasonal allergic rhinitis, *Ann Allergy Asthma Immunol* 87(1):22-26, 2001.

National Highway Traffic Safety Administration (NHTSA) notes: Antihistamines and driving-related behavior: a review of the evidence for improvement . . . including commentary by Runge JW, *Ann Emerg Med* 36(4):388-390, 2000.

Newer antihistamines, *Med Lett Drugs Ther* 43(1103):35, 2001.

'Non-sedative' drugs cause drowsiness in the workplace, *Occup Health* 52(6):7, 2000.

Offering advice on non-sedating antihistamines, *Pract Nurse* 19(9):468, 2000.

Simons FER, Fraser TG, Maher J, et al: Central nervous system effects of H_1-receptor antagonists in the elderly, *Ann Allergy Asthma Immunol* 82(2):157-160, 1999.

Stearn R: Help relieve the misery caused by allergy, *Pract Nurs* 17(6):369-372, 376, 1999.

Strenkoski-Nix LC, Ermer J, DeCleene S, et al: Pharmacokinetics of promethazine hydrochloride after administration of rectal suppositories and oral syrup to healthy subjects, *Am J Health Syst Pharm* 57(16):1499-1505, 2000.

Internet Resources

American Academy of Allergy, Asthma, and Immunology. Available online at http://www.aaaai.org/.

National Institute of Allergy and Infectious Diseases (NIAID), National Institutes of Health. Available online at http://www.niaid.nih.gov/default.htm.

CHAPTER

54

Expectorants, Antitussives, Decongestants, and Mucolytics

LYNN ROGER WILLIS • KATHLEEN GUTIERREZ

 Visit http://evolve.elsevier.com/Gutierrez/ for additional information.

KEY TERMS

Antitussives, p. 886

Decongestants, p. 888

Expectorant, p. 885

Mucolytic, p. 889

Productive cough, p. 884

Rhinitis, p. 884

Rhinitis medicamentosa, p. 888

OBJECTIVES

- Understand the origin of symptoms that are treated with expectorants, antitussives, decongestants, and mucolytics.
- Identify the mechanisms of action of these drugs.
- Consider likely adverse reactions to these drugs.
- Develop a patient teaching strategy for patients who use these drugs.
- Create a nursing care plan for a patient taking an expectorant, antitussive, and/or decongestant.

PHYSIOLOGY • Origin of Secretions

Nasal congestion results when the blood vessels in the nasal passages become dilated as a result of infection, inflammation, allergy, or emotional upset. Dilation increases capillary permeability allowing fluid to escape into the nasal passageway.

Respiratory secretions in the trachea, bronchi, and bronchioles originate from the goblet cells and bronchial glands. The goblet cells lie on the surface, making up part of the epithelial layer. The tracheal epithelium consists of about 20% goblet cells, and the bronchiolar ep-ithelium consists of 2% goblet cells. These cells produce a gelatinous mucus that they periodically secrete. It is unknown what factors normally control the goblet cells, but chronic exposure to irritants increases their size, number, and activity. An example is the phlegm coughed up by smokers. The bronchial glands lie several layers beneath the epithelium. The grapelike (acinar) cells are controlled by the cholinergic nervous system; when stimulated, acinar cells secrete a plentiful watery fluid into a duct that empties onto the surface.

PATHOPHYSIOLOGY

COMMON COLD

Viruses that cause the common cold include the rhinovirus (90% of patients), influenzae, parainfluenza, respiratory syncytial virus, corona virus, adenovirus, echovirus, and Coxsackie virus. These viruses infect the mucous membranes of the nose and eyes. The virus is usually delivered to those sites by contaminated hands.

Viral replication in the nasopharynx produces complaints of "being all stuffed up and having a runny nose," and is associated with varying degrees of nasotracheal inflammation resulting from dilation of the blood vessels in the nasal mucosa. The dilation engorges the mucous membranes with blood and increases the secretion of mucus. Characteristically, the copious nasal discharge progresses from being clear and watery to thick and sticky within 24 hours. The infection generally also includes a scratchy throat, nonproductive cough, loss of taste and smell, and sneezing.

RHINITIS

Allergic **rhinitis** is a type I hypersensitivity reaction to inhaled or ingested allergens. The antigen (e.g., pollen, dust, mold, animal dander) initially stimulates production of immunoglobulin E (IgE) antibodies that attach to receptors on mast cells and basophils in the nasal mucosa. Repeated exposure to the antigen causes release of several mediator substances, including histamine. The result is vasodilation, increased capillary permeability, smooth muscle contraction, and eosinophilia. Symptoms of rhinitis include itchy, watery, puffy eyes, nasal congestion, coughing, and sneezing.

Idiopathic rhinitis is thought to be related to an abnormal autonomic responsiveness that results in intermittent vascular engorgement of the nasal mucosa. The signs and symptoms seen might be related to an allergic response or to neurovascular imbalance.

Allergic rhinitis may be seasonal or perennial, depending on climate and individual response to offending antigens. Seasonal responses are usually caused by grasses, trees, and weeds. Perennial responses are usually caused by animal dander, molds, or dust mites. Signs and symptoms of allergic rhinitis include nasal stuffiness and congestion, pale, boggy mucous membranes, nasal polyps, sneezing (often paroxysmal), watery eyes, dark circles under the eyes (allergic shiners), plugged ears, fatigue, scratchy throat, and postnasal drip. A transverse nasal crease from rubbing the nose upwards (allergic salute) is common in children.

COUGH

Coughing provides a way of keeping the airway clear. Coughs occur with colds when the mucous membranes in the airway become dry and irritated, or when mucus from swollen membranes in the nose and throat trickles into the airway (postnasal drip). The irritation stimulates afferent fibers in the vagus (cranial nerve X), trigeminal (cranial nerve V), glossopharyngeal (cranial nerve IX), or phrenic nerves, which convey information to the cough center in the medulla. Efferent fibers from the cough center, in turn, carry motor impulses to the larynx and muscles of the diaphragm, chest wall, and abdomen to produce a cough.

A cough that loosens and expels mucus and phlegm is termed productive and should not be suppressed. Suppression of a **productive cough** leaves the mucus and phlegm to accumulate and become a potential breeding ground for bacteria. A dry, nonproductive cough, however, can and should be suppressed when it becomes an annoying source of pain or discomfort.

TABLE 54-1						
Pharmacokinetics of Selected Expectorants, Antitussives, Decongestants, and Mucolytics						
Drug	*Route*	*Onset*	*Peak*	*Duration*	*PB (%)*	$t_{1/2}$
Expectorants						
guaifenesin	po	30 min	UA	4-6 hr	UA	UA
Antitussives						
benzonatate	po	15-20 min	UA	3-8 hr	UA	UA
codeine	po	<30 min	60-90 min	4-6 hr	30-35	3 hr
dextromethorphan	po	15-30 min	UA	3-6 hr	UA	3.4 hr*
diphenhydramine HCl	po	15-60 min	1-2 hr	4-8 hr	80-85	2.4-9.3 hr
hydrocodone	po	Rapid	30-90 min	4-8 hr	30-35	4 hr
Decongestants						
ephedrine	IN	1-2 min	1 hr	3 hr	UA	UA
naphazoline	IN	<10 min	UK	2-6 hr	UA	UA
oxymetazoline	IN	1-2 min	5-10 min	Up to 12 hr	UA	UA
phenylephrine	IN	1-2 min	5-10 min	30-240 min	UA	2.6 hr
propylhexedrine	IN	0.5-5 min	UA	0.5-2 hr	UA	UA
pseudoephedrine	po	15-30 min	30-60 min	4-6 hr†	UA	4.3 hr
tetrahydrozoline	IN	1-2 min	UA	4-8 hr	UA	UA
xylometazoline	IN	1-2 min	5-10 min	5-6 hr	UA	UA
Mucolytics						
acetylcysteine	Inh	Rapid	UA	Brief	UA	UA
dornase alpha	IV	15 min	3 days	UA	UA	UA

IN, Intranasal formulations usually in the form of drops or sprays; *Inh,* inhaled formulation; *IV,* intravenous; *PB,* protein binding; $t_{1/2}$, elimination half-life; *UA,* unavailable.
*29.5 hours in poor biotransformers of the drug.
†The duration of action for sustained-action formulations of pseudoephedrine is 8 to 12 hours.

Sometimes all that is necessary to suppress a cough is for the patient to suck on a piece of hard candy or a "cough drop." Decongestant drugs can often relieve a cough simply by stopping postnasal drip. When the simple remedies fail, a cough suppressant (antitussive drug) can be used. Expectorants may be helpful by helping to keep the airway moist and relieving the irritation that may be causing a cough.

 DRUG CLASS • Expectorants

guaifenesin (Anti-Tuss, Halotussin, Humibid, Robitussin, and many others)

MECHANISM OF ACTION

An **expectorant** stimulates the production and flow of airway mucus. In the case of coughs caused by the dry, scratchy throat during a cold, an increase in mucus flow lubricates the airway and may relieve the cough. Guaifenesin stimulates the production of airway mucus by irritating the stomach lining and setting off the same neuronal response that promotes mucus flow and salivation

when nausea develops. Indeed, high doses of guaifenesin predictably cause nausea and vomiting.

USES

Guaifenesin is the only expectorant recognized by the Food and Drug Administration as safe and effective for use in OTC cough and cold remedies. Even so, the use of expectorants is controversial. The controversy stems partly from a lack of objective evidence that expectorant drugs are effective and partly from confusion concerning the expected effect of an expectorant drug. By one definition, an expectorant should promote the expulsion of mucus, phlegm, and fluid from the lungs and bronchial passages; that is, it should enhance the productiveness of a cough. By another, it should relieve a dry, irritating cough by causing the secretion of soothing and protective airway mucus. There is little evidence to suggest that expectorant drugs are any better than placebo either for promoting the expulsion of phlegm or for relieving a cough. Indeed, some authorities maintain that proper hydration with water alone should ensure the adequate production of airway mucus; hence, the old-time admonition to drink plenty of fluids when the cold virus strikes still stands.

Guaifenesin is used for the symptomatic management of coughs associated with the common cold, laryngitis, bronchitis, pharyngitis, pertussis, influenza, and measles. It is also used for coughs provoked by chronic paranasal sinusitis in patients who are unresponsive to increased fluid intake. Guaifenesin may be found in combination with analgesics and antipyretics, antihistamines, and decongestants. Many cough remedies also contain guaifenesin; but, given that an expectorant promotes the production and expulsion of airway mucus, and coughing facilitates the expulsion, it makes

no therapeutic sense to combine an expectorant and a cough suppressant.

PHARMACOKINETICS

The pharmacokinetic characteristics of expectorants are listed in Table 54-1. Guaifenesin is well absorbed from the GI tract after oral administration. Distribution sites are unknown, but its metabolites are biotransformed and eliminated through the kidneys.

ADVERSE REACTIONS AND CONTRAINDICATIONS

Adverse reactions associated with guaifenesin include nausea, vomiting, diarrhea, and abdominal pain. The nausea and vomiting derive from local irritation of the stomach, which in itself promotes the flow of airway mucus. Dizziness, headache, rashes, and urticaria have also been noted. Guaifenesin is contraindicated in patients with known allergy or hypersensitivity to the drug.

In general, expectorants should not be used for a persistent cough associated with smoking, asthma, or emphysema, or if excessive secretions accompany the cough. Safe use of expectorants during pregnancy has not been established, although guaifenesin has been used in that setting without adverse reactions.

DRUG CLASS • Antitussives

Nonopioids

benzonatate (Tessalon Perles, Tessalon✱)

diphenhydramine (Allerdryl,✱ Benadryl, Compoz, Sominex, and many others)

dextromethorphan (Balminil DM,✱ Benylin DM,✱ Robitussin Cough Calmers, Koffex DM,✱ and many others)

Opioids

codeine (Paveral,✱ generic)

hydrocodone

hydromorphone

MECHANISM OF ACTION

Tussis is the Latin word meaning cough, and cough suppressants are known as **antitussives**. Antitussives act either centrally or peripherally to suppress coughs. The centrally acting drugs, codeine, hydrocodone, hydromorphone, dextromethorphan, and diphenhydramine suppress the cough reflex by acting directly on the cough center in the medulla of the brain. The mechanism by which the suppression occurs is not known. All of the opioid drugs (see Chapter 13) suppress coughs,

but codeine, hydrocodone, and hydromorphone are the only opioids officially indicated for cough suppression. Of these, codeine is the most widely used because of its more favorable adverse-reaction profile and for its lower potential for causing dependence.

Benzonatate is related to the local anesthetic, procaine. Benzonatate acts peripherally at the site of the irritation that is producing the cough by anesthetizing the stretch, or cough, receptors of vagal afferent nerve fibers in the respiratory tract.

USES

Antitussives are most appropriately used to suppress dry, hacking, nonproductive coughs. They should not be used to suppress productive coughs, because the cough provides the means for clearing the airway and lungs of mucus and phlegm that would otherwise accumulate there.

Codeine, dextromethorphan, and diphenhydramine are available without prescription in most states in the United States, and literally scores of over-the-counter remedies for cough, cold, and allergy contain one or another of these three drugs. Benzonatate is available OTC in Canada, but not in the United States.

Codeine once was the most widely used OTC antitussive, but fears of abuse and addiction have caused its popularity to wane. Indeed, in recent years, many states have enacted laws severely restricting the OTC availability of codeine-containing cough remedies. Actually, the risk of dependence with codeine is much less than that for morphine or the other opioids, and it is virtually nonexistent when the drug is used in recommended doses for short periods. Nevertheless, neither dextromethorphan, diphenhydramine, nor benzonatate has the potential for causing dependence and have largely replaced codeine or the other opioids as the antitussive drugs of choice. Of the three, dextromethorphan is by far the most widely used.

PHARMACOKINETICS

The pharmacokinetics of the various antitussives are similar overall (see Table 54-1). The onset of most of the drugs occurs in 15 to 30 minutes after oral administration, peak action occurs in 30 to 90 minutes, and the duration of action ranges between 3 to 8 hours.

Interestingly, dextromethorphan and codeine are biotransformed by the cytochrome P450 2D6 (CYP2D6) system, which is subject to genetic polymorphism (see Chapter 1). Accordingly, about 7% of whites, and a lesser fraction of Asians and Africans biotransform these drugs much more slowly than the rest of the population. The elimination half-life of dextromethorphan in poor biotransformers of the drug may be prolonged by as much as a factor of 8, but because the adverse reaction profile for dextromethorphan is so favorable, adverse effects and toxicity are rarely a problem. In contrast, genetic polymorphism can pose a problem with codeine, but only in analgesic doses, which normally exceed the antitussive dosage by a factor of 3. In short, genetic polymorphism in the biotransformation of dextromethorphan and antitussive doses of codeine does not pose a clinically significant problem for patients.

ADVERSE REACTIONS AND CONTRAINDICATIONS

Drowsiness and constipation are the adverse reactions most often reported with opioid antitussives. The general spectrum of adverse effects and contraindications for opioids are discussed in detail in Chapter 13. The occurrence and severity of adverse effects caused by opioid antitussive drugs are related to dosage and generally include sedation, confusion, and hypotension.

The most serious adverse effects of these drugs are associated with overdose or hypersensitivity and include respiratory depression, laryngeal edema, and anaphylaxis. Opioids are contraindicated in patients with known hypersensitivity to the drug and during pregnancy and lactation.

Nonopioid antitussives include several chemical classifications and vary in the adverse reactions that they produce. The antitussive dosage of diphenhydramine (which is the same as for relief of allergy symptoms) predictably causes drowsiness and dry mouth and, in some patients, blurred vision and photosensitivity. The drug is contraindicated in asthma and in patients who are allergic to diphenhydramine.

Benzonatate rarely causes adverse effects, though some patients have reported experiencing constipation, confusion, and bronchospasm. Patients who are allergic to ester-type local anesthetics (see Chapter 16) may also be allergic to benzonatate. The drug is contraindicated where allergy is known and if the cough to be treated is productive.

Dextromethorphan causes few adverse reactions. Some people may experience nausea, dizziness, and sedation. The drug is contraindicated for patients with hypersensitivity and those taking monoamine oxidase inhibitors or selective serotonin reuptake inhibitors. Antitussives containing alcohol should be avoided in patients with a known alcohol intolerance. Many antitussives contain sugars and should be used carefully in patients with diabetes mellitus. The safety of dextromethorphan for use during pregnancy and lactation or in children under the age of 2 years has not been established.

INTERACTIONS

CNS depressants, alcohol, sedative-hypnotics, and antidepressants provide additive CNS depression when they are used concurrently with opioid and nonopioid antitussives.

There are many drug-drug interactions with dextromethorphan. Concurrent use with monoamine oxidase inhibitors or selective serotonin reuptake inhibitors results in serotonin syndrome (e.g., excitation, confusion, hypotension, and hyperpyrexia). Additive CNS depression has been noted with concurrent use of antihistamines, alcohol, sedative-hypnotics, other antidepressants, or opioids. Quinidine may increase the blood levels and adverse effects of dextromethorphan.

DRUG CLASS • Decongestants

desoxyephedrine (Vicks Inhaler)

ephedrine (Kondon's Nasal Jelly, Pretz-D, and combinations)

naphazoline (Privine)

oxymetazoline (Afrin, Allerest 12 Hour Nasal Spray, and many others)

phenylephrine (Cheracol Nasal Spray, Nafrine, ✽ Neo-Synephrine, Sinex)

propylhexedrine (Benzedrex Inhaler)

pseudoephedrine (Afrin Extended-Release Tablets, Drixoral, Novafed, Sudafed, Sudafed-SA)

tetrahydrozoline (Tyzine)

xylometazoline (Neo-Synephrine II Long-Acting)

MECHANISM OF ACTION

Decongestants are sympathetic nervous system drugs (see Chapter 12). They relieve nasal stuffiness and conjunctival redness and swelling by constricting blood vessels in swollen nasal membranes, decreasing local blood flow and swelling. The vasoconstriction is mediated through stimulation of alpha$_1$ receptors on vascular smooth muscle. When nasal swelling is relieved, breathing passages open.

The decongestant drugs are classified as direct acting, as indirect acting, or as having mixed action. Direct-acting decongestants stimulate alpha$_1$ receptors by binding directly to the receptors. Examples of direct-acting decongestants include phenylephrine, oxymetazoline, xylometazoline, and tetrahydrozoline. Indirect-acting decongestants are taken up into adrenergic nerve endings where they release the neurotransmitter norepinephrine, which stimulates the alpha$_1$ receptors. Mixed-action decongestants do both. Ephedrine and pseudoephedrine are examples of mixed-acting decongestants.

All of the drugs in this class are available in OTC remedies for colds and allergies as well as in prescription products. Several are also the active ingredients in ophthalmic solutions (see later discussion in this section).

USES

Decongestants are used to relieve symptoms associated with rhinitis, allergies, sinusitis, and colds. They have also been used as adjuncts for middle ear infections because they decrease congestion around the eustachian tubes. Eustachian tube dysfunction and ear pain during air travel are also responsive to decongestants.

Decongestants are available in systemic (oral) and topical dosage forms for nasal and ophthalmic use. The orally active decongestants are ephedrine, phenylephrine, and pseudoephedrine. Of these, pseudoephedrine is the most widely marketed. Ephedrine is considered obsolete because of its propensity to cause numerous adverse reactions, but it is still available in OTC remedies. Topical intranasal formulations include sprays and drops (naphazoline, oxymetazoline, phenylephrine, tetrahydrozoline, and xylometazoline), and inhalers (desoxyephedrine, propylhexedrine). Decongestants for ophthalmic use include naphazoline, oxymetazoline, phenylephrine, and tetrahydrozoline (see Chapter 65).

PHARMACOKINETICS

Topically applied decongestants have an onset of action within minutes and varying durations of action, depending on the individual drug (see Table 54-1). The oral absorption of phenylephrine is erratic because of poor bioavailability. Short-acting decongestants, such as phenylephrine and naphazoline, are effective for up to 4 hours. Long-acting decongestants, such as oxymetazoline, are effective for 12 hours or more.

ADVERSE REACTIONS AND CONTRAINDICATIONS

Stinging, burning, and drying of nasal mucosa may occur with the use of nasal decongestant drops or sprays. Prolonged use of a topical nasal decongestant (more than 3 to 5 days) may produce chronic congestion (i.e., **rhinitis medicamentosa**, "rebound" congestion). After more than 3 days of continuous use, response to these drugs becomes blunted (tolerance), leading to increased use, often on an hourly basis. Cessation results in marked rebound congestion, presumably due to reflex vasodilation and an erythematous mucosa. The congestion resolves in 2 or 3 weeks if the use of topical decongestants is stopped.

Rebound congestion normally does not occur with oral decongestants, but can also be a problem with topical ophthalmic decongestants (e.g., Visine). In that case, the congestion does not involve swollen nasal passages but engorged conjunctiva, which reddens the eyes. In either case, the rebound congestion appears as the decongesting effect of the drugs wear off, leading the user to conclude that it is time for another dose. In fact, the drug has set the stage for the congestion to recur.

Orally administered (systemic) decongestants can cause peripheral vasoconstriction, tachycardia, and elevated blood pressure. Men with benign prostatic hyperplasia (BPH) may notice increased difficulty voiding urine after taking a systemic decongestant. Mild CNS stimulation may also occur in the form of restlessness, nervousness, tremors, headache, and insomnia. Excessive

TABLE 54-2		
Drug-Drug Interactions of Selected Antitussives, Decongestants, and Mucolytics*		
Drug	*Interactive Drugs*	*Interaction*
Antitussives		
codeine, hydrocodone, diphenhydramine, dextromethorphan	Alcohol, antidepressants, antihistamines, opioids, sedative-hypnotics	Additive CNS depression
diphenhydramine	Tricyclic antidepressants, quinidine, and disopyramide	Additive anticholinergic properties
	MAO inhibitors	Intensify and prolong anticholinergic actions
dextromethorphan	MAO inhibitors	Serotonin syndrome, hypotension, hyperpyrexia
	SSRIs, quinidine	Increased blood levels and adverse effects of dextromethorphan
Decongestants		
desoxyephedrine, ephedrine, naphazoline, oxymetazoline, phenylephrine, propylhexedrine, tetrahydrozoline, xylometazoline	Tricyclic antidepressants, ergonovine, oxytocin	Increased cardiovascular effects of decongestant
	guanethidine, phenothiazines	Decreased effect of interactive drug
	Beta blockers	Mutual inhibition
	digoxin, theophylline	Increased risk of arrhythmias
	MAO inhibitors, methyldopa, furazolidone	Increased vasopressor effects

CNS, Central nervous system; *MAO,* monoamine oxidase; *SSRIs,* selective serotonin reuptake inhibitors.
*There are no significant drug-drug interactions with expectorants such as guaifenesin.

doses of systemic decongestants worsen the peripheral and central symptoms and may lead to life-threatening stroke or myocardial infarction. Another systemic decongestant, phenylpropanolamine, which was widely used in over-the-counter cold and allergy remedies and as an appetite suppressant, was ultimately withdrawn from the market after several stroke-related fatalities occurred from overdose.

Decongestants are contraindicated in patients who are concurrently using monoamine oxidase inhibitors. They should be used with caution by patients who have heart disease, hypertension, advanced arteriosclerosis, insulin-dependent diabetes mellitus, or hyperthyroidism. Overdose in patients more than 60 years old may result in hallucinations, CNS depression, and seizures.

INTERACTIONS

There are extensive drug interactions with decongestants. Table 54-2 provides an overview of specific interactions. Many of the interactions are related to drug effects on the cardiovascular or autonomic nervous systems. Concurrent use of drugs that acidify urine (e.g., ammonium chloride) decreases the therapeutic effects of pseudoephedrine by increasing its rate of elimination in the urine.

DRUG CLASS • Mucolytic Drugs

acetylcysteine (Mucomyst)

dornase alfa (Pulmozyme, DNase)

MECHANISM OF ACTION

Mucolytic drugs reduce the viscosity of mucus in conditions where accumulated mucus in the airway has become viscous and congealed. In cystic fibrosis, bronchiolar secretions become thickened and viscous because strands of DNA from deteriorating inflammatory cells accumulate in the mucus. Dornase alfa, which hydrolyzes DNA in the sputum, and acetylcysteine, which is believed to break disulfide bonds, liquefies the mucus and promotes its expulsion from the airway by the ciliary activity of airway cells (Figure 54-1).

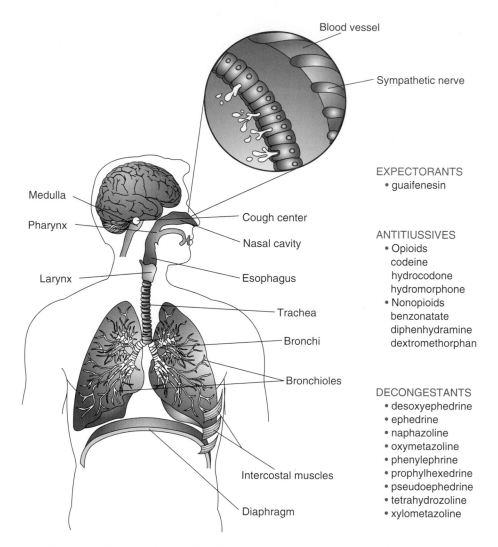

FIGURE 54-1 Sites of drug action for upper respiratory disorders. Drugs used to manage upper respiratory disorders fall into four classes: expectorants, antitussives, decongestants, and mucolytic drugs. Antitussive drugs act centrally in the cough center or peripherally at the site of irritation to suppress coughing. Expectorants stimulate the flow of respiratory tract secretions. Decongestants stimulate alpha receptors, causing vasoconstriction, reduced blood flow, reduced fluid exudation, and shrinkage of edematous membranes. Mucolytic drugs reduce sputum viscosity.

USES

Dornase alfa helps reduce the incidence of respiratory infections and improve pulmonary function in patients with cystic fibrosis. Dornase alfa is not a replacement for other components of therapy for cystic fibrosis.

Acetylcysteine is used as an adjunctive treatment for patients with abnormally thick mucus secretions such as those with acute and chronic bronchopulmonary disease, atelectasis from mucus obstruction, and cystic fibrosis. Recent clinical studies of acetylcysteine place its value and effectiveness as a mucolytic agent in doubt, but acetylcysteine has an additional use unrelated to mucolysis. Administered orally in large doses, acetylcysteine provides an effective treatment for preventing potentially fatal hepatotoxicity from acetaminophen overdose (see Chapter 14).

PHARMACOKINETICS

The onset of the effects of dornase alfa occurs within 15 minutes of nebulized administration. There is minimal systemic absorption after inhalation. Peak effects are not noted for 3 days, and the duration of action is unknown. It is unknown whether dornase alfa crosses the placenta or is excreted in breast milk.

Acetylcysteine is inhaled through a nebulizer or is instilled as a solution directly into the airway. The liver inactivates absorbed acetylcysteine.

ADVERSE REACTIONS AND CONTRAINDICATIONS

Adverse reactions to dornase alfa are uncommon, but voice alteration, pharyngitis, rash, chest pain, and allergic reactions may occur. There are no known contraindications or drug interactions involving dornase alfa.

Acetylcysteine can trigger bronchospasm in susceptible patients. For this reason, the drug is usually administered with or immediately after a bronchodilator. The most common adverse reaction to acetylcysteine includes a burning in the back of the throat, stomatitis, nausea, rhinorrhea, and epistaxis.

APPLICATION TO PRACTICE

ASSESSMENT
History of Present Illness

Attention should be given to obtaining a health history that includes environmental aspects and patient comfort. Ask if the patient has had nasal congestion or discharge, sneezing, sore throat, headache, itchy eyes, tearing, earache with decreased hearing, upper respiratory tract infection, or allergies. The sensation of postnasal drip is influenced more by the thickness of the drainage than the quantity. Ask the patient about the duration and extent of nasal congestion and about factors that precipitate or relieve the symptoms. Ask if there are times when symptoms are more pronounced under certain weather conditions, if they occur year round, or if they occur only in a particular season.

Malaise, pharyngitis, laryngitis, cough, headache, and substernal tightness and burning are common complaints in the patient with a common cold. There may be a history of a nonproductive cough or an overactive cough that interrupts the patient's sleep or produces muscular pain. The type, severity, and frequency of the cough should be assessed. Inquire about factors that trigger or relieve the cough.

Obtain a smoking history from the patient. Determine how long the patient has smoked and how many packs per day. If the patient does not smoke at present, ask if he or she has ever smoked. Information regarding the use of chewing tobacco should also be elicited.

Ask the patient with allergic rhinitis about itching of the nose, eyes, and oropharynx—the predominant symptoms. A watery discharge from the eyes is common. Nonnasal allergic symptoms such as shortness of breath or GI distress may also be present.

There is no sneezing with idiopathic rhinitis. Rhinorrhea associated with idiopathic rhinitis is watery, and the patient may indicate that the episodes are initiated by cold air, odors, nasal irritants, and stress.

Health History

Because many respiratory problems are associated with pollutants such as asbestos, fumes, organic dust particles, and chemicals, obtain information about the patient's occupation and geographic environment.

In addition, determine whether there is a family history of allergy, prior allergy testing, or treatment of allergies.

Lifespan Considerations

Perinatal. Nasal stuffiness and epistaxis are fairly common during pregnancy. They are the result of estrogen-induced edema and vascular congestion of the nasal mucosa. Respiratory depression in the fetus is a theoretic possibility if a woman with severely impaired renal function chronically takes dextromethorphan during and up to the time of delivery.

Pediatric. The common cold is the most prevalent infectious disease among children of all ages. Three annual waves of the common cold typically occur in children, with the greatest incidence occurring with the opening of school. The more severe cases with a tendency toward complications occur in midwinter. Another round of mild cases of the common cold also occurs in the spring.

Cold symptoms in a young child can pose additional problems. The obstruction of the upper airways cause difficulty in sucking, consumes energy, and increases oxygen needs. Restlessness, malaise, and anorexia result. Crankiness and an acetone breath odor appear because of secondary dehydration. A mild degree of ketoacidosis develops when fever is present. Viral enteritis may be present and accounts for the associated diarrhea.

Older Adults. In the standard medical model of diagnosis, there is a 1:1 correspondence between clinical signs and symptoms and a pathologic process. However, it is believed that the medical model does not accurately define the presentation of many illnesses in the older adult. Older adults and people with chronic debilitating diseases are especially vulnerable to complications associated with upper respiratory disorders.

Cultural/Social Considerations

Choices between ethnomedical options and interventions of Western medicine vary among ethnic groups and vary from one patient experience to another. At any given time, treatment of the common cold and other upper respiratory tract disorders may reflect exclusive use of traditional herbal remedies or a combination of herbs and Western medicine. In addition, it is often said that if families would familiarize themselves with herbs, their medicinal properties, and their uses, many visits to the health care provider would be saved. Herbs, no matter what their modern name and how unorthodox they are said to be, continue to be the treatment of choice by those who value their effects (see Chapter 8).

Societal and pharmaceutical industries encourage approximately 90% of patients to treat symptoms of upper respiratory tract infection (URI) at home. With adults experiencing an average of two to four colds a year and colds occurring more commonly in families with children, over $500 million is spent on OTC preparations (see the Case Study: Common Cold with Rhinorrhea).

Physical Examination

For the patient with a common cold, the nasal mucosa and pharynx may appear mildly swollen and erythematous. The edema may partially or totally occlude the nasal passages. A watery or thick, yellow nasal discharge and mild lymphadenopathy can be noted. Although fever is uncommon in adults with a common cold, it frequently occurs in children. Therefore, the patient's temperature should be taken.

The nasal mucosa of the patient with allergic rhinitis may appear pale, boggy, and edematous, or it may have a bluish color. The patient's sense of smell may be reduced. Sneezing is common. "Allergic shiners," the bluish discoloration of the lower eyelids due to chronic nasal congestion, are a common finding. Nasal polyps may be noted, especially in patients with perennial rhinitis. The gesture that allergic children often display of repeatedly lifting the tip of the nose with an open palm (allergic salute) can cause a permanent transverse crease above the tip of the nose that may be seen in adulthood. Postnasal drip, which may be evident by strands of stringy mucus down the back of the pharynx, can cause frequent throat clearing and coughing. Cervical adenopathy may or may not be present.

In idiopathic rhinitis, the nasal mucosa varies from bright red to a bluish hue. If a nasal discharge is present, note the amount, color, and thickness. Clear drainage suggests a diagnosis of idiopathic, allergic, or nonallergic rhinitis, whereas thick and discolored (yellow, brown, green) drainage suggests bacterial or viral infection.

Assess the patient's breath sounds. A dry, nonproductive cough does not produce sputum and is not associated with chest congestion. A productive cough is related to chest congestion, with a small amount of sputum produced. In some patients the cough can be severe and debilitating.

Laboratory Testing

The patient's history and physical examination are the two most important aspects of assessing the patient with a cough and cold. Laboratory testing is not usually indicated for the patient with a common cold or rhinitis. The throat culture is usually negative for streptococcal organisms or other bacterial causes of the illness. A nasal smear may be done to help identify the cause of signs and symptoms.

If leukocytosis is present, it indicates a disorder other than the common cold. An eosinophil smear should be examined if the diagnosis of allergy is uncertain. In patients with idiopathic rhinitis, the nasal smear may also help rule out allergic rhinitis.

GOALS OF THERAPY

Treatment goals for the patient with an upper respiratory disorder includes strategies that will prevent, minimize, or help correct symptoms. Treatment should be directed toward alleviating the unpleasant symptoms until the illness has had a chance to run its course.

INTERVENTION

Because the common cold is an acute URI of viral origin, there is no justification for the use of antibiotics, and because there is no cure for the cold, treatment is simply symptomatic (Box 54-1). Antibiotics are appropriate only if a bacterial infection is present.

Administration

The characteristics of the patient's cough (frequency, severity, productive, sputum volume, viscosity, and difficulty raising sputum) should be assessed before administration of an antitussive or mucolytic drug. The patient should also be monitored for adverse reactions and hypersensitivity responses.

Antitussives should be used with caution in young children because they can depress the cough reflex, leading to aspiration. Caution should also be used with combination cough and cold products. Many of these products contain aspirin, which has been associated with Reye's syndrome.

Administer antitussive syrups undiluted. Part of the perceived therapeutic benefit of syrups stems from their soothing effects on pharyngeal mucosa. However, adequate fluid intake following administration of a cough syrup enables the drug to circulate to the cough center where it acts. It is worth noting that many patients expect to receive a "syrup" formulation for cough suppression. Thus, using a syrup formulation may provide some psychologic benefit.

BOX 54-1	Save Yourself a Trip

There are more than 200 viruses that cause many of us to come down with a cough and cold. Viruses are elusive little creatures that *cannot be killed by traditional antibiotics*. A cold virus is killed by the body's own immune system, and it usually takes a week or two to do so.

PREVENTION

Even though there is no cure for colds, you may be able to avoid getting sick.
* Wash your hands often, especially when you are around people who have colds.
* Keep hands away from your mouth, nose, and eyes.
* Eat well and get plenty of sleep and exercise to keep up resistance.
* Reduce stress as much as possible.
* Stop smoking.
* Although there is no hard evidence to prove it, chicken soup, garlic, and vitamin C may be helpful in improving cold symptoms and boosting the immune system. As Grandma used to say, "They can't hurt."

SELF-TREATMENT

As miserable as we feel, most of us will recover completely without medical assistance. Home treatment will help relieve symptoms and prevent complications.
* *Get plenty of rest*. Your body needs the time to recover. Let your body be your guide in determining how much to restrict your activities.
* *Avoid tobacco and alcohol*. If that is impossible, at least cut back. Smoking will further irritate your airways and increase your risk of getting bronchitis and pneumonia. Alcohol causes you to become dehydrated and slows your recovery.
* *Drink extra fluids,* at least one glass of water or juice every hour you are awake. Hot liquids soothe the throat and help loosen secretions and relieve nasal congestion.
* *Use disposable tissues* instead of handkerchiefs. Research has shown that cold viruses can live for hours on handkerchiefs.
* *Use a decongestant* like pseudoephedrine (Sudafed) to help relieve congestion. If you have high blood pressure, do not use a decongestant without first checking with the health care provider.
* *Humidify* the bedroom when sleeping, making sure that the water reservoir and filter is cleaned regularly. Take hot showers to relieve nasal stuffiness.
* *Use a single-ingredient OTC cough suppressant* if your cough is dry. A cough suppressant should not be used when your chest is full of mucus. An expectorant would be appropriate when your chest is full of mucus.
* *Use an OTC pain and fever drug* such as acetaminophen (i.e., Tylenol) or ibuprofen (i.e., Motrin or Advil) to relieve fever, headache, and muscle aches. *Do not give aspirin to children or teens under age 20.*
* *Irrigate your sinuses*. It removes mucus that contributes to sinus infections and helps to relieve congestion caused by allergies. Obtain a rubber "nose" syringe at your pharmacy or you may use the nasal attachment to a Water-Pic. Make up a salt-water solution as follows:
  1 cup of warm water
  $\frac{1}{4}$ teaspoon of table salt or sea salt
  $\frac{1}{4}$ teaspoon of baking soda.
  Irrigate 2 to 3 times daily using $\frac{1}{2}$ cup for each side of your nose. Be sure to blow your nose carefully after irrigating. If you are provided with a steroid nasal spray (for allergies) be sure to use it as instructed but after the irrigation is complete.
* *Self-treatment for sore throat and to soothe the throat when coughing:* There are several things you can try: You may gargle with warm salt water ($\frac{1}{4}$ teaspoon salt in 8 ounces warm water); use zinc throat lozenges as directed on the package, suck on hard candy, or sip the "sore throat toddy" using the following recipe:
  2 cups of hot water
  $\frac{1}{2}$ cup honey
  $\frac{1}{2}$ cup lemon juice
  $\frac{1}{4}$ teaspoon each of ground cinnamon, ginger, and cloves
* *Purchase a new toothbrush* to avoid reinfecting yourself.

Make an Appointment with Your Health Care Provider If You Have

* *Severe chest pain* or difficulty swallowing.
* *A fever* of 104° F or higher that does not come down within 2 hours after taking fever-reducing drugs, or a fever that stays high; for example, a fever of
  102° F or higher for 2 full days
  101° F or higher for 3 full days
  100° F or higher for 4 full days
* *Ear pain* that is more than just stuffiness, especially if it is on one side and lasts more than 24 hours.
* *Nasal discharge* that changes from clear to yellow, green, gray, or rust-colored after 7 to 10 days and is accompanied by other worsening symptoms. Mucus is normally yellow or green at the start of a cold.
* *A rash* that covers most of your body.
* *A cold or a cough that lasts 10 days or more with no improvement* or a cough that contains bloody mucus.

EVIDENCE-BASED PRACTICE
Antiviral Drugs to Treat the Common Cold

Setting

Approximately 31 episodes of the common cold occur per 100 persons per year (counting only colds that lead to medical attention or at least 1 day of restricted activity). The common cold is a short and usually mild illness for which preventive and treatment interventions have been under development since the mid-1940s. As our understanding of the disease has increased, more antiviral drugs have been developed.

Objective of Literature Review

To synthesize the results of published and unpublished randomized controlled trials of the effects of experimental antiviral drugs developed to prevent or minimize the impact of the common cold.

Investigators searched the electronic databases, corresponded with researchers, and hand-searched the archives of the Medical Research Center's Common Cold Unit.

Criteria for Inclusion of Studies in Review of Literature

Investigators included original reports of randomized and quasi-randomized trials assessing the effects of antiviral drugs on volunteers who were artificially infected and on individuals exposed to cold viruses in the community.

Data Extraction and Analysis

Two investigators reviewed 241 studies (contained in 230 reports) that took place in experimental or community settings and which assessed the effects of interferons, interferon-inducers, and other antiviral drugs on subjects who had artificially infected or naturally occurring common colds.

Results of Review

Intranasal interferons were shown to be highly efficacious in preventing experimentally induced colds and natural colds, and are also significantly more effective than placebo in altering the course of experimentally induced colds. Nevertheless, their safety profile makes compliance difficult (e.g., prolonged prevention of community colds with interferons caused blood-tinged nasal discharge). Dipyridamole (Persantine), ICI 130, 685, palmitate (Infuvite), and pleconaril appear to have important antiviral properties and are well tolerated. The evidence of effectiveness of other compounds in the treatment of experimentally induced or natural colds is meager.

Investigators' Conculsions

To date, there are FDA approved effective antiviral drugs for the common cold. Interferons have no place in everyday use because prolonged intranasal administration causes a clinical picture not indistinguishable from the common cold. The effects of experimental antiviral drugs in preventing the common cold should undergo further evaluation. Since many factors contribute to the cause of the common cold, future research efforts should focus on non–virus-specific compounds.

Capsule formulations (e.g., benzonatate perles) should not be opened or chewed. When opened or chewed, the local anesthetic effects numb oral mucosa. Enteric-coated tablets are swallowed whole, without chewing or crushing and should be taken with a full glass (8 ounces) of liquid.

The patient in whom an opioid antitussive is being used should have his or her cough and sputum checked to ensure that the secretions have not thickened. Although the dosage of an opioid antitussive is less than that used for pain, the patient's level of consciousness and respiratory depth and rate should be checked before administration. The patient should also be observed during treatment for the development of constipation.

A bronchodilator should be provided before the administration of acetylcysteine. When 25% of the drug remains in the nebulizer, it should be diluted with an equal amount of normal saline solution to minimize reconcentration. A suction apparatus should be available for patients with an ineffective cough. Adequate patient hydration helps decrease the viscosity of the sputum. To prevent drug-induced irritation of oral and pharyngeal membranes, the patient taking acetylcysteine should rinse his or her mouth after treatment.

The patient's history should be checked for possible contraindications before the use of decongestants. Decongestants can be administered as drops, nasal sprays, or oral inhalation, or they may be taken orally. Topical nasal decongestants should not be used for more than 3 to 5 days because of the high risk of rhinitis medicamentosa.

To minimize systemic absorption of topical decongestants, the nasal spray should be used with the patient in an upright position, squeezing the drug into each nostril. Nasal drops are administered with the head tilted back over the edge of a bed or chair. Do not touch the dropper to the nares. The recommended number of drops is instilled into each nostril with the patient breathing through the mouth. The head should remain tilted backward for 3 to 5 minutes. Give nasal decongestants to infants 20 to 30 minutes before feeding.

Nasal decongestants are usually dilute, aqueous solutions prepared specifically for intranasal use. Some of these drugs (e.g., phenylephrine) are also available for ophthalmic use. The two formulations cannot be used interchangeably. Be sure to use the drug formulation and concentration that has been ordered. Some drug formulations are available in several concentrations.

Education

The best preventive measures to avoid catching a cold are to avoid exposure to others who are ill, engage in good handwashing, and keep the hands away from the face. A proactive approach to avoidance of coughs and colds is to send educational materials to patients at the beginning of the URI season. Unnecessary office visits and telephone calls have been reduced by as much as 30% to 40% through well-designed educational efforts.

Because many patients self-treat coughs, colds, and rhinitis, it is important to discuss the dangers of indiscriminate use of OTC expectorants, antitussives, and decongestants. Patients should be helped to understand which symptoms may be relieved with self-treatment and those for which self-treatment is ill-advised. Instruct the patient to choose OTC remedies appropriate for their symptoms and to read product labels. Hundreds of OTC products contain two or more ingredients. Consult the health care provider or pharmacist for help in choosing an appropriate remedy for a specific symptom.

Relief from cold symptoms and avoidance of complications are facilitated by rest, fluids, analgesia, and perhaps inhalation of steam. For some patients a nasal irrigation may be helpful in relieving congestion (see Box 54-1). Vitamin C has no proven role in the prevention or alleviation of symptoms of the common cold. Recommend that at least eight glasses or more (1500 to 2000 mL) of liquids be taken per day. Talk with the patient about the benefits of a balanced diet. They should be advised about the need for additional rest and sleep during periods of illness. Advise patients to stop smoking. Limiting talking, maintaining adequate environmental humidity, and chewing sugarless gum or sucking on hard candy help alleviate the discomfort caused by a nonproductive cough. Instruct the patient to contact the health care provider if a cough persists for more than

1 week or if it is accompanied by fever, rash, persistent headache, or sore throat.

Instruct patients about the correct administration and use of nasal sprays or drops. Advise them that nasal decongestants used for more than 3 to 5 days or in excessive amounts may produce rebound nasal congestion. Teach the patient to blow the nose gently before instilling nasal solutions or sprays. Avoid contamination of nasal droppers or spray tips. Administration devices should be rinsed in hot water after use and allowed to dry.

Patients should be advised to minimize caffeine intake because it may cause increased nervousness, tremors, or insomnia in the presence of decongestants. The patient should discontinue the drug and contact the health care provider if headache, nausea, vomiting, irregular pulse, extreme nervousness or restlessness, confusion, delirium, or muscle tremors occur. Drowsiness is a common adverse effect of many cough and cold preparations. The patient should be advised to use caution when driving or operating machinery.

Patients should be instructed in proper cough techniques. Patients with a dry, hacking cough are encouraged to take fluids freely to promote thin, easily raised sputum. Although the risk is small, opioid antitussives carry a risk of habituation and dependency, and the recommended dosage should not be exceeded. Increasing the dose does not appreciably increase antitussive efficacy. The potential for abuse, however, is increased with an increase in dosage. Coughs that last longer than 1 week or which are accompanied by fever, rash, or headache require further evaluation.

Teach patients that opioid adverse effects (i.e., respiratory depression) are potentiated by concurrent use of barbiturates or alcohol. The alcohol content of some antitussives can be as high as 40%. Opioids also tend to cause constipation. Teach measures that will help prevent or alleviate constipation.

EVALUATION

Treatment with these drugs is successful if symptoms are relieved. The effectiveness of expectorants is demonstrated by an ability of the patient to effect a productive cough with increased sputum clearance. Antitussives should produce cough suppression, a decrease in the frequency and duration of coughing spells, and improvement in the patient's ability to sleep.

The effectiveness of decongestants is dramatic, with efficacy noted within a short time. The patient often reports that he or she can breath easier, postnasal drip is relieved, and nasal discharge and sneezing are reduced. Rhinitis medicamentosa is avoided.

The effectiveness of a mucolytic drug is demonstrated by decreased sputum viscosity and increased productivity.

CASE STUDY　*Common Cold with Rhinorrhea*

ASSESSMENT

HISTORY OF PRESENT ILLNESS

JE is a 27-year-old woman who came in today with complaints of a "stuffy head" and a dry, hacking cough that is keeping her and her partner awake at night. She has had symptoms for 3 days and they are interfering with her work performance. She is requesting a diagnosis so that she purchases the "right medicine at the drug store." She reports that fellow workers have been sick all winter with "head colds," and at her place of work (a day care center), 12 children have been absent because of coughs and colds.

HEALTH HISTORY

JE has a history of seasonal allergic rhinitis, which she treats each spring by avoiding suspected allergens as much as possible. She self-treats with OTC antihistamines only if the sneezing becomes uncontrollable. She denies having a history of cardiovascular disease, hypertension, hyperthyroidism, or diabetes mellitus. JE also denies having drug or food allergies and using home remedies. She denies using other drugs at this time.

LIFESPAN CONSIDERATIONS

JE believes that she finally has a position in a stable company that will maximize her contributions and also provide her with long-lasting career opportunities.

CULTURAL/SOCIAL CONSIDERATIONS

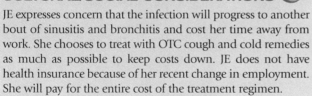

JE expresses concern that the infection will progress to another bout of sinusitis and bronchitis and cost her time away from work. She chooses to treat with OTC cough and cold remedies as much as possible to keep costs down. JE does not have health insurance because of her recent change in employment. She will pay for the entire cost of the treatment regimen.

PHYSICAL EXAMINATION

JE's blood pressure is 116/72 mm Hg, temperature 99.2° F, pulse 88, respirations 24. Tympanic membranes without bulging or retraction, landmarks are visible. Nasal passages have clear discharge. Oropharynx slightly reddened with clear mucus present. No palpable sinus tenderness or cervical adenopathy. Breath sounds are clear bilaterally.

LABORATORY TESTING

Quick strep test was negative; back-up throat culture sent to the laboratory.

PATIENT PROBLEM(S)

Common cold with rhinorrhea.

GOALS OF THERAPY

Relieve uncomfortable symptoms until illness has had chance to run its course.

CRITICAL THINKING QUESTIONS

1. What factor(s) lead the health care provider to a diagnosis of common cold rather than seasonal rhinitis?
2. The health care provider orders guaifenesin 600 mg tabs 2 po bid and phenergan with codeine one teaspoon po every 4 to 6 hours as prn for cough. What is the mechanism of action of these drugs?
3. What is the most important information for JE to have regarding self-treatment for her illness?
4. What patient teaching is required regarding the use of a cough syrup?
5. Under what circumstances is an antitussive drug warranted?

Bibliography

Chow AW: Acute sinusitis: current status of etiologies, diagnosis, and treatment, *Curr Clin Top Infect Dis* 21:31-63, 2001.

Corey JP, Houser SM, Ng BA: Nasal congestion: a review of its etiology, evaluation, and treatment, *Ear Nose Throat J* 79(9):690-693, 2000.

Galant SP, Wilkinson R: Clinical prescribing of allergic rhinitis medication in the preschool and young school-age child: what are the options? *Biodrugs* 15(7):453-463, 2001.

Osguthorpe JD: Adult rhinosinusitis: diagnosis and management, *Am Fam Physician* 63(1):69-76, 2001.

Schroeder K, Fahey T: Should we advise parents to administer over the counter cough medicines for acute cough? Systematic review of randomised controlled trials, *Arch Dis Child* 86(3):170-175, 2002.

Schroeder K, Fahey T: Systematic review of randomised controlled trials of over the counter cough medicines for acute cough in adults, *BMJ* 324(7333):329-331, 2002.

Wallis C: Mucolytic therapy in cystic fibrosis, *J R Soc Med* (94 Suppl)40:17-24, 2001.

Internet Resources

American College of Allergy, Asthma, and Immunology maintains a website for patients and professionals. Available online at http://www.allergy.mcg.edu/home.html.

The Medical Letter: OTC cough remedies. Available online at http://www.medicalletter.com/#1100.

The National Institute of Allergy and Infectious Disease commissioned a report on allergies and their treatment. Available online at http://www.theallergyreport.org/.

CHAPTER

55

Pituitary Drugs

MICHAEL R. VASKO • KATHLEEN GUTIERREZ

 Visit **http://evolve.elsevier.com/Gutierrez/** for additional information.

KEY TERMS

Acromegaly, p. 905

Anterior pituitary, p. 899

Diabetes insipidus, p. 903

Dwarf, p. 905

Gigantism, p. 905

Hormone, p. 897

Negative feedback regulation, p. 898

Posterior pituitary, p. 899

Syndrome of inappropriate ADH (SIADH), p. 903

Target tissues, p. 897

OBJECTIVES

- Identify the two parts of the pituitary gland.
- Describe the function of the two hormones of the neurohypophysis (posterior pituitary).
- Describe the function of the hormones of the adenohypophysis (anterior pituitary).
- Describe the use of antidiuretic hormone.
- Identify the source and use of growth hormones.
- Develop a nursing care plan for the patient receiving drug therapy for diabetes insipidus, for growth hormone deficiency, or to suppress excessive release of growth hormone.

 PHYSIOLOGY • Endocrine System

A **hormone** is a substance synthesized by a specific cell type and released into the circulation to act on target tissues elsewhere in the body, thereby producing a physiologic or biochemical response. An example is thyrotropin (thyroid-stimulating hormone, or TSH), which is synthesized in the anterior pituitary, released into systemic circulation, and taken up by the thyroid gland, where it stimulates production of thyroid hormones (see Chapter 56).

Organs producing hormones that enter systemic circulation are called endocrine glands—pancreas, adrenals, thyroid, parathyroids, testes, ovaries, and pituitary. Tissues affected by hormones from endocrine glands are designated **target tissues.** For example, the thyroid gland is a target tissue for TSH. Other tissues do not respond to this hormone.

Hormones fall into two categories based on their chemical composition. One type, the steroid hormones that are derived from cholesterol, includes hormones of the adrenal gland (e.g., cortisol, cortisone, aldosterone, and corticosterone) and hormones of the sex glands (androgens, estrogens, and progestins). Hormones of the second type are peptides or proteins formed from amino acids. Examples of amino acid derivatives are triiodothyronine and thyroxine, which are formed in the thyroid by iodinating tyrosine.

Peptides and proteins are different in size, and peptides contain fewer amino acids than proteins. Peptides and proteins are similar chemically in that both are formed by peptide bonds linking carboxyl and amino groups of adjacent amino acids. Examples of peptide hormones are the releasing factors produced in the hypothalamus (e.g., thyrotropin-releasing hormone, composed of three amino acids) and the posterior pituitary hormones, oxytocin and antidiuretic hormone (ADH; also known as vasopressin), which are each composed of nine amino acids. Protein hormones are larger as exemplified by luteinizing hormone (LH) and follicle-stimulating hormone (FSH), both of which have molecular weights near 30,000 Daltons (atomic mass units).

Hormones are potent agents capable of exerting profound effects on metabolism. To remain healthy the body must ensure that hormones act only where and when they are needed and that they are present at the proper concentrations. The time of appearance and the concentration of a hormone in the blood may be regulated by controlling its rate of synthesis, release from storage sites, degradation, and clearance from the body. Several hormones are stored after synthesis and are released from storage sites only when the proper stimulus is received. For example, triiodothyronine and thyroxine are stored in a complex with thyroglobulin in the thyroid gland. Insulin is stored in granules within beta cells of the pancreas. In these cases, when the endocrine gland is stimulated to release hormone, the stored hormone is released first. Then, if required, newly synthesized hormone is released into the blood.

Regulation of synthesis and release of many hormones involves interactions between the CNS and the endocrine glands. For example, the hypothalamus in the brain controls the pituitary gland, which regulates production of hormones by the ovaries, testes, thyroid, and adrenal glands. This system is called **negative feedback regulation** (Figure 55-1).

Controlling a hormone's location of action is accomplished by one of two localization mechanisms. The first one restricts distribution of the hormone. Examples

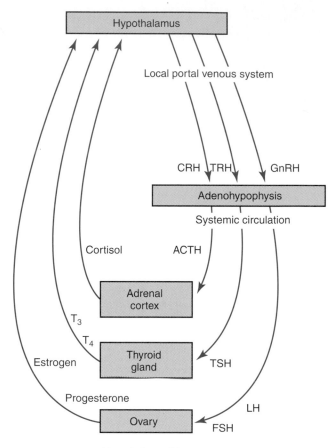

FIGURE 55-1   Regulation of hormone synthesis by negative feedback loops. Each arrow indicates a hormone, its source, and its target tissue. Hypothalamic synthesis of individual releasing factors is suppressed by high blood concentrations of appropriate final hormone. For example, cortisol suppresses corticotropin-releasing hormone (*CRH*) synthesis and release, thereby blocking further cortisol synthesis. Other loops are similarly regulated. *ACTH*, Adrenocorticotropic hormone; *FSH*, follicle-stimulating hormone; *GnRH*, gonadotropin-releasing hormone; *LH*, luteinizing hormone; T_3, triiodothyronine; T_4, thyroxine; *TRH*, thyrotropin-releasing hormone.

include the releasing factors synthesized in the hypothalamus that are secreted into local portal veins (transporting the hormones directly to the anterior pituitary) and not into general circulation.

The second mechanism localizes the effect of widely released hormones. These hormones interact with specific receptors found only in their target tissues. A specific receptor is required for hormone activity. For example, TSH receptors are found in the thyroid gland but not in most other organs. Therefore, even though TSH is released into general circulation, it acts only on the thyroid.

Hormone receptors may be within cells. For example, steroids and thyroid hormones affect target cells by interacting with intracellular receptors, such as those discussed in Chapter 1. Steroid hormones are bound to specific receptors that transport the hormones through the cytoplasm of the cell and into the nucleus, where the final effect of the hormone is produced. Thyroid hormones likewise move to the nucleus of target cells, where they bind to specific receptors and ultimately alter protein synthesis in cell.

In contrast to the receptors for steroids and thyroid hormones, receptors for peptide and protein hormones are on the external surface of cell membranes. Therefore the peptide and protein hormones need not enter cells to become effective. One mechanism by which these externally bound hormones act is by releasing an internal regulator, or second messenger. Second messengers include cyclic adenosine monophosphate (cAMP), calcium ions, and inositol 1,4,5-trisphosphate (IP_3).

Although the pituitary gland consists of less than 1 g of tissue at the base of the brain, it is the primary regulator of the endocrine system, controls normal growth, and regulates water balance. The pituitary gland is divided into two portions with different tissue compositions and embryologic origins: the **anterior pituitary** (or adenohypophysis) and the **posterior pituitary** (or neurohypophysis).

POSTERIOR PITUITARY

The posterior pituitary gland is composed of nerve fibers that arise from the hypothalamus during fetal development. In adulthood, close contact between the CNS and the posterior pituitary is maintained by the nerve fibers that run from the hypothalamus through the hypophyseal stalk to the posterior pituitary (Figure 55-2). Two peptide hormones closely related in structure, ADH and oxytocin, are released by the posterior pituitary. These hormones are synthesized in the hypothalamus and transported in secretion granules down the axons to the posterior pituitary. The granules accumulate at the nerve fiber terminals in the posterior pituitary, where their release into systemic circulation is regulated by nerve impulses from the hypothalamus. Damage to the hypophyseal stalk impairs transport of secretory granules to the posterior pituitary and interferes with appropriate release of the hormones.

Neurohypophyseal Hormones

The target organs of oxytocin are breast myoepithelium and smooth muscle of the uterus, especially during the second and third stages of labor. The effects of oxytocin on these tissues are discussed in Chapter 60. Oxytocin also causes milk ejection by stimulating contraction of the breast myoepithelium. The regulation of oxytocin release is a particularly good example of the close interaction of

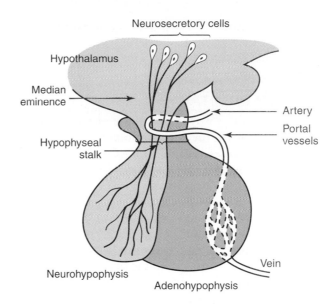

FIGURE 55-2 Anatomy of the pituitary gland.

the CNS with pituitary function. Suckling by the infant induces afferent nerve impulses from the breast to the brain, which causes more oxytocin to be synthesized and the stored hormone to be released. A similar reflex loop may operate in parturition when dilation of the cervix is thought to stimulate synthesis and release of oxytocin.

ADH acts primarily on renal tubular epithelium. It increases permeability of the renal collecting duct to water by causing a protein called aquaporin-2 to associate with the cell membrane; this movement creates a pore or channel through which water may pass. This action allows water to be reabsorbed and the urine to become concentrated. Other target tissues such as smooth muscle of blood vessels and of the GI tract may respond to concentrations of ADH that are higher than normal. The action of ADH on these tissues cause vasoconstriction and increased GI motility, respectively.

Secretion of ADH is regulated mainly in response to plasma osmolarity, the concentration of solute molecules that increase osmotic pressure. Dehydration causes the effective osmotic pressure of blood to increase. Osmoreceptors in the hypothalamus respond to this change by stimulating the neurohypophysis to secrete ADH. In turn, ADH causes the kidneys to conserve body water and prevent or slow further dehydration. Recovery from dehydration is aided further by stimulation of the thirst center, which usually leads to increased fluid intake. Reduction in the effective plasma volume caused by hemorrhage or reduced cardiac output stimulates ADH release and promotes antidiuresis (water retention).

In addition to these physiologic controls, certain drugs may also influence ADH secretion. Acetylcholine, barbiturates, nicotine, morphine, and bradykinin cause release of ADH in healthy subjects. Ethanol or phenytoin may promote diuresis by inhibiting ADH release.

ANTERIOR PITUITARY

The anterior pituitary is regarded as the master gland of the endocrine system. The anterior pituitary secretes several peptide hormones, most of which directly stimulate secretion by the adrenal glands, thyroid gland, and reproductive organs (Table 55-1).

Although the anterior pituitary is a true secretory tissue that synthesizes and releases its hormones, control of those secretions lies in the brain. Small polypeptides called neurohormones or releasing factors are synthesized in the median eminence of the hypothalamus and released into the portal venous system (see Figure 55-2), which carries them directly to the anterior pituitary, where the neurohormones act on a specific type of tar-

get cell to stimulate or inhibit synthesis and release of the proper hormone.

Damage to the pituitary may cause it to produce insufficient amounts of hypophyseal hormones, a condition called panhypopituitarism. Adults who have this syndrome require replacement therapy with thyroid hormones, adrenal steroids, and appropriate sex steroids. Children who have panhypopituitarism may also exhibit reduced growth because of a lack of growth hormone.

Growth Hormone

Growth hormone regulates the length of the long bones of the skeleton, which determines adult height. In addition, the hormone is a potent anabolic agent that causes many tissues to increase cell size and numbers. This anabolic action results from changes produced in protein, carbohydrate, and fat metabolism. The hormone increases amino acid transport into cells and elevates cellular protein synthesis. Growth hormone also antago-

TABLE 55-1

Physiologic Action of Adenohypophyseal Hormones

Descriptive Name	Other Names	Hypothalamic Factors	Target Tissue	Target Tissue Response
Adrenocorticotropic hormone	ACTH	Corticotropin-releasing hormone (CRH)	Adrenal cortex	Increased steroid synthesis
Follicle-stimulating hormone	FSH	Gonadotropin-releasing hormone (GnRH) FSH-releasing hormone (FRH and FSH-RH)	Ovary Seminiferous tubules	Increased estrogen production Maturation
Growth hormone	GH Somatotropin	Growth hormone–releasing hormone (GHRH) Somatostatin	Whole body	Increased anabolism, cell size, and cell numbers
Lipotropin	LPH	Corticotropin-releasing hormone (CRH)	Unknown	Unknown
Luteinizing hormone	Interstitial cell–stimulating hormone LH	Gonadotropin-releasing hormone (GnRH) Luteinizing hormone–releasing hormone (LH-RH)	Ovary Leydig's cells	Ovulation; formation of corpus luteum Increased androgen synthesis
Alpha melanocyte-stimulating hormone	Alpha MSH	Corticotropin-releasing hormone (CRH)	Melanocytes	Disperse pigment in melanocytes
Beta melanocyte-stimulating hormone	Beta MSH	Corticotropin-releasing hormone (CRH)	Unknown	Unknown
Prolactin	PRL	Dopamine	Breast	Milk formation
Thyroid-stimulating hormone	Thyrotropin, TSH	Thyrotropin-releasing hormone (TRH)	Thyroid gland	Increased triiodothyronine (T_3) and thyroxine (T_4) synthesis

nizes the action of insulin; this action tends to decrease glucose uptake and carbohydrate use, thus elevating liver glycogen and blood glucose levels. Finally, growth hormone increases the mobilization of fats for energy, which leads to a rise in blood levels of free fatty acids.

Many actions of growth hormone are mediated by peptides called insulin-like growth factors (IGFs), formerly called somatomedins. Growth hormone stimulates production of IGF-I and IGF-II in liver and at the cartilaginous growing plate of bone. In addition to stimulating skeletal growth, these peptides have insulin-like actions on other tissues.

The secretion of growth hormone is regulated by two hormones from the hypothalamus; one stimulates release and the other inhibits it. The releasing hormone, gonadotropin hormone–releasing hormone (GHRH), is a protein containing about 40 amino acids. The inhibitory factor is a smaller, 14–amino acid peptide called somatostatin. In addition to regulating growth hormone release, somatostatin may also influence TSH and adrenocorticotropic hormone (ACTH) release from the pituitary. Somatostatin is found in other tissues, such as the gut and the pancreas, and can block the release of insulin, glucagon, and gastrin at those sites.

Prolactin

Prolactin is released from the anterior pituitary and is important in development of the ductus and lobuloepithelium of the breast. After birth, the prolactin level in males declines and remains low, whereas the level in females varies with their menstrual cycle. During pregnancy, the prolactin level rises and can remain elevated after parturition if the mother is lactating. The suckling response of the child promotes prolactin release from the pituitary. Prolactin is negatively regulated by dopamine, which is released into the portal circulation and acts on D_2 receptors on lactotropes in the anterior pituitary. Drugs that block D_2 receptors (e.g., antipsychotics) can result in hyperprolactinemia, whereas D_2 receptor agonists can inhibit secretion.

Hyperprolactinemia occurs with the use of dopamine antagonists, with diseases of the hypothalamus or pituitary (including tumors), or in some instances with renal failure. Women with an excess of prolactin may have amenorrhea, galactorrhea, or infertility; men may be impotent or infertile and may have loss of libido. Treatment of this condition is covered in Chapter 61.

Gonadotropic Hormones

The gonadotropic hormones of the adenohypophysis are follicle-stimulating hormone (FSH), luteinizing hormone (LH), and prolactin. Both FSH and LH regulate maturation and function of male and female sexual organs. Release of these two hormones from the adenohypophysis is controlled by gonadotropin-releasing hormone (GnRH), which is produced in the hypothalamus. The clinical uses of GnRH are covered in Chapter 61.

In the pubertal male, FSH causes the seminiferous tubules to mature, and LH increases the number of testicular interstitial cells and stimulates their secretion of androgens. These androgens are the steroid hormones that complete the maturation process, leading to the production of viable sperm and the development of secondary male sexual characteristics. In the maturing female, FSH and LH are produced in greater quantities at puberty and stimulate ovarian estrogen production. Estrogens, the female steroid hormones, cause the female secondary sex characteristics to develop.

In addition to their role in development, FSH and LH control the menstrual cycle in women (Figure 55-3). Regulation of this function involves the hypothalamus, adenohypophysis, ovaries, and endometrium (uterine lining). The first event in the cycle is a rise in the concentration of FSH in the blood. In response, one of the hundreds of primordial ovarian follicles begins to develop. As the follicle matures under the influence of FSH, it begins to produce increasing amounts of estrogens, which greatly increase adenohypophyseal secretion of LH. This surge in LH secretion at midcycle is the primary trigger for ovulation, the release of an ovum from the mature follicle. The uses of LH and FSH to treat infertility are covered in Chapter 61.

In the second half of the menstrual cycle, LH causes the follicle (from which an ovum was released) to develop into a thickened, secretory tissue called the corpus luteum. The corpus luteum secretes large quantities of progesterone, another steroid hormone. By about day 21 of the cycle, the large quantities of circulating estrogen and progesterone inhibit adenohypophyseal secretion of FSH and LH (see Figure 55-3), and the corpus luteum begins to involute. Steroid hormone production falls rapidly as the corpus luteum fails and brings about the final stage in the cycle, the collapse of the endometrial lining.

During menses the inner uterine surface is denuded, and the endometrium rapidly collapses to about 65% of its former thickness. About 70 mL of blood and serum is lost along with necrotic and dissolving tissue during a typical menstrual period. Normally this blood does not clot, because fibrinolysin is in the fluid. Fibrinolysin is an enzyme that digests the fibrin matrix on which blood clots form. Despite the favorable environment for bacterial growth, the uterus is resistant to infection during menstruation, partly because of the many leukocytes present in menstrual fluid.

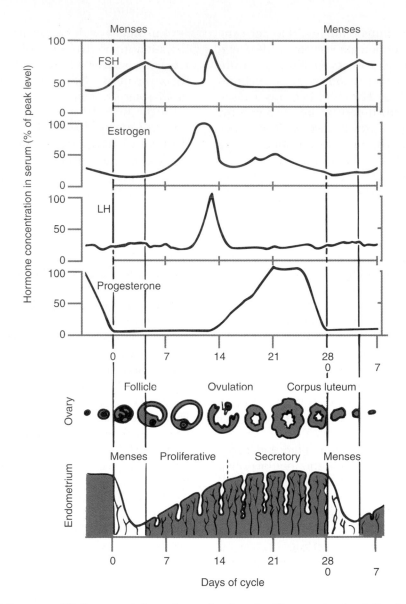

FIGURE 55-3 Pituitary regulation of menstrual cycle. Changes in circulating hormone levels are correlated with ovarian follicle and endometrial alterations. *FSH*, Follicle-stimulating hormone; *LH*, luteinizing hormone.

Proopiomelanocortin Hormones

When corticotropin (adrenocorticotropic hormone, or ACTH) is released by the anterior pituitary, it stimulates the adrenal cortex to synthesize and release cortisol (a major adrenocortical steroid hormone) as well as other glucocorticoids and minor amounts of sex steroids (see Chapter 57).

Cortisol blood levels are monitored by the hypothalamus, which adjusts the rate of release of corticotropin-releasing hormone (CRH) into the portal venous system to the adenohypophysis, thereby controlling the release of ACTH. When cortisol levels become too high, the hypothalamus reduces CRH release. The adenohypophysis, lacking appropriate stimulation, reduces ACTH production, and the blood level of ACTH falls. The adrenocortical production of cortisol falls because of the lowered ACTH level. Blood levels of cortisol thus are prevented from exceeding an upper limit. Conversely, when cortisol levels in blood fall too low, the hypothalamus prevents a dangerously low level from developing by releasing CRH into the portal venous system to stimulate release of ACTH from the adenohypophysis. In response to the increased ACTH concentration, the adrenal cortex elevates cortisol production. This intricate regulatory sequence is an example of a negative feedback loop, a regulatory mechanism whereby the product of a reaction sequence inhibits operation of the sequence and keeps the concentration of the product between fixed limits (see Figure 55-1).

The other hormones in this family include alpha and beta melanocyte-stimulating hormone as well as beta and gamma lipotropins. Although alpha-MSH stimulates melanocytes, the physiologic function of the other hormones is not well understood.

Thyroid-Stimulating Hormone

Negative feedback regulation applies not only to the adrenal cortex and the ovary but also to the thyroid gland (see Figure 55-1). The hormone TSH is discussed in Chapter 56.

PATHOPHYSIOLOGY • ADH Deficiency or Excess

When the hypothalamic region responsible for synthesis of ADH is destroyed or when the hypophyseal stalk above the median eminence is separated, ADH is significantly reduced or absent (see Figure 55-2). In these cases, urinary concentration is impossible, and a large volume of dilute, sugar-free urine is produced. This condition is called **diabetes insipidus** and differs from diabetes mellitus, which arises from the inability to use blood glucose or to release insulin.

Diabetes insipidus is not life threatening unless severe electrolyte imbalances develop. If the patient has a functional thirst center and can balance excessive fluid losses with high fluid intakes, severe imbalances usually do not occur. When a person is unconscious and unable to take in adequate fluids, however, severe dehydration may set in before the condition is noticed. Thus, after head injuries or surgery to the hypothalamic region, health care personnel must monitor urinary specific gravity and the blood sodium level along with fluid intake and urinary volumes to detect excessive diuresis and resultant dehydration.

In many patients with trauma to the hypothalamus or the hypophyseal stalk, the resultant diabetes insipidus may be transitory. In patients whose condition is chronic, reversal of symptoms can be achieved by replacement therapy (using a form of ADH) or drug therapy (using thiazide diuretics, for instance). This form of diabetes insipidus is called central diabetes insipidus because it arises from a lack of secretion of ADH from the neurohypophysis. The symptoms of diabetes insipidus may also arise if the neurohypophysis is producing normal amounts of ADH but the kidney responds poorly or not at all to ADH. This syndrome, called nephrogenic diabetes insipidus, may be treated with thiazide diuretics but is resistant to therapy with ADH. Although nephrogenic diabetes insipidus may arise as a genetic disease, it also may be induced by drugs such as lithium that impair the ability of the kidney to react to ADH.

The **syndrome of inappropriate ADH (SIADH)** secretion is a rare condition in which patients show symptoms of water intoxication, including hyponatremia (low sodium level in the blood and low serum osmolality). Despite these conditions, the kidneys continue to excrete sodium. The symptoms of SIADH are caused by release of more ADH than is appropriate for response to normal osmotic regulatory signals. In most patients with SIADH, the excess ADH is released by a tumor such as a bronchogenic carcinoma. Other less common causes of SIADH are CNS disorders (including head injuries or infections), extreme physical stress (such as surgery), or extreme emotional stress. A variety of drugs, including carbamazepine, chlorpropamide, antipsychotics, antidepressants, and thiazide diuretics, occasionally trigger SIADH.

Treatment of SIADH usually is aimed directly at removing the cause of the condition, such as removing the tumor or discontinuing the drug thought to precipitate the disorder. Fluid restriction, infusion of hypertonic saline, and use of diuretics all may help control the fluid and electrolyte imbalances associated with SIADH. If the cause of excessive ADH cannot be completely removed, symptoms may be relieved by administering demeclocycline, a tetracycline (see Chapter 28) that renders the kidneys less sensitive to ADH.

DRUG CLASS • Posterior Pituitary Replacement Drug

desmopressin acetate (DDAVP, Stimate)

MECHANISM OF ACTION

The synthetic vasopressin analog desmopressin has the same actions on renal ADH receptors as the missing natural hormone. Desmopressin therefore enables the kidneys to concentrate urine and conserve body water.

USES

Central diabetes insipidus is caused by a deficiency in ADH and therefore can be treated by replacement therapy with desmopressin. This drug is also used for renal failure (Chapter 47), but is not effective in nephrogenic diabetes insipidus.

PHARMACOKINETICS

When used to treat central diabetes insipidus, desmopressin is most commonly administered intranasally. The onset of action by this route is about an hour, and the duration is from 8 to 20 hours. Desmopressin may also be used intravenously, primarily for unconscious patients.

ADVERSE REACTIONS AND CONTRAINDICATIONS

Mild hypertension may be caused by the weak vasoconstrictor action of the drug. Effects on intestinal smooth muscle may cause stomach or intestinal cramping. Local effects may include rhinitis (with the intranasal dosage form) and phlebitis (with an intravenous injection).

Water retention is an expected result of taking the drug, but occasionally with long-term therapy, water intoxication and hyponatremia may arise.

INTERACTIONS

DDAVP used in the presence of chlorpropamide, clofibrate, or carbamazepine may elicit an enhanced diuretic response. Demeclocycline, lithium, or norepinephrine may diminish the antidiuretic response to desmopressin.

 DRUG CLASS • Miscellaneous Drugs Used to Treat Diabetes Insipidus

Thiazide Diuretics

chlorpropamide

clofibrate

MECHANISM OF ACTION

Thiazide diuretics are commonly used to increase urine flow (see Chapter 46). Paradoxically, thiazide diuretics are effective in some cases of central diabetes insipidus, especially when combined with another oral agent listed in this section. The effectiveness of thiazide diuretics is based on their ability to block electrolyte reabsorption, resulting initially in increased sodium and water excretion. The kidneys respond to this change by reabsorbing more water by mechanisms that do not depend on ADH. Moderate salt restriction may enhance the action of these drugs.

When chlorpropamide is used to treat diabetes insipidus, the action sought is a direct sensitization of the kidneys to ADH so that lower than normal levels of ADH cause nearly normal water reabsorption. Alone or with a thiazide diuretic, chlorpropamide usually reduces urine volume.

Clofibrate may be effective in treating diabetes insipidus, either alone or combined with a thiazide diuretic, because clofibrate increases release of ADH from the posterior pituitary and also potentiates the action of ADH on the kidney.

USES

In addition to their use to treat diabetes insipidus, thiazides are commonly used diuretics (see Chapter 46); chlorpropamide is an oral hypoglycemic drug (see Chapter 58); and clofibrate is an antilipemic drug (see Chapter 42).

PHARMACOKINETICS

Each of these drugs is orally administered; this provides convenience for patients using them long-term. For other information, see the chapters noted above, under Uses.

ADVERSE REACTIONS AND CONTRAINDICATIONS

Doses of thiazides used to treat diabetes insipidus are the same as those used for other indications. The most common side effect is potassium depletion, which in extreme cases may induce arrhythmia and impair neuromuscular, GI, or renal function.

Chlorpropamide is used at similar doses to treat diabetes mellitus or diabetes insipidus. The major potential result of toxicity is hypoglycemia.

Clofibrate may produce nausea or, in rare cases, muscle cramps and weakness.

INTERACTIONS

The most important interactions for thiazides relate to their tendency to cause potassium loss. For other interactions, refer to the chapters noted under Uses.

PATHOPHYSIOLOGY • Growth Hormone Deficiency or Excess

Deficiency of growth hormone in childhood results in loss of IGF-I activity, which causes the adult height to be well below average. A person with growth hormone deficiency may be referred to as a **dwarf**.

In addition to the obvious effects on stature, growth hormone deficiency is linked to reduced mass of the left ventricle such that these patients show poor left ventricular function on exercise. Treatment by replacement therapy with growth hormone corrects both aspects of the disease.

Acromegaly and **gigantism** are produced by excessive growth hormone, but the age of onset causes significant differences in the manifestations of the disease. Excessive growth hormone from an early age produces the rare condition of gigantism; growth rates up to 3½ inches per year have been observed.

Acromegaly results if excessive growth hormone production continues past puberty (i.e., after the plates of the long bones have joined and normal skeletal growth has halted). In this condition, only those tissues still able to grow and expand respond to growth hormone. This results in thickened fingers, coarse facial features, and a massive lower jaw. Less obvious changes include myocardial hypertrophy occurring with various signs of cellular damage in the heart. Some of these changes can be reversed by lowering growth hormone or IGF-I levels.

Gigantism and acromegaly are both caused by pituitary neoplasms that secrete excessive amounts of growth hormone. Consequently, therapy is designed to destroy or remove the tumor. Successful treatment arrests progressive symptoms of the disease but does not erase existing deformations. When removal or destruction of the tumor is impossible or only partially successful, dopamine receptor agonists such as bromocriptine and cabergoline may inhibit release of growth hormone in patients with acromegaly. For a discussion of dopamine receptor agonists see Chapter 23. Other drugs to treat growth hormone deficiency are summarized in Table 55-2 and discussed later in the chapter.

TABLE 55-2

Drugs Affecting Growth Hormone

Generic Name	Brand Name	Comments
bromocriptine	Parlodel	Derivative of ergot alkaloids that is a dopamine receptor agonist and suppresses growth hormone secretion
cabergoline	Dostinex	Long-acting dopamine receptor agonist
lanreotide	Somatuline LA	Analog of somatostatin
octreotide	Sandostatin, Sandostatin-LAR	Analog of somatostatin that suppresses intestinal hormones, insulin, glucagon, and growth hormone
sermorelin	Geref	Form of growth hormone–releasing hormone that stimulates release of growth hormone from intact pituitaries
somatrem	Protropin	Recombinant protein that differs from natural human growth hormone by one amino acid; used as replacement therapy
somatropin	Genotropin, Humatrope, Nutropin, Saizen, Serostim	Recombinant protein that is identical to natural human growth hormone; used as replacement therapy

DRUG CLASS • **Growth Hormones**

sermorelin (Geref)

somatrem (Protropin)

somatropin (Genotropin, Humatrope, Nutropin, Saizen, Serotim)

MECHANISM OF ACTION

Recombinant growth hormone stimulates growth by the same physiologic mechanisms as natural growth hormone, including stimulating production of IGF-I. Human growth hormone extracted from human pituitaries has not been used since 1985 because of the risk of transmitting Creutzfeldt-Jakob disease.

USES

Slow or inadequate growth may arise from many causes, but only that form caused by growth hormone deficiency is appropriately treated with growth hormone. The standard preparations for therapy are prepared by recombinant DNA techniques. Recombinant somatotropin has the same amino acid sequence as the natural human hormone (see Table 55-2). Somatrem is a recombinant form that has one more amino acid than natural growth hormone but has the same action as the natural hormone. Children or adolescents with pituitary dwarfism who receive growth hormone typically show an immediate increase in growth and may increase 12 inches or more in height over several years of treatment. Ultimately, resistance to the protein develops and growth tapers off.

PHARMACOKINETICS

Growth hormone, as a peptide, is susceptible to degradation by gastric acid and thus cannot be given orally. When given subcutaneously or intramuscularly the hormone has a half-life in serum of 5 hours or less, but the duration of measurable metabolic effects may be as long as 2 days. Growth hormone is cleared by hepatic mechanisms.

ADVERSE REACTIONS AND CONTRAINDICATIONS

Growth hormone causes few adverse reactions in most patients. In predisposed individuals, prolonged treatment with growth hormone may precipitate diabetes mellitus, because many actions of growth hormone antagonize those of insulin. Hypothyroidism will interfere with the response to growth hormone.

Growth hormone should not be given to adolescents whose epiphyses have sealed because stimulation of further natural growth will not occur. These preparations should not be used to enhance size or bulk in healthy young athletes because the risks outweigh the minimal benefits.

INTERACTIONS

Glucocorticoids may antagonize the growth stimulation produced by growth hormone. This effect is more pronounced with long-term dosing of glucocorticoids.

 DRUG CLASS • **Somatostatin**

lanreotide (Somatuline LA)

octreotide (Sandostatin, Sandostatin-LAR)

MECHANISM OF ACTION

These drugs mimic the actions of natural somatostatin as well as suppress the secretion of growth hormone and insulin-like growth factor (see Table 55-2). Somatostatin analogs are agonists at somatostatin receptors (SSTRs) and have high affinity at peripheral receptors. They also suppress the release of serotonin and other hormones including secretin, glucagons, insulin, and LH.

USES

Lanreotide and octreotide are used to treat disorders resulting from excessive growth hormone, namely acromegaly and gigantism. These drugs also are used to treat GI tumors. Octreotide is used as prophylaxis for patients undergoing pancreatic surgery and as an adjunct for patients with gastroesophageal bleeding. It also is used to treat diarrhea resulting from AIDS or cancer chemotherapy.

PHARMACOKINETICS

These drugs are usually given by intramuscular injection, although octreotide can be given by other parenteral routes. Octreotide is typically administered three times a day, but a slow-release formulation injected approximately once a month is available. Lanreotide is a longer-acting analog, which is injected every 10 to 14 days. The half-lives of octreotide and lanreotide are approximately 90 minutes and 5 days, respectively. These drugs are moderately bound to plasma proteins.

They are biotransformed by the liver and have a significant renal elimination.

ADVERSE REACTIONS AND CONTRAINDICATIONS

The most common adverse reactions to these drugs include nausea, vomiting, diarrhea, and abdominal pain. Irritation can occur at injection sites. A significant number of patients taking octreotide develop gallstones. Other less frequent adverse effects include headache, dizziness, and fatigue. Hypothyroidism and alteration of blood glucose also can occur. Lanreotide is contraindicated for women during pregnancy. These drugs should be given with caution to patients with diabetes mellitus or hypothyroidism.

INTERACTIONS

These drugs can reduce the absorption of other medications, especially cyclosporine.

APPLICATION TO PRACTICE

ASSESSMENT
History of Present Illness

When eliciting the patient's history of present illness, be alert to the time of onset, sequence of events, changes in complaints, and description of symptoms. Ask the patient about polyuria, polydipsia, polyphagia, symptoms of hyperglycemia, weight gain or loss, changes in body size or composition (including hat size), and nipple discharge. Symptoms need to be recorded regarding location, severity, tempo, and quality, as well as aggravating or alleviating factors.

Health History

Asking about previous illnesses helps the patient to recall past events of medical-surgical, psychiatric, or obstetric significance. Ask about previous hospitalizations, childhood and adult illnesses, surgical procedures, head injury, and trauma. A history of head trauma or visual changes is valuable in evaluating pituitary causes of polyuria. A menstrual and fertility history should also be noted. It is also important to inquire about sexual growth and development (axillary and pubic hair growth, genital development), menstrual patterns, and fertility status.

Elicit information from the patient about family members' illnesses, state of health or cause of death, and age. Identify any disorders occurring in family members that may relate to the patient's reports of symptoms (e.g., diabetes mellitus, thyroid disease, anemia, epilepsy, headaches, strokes, kidney disease, mental illness, and other conditions).

Ask the patient about the use of carbamazepine, chlorpropamide, antipsychotics, antidepressants, and thiazide diuretics because these drugs occasionally trigger SIADH. The patient should also be questioned about hypersensitivity to corticosteroids or porcine products.

Lifespan Considerations

Perinatal. A threefold increase in circulating levels of endogenous ADH has been reported during the last trimester of pregnancy and in labor compared with the nonpregnant state. Although such occurrences are infrequent, induction of uterine activity has been reported after intramuscular or intranasal administration of ADH. The intravenous use of desmopressin has also been reported to cause uterine contractions. Desmopressin has not been shown to produce tonic uterine contractions that could be deleterious to the fetus or threaten a pregnancy. However, it is classified as a category C drug and should be used during pregnancy only when clearly indicated.

Pediatric. The use of pituitary drugs in children older than 6 months of age is fairly safe. Because of the immaturity of the negative feedback mechanisms in children, the plasma levels of exogenous pituitary hormones might be difficult to regulate. Because children are more susceptible to fluid volume disturbance, drug therapies should be carefully chosen.

Although children who have a deficiency of growth hormone are normal at birth, growth progressively deviates from normal patterns, often beginning in infancy. Boys are affected more often than girls by a ratio of 3:1. The extent of the growth hormone deficiency may be complete or partial, but the cause is unknown. The disorder is frequently associated with deficiencies of other pituitary hormones such as TSH and ACTH. Thus it appears that the disorder is probably caused by hypothalamic deficiency. It has also been noted that there is a higher than average frequency in some families, which suggests a possible genetic cause in a number of instances.

Growth hormone has great potential for misuse, primarily because of its real and perceived effects on body size and composition. Enhanced athletic performance is the most commonly desired result.

Older Adults. Growth hormone is useless for stimulating linear growth in adults because of the closure of epiphyseal plates. Yet adult athletes often seek growth hormone to increase muscle mass and decrease body fat in a manner undetectable by current drug testing programs.

Owing to the age-related decline in hepatic and renal functioning, older adults are at higher risk for drug overdose. Older adults taking pituitary drugs should have routine monitoring of hepatic and renal functioning.

Cultural/Social Considerations

In general, pituitary disorders do not, in and of themselves, cause or produce significant cultural or social dysfunction. However, the disorders treated by pituitary drugs are often observable and might cause the patients some degree of social discomfort. Treatment is more likely to alleviate the social discomfort associated with pituitary-related illnesses than to add to it (see the Case Study: Diabetes Insipidus).

Physical Examination

In general, a complete physical examination should be performed on the patient with pituitary disorders. Pay special attention to the status of the patient's renal, cardiovascular, and respiratory systems, as well as his or her fluid and electrolyte balance. A thorough neurologic examination should be performed. The blood pressure should be checked with the patient lying down and standing. An accurate intake and output record should be kept, and the patient should be monitored for edema. The patient's height and weight is noted and compared with growth charts for children or with standardized tables for adults. The patient with suspected growth abnormalities should also have his or her hat and ring size, heel pad thickness, and soft tissue volume noted.

Laboratory Testing

Laboratory tests used to diagnose or monitor the patient with a pituitary disorder include urine specific gravity and osmolarity and screens of urine for FSH and LH, 17-ketosteroids, and 17-hydroxycorticosteroids. Other tests that may also be performed include serum electrolytes; blood sugar; testing for hormones such as ADH, cortisol, growth hormone, PRL, and somatomedin-C; thyroid function; and cortisol stimulation. CT or MRI scans can be used to visualize anatomic structures.

GOALS OF THERAPY

Because pituitary disorders are so rare and their treatment advances so rapid, consultation with a specialist in endocrinology is usually indicated. However, the overall goal of therapy is to bring the plasma levels of the affected hormone or hormones to within a normal range. With hormone excess, the relevant goal is to suppress the production of that hormone. With hormone deficits, the goal is to replace the deficient hormone and maintain or improve existing system functioning.

INTERVENTION
Administration

The use and dosages of pituitary drugs is determined on an individual basis, because the responsiveness of affected tissues varies. The drug should be administered as directed, and the patient monitored for allergic and adverse reactions. With a few exceptions, most pituitary drugs are available for parenteral use only. Because pituitary drugs are very potent, extra care is needed when preparing the drugs for use to prevent drug overdose.

Anterior Pituitary Hormones. Patients allergic to porcine products should receive an intradermal test dose before therapeutic or diagnostic dosages of corticotropin are given. Hypersensitivity reactions (i.e., wheezing, rash or hives, bradycardia, irritability, seizures, nausea, and vomiting) are more likely to occur when the drug is administered subcutaneously or during prolonged therapy. Additionally, patients on prolonged corticotropin therapy should routinely have hematologic, electrolyte, serum, and urine glucose values evaluated. Blood or urine glucose levels should be monitored periodically throughout therapy for patients on somatrem or somatropin.

Growth hormone drugs must be refrigerated before and after they are reconstituted with bacteriostatic water for injection. The solution should be clear after reconstitution and used within 14 days. The patient's height and weight, thyroid function, and glucose tolerance should be checked at regular intervals. Somatropin injections are administered at least 48 hours apart.

Posterior Pituitary Drugs. Desmopressin acetate is administered through a flexible nasal catheter used to measure the liquid. Once the drug is drawn into the catheter, one end is placed in the patient's nose and the other end in the patient's mouth. The patient then blows into the catheter to deposit the drug in the nasal passageways.

Lypressin should be administered by holding the bottle upright; the patient should be in a vertical position with the head upright. No more than three sprays should be taken at any one time. The two drugs should not be inhaled.

Hormone-Suppressant Drugs. Blood pressure should be monitored before and frequently during drug therapy. Advise the patient to remain supine during and for several hours after the first dose, because severe hypotension may occur. Ambulation and transfer should be supervised during initial dosing to prevent injury from the hypotension.

The preferred injection sites for octreotide are the hip, thigh, and abdomen. The injection sites should be rotated, and multiple injections to one site within a short time period should be avoided. The drug should be allowed to reach room temperature before administration to minimize local reactions at the injection site. The injections should be administered between meals and at bedtime.

Education

Proper planning is important for the patient receiving pituitary hormone therapy. The amount of instruction can vary, based on the treatment plan. For example, when the patient is a child it is important to make sure the family has a responsible caregiver who will ensure compliance with the treatment plan. In addition to teaching injection techniques, let the patient and caregivers know how and where to get the drugs and supplies for giving injections.

It is important to advise the patients and caregivers what to expect from the treatment and what changes should be reported to the health care provider. Routine

monitoring of drug and hormone levels should be stressed. Most of the drugs have a very short half-life, so it is important to ensure that the patient is compliant with drug administration.

Teaching plans must include information about the consequences of abruptly discontinuing treatment, physical changes to expect, and physical changes that must be brought to the attention of the health care provider. The patient should be advised to wear or carry medical alert identification, and advised to avoid the use of OTC drugs and to consult with the health care provider before adding any other drug to the treatment regimen.

A patient taking corticotropin should be advised to avoid immunizations that use live vaccines, because this drug decreases immunity. The patient should be instructed to notify the health care provider if fever, sore throat, muscle weakness, sudden weight gain, or edema develops. A dietitian can provide information about

---

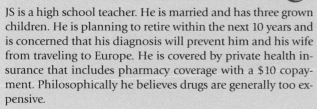

CASE STUDY *Diabetes Insipidus*

ASSESSMENT

HISTORY OF PRESENT ILLNESS

JS is a 53-year-old white man who comes to the outpatient clinic with complaints of increased thirst (particularly for ice-cold water) for the past 2 to 3 weeks and increased urination that keeps him up at night. He adds that epigastric fullness and anorexia is a problem. He has had an unintentional weight loss of 15 pounds over the last 2 to 3 weeks.

HEALTH HISTORY

JS's health history is positive for a broken nose with an obstructed right naris. He denies a history of brain tumor, head trauma, transient ischemic attack, stroke, or granulomatous disease. He has no known drug or food allergies and denies use of prescription or OTC drugs. He has frequent, severe episodes of allergic rhinitis.

LIFESPAN CONSIDERATIONS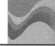

JS has no significant age-related changes in hepatic, renal, or cardiac functioning.

CULTURAL/SOCIAL CONSIDERATIONS

JS is a high school teacher. He is married and has three grown children. He is planning to retire within the next 10 years and is concerned that his diagnosis will prevent him and his wife from traveling to Europe. He is covered by private health insurance that includes pharmacy coverage with a $10 copayment. Philosophically he believes drugs are generally too expensive.

PHYSICAL EXAMINATION

JS is restless. His skin and mucous membranes are dry; skin turgor is poor. Blood pressure is 104/62 mm Hg, pulse 100, respirations 20.

LABORATORY TESTING

Urine specific gravity 1.001 with an osmolality of 175 mOsm/kg. Total 24-hour urinary output is 10.4 L. Serum sodium is 129 mEq/L; serum osmolality is 350 mOsm/kg; BUN 20 mg/dL; creatinine 1.5 mg/dL. Head MRI scan is unremarkable.

PATIENT PROBLEM(S)

Diabetes insipidus.

GOALS OF THERAPY

Restore renal function and prevent dehydration and hyponatremia.

CRITICAL THINKING QUESTIONS

1. The health care provider orders desmopressin intranasally at bedtime. What is the mechanism of action of desmopressin?
2. Why is desmopressin the preferred drug for JS?
3. What are the adverse reactions to desmopressin?
4. What laboratory testing is needed to monitor desmopressin therapy?
5. What instruction is needed for JS to properly administer desmopressin?

sodium-restricted diets that are high in vitamin D, protein, and potassium.

Advise patients taking drugs that cause drowsiness to use caution when driving or engaging in activities requiring alertness until the drug response is known. Caution the patient to avoid concurrent alcohol and OTC drug use during the course of treatment without first checking with the health care provider.

EVALUATION

Evaluation of treatment outcomes can be accomplished in a number of different ways. If the goal is to bring the hormone level to the normal range, routine monitoring of the plasma level of the drug and the affected hormone(s) is sufficient. But if the goal of treatment is to produce organ change, specific organ monitoring is needed. For example, if synthetic ADH is given for the treatment of diabetes insipidus, close monitoring of urine osmolarity and volume is vital. Finally, because of the integration of the endocrine system, it is important to evaluate the function of the other endocrine glands (e.g., by monitoring the blood glucose level).

A patient's clinical response to growth hormone can be evaluated by the child's attainment of normal adult height. The patient should be monitored for development of neutralizing antibodies if the growth rate does not exceed 2.5 cm in 6 months.

The effectiveness of treatment with desmopressin can be evaluated when the following are observed: decreased urinary output, increased urine specific gravity, decreased signs of dehydration, and decreased thirst. The patient should, however, be monitored for symptoms of water intoxication (e.g., drowsiness, listlessness, or headache).

Serum growth hormone levels and insulin-like growth factor concentrations should be monitored periodically during therapy. The effectiveness of therapy can be demonstrated by a decrease in galactorrhea in 6 to 8 weeks and by a decreased serum level of GH in patients with acromegaly.

The effectiveness of treatment with octreotide can be demonstrated by a relief of symptoms and suppressed tumor growth in patients with pituitary tumors associated with acromegaly.

Bibliography

Birmingham J: Growth hormone therapy in adults: what case managers need to know, *Case Manager* 12(2):57-63, 2001.

Dorton AM: The pituitary gland: embryology, physiology, and pathophysiology, *Neonatal Netw* 19(2):9-17, 70-74, 2000.

Growth hormone treatment outcome, *Nurses Drug Alert* 25(8):60-61, 2001. Levine LS, Boston BA: Effect of inhaled corticosteroids on the hypothalamic-pituitary-adrenal axis and growth in children, *J Pediatr* 137(4):450-454, 2000.

Maghnie M, Cosi G, Genovese E, Manca-Bitti ML, Cohen A, Zecca S, et al: Central diabetes insipidus in children and young adults, *N Engl J Med* 343(14):998-1007, 2000.

Settle M: Endocrine series #5. The hypothalamus, *Neonatal Netw* 19(6):9-14, 2000.

Tiedje LB: Toward evidence-based practice. Pituitary-adrenal and autonomic responses to stress in women after sexual and physical abuse in childhood. Commentary on Heim C, Newport DJ, Heit S, et al: Pituitary-adrenal and autonomic responses to stress in women after sexual and physical abuse in childhood, *JAMA* 284(5):592-597, 2000. *MCN Am J Matern Child Nurs* 26(6):344, 2001.

Vimalachandra D, Craig JC, Cowell CT, Knight JF: Growth hormone treatment in children with chronic renal failure: a meta-analysis of randomized controlled trials, *J Pediatr* 139(4):560-567, 2001.

Woodrow P: Head injuries: acute care, *Nurs Stand* 14(35):37-46, 2000.

Internet Resources

http://www.diabetesinsipidus.maxinter.net/.
http://www.emedicine.com/ped/topic2634.htm.
http://www.ndif.org/.
http://www.niddk.nih.gov/health/endo/pubs/acro/acro.htm.
http://www.nlm.nih.gov/medlineplus/ency/article/000377.htm.

CHAPTER

56

Thyroid and Parathyroid Drugs

MICHAEL R. VASKO • KATHLEEN GUTIERREZ

 Visit **http://evolve.elsevier.com/Gutierrez/** for additional information.

KEY TERMS

Chvostek's sign, p. 927

Cretinism, p. 914

Euthyroid state, p. 917

Follicular cells, p. 912

Graves' disease, p. 920

Hyperparathyroidism, p. 926

Hyperthyroidism, p. 920

Hypoparathyroidism, p. 926

Hypothyroidism, p. 914

Iodism, p. 925

Myxedema, p. 914

Trousseau's sign, p. 927

OBJECTIVES

- Compare and contrast the mechanism of action of thyroid and parathyroid hormones.
- Differentiate the physiologic and pathophysiologic changes that occur with excess and insufficient thyroid or parathyroid hormones.
- Discuss the rationale for therapy of hyperthyroidism.
- Describe the classes of drugs used for the treatment of hypothyroidism and hypoparathyroidism.
- Identify the goals of therapy for patients with thyroid and parathyroid disorders.
- Develop a nursing care plan for the patient receiving drug therapy for hypothyroidism or hyperthyroidism.
- Develop a nursing care plan for the patient receiving drug therapy for hypoparathyroidism or hyperparathyroidism.

911

PHYSIOLOGY • Thyroid Hormones

The thyroid gland and parathyroid glands are highly vascular organs that lie across the trachea in the region of the larynx (Figure 56-1). **Follicular cells** in the thyroid gland contribute to normal development and regulate the basal metabolic rate for most tissues in the body by synthesizing and releasing the iodine-containing hormones triiodothyronine (T_3) and thyroxine (T_4) into general circulation. These hormones then act through high-affinity receptors in cell nuclei to regulate expression of genes and modulate the primary function of cells by changing the pattern of protein synthesis. The receptor for thyroid hormones is in the same family of receptors used by adrenal steroids, vitamin D, and vitamin A. Tissues especially sensitive to thyroid hormones include skeletal muscle, heart, liver, and kidneys. The basal metabolic rate in these tissues is strongly stimulated by thyroid hormones, and clinically observed signs of these effects include rapid heartbeat and increased cardiac output. Other organs, including the brain, also respond to thyroid hormones, but to a lesser degree.

The thyroid also produces another hormone, calcitonin. This hormone regulates calcium levels in the body and acts in opposition to parathyroid hormone (see later in the chapter). It is released in response to a high level of calcium in the blood; conversely, secretion of the hormone is shut off when the calcium concentration is low.

REGULATION OF SYNTHESIS AND RELEASE OF THYROID HORMONES

The level of thyroid hormone in the blood is regulated in part by the negative feedback system, which holds TSH levels low when thyroid hormone levels are high, but elevates TSH levels when thyroid hormone levels are low. Thyroid-stimulating hormone (TSH) from the anterior pituitary stimulates each step of thyroid hormone synthesis described below.

The first step in synthesizing T_4 and T_3 is iodine uptake by follicular cells (Figure 56-2). The iodide level in blood is normally low, so follicular cells must concentrate iodide to carry out the synthetic reactions required to make T_4 and T_3. The active transport of iodide into the cells is stimulated by TSH. The normal concentration of iodide in the thyroid is 20 to 50 times that found in

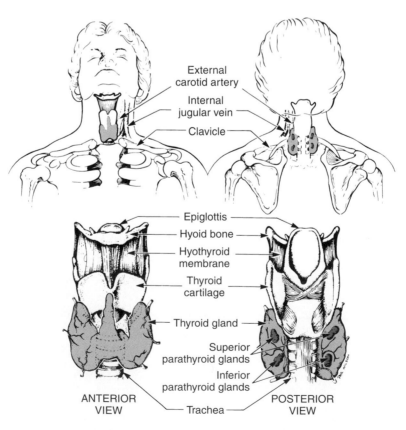

FIGURE 56-1 Anatomic location of thyroid and parathyroid glands.

plasma. In the second step of thyroid hormone synthesis, iodide is oxidized to its active form by thyroid peroxidase, an enzyme formed in follicular cells. This activation step takes place on the apical surface of the cell in microvilli protruding into colloid that fills the thyroid follicle. Once activated, iodide is attached to tyrosine molecules contained within the peptide chains of thyroglobulin in a process called organification. Thyroglobulin is a large protein synthesized in follicular cells and extruded into follicles, and it is the major protein component of colloid. This process results in monoiodotyrosyl or diiodotyrosyl residues in thyroglobulin.

The third step involves a coupling reaction in which two molecules of diiodotyrosyl combine to produce one molecule of thyroglobulin-bound T_4, or one molecule each of diiodotyrosyl and monoiodotyrosyl combine to yield one molecule of T_3. These reactions are catalyzed by thyroid peroxidase and regulated by TSH. Thyroglobulin is primarily a storage depot for thyroid hormones as well as monoiodotyrosyl and diiodotyrosyl residues. In healthy persons, each molecule of thyroglobulin contains two molecules of T_4, whereas a single molecule of T_3 occurs in about one of three molecules of thyroglobulin within the follicles.

When release of thyroid hormones is required, TSH stimulates microvilli of the follicular cells to move droplets of colloid into the cell. The colloid droplets fuse with lysosomes inside the cells to form vesicles called phagolysosomes (see Figure 56-2). The low pH and protein-digesting enzymes from the lysosomes break thyroglobulin down to amino acids. This process releases T_3, T_4, and the monoiodotyrosyl and diiodotyrosyl residues into the cell. The thyroid hormones T_3 and T_4 are transported to the cell surface and released into the blood. However, the monoiodotyrosyl and diiodotyrosyl residues are retained within the cell, and the iodide they contain is reclaimed for use in new hormone synthesis. Persons who lack the salvage pathway lose excessive iodide in urine and ultimately fail to produce sufficient thyroid hormones.

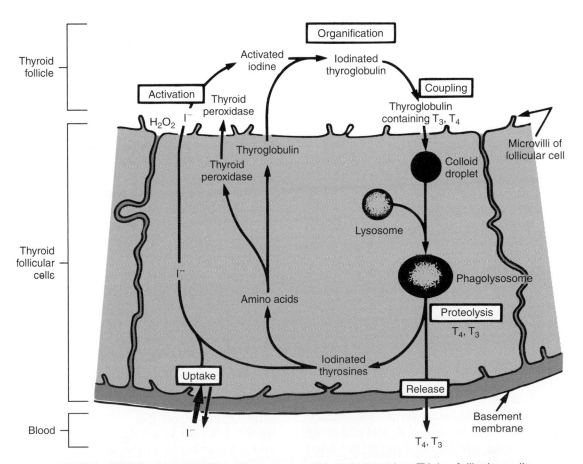

FIGURE 56-2 Synthesis of triiodothyronine (T_3) and thyroxine (T_4) by follicular cells within the thyroid gland. Single follicular cell is depicted. Cell base is in close contact with blood, and cell apex is in contact with colloid. These cells surround areas of colloid to form thyroid follicles. Parafollicular cells of thyroid gland do not directly contact colloid.

Once in the blood, thyroid hormones are rapidly and almost completely bound to a special alpha-globulin called thyroid-binding globulin (TBG). A less important carrier is prealbumin. Very little thyroid hormone is bound to plasma albumin in normal persons because the thyroid hormones are so tightly bound to TBG. However, the amount of thyroid hormone that may be bound to TBG is limited. TBG can bind about 2.5 times more hormone than it ordinarily carries. When that limit is reached, the excess hormone is bound to albumin and prealbumin. These proteins bind the hormone less tightly than TBG but have nearly unlimited capacity for hormones. The binding of thyroid hormones to plasma proteins prevents the metabolism of the hormones. Furthermore, only free (unbound) hormone is active.

The relative distribution of T_3 and T_4 differs within the body. T_4 is much more abundant than T_3 in the thyroid and the blood. The thyroid gland normally releases 70 to 90 mg of T_4 daily and only 15 to 30 mg of T_3, but T_4 is rapidly converted to T_3 in most tissues. Thus the most abundant form of thyroid hormone in target cells is T_3. This hormone is also the primary thyroid hormone that binds to nuclear receptors, setting off the metabolic events characteristic of thyroid action. For these reasons, T_3 is the most important metabolic regulator from the thyroid. In addition to being converted to T_3, T_4 may be converted to an alternate form called reverse T_3, which contains a different arrangement of iodine atoms than T_3 and is metabolically inactive.

PATHOPHYSIOLOGY • Hypothyroidism

Hypothyroidism occurs when the production of thyroid hormones is insufficient to meet the body's demands. Mild hormone deficiencies produce minimum disease with vague symptoms, sometimes making the condition difficult to diagnose. Untreated patients may ultimately develop characteristic signs and symptoms related to slowed metabolic rates and changes in the CNS (Table 56-1). The severe form of the disease is called **myxedema**, which may progress to a life-threatening coma with a profoundly lowered metabolic rate, depression of CNS functions, and hypoventilation. Although the typical patient with hypothyroidism is a woman over age 50, the disease can occur at any age and in either gender. Most cases occur in patients who are between the ages of 30 and 60. Hypothyroidism is at least twice as prevalent as hyperthyroidism, but treatment is relatively straightforward.

Most patients with hypothyroidism have primary thyroid atrophy. In North America, Hashimoto's thyroiditis (chronic lymphocytic thyroiditis, autoimmune thyroiditis) is a common cause. Prior treatment with radioiodine or thyroidectomy also is a common cause of hypothyroidism. This disorder may also coexist with other autoimmune disorders such as rheumatoid arthritis, systemic lupus erythematosus, or pernicious anemia. In primary hypothyroidism, the thyroid gland enlarges in an attempt to compensate for the inadequacy, and a goiter is formed. Insufficient quantities of thyroid hormones result in an overall decrease in the basal metabolic rate and in a variety of system manifestations (see Table 56-1).

Hypothyroidism may arise for reasons other than primary failure of the thyroid gland. For example, if the pituitary fails to release adequate TSH, too little thyroid hormone is made, and secondary hypothyroidism develops. Rarely, patients with hypothalamic damage fail to produce thyrotropin-releasing hormone (TRH), which is required to stimulate TSH production in the pituitary. This condition is called tertiary hypothyroidism. In this instance patients may be given either TRH or TSH as replacement therapy (Table 56-2).

Hypothyroidism may develop in newborns because of an embryologic or genetic defect that arrests thyroid development or prevents its function (congenital hypothyroidism). A child lacking adequate thyroid function during fetal development may appear nearly normal at birth because much of fetal development can be supported by maternal T_4, which readily crosses the placenta and enters the fetal brain. If the disease is not detected soon after birth, however, irreversible brain damage and associated physical signs develop. Congenital hypothyroidism (also called **cretinism**) can be treated by hormone replacement if the disease is recognized early.

Hypothyroidism that develops after the neonatal period but before puberty is called juvenile hypothyroidism. The most prominent early sign of juvenile hypothyroidism is stunted growth. If not treated appropriately, juvenile hypothyroid patients exhibit not only arrested growth but also other signs and symptoms associated with adult forms of the disease.

The diagnosis of primary hypothyroidism requires showing that a patient has lower than normal thyroid

TABLE 56-1

Thyroid Disorders

Condition	Symptoms	Physical Appearance
Hypothyroidism, adult onset (also called myxedema and Gull's disease)	Diminished vigor and muscle weakness Reduced mental acuity Emotional changes, especially depression Slow relaxation of deep tendon reflexes Muscle cramps Constipation Decreased appetite Abnormal menses in females Slow pulse and enlarged heart Tendency to gain weight Lowered basal metabolic rate	Puffy face and eyes Thin, coarse hair and eyebrows Dry, scaly, cold, and slightly yellow skin Enlarged tongue Slow, husky speech Dull or slow-witted appearance
Hypothyroidism, congenital (cretinism)	Absence of distal femoral and proximal tibial epiphyses Slowed brain development	Essentially normal at birth Slightly longer and heavier than normal
At 3 months with no treatment	Lethargy Feeding difficulty Constipation Persistent neonatal jaundice Respiratory distress Hoarse cry Intermittent cyanosis	Enlarged tongue Puffy face and thick neck Poor muscle tone Depressed nasal bridge with broad, flat nose Distended abdomen Umbilical hernia Short legs
Hyperthyroidism (also called thyrotoxicosis or Graves' disease)	Cardiac arrhythmia Enlarged thyroid gland Rapid pulse rate Increased basal metabolic rate Muscle weakness and wasting Fine tremor Heat intolerance Weight loss in most patients	Restlessness or nervousness Abrupt actions and speech Warm, moist palms Loosening of fingernails from nailbeds Bulging eyes with sclera visible all around iris White, unpigmented patches on skin (vitiligo)

hormone levels and an elevated level of TSH in the blood. Direct TSH determinations are commonly used, along with one of the measures of T_3 or T_4 in serum. Thyroidal uptake of iodine is also reduced in hypothyroidism, but this test is seldom useful in diagnosing the disease, because thyroidal uptake is affected by intake of iodine, which may come in food or drugs. The patient may be unaware that iodine is being taken. For example, potassium iodide, used as an expectorant, is a constituent of several prescription cough medicines.

Secondary and tertiary hypothyroidism may be distinguished from primary hypothyroidism by measuring the level of TSH. In primary hypothyroidism, TSH is elevated by the natural action of the negative feedback system attempting to elevate thyroid hormone levels, but TSH levels are low or undetectable in the other two forms of hypothyroidism. Secondary and tertiary hypothyroidism may be distinguished from each other by the protirelin (TRH) test, which measures the ability of the hypophysis to respond to its normal regulatory hormone. If TSH rises after TRH is given, the implication is that the hypothalamus is defective, and both the hypophysis and the thyroid could function normally if properly stimulated.

TABLE 56-2

Drugs for Thyroid Replacement Therapy or Diagnosis

Generic Name	Trade Name	Comments
Thyroid Hormones		
levothyroxine	Eltroxin, ✽ Levo-T, Levothroid, Levoxyl, Novothyrox, Unithroid	This pure form of T₄ is the preferred therapy for hypothyroidism. Intravenous form is used for myxedema coma.
liothyronine	Cytomel, Triostat	This pure form of T₃ may be used for adult hypothyroidism but not for cretinism, because T₃ may not cross the blood-brain barrier as well as T₄.
liotrix	Thyrolar	This combination of pure T₄ and T₃ in a 4:1 ratio may be used for hypothyroidism.
thyroid hormone	Thyrar	This crude preparation from thyroid glands contains variable amounts of T₄ and T₃. Dosage is difficult to adjust and maintain.
Adenohypophyseal Hormones		
protirelin	Thyrel, Relefact TRH ✽	This synthetic tripeptide identical to natural TRH is used for diagnosis.
thyrotropin	Thyrogen	Thyrotropin is natural TSH extracted from animals. It is used for diagnosis.

✽ Available only in Canada.

DRUG CLASS • Thyroid Hormones

desiccated thyroid USP (Armour Thyroid)

levothyroxine (Levo-T, Levothroid, Levoxyl, Novothyrox, Synthroid, Unithroid, Eltroxin,✽ PMS-Levothyroxine Sodium✽)

liothyronine (Cytomel, Triostat)

liotrix (Thyrolar)

MECHANISM OF ACTION

Thyroid hormones used in replacement therapy have exactly the same actions as the hormones naturally produced in the body. Basal metabolic rates are increased by actions on nuclear receptors in skeletal muscle as well as in the heart, liver, lungs, intestines, and kidneys. They promote gluconeogenesis, thus increasing the utilization and mobilization of glycogen stores. The drugs also stimulate protein synthesis, cell growth, and differentiation as well as aid in the development of the CNS.

USES

Thyroid hormones are primarily used to treat thyroid deficiency. They also have a role in control of goiter and thyroid carcinoma. They may also occasionally be used for diagnosis. Thyroid hormones should never be used in weight-loss programs.

Patients with myxedemic coma must be treated aggressively with thyroid hormones, glucocorticoids, and other supportive measures. Rapid replacement with thyroid hormones is necessary. Levothyroxine (T₄) is the preferred drug for replacement therapy of hypothyroidism. Liothyronine is a pure synthetic form of the natural thyroid hormone T₃. Liotrix is a thyroid preparation that contains both pure synthetic T₄ and T₃ in the ratio of 4:1. This mixture was designed to produce normal thyroid function tests when therapy is adequate, but there is little evidence that liotrix has any clinical advantage over levothyroxine. Thyroid USP is a defatted extract of whole thyroid glands. It contains T₄ and T₃ in the natural ratio of 2.5:1.

PHARMACOKINETICS

When it is given orally, levothyroxine is variably absorbed (48% to 79%) from the GI tract, whereas liothyronine is well absorbed. Both are distributed to the whole body. The onset of action is 48 hours, and peak effects are observed in 24 to 72 hours for liothyronine (T₃) and in 1 to 3 weeks for levothyroxine (T₄). Because of strong binding to plasma proteins (99%) levothyroxine has a serum half-life of about 7 days, making the serum level stable with once-daily dosing. The half-life of liothyronine is less than 1 to 2 days, making it less desirable for long-term therapy. Liothyronine and levothyroxine are biotransformed by the liver to glucuronide and sulfate derivatives, which then are eliminated in bile. No significant reuptake of the hormones occurs from the gut. Levothyroxine also is converted to T_3 by peripheral tissues. Other hormone destruction occurs in the target tissues, where the hormones are deiodinated and transformed to reverse T_3 and other inactive products.

ADVERSE REACTIONS AND CONTRAINDICATIONS

There are few adverse reactions to levothyroxine or liothyronine other than those indicating overdosage. The most common adverse reactions include irritability, insomnia, nervousness, headache, weight loss, and tachycardia. The adverse effects are essentially those of hyperthyroidism. In patients who have been newly diagnosed as having hypothyroidism, thyroid hormones are started at low dosages and increased gradually until the **euthyroid state** (normal levels of thyroid hormones) is achieved. These gradually increasing doses are used because a sudden return to adequate thyroid hormone levels produces acute stress on several body systems. Although rare, some older adults or predisposed patients are at risk for angina pectoris, coronary occlusion, or stroke, even with low dosages. Another difficulty may be relative adrenal insufficiency, which arises in patients who have inadequate pituitary function causing secondary hypothyroidism and secondary adrenal insuffi-

ciency. If thyroid hormone therapy is started in these patients without also restoring adequate glucocorticoid levels, they may experience a dangerous adrenal crisis. Overdosage with thyroid hormones produces signs of hyperthyroidism (see Table 56-1).

A few patients may be allergic to the tartrazine dye used in the yellow (100 mcg) or green (300 mcg) levothyroxine tablets. Although the incidence of tartrazine sensitivity in the general population is low, it is frequently found in patients who have aspirin hypersensitivity.

INTERACTIONS

Catecholamines must sometimes be given to combat the shock-like symptoms found in myxedemic coma. Patients so treated are especially at risk for developing an arrhythmia, because catecholamines and thyroid hormones both tend to cause this dangerous adverse reaction. Cholestyramine or colestipol may impede oral absorption of thyroid hormones; dosages can be adjusted based on thyroid function tests. Coumarins or other anticoagulants may be influenced by thyroid function; dosages can be adjusted based on prothrombin times. Desiccated thyroid has been shown to increase insulin or oral hypoglycemic requirements in patients with diabetes mellitus.

APPLICATION TO PRACTICE

ASSESSMENT
History of Present Illness

The patient with hypothyroidism most often complains of cold intolerance; coarse, dry skin; decreased sweating; swelling of the eyelids; and lethargy. Frequent complaints also include anorexia, constipation, hair loss, hoarseness or aphonia, swelling of the legs or face, and memory impairment.

Health History

When obtaining a health history, the health care provider elicits information from the patient related to congenital anomalies, stress, trauma, infection, and radiation exposure. Furthermore, information about comorbid diseases such as rheumatoid arthritis, systemic lupus erythematosus, and pernicious anemia should be elicited. Preexisting conditions presently treated with thyroid hormones must be included. A family history positive for thyroid abnormalities is important to note.

Lifespan Considerations

Perinatal. Pregnant women and newborns should be monitored for potential thyroid abnormalities as a basic standard of care, although hypothyroidism is un-

common in pregnancy. However, if the condition is left untreated, there is an increased risk of stillbirths, abortions, and congenital abnormalities. Fetal thyroid hormone production starts in the twelfth week of gestation. A low T_4 level in the mother during the first trimester may result in impaired fetal brain development.

Fetal thyroid state can be monitored by measuring thyroid hormones in amniotic fluid. Neonatal hypothyroidism occurs independently of maternal thyroid disease and is routinely screened via TSH testing 5 to 7 days after birth. If mothers who are taking thyroid hormones wish to breast-feed, infant thyroid hormone levels should be monitored.

Pediatrics. Thyroid disease may be congenital, causing onset to occur between birth and 2 years of age. If the condition is left untreated, it affects growth and development, causing mental retardation. The incidence rate of congenital hypothyroidism is approximately 1 in 4000; a 1% to 3% prevalence is reported in schoolchildren. Cretinism results when thyroid hormone deficiency during fetal or early neonatal life goes untreated. Such deficiency may be related to maternal iodine deprivation or congenital thyroid abnormalities.

Acquired hypothyroidism may result from thyroiditis caused by pituitary deficiency; operative removal of the thyroid gland; or other, unknown causes. Hypothyroidism occurring after 18 months of age is associated with reversible mental slowness. Between the ages of 1 and 5 years, the cause of hypothyroidism is usually maldeveloped or ectopic thyroid tissue.

Prompt diagnosis and treatment of hypothyroidism in children is necessary to prevent developmental retardation. Ossification of the epiphyses as well as brain growth and development are particularly affected. A delay of only 3 months in treatment of neonatal hypothyroidism causes irreversible mental retardation.

Thyroid disease is the most common endocrine disorder of adolescence. During adolescence, the prognosis of thyroid disease is usually good with appropriate therapy.

Older Adults. The clinical manifestations of hypothyroidism in the older adult are often subtle and can be mistakenly attributed to normal changes of aging. Hypothyroidism can manifest as carpal tunnel syndrome, dementia, pernicious anemia, or elevated cholesterol in addition to the common signs and symptoms previously discussed. Because clinical symptoms of thyroid disease are unreliable in this age group, routine laboratory screening is recommended.

Cultural/Social Considerations

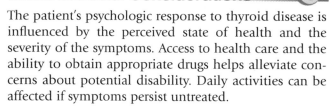

The patient's psychologic response to thyroid disease is influenced by the perceived state of health and the severity of the symptoms. Access to health care and the ability to obtain appropriate drugs helps alleviate concerns about potential disability. Daily activities can be affected if symptoms persist untreated.

Physical Examination

The physical examination should include an assessment of vital signs; height and weight; cardiac rhythm and regularity; skin color, temperature, and texture; and the texture of hair and nails. In hypothyroidism, there may be a notable loss of the outer third of the eyebrow. Vision, deep tendon reflexes, and mental status should also be evaluated.

Assessment of other body systems should include the presence or absence of tremor, pain, and proximal muscle weakness as well as the presence of periorbital or peripheral edema, slow speech, and hoarseness.

Laboratory Testing

T_3 and T_4 levels may remain within a broad range of normal, even when the patient has true but mild hypothyroidism. A slight elevation of TSH assay is also present. The serum TSH value, however, may be mis-

leading in patients who have pituitary or hypothalamic hypothyroidism.

The T_4 level should not be relied on to define the patient's thyroid status. Although the values may fall within the normal range for the population as a whole, they can be abnormal for the individual. There are many drugs and other disorders that produce falsely low T_4 values. Falsely low values may result from reduced serum thyroxine–binding globulins (e.g., nephrotic syndrome, protein loss by the gut, or glucocorticoids) or displacement of T_4 from binding proteins (e.g., high-dose salicylates, the use of furosemide in patients with renal failure, or phenytoin).

Antimicrosomal antibodies are present in the sera of 90% of middle-aged patients but may be negative in young patients. Antithyroglobulin antibodies are noted a few years after the antimicrosomal antibodies are found. The elevation presumably represents a response to antigens leaking from the damaged thyroid.

GOALS OF THERAPY

The primary goal in the management of hypothyroidism is to restore the patient to a euthyroid state and to maintain plasma TSH levels in the low-normal range. Relief of the symptoms of hypothyroidism is also a treatment goal. Management includes the gradual replacement of thyroid hormones and a low-calorie diet to promote weight loss. Lifelong therapy should be expected.

Thyroid hormone replacement is the only treatment available for hypothyroidism. Levothyroxine provides standardized, predictable effects, thereby preventing the wide variety of symptomatic and metabolic disturbances associated with insufficient thyroid production. However, the patient's response is greatly affected by age, the cause and duration of the goiter, and the degree of nodularity.

Patients with signs and symptoms of hypothyroidism whose TSH levels are greater than 15 mU/L and who have T_4 levels below normal values can be effectively treated with thyroid hormone replacement. Patients with mild or no symptoms of hypothyroidism, moderately elevated TSH levels (6 to 15 mU/L), and T_4 levels within normal limits should be treated earlier rather than later for subclinical hypothyroidism. Thyroid hormone replacement is not required in patients with TSH levels that are within the normal limits and T_4 levels that are low or low-normal.

INTERVENTION
Administration

Blood pressure and apical pulse should be assessed before and periodically during therapy. Overdosage of thyroid hormone is manifested as signs and symptoms of hyperthyroidism. Assess for tachycardia, chest pain, nervousness, insomnia, diaphoresis, tremors, weight loss. Monitor the blood TSH level, blood pressure, and pulse throughout therapy. If the pulse rate in an adult is more than 100 beats per minute, withhold the dose and contact the health care provider. The usual intervention is to withhold the thyroid hormone for 2 to 6 days. Acute overdose is treated by induction of emesis or gastric lavage.

Education

The patient should receive an explanation of the disorder and understand that treatment for hypothyroidism is lifelong. Response to treatment usually takes several weeks to manifest, and maximal response is usually not seen for several months.

Patients should be instructed to take levothyroxine exactly as directed, on an empty stomach, and at the same time each day. Administration before breakfast helps pre-

---

CASE STUDY  *Hypothyroidism*

ASSESSMENT

HISTORY OF PRESENT ILLNESS

JC is a 35-year-old part-time secretary and mother who arrived at the clinic accompanied by her husband. She complains of cold intolerance; coarse, dry skin; decreased sweating; swelling of the eyelids, face, and legs; lethargy; anorexia; constipation; hair loss; hoarseness; and memory impairment. She also reports that she is gaining weight although she is eating little. In addition, she states her neighbor thinks she is on "some kind of downers" because of the lethargy.

HEALTH HISTORY

JC denies a history of previous thyroid disorders but reports that her mother developed an "underactive thyroid" at age 33. She denies a history of surgery or neurologic, musculoskeletal, or other hormonal disorders. She notes an allergy to aspirin.

LIFESPAN CONSIDERATIONS

JC's husband reports that she thinks she may be pregnant because her periods are less frequent and decreased in amount.

CULTURAL/SOCIAL CONSIDERATIONS

JC's husband describes his wife as a normally outgoing, well-organized individual, who finishes projects she starts and coordinates family activities very well. Over the last 3 months, he reports, she has become unorganized and does not finish projects or activities she has started. He also reports that she does not like to take medicine of any kind. He has noticed her wearing long pants and a sweater even though it is summertime. They have been arguing recently because she wants the windows closed; he gets hot and wants them open. JC's husband is a bank executive. He reports that the family is enrolled in a health plan that covers clinic visits and hospitalizations. The prescription drug plan requires a copayment for prescription drugs. He believes that the insurance premiums are reasonable and the plan supports their health care needs.

PHYSICAL EXAMINATION

JC is 5'7" tall and weighs 133 pounds (10 to 15 pounds more than her usual weight). Her blood pressure is 116/62 mm Hg (BP 1 year ago 130/80 mm Hg), apical pulse 66 and regular, respirations 18, temperature 98.2° F. No bruits are noted over the thyroid gland. JC is able to close her eyelids completely, and her visual fields are unimpaired. Her skin, hair, and nails are dry and brittle. She has hypoactive deep tendon reflexes. Her decreased attention span is evident.

LABORATORY TESTING

JC's diagnostic workup reflects a high TSH level and a decreased T_4. The free T_4 level is low and the T_3 is elevated. Her cholesterol, CK, LDH, AST, and sodium levels are elevated. A pregnancy test reveals that she is not pregnant.

PATIENT PROBLEM(S)

Hypothyroidism.

GOALS OF THERAPY

Restore a euthyroid state by returning plasma thyroid function level to a normal range; provide symptom relief while waiting for therapeutic effectiveness of drug to be achieved.

CRITICAL THINKING QUESTIONS

1. The health care provider starts JC on levothyroxine 50 mcg by mouth daily. What is the mechanism of action of this drug?
2. Approximately how long will it take for JC to notice the effectiveness of the drug?
3. Of which adverse effects of levothyroxine should JC be aware?
4. Because of JC's aspirin allergy, what other concerns should the health care provider have?
5. What are the goals of levothyroxine therapy for JC?

vent insomnia. If a dose is missed, it should be taken as soon as it is remembered. The health care provider should be notified if more than two or three doses are missed. However, because of levothyroxine's long half-life, in some cases, the forgotten doses may be taken all at once. The drug should not be discontinued without first consulting the health care provider. A levothyroxine suspension is readily available for patients who cannot or will not swallow whole tablets. It can be given by spoon or dropper. A crushed tablet may be sprinkled over a small amount of cooked cereal or applesauce.

Because the bioavailability of levothyroxine may differ between preparations, the patient should be cautioned not to change brands of levothyroxine when refilling prescriptions. The concurrent use of other OTC drugs should be avoided unless otherwise instructed. Additive CNS and cardiac stimulation may occur with decongestants. Patients with diabetes mellitus should monitor glucose levels carefully because an adjustment in diet or insulin dosage may be needed with the expected change in metabolism.

Teach the patient and family how to take the pulse. A resting pulse rate over 100 beats per minute may indicate overdosage. In this case the drug should be withheld and the health care provider notified. Instruct female patients to keep a record of their menstrual cycles because irregularities may occur. Remind the patient to inform all health care providers of all drugs being used. Regular use of thyroid replacement hormones may contribute to interactions with other drugs. Encourage the patient to wear a medical alert identification tag or bracelet stating that thyroid hormones are used regularly.

The importance of follow-up should be stressed. Thyroid function tests should be performed regularly during the initial phase of treatment and at least yearly throughout therapy.

EVALUATION

The patient's clinical response to levothyroxine can be evaluated by resolution of signs and symptoms of hypothyroidism. The expected response includes weight loss, an increased sense of well-being, and greater energy levels. The texture and characteristics of hair, skin, and nails should normalize, and constipation should be corrected.

The TSH and serum T_4 levels can be used to monitor the treatment effectiveness. If the serum T_4 level is low but the TSH is normal, measurement of the level of free T_4 is warranted. Persistent clinical and laboratory evidence of hypothyroidism despite adequate replacement indicates poor patient compliance, poor absorption, excessive fecal loss, or inactivity of the formulation. Intracellular resistance to thyroid hormones is rare.

PATHOPHYSIOLOGY • Hyperthyroidism

Hyperthyroidism occurs when excess thyroid hormones are released into circulation. Hyperthyroidism is rare in children and is most common in adults in the third or fourth decade of life. Women are affected more often than men, but the reasons are unclear. The disease ranges from mild forms displaying few of the symptoms shown in Table 56-1 to a severe condition called thyroid storm, in which death may result from an abrupt rise in body temperature and vascular collapse. Increased thyroid hormone production may result from hyperfunction of the entire gland or from excessive output of one or more small nodules within the thyroid. A rare cause of hyperthyroidism is excess TSH, either from the pituitary gland or from a tumor.

The most common cause of hyperthyroidism is **Graves' disease** (toxic diffuse goiter). Graves' disease accounts for about 85% of cases of hyperthyroidism. Many patients with this condition display exophthalmos (bulging eyes). Because many patients also have enlarged thyroid glands, another common name for this condition is exophthalmic goiter. Graves' disease is a form of autoimmune disease. In this condition, certain IgG antibodies are formed that stimulate the TSH receptor, causing overproduction of thyroid hormones.

Another form of hyperthyroidism, toxic multinodular goiter (TMNG), produces the same general symptoms as Graves' disease, except that eye symptoms are rare. Other causes of hyperthyroidism include thyroid tumors and thyroiditis.

Hyperthyroidism produces a state of hypermetabolism, including increased heat production, motor activity, and sympathetic nervous system activity (see Table 56-1). Excessive thyroid hormones affect carbohydrate, protein, and fat metabolism. There is an increased absorption of glucose and diminished sensitivity to exogenous insulin. Protein breakdown can exceed protein synthesis, resulting in a negative nitrogen balance. Synthesis, mobilization, and breakdown of fats are increased. The net effect is lipid depletion and a chronic state of protein-energy malnutrition. Excess thyroid hormones also increase heart rate and stroke volume, thus increasing cardiac output and peripheral blood flow. Systolic blood pressure also is elevated.

Hyperthyroidism is characterized by elevated levels of serum T_4, serum T_3, free T_4, and free T_3 in most patients. Thus diagnostic tests that directly measure one of these parameters (serum T_4 or serum T_3 testing) are often used. The level of TSH is low for most forms of hyperthyroidism because high circulating levels of T_4 and T_3 suppress the regulatory factors in the hypothalamus and pituitary. Radioactive iodine uptake also may be measured and is useful in distinguishing among various forms of hyperthyroidism.

 DRUG CLASS • Antithyroid Drugs

methimazole (Tapazole)

propylthiouracil (PTU, Propyl-Thyracil✱)

MECHANISM OF ACTION

Propylthiouracil and methimazole inhibit the synthesis of thyroid hormones, blocking each step in synthesis except iodide uptake (Table 56-3). Propylthiouracil, but not methimazole, also inhibits the conversion of T_4 to T_3 in peripheral tissues. Methimazole can antagonize the inhibition caused by propylthiouracil if they are taken together. Because these compounds are primarily enzyme inhibitors, they do not directly destroy thyroid tissue but only prevent its excessive action.

The action of these drugs on the thyroid gland is rapid, and reduced hormone synthesis occurs within hours. However, observable clinical response to the drugs does not appear for days or weeks, the period required for stored thyroid hormones to be depleted. A patient's condition may be maintained for months by therapy with methimazole or propylthiouracil, provided the hyperthyroidism is well controlled during that time. After about 1 year, the drug is usually withdrawn and thyroid function is reevaluated. Many patients remain euthyroid after the drug is discontinued, and no further therapy may ever be required.

USES

Propylthiouracil and methimazole are used in most patients to manage manifestations of hyperthyroidism. They are first-line drugs used in the treatment of thyrotoxicosis, helping maintain normal metabolism until the natural course of the disease produces a spontaneous remission.

PHARMACOKINETICS

Both propylthiouracil and methimazole are well absorbed from the GI tract and concentrate in the thyroid

TABLE 56-3

Drugs Used to Treat Hyperthyroidism

Generic Name	Brand Name	Comments
Thioamides		
methimazole	Tapazole	Inhibits thyroid hormone synthesis but not release
propylthiouracil	PTU, Propyl-Thyracil ✱	Inhibits thyroid hormone synthesis but not release as well as conversion of T_4 to T_3 in peripheral tissues
Beta-Adrenergic Receptor Antagonist		
propranolol	Inderal	Controls symptoms of hyperthyroidism but does not lower T_4 and T_3 release from thyroid See Chapter 12 for discussion of beta adrenergic receptor blockers
Iodine		
potassium iodide	Lugol's Solution, Pima, SSKI, Thyro-Block ✱	Produces short-term inhibition of thyroid hormone synthesis by direct action on thyroid
sodium iodide ^{131}I	Iodotope	This radioactive nuclide is concentrated in thyroid and releases radiation that destroys thyroid tissue

✱ Available only in Canada.

gland. The onset of the effects of propylthiouracil occurs in 10 to 21 days compared with 1 week for methimazole. Propylthiouracil has a moderate degree of binding to plasma proteins (75%), whereas methimazole does not have significant binding. Methimazole has a longer half-life (4 to 6 hours) than propylthiouracil (75 minutes). The actions of methimazole peak in 4 to 10 weeks in contrast to propylthiouracil, which may take up to 6 to 10 weeks to peak. Elimination of the drugs and their metabolites is primarily through the kidneys. Propylthiouracil and methimazole are transported across placental membranes, but only about 25% of the serum concentration of propylthiouracil crosses the placenta compared with that of methimazole.

ADVERSE REACTIONS AND CONTRAINDICATIONS

Common reactions to these drugs include fever, itching, and skin rash. Blood dyscrasias or peripheral neuropathy may occur. Propylthiouracil is especially associated with pain and swelling of joints or with a lupuslike syndrome. Methimazole may cause dizziness or alterations in taste. Patients who have had allergic or other severe reactions to either of these drugs should not receive them again. Patients with impaired hepatic function may require reduced dosages.

Agranulocytosis is the most feared adverse reaction to propylthiouracil and methimazole, occurring in 0.2% of patients. It usually develops within 90 days of starting therapy and is characterized by high fever, bacterial pharyngitis, and an absolute granulocyte count below 250/mm^3. Fortunately, the patient's white blood cell count normalizes in 7 to 10 days once the drug has been stopped. Overdosage with these drugs results in hypothyroidism (see Table 56-1).

INTERACTIONS

Any preparation containing iodine may interfere with the antithyroid action of propylthiouracil and methimazole. Such agents include amiodarone, iodine solution, potassium iodide, and many contrast imaging dyes. Coumarins or other anticoagulants may be influenced by thyroid function; dosages can be adjusted based on prothrombin times. Digitalis dosage may be influenced by thyroid status. Dosages of the cardiac glycoside may require reduction as hyperthyroidism is brought under control.

DRUG CLASS • Iodine

calcium iodide (Calcidrine)

potassium iodide (saturated solution of potassium iodide [SSKI], Lugol's Solution, Pima, Quadrinal, Thyro-Block❋)

sodium iodide ^{131}I (Iodotope)

MECHANISM OF ACTION

Iodide is required for synthesis of thyroid hormones, but high concentrations of iodide suppress continued uptake by the thyroid gland and thus slow synthesis of thyroid hormones. Iodide also inhibits the synthesis of iodotyrosines and inhibits the release of thyroid hormone. Suppression of hormone synthesis is not complete with iodine administration, and many patients return to the hyperthyroid state even with continued high dosages. The destructive beta rays of iodine-131 (^{131}I) act almost exclusively on the parenchymal cells of the thyroid to reduce hormone synthesis. There is little or no damage to surrounding tissues.

USES

Iodide is seldom used today for long-term suppression of a hyperactive thyroid gland, but it is still used to prepare a hyperthyroid patient for surgery. Iodide not only suppresses thyroid function but also reduces vascularization of the gland, thus reducing surgical risk. Iodide also is used with antithyroid drugs to treat hyperthyroid crisis. Potassium iodide may be used to block the thyroidal uptake of radioactive isotopes of iodine in a radiation emergency.

Radioactive iodine is used to treat hyperthyroidism and for diagnosis. The use of radioactive iodine allows the thyroid to be functionally destroyed without resorting to surgery. Nearly all patients treated with radioactive iodine ultimately become hypothyroid and require replacement therapy with thyroid hormones.

PHARMACOKINETICS

Iodide and ^{131}I are readily absorbed from the GI tract and taken up by the thyroid gland. The effects of iodide are rapid and occur within 24 hours but do not reach their maximal effect until 10 to 15 days after therapy is started. The onset action of ^{131}I occurs in 3 to 6 days, and the isotope has a half-life of 8 days. Over 99% of its radiant energy is expended within 56 days.

ADVERSE EFFECTS AND CONTRAINDICATIONS

The major adverse reaction to iodide therapy is hypersensitivity, which may include angioedema, swelling of the larynx, skin lesions, and symptoms analogous to serum sickness (fever, eosinophilia, etc.). The major adverse reaction to ^{131}I is iatrogenic hypothyroidism. The development of hypothyroidism is so characteristic that it is considered a consequence of therapy rather than a true adverse reaction. Hypothyroidism develops in at least 50% of patients within the first year of ^{131}I therapy, with an annual increase of 2% to 3% each year. Consequently, within 10 to 20 years, nearly all patients will become hypothyroid. For this reason, it is mandatory that patients receive close, lifelong follow-up care. Radioactive iodide treatment is contraindicated during pregnancy.

TOXICITY

Iodide toxicity is dose dependent, and early manifestations have symptoms analogous to a bad cold. Patients have irritation of the mouth and throat, with a lingering brassy taste, headaches, cough, sneezing, and increased salivation. As the dosage increases, there is considerable GI irritation, enlarged glands, skin lesions, and pulmonary edema.

INTERACTIONS

Propranolol and antithyroid drugs hasten the control of hyperthyroidism while the patient awaits the full effects of ^{131}I.

APPLICATION TO PRACTICE

ASSESSMENT
History of Present Illness

The patient with hyperthyroidism most often reports anxiety, diaphoresis, fatigue, hypersensitivity to heat, nervousness, and palpitations. The patient may also voice confusion about losing weight in spite of an increased appetite. Anorexia and constipation are infrequent. Often, there are reports of problems with the eyes such as difficulty focusing. The patient may also note peripheral edema, diarrhea, and oligomenorrhea or amenorrhea.

Health History

The patient with hyperthyroidism may have a history of atrial fibrillation, angina, or heart failure. Sufficient information about the patient's history should be obtained to help distinguish hyperthyroidism from anxiety (especially at menopause) or other diseases associated with hypermetabolic states (e.g., pheochromocytoma and acromegaly). Myasthenia gravis causes some of the same ophthalmoplegic signs as that of hyperthyroidism. Orbital tumors can cause exophthalmos.

Lifespan Considerations

Perinatal. Minor changes in thyroid function occur during pregnancy. High estrogen levels during pregnancy stimulate the liver to increase its production of TBGs. Increased globulin levels result in the elevation of T_3 and T_4 levels; elevated T_4 levels last 6 to 12 weeks postpartum. Serum concentrations of free T_3 and T_4 are essentially unchanged. The serum level of TSH is normal to slightly low during pregnancy. Human chorionic gonadotropin (hCG) produced by the placenta has weak thyroid-stimulating activity.

Pediatric. Neonatal hyperthyroidism results from the transfer of maternal thyroid-stimulating immunoglobulin (TSI) to the fetus. It is usually transient, lasting only 1 to 3 months, because the half-life of neonatal TSI is approximately 2 weeks. TSI stimulates the fetal thyroid to produce thyroid hormones, causing fetal or neonatal hyperthyroidism. Neonatal hyperthyroidism depends on maternal TSI and not on the mother's thyroid status. Therefore infants of euthyroid women with a previous history of hyperthyroidism are also at risk.

Measurement of the maternal TSI level is useful in predicting the likelihood of neonatal hyperthyroidism.

Older Adults. Hyperthyroidism frequently goes undetected in older persons for several reasons. The patient has fewer diagnostic signs and symptoms, coexisting diseases may mask symptoms, and the symptoms commonly present in the younger population may be absent in older adults. Confirmation of hyperthyroidism therefore relies heavily on laboratory test results.

Symptoms of hyperthyroidism in the older adult are often atypical. Only about 25% of older adults have the classic hyperactivity, restlessness, and nervous appearance. The older adult may or may not have tachycardia or moist, flushed skin. Classic eye manifestations are rare. The most frequent patient reports relate to anorexia and a loss of ambition. Weight loss is the most frequent objective finding. An enlarged thyroid is present in 80% of those affected. More than 75% of patients have cardiovascular symptoms such as palpitations, heart failure, atrial fibrillation, and angina pectoris.

Laboratory reports indicate there is an age-related decrease in T_3 levels in healthy older adults. T_3 levels decrease by age 60 in men. Levels in women do not show a consistent decrease until age 70 or 80. The normal decrease in T_3 levels makes the diagnosis of mild hyperthyroidism difficult. Circulating T_4 levels also decrease modestly with age. The reduction may be caused by reduced metabolism of the aging thyroid gland, where most T_4 is produced. There is also an age-related increase in TSH levels.

Cultural/Social Considerations

The wide variation in the signs and symptoms of hyperthyroidism may affect the patient's activities of daily living. Workplace relationships may be affected because of the hyperactive state of the patient. Mood swings, irritability, decreased attention span, and manic behavior may be exhibited. Although the patient may not be aware of some of the mood changes, fellow employees and family members can usually note them.

Physical Examination

Generally, the patient with hyperthyroidism is nervous and thin. Muscle wasting may be evident. Vital signs reflect tachycardia, irregular pulse, and a widened pulse pressure. The skin is moist and velvety and may show increased pigmentation or vitiligo. Hair is often fine and thin. Spider angiomas and gynecomastia may also be evident. Lid lag may be present with a lack of accommodation on examination. Exophthalmos may also be evident, and the patient may appear to stare. In severe cases, the patient may be unable to close the eyelids and must have the lids taped shut to protect the eyes.

An examination of the neck reveals an enlarged thyroid gland that is either smooth or nodular and symmetric or asymmetric. A thyroid bruit may be noted on auscultation, although absence of a bruit or of changes in the appearance of the neck does not rule out hyperthyroidism. Auscultation of heart sounds may reveal evidence of paroxysmal atrial fibrillation, a harsh pulmonary systolic murmur, and the presence of an S_3 heart sound.

Deep tendon reflexes are hyperactive, and fine tremors of the fingers and tongue may be present. Mental status changes range from mild exhilaration to delirium. In the elderly patient, however, apathy, lethargy, and depression may be evident.

Laboratory Testing

Laboratory diagnosis of hyperthyroidism is generally straightforward. All forms of hyperthyroidism (except that caused by a rare pituitary TSH-secreting tumor) are associated with low or undetectable serum TSH concentrations. In addition, most patients have elevated circulating levels of T_3, T_4, and free T_4. The 24-hour radioactive iodine uptake test is neither sensitive nor specific for hyperthyroidism. It is, however, useful in distinguishing hyperthyroidism that may develop during the postpartum period from postpartum thyroiditis and in confirming the diagnosis of subacute thyroiditis.

If the patient has only one or two characteristic signs and symptoms of hyperthyroidism, the pretest probability of this condition is low, and no testing is required. However, if the health care provider is com-

pelled to test, the free T_4 level is a better reflection of the patient's true hormonal status. If the patient exhibits five or more characteristic signs and symptoms, the ultrasensitive TSH is probably the best indicator of patient thyroid status.

GOALS OF THERAPY

The treatment goal for hyperthyroidism is to reduce the levels of circulating thyroid hormones in anticipation of a spontaneous remission and a euthyroid state. Reducing the uncomfortable signs and symptoms is also important.

Historically, surgery was the first-line treatment for hyperthyroidism. It is not used as frequently today but may be appropriate for children, adolescents, pregnant women unable to tolerate propylthiouracil (PTU), and adults who are unresponsive to antithyroid drugs and who refuse radioactive iodine. Antithyroid drugs and radioactive iodine have replaced surgery as the treatments of choice. Although these drugs are generally safe and effective, none of them are perfect. They do, however, provide satisfactory outcomes for most patients.

The primary drugs used in the treatment of hyperthyroidism include the thioureylenes PTU or methimazole. The advantage of using antithyroid drugs is that they provide an opportunity for the patient to have a spontaneous remission, thus allowing him or her to avoid lifelong drug treatment regimens. However, the disadvantage is that permanent remission occurs in only about 30% of patients. Continuous and repeated therapy is usually required.

The indications and adverse effects of both PTU and methimazole are essentially the same. However, for bothersome symptoms, long-acting beta blockers (propranolol, metoprolol, atenolol, nadolol) (see Chapter 11) are usually given as adjunctive therapy until the drug restores the patient to a euthyroid state. The long-acting form of propranolol is preferred to the standard formulation of propranolol, which has a short duration of action.

Because hyperthyroidism usually remits during pregnancy, it is usually controlled with low doses of an antithyroid drug. It may even be possible to stop antithyroid drug therapy. However, the disease may relapse or worsen after delivery. PTU is the drug of choice for pregnant hyperthyroid women because of its limited placental transfer and low potency; however, both drugs are in pregnancy category D. Another reason PTU is the drug of choice during pregnancy is the reported development of scalp defects in fetuses exposed to methimazole in utero.

Radioactive iodine is concentrated only in areas of the thyroid that are functional. Suppressed perinodular areas are spared radiation exposure. Therefore hypothyroidism, though still possible, is less of a problem. There are several advantages to using [131]I. First, no other body tissues are exposed to detectable amounts of ionizing radiation. Because this drug is taken orally, it is easy to administer. The health care provider should administer it only after stopping any other antithyroid drugs. Should a remission occur, lifelong follow-up is indicated. If a remission is not achieved, the patient may require a second course of antithyroid therapy or radioactive iodine.

The economic factor alone makes PTU less desirable than methimazole. Even at minimal recommended dosages, the cost of a 30-day supply of PTU is approximately three times that of methimazole.

INTERVENTION
Administration

Antithyroid drugs should be administered at the same time each day in equally divided doses. Overdose with an antithyroid drug produces clinical hypothyroidism. Assess for tingling of fingers and toes. Monitor the patient's weight. Inspect the skin for changes or hair loss. Monitor the CBC count with differential as well as thyroid and liver function tests during therapy.

Education

The patient and family should be taught about the therapeutic and adverse effects of thyroid hormones and antithyroid drugs on the body. Methimazole and PTU may be taken without regard to meals but should be taken the same way each time, either always with meals or always on an empty stomach. If more than one dose per day is prescribed, it is best to space doses evenly throughout the day. Work with the patient to develop a satisfactory dosing schedule. If a dose is missed, the patient should be instructed to take it when it is remembered. If it is almost time for the next dose, both doses should be taken. The health care provider should be contacted if more than one dose is missed. Instruct the patient to also report any signs of agranulocytosis, such as fever, chills, sore throat, and unexplained bleeding or bruising.

Advise the patient taking an oral solution of iodide (i.e., potassium iodide [SSKI]) to dilute the drug in a full 8-ounce glass of water, juice, milk, or beverage of choice. Tablet formulations should be swallowed whole. Patients taking the uncoated tablet form should be taught to dissolve each tablet in half a glass (4 ounces) of water or milk and to then drink the entire beverage to get the full dose. Inform the patient that a metallic taste in the mouth may be noticed.

Signs of **iodism** (excessive iodine intake) include a metallic taste in the mouth, sneezing, a swollen and tender thyroid gland, vomiting, and bloody diarrhea. Concomitant excessive use of OTC drugs containing iodine (e.g., asthma or cough preparations) may contribute to iodism.

The radiation dosage of ^{131}I is not high, but those preparing or administering the drug should be careful to avoid spilling the mixture on themselves or on countertops. Wear rubber gloves when preparing the drug. Adverse reactions are rare but include soreness over the thyroid gland and, in rare cases, difficulty swallowing and breathing because of gland enlargement. Eventually, many patients who have taken ^{131}I develop hypothyroidism.

Signs and symptoms of hyperthyroidism and hypothyroidism should also be discussed. Adverse reactions may not appear for days to weeks after starting therapy; remind the patient to report any new adverse reactions to the health care provider.

Encourage the patient to return as instructed for follow-up visits and to notify the health care provider of all drugs being used. Instruct the patient as to the importance of using contraceptive measures and the need to avoid pregnancy. Have the patient notify the health care provider if they become pregnant while taking these drugs. Have the patient wear a medical alert identification tag or bracelet.

PHYSIOLOGY • Parathyroid Hormones

The function of the parathyroid gland is to secrete parathyroid hormone (PTH), the hormone responsible for maintaining the blood calcium level above the critical threshold required for body function. Parathyroid hormone is synthesized from a prohormone and is stored in the cells of the parathyroid gland or broken down by proteases before secretion. Parathyroid hormone secretion is regulated by calcium concentration in the blood. Calcium binds to a receptor (sensor) on cells in the parathyroid gland, which results in a decrease in the secretion of parathyroid hormone and a greater amount of the hormone broken down in the cell. As the calcium concentration in the blood falls, secretion of parathyroid hormone is stimulated, less is broken down, and calcium is mobilized.

Parathyroid hormone stimulates osteolysis by osteoclasts that release calcium and phosphate into extracellular fluid. It increases the renal tubular reabsorption of calcium and decreases the renal tubular reabsorption of phosphate. Parathyroid hormone also increases the synthesis of the active form of vitamin D, called calcitriol, from its precursor through activation of a specific enzyme in the kidney. Calcitriol directly enhances absorption of calcium in the intestines. All of these actions tend to raise calcium concentration in blood.

Alteration of parathyroid gland function produces **hypoparathyroidism** (i.e., hypocalcemia) or **hyper-**

parathyroidism (HPT) (i.e., hypercalcemia). Although they are not as common as thyroid disorders, parathyroid disorders can be life threatening, depending on their severity.

PATHOPHYSIOLOGY • Hypoparathyroidism

Hypoparathyroidism usually results from the inadvertent removal of the parathyroid glands during a thyroidectomy or parathyroid surgery, but idiopathic forms (those with an unknown cause) of the disease exist. Pseudohypoparathyroidism is a rare condition in which the target organs fail to respond to parathyroid hormone. Hypoparathyroidism leads to hypocalcemia. This electrolyte imbalance produces symptoms such as paresthesis, muscle spasms, tetany, and seizures (see Table 56-4). In theory, the parathyroid hormone could be used to raise blood calcium levels in conditions where blood levels are abnormally low; however, administration of one of the forms of vita-

min D, with or without calcium, is the preferred treatment. Refer to Chapter 63 for a discussion of calcium preparations, vitamin D preparations, and drugs to treat osteoporosis.

A synthetic fragment of parathyroid hormone, teriparatide, retains full biologic activity and is used as a diagnostic drug for hypoparathyroidism. Teriparatide is infused, and urinary cyclic adenosine monophosphate and phosphate are measured to detect the response of a target organ to the hormone. Hypoparathyroidism is a deficiency in parathyroid hormone production, but the target organs respond to exogenous parathyroid hormone.

TABLE 56-4

Symptoms of Altered Calcium Balance

Hypercalcemia	Hypocalcemia	Hypercalcemia	Hypocalcemia
Early Symptoms		**Late Symptoms**	
Central Nervous System		*Central Nervous System*	
Depression	Hyperreflexia	Confusion	Convulsions
Headache	Muscle spasms	Drowsiness	Delusions
Irritability	Paresthesias		
Tiredness or weakness	Positive Chvostek's sign		
Gastrointestinal Tract		*Cardiovascular*	
Anorexia		Arrhythmia	Arrhythmia
Constipation		Hypertension	Tachycardia
Dry mouth			Vasospasm
Other		*Gastrointestinal Tract*	
Increased thirst		Nausea	
Metallic taste		Vomiting	
		Other	
		Sensitivity to light	Difficulty breathing
		Large urine volume	Laryngospasm
			Tetany/muscle spasm
			Loss of hair
			Cataracts

APPLICATION TO PRACTICE

ASSESSMENT
History of Present Illness

Patients with acute hypocalcemia may report muscle cramps as well as tingling of the circumoral area, hands, and feet. Symptoms of a chronically low serum calcium level include blurring of vision, personality changes, and anxiety.

Health History

An interview with the patient about his or her health history should elicit information regarding pancreatitis, osteomalacia, renal failure, malabsorption syndrome, a low calcium level, or a history of neck surgery. Be sure to ask about all drugs, vitamins, and herbal remedies the patient is using.

Lifespan Considerations

Perinatal. Hypoparathyroidism in pregnancy is relatively uncommon. However, more pregnant patients are diagnosed with symptomatic hypoparathyroidism than nonpregnant patients. This finding probably reflects the lack of routine screening of calcium levels rather than an increased severity of the disease. An intact PTH level is not altered by pregnancy; therefore diagnosis of hypoparathyroidism during pregnancy is similar to that of nonpregnant patients.

The fetus or neonate may have hypoparathyroidism resulting from maternal hypercalcemia; 25% of these cases result in fetal death, 50% result in tetany, and 2% of neonates have a congenital absence of parathyroid glands and thymus, which may cause early death.

Pediatric. Clinical manifestations of hypoparathyroidism in children result from hypocalcemia. The signs and symptoms include tetany; generalized tonic-clonic, absence, and simple partial seizures; carpopedal spasms; muscle cramps or twitching; paresthesias; and respiratory stridor. The skin can be dry and coarse. Maculopapular skin eruptions and eczematous dermatitis can occur. The hair is often brittle, and there may be areas of alopecia. Nails are thin and brittle, and there is dental and enamel hypoplasia.

Children with pseudohypoparathyroidism are short and have round faces with short, thick necks. The fingers and toes are stubby with dimpled skin over the knuckles. Calcium deposits in subcutaneous soft tissue is common. Mental retardation is a more prominent feature of pseudohypoparathyroidism than of the idiopathic form. Mood swings, memory loss, depression, and confusion can also occur.

Candidiasis of the nails and mouth occurs with the idiopathic form but seldom with pseudohypoparathy-roidism. Furthermore, papilledema, thought to be related to increased intracranial pressure, may occur in the idiopathic form but is rare in pseudohypoparathyroidism.

Older Adults. Older adults may be susceptible to hypoparathyroidism because of dietary deficiencies of calcium and vitamin D or because of decreased activity and lack of exposure to sunshine. Secondary causes of hypoparathyroidism that may occur more often in older adults include cancer of the prostate, pancreatitis, and liver or renal disease. Older adult patients are more susceptible to osteoporosis with the potential for spontaneous fractures.

Cultural/Social Considerations

Prolonged hypocalcemia may produce changes in the skin, hair, muscle coordination, and pain from ulcers or pancreatitis. These problems adversely affect the patient's self-esteem and ability to perform the activities of daily living (see the Case Study: Hypoparathyroidism).

Physical Examination

Acute hypocalcemia causes tetany with muscle cramps, irritability, carpopedal spasm, and seizures. In most cases, the neuromuscular irritability caused by a low calcium level may be demonstrated by tapping over the facial nerve just in front of the ear. A unilateral contraction of facial muscles occurs (**Chvostek's sign**). Carpopedal spasms may be induced by placing a blood pressure cuff on the arm and inflating it above systolic pressure (**Trousseau's sign**) for a period of 3 minutes. Deep tendon reflexes may be hyperactive.

Slit-lamp examination of the eyes may show early posterior lenticular cataract formation. Papilledema may be noted. A chronically low level of calcium may be associated with dental abnormalities (pitting or delayed eruptions) or subcutaneous calcifications. Prolonged hypocalcemia causes changes in the skin, hair, nails, and teeth, as well as the lenses of the eyes. If the condition is left untreated, cataracts may develop within a few years. The skin becomes coarse, dry, and scaly. Alopecia may develop with patchy or absent eyelashes and eyebrows. The nails become thin and brittle with transverse grooves. Dentition may be delayed and hypoplastic.

Laboratory Testing

True hypoparathyroidism is associated with a low level of intact PTH in light of low total and ionized calcium concentrations. Serum and urinary calcium levels are low, whereas serum and urinary phosphate levels are high. The alkaline phosphatase level is normal. Serum calcium is largely bound to serum albumin. Therefore the serum calcium level should be corrected for serum albumin level using the following formula:

$$\text{Corrected serum calcium} = \\ \text{Serum calcium mg/dL} + (0.8 \times [4.0 - \text{Albumin in g/dL}])$$

An ECG may be necessary to evaluate the heart rhythm and the QT interval. Radiographic tests may be used to determine the presence of renal calculi, fractures, bony tumors, osteoporosis, or tuberculosis.

GOALS OF THERAPY

Regardless of the cause of hypoparathyroidism, the primary goals are twofold: maintain the serum calcium level in a slightly low range, but not so low as to be symptomatic. In keeping the calcium level on the low side of normal, long-term complications such as renal stones and ectopic calcifications are avoided.

Calcium carbonate is the most efficient form of calcium available and is the drug of choice in the treatment of chronic hypocalcemia related to hypoparathyroidism. It is also less expensive than other formulations. Calcium carbonate is a weak phosphate binder that is also helpful in controlling the serum phosphate level associated with renal failure.

Therapy with vitamin D should be started as soon as oral calcium is begun. The vitamin D drug of choice for chronic hypoparathyroidism is ergocalciferol (vitamin D_2). With proper dosages the patient's serum calcium level can be maintained within normal limits. Ergocalciferol provides a more stable serum calcium level than do shorter-acting formulations of vitamin D. Dihydrotachysterol has a shorter duration of action than ergocalciferol and is more effective in the mobilization of calcium from bone.

The treatment of choice for hypoparathyroidism during pregnancy consists of calcium and vitamin D. It should be noted that if hypoparathyroidism during pregnancy remains untreated, a high maternal and fetal mortality ensues. Further neonatal hyperparathyroidism may develop in response to the hypocalcemia. Breast-feeding may cause hypervitaminosis D in the infant because vitamin D is eliminated in the breast milk.

Calcium is given to neonates to treat tetany, to overcome cardiac toxicity of hyperkalemia, for cardiopulmonary resuscitation, and to treat the acute symptoms of lead colic. As in the management of the adult, the goal is the maintenance of normal serum calcium levels. Some children may be treated with oral calcium salts alone. Others may also require supplemental vitamin D. Close follow-up is crucial to the well-being of the child. Serum calcium and phosphorus levels should be checked twice weekly during initial therapy and then monthly thereafter.

INTERVENTION
Administration

Oral calcium preparations should be taken 2 to 3 hours after eating. Calcium tablets should be chewed well before swallowing and followed by a full glass of water.

Intravenous calcium must be administered at room temperature, slowly into a large vein to avoid local trauma and arrhythmia, according to the manufacturer's instructions. Too rapid administration may contribute to arrhythmia and cardiac arrest. Monitor for hypotension, dizziness, flushing, a sensation of warmth, nausea, vomiting, and a tingling sensation. Slow or temporarily halt the infusion if the patient displays symptoms or complains of discomfort. Keep the patient recumbent after injection to prevent postural hypotension. It is essential to monitor the ECG to detect QT changes and inverted T wave abnormalities.

Infiltration of intravenous calcium may contribute to severe tissue damage that requires skin grafting. Determine that the intravenous site is patent before administering the drug. Check the infusion and infusion site frequently for extravasation, necrosis, or sloughing. Thromboses of peripheral veins also may occur with intravenous administration of calcium.

Monitoring of the serum calcium level at regular intervals, at least every 3 months, is important. The urine calcium level with spot urine determinations should also be monitored and kept below 30 mg/dL if possible.

The adverse effects of vitamin D preparations are essentially those of hypercalcemia and result from overdosing. The effects include ataxia, fatigue, irritability, seizures, somnolence, tinnitus, hypertension, gastrointestinal distress or constipation, and hypotonia in infants. Other symptoms of overdose include headache, increased thirst, a metallic taste in the mouth, nausea, vomiting, and fatigue. Assess the patient for these adverse effects. Ongoing assessment is important because it may be difficult to distinguish adverse effects from those accompanying renal failure or chronic disease.

Monitor blood pressure, pulse, intake, and output as well as BUN, serum creatinine, serum calcium, serum phosphorous, and serum alkaline phosphatase levels. Obtain a urine sample as directed by the health care provider.

Education

The patient taking calcium preparations should be taught to avoid taking enteric-coated drugs within 1 hour of the calcium preparation. Doing so will result in premature dissolution of the tablets. Encourage patients to drink a full 8-ounce glass of water or juice when taking an oral calcium supplement. Instruct patients to take doses 1 to 1.5 hours after meals unless directed otherwise by the health care provider. Patients taking the syrup form should take the drug before meals. The syrup can be mixed with water or fruit juice for infants or small children. Calcium carbonate may be used to bind phosphate in patients with renal failure. When used for this purpose, the health care provider may want it taken with meals.

Calcium carbonate should not be taken concurrently with foods containing large amounts of oxalic acid (e.g., spinach, Swiss chard, rhubarb, beets) or phytic acid (e.g., brans, whole grain cereals) (see Appendix A). The concurrent administration of dairy products (containing phosphorus) may produce a milk-alkali syndrome manifested as headache, confusion, nausea, and vomiting.

The patient should also be taught that calcium preparations might cause constipation; thus patients should be encouraged to increase bulk and fluid in the diet and to increase mobility. Severe constipation may indicate toxicity, necessitating contact with the health care provider.

Advise patients to avoid bonemeal or dolomite as a source of calcium. These preparations have been associated with high levels of lead and may contribute to lead poisoning. Remind the patient not to increase or decrease the dosage of calcium without consulting with the health care provider.

Remind them to inform all health care providers of all drugs being used and to avoid taking any drugs not previously approved by the provider. Have the patient avoid antacids containing magnesium and other substances containing calcium, phosphorus, or vitamin D unless discussed first with the health care provider. Warn patients taking vitamin D preparations to avoid driving or operating machinery if fatigue, somnolence, vertigo, or weakness develop.

EVALUATION

The effectiveness of drug therapy for hypoparathyroidism will be evidenced by resolution of hypoparathyroid symptoms and an increase in the serum calcium level to a more normal range.

PATHOPHYSIOLOGY • Hyperparathyroidism

Primary hyperparathyroidism is defined as hypercalcemia resulting from excessive production of parathyroid hormone. The symptoms exhibited by patients with hypercalcemia are outlined in Table 56-4. Many patients with this condition show decreases in bone calcification as a result of the action of parathyroid hormone. These patients excrete large amounts of calcium, and renal stones are common. Hypersecretion of parathyroid hormone from any cause can lead to a bone disorder known as osteitis fibrosa cystica generalisata. Excessive PTH increases osteoclastic activity and decreases osteoblastic activity. This results in the release of calcium and phosphorus into the circulation and decalcification of bone. However, only 33% of patients who have HPT show minor degrees of decalcification.

Secondary hyperparathyroidism is a response to vitamin D deficiency or the hypocalcemia of chronic renal disease. Increased quantities of PTH act directly on the kidneys. Calcium resorption (not reabsorption) and phosphate elimination increase in the renal tubules. Under ordinary circumstances, the serum calcium level is maintained within a narrow range despite large swings in calcium absorption during the day. These variations contribute to an elevated serum calcium level and a low phosphorus level.

No specific inhibitors of parathyroid release are available for clinical use; thus therapy consists primarily of surgery to remove the source of excess parathyroid hormone synthesis. The drugs discussed below do not specifically reduce the level of parathyroid hormone but rather treat the hypercalcemia.

DRUG CLASS • Drugs Used to Treat Hypercalcemia

calcitonin (Calcimar, Miacalcin)

clodronate (Bonefos✱)

edetate disodium (Disotate, Endrate)

plicamycin or mithramycin (Mithracin)

Biphosphonates such as etidronate can be used as adjunct treatments for hypercalcemia, and these are dis-

cussed in Chapter 63. Loop diuretics are also used to enhance excretion of calcium, and these drugs are discussed in detail in Chapter 46.

MECHANISM OF ACTION

Calcitonin lowers serum calcium by slowing bone resorption of calcium. Clodronate is a biphosphonate

TABLE 56-5		
Drugs Used to Treat Hypercalcemia		
Generic Name	*Brand Name*	*Comments*
salmon calcitonin	Calcimar Miacalcin	Used to rapidly reduce calcium levels Used in diseases of bone remodeling (Paget's disease)
clodronate	Bonefos ✹	Used to reduce high calcium levels caused by cancer
edetate disodium	Disotate Endrate	Strong chelating drug that removes excess calcium from system on short-term basis
plicamycin (mithramycin)	Mithracin	Potent antineoplastic drug that may prevent effect of parathyroid hormone on osteoclasts

✹ Available only in Canada.

that binds to hydroxyapatite and thus inhibits calcium crystals from forming. This drug, which is only available in Canada, also prevents bone resorption. Edetate disodium is a strong chelator of calcium, forming soluble complexes excreted readily by the kidneys. Plicamycin is an antineoplastic agent that is very effective in lowering the serum calcium level. Plicamycin inhibits the action of parathyroid hormone on osteoclasts presumably by inhibiting RNA synthesis in response to the hormone.

USES

Calcitonin is used to decease calcium and phosphate concentrations in patients with hyperglycemia (Table 56-5). It is used to treat disorders of bone remodeling (e.g., Paget's disease), in which excessive bone resorption leads to fragile bones. Calcitonin also is used to control postmenopausal osteoporosis, along with vitamin D and calcium supplements. Clodronate and plicamycin are used to treat hypercalcemia resulting from cancer, especially malignancies of the bone. Plicamycin also is used as an antineoplastic agent in tumors of the testes. Edetate disodium is used for emergency treatment of hypercalcemia. The drug may also be used for treatment of digitalis toxicity, but digoxin immune Fab is the preferred drug.

PHARMACOKINETICS

Calcitonin usually is administered by subcutaneous or intramuscular injections. A metered spray for intranasal administration makes the use of this drug convenient for chronic use by outpatients. Oral absorption of clodronate is poor (3%), so the drug is usually administered intravenously. The onset of action after intravenous administration is approximately 2 days; continuing effects last for 4 to 6 days. Clodronate is not biotransformed but rather is excreted unchanged in the urine.

Edetate disodium is given by intravenous infusion with constant monitoring of serum calcium. Edetate is not biotransformed, and up to 95% of a dose appears in urine within 1 day. The onset of the hypocalcemic effect of plicamycin occurs 24 to 48 hours after intravenous administration, and the drug's duration of action is 1 to 2 weeks. The dosage of plicamycin is about one tenth that used for antineoplastic therapy; thus the adverse effects are proportionately lower.

ADVERSE REACTIONS AND CONTRAINDICATIONS

Many patients experience nausea, swelling of the hand, urticaria, and occasional inflammatory reactions when calcitonin is injected. Because the hormone is a peptide and is administered in a gelatin solution, allergic reactions may occur. Synthetic human calcitonin may be less likely than salmon calcitonin to cause allergic reactions. Intranasal administration of calcitonin causes few systemic adverse effects but commonly causes nasal effects such as dry membranes, itching, irritation, crusting, or bleeding. Clodronate and plicamycin produce gastrointestinal side effects including nausea, vomiting, and diarrhea. Clodronate also can cause renal dysfunction, dry mouth, muscle cramps, and rarely nonlymphocytic leukemia or convulsions.

The most serious adverse reaction to edetate disodium is thrombophlebitis at the injection site. Dizziness may occur as well as GI signs including cramps and diarrhea. With the dramatic decrease in calcium, patients risk cardiac, renal, or neurologic damage. The drug is not usually given to patients who have preexisting renal problems. The most serious adverse effect of plicamycin is a bleeding syndrome resulting from hematologic abnormalities. The drug can also produce fever, drowsiness, weakness, headache, and skin rashes.

TOXICITY

Overdosage of calcitonin may cause hypocalcemia, but the effect is mild and short lived. In contrast, acute overdoses of edetate disodium can cause severe hypocalcemia. Calcium ion replacement may be necessary.

INTERACTIONS

Calcium or vitamin D preparations may antagonize the actions of the antihypercalcemic drugs. Digoxin effects are reduced when serum calcium is lowered.

APPLICATION TO PRACTICE

ASSESSMENT
History of Present Illness

The patient with hyperparathyroidism may report problems related to the musculoskeletal system that include simple back pain, joint pains, painful shins, or muscle spasms. Depression or anxiety, arthralgias, nausea, and vomiting may also be noted. Complaints of constipation, abdominal pain, ulcers, muscle weakness, and fatigue are also frequent.

Health History

When interviewing the patient, the examiner should include questions about a history of calcium oxalate or calcium phosphate renal calculi, thyroid disease or surgery, neck dissection, renal failure, or adrenal insufficiency (Addison's disease). The patient may also note a personal history of sarcoidosis, milk-alkali syndrome, multiple myeloma, cancer with metastasis, or seizures that required therapy.

Lifespan Considerations

Perinatal. Hypercalcemia during pregnancy is rare. Only about 80 cases have been described in the medical literature. More pregnant patients are diagnosed with symptomatic hypercalcemia than nonpregnant patients; this probably reflects the lack of routine screening of calcium levels rather than an increased severity of the disease. An intact PTH level is not altered by pregnancy, and therefore the evaluation of hypercalcemia during pregnancy is similar to that of nonpregnant patients.

The treatment of choice for primary hypercalcemia during pregnancy is parathyroidectomy. Surgery is usually performed during the second trimester, when fetal body systems are developed, but before the third trimester, when a greater chance of premature labor exists. When parathyroidectomy is contraindicated, oral phosphate therapy may be appropriate for some patients. Treatment with hormones or biphosphates is contraindicated.

Pediatric. Parathyroid hormone excess manifested by hypercalcemia is very rare in children. When it is present, the clinical manifestations include renal colic, bone pain and bone masses, and osteoporosis.

Older Adults. Older adults may exhibit signs of hypercalcemia such as progressive hypertension, lethargy, drowsiness, depression, and GI discomfort. Radiation therapy to the neck or chest as well as a history of lithium use may precipitate the disorder.

Cultural/Social Considerations

The notion that the patient with hypercalcemia has difficulty with "bones, stones, abdominal groan, psychic moans, and fatigue overtones" is common. These problems affect the patient's ability to carry out activities of daily living. The variety of signs and symptoms cause the patient to seek medical attention numerous times over the course of the disease.

Physical Examination

The physical examination should include vital signs, height and weight, and skin color and texture. The eyes should be examined for corneal changes related to precipitation of calcium in the corneas (band keratopathy), conjunctivitis, papilledema, blepharospasm, and photophobia.

Intense pruritus may accompany severe hypercalcemia with evidence of broken skin surfaces. In hyperparathyroidism associated with renal failure, calcium also precipitates in the soft tissues, especially around the joints. Bony tenderness may be noted on palpation.

Laboratory Testing

The hallmarks of primary hypercalcemia are the elevated ionized or total serum calcium level and an elevated PTH level. The PTH-C (C-terminal fragment) level is also elevated. The C assay tends to have a higher value and is more widely accepted as an indicator of hyperparathyroidism. The sodium phosphorus level tends to be low. The results are then correlated with the patient's clinical picture.

Most patients with primary hypercalcemia show no evidence of bone disease. However, with untreated, long-standing hyperparathyroidism, extensive bone erosion results. The bone resorption is readily demonstrated in the cortex of the phalanges. In a small number of patients who have significant osteitis, serum alkaline phosphatase levels are also elevated. The elevation reflects osteoblastic activity.

Because of the effects of PTH, the bicarbonate level is reduced and the serum chloride level is elevated. The concentration of cyclic adenosine monophosphate (cAMP) in the urine is also increased. The urinary calcium level may be normal or elevated. Its measurement is used in the diagnosis of familial benign hypercalcemia. However, marked hypercalciuria may suggest a non–PTH-related hypercalcemia. Other causes of hypercalcemia can be readily identified by other clinical manifestations or by laboratory studies.

GOALS OF THERAPY

The primary treatment objective for hypercalcemia is to control the underlying disease. Management is aimed at reducing the serum calcium level.

There is no totally acceptable medical treatment regimen for hypercalcemia. Surgical removal of the abnormal parathyroid gland has been the treatment of choice in symptomatic patients. Symptomatic patients are usually dehydrated; therefore hydration with isotonic saline is the first step in treatment. In addition, calcium intake is restricted and electrolyte deficits (i.e., potassium and magnesium) are corrected. When expansion of plasma volume has been accomplished, a loop diuretic such as furosemide is given to promote urinary elimination of calcium. If it is used too early in treatment, however, furosemide may further dehydrate the patient and worsen the hypercalcemia. Therefore it should be used only after circulatory volume has been restored. Thiazide diuretics should not be used, because they decrease the elimination of calcium and worsen the hypercalcemia.

Hypocalcemic drugs such as etidronate, pamidronate, and salmon calcitonin have been used with some success in the management of mild hypercalcemia. Because of the adverse GI effects and possibility of bone pain, neither etidronate nor pamidronate are drugs of choice for the treatment of hypercalcemia. Salmon calcitonin has fewer adverse GI effects and may therefore be more desirable. Calcitonin may also be given subcutaneously or by nasal spray and would be appropriate for patients with low weight and small body frame.

Glucocorticoids have been effective for hypercalcemia associated with sarcoidosis and hypervitaminosis D. They are not useful for hypercalcemia that occurs

with hyperparathyroidism or with production of a PTH-related hormone. At present, no PTH-inhibiting drug is available.

Hypercalcemic states have also been reduced with the administration of phosphate. Phosphate promotes the deposition of calcium in the bone and soft tissues. Phosphate use is discouraged, however, because of the risk of fatal calcifications in the lungs, kidneys, and other soft tissues.

Patients receiving cardiac glycosides should be given hypocalcemia therapy with caution because of an increased risk for cardiac glycoside toxicity.

Conjugated estrogen has been used in some patients to reduce bone resorption and serum calcium levels. In many patients, estrogen therapy helps stabilize the disease. However, a history of estrogen-receptor–positive breast cancer contraindicates this therapy option. In addition, for patients who refuse surgery or who are not candidates, drugs that suppress PTH-mediated bone turnover may be useful.

INTERVENTION
Administration

Etidronate should be administered on an empty stomach at least 2 hours before or after a meal. Intravenous etidronate is diluted in normal saline and administered over 2 hours. The patient should be monitored for bone pain and reports of adverse gastrointestinal effects. The serum phosphate level usually returns to normal 2 to 4 weeks after therapy is begun. With long-term therapy (over 3 months), the risk of fractures increases. Etidronate may cause systemic reactions including tetany.

Allergy testing is usually done before initiating salmon calcitonin therapy. If the skin test produces a wheal, the drug should not be given. If more than 2 mL of salmon calcitonin is to be administered, an intramuscular route is preferred. To minimize the flushing effect of the drug, it should be given at bedtime. Injection sites should be rotated.

The patient should follow up with the health care provider to monitor serum calcium, phosphorus, alkaline phosphatase, and PTH levels. These levels should normalize within a few months of the start of therapy. Periodic monitoring of urine for casts should also be performed.

Vigorous saline hydration (i.e., maintaining a urine output of 2000 mL per 24 hours) should be undertaken concurrently with pamidronate therapy but should be initiated cautiously with patients with underlying heart failure. Advise the patient to notify the health care provider of pain at the infusion site or if bone pain becomes severe or persistent.

Education

Patients should be advised to take the hypocalcemia drug as directed. If a dose is missed but remembered within 2 hours of the next dose, it should be taken. Patients should be advised not to double up doses. Patients should be informed that calcium supplements, antacids, and iron might decrease the absorption of etidronate, antagonizing the drug's beneficial effects. The correct technique for subcutaneous injection should be included in patient teaching. The patient should be reassured that the flushing and warm sensation following injection is transient and usually lasts about 1 hour. Nausea following injection tends to decrease with continued therapy.

Teach the patient to watch for signs of hypocalcemic tetany with the first several doses of hypocalcemic drugs. Nervousness, irritability, paresthesia, and muscle twitching should be immediately brought to the attention of the health care provider. Signs of hypercalcemic relapse (e.g., bone or flank pain, renal calculi, anorexia, nausea, vomiting, thirst, and lethargy) should be promptly reported.

EVALUATION

A lowered serum calcium level and fewer complaints of bone pain and fractures will evidence the effectiveness of drug therapy.

CASE STUDY  *Hypoparathyroidism*

ASSESSMENT

HISTORY OF PRESENT ILLNESS

SM is a 47-year-old divorced man who has returned to the surgical clinic after having a total thyroidectomy 3 days ago at the ambulatory surgery center. He is complaining of lethargy, irritability, muscle cramps, and circumoral tingling.

HEALTH HISTORY

SM has a 10-year history of alcohol abuse, consuming one to two six-packs of beer daily. He has had no alcohol in the last 8 months since joining Alcoholics Anonymous. Because of his alcohol abuse, he developed chronic gastroenteritis. He has curtailed his intake of calcium because it contributes to diarrhea, and he admits that he does not follow a balanced diet. He has no allergies and takes no drugs.

LIFESPAN CONSIDERATIONS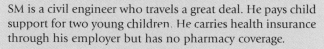

No specific developmental considerations for SM at this time.

CULTURAL/SOCIAL CONSIDERATIONS

SM is a civil engineer who travels a great deal. He pays child support for two young children. He carries health insurance through his employer but has no pharmacy coverage.

PHYSICAL EXAMINATION

SM is 5'9" tall and weighs 155 pounds. Blood pressure is 136/88 mm Hg, apical pulse 88, respirations 24, temperature 98.6° F. Surgical incision does not show redness, edema, or exudate. Wound edges are approximated, and staples remain in place. Breath sounds clear on auscultation. Chvostek's test is positive, Trousseau's sign is present,

and deep tendon reflexes are hyperactive. Skin is warm, dry, and scaly.

LABORATORY TESTING

Serum calcium level is 7.8 mg/dL (Norm 8.8 to 10.0 mg/dL). Ionized calcium value 4 mg/dL (Norm 4.4 to 5.4 mEq/L). Total plasma proteins (albumin and globulins) 5 g/dL (Norm 6 to 8 g/dL). Serum phosphorous level 5.0 mg/dL (Norm 2.7 to 4.5 mg/dL). Serum magnesium level 1.0 mEq/L (Norm 1.3 to 2.1 mEq/L). BUN, creatinine, and electrolyte levels within normal limits.

PATIENT PROBLEM(S)

Hypoparathyroidism.

GOALS OF THERAPY

Maintain serum calcium levels in a slightly low but asymptomatic range; prevent long-term complications such as renal stones and ectopic calcifications.

CRITICAL THINKING QUESTIONS

1. The health care provider orders calcium carbonate 600 mg with vitamin D 250 IU po bid 1 to 2 hours after meals. What is the mechanism of action of these drugs?
2. Where in the GI tract is calcium absorbed?
3. Which laboratory tests are necessary before calcium therapy?
4. Which adverse reactions are common with oral calcium supplements?
5. Which physical examination findings suggest hypocalcemia?

Bibliography

Barnett ML: Hypercalcemia, *Semin Oncol Nurs* 15(3):190-201, 1999.

Clement B: Parathyroid pathophysiology, *Semin Perioper Nurs* 7(3):186-92, 1998.

Czenis AL: Thyroid disease in the elderly, *Adv Nurse Pract* 7(9):38-46, 1999.

Dahlen R: Managing patients with acute thyrotoxicosis, *Crit Care Nurse* 22(1):62-69, 2002.

Diehl K: Thyroid dysfunction in pregnancy, *J Perinat Neonatal Nurs* 11(4):1-12, 1998.

Elliott B: Diagnosing and treating hypothyroidism, *Nurse Pract* 5(3):92-94, 99-105, 2000.

Harrell GB, Murray PD: Diagnosis and management of congenital hypothyroidism, *J Perinat Neonatal Nurs* 11(4):75-85, 1998.

Jordan S, White J: The immune system: hyperthyroidism, *Nurs Times* 94(24):48-51, 1998.

Kirsten D: The thyroid gland: physiology and pathophysiology, *Neonatal Netw* 19(8):11-26, 37-40, 2000.

Schilling JS: Hyperthyroidism: diagnosis and management of Graves' disease, *Nurse Pract* 22(6):72, 75, 78, 96-97 passim, 1997.

White J, Jordan S: The endocrine system: hypothyroidism, *Nurs Times* 94(29):50-53, 1998.

Woeber KA: Update on the management of hyperthyroidism and hypothyroidism, *Arch Intern Med* 160(8):1067-1071, 1206-1207, 2000.

Internet Resources

Adult hypothyroidism. Available online at http://www.medstudents.com.br/english.htm.

Thyroid disorder. Available online at http://www.merck.com/pubs/mmanual/section2/chapter8/8a.htm.

Adrenalcortical Steroids and Drugs Affecting the Adrenal Cortex

JOSEPH A. DiMICCO • KATHLEEN GUTIERREZ

 Visit http://evolve.elsevier.com/Gutierrez/ for additional information.

KEY TERMS

Addison's disease, p. 938

Adrenocorticotropic hormone (ACTH), p. 936

Aldosterone, p. 936

Cortisol, p. 936

Cushing's syndrome, p. 938

Glucocorticoids, p. 936

Gluconeogenesis, p. 937

Hypokalemia, p. 939

Mineralocorticoids, p. 936

Secondary adrenal insufficiency, p. 938

OBJECTIVES

- Describe the two types of hormones produced in the adrenal glands.
- Distinguish mineralocorticoid effects from glucocorticoid effects.
- Contrast the use of corticosteroids in replacement therapy and in the treatment of inflammation and immune disorders.
- Compare and contrast the antiinflammatory and sodium-retaining activity of the systemic glucocorticoids.
- Describe the adverse effects associated with long-term glucocorticoid use.
- Describe drugs used to suppress and to stimulate the activity of the adrenal cortex and indicate their therapeutic uses.
- Develop a nursing care plan for patients receiving glucocorticoids.

PHYSIOLOGY • Adrenal Cortex

The human adrenal gland is divided into two functional units: the adrenal medulla and the adrenal cortex. These regions of the gland differ in embryologic origin, type of cells composing the tissue, and hormones produced (Figure 57-1). The adrenal cortex is composed of lipid-rich secretory tissue. Three distinct layers within the cortex may be distinguished histologically. These regions differ in cellular arrangement, in the major steroid hormone produced, and in the regulation of steroid synthesis.

The outer layer, or zona glomerulosa, is where the precursor cholesterol is converted to steroid hormones called **mineralocorticoids**. These hormones cause the kidneys to retain sodium and associated water but promote potassium loss. Regulation of mineralocorticoid synthesis and secretion involves the renin-angiotensin system discussed in Chapter 41 (Figure 57-2). Briefly, the trigger for this feedback system is in the kidneys, where lower blood levels of sodium or lower intravascular volume causes a release of the enzyme renin into the blood. Renin converts angiotensinogen, a protein from the liver, into angiotensin I. The angiotensin-converting enzyme found in the blood and lungs rapidly converts angiotensin I to angiotensin II. Angiotensin II then stimulates the adrenocortical zona glomerulosa to secrete mineralocorticoids, the most important of which is **aldosterone**. Aldosterone produces its major effects by acting at mineralocorticoid receptors in the kidneys. Stimulation of these receptors by aldosterone leads to reduced excretion of sodium and water and increased excretion of potassium. As a result, plasma volume expands and, therefore, the secretion of renin decreases. When the concentration of renin falls, production of angiotensin II slows, aldosterone secretion by the adrenal gland falls, and the kidneys once again begin to rid the body of accumulated sodium.

The inner two layers of the adrenal cortex, the zona fasciculata and zona reticularis, convert cholesterol to steroids with other activities, the principal ones being **glucocorticoids**. The primary glucocorticoid is **cortisol**, or hydrocortisone. (The inner layers of the adrenal cortex also produce small amounts of sex steroids, but the primary sources of these hormones are the ovaries in women and the testes in men.) The synthesis of cortisol is regulated by the pituitary gland and the hypothalamus through a negative feedback mechanism (described in Chapter 55). Cortisol is the key to the regulation of steroid synthesis in the zona fasciculata and zona reticularis. Corticotropin (also known as **adrenocorticotropic hormone** or **ACTH**) from the pituitary stimulates the synthesis of cortisol and other steroids by these regions of the adrenal cortex. Cortisol in the bloodstream inhibits the release of corticotropin from the pituitary, thus completing the negative feedback loop. Cortisol and other endogenous

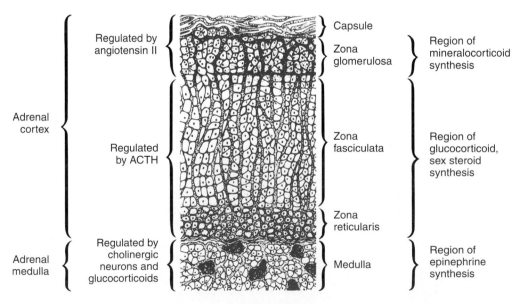

FIGURE 57-1   Regions of the adrenal gland. Each distinct zone of the adrenal gland synthesizes specific hormones and is controlled by specific regulators. The medulla (center of adrenal gland) is thicker than shown in this cross section. *ACTH,* Adrenocorticotropic hormone.

glucocorticoids are secreted cyclically, with the largest amount produced in the morning and the smallest amount during the evening hours (in people on a normal day-night schedule).

Glucocorticoids have powerful and widespread physiologic effects on varied aspects of metabolism, many of which are designed to help the organism survive acute stress. The primary metabolic effect is stimulation of **gluconeogenesis** (the formation of glucose) by actions on peripheral tissues and the liver. In striated muscle, glucocorticoids stimulate the breakdown of muscle protein. The result is an increase in circulating levels of amino acids and an overall depletion of muscle protein, which ultimately is expressed as a negative nitrogen balance (more nitrogen is excreted than is absorbed in the diet). In the liver, glucocorticoids increase activities of enzymes that convert amino acids to glucose. Much of this excess glucose is then stored in the liver as glycogen. In addition, amino acids are the source of precursors for synthesis of fat, which is also increased by glucocorticoids.

In addition to their metabolic effects, glucocorticoids have the potential to suppress the immune system and inflammatory responses in a variety of important ways. At high physiologic concentrations, glucocorticoid ac-

tivity suppresses the inflammatory response, whether the initiating event is an infection, physical or chemical injury, or an immune reaction. Inflammation and an immune response are closely linked. The inflammatory response focuses on the local release of humoral agents to affect a given site. The immune response refers to the mobilization and interactions of the various immune cells, such as lymphocytes, macrophages, neutrophils, eosinophils, basophils, and mast cells. Inflammation is a nonspecific response of tissues to a stimulus or insult and includes the migration of leukocytes to the area and their release of various humoral agents. These humoral agents include complement 5a, leukotrienes, interleukin-8, and transforming growth factor beta. These agents not only have effects of their own but also serve to attract more leukocytes to the inflammatory site, augmenting the inflammatory response. Glucocorticoids inhibit the access of leukocytes to inflammatory sites, interfere with their function, and suppress the production and effects of humoral agents. Glucocorticoids suppress the activity of lymphoid tissue and inhibit proliferation so that the number of circulating lymphocytes is reduced. Because of these and other effects, glucocorticoids can dramatically suppress troublesome or even life-threatening

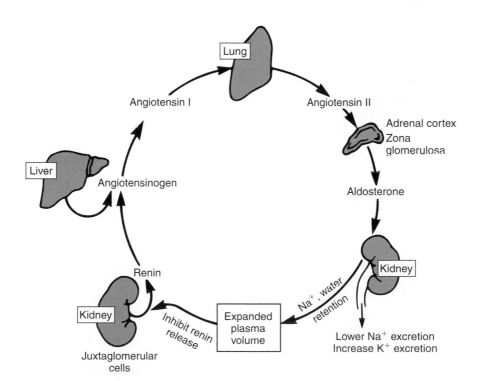

FIGURE 57-2 Negative-feedback loop regulating mineralocorticoid synthesis and release. The kidneys are involved in regulating synthesis and release of aldosterone, the primary natural mineralocorticoid. Renin is released from juxtaglomerular cells in the kidneys to set a cascade in motion, and the kidneys are ultimate targets of aldosterone. Expanded plasma volume, which results when the kidneys retain sodium ion (Na^+) and water, is a regulator that halts renin release. K^+, Potassium ion.

symptoms resulting from inflammatory or immune responses seen in a wide range of pathologic conditions (see later section on Uses). However, to achieve this effect, glucocorticoids must be given at relatively high doses that produce activity much greater than that seen physiologically. Therefore, their prolonged systemic use at the higher-than-physiologic levels that are required leads to serious adverse effects. In addition to direct effects, glucocorticoids have permissive activities that allow the body to deal successfully with stress or trauma. For example, cortisol sensitizes arterioles to norepinephrine, allowing the catecholamine to increase blood pressure. In the liver, cortisol must be present before epinephrine and glucagon can stimulate breakdown of liver glycogen to glucose, releasing the sugar as an energy source for peripheral muscle.

Adrenal Insufficiency

Failure of the adrenal cortex may be life threatening, particularly under conditions of stress. If failure is sudden, which might occur after adrenal injury or thrombosis, death can occur within hours. Early symptoms of acute adrenal insufficiency include confusion, restlessness, nausea, and vomiting. Circulatory collapse, deep shock, and death may follow rapidly.

If synthesis of glucocorticoids is reduced but not halted, patients who are not under stress or traumatized may not be in immediate danger, but will nonetheless show effects of inadequate amounts of glucocorticoids. This chronic primary adrenal insufficiency is called **Addison's disease.** Symptoms include weakness, weight loss, dehydration, hypotension, hypoglycemia, and anemia. Most patients with Addison's disease also display increased skin pigmentation. This unusual or excessive tanning is caused by a direct effect on melanin-containing skin cells by the long-term excess of ACTH, which is secreted by the hypophysis in response to the elevated levels of corticotropin-releasing hormone induced by low blood levels of cortisol.

Symptoms similar to those of Addison's disease are produced when the adenohypophysis is diseased or destroyed and no longer produces adequate ACTH. Without ACTH, the zona reticularis and zona fasciculata do not synthesize cortisol, and over time these adrenal tissues atrophy. This condition is known as **secondary adrenal insufficiency.** One characteristic that often visibly distinguishes these patients from those with Addison's disease is the absence of excessive pigmentation. In secondary adrenal insufficiency, the hypophysis does not release large quantities of ACTH, and the skin is not darkened.

Effects of Excessive Glucocorticoids

Overproduction of cortisol, a condition called **Cushing's syndrome,** may be induced by a variety of factors.

Some patients have high cortisol production from tumors of the adrenal cortex, which may synthesize massive amounts of the steroid. Other patients have increased cortisol synthesis because of excessive circulating levels of ACTH, which keep the zona fasciculata and zona reticularis maximally stimulated to produce glucocorticoids. The condition predominantly affects women in an 8:1 ratio compared to men. The average age of onset of Cushing's syndrome is between ages 20 and 40, but it may occur up to age 60.

Excess ACTH usually comes from a tumor of the hypophysis, but occasionally it comes from some unusual source. Excesses can arise from the ectopic production of ACTH by a tumor of the lung, adrenal gland, GI tract, or pancreas, tissues which would not ordinarily be expected to synthesize ACTH. Adrenal tumors are usually unilateral and are responsible for approximately 25% of all cases of Cushing's syndrome. In adults, approximately 50% of these tumors are malignant. The remainder of the cases result from bilateral adrenal hyperplasia caused by pituitary or nonendocrine tumors that produce excessive ACTH. Most often, however, Cushing's syndrome is caused by administration of high doses of glucocorticoids.

The symptoms of Cushing's syndrome can be predicted from the metabolic actions of cortisol. Certain fat stores, especially those on the face and shoulders, are increased as a result of stimulation of fat deposition at these sites. The extremities may be weak and, in more advanced cases, may be thin because of the muscle-wasting effects of the hormone. The skin is fragile and easily bruised as a result of protein breakdown in that tissue. Examination of the skin on the trunk may reveal striae, or stretch marks, over areas where fat deposition is most pronounced. Many patients also have superficial fungal infections of the skin, related in part to the fragility of the skin and also to the reduced host immune response caused by the excess steroid. Bone thinning occurs because of changes in calcium metabolism; compression fractures of the spine may occur relatively easily. Diabetes mellitus may be precipitated from the increased insulin demand caused by excess cortisol. Hypertension is common in these patients, and atherosclerosis may occur. Mood changes are also common and may be extreme. Psychosis may be precipitated.

Effects of Excessive Mineralocorticoid (Hyperaldosteronism)

Tumors of the adrenal gland may produce excessive amounts of aldosterone or, less often, other mineralocorticoids. In these patients, two types of symptoms appear: those associated with hypertension and those associated with Cushing's syndrome (low blood potassium concentration). Hypertension is caused by sodium and water retention arising from excess aldosterone acting on the kidneys, whereas the muscle weakness associated with hypokalemia is a result of the potassium-wasting action of the steroid in the kidneys. Treatment involves surgical removal of the tumor when possible. Spironolactone, an aldosterone antagonist, may also be used (see Chapter 46).

Effects of Mineralocorticoid Deficiency

When the adrenal gland fails, mineralocorticoid action is lost. As a result, salt balance becomes deranged. Survival requires replacement of the lost hormone activity.

Effects of Excessive Adrenal Production of Sex Steroids

Sex steroids produced in the adrenal cortex are normally of minor importance because the adrenal output is small compared with that of the gonads; however, under certain conditions, sex steroid overproduction in the adrenal glands may cause a devastating endocrine imbalance. For example, a woman with an androgen-producing adrenal tumor may undergo masculinization, including development of secondary male sex characteristics and suppression of the menstrual cycle. A man with an estrogen-producing tumor may develop breast tenderness or loss of libido. A child may show precocious sexual development.

DRUG CLASS • Glucocorticoids

betamethasone (Beta-Val, Celestone, Diprosone, Valisone)

budesonide (Pulmicort, Rhinocort)

dexamethasone (Decadron, Dexacort, Maxidex)

hydrocortisone (Anucort, Anusol-HC, Cortef, Cortenema, Cortifoam, Hydrocortone, Locoid, Proctocort)

methylprednisolone (A-Methapred, Medrol)

prednisolone (Delta-Cortef, Econopred, Inflamase, Ocu-Pred-A, Pediapred, Pred Mild, Predair)

prednisone (Deltasone)

triamcinolone (Aristocort, Aristospan, Azmacort, Kenacort, Nasacort AQ)

For other drugs of this class, see Table 57-3.

MECHANISM OF ACTION

As with other steroid hormones and drugs, glucocorticoids are thought to act primarily by turning on or off the expression of different genes. Glucocorticoids enter a target cell and bind to specific receptors in the cell cytoplasm. The binding of the glucocorticoid activates the receptor, which allows the complex to enter the nucleus. In the nucleus the complex binds to selected DNA sites known as glucocorticoid response elements (GREs). This promotes or inhibits the transcription of specific mRNAs. In turn, the synthesis of the respective proteins is promoted or inhibited. A considerable delay may occur between uptake of the steroid into the cell and appearance of the effect in the target cell. More time may elapse before the effect ends and the steroid is destroyed.

The dosages of steroids used clinically provide much more than the natural level of glucocorticoid activity. As a result, many of the effects produced are very different from the physiologic effects of naturally occurring hormones. These pharmacologic (rather than physiologic) effects are achieved when glucocorticoids are required to treat disorders unrelated to adrenocortical function, such as allergic reactions, autoimmune diseases, asthma, and inflammation (see section on Uses).

Cortisol and cortisone, the naturally occurring glucocorticoids, have relatively low affinity for the mineralocorticoid receptor but still may produce some salt and water retention. Other glucocorticoids have relatively less mineralocorticoid activity.

USES

Glucocorticoids are used in two very different ways. First, glucocorticoids are given when the adrenal glands are unable to produce the normal amounts of endogenous glucocorticoids (adrenal insufficiency). In this case, glucocorticoids are administered systemically at doses calibrated to replicate the physiologic activity seen normally. This approach, called replacement therapy, will generally use one of the glucocorticoids listed in Table 57-1. Examples of replacement therapy include the use of cortisol to treat Addison's disease or secondary adrenal insufficiency. Dosages of adrenal steroids used in replacement therapy are relatively low because they are intended to replace only amounts of the hormone that are normally present. Because the normal daily production of cortisol is about 15 to 25 mg, the daily replacement dose is calculated to achieve the level of activity produced by that amount of cortisol. Wide variations in dosage exist because stress and other factors affect steroid requirements. The dosage must be adjusted to each patient's needs and monitored to ensure continued success of the therapy. Successful treatment of adrenal insufficiency is often obtained with hydrocortisone or cortisone, natural glucocorticoids with sufficient mineralocorticoid activity to maintain sodium balance for many individuals. Other patients may require additional supplementation with a mineralocorticoid such as fludrocortisone. When done properly, replacement therapy is not complicated by adverse reactions because its goal is to replicate the physiologic effects of the missing endogenous hormones. Patients who receive corticosteroids as replacement therapy would normally continue to receive them for life.

Glucocorticoids are usually administered at much higher doses (or local concentrations, if used topically) to suppress inflammation and immune responses. This action is the basis for the therapeutic effect of glucocorticoids in the treatment of a wide variety of diseases and conditions, many of which are detailed in the paragraphs that follow. However, it is important to remember that the reactions that are suppressed by glucocorticoids are generally symptoms of an underlying disorder that these drugs rarely cure. Instead, their prolonged systemic use may lead to serious adverse effects (see later discussion) because glucocorticoid activity greatly in excess of physiologic levels is the desired therapeutic goal.

Allergic States. Glucocorticoids may be used as adjunct therapy in treating acute, severe episodes of asthma, angioedema, transfusion reactions, and serum sickness. Local application is often employed to limit the action of the drug. Inhaled glucocorticoids have become a preferred prophylactic treatment of chronic asthma to suppress inflammation of the bronchioles.

Dermatologic Disorders. Various types of dermatitis and pemphigus are treated with glucocorticoids. Topical glucocorticoids are used for keloids, lichen planus, lichen simplex chronicus, discoid lupus, and severe psoriasis. Dermatologic allergic reactions, such as severe reactions to poison ivy, can be blunted with oral or topical glucocorticoids.

Gastrointestinal Disorders. Inflammatory bowel diseases, including ulcerative colitis, regional enteritis (Crohn's disease), and ulcerative proctitis, are treated with glucocorticoids.

Hematologic Disorders. Large doses of glucocorticoids suppress the immune processes, destroying blood cells in the acute phases of autoimmune hemolytic anemia and thrombocytopenia. Lower dosages maintain remission.

Joint Inflammation. Injection of glucocorticoids directly into inflamed joints gives symptomatic relief in patients who have bursitis.

Neoplastic Diseases. Glucocorticoids are administered with antineoplastic drugs to produce remissions for patients who have leukemia or lymphoma. The antilymphocytic action of glucocorticoids aids in destroying lymphoid cancers.

Ophthalmic Diseases. Steroids may be applied directly to the eye to treat allergic conjunctivitis, chorioretinitis, iritis, iridocyclitis, and keratitis. The antiinflammatory action reduces permanent eye damage and controls acute symptoms.

Rheumatic Diseases. Acute inflammatory episodes of various types of arthritis (ankylosing spondylitis, psoriatic arthritis, rheumatoid arthritis) respond to glucocorticoids. Modest dosages are sometimes used to maintain inhibition of the inflammatory and autoimmune pro-

---

TABLE 57-1

Adrenocortical Drugs Used for Replacement Therapy

Generic Name	Brand Name	Description
betamethasone	Celestone✱	Synthetic glucocorticoid with little or no mineralocorticoid action; used with mineralocorticoid
cortisone	Cortone✱	Natural hormone with both glucocorticoid and mineralocorticoid action
fludrocortisone	Florinef✱	Synthetic steroid with strong mineralocorticoid action; used with glucocorticoid for replacement therapy
hydrocortisone (cortisol)	Cortef✱	Major natural glucocorticoid in humans with some mineralocorticoid activity
triamcinolone	Aristocort,✱ Kenacort✱	Synthetic glucocorticoid with little or no mineralocorticoid action; used with mineralocorticoid

✱ Available only in Canada.

cesses. Glucocorticoids are used to control flares of systemic lupus erythematosus.

PHARMACOKINETICS

The chemical form of a steroid determines the pharmacokinetics of the preparation. Most corticosteroids are relatively insoluble in water and form suspensions that are not suitable for intravenous administration. In contrast, sodium phosphate and sodium succinate derivatives of several glucocorticoids are quite water soluble; these are the forms that must be used when intravenous administration of an adrenal steroid is required.

Administered intramuscularly as suspensions, many glucocorticoids are dissolved and absorbed slowly from the injection site, producing a relatively long duration of action, which may be an advantage for control of certain conditions.

Oral preparations are commonly used for systemic glucocorticoid therapy because they are well absorbed from the GI tract. Peak plasma concentrations are reached in 1 to 2 hours. Glucocorticoids are lipophilic and readily cross cell membranes. Cortisone and prednisone are converted to their active forms, hydrocortisone and prednisolone, by the liver. Hydrocortisone and prednisolone bind to a plasma protein, corticosteroid-binding globulin (CBG), and albumin, which keeps them from being readily cleared from the plasma. Generally, the other glucocorticoids are also highly bound to these plasma proteins, a phenomenon which prolongs their duration of action. Only the unbound portion is active.

A major factor in the overall potency of the various glucocorticoids is their relative rate of biotransformation by the liver. The intermediate- and long-acting glucocorticoids have structural modifications that not only decrease their mineralocorticoid activity but also slow their rate of biotransformation (Table 57-2). For systemic use in treating inflammatory conditions, the intermediate-acting glucocorticoids are generally preferred because they have low mineralocorticoid activity and can be administered in a way to lessen adverse reactions. Prednisone remains the most commonly used glucocorticoid of this group because of its long history of reliable use and low cost.

Severe liver disease has multiple effects on bioavailability of glucocorticoids. In this setting, hydrocortisone and prednisolone are preferred over cortisone or prednisone because they do not require hepatic biotransformation into an active form. In general, severe liver disease increases the biologic and toxic effects of glucocorticoids. The hypoalbuminemia of severe liver disease increases the free concentration of most glucocorticoids, and their biotransformation may also be impaired.

Glucocorticoids are also biotransformed by the placenta in pregnant women, limiting exposure of the fetus. However, very high doses of glucocorticoids can still suppress fetal adrenal function.

Because the action of glucocorticoids depends on the promotion or inhibition of new protein synthesis, the onset of action is in hours to days and the duration of action is in days to weeks. The glucocorticoids used systemically vary in their duration of action, depending not only on the chemical characteristics of the glucocorticoid but also on the formulation and route of administration. Oral glucocorticoid therapy usually begins with one or more daily doses to control symptoms. When symptoms are under control, treatment can often be continued with alternate-day administration of prednisone, prednisolone, or methylprednisolone. The advantage of alternate-day therapy is that the suppression of the hypophyseal-pituitary-adrenal

---

TABLE 57-2

Pharmacokinetics of Selected Glucocorticoids Used for Systemic Administration

Steroids	Glucocorticoid Activity Relative to Hydrocortisone	Mineralocorticoid Activity Relative to Hydrocortisone	Biologic Half-Life*
Short Acting			
hydrocortisone (Cortisone)	1 (0.8)	1 (0.8)	8-12 hr
Intermediate Acting			
methylprednisolone, prednisolone, prednisone, triamcinolone	4-5	<1	18-36 hr
Long Acting			
betamethasone, dexamethasone	20-30	0	36-54 hr

*Refers to the persistence of the agent in tissues; this relates more closely to duration of action than plasma half-life because of the mechanism of action of steroids.

axis is lessened, thus maintaining growth rate in children and reducing bone loss in all individuals.

A number of glucocorticoids have been developed specifically for local administration. Glucocorticoids formulated for such use are listed in Table 57-3. Local uses of glucocorticoids include bronchial inhalation for asthma; dental pastes; various creams, ointments, and other preparations for use on the skin; nasal sprays; drops for the eyes and ears; and ointments and suppositories for rectal administration.

TABLE 57-3

Glucocorticoids in Preparations for Nonsystemic Use

Generic Name	Brand Name	Potency Rankings (Where Applicable)
Inhalation (Aerosols, Powders, Suspensions): Airway Inflammation, Asthma		
beclomethasone	Beclovent, Beclodisk, Vanceril	
budesonide	Pulmicort Nebuamp, Pulmicort Respules, Pulmicort Turbuhaler	
dexamethasone	Decadron Respihaler	
flunisolide	AeroBid, AeroBid-M, Bronalide	
fluticasone	Flovent, Flovent Disk, Flovent Rotadiskus	
triamcinolone	Azmacort	
Nasal (Aerosols, Solutions, Suspensions): Rhinitis, Polyps		
beclomethasone	Beconase, Vancenase	
budesonide	Rhinocort, Rhinocort Turbuhaler	
dexamethasone	Dexacort Turbinaire	
flunisolide	Nasalide, Nasarel, Rhinalar	
fluticasone	Flonase	
mometasone	Nasonex	
triamcinolone	Nasacort AQ	
Ophthalmic (Ointments, Solutions, Suspensions): Allergy, Inflammation		
dexamethasone	AK-Dex, Baldex, Decadron, Dexaire, Dexotic, Maxidex, Ocu-Dex, Spersadex	
fluorometholone	Eflone, Flarex, Fluor-Op, FML S.O.P.	
medrysone	HMS Liquifilm	
prednisolone	AK-Tate, Econopred, Ocu-Pred-A, Predair A, Pred Forte, Pred Mild, Ultra Pred	
rimexolone	Vexol	
Otic (Solution): Inflammation of External Auditory Meatus		
dexamethasone	Decadron	
Rectal (Enemas, Foams, Suppositories): Ulcerative Colitis, Hemorrhoids, Proctitis		
hydrocortisone	Anucort-HC, Anu-Med HC, Anuprep HC, Anusol-HC, Anuzone-HC, Cort-Dome, Cortenema, Cortifoam, Cortiment, Proctocort, Proctosol-HC, Rectocort, Rectosol-HC	Low
Topical (Ointments, Creams, Aerosol Sprays, Gels, Lotions, Solutions): Skin Disorders and Oral Lesions		
alclometasone	Aclovate	Low
amcinonide	Cyclocort	High
betamethasone	Alphatrex, Beben, Betatrex, Celestoderm-V, Dermabet, Diprolene, Diprosone, Ectosone, Maxivate, Metaderm, Occlucort, Topisone, Uticort, Valisone, Valnac	Medium to very high

ADVERSE REACTIONS AND CONTRAINDICATIONS

Glucocorticoid dosages that are higher than physiologic levels lead to altered metabolism of a number of tissues and organs. These changes include muscle wasting from the negative nitrogen balance induced by glucocorticoids and increased fat tissue, especially in the central portion of the body and around the face. The result is a typical cushingoid appearance: moon face, thin limbs, and fat on the trunk of the body. Other effects of glucocorticoids include changes in behavior and personality, usually marked by euphoria, but occasionally psychotic episodes are seen. Growth is suppressed in children. Long-term use of glucocorticoids leads to osteoporosis. Osteonecrosis is also more common. The metabolic effects of glucocorticoids can lead to impaired glucose tolerance and frank diabetes mellitus.

Adverse actions of high-dose glucocorticoids severely limit their long-term use. High doses of glucocorticoids administered for a few days have relatively few adverse effects. However, even low doses of glucocorticoids used clinically may inhibit the normal release of ACTH from the pituitary (see Chapter 55). If these doses are given for a prolonged period, the chronic lack of ACTH causes atrophy of the adrenal cortex. Therefore, glucocorticoids cannot be abruptly discontinued after prolonged therapy, because the adrenal glands no longer produce cortisol and need time to recover under the influence of ACTH. The dosage must be gradually tapered to allow the adrenal gland to resume functioning, thereby avoiding an adrenal crisis.

Because pharmacologic doses of glucocorticoids suppress inflammatory and immune responses, patients be-

---

TABLE 57-3

Glucocorticoids in Preparations for Nonsystemic Use—cont'd

Generic Name	Brand Name	Potency Rankings (Where Applicable)
Topical (Ointments, Creams, Aerosol Sprays, Gels, Lotions, Solutions): Skin Disorders and Oral Lesions—cont'd		
clobetasol	Cormax, Temovate	Very high
clocortolone	Cloderm	Low
desonide	DesOwen, Tridesilon	Low
desoximetasone	Topicort	Medium to high
dexamethasone	Aeroseb-Dex, Decaderm, Decadron, Decaspray	Low
diflorasone	Florone, Maxiflor, Psorcon	High to very high
fluocinolone	Bio-Syn, Fluocet, Fluonid, Flurosyn, Synalar, Synemol	Medium to high
fluocinonide	Fluocin, Licon, Lidex, Lidex-E	High
flurandrenolide	Cordran, Cordran SP, Drenison	Low to medium
fluticasone	Cutivate	Medium
halcinonide	Halog, Halog-E	High
halobetasol	Ultravate	Very high
hydrocortisone	Acticort, Aeroseb-HC, Ala-Cort, Allercort, Alphaderm, Anusol-HC 1, Bactine, CaldeCORT, Carmol-HC, Cetacort, Cortate, Cort-Dome, Cortaid, Corticaine, Cortifair, Cortril, Delacort, DermiCort, Dermtex HC, Dermarest DriCort, Emo-Cort, FoilleCort, Gly-Cort, Gynecort, Hydro-Tex, Hytone, LactiCare HC, Lanacort, Lemoderm, Locoid, MyCort, Nutracort, Orabase-HCA, Pandel, Penecort, Pentacort, Rederm, Rhulicort, Synacort, Texacort, Westcort	Low to medium
mometasone	Elocon	Medium
prednicarbate	Dermatop	
triamcinolone	Aristocort, Flutex, Kenac, Kenalog, Kenalog in Orabase, Kenonel, Oracort, Oralone, Triacet, Trianide, Triderm	Medium to high

ing treated will be more susceptible to infection. Furthermore, many clinical signs and symptoms that signal important problems may be suppressed or absent in a patient on glucocorticoids, leading to missed or inaccurate diagnosis of the patient's disorder.

Glucocorticoids are classified in the Food and Drug Administration (FDA) pregnancy category C. Glucocorticoids are found in breast milk; however, as long as the mother is taking small doses of glucocorticoids, the small amount in the breast milk poses no risk for her infant.

TOXICITY

Toxic reactions to long-term glucocorticoid therapy are listed in Table 57-4. The frequency of adverse effects is related to the duration of therapy. Any glucocorticoid, if given in high enough dosages, will produce Cushing's syndrome. This toxicity is one of the most common reactions seen with glucocorticoid therapy. For these patients the steroid dosage should be reduced, if allowed by the severity of the condition being treated. Although usual replacement doses slightly exceed normal daily production of steroids, these doses would not be expected to cause Cushing's syndrome.

INTERACTIONS

A number of clinically important adverse drug interactions occur with glucocorticoids. Drugs that slow the biotransformation or clearance of glucocorticoids include antibiotics, cyclosporine, estrogen, isoniazid, and ketoconazole. The dosage of glucocorticoids should be decreased.

Drugs that increase the biotransformation or clearance of glucocorticoids include aminoglutethimide, carbamazepine, cholestyramine, phenobarbital, phenytoin, and rifampin. The dosage of glucocorticoids should be increased.

Glucocorticoids affect biotransformation or clearance of some other drugs, requiring adjustment of their dosages. These drugs include antianxiety drugs, antipsychotics, anticholinesterases, anticoagulants, antihypertensive drugs, cyclosporine, hypoglycemic drugs, live or killed virus vaccines, pancuronium, salicylates, and sympathomimetic drugs.

TABLE 57-4

Undesirable Glucocorticoid Effects

Common	*Sporadic*
Early Effects (Days to Weeks)	
Weight gain from changes in lipid metabolism	Anaphylactoid reactions; hypersensitivity reaction
Mood changes; euphoria most common, also increased appetite, insomnia; uncommonly, psychoses	Hypertriglyceridemia from changes in lipid metabolism
Glucose intolerance from gluconeogenic effects; resulting diabetes usually mild and reversible	Peptic ulcers may be induced or masked by glucocorticoids
Transient adrenal suppression of physiologic feedback on hypothalamic-pituitary-adrenal axis	Acute pancreatitis may result from changes in lipid metabolism
Potassium/sodium changes glucocorticoids with mineralocorticoid activity may cause decreased serum potassium and increased sodium concentrations	
Later Effects (Months to Years)	
Central obesity; classic cushingoid appearance from altered lipid metabolism	Aseptic necrosis of bone most commonly affects femoral head
Skin fragility from inhibitory effects on synthesis of collagen and extracellular matrix; also, changes in hair	Cataracts; cause unknown; seen with systemic or local therapy
Myopathy from protein break down; more pronounced with fluoride derivatives such as triamcinolone	Glaucoma from interference with normal aqueous outflow; greater risk in diabetic patients
Osteoporosis from increased bone resorption; patients with arthritis and postmenopausal women at greatest risk	Hypertension; more of a problem with cortisone and hydrocortisone, which have significant mineralocorticoid activity
Growth failure from inhibition of growth hormone action; limits use in children	Opportunistic infections from suppression of immune functions

DRUG CLASS • Mineralocorticoids

fludrocortisone (Florinef)

MECHANISM OF ACTION

Fludrocortisone binds to renal mineralocorticoid to promote the reabsorption of sodium and water and the excretion of potassium. Fludrocortisone has minimal activity at glucocorticoid receptors.

USES

Fludrocortisone is used for replacement of mineralocorticoid activity where normal aldosterone synthesis is absent or impaired in cases of adrenocortical failure.

PHARMACOKINETICS

Fludrocortisone is well absorbed and highly bound to plasma proteins. A single dose has a duration of action of 1 to 2 days and is eliminated by both hepatic biotransformation and renal excretion.

ADVERSE REACTIONS AND CONTRAINDICATIONS

Fludrocortisone may cause typical signs of mineralocorticoid excess, including edema and low potassium. It should be used with caution in patients with heart failure or hypertension. Rarely, fludrocortisone may cause anaphylaxis.

INTERACTIONS

Interactions with fludrocortisone are often associated with electrolyte changes caused by the drug. For example, hypokalemia caused by fludrocortisone can increase the toxicity of cardiac glycosides and increase the risk with other drugs that cause hypokalemia, including many diuretics and beta receptor agonists used as bronchodilators. Drugs or foods that contain large amounts of sodium may cause hypernatremia because the kidneys, under the influence of fludrocortisone, may be unable to clear the excess sodium.

Inducers of hepatic enzymes may increase biotransformation of fludrocortisone, necessitating an increase in dosage of fludrocortisone. Rifampin and phenytoin have been reported to cause this effect.

 DRUG CLASS • Adrenocortical Inhibitors

aminoglutethimide (Cytadren)
metyrapone (Metopirone)
mitotane (Lysodren)

MECHANISM OF ACTION

Aminoglutethimide blocks the first step in the synthesis of all steroid hormones from cholesterol. Therefore, aminoglutethimide not only blocks all steroid synthesis in the adrenal cortex, but also inhibits the synthesis of steroid hormones by the testes and ovaries. Metyrapone, however, blocks the enzyme responsible for the last step of the synthesis of cortisol, so that levels of only this steroid are reduced. In healthy persons the fall in blood cortisol level stimulates the hypothalamus and, in turn, the pituitary gland, with the result that ACTH is released into the blood. Under the influence of ACTH, early steps in steroid synthesis proceed, but metyrapone prevents cortisol from being formed in normal amounts. Therefore steroid precursors accumulate and are excreted in urine.

Mitotane is a toxic drug specific for adrenal cortical cells. Therefore, unlike the other drugs, the suppression of adrenal function caused by mitotane is irreversible because the drug destroys the adrenal cortex. Clinical response to treatment may be assessed by measurement of morning plasma cortisol levels or 24-hour urinary corticosteroid metabolites (usually 17-hydroxycorticosteroids).

USES

Aminoglutethimide is used in the management and treatment of Cushing's disease. Because it inhibits the synthesis of steroids in other tissues besides the adrenal cortex, it is also employed in the treatment of breast and prostate cancer (see Chapter 37).

Metyrapone is used to test the ability of the pituitary gland to increase ACTH release in the diagnosis of different variants of Cushing's syndrome and adrenal insufficiency, and is used infrequently in the short-term management of Cushing's syndrome. While metyrapone is being administered, cortisol synthesis falls dramatically.

If no precursors accumulate under these conditions, it is concluded that the pituitary gland failed to produce ACTH. If the metyrapone test is administered to a person with adrenal insufficiency, a danger exists of precipitating an adrenal crisis because in such a patient metyrapone may stop cortisol synthesis altogether.

Mitotane is used in the treatment of adrenocortical carcinoma and Cushing's syndrome.

PHARMACOKINETICS

Aminoglutethimide is rapidly and completely absorbed from the GI tract, but its effect to suppress adrenal function is not seen for several days after administration. The drug is both biotransformed in the liver and excreted unchanged by the kidneys. Aminoglutethimide has a plasma half-life of 12.5 hours initially, but because the drug induces the hepatic enzymes responsible for its own biotransformation, the half-life may fall to 7 hours with repeated administration.

Metyrapone is well absorbed from the GI tract but is rapidly cleared from the circulation by hepatic biotransformation (plasma half-life is 20 to 30 minutes). Its peak effects occur within 24 hours after administration.

Only about 40% of an oral dose of mitotane is absorbed. However, the drug has a very long half-life (3 weeks or longer) and may still be measurable in the circulation 6 to 9 weeks after the last dose. Effects may be seen within 2 to 3 days after initiation of treatment with mitotane.

ADVERSE REACTIONS AND CONTRAINDICATIONS

Aminoglutethimide may cause blurred vision, drowsiness, weakness, and skin rash with itching. In some patients, decreased blood pressure, dizziness, loss of appetite and nausea may occur. Most of these effects are reduced after the first few weeks of continued therapy. Aminoglutethimide should not be given to pregnant patients.

Metyrapone may produce many of the same reactions: headache, rash, drowsiness, and nausea. Long-term use of metyrapone is limited in large part by the potential for more serious effects, including bone marrow depression, edema, and hypokalemic alkalosis.

Mitotane produces typical signs of adrenal insufficiency in 40% to 80% of treated patients. These signs may include darkening of skin, tiredness, drowsiness, dizziness, loss of appetite, depression, and nausea and vomiting. Less frequently, double or blurred vision or allergic reactions may occur. Administration of mitotane should be avoided during pregnancy, especially during the first trimester.

INTERACTIONS

Aminoglutethimide induces hepatic enzymes and may increase the rate of clearance of other drugs that are eliminated primarily by biotransformation in the liver. Conversely, concurrent treatment with one of many drugs that induce hepatic enzymes may decrease the effectiveness of metyrapone. The CNS depression caused by mitotane is additive with that of other drugs producing this effect.

DRUG CLASS • Adrenocortical Stimulants

corticorelin ovine triflutate (Acthrel)
cosyntropin (Cortrosyn)

MECHANISM OF ACTION

Cosyntropin is a synthetic version of ACTH that contains the first 24 of the 39 amino acids found in natural ACTH. Like natural ACTH, this synthetic form of ACTH directly stimulates the adrenal cortex to synthesize adrenal steroids. Corticorelin ovine triflutate is a form of corticotropin-releasing hormone (CRH) that is related to human CRH and has the same ability to cause release of ACTH from the anterior pituitary gland in humans.

USES

Cosyntropin can be used diagnostically to distinguish between Addison's disease and secondary adrenal insufficiency that results from pituitary dysfunction. Normal adrenal glands respond to ACTH by synthesizing and releasing cortisol into the bloodstream, where it may be measured. In Addison's disease the adrenal gland cannot respond to ACTH, and no excess cortisol is produced. In patients who have low pituitary function, the adrenal gland may be suppressed and may respond less rapidly to ACTH than would a normal gland. Cosyntropin has replaced the natural ACTH purified from animal pituitaries (Acthar gel) because it is much less likely to cause allergic reactions.

Corticorelin ovine triflutate is used to identify the source of high ACTH levels. The drug induces release of ACTH from the pituitary, but tumors or other ectopic sites of ACTH production usually do not respond. Thus persons with normal pituitary function or with oversecretion from the pituitary show a rise in ACTH and cortisol after administration of corticorelin ovine. Production of ACTH or cortisol is not changed in response to corticorelin ovine when the primary source of ACTH is a tumor.

PHARMACOKINETICS

Because they are peptides, corticorelin and cosyntropin are not effective orally and must be given by injection. Both are rapidly cleared from the circulation and produce peak increases in plasma cortisol 30 to 60 minutes after administration.

ADVERSE REACTIONS AND CONTRAINDICATIONS

The principal adverse reactions that are possible with either drug are a consequence of increased secretion of adrenal corticosteroids. Corticorelin may produce flushing after intravenous injection; shortness of breath, hypotension, and tachycardia have also been reported. Usually these effects are transient, lasting from 5 to 30 minutes. Although less antigenic than native ACTH, cosyntropin may still produce allergic reactions and anaphylaxis in rare cases.

INTERACTIONS

Corticorelin may produce severe hypotension in the presence of heparin. Concurrent use of these agents should be avoided.

APPLICATION TO PRACTICE

ASSESSMENT

The patient may exhibit signs and symptoms consistent with either adrenal insufficiency or excessive glucocorticoid levels. Therefore, the health care provider should be watchful for the wide spectrum of abnormal findings indicating the need to initiate, maintain, reduce, or increase the dosage of the adrenal hormone. Adrenal hormone dosing varies from person to person and changes even for the same individual from time to time. A thorough assessment allows for more informed decisions to be made about the dosage required.

History of Present Illness

For the patient with adrenal insufficiency, ask questions about changes in activity levels because lethargy, fatigue, and muscle weakness are often present. Information about a patient's history of GI problems such as anorexia, nausea, vomiting, weight loss, diarrhea, and abdominal pain should also be elicited. Ask about salt craving because it is often a symptom of adrenal hypofunction. Associated low androgen levels may result in the loss of body, axillary, and pubic hair. Female patients may report menstrual changes related to weight loss and hormonal imbalances, and men may note impotence.

Patients with hypercortisolism (Cushing's syndrome) come in with a variety of complaints. Ask about changes in activity or sleep patterns; changes in body appearance or skin integrity; or fatigue, muscle weakness, and easy bruising. Because osteoporosis is a common occurrence in hypercortisolism, patients should be asked if they have bone pain or a history of fractures. A history of frequent infections or frequent bruising may also be noted. Mental symptoms such as emotional lability, irritation, confusion, and depression may be present and identified by a family member.

When glucocorticoids are used to treat inflammatory disorders or to prevent transplant rejection, the patient should be questioned about the occurrence of symptoms associated with the primary disorder or rejection. The focus of specific questions to ask should be guided by a knowledge of the signs and symptoms of normal versus abnormal function of the body system being treated. Judgments about the potential consequences of glucocorticoids versus an exacerbation of the inflammatory disorder are made only after careful review of the patient's health history.

Health History

The patient's health history helps to identify potential causes of adrenal insufficiency. Inquire whether the patient has had intracranial surgery or radiation therapy to the head or abdomen. Significant medical problems such as tuberculosis, diabetes mellitus, heart failure, or peptic ulcer disease should be noted because these conditions develop from or may be exacerbated by administration of glucocorticoids.

Elicit a complete health history from the patient, including allergies, and concomitant disease(s). All past and current drug use should be recorded, especially the use of anticoagulants and cytotoxic drugs. Although glucocorticoids are often used to treat allergic reactions, patients can develop an allergic reaction to the synthetic glucocorticoid preparations. Determination of concurrent or recent drug therapy is also important because many drugs use the same biotransformation pathways as the glucocorticoids.

Determining what the patient perceives to be a stressful situation and how that patient reacts under stressful conditions is also important. During periods of increased stress, the body requires additional amounts of adrenal hormones to achieve the same physiologic effects.

Lifespan Considerations

Perinatal. Couples who have a history of adrenal hormone disorders who are thinking about conception must consider the potential consequences to both the mother and fetus. Glucocorticoids taken for physiologic replacement therapy should not affect the pregnant woman or the fetus. However, maintaining exact physiologic drug requirements during pregnancy is difficult given the increased stress and the physical changes of pregnancy (see Chapter 2). Relative overdosage with glucocorticoids causes sodium and water retention, resulting in elevated blood pressure and edema for some women. Any blood pressure elevations and peripheral edema associated with pregnancy may be worsened.

Infants born to mothers receiving high dosages of glucocorticoids are monitored closely immediately after birth for signs and symptoms of adrenal insufficiency. Supplemental doses of steroids may be required temporarily by the newborn. The health care provider determines whether the infant's adrenal glands can be stimulated naturally through the gradual withdrawal of exogenous steroids.

Pediatrics. Managing corticosteroid replacement therapy in children is difficult because of their age and the need for physical growth. The most significant problem related to glucocorticoid replacement therapy is suppression of the growth hormone (GH), which results in failure of the child to reach normal adult stature. Although regulation of GH arises from alternate mechanisms, GH release is decreased with hypothalamus-pituitary-adrenal (HPA) suppression. Health care providers should closely monitor the growth of the child, attempting to maintain the child's growth in the 50th percentile for similar age groups. Supplemental doses of GH are controversial but, when required, may be used during predicted high-growth periods to stimulate normal development.

Older Adults. The use of glucocorticoids in older adults poses many challenges. Although the mechanisms of action are similar for both young and older adults, normal physiologic changes and pathophysiologic changes common with aging make dosing difficult. Normal changes of aging such as weakness, fatigue, anorexia, and sparse hair are also seen in adrenal insufficiency. Slight-to-moderate immunosuppression, development of cataracts, redistribution of body mass, changes in vessel compliance, decreased glucose tolerance, alterations in GI functioning, and thinning of the skin are also associated with normal changes of aging and may be difficult to distinguish from the signs and symptoms of adrenal insufficiency. Additionally, many older adults have preexisting fluid and sodium retention associated

with hypertension and heart failure. The added burden of glucocorticoids increases fluid and sodium retention, leading to further pathology. When used in the older adult, the corticosteroid dose is usually reduced because of the decreased muscle mass, plasma volume, hepatic biotransformation, and renal elimination.

Cultural/Social Considerations

Question the patient about past experiences with glucocorticoid therapy to determine adverse as well as beneficial effects of the drug therapy. Did the patient feel better while under treatment? What therapeutic and adverse reactions occurred? How did the patient feel emotionally? What happened when the patient was weaned off the drug? If the health care provider suspects that the patient will not comply with the treatment plan, the issue should be discussed and alternate measures for treatment explored.

Depending on the degree of insufficiency, the patient may appear lethargic, apathetic, depressed, confused, or psychotic. The family may report that the patient is emotionally labile and forgetful. Such changes place serious stressors on family relationships (see the Case Study: Adrenal Insufficiency).

Patients with hypercortisolism may also have difficulty coping with their health care problems. The changes in physical appearance contribute to an altered body image and social isolation.

Physical Examination

Assess vital signs and blood pressure (including orthostatic readings), weight, history of any weight gain or loss, and dependent areas for edema. Assess for nausea and vomiting and perform a mental status examination. Watch the skin for striae (reddish-purple lines), thin skin, unusual or excessive bruising, change in skin color, change in amount of hair growth, and acne. Monitor height and growth pattern in children receiving long-term therapy.

The clinical manifestations of adrenal insufficiency vary from patient to patient, and the severity of signs is related to the degree of hormone deficiency. Thorough assessment of the skin, mucous membranes, knuckles on the hand, areolae, and surgical scars is essential. Increased pigmentation, especially over skin folds and pressure areas, is a classic sign of insufficiency. With primary adrenal insufficiency, areas of decreased pigmentation may be noted because of the autoimmune destruction of melanocytes. In secondary disease, there is no change in skin pigmentation.

Hypoglycemia may be noted because of impaired gluconeogenesis. The patient should be observed for diaphoresis, tachycardia, and tremors. With primary insufficiency, cortisol and aldosterone deficiencies result in volume depletion; therefore, the patient should be examined for evidence of dehydration. A deficiency of aldosterone may manifest as hyperkalemia and arrhythmias.

The physical examination of the patient with an inflammatory disorder focuses on the abnormalities associated with the particular primary disease causing inflammation. Measures indicating fluid balance status are also assessed, including neck vein distention, peripheral edema, lung sounds, mucous membranes, and skin turgor. Evaluation of eyes and vision for glaucoma or cataracts is important in early detection and interventions of complications.

Thorough assessment of the skin and musculoskeletal system is essential for anyone taking high doses of glucocorticoids. Physical changes resulting from glucocorticoid therapy include muscle wasting and weakness, redistribution of fatty tissue to central areas of the body (moon face, buffalo hump, truncal obesity), striae, thin and fragile skin that bruises easily, acneiform eruptions, hirsutism, and poor wound healing.

Laboratory Testing

Laboratory findings associated with adrenal insufficiency include a low serum cortisol level (between 8 and 9 AM); elevated serum potassium (reflected as peaked T waves, a widening QRS complex, and an increase in the PR interval), calcium, blood urea nitrogen (BUN) and creatinine levels; and decreased fasting blood glucose level. There is an elevated ACTH level with moderate neutropenia, eosinophilia, relative lymphocytosis, and anemia. Plasma ACTH and melanocyte-stimulating hormone levels are elevated because of the loss of the HPA feedback system.

Plasma cortisol levels are drawn at various times throughout the day and evening to determine whether the normal diurnal pattern of a rise in the early morning (peaking between 8 and 9 AM to 7 to 25 mcg/dL) and a fall in the evening (less than 10 mcg/dL) to almost undetectable levels near midnight is evident. Levels lower than expected suggest some form of adrenal insufficiency. Cortisol levels of less than 5 mcg/dL between 8 and 9 AM are considered diagnostic. Care providers should be familiar with the sleep patterns of the patient because the expected diurnal pattern changes when the person habitually works throughout the night and sleeps in the daytime.

It is important to note that although basal cortisol and ACTH levels may be helpful, definitive stimulation testing is required to confirm a diagnosis of adrenal insufficiency. Cortisol samples are drawn at baseline and again 45 minutes after an intramuscular injection of cosyntropin. A diagnosis of adrenal insufficiency is likely if levels fail to rise at least 10 mcg/dL. Plasma

ACTH levels are higher than normal with primary adrenal insufficiency.

Dexamethasone testing serves as an initial screening method for hypercortisolism. Plasma cortisol levels are measured the morning following a midnight oral dose of dexamethasone. Normally, plasma cortisol levels are less than 5 mg/dL. Further definitive testing for Cushing's syndrome is required if plasma levels are higher than 5 mg/dL.

Patients receiving glucocorticoids for the antiinflammatory or immunosuppressive properties no longer exhibit the normal diurnal pattern of cortisol secretion. Thus, serum cortisol levels are not helpful in estimating the therapeutic benefits of synthetic steroids in suppressing inflammatory reactions.

Bone density studies reveal the amount of bony matrix loss for patients receiving long-term therapeutic glucocorticoid therapy. Upper and lower GI imaging aids in the assessment for potential ulcerations in the mucosal lining caused by glucocorticoid drugs.

GOALS OF THERAPY

The treatment goal for the patient with adrenal insufficiency is to reduce signs and symptoms to a tolerable level. Reasonable goals for drug therapy should be set in collaboration with the patient.

Adrenal insufficiency, whether caused by Addison's disease, surgical removal of the adrenal glands (adrenalectomy), or inadequate corticotropin-releasing hormone secretion, requires replacement of both glucocorticoids and mineralocorticoids. Hydrocortisone and cortisone are usually the drugs of choice because they have greater mineralocorticoid activity compared with other glucocorticoids. If additional mineralocorticoid activity is required, fludrocortisone is most convenient because it can be given by mouth.

Treatment of secondary adrenal insufficiency includes the administration of either the hypothalamic-releasing factor (i.e., CRH) or pituitary-stimulating hormone (i.e., ACTH) that signal the release of adrenal hormones. However, drugs for hypothalamic and pituitary hormones are expensive and must be administered parenterally.

Antiinflammatory and immunosuppressive therapy is aimed at maintaining the lowest glucocorticoid dosage possible without the recurrence of symptoms of the original disorder.

INTERVENTION

Update immunizations before the start of therapy of glucocorticoid therapy if possible. Instruct the patient to avoid immunizations during therapy and for at least 3 months after therapy and to check with the health care provider if they have questions. Instruct the patient to avoid contact with anyone who has received oral polio vaccine recently or to wear a mask that covers the nose and mouth if contact is unavoidable.

Administration

Adverse drug reactions are lessened when the dosage of glucocorticoid is at the lowest level possible. Giving the drug early in the morning or using an alternate-day therapy (ADT) regimen is helpful in minimizing adverse effects.

When used for adrenal insufficiency, glucocorticoids are administered orally twice daily—in the early morning and late afternoon—to simulate natural glucocorticoid diurnal rhythms. Ideally, the drug is taken between 6 and 9 AM with the second dose given between 4 and 6 PM. Patients who routinely work during the night may need to make scheduling adjustments.

There are several different schedules that can be used for administering glucocorticoids for acute disorders (Table 57-5). Acute disorders requiring systemic glucocorticoids respond best to large amounts of the drug given in divided daily doses, usually over 4 to 10 days.

Once the desired response is achieved or the acute situation resolved, the daily dosage is tapered.

For patients requiring long-term corticosteroid therapy, ADT is the preferred choice of therapy. Only short-acting glucocorticoids (e.g., prednisone, prednisolone, methylprednisolone) are used. ADT lessens HPA-axis suppression. Surprisingly, higher dosages of glucocorticoids given on alternate days leads to fewer adverse effects than lower dosages given daily.

When a glucocorticoid is injected into a joint or soft tissue, the patient is advised to limit activities involving the injected joint or tissue for 1 to several days. Limiting activities may be somewhat difficult for the patient because, after injection, the affected area begins to feel better and the patient is tempted to return to his or her regular activities, causing additional stress on the tissue or joint. Too much use too soon may stress the joint.

Use care in moving and positioning immobilized patients receiving long-term therapy to prevent fractures and bruising. Pad the side rails as appropriate. Avoid using adhesive tape on fragile skin.

TABLE 57-5

Examples of Burst Schedules

Example 1: Hydrocortisone Therapy (used when short-term, high-dose therapy is needed, followed by tapering and discontinuance)

	Day 1 SUN	Day 2 MON	Day 3 TUES	Day 4 WED	Day 5 THURS	Day 6 FRI	Day 7 SAT
Morning	40 mg	40 mg	40 mg	40 mg	40 mg	20 mg	None
Noon	40 mg	20 mg	None	None	None	None	None
Evening	40 mg	40 mg	40 mg	20 mg	None	None	None

Example 2: Prednisone Taper (used when short-term, high-dose therapy is needed, followed by tapering and discontinuance)

	Day 1	Day 2	Day 3	Day 4	Day 5	Day 6	Day 7
Morning	50 mg	50 mg	40 mg	40 mg	40 mg	30 mg	30 mg

	Day 8	Day 9	Day 10	Day 11	Day 12	Day 13	Day 14
Morning	30 mg	20 mg	20 mg	10 mg	10 mg	10 mg	10 mg

Example 3: Methylprednisolone Therapy (used when changing to alternate-day therapy)

	Day 1 SUN	Day 2 MON	Day 3 TUES	Day 4 WED	Day 5 THURS	Day 6 FRI	Day 7 SAT
Morning	32 mg	32 mg	32 mg	16 mg	16 mg	16 mg	16 mg
Evening	32 mg	32 mg	32 mg	16 mg	16 mg	16 mg	None

	Day 8 SUN	Day 9 MON	Day 10 TUES	Day 11 WED	Day 12 THURS	Day 13 FRI	Day 14 SAT
Morning	16 mg	16 mg	8 mg	8 mg	8 mg	None	8 mg
Evening	None	None	None	None	None	None	None

	Day 15 SUN	Day 16 MON	Day 17 TUES	Day 18 WED	Day 19 THURS	Day 20 FRI	Day 21 SAT
Morning	None	8 mg	None	8 mg	None	8 mg	None
Evening	None	None	None	None	None	None	None

Education

Educational needs are extensive for the patient taking glucocorticoids. Patients must be taught that hormone replacement is lifelong. In addition, a diagnosis of adrenal insufficiency requires significant participation by the patient in the treatment plan. By identifying potential emotional and environmental stressors and discussing possible interventions, the health care provider helps alleviate the anxiety surrounding chronic illness and minimizes crises.

Review the anticipated benefits and possible adverse effects of drug therapy. With short-term use (7 to 10 days, or less), adverse effects may be minimal, if noticeable. With long-term use, some adverse effects usually develop. Instruct the patient to report any new adverse reactions.

Instruct the patient to take oral doses of glucocorticoids with meals or a snack to lessen gastric irritation. Some health care providers prescribe antacids or other drugs prophylactically to lessen the risk of ulceration. Instruct the patient to avoid alcoholic beverages while taking this drug because the combination contributes to increased stomach irritation.

For missed doses, when the dosage regimen is once every other day, the patient should take the missed dose as soon as remembered, if remembered on the day it was to be taken. If not remembered until the next day, the patient should take the dose, then readjust the dosage schedule to be every other day from the day the most recent dose was taken. Instruct the patient to not double up for missed doses.

For missed doses, when the dose is taken once a day, the patient should take the missed dose as soon as remembered unless not remembered until the next day. In that case, the patient should omit the missed dose and resume the regular dosing schedule. Instruct the patient not to double up for missed doses.

For missed doses, when the drug is taken more than once a day, the patient should take the missed dose as soon as remembered. If not remembered until the next dose is due, the patient should take both doses at that time and resume the regular dosing schedule.

Warn patients receiving long-term therapy to take doses every day as ordered, even if they are sick. Failure to take ordered doses, even for a few days, may result in adrenocortical insufficiency in susceptible patients. Remind the patient not to discontinue long-term steroid therapy without consulting the health care provider; tapering the dosage may be necessary. Also warn the patient not to increase or decrease the dosage without consulting the health care provider. Remind the patient to inform all health care providers of all drugs being used and not to take any drugs unless approved by the health care provider. Advise the patient not to share drugs with others and to keep all drugs out of the reach of children.

If weight gain associated with glucocorticoids is excessive, advise the patient about weight reduction diets; consult the health care provider about a possible change in glucocorticoid or dose. Other dietary modifications may include decreasing sodium intake and increasing potassium intake.

Instruct the patient to notify the health care provider if any of the following develop: blood in stool; black, tarry stools; mood changes, depression, or insomnia; changes in vision, headache, or weight gain in excess of 2 pounds per day or 5 pounds per week; menstrual irregularities; irregular heartbeat; excessive fatigue; severe or persistent stomach or abdominal pain; or any serious injury or infection. Instruct the patient to avoid rough activities to prevent the skin from becoming easily bruised. Warn patients who have diabetes to monitor blood glucose levels carefully because glucocorticoids increase blood glucose levels; a change in diet or insulin may be necessary.

Patients should be instructed to avoid becoming fatigued, even if steroid therapy has resulted in increased energy levels. A normal exercise regimen is required to prevent excessive muscle wasting and to help maintain bone mass; however, it should be interspersed with adequate rest periods.

Large doses of glucocorticoids increase susceptibility to infection and mask the symptoms of infection. Warn the patient about this adverse effect. Instruct the patient to notify the physician of fever, cough, sore throat, malaise, and injuries that do not heal. Instruct the patient to avoid contact with individuals with active infections. Treatment for even minor infections should be initiated quickly. Instruct the patient to avoid skin testing, unless approved by the health care provider, and to avoid contact with anyone who has measles or chicken pox.

Patients should be taught that when drug levels are maintained at near-normal physiologic levels, no dietary alterations are necessary. Dietary sodium intake should remain constant after the requirements for mineralocorticoid replacement have been determined. However, should drug dosages exceed physiologic levels, patients may need to limit foods high in sodium to prevent fluid retention, edema, and hypertension. A shift of sodium intake in either direction may require a concomitant change in the dosage of mineralocorticoid replacement. Abrupt decreases in sodium intake can precipitate an adrenal crisis. In climates where there is great variation in temperatures, mineralocorticoid dosage may need to be adjusted.

Menstrual difficulties may develop with long-term therapy. Instruct women to keep a record of menstrual periods. Counsel about contraceptive methods as appropriate. Warn the patient to notify the physician if pregnancy is suspected.

Encourage the patient receiving long-term therapy to wear a medical identification tag or bracelet indicating that glucocorticoids are being used.

EVALUATION

With adequate treatment, blood pressure and other vital signs stabilize; fluid, electrolyte, and blood glucose levels of the patient with adrenal insufficiency return to normal; appetite and physical strength improve; and weight is regained. Additionally, the patient has minimal to no signs and symptoms of overtreatment.

Patients should have adequate knowledge about the disease, appropriate treatment plans, the potential for complications, and when to contact the health care provider. Finally, the patient should be aware of the potential need to make dosage adjustments in drug therapy.

CASE STUDY — *Adrenal Insufficiency*

ASSESSMENT

HISTORY OF PRESENT ILLNESS

PK is a 4-year-old boy accompanied to the clinic by his parents. PK has been well and developing normally until approximately 1 week ago. He is complaining of stomachache, muscle weakness, diarrhea, irritability, and is unable to keep up with his 5-year-old brother in play. He also complains of headache, and his mother states that he is frequently sweaty. He has not been eating well for several weeks, and his mother believes he has lost weight. For the past week, PK frequently asks to lie down and refuses to play with his brother. The parents have seen no evidence of seizure activity.

HEALTH HISTORY

Other than insignificant acute illnesses, PK has been seen only for regularly scheduled well-child examinations. He has no known allergies to drugs, foods, or environmental elements. Family history is noncontributory.

LIFESPAN CONSIDERATIONS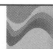

PK is more susceptible to HPA-axis suppression and decreased secretion of growth hormone with treatment. The lowest possible dosage of glucocorticosteroid will need to be used in an attempt to maintain PK's growth within the 50th percentile of children his age.

CULTURAL/SOCIAL CONSIDERATIONS

Because PK is not yet in school and stays at home with his mother during the day, adapting his schedule to allow for his increased appetite, nutritional needs, needs for rest, and administration of drugs is not problematic. PK and his 5-year-old brother live with both parents in a middle-class neighborhood. The father works full-time, and the mother is able to stay home with the boys. All family members are covered by an HMO through the father's employment. All prescription drugs are $5.00 per prescription, regardless of the drug cost.

PHYSICAL EXAMINATION

PK is irritable but cooperates with the examination. Vital signs are within normal limits except blood pressure, which is slightly lower than expected for his age. Weight is down 2 pounds since his last visit 2 months ago. Pupils are equal, round, and reactive to light and accommodation. Skin is smooth, warm, pale, and moist with elastic turgor and with no evidence of infection or purpura. Lungs are clear to auscultation. Heart rate and rhythm are regular, without murmurs. Abdomen is slightly distended and tender to deep palpation in all four quadrants. No nuchal rigidity elicited. Gait is symmetric and equal.

LABORATORY TESTING

Serum sodium 134 mEq/L; serum potassium 5.0 mEq/L; serum calcium 12 mg/dL; BUN, 19 mg/dL; fasting blood glucose 62 mg/dL. CBC count shows moderate neutropenia, lymphocytosis, and hemoconcentration.

PATIENT PROBLEM(S)

Adrenal insufficiency.

GOALS OF THERAPY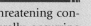

Replace adrenal hormones to prevent life-threatening consequences associated with the lack of naturally occurring corticosteroids.

CRITICAL THINKING QUESTIONS

1. The health care provider orders prednisone and fludrocortisone. What is the mechanism of action of these drugs?
2. What is the advantage of using alternate-day therapy (ADT) with systemic glucocorticoids?
3. What are the early and late adverse effects of long-term prednisone administration?
4. What is the primary goal of glucocorticoid therapy for PK?
5. Considering the natural diurnal release of adrenal hormones, at what times should the prednisone be given?
6. What safety instructions should be provided to PK's parents?

Bibliography

Bello CE, Garrett SD: Therapeutic issues in oral glucocorticoid use, *Lippincott's Prim Care Pract* 3(3):333-344, 1999.

Brenner ZR, Cannito M: Administering steroids successfully, *Nurs 1998* 28(3):34-38, 1998.

Chaffman MO: Topical corticosteroids: a review of properties and principles in therapeutic use, *Nurse Pract Forum* 10(2):95-105, 1999.

Segatore M: Corticosteroids and traumatic brain injury: status at the end of the decade of the brain, *J Neurosci Nurs* 31(4):239-250, 1999.

Internet Resources

http://www.aafp.org/afp/980800ap/zoorob.html.
http://www.corticosteroid.com/.
http://www.healthwell.com/healthnotes/Drug/Corticosteroids.cfm.
http://www.hon.ch/Library/Theme/Allergy/Glossary/corticosteroid.html.
http://www.njc.org/medfacts/corticosteroids.html.
http://www.nlm.nih.gov/medlineplus/druginfo/corticosteroidsglucocorticoide202018.html.

Drugs to Treat Diabetes Mellitus

JOSEPH A. DiMICCO • KATHLEEN GUTIERREZ

 Visit http://evolve.elsevier.com/Gutierrez/ for additional information.

KEY TERMS

Beta (B) cells, p. 959

Diabetes mellitus, p. 956

Gestational diabetes mellitus (GDM), p. 957

Glucagon, p. 959

Glucosuria, p. 957

Hyperglycemia, p. 959

Hypoglycemia, p. 959

Impaired fasting glucose, p. 957

Impaired glucose tolerance, p. 957

Insulin, p. 959

Ketoacidosis, p. 957

Lipoatrophy, p. 963

Nephropathy, p. 958

Neuropathy, p. 958

Polydipsia, p. 957

Polyphagia, p. 957

Polyuria, p. 957

Retinopathy, p. 958

Type 1 diabetes mellitus, p. 956

Type 2 diabetes mellitus, p. 956

OBJECTIVES

- Identify the five types of diabetes mellitus.
- Discuss the differences among type 1 diabetes, type 2 diabetes, and gestational diabetes.
- Explain the advantages of the different forms of insulin.
- Explain the mechanisms of action and uses of different classes of oral antidiabetic drugs.
- Develop a nursing care plan for a patient with diabetes mellitus.
- Develop a teaching plan for a patient with diabetes mellitus.

PATHOPHYSIOLOGY • Diabetes Mellitus

There are five distinct types of **diabetes mellitus** based on the classification system developed by the National Diabetes Data Group (NDDG) and the World Health Organization (WHO). They include type 1, type 2, gestational diabetes, impaired glucose tolerance, and others (e.g., impaired fasting glucose, endocrinopathies). Different clinical presentations as well as different genetic and environmental etiologic factors among the five types permit discrimination among them. This heterogeneity has important implications not only for patient treatment but also for biomedical research.

TYPE 1 DIABETES MELLITUS

In diabetes mellitus, insulin action is lost. If all insulin production ceases, the disease is called **type 1 diabetes mellitus;** it has also been called insulin-dependent diabetes mellitus or juvenile-onset diabetes and, as the name implies, it primarily affects the young. This form of diabetes accounts for only about 8% of all diabetes mellitus cases in the United States. Type 1 diabetes encompasses the vast majority of cases that are primarily ascribable to an autoimmune process and those for which a cause is unknown. It does not include forms of beta cell destruction or failure for which a non–

autoimmune-specific cause can be assigned (e.g., cystic fibrosis). Most type 1 diabetes is characterized by the presence of islet cell, GAD, IA-2, IA-2 beta, or insulin autoantibodies that identify the autoimmune process leading to beta cell destruction. At least one, though usually more, of these autoantibodies is present in 85% to 90% of patients when fasting hyperglycemia is initially detected. The disease has strong human lymphocytic antigen (HLA) associations; it is linked to DQA and B genes and influenced by the DRB genes. These HLA-DR/DQ alleles can be either predisposing or protective. However, in some patients, no evidence of autoimmunity is present. These cases are classified as type 1 idiopathic (see Table 58-1 for comparison of type 1 and type 2).

TYPE 2 DIABETES MELLITUS

If insulin production continues but is insufficient to meet the body's demands, the disease is called **type 2 diabetes mellitus,** or adult-onset diabetes. Type 2 diabetes is usually found in persons who are older than 40 years of age or obese. It appears more often in women with prior gestational diabetes (see later in chapter) and persons with hypertension or hyperlipidemia. It is also

---

TABLE 58-1

Comparison of Type 1 and Type 2 Diabetes Mellitus

Feature	Type 1	Type 2
Also known as	Insulin-dependent	Non–insulin-dependent
Etiology	HLA-DR3, HLA-DR4 antigens	Strong genetic predisposition
Incidence rate	10% of diabetic population	85%-90% of diabetic population
Age at onset	Usually under age 30, but may occur at any age	Usually over age 40
Onset of symptoms	Sudden, symptomatic	Insidious, usually asymptomatic
Manifestations	Polyuria, polyphagia, polydipsia, fatigue	Frequently none
Endogenous insulin	Absolute deficit	Relative deficit
Insulin resistance	No	Yes
Insulin receptors	Normal	Defective or decreased
Body weight at diagnosis	Nonobese	Obese in 85% of patients
Prone to ketoacidosis	Yes (DKA)	Usually resistant (HHNS)
Susceptible to infection	Yes	Yes
Poor wound healing	Yes	Yes
Drug management	Yes, insulin	Yes, oral drugs*
Dietary regimen	Yes, essential	Yes, essential
Weight loss program	No, in most cases	Yes, in many cases
Exercise program	Yes	Yes

DKA, Diabetic ketoacidosis; *HHNS,* hyperglycemic, hyperosmolar nonketotic syndrome
*Insulin may be required in 20% to 30% of patients with type 2 diabetes if diet, weight loss, and exercise are ineffective.

more often associated with a strong genetic predisposition than type 1 diabetes. However, the specific role of genetics in type 2 diabetes is complex and not clearly identified. Diabetes in these patients involves insulin resistance; although the insulin concentration in the blood may be normal, the target tissues are unresponsive to insulin. More than 90% of all cases of diabetes mellitus in the United States are type 2.

GESTATIONAL DIABETES

Gestational diabetes mellitus (GDM) is defined as any degree of glucose intolerance with onset or first recognition during pregnancy. The definition applies whether insulin or diet modification only is used for treatment and even if the diagnosis persists after pregnancy. During normal pregnancy, changes in maternal metabolism are brought about by endogenous and placental hormones. These changes permit the steady transport of glucose to the fetus for growth and development but frequently, especially in early pregnancy, these changes can result in a fasting hypoglycemic state. In addition, there is progressive insulin resistance as the pregnancy progresses. This resistance is caused by rising placental hormones and other factors that result in increased blood sugar levels after meals. The pregnant woman who has limited pancreatic reserves and is unable to boost her insulin production to offset this insulin resistance develops GDM. This disorder usually resolves after delivery, but the woman then has a greater risk for developing type 2 diabetes.

IMPAIRED GLUCOSE TOLERANCE/ IMPAIRED FASTING GLUCOSE

Impaired glucose tolerance and impaired fasting glucose refer to a metabolic stage between normal glucose homeostasis and diabetes. Diagnosis of these abnormalities is based on glucose levels. **Impaired glucose tolerance** is defined as fasting glucose levels above 110 mg/dL but below 126 mg/dL. **Impaired fasting glucose** refers to a fasting plasma glucose level above 110 mg/dL but below 140 mg/dL. Although it is recognized that these ranges are somewhat arbitrary, they are near the level above which acute-phase insulin secretion is lost in response to intravenous administration of glucose.

Assigning a type of diabetes to a patient often depends on the circumstances present at the time of diagnosis, and many patients do not easily fit into a single class.

METABOLIC DERANGEMENTS

Significant metabolic derangements occur when insulin action is lost. Without insulin, less glucose is used in muscle and fat cells, and more glucose is released into the circulation by the liver. Muscle cells, starved for energy sources, break down protein and release amino acids into the blood. The liver converts a portion of these amino acids into glucose and returns it to the blood. These processes contribute to the persistently elevated level of glucose in blood. When the glucose level in the blood exceeds about 160 mg/dL, glucose begins to appear in the urine (a condition called **glucosuria**).

The most common early symptoms of diabetes mellitus result directly from osmotic and metabolic changes. Patients often first note a feeling of constant fatigue because energy production in body cells is impaired. Increased frequency of urination (**polyuria**), often first noticed at night, occurs because excess glucose in the urine produces osmotic diuresis (i.e., more water must be excreted to carry out the high concentration of glucose). As urine output increases, most patients develop excessive thirst (**polydipsia**), which results from the body's efforts to maintain normal hydration despite excessive fluid losses through the kidneys. Some patients develop urogenital infections, which are made more likely by the high level of glucose. Hypotension may develop as a result of decreased plasma volume. The alterations in metabolism caused by insulin deficiency and the relative excess of catabolic hormones (catecholamines and steroids) ultimately result in excessive protein and fat breakdown. Protein catabolism and potassium loss from polyuria contribute to complaints of weakness. Starvation resulting from tissue breakdown causes excessive hunger (**polyphagia**). Protein is metabolized to amino acids and then to glucose, whereas fats are converted to free fatty acids and then to ketone bodies that are released into the circulation. These excess breakdown products may cause a patient to become ketotic or acidotic.

Ketoacidosis is a serious, acute complication of diabetes mellitus seen primarily in patients with type 1 diabetes who have little or no endogenous insulin production. These patients are sometimes called ketosis-prone diabetic patients. Patients with type 2 diabetes who produce enough insulin to suppress lipid breakdown are resistant to ketosis but may still experience ketoacidosis, especially if the system is stressed by an infection or a stroke. The symptoms of ketoacidosis include hyperglycemia, osmotic diuresis with fluid depletion, and acidosis (Table 58-2). Ketones are detected in blood. Ketoacidotic coma is associated with mortality rates of 3% to 30%. The mortality rate is highest when treatment is delayed, so the key to survival is early recognition of the signs. Treatment involves controlling hyperglycemia with insulin and treating the fluid and electrolyte imbalances appropriately, often with fluids containing potassium. If the ketoacidosis has been precipitated by an infection, stroke, or heart attack, these underlying conditions must also be controlled to regain control of the diabetes.

TABLE 58-2

Differential Diagnosis of Diabetic Coma and Hypoglycemic Reactions

	Diabetic Ketoacidosis	*Hypoglycemia*
History	Onset of symptoms usually occurs over days	Onset of signs and symptoms related to type of drug used
		Regular insulin overdose producing signs and symptoms more rapidly than longer-acting insulins or oral drugs
Precipitating factors	Untreated diabetes	Insulin overdose
	Infection or disease in patient with previously controlled diabetes	Skipping meals
	High degree of emotional stress	Excessive exercise before meals
Symptoms	Headache	Nervousness
	Thirst	Hunger
	Kussmaul breathing*	Sweating
	Nausea and vomiting	Weakness
	Abdominal pain	Stupor
	Constipation	
Signs	Facial flushing	Pallor
	Air hunger	Shallow respirations
	Soft eyeballs	Normal eyeballs
	Normal or absent reflexes	Babinski's reflex may be present
	Breath that smells like acetone (sweet)	Seizures
Blood glucose level	High (greater than 250 mg/dL)	Low (less than 60 mg/dL)
Blood CO_2	Low	Normal
Urine glucose	Positive	Negative
Urine acetone	Positive	Negative

*Kussmaul breathing is characterized by a very deep, gasping type of respiration.

Any diabetic person may become comatose as a result of dehydration. As the plasma becomes hyperosmolar (i.e., having a higher solute concentration than normal for blood), water is pulled from body tissues, and severe water and electrolyte imbalances occur. Patients in this type of hyperosmolar, hyperglycemia, nonketotic coma tend to be older than 60 years of age and tend to have an even higher mortality rate than patients in ketoacidotic coma.

In addition to the possibility of these acute events, patients with diabetes are at risk for long-term pathologic changes in blood vessels, nerves, and kidneys. Retinal hemorrhages may destroy sight (**retinopathy**).

Other vessels may also be affected, although those changes are not so easily observed early in the disease. At later stages, circulation to the limbs may be impaired. Pathologic changes also occur in the kidneys. First, the glomerular filtration rate is affected; the next change results in glomerulosclerosis, which thickens the capillary basement membranes (**nephropathy**). Nephrotic syndrome with protein loss in urine and frank kidney failure is a late complication of diabetes. Late in the disease, nerve function is impaired, and therefore the patient may lose feeling in his or her limbs or other parts of the body (**neuropathy**). Sexual impotence is common among diabetic men.

PHYSIOLOGY • Regulation of Glucose Metabolism

The pancreas is an exocrine gland that supplies digestive juices to the small intestine. However, within the pancreas lie discrete clusters of cells with different functions from those of most pancreatic cells. These cell clusters, called the islets of Langerhans, contain several types of endocrine cells. Three of these cell types release peptide hormones that affect glucose metabolism. Alpha (A) cells synthesize and release the peptide hormone **glucagon**, beta (B) cells synthesize and release insulin, and D cells synthesize somatostatin.

INSULIN AND GLUCOSE METABOLISM

Insulin is the primary hormone regulating glucose metabolism. Insulin stimulates glucose uptake by the glucose transporter GLUT 4 in fat and muscle cells, and promotes the conversion of glucose to the storage carbohydrate glycogen in liver and muscle cells (Table 58-3). The body seldom relies on a single mechanism to control an important physiologic function. This rule applies to the regulation of glucose levels. Therefore insulin does not work alone, and its metabolic actions must always be considered in relation to the actions of other hormones. For example, an elevated blood glucose level after a meal stimulates insulin release from the pancreas. Blood glucose is thereby reduced because insulin stimulates the uptake and use of glucose for energy in fat and muscle cells as well as the storage of glucose in the liver. However, the blood glucose level should never fall too low because, unlike other tissues of the body, the brain needs a constant and steady supply of glucose to function normally. Therefore, as the blood glucose level falls in response to insulin, glucagon release from A cells of the pancreas is stimulated. Glucagon in many ways directly opposes the action of insulin in glucose metabolism (see Table 58-3). Glucagon stimulates the liver to break down glycogen and amino acids so that glucose is released into the blood. Glucagon also inhibits the uptake of glucose by muscle and fat cells. By balancing the action of these hormones, the body protects itself from high blood glucose (**hyperglycemia**) and low blood glucose (**hypoglycemia**).

Even the concept of metabolic balance achieved with two antagonistic hormones does not adequately describe glucose regulation. For example, the polypeptide hormone somatostatin released from D cells of the pancreas inhibits release of insulin and glucagon from islet cells. Other hormones antagonize the peripheral effects of insulin. Cortisol (an adrenocortical glucocorticoid) and epinephrine (a catecholamine released by the adrenal medulla) concentrations are elevated during times of stress, thus antagonizing the actions of insulin in muscle or fat cells (see Table 58-3). The overall function of cortisol and epinephrine is to increase blood glucose levels.

TABLE 58-3

Metabolic Actions of Insulin and Insulin-Opposing Hormones

Tissue/Metabolic Process	Insulin	Glucagon	Epinephrine	Cortisol	Growth Hormone
Liver					
Glycogen formation	↑	↓	↓	↑	—
Glucose formation from amino acids	↓	↑	—	↑	↓
Glucose formation from glycogen	↓	↑	↑	—	—
Skeletal Muscle					
Glucose uptake or use	↑	↓	↓	↓	↓
Amino acid uptake	↑	—	—	—	↑
Protein synthesis	↑	↓	—	↓	↑
Glucose release from glycogen	↓	↑	↑	—	—
Fat Cells					
Synthesis of storage lipids	↑	↓	↓	↓	↓
Release of free fatty acids from stored lipids	↓	↑	↑	↑	↑
Blood					
Glucose level	↓	↑	↑	↑	↑
Free fatty acid level	↓	↑	↑	↑	↑

↑, Increased effect; ↓, decreased effect; —, minimal effect.

Growth hormone also increases blood glucose primarily by lowering glucose uptake in muscle cells.

ROLE OF INSULIN IN FAT AND PROTEIN METABOLISM

Although insulin is most often considered a regulator of glucose metabolism, it also regulates fat and protein metabolism (see Table 58-3). Insulin directly stimulates synthesis of storage lipid within fat cells, blocks breakdown and release of stored lipids, and promotes protein synthesis by stimulating amino acid uptake and directly stimulating protein synthetic processes.

The action of insulin on fat and protein metabolism is opposed by other hormones (see Table 58-3). For example, epinephrine, glucagon, cortisol, and growth hormone stimulate the breakdown of fat in fat cells, thereby directly opposing the action of insulin in that tissue. Therefore these hormones tend to raise the blood content of free fatty acids and other breakdown products of lipids. In addition, glucagon and cortisol block protein synthesis in direct opposition to insulin action. Growth hormone differs from the other insulin-opposing hormones in that growth hormone directly stimulates protein synthesis in many body tissues. An understanding of this delicate balance of hormonal actions is important to appreciate the origin of some of the metabolic derangements that occur with diabetes mellitus.

REGULATION OF INSULIN SECRETION

The B cells of the pancreas must respond to the changing level of glucose in the blood and release insulin when needed (and in the amount needed) to handle the glucose load. The primary glucose sensor is a glucose transporter called GLUT 2. The GLUT 2 transporter has a higher threshold than other glucose transporters in the body, which means that a relatively high level of glucose is needed before this transporter operates. Such a level is expected after meals.

When the GLUT 2 transporter begins to operate, glucose enters the B cell of the pancreas and is metabolized to generate energy in the form of adenosine triphosphate (ATP). This chemical causes a potassium channel in the cell membrane to close. This closing of the potassium channel leads to depolarization of the cell, which alters the membrane permeability to several ions. The crucial change that triggers insulin release is the opening of a calcium channel, which raises the level of calcium in the B cell. It is this increase in calcium that finally causes release of insulin from the cell into the bloodstream. The pancreas stores the equivalent of about 200 units of insulin ready for release on demand.

In addition to stimulating release of stored insulin, glucose stimulates synthesis of new insulin. Insulin naturally complexes with other molecules of insulin in clusters of six (called hexamers) in the presence of zinc; it is thought to be stored in B cells in this form. Once these clusters are secreted and the local concentration of insulin falls, the hexamers break apart for insulin to circulate and act as individual molecules, or monomers.

DRUG CLASS • Insulin and Insulin Analogs*

Ultra-Short-Acting Insulin
insulin aspart (Novolog)

insulin lispro (Humalog)

Short-Acting Insulin
buffered insulin human (Vesulosin)

insulin human (Humulin R, Novolin R)

regular insulin, pork (Regular Iletin II, Regular Insulin)

Intermediate-Acting Insulin
isophane insulin suspension (NPH insulin), pork (NPH Iletin II, NPH Purified Insulin)

isophane insulin, human (Humulin N, Novolin N)

Insulin zinc suspension, pork (Lente, Lente Iletin II)

insulin zinc suspension, human (Humulin L, Novolin L)

Long-Acting Insulin
extended insulin human zinc suspension (Humulin U)

insulin glargine (Lantus)

Combination Insulins
insulin human 50% + Isophane insulin, human 50% (Humulin 50/50)

insulin human 70% + Isophane insulin, human 30% (Humulin 70/30, Novolin 70/30)

MECHANISM OF ACTION
As described above, insulin is a naturally occurring hormone that acts by binding to its own unique receptors to regulate a host of processes that together regulate glucose levels and relevant aspects of metabolism. Two types of

*Additional preparations are available in Canada.

insulin are available in the United States: human and pork. Human insulin has become the standard and comes from two sources. Semisynthetic human insulin is prepared by converting pork insulin to the human form by chemically changing the one differing amino acid. Human insulin is also made by recombinant DNA techniques; human genes for insulin are inserted into bacteria, which then produce large amounts of the protein to be processed and purified. Insulin and insulin analogs (aspart, lispro, and glargine), which differ from human insulin by only one or a few amino acids, are thought to act in exactly the same way and produce similar effects.

Pork insulin is obtained from the pancreas of pigs slaughtered for food. (Beef insulin has been used in the past and is still used in Canada but is no longer available in the United States.) Preparations of pork insulin may also contain proinsulin as a contaminant. However, the pork insulin preparations in use today are usually highly purified and thus contain much less proinsulin. The key difference among all these products is not how they act or what effects they produce, but the differences in their onset and duration of action (see Pharmacokinetics).

USES

Insulin is used primarily for the treatment of type 1 diabetes mellitus, the condition in which B cell function is lost and insulin production is very low or absent. Insulin may also be used in cases of type 2 diabetes mellitus that cannot be controlled by diet or oral hypoglycemic drugs (discussed later).

PHARMACOKINETICS

Insulin must be used by injection because it is a protein and therefore would be destroyed in the GI tract. Any of the available insulin preparations can be given subcutaneously, and this is the usual route of administration; only regular insulin can be given intravenously. A recent advance that has been successfully employed in selected patients is the use of subcutaneous infusion pumps to deliver insulin by constant or variable infusion. Other routes of delivery (e.g., inhalation) are currently under investigation but have so far proven impractical.

Insulin is available in ultra-short-acting, short-acting, intermediate-acting, and long-acting preparations (Table 58-4). These differences result from differences in the rates of absorption. The rate of absorption is determined primarily by the type of insulin but is also affected by the site and volume of injection as well as other factors. In its natural form insulin is rapidly absorbed from subcutaneous administration sites and, once in the bloodstream, has a half-life of only 5 to 6 minutes. Insulin biotransformation takes place primarily in the liver (about 50%) and secondarily in the kidneys (25%), muscles, and other tissues.

The ultra-short-acting insulins lispro and aspart are slightly modified from regular insulin so that they do not readily form hexamers (see earlier in the chapter). Because of this they are more rapidly absorbed and have the most rapid action; onset of action occurs in only 15 minutes and peak effect is reached in 30 to 90 minutes. Thus these analogs can provoke hypoglycemia very rapidly if

---

TABLE 58-4

Pharmacokinetics of Different Insulin Preparations after Subcutaneous Injection

Type	Onset	Peak	Duration
Ultra-Short-Acting			
Insulin lispro	15 min	30-90 min	2-4 hr
Insulin aspart			
Short-Acting			
Regular insulin	30-60 min	2-4 hr	5-7 hr
Insulin human			
Intermediate-Acting			
Isophane insulin	2-4 hr	6-12 hr	18-28 hr
Insulin zinc suspension			
Long-Acting			
Extended insulin human zinc suspension	4-6 hr	18-24 hr*	36 hr
Insulin glargine			
Combination Insulins			
Pre-mixed combination: 70/30 regular/isophane	30 min	4-8 hr	24 hr

*NOTE: No clear peak evident for insulin glargine because of constant and slow rate of absorption.

adequate calories are not consumed immediately after the injection. These drugs are available as clear solutions; they are never used alone but always employed in combination with the longer-acting insulin preparations discussed below.

Short-acting insulin preparations are clear solutions of crystalline zinc insulin—the so-called regular insulin, similar to the form in which it is stored in the B cell. The effect of these preparations begins about 30 minutes after subcutaneous injection, peaks in 2 to 4 hours, and lasts 6 to 8 hours. Regular insulin, which may be human or pork, is the only insulin preparation that may also be administered intravenously. When given in this manner, insulin produces a rapid fall in blood glucose levels to a nadir in 20 to 30 minutes. In the absence of a sustained intravenous infusion, insulin is rapidly cleared and the glucose level returns to baseline in about 2 to 3 hours.

Intermediate- and long-acting insulins are cloudy suspensions, formulated to dissolve more slowly when administered subcutaneously. They are modified by adding protamine (a large, insoluble protein), zinc, or both to slow absorption and prolong drug action. Intermediate-acting insulins have similar pharmacokinetic profiles. The effects appear within 1 to 2 hours, peak in 6 to 12 hours, and last for 18 to 28 hours.

The long-acting insulin preparation (formerly called Ultralente when available as an animal product) is a zinc suspension with onset in 4 to 6 hours, peak effect in 16 to 24 hours, and duration of action of 18 to 36 hours. The half-life of long-acting insulins makes it difficult to determine the optimal dosage, because several days of treatment are required before a steady-state concentration of circulating insulin is achieved. Insulin glargine is an analog of insulin that forms very stable hexameric complexes. As a result, insulin glargine is absorbed very slowly without the initial peak typical of other insulin preparations. Because of this lack of a peak, insulin glargine is less likely to cause hypoglycemia; otherwise, its pharmacokinetic profile is similar to the long-acting insulin preparation.

Pork and human insulins differ slightly in their pharmacokinetics. For example, human insulin preparations have a slightly shorter duration of action than corresponding pork insulin preparations. Dosages may require slight adjustment when switching from one preparation to another.

ADVERSE REACTIONS AND CONTRAINDICATIONS

Insulin therapy is associated with two important acute adverse effects. If insulin activity is inadequate, the person may go into a coma as a result of uncontrolled metabolic derangements; blood glucose concentration will be high, and diabetic ketoacidosis (DKA) or hyper-osmolar coma may result. If insulin overdosage occurs or if a patient does not eat or exercises excessively, the patient may lapse into coma resulting from hypoglycemia. It is critical for health care professionals to be able to differentiate between these conditions. The distinguishing symptoms are outlined in Table 58-2.

Hypoglycemia is a more likely adverse effect of insulin when strict glucose control is attempted. Strict control is usually not attempted with children, because hypoglycemia has the potential to damage developing brains. Strict control is also contraindicated for older adults and patients with severe renal disease because hypoglycemia places these patients at greater risk.

Conscious patients receive an orally administered form of glucose to treat hypoglycemia, whereas unconscious patients are given either a glucagon injection or glucose intravenous infusion (see later in the chapter). Treatment of diabetic coma requires administration of insulin to lower blood glucose concentration.

Many patients receiving insulin therapy have insulin antibodies in their blood. These antibodies may contribute to insulin resistance in some patients. Human

---

TABLE 58-5

Drugs Influencing Blood Glucose Level

Drugs Elevating Blood Glucose Levels

allopurinol	adrenocorticotropin hormone (ACTH)
Amphetamines	
Beta blockers	asparaginase
caffeine (in large quantities)	Carbonic anhydrase inhibitors
cyclophosphamide	Calcium-channel blockers
diazoxide	Decongestants
Estrogens	epinephrine
glucagon	furosemide
Glucocorticosteroids	Glucose gel/tablets
lithium	Growth hormone
morphine	Marijuana
nicotinic acid	Nicotine (cigarette smoking)
phenytoin	Oral contraceptives
Thiazide diuretics	pentamidine
	Thyroid hormones

Drugs Decreasing Blood Glucose Levels

Alcohol	allopurinol*
Anabolic steroids	Beta blockers
clofibrate*	chloramphenicol*
fenfluramine	guanethidine
Histamine-2 antagonists	insulin
isoniazid	Monoamine oxidase inhibitors
Oral anticoagulants*	Oxyphenbutazone*
oxytetracycline	pentamidine
phenylbutazone*	probenecid
Salicylates*	Sulfonamides*

*Interaction with sulfonylurea drugs only.

insulin and purified pork insulin are less antigenic than unpurified pork insulin. Patients treated with unpurified pork insulin may be switched to one of these forms to help control allergic reactions associated with insulin therapy.

Insulin may also provoke the atrophy of subcutaneous fat near injection sites. This lipoatrophy leads to the formation of hollows (depressions in the skin). Careful rotation of injection sites minimizes this effect. Lipoatrophy is less common with the highly purified insulin preparations.

TOXICITY

Insulin overdose produces hypoglycemia that in severe cases results in convulsions or coma. The very young and older adults are especially at risk for developing this condition.

INTERACTIONS

Alcohol tends to enhance the hypoglycemic action of insulin. Thus the risk of hypoglycemic reactions may be greater but is usually minimal unless alcohol is consumed in a moderate to high amount and without food.

Beta-adrenergic drugs or corticosteroids may antagonize some of the actions of insulin (Table 58-5) such that insulin dosages may require adjustment either up or down. Beta blockers may cause additional problems by masking the warning signs of acute hypoglycemia.

DRUG CLASS • Sulfonylureas and Related Drugs

First-Generation Sulfonylureas

   acetohexamide (Dymelor, Dimelor)

   chlorpropamide (Diabinase)

   tolazamide (Tolinase)

   tolbutamide (Orinase, Mobenol)

Second-Generation Sulfonylureas

   gliclazide (Diamicron✢)

   glimepiride (Amaryl)

   glipizide (Glucotrol)

   glyburide (Micronase, Diabeta, Euglucon, Glynase)

Sulfonylurea-like Drugs

   nateglinide (Starlix)

   repaglinide (Prandin)

MECHANISM OF ACTION

Sulfonylureas and related drugs act by blocking the ATP-sensitive potassium channel in the membranes of B cells. This action depolarizes the cell and stimulates release of insulin. The second-generation sulfonylureas and repaglinide are many times more potent than first-generation sulfonylureas. For example, 5 mg of glyburide or glipizide has an effect equivalent to that of 250 mg of chlorpropamide or tolazamide. At the dosages given to patients, clinical effects are similar. Drugs in this class are commonly referred to as oral hypoglycemics and have the potential to cause the blood glucose level to fall below normal (see Adverse Reactions and Contraindications).

USES

These drugs are useful only for patients who produce some insulin on their own (i.e., patients with type 2 diabetes mellitus) and are usually employed therapeutically in combination with diet and exercise. Clinical studies of patients with type 2 diabetes mellitus have shown that many have normal or even above-normal insulin levels. However, the cells of these patients are resistant to the action of insulin. Therefore insulin action is lost not because insulin is missing but rather because target cells fail to respond normally. Sulfonylureas also may diminish hepatic glucose production and may directly increase tissue responsiveness to insulin. These actions tend to diminish fasting plasma glucose concentrations and improve glucose use by fat and muscle cells. The effectiveness of sulfonylureas in obese patients with type 2 diabetes mellitus is enhanced by caloric restriction and weight loss. This dietary manipulation also tends to increase the responsiveness of target cells to insulin.

Repaglinide and nateglinide have relatively short durations of action (see later in the chapter) and are therefore useful in reducing hyperglycemia at mealtimes without the prolonged action that may lead to hypoglycemia later. They are usually taken 1 to 30 minutes before eating.

PHARMACOKINETICS

Sulfonylureas and related drugs are well absorbed when given orally, although food may delay absorption of some of the drugs. These drugs bind extensively to serum proteins. The sulfonylureas differ from one another primarily in onset and duration of action (Table 58-6), which is strongly influenced by their hepatic biotransformation. For example, tolbutamide is relatively short-acting

| TABLE 58-6 |

Pharmacokinetics of Sulfonylureas and Related Drugs

Generic Name	Brand Name	Time to Peak Effect	Duration of Action
First-Generation Sulfonylureas			
acetohexamide	Dymelor, Dimelor ✲	2-6 hr	8-24 hr
chlorpropamide	Diabinase, Apo-Chlorpropamide ✲	2-4 hr	24-72 hr
tolazamide	Tolinase	3-4 hr	12-24 hr
tolbutamide	Orinase, Apo-Tolbutamide, ✲ Mobenol	3-4 hr	6-12 hr
Second-Generation Sulfonylureas			
gliclazide	Diamicron	4-6 hr	24 hr
glimepiride	Amaryl	2-3 hr	24 hr
glipizide	Glucotrol	1-3 hr (extended release: 6-12 hr)	12-24 hr
glyburide	Micronase, Diabeta, Euglucon, Glynase, Apo-Glyburide ✲	2-5 hr	16-24 hr
Related Drugs			
nateglinide	Starlix	1 hr	4 hr
repaglinide	Prandin	1 hr	4 hr

because it is quickly converted to an inactive product. In contrast, acetohexamide and tolazamide must be converted to active products before they become effective. Hence they are intermediate in action onset. Chlorpropamide, the longest-acting member of the class, is tightly bound to plasma protein, slowly biotransformed, and excreted in urine.

Glyburide, glipizide, and glimepiride are extensively biotransformed, and they are excreted primarily in urine; a small amount is also excreted in bile. Repaglinide and nateglinide are also extensively biotransformed in the liver, and most of the drug is eliminated in bile; only minor amounts are found in urine.

ADVERSE REACTIONS AND CONTRAINDICATIONS

Hypoglycemia is a common adverse effect with sulfonylureas and other related drugs. It is estimated that about 20% of treated patients will experience hypoglycemia within 6 months. For some of these patients hypoglycemia may occur only at night and cause no noticeable symptoms; for others the symptoms may be more frequent and obvious. Hypoglycemia indicates a need for dosage adjustment or change of medication. Nateglinide, the newest of these drugs, has been reported to produce fewer instances of hypoglycemia than the others, but experience is too limited to determine whether this is indeed the case.

Other adverse reactions to sulfonylureas include GI tract distress, flushing, and neurologic symptoms such as dizziness, drowsiness, or headache. Allergy to the drugs occurs in some patients; skin reactions are the most common sign. The incidence rate of these types of reactions is reported to be less than 5% of patients treated.

Weight gain is another common adverse effect of sulfonylureas, especially if these drugs must be combined with insulin. Gliclazide, glimepiride, and repaglinide may cause less weight gain than other drugs in this class.

Repaglinide and nateglinide cause symptoms similar to upper respiratory infections such as cough, runny nose, sneezing, and sore throat. Bronchitis and shortness of breath may also be observed.

Sulfonylureas and related drugs are never to be given to patients with type 1 diabetes mellitus, patients with type 2 diabetes mellitus who are prone to diabetic ketoacidosis, or pregnant patients. These drugs are also not intended for use during metabolic stress, such as that attending serious acute infections, major surgery, trauma, or severe burns. Insulin therapy is indicated for these conditions.

TOXICITY

Hypoglycemia is a danger with sulfonylureas and may be caused by drug overdose, drug interactions, altered drug biotransformation, or the patient's failing to eat. In some instances coma has been reported. Sulfonylureas should not be used when renal or liver function is inadequate; normal function of those organs is required for biotransformation and elimination of sulfonylureas. Repaglinide and nateglinide should also be used cautiously in patients with hepatic impairment. Older adult patients also occasionally show excessive hypoglycemic reactions to these drugs.

INTERACTIONS

Sulfonylureas can be found in many drug interactions that can have serious consequences for the patient. The major interactions occur with ethyl alcohol, phenylbutazone, sulfonamides, salicylates, phenothiazines, and thiazides.

Patients receiving sulfonylureas should avoid alcoholic beverages. Several interactions between alcohol and sulfonylureas are possible. Some patients receiving sulfonylureas develop a disulfiram-like reaction when they ingest alcohol. The most striking symptoms of this reaction are unpleasant flushing and severe headache. Other patients taking sulfonylureas become hypoglycemic when they ingest alcohol; ethanol acts as a hypoglycemic drug in some people.

Hypoglycemia can result when one of several drugs is given to a patient taking sulfonylureas, most importantly the antiinflammatory drugs phenylbutazone and salicylates and the sulfonamide antibiotics. These three types of drugs are all tightly bound to plasma proteins and may displace sulfonylureas, which also tend to be highly bound to plasma proteins. Thus the blood concentration of free sulfonylurea is elevated. Because the free drug is the active form, the result is an enhancement of the hypoglycemic effect of the sulfonylurea. In addition to this mechanism, phenylbutazone may block excretion of the active metabolite of acetohexamide, an action that also tends to increase hypoglycemia. Sulfonamides may inhibit the metabolic breakdown of tolbutamide and thereby enhance its hypoglycemic action. The hypoglycemic effect of glipizide, glyburide, and tolbutamide is also increased by the antifungal agents fluconazole and miconazole.

Phenothiazines, such as chlorpromazine, may impair the effectiveness of sulfonylureas. Chlorpromazine inhibits the release of insulin from B cells and elevates adrenal production of epinephrine, a hormone that can raise blood glucose levels (see Table 58-5). These actions of chlorpromazine directly antagonize the hypoglycemic action of sulfonylureas.

Thiazide diuretics possess hyperglycemic activity in addition to their diuretic actions; thus they may impair diabetes control with sulfonylureas.

Beta-adrenergic blocking drugs diminish the intensity of the symptoms of hypoglycemia. Thus patients may become profoundly hypoglycemic before they realize it.

DRUG CLASS • Biguanides

metformin (Glucophage, Glucophage XR, Apo-Metformin, Glycon, others)

MECHANISM OF ACTION

Metformin, the only drug in this class currently available, is thought to increase the ability of insulin to bind to peripheral tissues, thus increasing glucose uptake by muscle and other tissues. Metformin is effective only for patients who produce insulin. One advantage of metformin over sulfonylureas is that it almost never causes hypoglycemia when used alone.

USES

Metformin is used only for the treatment of type 2 diabetes mellitus and administered alone or in combination with another oral antidiabetic drug and/or insulin.

PHARMACOKINETICS

Metformin is slowly absorbed after oral doses. Food delays absorption and reduces the total amount of drug absorbed. Bioavailability is generally low. Absorbed drug is not significantly bound to plasma proteins. Metformin is excreted unchanged primarily in urine and has a half-life of 4 to 9 hours.

An extended release preparation of metformin is now available.

ADVERSE REACTIONS AND CONTRAINDICATIONS

The most common adverse reactions to metformin are gastrointestinal, including anorexia, flatulence, metallic taste, nausea, stomach pain, vomiting, or weight loss. Some of these are transient and may be minimized by using small doses initially and increasing the dosage gradually.

Metformin is not sufficient during traumatic disease or injury in a diabetic patient; insulin is usually required. Giving metformin to patients with significant cardiorespiratory insufficiency, heart failure, heart attack, or severe liver or renal disease or to patients who are prone to lactic acidosis should also be avoided. In all of these conditions, the risk of potentially fatal lactic acidosis is increased. For the same reason, administering metformin to patients with renal failure or impairment as well as to those undergoing angiography or pyelography should be avoided, because the contrast medium used in these procedures may increase the risk of lactic acidosis.

TOXICITY

Overdoses of metformin may cause hypoglycemia and fatal lactic acidosis.

INTERACTIONS

Patients taking metformin should avoid alcoholic beverages to prevent excessive risk of hypoglycemia or lactic acidosis. Amiloride, cimetidine, digoxin, morphine, procainamide, quinidine, quinine, ranitidine, triamterene, trimethoprim, and vancomycin may block renal secretion of metformin and increase its plasma level. Furosemide may increase oral absorption of metformin. The result of both types of interaction is increased blood concentration of metformin; dosages of metformin may require reduction.

 DRUG CLASS • Thiazolidinediones

pioglitazone (Actos)

rosiglitazone (Avandia)

MECHANISM OF ACTION

Rosiglitazone and pioglitazone act primarily on target tissues of insulin to decrease insulin resistance. Their mechanism appears to involve activation of insulin responsive genes concerned with lipid and carbohydrate metabolism. They do not stimulate insulin release but instead depend on the presence of insulin to achieve their desired clinical effect.

USES

Rosiglitazone and pioglitazone are indicated only for the treatment of type 2 diabetes mellitus. The drugs may be added to a regimen of diet and exercise to achieve adequate control, and may be used in combination with insulin or a sulfonylurea.

PHARMACOKINETICS

Thiazolidinediones are well absorbed orally, usually within about 2 hours. However, because their mechanism of action involves activating genes and altering protein synthesis, maximal clinical response is not seen for 6 to 12 weeks. The drugs are biotransformed by liver enzymes and should not be used in the presence of significant hepatic disease.

ADVERSE REACTIONS AND CONTRAINDICATIONS

Rosiglitazone and pioglitazone appear not to produce significant hypoglycemia, probably because of their mechanism of action. However, they are known to cause fluid retention and increased plasma volume. Therefore these drugs are contraindicated for patients with moderate to severe heart failure. Dizziness, headache, nausea, weight gain, and generalized weakness have also been noted in a significant number of treated patients. In addition, peripheral edema and jaundice, though rare, have been documented and may signal a dangerous reaction; jaundice could indicate the onset of liver damage. Troglitazone, a related drug, was withdrawn from the market after causing fatal hepatotoxicity and liver failure.

As with all oral antidiabetic drugs, the thiazolidinediones are contraindicated for women during pregnancy.

INTERACTIONS

Ketoconazole is known to interfere with the metabolism of pioglitazone. Practical experience with these drugs is currently too limited to permit a clear picture of other potential drug interactions.

 DRUG CLASS • Alpha-Glucosidase Inhibitors

acarbose (Precose)

miglitol (Glyset)

MECHANISM OF ACTION

Acarbose and miglitol are inhibitors of intestinal enzymes that break complex carbohydrates into smaller molecules such as glucose. Alpha glucosidases are the primary enzymes inhibited. The results of the reversible inhibition of these enzymes include slowed digestion of complex carbohydrates and decreased hyperglycemia after eating.

USES

Use of acarbose or miglitol is indicated for type 2 diabetes mellitus when adequate control cannot be maintained by diet alone. If needed, these drugs may also be combined with a sulfonylurea. They are generally taken at the beginning of meals.

PHARMACOKINETICS

Acarbose is only minimally absorbed from the GI tract; thus it tends to stay at its site of action, the intestinal lumen. Some of the drug is eventually biotransformed and absorbed, but most is eliminated unchanged in the feces.

Miglitol is absorbed after oral dosage and eliminated almost exclusively by the kidneys. There is no significant biotransformation of this drug.

ADVERSE REACTIONS AND CONTRAINDICATIONS

GI adverse effects are the most common reactions to acarbose and miglitol. Symptoms include abdominal pain, diarrhea, and flatulence. Nearly all treated patients report one or more of these symptoms, but for many these diminish with time.

TOXICITY

Acarbose or miglitol overdose should not cause hypoglycemia but should be expected to cause more profound interference with digestive processes, including worsened diarrhea and other GI symptoms.

INTERACTIONS

Corticosteroids and thiazide diuretics may interfere with control of hyperglycemia when administered with acarbose. Intestinal adsorbents such as activated charcoal may interfere with the actions of acarbose or miglitol. Digestive enzyme preparations often contain carbohydrate-splitting enzymes and would thus directly antagonize the effects of both acarbose and miglitol.

Miglitol has a dramatic effect on the pharmacokinetics of propranolol and ranitidine, reducing the bioavailability by 40% to 60%.

 DRUG CLASS • Antihypoglycemic Drugs

dextrose (glucose, Glutose, Insta-glucose)

diazoxide (Proglycem)

glucagon (Glucogen, Glucagon)

octreotide (Sandostatin)

Oral or intravenous dextrose is commonly used in the treatment of hypoglycemia. In low concentrations (2.5% to 11.5%) it provides hydration and calories. Higher concentrations (up to 70%) are used to treat hypoglycemia and, in combination with amino acids, are used for parenteral nutrition. Dextrose is available as an oral gel, chewable tablets, and in solution for injection. It is well absorbed, widely distributed, and rapidly utilized. It is metabolized to carbon dioxide and water. When the renal threshold is exceeded, dextrose is excreted unchanged by the kidneys. The most common adverse effect is local pain and irritation at the intravenous site, but other possible reactions include fluid overload, hypokalemia, hypomagnesemia, and hypophosphatemia.

Diazoxide is a vasodilator that also produces hyperglycemia by interacting with the ATP-sensitive potassium channels on pancreatic B cells to promote their opening. Thus diazoxide acts in a way opposite to that of sulfonylureas—by inhibiting the release of insulin and decreasing peripheral utilization of glucose. It is also used in the management of hyperinsulinism in infants and children. It is not indicated for the treatment of functional hypoglycemia. The most commonly reported adverse effects of diazoxide include a decrease in urine output, resulting in edema of the hands and lower extremities, weight gain, and heart failure in susceptible individuals. Diazoxide is discussed in detail in Chapter 39.

Glucagon is also available in an emergency kit to be used in the acute treatment of severe hypoglycemia, particularly in diabetic patients who have overdosed with insulin and are unconscious. It is useful, though, only if liver glycogen is available for use; thus it is ineffective in chronic hypoglycemic states or starvation and adrenal insufficiency. Glucagon is a peptide hormone secreted by the A cells in response to hypoglycemia. It maintains the plasma glucose level by stimulating hepatic glycogenolysis and gluconeogenesis. Glucagon affects carbohydrate metabolism in a manner opposite that of insulin. It promotes the breakdown of glycogen, reduces glycogen synthesis, and stimulates the biosynthesis of glucose and thus raises plasma glucose levels. Glucagon must be given parenterally and is generally administered by intravenous or intramuscular injection to achieve a rapid effect. Before administration of glucagon, a rapid blood glucose test should be administered to confirm the hypoglycemia.

Octreotide acts like naturally occurring somatostatin to inhibit the release of a range of hormones from a wide range of different types of endocrine cells located throughout the body. Octreotide is used in the treatment of diarrhea associated with endocrine tumors, including carcinoid (a serotonin-secreting tumor) and VIPoma (a tumor secreting vasoactive intestinal polypeptide, or VIP) (see Chapter 49). The drug is also effective in suppressing the secretion of growth hormone from the pituitary. Recently octreotide has been suggested to be useful in the emergency treatment of sulfonylurea-induced hypoglycemia, presumably by suppressing the release of insulin from pancreatic B cells. Octreotide is a peptide analog of somatostatin and has a longer duration of action (up to

12 hours). Because it is a peptide, it must be given by injection. The drug has been reported to cause arrhythmia, bradycardia, acute abdominal pain, and nausea and vomiting. Octreotide may also cause either hyperglycemia or hypoglycemia. The drug should not be given to patients with gallbladder disease or gallstones. Octreotide may interact with insulin as well as any of the antidiabetic or antihypoglycemic drugs to produce marked hyperglycemia or hypoglycemia. Overdose of octreotide may provoke abdominal cramps and decreased heart rate.

APPLICATION TO PRACTICE

ASSESSMENT

When the patient arrives at the office or acute care setting, information about the reason for the visit must be obtained. Inquire about the patient's risk factors for diabetes (Box 58-1). If there is a history of diagnosed diabetes, the patient should be questioned as to the type and how long it has been since the original diagnosis was made. The patient should be asked about specific symptoms and how long they have been present. Subjective information to be sought from the patient includes complaints of fatigue, polyuria, polydipsia, polyphagia, blurry vision, dry or itchy skin, and history of obesity. Information regarding recent stressors, life changes, and any other precipitating factors should also be elicited from the patient. Dietary restrictions, the degree to which self–blood glucose monitoring is done, activity levels, and the extent of patient education regarding diabetes should be ascertained as well. Additionally, the patient should be asked about other drugs taken that may affect blood glucose level (see Table 58-5) and identify risk factors for atherosclerosis, such as cigarette smoking, hypertension, obesity, hyperlipidemia, and a family history of these disorders (see the Case Study: Insulin-Dependent Type 2 Diabetes Mellitus).

The following questions may guide the health care provider in assessing complications of diabetes:

- Does the patient experience intermittent claudication (leg pain) when walking or exercising?
- Has there been a noticeable change in color, temperature, tingling or pain in the extremities?
- Has the patient experienced blurred or double vision, blind spots, or floaters within the field of vision?
- When eating, are there feelings of fullness, followed by bloating and flatus?
- Has there been difficulty voiding?

Health History

Obtaining a complete health history is important when assessing the patient with diabetes. History of major illnesses, childhood illnesses, surgical operations, social habits, and immunizations should be obtained.

Obtaining information about the family history of diabetes, heart disease, and stroke is particularly important. Women should be asked about gestational history, including information about hyperglycemia, delivery of an infant weighing more than 9 pounds, toxemia, stillbirth, polyhydramnios, or other complications of pregnancy. Finally, cigarette smoking, excessive alcohol intake, fatigue, emotional upset, and some OTC drugs may exacerbate hyperglycemia.

The frequency, severity, and cause of acute complications (such as ketoacidosis and hypoglycemia), as well as precipitating factors such as accompanying illness or infection should be included in the history. Prior infections, particularly of the skin, foot, dental, and urogenital tracts, can put the patient at risk for future problems and should therefore be noted. Symptoms and treatment of chronic complications associated with diabetes, such as eye, heart, kidney, nerve, and sexual function, as well as peripheral vascular and cerebrovascular disease, should also be elicited from the patient.

Lifespan Considerations

Perinatal. Gestational diabetes develops in 1% to 3% of pregnant women (Table 58-7). Native Americans and Hispanics show an increased incidence (up to 10%); African Americans are also more prone to GDM than whites. Pregnancy-related morbidity and mortality in patients with diabetes has been significantly reduced over the past decade. However, the mortality risk remains higher in the diabetic population than in the nondiabetic population. Intensive antepartum surveillance of diabetic pregnancies is crucial.

BOX 58-1 | **Risk Factors for Diabetes**

African-American, Asian-American, Hispanic, Native American, or Pacific Islander heritage

Family history of diabetes in a first-degree relative (i.e., parents or siblings)

Gestational diabetes or giving birth to a child weighing more than 9 pounds

History of a fasting blood glucose level of 110 to 125 mg/dL

Hypertension (i.e., blood pressure greater than 140/90 mm Hg)

Truncal obesity; body mass index over 27 kg/m²

Hypertriglyceridemia (over 250 mg/dL) or a low HDL level (less than 40 mg/dL)

Pediatric. Insulin is almost always required with a diagnosis of pediatric diabetes. Insulin dosage can be difficult to regulate in pediatric and adolescent patients because calorie intake, activity levels, and hormonal levels fluctuate significantly. The adolescent who has diabetes must contend with peer pressure, teenage dietary practices, and growth spurts. As a general rule, the earlier the onset of diabetes, the more years there are for complications to develop.

Older Adults. Most older adults have type 2 diabetes associated with age-related impairment of both pancreatic beta cells and insulin action. The older adult is more likely to be overweight and have lower activity levels that lead to insulin resistance. In addition, factors that predispose the older adult to diabetes may exist, including comorbid illnesses and the use of hyperglycemia-inducing drugs.

Cultural/Social Considerations

Although patients with diabetes are not at greater risk for psychologic problems, they are at risk for cultural and social complications from their illness. Women with type 1 diabetes are at higher risk for eating disorders such as anorexia nervosa and bulimia, and patients with long-standing diabetes have an increased risk for depression and anxiety. A diagnosis of diabetes can be very frightening for those who have preconceived ideas about the disease. Compliance may be dependent on the person's ability to make necessary lifestyle changes.

Stress is thought to play a major role in the management of diabetes. Not only does stress cause a change in

---

TABLE 58-7

Criteria for Diagnosis of Gestational Diabetes*

	mg/dL
100-g Glucose Load	
Fasting	95
1 hour	180
2 hours	155
3 hours	140
75-g Glucose Load	
Fasting	95
1 hour	180
2 hours	155

*Two or more of the venous plasma elevations must be met or exceeded for a positive diagnosis. Test should be performed in the morning after an overnight fast between 8 and 14 hours and after at least 3 days of unrestricted diet (>150 g of carbohydrates daily) and unlimited physical activity. The patient should remain seated during testing; smoking and tobacco use should be prohibited, because both can lead to falsely elevated values at 2 hours. Strenuous exercise, in contrast, can lead to falsely decreased values.

---

eating or exercise behaviors, but it also exhibits a physiologic response that directly affects the blood glucose level. For this reason, inquiries about stressful events should be a routine part of a patient's evaluation.

For many people the thought of injections can be overwhelming and frightening. Special consideration may need to be given to those who fear needles. Compliance may be minimal if the patient cannot overcome the fear.

Many people with diabetes find it difficult to comply with recommended meal plans. Because eating is such a social activity, many people lack the support they may need to persist in a regimented manner. Ethnic and cultural variations of meal patterns also influence the treatment plan. Evaluation of the patient's educational level is vital if patient teaching and treatment regimens are to be successful.

Physical Examination

A complete physical examination should be performed with initial or interim evaluations. Because patients with diabetes are at greater risk for eye, kidney, nerve, heart, and vascular complications, a head-to-toe assessment should be performed, in which the examiner looks for manifestations of disease progression and complications.

Clinical manifestations of retinopathy include tortuosity (beading of the retinal blood vessels), pinpoint hemorrhages, or exudates on the retinal surface. Retinopathy may lead to blindness.

Manifestations of neuropathy include decreased sensation, decreased reflexes, and positional blood pressure changes. Neurologic manifestations are assessed by evaluating reflexes, vibratory sense, and response to sharp and dull stimuli. Decreased peripheral circulation manifests as decreased skin temperature and weak posterior tibial or dorsalis pedis pulses. Neuropathy may lead to amputations. Skin turgor should also be assessed to determine the state of dehydration. In children, growth and maturity should be evaluated. Insulin injection sites should also be assessed in the patient with type 1 diabetes.

The presence of fruity odor on the breath may be detected if the patient is experiencing ketoacidosis. The level of consciousness is determined by the patient's orientation and response to stimulation. Vital signs, including blood pressure and weight, should also be noted at each visit.

Laboratory Testing

Blood testing is done to establish a diagnosis of diabetes, determine glycemic control, and determine the extent of associated complications and risk factors. The revised criteria for the diagnosis of diabetes are shown in Box 58-2. All women should be screened for GDM between the twenty-fourth and twenty-eighth week of gestation. If it is suspected that glucose intolerance exists, full diagnostic glucose tolerance testing should be performed (see Figure 58-1). Other laboratory testing for diagnosis

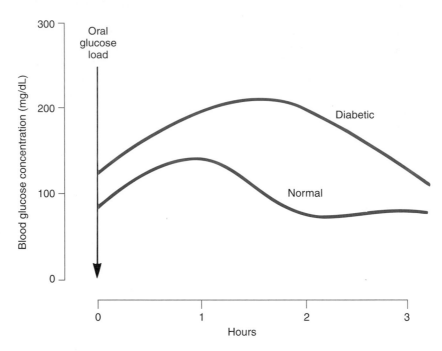

FIGURE 58-1 Typical results of glucose tolerance test for normal and diabetic patients. Test is performed preferably in ambulatory patients in the morning before breakfast. About 75 g of glucose is given orally in solution, and blood is drawn at appropriate intervals (before glucose and 60, 90, 120, and 180 minutes after glucose is administered) and analyzed for glucose concentration.

or monitoring may include electrolytes, blood urea nitrogen (BUN), serum creatinine, microalbuminuria, glycosylated hemoglobin levels, pH, CO_2, and lipid levels.

Connecting peptide (C-peptide) has also been used to diagnose type 1 diabetes. This peptide is formed during the conversion of proinsulin to insulin in B cells. Because C-peptide and insulin are formed in equal amounts, this test indicates the amount of endogenous insulin production. Normally a strong correlation exists between levels of insulin and C-peptide, except possibly in obese persons and in the presence of islet cell tumors. Patients with type 1 diabetes usually have no or low concentrations of C-peptide, whereas patients with type 2 diabetes tend to have normal or elevated levels.

Glycosylated hemoglobin (HbA_{1c}) levels help determine the amount of glycosylated hemoglobin (glycohemoglobin) bound to glucose molecules. The amount of glycosylated hemoglobin found and stored by the red blood cell depends on the amount of glucose available over the cell's 120-day life span. A normal range for nondiabetic persons is 4% to 6%. Values are increased in patients whose diabetes is poorly controlled and those with newly diagnosed diabetes. In these instances, HbA_{1c} levels comprise 8% to 12% of the total hemoglobin. With optimal insulin control, HbA_{1c} levels return toward normal.

The HbA_{1c} test helps to determine the adequacy of dietary or insulin therapy, determines the duration of hyperglycemia in new cases of juvenile-onset diabetes with

---

BOX 58-2 | **Criteria for Diagnosis of Diabetes Mellitus***

1. Symptoms of diabetes plus casual plasma glucose concentration above 200 mg/dL. (Casual is defined as any time of day without regard to time since last meal.)

OR

2. Fasting plasma glucose level above 126 mg/dL. (Fasting is defined as no calorie intake for at least 8 hours.)

OR

3. Result of 2-hour oral glucose tolerance test exceeds 200 mg/dL. (The test should be performed as described by the WHO, using a glucose load containing the equivalent of 75 g anhydrous glucose dissolved in water.)

*In the absence of unequivocal hyperglycemia with acute metabolic decompensation, these criteria should be confirmed by repeat testing on a different day. The third measure is not recommended for routine clinical use. Levels above those identified provide a provisional diagnosis of diabetes. The diagnosis must be confirmed. A fasting plasma glucose level between 110 and 126 mg/dL is considered impaired fasting glucose. The corresponding result for an oral glucose tolerance test between 140 and 200 mg/dL is considered impaired glucose tolerance.

acute ketoacidosis, and provides a sensitive estimate of glucose imbalance in mild cases of diabetes. In addition, it may be used as a mechanism for determining the effectiveness of old and new forms of therapy, such as oral hypoglycemia drugs, single or multiple insulin injections, and B cell transplantation. At the present time it is not used to diagnose diabetes. These test results are not affected by time of day, dietary intake, exercise, recently administered diabetic drugs, emotional stress, or patient cooperation.

A fasting lipid profile (total cholesterol, high- and low-density lipoprotein cholesterol, and triglycerides) helps to determine the risk for cardiovascular complications (see Chapter 42). Serum creatinine and BUN levels should be measured in all adults, especially to determine the degree of renal dysfunction or damage when proteinuria is present. Microalbuminuria may be used to de-

tect early renal damage. Alterations in these results should be taken into account when drug treatment is planned, because the kidneys eliminate many drugs. A urinalysis should include ketones, glucose, protein, leukocyte esterase, and nitrates. A culture should be obtained if microscopic findings are abnormal or if symptoms are present.

In addition, thyroid function tests should be included because diabetes is associated with thyroid disease. Retinal photographs provide an effective means to document retinal status and are performed following a diagnosis of type 2 diabetes or 5 years after a diagnosis of type 1 dia-

---

EVIDENCE-BASED PRACTICE
Management of Patients with Diabetes Mellitus

Setting

Diabetes mellitus is a common chronic disease characterized by pancreatic insufficiency and decreased insulin receptivity, resulting in possible hyperglycemia and end-organ complications such as accelerated atherosclerosis, neuropathy, nephropathy, and retinopathy. Patients with the disorder are increasingly managed in primary care settings. Different systems have been proposed to manage the care of these patients.

Objectives of Literature Review

To assess the effectiveness of different interventions targeted at health care providers, or the structure in which they deliver care, on the management of patients with diabetes in primary care, outpatient, and community settings.

Investigators searched the electronic databases of the Cochrane Effective Practice and Organization of Care Group specialized register, the Cochrane Controlled Trials Register, MEDLINE, EMBASE, Cinahl, and reference lists of relevant articles.

Criteria for Inclusion in Review of Literature

Investigators included randomized clinical trials (RCTs), controlled clinical trials, controlled before-and-after studies, and interrupted time series analyses of professional, financial, and organizational strategies aimed at improving care for people with type 1 or type 2 diabetes mellitus. The subjects included physicians, nurses, and pharmacists. The outcomes included objectively measured performance of the health care provider or patient outcomes, and self-report measures with known validity and reliability.

Data Extraction and Analyses

Two investigators independently extracted data and assessed the quality of 41 studies involving more than 200

practices and 48,000 patients. Twenty-seven of the studies were RCTs, 12 were controlled before-and-after studies, and 2 were interrupted time series studies. The studies varied in terms of interventions, subjects, settings, and outcomes. The methodologic quality of the studies was often poor. In all studies the intervention strategy was multifaceted. In 12 of the studies the interventions were targeted at health care providers, 9 studies targeted the organization of care, and 20 studies targeted both. Patient education was added to the health care provider and organizational interventions in 15 of the studies.

Results

A combination of professional interventions improved process outcomes. The effect on patient outcomes remained less clear because these were rarely assessed. Arrangements for follow-up (organizational intervention) also showed a favorable effect on process outcomes. Multiple interventions in which patient education was added or in which the role of the nurse was enhanced also reported favorable effects on patients' health outcomes.

Investigators' Conclusions

Investigators concluded that a multfaceted interventional approach enhanced the performance of health care providers in managing patients with diabetes. Organizational interventions that improved prompt recall and review of patients (e.g., centralized computer tracking systems or regular contact by the nurse) likewise improved management of the patient with diabetes. The addition of patient-oriented interventions led to better patient outcomes. Nurses played an important role in patient-oriented interventions and facilitated adherence to treatment through regular patient education.

Renders C, Valk, G, Griffin S, et al: *Interventions to improve the management of diabetes mellitus in primary care, outpatient, and community settings* (Cochrane Review). In *The Cochrane Library*, Issue 2, Oxford, 2002, Update Software.

betes. Nerve conduction tests may be performed when abnormalities such as tingling, numbness, or pain are noted.

GOALS OF THERAPY

To the extent that complications of diabetes are related to hyperglycemia, the goal of treatment includes normalizing both fasting and postprandial blood glucose concentrations. Treatment interventions aimed at lowering blood glucose levels to or near normal levels in all patients is mandated by the following proven benefits: (1) the risk of DKA and HHNC, and their accompanying morbidity and mortality, is markedly reduced; (2) the symptoms of polyphagia, polydipsia, polyuria, weight loss, and fatigue may be decreased; (3) the development or progression of diabetic retinopathy, nephropathy, and neuropathy are greatly reduced; and (4) near-normal blood glucose levels are associated with a reduction of plasma lipid levels.

INTERVENTION

The treatment regimen is individualized and based in part on the type of diabetes and motivation level of the patient. Consideration should be given to the patient's age, health care beliefs and convictions, school or work schedule and conditions, degree of physical activity, eating patterns, social situation and personality, cultural variables, and presence of complications of diabetes or other comorbid conditions. Implementation of the plan requires that each aspect be understood, reasonable, and agreed upon by the patient and the health care provider.

Administration

Oral Antidiabetic Drugs. Oral antidiabetic drugs may be administered once in the morning or in divided doses. The drug should be administered with meals to ensure best diabetic control and minimize gastric irritation. The drug should not be taken after the last meal of the day to avoid hypoglycemia episodes during the night. Tablets may be crushed and taken with fluids, applesauce, or pudding if the patient has difficulty swallowing.

Insulins. The challenge of insulin therapy is to coordinate insulin administration with the changing requirements for glucose through the course of a normal day. In all cases the principle is the same: doses of insulin must be timed such that the patient is protected from hyperglycemia at any time and from hypoglycemia during peak periods of insulin action. Injecting insulin formulations at different times, as well as carefully controlling and scheduling food intake, usually achieves this accordingly. Studies suggest that many of the late pathologic changes associated with diabetes may be delayed or reduced in severity by strict control of the blood glucose level in diabetes.

Insulin is available in different types and strengths and is taken from different species. Check the type, species, dose, and expiration date before administration.

The various types of insulins should not be interchanged without first contacting the health care provider. Only short-acting insulin (e.g., regular insulin) is used for patients on so-called sliding scale insulin regimens and for intravenous administration.

Short-acting and longer-acting insulins are often combined and injected together to provide higher insulin levels just after meals (from the rapidly absorbed component) and lower levels later. Short-acting (i.e., regular) and intermediate-acting insulins may be mixed in the same syringe and used immediately or stored for later use. However, some mixtures of insulin in a syringe must be administered within a few minutes of drawing them up. Consult with the pharmacist for specific information. Regular insulin (which is clear) is always drawn up first, followed by intermediate-acting insulin (which is cloudy). Different intermediate- or longer-acting suspensions are never mixed together in one syringe.

Intermediate-acting and longer-acting insulin multidose vials must be gently but thoroughly rolled between the palms to mix the suspension before withdrawing the required dose. The bottle should not be shaken vigorously because the protein molecules become denatured by the whipping action. Frothing or foaming of the solution indicates the start of protein breakdown.

Insulin Injection Technique. Only use insulin syringes to draw up the required dose. Insulin is ordered in "units" rather than other units of measurement such as milligrams or grams. U-100 insulin syringes (i.e., 100 units of insulin/mL) are ordinarily used, but the unit markings on the insulin syringe must match the insulin vial's "units/mL" designation. Smaller syringes are available for doses less than 50 units.

Insulin is most often given subcutaneously. Injection sites include the subcutaneous tissues of the upper arm, abdomen, anterior and lateral aspects of the thigh, and the buttocks. In general, insulin injected into the abdomen is absorbed the fastest; insulin injected into the arm absorbed more slowly; and insulin is absorbed slowest when injected into the thigh. Most health care providers are taught to inject insulin at a 90-degree angle. In patients with less subcutaneous tissue a 45-degree angle may be used to avoid an inadvertent intramuscular injection. Aspiration before administration is not required. Apply moderate pressure to the administration site but do not rub. Exercise increases the rate of absorption from injection sites and should be taken into consideration when choosing a site.

The insulin should be at room temperature, and injection sites should be rotated to minimize disfiguring lipoatrophy that slows insulin absorption. In emergency situations, regular insulin may be given intravenously. Insulin cannot be taken orally, because it is a protein that would be destroyed by proteolytic enzymes in the stomach.

Insulin Delivery Systems. There are a variety of insulin delivery systems on the market. In the acute setting during periods of illness or stress, a continuous intravenous infusion of regular insulin may be required.

Jet injectors are available for patients afraid of needles or unable to use syringes. These devices deliver insulin in a fine, pressurized stream through the skin without the use of a needle but may traumatize the tissues if used incorrectly. Typically the onset and peak action of the insulin occurs earlier when these devices are used, thus requiring caution by the patient.

Penlike devices with insulin-containing cartridges are available to be inserted into a penlike holder. After the attachment of a disposable needle, insulin is injected by selecting a dose and depressing a button once. Although needles are used for the injection, there is no need for insulin to be drawn from multidose vials; this adds to the convenience and accuracy of administration. The penlike devices may be useful for patients who need multiple daily injections and for those who are visually or neurologically impaired.

Subcutaneous insulin pumps are available as an alternative to conventional injections and ordinarily provide excellent glucose control, but they require strong patient motivation to learn to use them. Only buffered insulin is used in insulin pumps. The pumps deliver a constant basal rate of insulin throughout the day and night and have the capability of delivering a bolus of insulin at mealtime. The needle, attached to a syringe via a long strip of plastic tubing, remains indwelling in the subcutaneous tissue of the abdomen. Patients program the pump to deliver the optimal amount of insulin, based on self-monitoring of blood glucose levels. Patients must be alert to tenderness and erythema at the insertion site, which may indicate infection or abscess.

Insulin Handling and Storage. Vials in current use should be kept at room temperature to minimize irritation at the injection site caused by cold insulin. Insulin can be safely kept at room temperature for up to 1 month; afterward it should be discarded. Constant refrigeration is not needed for most insulin, although extra bottles of insulin should be refrigerated (not frozen) until needed for up to 1 month.

Documentation. Record insulin administration in the patient's record, and be sure to include the injection site, date, and time. If local irritation is severe or persistent, contact the health care provider about a change in type of insulin.

Education

The most important part of diabetes management, in addition to compliance with the treatment plan, is patient education. Compliance is enhanced when the patient understands and can use the information provided. Except during periods of acute illness, the educational needs of the patient with diabetes should be given high priority. Although comprehensive diabetes management education is beyond the scope of this text except as it relates to drug therapy, it is important to teach a few of the basic principles. As always, principles of teaching and learning must be applied.

Educational materials should be written or adapted to the patient's learning ability, lifestyle, and cultural and social variables. In most instances, the use of printed materials encourages the patient to review the information or procedures at a later date. Family members or other support systems should be included in the educational plan so they can act as a resource and help the patient with compliance.

Support groups help with the development of realistic expectations. In rural communities where support groups may not be available, regional or national organizations are usually accessible for resource information and support. In addition, nurse educators, dietitians, physical therapists, and behaviorists who specialize in the care of diabetic patients are good resources and should be consulted when educating a patient about diabetes. In relation to diabetic control in general, the patient must be taught about the disease, drug therapy, blood glucose monitoring techniques, the importance of meal planning, exercise, the signs and symptoms of hyperglycemia and hypoglycemia, how to cope with sick days and insulin reactions, and when to seek professional attention.

Oral Drugs. Advise the patient to take the drug as ordered, even if he or she is not feeling well. If a dose is missed, instruct the patient to take it as soon as he or she remembers. If it is almost time for the next dose, omit the missed dose and resume the regular dosing schedule; the patient should not double up for missed doses. Advise the patient taking acarbose or miglitol to take it with the first bite of each meal.

Insulins. Review with the patient the importance of obtaining the correct concentration and type of insulin and the correct syringes. Instruct the patient not to switch the type or source of insulin without consulting the health care provider, because a change in dosage is often necessary. Also tell the patient to use the same brand of syringe at all times. Switching syringes may cause variations in level of blood glucose control as a result of the different volumes between the needle and the end of the calibrated syringe (dead space). Remind the patient to monitor the supply of insulin and syringes on hand to prevent running out unexpectedly. Review the manufacturer's instructions in teaching the patient how to prepare and use specialized insulin injectors.

Advise the patient not to use discolored insulins or those that appear grainy. Insulin deteriorates when it is exposed to excessive heat, light, or agitation and should always be inspected for clumping before each use. Extra vials of insulin should be available in case of breakage.

Glucose Monitoring. Blood glucose monitoring is recommended for patients with type 1 and type 2 diabetes; however, the supplies needed to maintain tight diabetes control can be costly. There are many blood glucose testing products available that are compact, easy to use, and reasonably priced. The cost of test strips for these products should be taken into account when putting a testing plan in place for the patient. Support groups and organizations may also be able to provide financial assistance or resources for those who cannot afford the high cost of glucose-monitoring supplies.

Patients are ordinarily taught to test glucose levels before each meal and at bedtime. The more closely blood glucose levels approach normal, the less likely complications are to develop (although strict control does not always ensure that complications will not occur). The development of blood glucose meters has made urine testing for glucose obsolete for most patients. Furthermore, urine glucose testing can be affected by fluid intake and many drugs. Testing, however, is irrelevant if the patient does not know what to do with the results.

Equipment Disposal. The patient should be taught proper syringe disposal, which varies from state to state. Unless the syringe is to be reused, it should be placed in a puncture-resistant container. The syringe is less likely to be reused by another individual if the plunger is removed from the syringe before disposal.

Disposable syringes and needles are designed for one-time use. However, some patients reuse the syringes and needles, usually for economic reasons. If the patient must reuse syringes and needles, review the importance of cleaning the needle and capping it between uses. A syringe and needle should be used, even if repeated, on only one person and never shared. Finally, the syringe and needle should be reused for a few injections only, not on a continuing basis. If skin irritation is a problem, the patient may want to use a new needle or syringe more often.

Syringe manufacturers cannot guarantee sterility of needles that are reused. However, insulin contains bacteriostatic additives that inhibit the growth of bacteria commonly found on skin. For some patients syringe reuse is not only safe but also economical. Immunosuppressed patients may be more at risk for infection than others; syringe reuse is therefore not appropriate for these individuals. In addition, needles become dull when used several times, causing injections to become painful. Cleansing needles to be reused with alcohol should be avoided, because the alcohol removes protective oils and contributes to development of dull needles.

Hypoglycemia. The patient should be taught the signs, symptoms, and proper treatment of hypoglycemia and when to notify the health care provider. Most hypoglycemic episodes are preventable by adhering to regularly scheduled meal times and snacks, careful timing of exercise, and proper drug dosing, regardless of whether insulin or oral antidiabetic drugs are used. Patients should be instructed to carry at least 15 g of a fast-acting carbohydrate to treat unexpected episodes of hypoglycemia. The following foods, among others, contain 15 g of fast-acting carbohydrate:

- 4 to 6 ounces of fruit juice (without added sugar)
- ½ cup of regular (not diet) carbonated beverage
- Six Life Savers candies
- Two or three squares of graham crackers
- 4 teaspoons of granulated sugar
- 1 cup of milk
- Six sugar cubes
- ½ cup of regular gelatin (not diet)

The patient should take one of the above food items followed by a complex carbohydrate and a protein so that the blood glucose level will be sustained. When the reaction is severe and the patient cannot swallow, a glucagon injection should be administered. Family members, roommates, and coworkers should be instructed in the use of glucagon for situations when the individual cannot be treated orally. All patients should be instructed to carry medical alert identification to alert others to their diabetes in case of emergency.

Meal Planning. For most people with diabetes, diet control is the key to managing this complicated disease, although it is also extremely difficult. Advise the patient that having diabetes does not mean they will have to give up all of the foods that they now enjoy. The current state of the diabetic diet is in flux and at this time there is no single diet that meets all of the needs of everyone with diabetes. There are some constants, however. All persons with diabetes should aim for healthy lipid levels and control of blood pressure.

People with type 1 and type 2 diabetes must control blood glucose levels by coordinating caloric intake with drug administration and exercise. Nutritional recommendations for patients with diabetes are similar to those of the American Heart Association, National Cancer Institute, Nutritional Committee for Recommendations for Children with Diabetes of the American Academy of Pediatrics, and U.S. Dietary Guidelines. However, the patient should have an individualized meal plan, including three meals and three snacks, and should know how to make daily meal choices.

The meal plan should be realistic and provide as much flexibility as possible to allow for integration into the individual's lifestyle. Calorie levels are individualized to the patient's weight, desired weight, and activity level. Adequate calories must be maintained for normal growth in children, for increased needs during pregnancy, and after illness. Low-fat meal principles should be enforced, and alternative cooking methods should be used. Sugar substitutes should be offered. High-fiber diets should be encouraged because fiber slows the absorption of glucose from the GI tract and reduces total cholesterol and low-density lipoprotein cholesterol. The patient should be encouraged to make appointments with the health care provider at regular intervals (i.e., usually every 3 months) to ensure that changes in lifestyle are noted and appropriate adjustments are made to the treatment program. Patients with weight loss goals and those whose drug dosages are in flux need more frequent follow-up.

The most common dietary method for controlling blood glucose levels is the use of diabetic exchange lists. More sophisticated methods include counting carbohydrate grams and using the so-called glycemic index to determine the impact of carbohydrates on blood sugar. If one of these approaches works to control glucose levels, there is no reason to choose another. Each of them can be effective, but because regulating glucose level is an individual situation, patients should get help from a dietary professional in selecting the best method.

Exercise. Regular exercise is recommended for all persons with diabetes. Patients should be taught the benefits of regular exercise and precautions to take while exercising. The benefits of exercise include better glycemic control, improved cardiovascular health, weight loss, decreased anxiety, improved self-image, and disease prevention. An exercise plan should always include a low-intensity warm-up and a postexercise cooldown. Aerobic exercise is the most beneficial type of exercise to achieve glycemic and cardiovascular benefits. The patient should be taught first to discuss the intensity, duration, and frequency of exercise with the health care provider, and the exercise regimen should then be individualized based on the patient's ability and health.

Exercise in extreme heat or cold should be avoided. It is important for the patient to understand that exercise during periods of poor metabolic control should be avoided and to carry at least 15 g of fast-acting carbohydrate at all times to treat hypoglycemia if it occurs unexpectedly. If the patient takes insulin, the blood glucose level should be monitored before, during, and after exercise. An exercise regimen carried out at a convenient time and location helps improve compliance with the exercise program.

Foot Care. The patient should be instructed to wear protective footwear and to inspect the feet daily as well as after exercise for evidence of skin breakdown. If the patient cannot perform the inspection, another sighted individual can be asked to do so. Regular inspections help to reduce the risk of complications related to neuropathy.

Stress Management. Stress management is important to properly control the blood glucose level. Any physical or emotional stress affects glycemic control, and the patient may require an increased dosage during this time. The patient may find it helpful to visit with a behaviorist to counteract any emotional stress that may be affecting the individual's health. Family members should be included as appropriate.

Travel Behavior. Patients with diabetes who travel must take their antidiabetic drugs or insulin and related equipment with them. They should be advised to carry extra insulin and syringes in separate, carry-on baggage should their luggage be misplaced while en route. Some states require prescriptions for syringes; suggest that patients carry an adequate supply for the entire trip. This is particularly important for international travel. A letter from the health care provider that lists the need for insulin and syringes should be carried, because this may help if the drug or equipment is lost in the event of any delays. The patient should talk to his or her pharmacist before the trip about any special considerations for insulin storage. Specially designed containers for insulin and syringes are commercially available.

Sick-Day Behavior. The patient should be instructed what to do when illness occurs. Blood sugar levels should be checked at least every 4 hours to detect hyperglycemia or hypoglycemia. The patient should consume 10 to 15 g of carbohydrates every hour. Liquids such as regular soda, popsicles, and sweetened gelatin are examples of sick-day foods that provide needed carbohydrates. The patient should also consume 8 ounces of water per hour to avoid dehydration. The health care provider should be notified if one or more of the following occur: blood glucose levels exceed 250 mg/dL, fever exceeds 101.1° F for more than 24 hours, the patient is unable to take food or fluids, breathing becomes shallow, or there is chest pain. It is important that the patient and family understand sick-day guidelines, because proper management can avoid hospitalization.

EVALUATION

The effectiveness of drug therapy for patients with diabetes is demonstrated by control of blood glucose levels without the appearance of hypoglycemia or hyperglycemic episodes. Additionally, the risk of DKA and HHNC (and the accompanying morbidity and mortality) is markedly reduced; the symptoms of polyphagia, polydipsia, polyuria, weight loss, and fatigue are decreased; the risk for retinopathy, nephropathy, and neuropathy are greatly reduced; and near-normalization of the blood glucose level is associated with a reduction of plasma lipid levels.

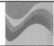

CASE STUDY — *Insulin-Dependent Type 2 Diabetes Mellitus*

ASSESSMENT

HISTORY OF PRESENT ILLNESS

VH is a 72-year-old black woman who is visiting the clinic today for 3-month follow-up of her type 2 diabetes mellitus. She reports having periods of hyperglycemia several times a week for the last 3 months but thought she was just tired. She follows an 1800-kilocalorie diabetic diet as learned in diabetes management class. She reports no signs or symptoms of UTI, skin breakdown, or recent vision changes.

HEALTH HISTORY

VH has a history of hemoglobinopathy, heart failure, hypertension, and previous transmetatarsal amputation of the left foot. Her last eye examination was 3 months ago. Retinopathy present. Present drugs: digoxin 0.25 mg po qd; gemfibrozil 600 mg po bid; metoprolol 50 mg po bid; naproxen 500 mg po bid; glipizide 10 XL mg po qd.

LIFESPAN CONSIDERATIONS

VH's husband attended diabetes management classes with her. She reports that he does all the shopping and cooking and follows the prescribed dietary regimen. VH and her husband are retired owners of a florist shop.

CULTURAL/SOCIAL CONSIDERATIONS

VH has three children who live out of state but are in contact once a month. She is active in a women's church group. She wears special orthotic shoes to accommodate a previous transmetatarsal amputation. Both husband and wife are on Social Security disability with military health care and pharmacy coverage. Her husband reports he is unsure of the accuracy of the glucose monitoring device currently in use. It is 5 years old.

PHYSICAL EXAMINATION

VH is 5'2" tall and weighs 143 pounds (up from 135 pounds 3 months ago). Her blood pressure is 170/96 mm Hg, pulse 88, respirations 16. Skin is warm and dry; mucous membranes dry; thyroid nonpalpable. S_3 heart sound present; bilateral pulses 2+. No evidence of skin breakdown in bilateral lower legs or feet; scar from transmetatarsal incision evident.

LABORATORY TESTING

Urinalysis shows trace protein, 250 mg/dL glucose. HbA_{1c} 9%; cholesterol 193 mg/dL; triglyceride 724 mg/dL. Fasting blood glucose level 268 mg/dL. SBGM indicates AM blood glucose readings consistently range from 200 to 220 mg/dL before meals and at bedtime.

PATIENT PROBLEM(S)

Insulin-dependent type 2 diabetes mellitus.

GOALS OF THERAPY

Control blood glucose at level that will minimize symptoms of hyperglycemia and yet avoid hypoglycemia. Prevent, postpone, and reverse complications associated with long-term history of diabetes mellitus.

CRITICAL THINKING QUESTIONS

1. The health care provider leaves the following orders: continue glipizide XL 10 mg po qd each morning; start Lantus insulin, 20 units at bedtime; replace glucose monitoring device and strips. What is the mechanism of action of glipizide XL and glargine insulin?
2. Of what adverse effects should VH be made aware?
3. What factor may have caused the health care provider to add glargine insulin to VH's treatment regimen?
4. Why must insulin be injected rather than taken by mouth?
5. What is the longest acting sulfonylurea?
6. If VH were to have a hypoglycemic episode, at what time(s) would it most likely occur?
7. What nursing intervention is appropriate if VH were to have a hypoglycemic episode?

Bibliography

Abramowicz M, editor: Insulin aspart, a new rapid-acting insulin, *Med Lett Drug Ther* 43:1115, 89-90, 2001.

Abramowicz M, editor: Insulin glargine (Lantus), a new long-acting insulin, *Med Lett Drug Ther* 43:1110, 65-66, 2001.

Bennett O: Cardiovascular problems in the diabetic patient, *Prof Nurse* 16(9):1339-1343, 2001.

Berardinelli C, Kupecz D: Drug news. Insulin glargine: a novel basal insulin analog, *Nurse Pract* 25(9):68, 74-75, 78, 2000.

Clarke P: Developments in insulin therapy and diabetes management, *J Diabetes Nurs* 5(2):56-58, 2001.

Cooper JW: Oral agent treatment of diabetes mellitus in older adults, *Ann Long Term Care* 6(13):414-422, 1998.

The Expert Committee on the Diagnosis and Classification of Diabetes Mellitus: Report of the Export Committee on the Diagnosis and Classification of Diabetes, *Diabetes Care* 23:1, S4-S19, 2000.

Hicks D: Recent developments in the management of type 2 diabetes, *Br J Community Nurs* 6(11):572, 574-575, 578-580, 2001.

Internet Resources

http://www.ahealthyme.com/topic/diabetesdrugs.
http://www.springnet.com/ce/p201a.htm#insulin.
http://www.springnet.com/ce/p201a.htm#nateglinide.

CHAPTER

59

Estrogens, Progestins, and Contraceptives

JOSEPH A. DiMICCO • KATHLEEN GUTIERREZ

 Visit http://evolve.elsevier.com/Gutierrez/ for additional information.

KEY TERMS

Corpus luteum, p. 978

Endometriosis, p. 983

Endometrium, p. 978

Estradiol, p. 978

Estrogens, p. 978

Estrone, p. 978

Follicle-stimulating hormone (FSH), p. 978

Gonadotropin-releasing hormone (GnRH), p. 978

Hormone replacement therapy (HRT), p. 979

Luteinizing hormone (LH), p. 978

Menopause, p. 979

Menstrual cycle, p. 978

Oral contraceptives, p. 979

Ovulation, p. 978

Postcoital contraceptives, p. 986

Progesterone, p. 978

Progestins, p. 978

Selective estrogen receptor modulators (SERMs), p. 983

OBJECTIVES

- Identify the physiologic changes that occur with the onset of menses and menopause.
- Describe the use and benefits of estrogens in hormone replacement therapy.
- Discuss the use of progestins alone or progestins in combination with estrogens as contraceptives.
- Explain the concept of selective estrogen receptor modulation.
- Identify the treatment goals for contraception and management of the menstrual cycle.
- Develop a nursing care plan for a patient receiving a drug discussed in this chapter.

PHYSIOLOGY • Menses and Menopause

The female reproductive system depends on a finely regulated interaction of hormones and endocrine tissues. The negative feedback loop that regulates the **menstrual cycle** involves the hypothalamus, the anterior pituitary, and the ovaries (see Chapter 55). The communication and interaction of these three components through a variety of hormones maintains female reproductive capacity.

The most important hormones regulating female reproduction are estrogens and progestins. **Estrogens** are steroids that influence a number of female reproductive tissues; **progestins** are steroids that specifically affect the uterine lining. Both hormones are produced primarily in the ovaries and, like all steroids, are derived from cholesterol. Progestins are formed first and are the precursors of androgens. Androgens, steroid hormones capable of producing masculinization (see Chapter 62), serve primarily as precursors of estrogen synthesis in women. Androstenedione is the androgen precursor of **estrone,** a circulating estrogen formed mostly in peripheral tissues and not in the ovaries. **Estradiol,** the most abundant circulating estrogen, is formed in the ovaries.

Although synthesis of both estrogens and progestins occurs primarily in the ovaries, this synthesis is ultimately under the control of the brain. The hypothalamus supplies **gonadotropin-releasing hormone (GnRH),** a peptide that acts directly on the anterior pituitary, stimulating the synthesis and release of **follicle-stimulating hormone (FSH)** and **luteinizing hormone (LH),** the major gonadotropins. In the process of normal reproductive cycling, FSH stimulates the maturation of an ovum and the formation of a follicle to nurture it. Under the influence of FSH, these follicular cells synthesize estradiol. Luteinizing hormone acts primarily on the mature follicle to cause release of the ovum; the ruptured follicle then develops into a structure called the **corpus luteum.** The corpus luteum secretes estradiol and **progesterone,** the endogenous progestin in humans.

At birth the ovary is already in an advanced stage of development and contains between 2 and 4 million oocytes, cells that will form ova. The primordial follicles containing oocytes are not quiescent before puberty but rather undergo a process called atresia, in which oocytes are destroyed and follicles are resorbed. At menarche, when menstrual cycles begin during puberty, an estimated 400,000 oocytes remain. Even after **ovulation** starts, atresia continues and is responsible for the destruction of more than 99% of the follicles present in the ovary.

As puberty begins, the immature ovaries are stimulated by increasing amounts of pituitary gonadotropins (i.e., FSH and LH). As a result, estrogen synthesis is promoted and estrogen levels in the blood rise. The pri-mary function of estrogens during early puberty is to promote development of the reproductive system. The uterus and fallopian tubes enlarge to adult proportions. The vagina enlarges, and the vaginal epithelium thickens and strengthens. In the breasts, estrogen promotes proliferation of tissues responsible for the production of milk.

The development of secondary sexual characteristics also depends on estrogens. These hormones promote increased deposition of fat, especially in the breasts and hips. Without estrogens, the typical contours of the female body do not develop.

Estrogens are also involved in regulating the start and the stop of the growth spurt characteristic of puberty. Along with other hormones, estrogen causes retention of calcium and phosphorus and thereby promotes bone growth. Estrogens also induce closure of the epiphyses. When this closure occurs, no further increase in height occurs.

HORMONES AFFECTING OVULATION

Ovulation requires proper functioning of the hypothalamus, anterior pituitary, and ovaries in the negative feedback loop described in Chapter 55. FSH and LH are required to act on the developing follicle before a mature ovum may be released to begin its journey down the fallopian tube to the uterus. Estrogen synthesis is required for its action on the follicle and for its ability to trigger the midcycle surge of LH from the anterior pituitary.

HORMONES AFFECTING ENDOMETRIAL FUNCTION

The uterus is composed of smooth muscle tissue (the myometrium) and the glandular epithelium, or **endometrium.** The endometrium, which nourishes and supports the fertilized ovum during development into an embryo and then a fetus, is controlled primarily by estrogens and progestins. Estrogens promote proliferation and thickening of the endometrium during the first half of the menstrual cycle, before ovulation occurs. Progesterone, which is formed in the corpus luteum of the ovary during the second half of the menstrual cycle, acts on both the endometrium and the myometrium. Progesterone reduces myometrial activity, preventing muscular contractions, and promotes development of the secretory capacity of endometrium. Actions on these two tissues aid in establishing the environment in which the fertilized ovum may implant successfully and begin development. Once implantation has occurred, progesterone continues to alter the endometrium, ultimately changing the tissue so that a second implantation becomes impossible.

HORMONES IN PREGNANCY

Pregnancy requires that a mature ovum be released from the ovary at the appropriate time, that the ovum be fertilized successfully within about 2 days of its release, and that the fertilized ovum be able to implant within the endometrium and draw nourishment to support the early stages of development. The most important hormone during these first days and weeks of pregnancy is progesterone. In a cycle in which fertilization of the ovum does not occur, levels of LH in the blood gradually decrease, causing the corpus luteum to degenerate and its production of progesterone to fall. Without adequate progesterone, the endometrium breaks down and is sloughed off as normally happens in menstruation at the end of the typical cycle in which pregnancy has not occurred.

To prevent sloughing of the endometrial lining and to maintain the pregnancy, the progesterone level must be maintained. Control of progesterone synthesis is exercised by cells of the fetus itself that develop into the placenta. A few days after implantation of the ovum in the endometrium, these fetal cells begin to produce a hormone called human chorionic gonadotropin (HCG); HCG acts like LH on the corpus luteum to keep it from degenerating and maintain its production of progesterone (see Chapter 61). Luteal progesterone is produced for about the first 10 weeks of pregnancy. By the fifth week of pregnancy the placenta has developed to where it begins to synthesize progesterone directly. Placental progesterone production increases during the remainder of the pregnancy, whereas production of progesterone by the corpus luteum eventually disappears.

MENOPAUSE

Eventually, the production of estrogen by the ovaries begins to decline gradually as the number of follicles dwindles. The menstrual cycle, including the development of follicles and menses, becomes irregular and eventually ceases. This period is called **menopause**, and is associated with many significant changes. Bone density is gradually lost, resulting in increased susceptibility to fractures. Hot and cold flashes often result because of circulatory changes, and inappropriate sweating may occur. Other vascular changes that may not be immediately obvious lead to an increased risk of atherosclerosis and mycardial infarction. Tissues lining the vagina may dry out and itch, and changes in the bladder may result in sudden incontinence. Most of these effects are a direct result of the reduced action of estrogen on different tissues. However, because of the reduction in the negative feedback usually exerted by circulating estrogen, excessive secretion of FSH and LH from the pituitary is common during menopause, which may have additional effects.

◣ DRUG CLASS • Estrogens

conjugated estrogens (Premarin)

dienestrol (Ortho Dienestrol)

esterified estrogens (Estratab, Menest)

estradiol (Estrace, Delestrogen, Estrofem, depGynogen, Depo-Estradiol, Dura-Estrin, Estragyn LA, FemPatch, Climara, Alora, Vivelle, others)

estrone (Aquest, Wehgen, Estragyn, Estrone, Oestrilin✶)

estropipate (Ogen)

ethinyl estradiol (Estinyl)

mestranol

MECHANISM OF ACTION

All of these drugs mimic the effects of estrogen in estrogen-sensitive target tissues. Like estrogen, the drugs enter cells and bind to cytoplasmic estrogen receptors. The bound receptor then enters the nucleus, where it binds with other proteins to form a complex. This complex then interacts with DNA to alter the expression of specific genes. Because different proteins are involved in different tissues, the exact nature of the estrogen receptor complex will vary. This means that stimulation of estrogen receptors may alter the expression of different genes in different tissues.

USES

The major use for estrogens is in postmenopausal women for **hormone replacement therapy (HRT)** and in birth control pills, or **oral contraceptives**. Estrogen is always combined with a progestin when given as a contraceptive (see section on oral contraceptives and Table 59-1) and is often used along with a progestin in HRT as well (Table 59-2). Systemic estrogen effectively treats the major adverse symptoms resulting from the loss of endogenous estrogen in menopause, including vasomotor symptoms (hot flashes and sweating) and *osteoporosis* (bone loss), and reduces the elevated risk of cardiovascular disease typically seen in postmenopausal women. Estrogen ther-

---

TABLE 59-1

Combination Oral Contraceptives

Combination (estrogen + progestin)	Type	Brand Names
ethinyl estradiol + desogestrel	Monophasic Triphasic	Desogen, Ortho-Cept Mircette
ethinyl estradiol + ethynodiol	Monophasic	Demulen, Zovia
ethinyl estradiol + levonorgestrel	Monophasic Triphasic	Alesse, Levlite, Levlen, Levora, Nordette Tri-Levlen, Triphasil, Trivora
ethinyl estradiol + norethindrone	Monophasic Biphasic Triphasic	Loestrin, Brevicon, Genora 1/35, Intercon, Necon 0.5/35, Necon 1/35, Ortho-Novum 1/35, Ovcon-35, Nelova 0.5/35E Necon 10/11, Nelova 10/11, Ortho-Novum 10/11, Jenest-28 Estrostep 21, Tri-Norinyl, Ortho-Novum 7/7/7
ethinyl estradiol + norgestimate	Monophasic Triphasic	Ortho-Cyclen Ortho Tri-Cyclen
ethinyl estradiol + norgestrel	Monophasic	Lo/Ovral, Ovral
mestranol + norethindrone	Monophasic	Genora 1/50, Intercon 1/50, Necon 1/50, Nelova 1/50M, Norethin 1/50M, Norinyl 1 + 50, Ortho-Novum 1/50

TABLE 59-2

Examples of Hormonal Replacement Therapy Regimens

Regimen	Component* (Estrogen + Progesterone Where Indicated)	Dosing Schedule
Continuous, combined	estrogen progestins	Daily Daily
Continuous, sequential	estrogen progestin	Daily Days 1-14
Cyclical, sequential	estrogen progestin	Days 1-25 Days 1-14 or 13-25
Cyclical, combined	estrogen and progestins	Days 1-25
Continuous	estrogen†	Days 1-30

*Estrogens commonly used: conjugated estrogen, estrone, micronized estradiol. Progestins commonly used: medroxyprogesterone, norethindrone, micronized progesterone.
†Estrogen-only dosage regimen for women who no longer have a uterus.

---

apy is also indicated for atrophy of vaginal and urethral tissue that occurs after menopause and in certain other settings; it can also be given locally as a vaginal cream or insert for this purpose.

Estrogens are also used for replacement therapy when the synthesis of endogenous estrogen is inadequate during puberty, when estrogen is required for normal growth and sexual development; menarche may not occur. This endocrine malfunction is one of several abnormalities that may be responsible for amenorrhea (the absence of menstrual cycles). Estrogen and estro-genic compounds are available in a variety of preparations for these purposes.

Systemic estrogen therapy is used in selected patients with metastatic breast cancer or advanced prostatic carcinoma. For more on the use of these and of other hormonal drugs in cancer chemotherapy, see Chapter 37.

The doses of estrogen used vary depending on the condition being treated. When used in replacement therapy, estrogen dosages tend to be low. Higher dosages are often used in oral contraceptives, and even higher doses are employed to treat conditions such as advanced breast cancer.

PHARMACOKINETICS

Estrogens and estrogenic drugs are generally well absorbed, and most are highly protein bound. Estradiol and estrone, the two naturally occurring steroid estrogens used clinically, do not persist long in the body because they are rapidly biotransformed by the liver and renally excreted. As steroids, these compounds are not water soluble, but they are soluble in oil and are often given by injection in such a form. When estradiol is given in this way, slower absorption and longer duration of action may be achieved by using the cypionate or the valerate ester of the natural steroid. Estradiol is absorbed orally if the drug crystals are reduced to particles 1 to 3 mm in diameter. However, because of rapid first-pass biotransformation, bioavailability is low, meaning that large oral doses must be given to produce systemic effects. Estradiol is also well absorbed transdermally, and patches are now available to deliver a dose of the drug slowly over a period of several days. Estrone is not well absorbed orally in its natural form but may be used orally if converted to piperazine sulfate (estropipate). Estrone is also the major component of various estrogen mixtures described as esterified or conjugated estrogens. These mixtures, which are isolated from the urine of pregnant mares (hence the name Premarin), are relatively cheap and are effective for many purposes. Estrogenic mixtures can also be taken orally, which makes them a convenient drug form for many patients.

Ethinyl estradiol is a synthetic steroidal estrogen that can be taken orally because it is relatively resistant to hepatic biotransformation. Ethinyl estradiol is more potent than naturally occurring estrogens. This drug has a relatively short duration of action (i.e., a plasma half-life of 12 to 24 hours) but still persists in the body longer than any of the natural estrogens. As with other steroidal estrogens, the duration of action of ethinyl estradiol is significantly prolonged by enterohepatic cycling, a phenomenon described in Chapter 1. Mestranol, another synthetic steroidal estrogen used only in oral contraceptives, acts primarily after its rapid conversion to ethinyl estradiol in the body.

Dienestrol is a nonsteroidal estrogen used only topically in a vaginal cream.

ADVERSE REACTIONS AND CONTRAINDICATIONS

Adverse reactions to estrogens include overreactions of certain reproductive tissues to the hormones. Breast tenderness is reported by many women who take estrogen. Estrogens stimulate endometrial proliferation, and treatment with estrogens alone increases the risk of endometrial cancer; estrogens given cyclically with progestins do not support endometrial hyperplasia, and the risk of endometrial cancer is reduced. Estrogens are not routinely given to breast cancer patients, because estrogens may promote growth of estrogen-sensitive tumors. Whether estrogen therapy increases the risk for development of breast cancer remains an unanswered question. However, it is clear that, if it exists, any increase in this risk is relatively small for most women.

Estrogens are often associated with acute adverse reactions such as nausea and vomiting, anorexia, and mild diarrhea. Malaise, depression, and excessive irritability are also related to estrogen therapy in some women. Estrogens promote salt and water retention and may therefore produce edema in some patients. Atherosclerosis is a definite risk for patients who take estrogens, especially if they have other high-risk factors such as cigarette smoking. Hypertension has been associated with estrogen use. Estrogen also enhances blood clotting mechanisms and thus may increase the risk of thromboembolic disorders in certain patients. All of these adverse effects are much more common at high doses.

Estrogens are thought to be responsible for most of the adverse reactions associated with combination oral contraceptives (see later section and Table 59-3). Estrogens are never given during pregnancy. Diethylstilbestrol (DES), a synthetic nonsteroidal estrogen no longer available, was once widely used to prevent spontaneous abortions. Not only was it later shown not to be effective for this purpose, but the children who were exposed in utero at the time of DES treatment also experienced serious adverse effects. Female children had a sharply increased incidence of vaginal adenosis and adenocarcinoma as adults, and males were prone to develop epididymal cysts. Therefore estrogens are contraindicated in known or suspected pregnancy.

Vaginal bleeding also precludes the use of estrogens, because the bleeding may signal conditions such as endometrial hyperplasia or carcinoma, which would be worsened by estrogens.

High doses of estrogens in women may produce any of the signs noted previously. Migraine headaches and vomiting triggered by effects in the CNS may also occur.

INTERACTIONS

Estrogens increase the risk of toxicity with hepatotoxic drugs. Both hepatotoxicity and nephrotoxicity of cyclosporine may be enhanced because estrogens inhibit biotransformation of cyclosporine. Ritonavir and other HIV protease inhibitors promote biotransformation of estrogens, so estrogens are cleared more rapidly from the body. Certain antibiotics may increase the clearance of estrogens subject to enterohepatic cycling because they kill the intestinal bacteria required for this to occur.

TABLE 59-3

Adverse Reactions to Oral Contraceptives

Adverse Reaction	Relation to Oral Contraceptives	Comments
Thromboembolic disorders	Risk increased two- to sevenfold in users over nonusers. Incidence rate about 100:100,000 woman years; fatalities 2:100,000 woman years.*	Obesity, family history of thromboembolic disorders, immobility, or group A blood type may increase risk. Women with blood type O have lower risk. Directly related to estrogen dosage.
Thrombotic stroke	Risk increased about three- to six-fold. Incidence rate about 25:100,000 woman years; fatalities 0.5:100,000 woman years.*	Hypertension increases risk.
Hemorrhagic stroke	Risk increased at least twofold. Incidence rate about 10:100,000 woman years.*	Hypertension and heavy smoking are strong risk factors.
Myocardial infarction	Risk increased about two-fold over nonusers when estrogen doses exceed 50 mg per day.	Synergistic increase in risk if oral contraceptives are used by patients who smoke.
Hypertension	About 15% of patients show increase in blood pressure. Clinical hypertension is less common.*	Risk is increased by age, obesity, and parity.
Gallbladder disease	Risk increased an estimated two-fold.*	Risk may be related to duration of use.
Liver disease	Up to 50% of patients show altered liver function. Incidence rate 10:100,000 woman years for jaundice. Tumors are rare.	Reversible. Dangerous for patients with preexisting liver disease (hepatitis or cholestasis). Liver tumors may be related specifically to mestranol.
Hepatocellular carcinoma	Risk of this rare tumor increases after 8 years of oral contraceptive use.	This tumor occurs in fewer than 1 woman per 1 million long-term users of oral contraceptives.
Carbohydrate metabolism	Many patients show impaired glucose tolerance.	Important only in prediabetic women who may become insulin dependent. Related to dose and potency of progestin.
Lipid metabolism	Many patients have increased serum triglyceride levels.	Reversible effect; relationship to coronary artery disease in these patients is unknown.
Melasma	3% to 4% of patients treated.	Reversible effect; increased sensitivity to sunlight also occurs.
Headaches	Increased or worsened in about 20% of patients.	Chronic headache may presage stroke.
Visual disturbances	Have been associated with use of oral contraceptives.	Temporary blindness, blind spots, and changes in field of vision have been reported.
Endometrial cancer	1 year of treatment confers 15 years of protective effect against endometrial cancer.*	Risk is increased by estrogens alone but is reduced by progestins.
Ovarian cancer	3 years of use confers up to 10 years protective effect.	Short-term use confers no protection that can be documented.
Cervical cancer	Risk is increased twofold after 5 years of use and continues to increase with longer use.	Frequency of coitus and number of sexual partners are also important risk factors.
Breast cancer	No clear relationship established.	Risk may depend on age or duration of use.
Benign fibrocystic breast disease	40% reduction in incidence rate for 2 years after use.*	Data based on estrogen doses of 50 mg or more; effect of low dosage unknown.
Permanent infertility	No relationship established.	Most patients quickly return to fertility when oral contraceptives are discontinued.
Outcome of later pregnancies	No increased risk to mother or fetus demonstrated.	Data are for pregnancies begun after oral contraceptives have been discontinued.

*Risks or benefits may be reduced with currently used products using lower doses of estrogens.

DRUG CLASS • Estrogen Antagonists and Selective Estrogen Receptor Modulators

clomiphene (Clomid, Milophene, Serophene)

raloxifene (Evista)

tamoxifen (Nolvadex)

toremifene (Fareston)

MECHANISM OF ACTION

As discussed for estrogens above, the interaction of an estrogen with its own receptor produces different effects in different tissues because once the estrogen binds to a receptor and enters the nucleus, it then binds to proteins to form a complex that can interact with DNA. Because different proteins are involved in different tissues, the transcription of different genes may be affected, or the expression of the same genes may be altered in different ways.

Clomiphene is an estrogen antagonist. Clomiphene binds to estrogen receptors in such a way that it produces no significant estrogenic action in any tissue. However, by occupying the receptors, clomiphene blocks the ability of endogenous estrogen to produce its usual effects. The use of clomiphene as an estrogen antagonist in the treatment of infertility is discussed in Chapter 61.

Selective estrogen receptor modulators (SERMs) also bind to the estrogen receptor but in a way that differs both from that of estrogens and from the estrogen antagonist clomiphene. This drug-receptor complex can still associate with the nuclear proteins in certain tissues to produce typical estrogenic effects. However, in other tissues, where different nuclear proteins are usually involved in the actions of estrogens, the same drug-receptor complex may fail to interact with available proteins to produce a complex with the usual estrogenic effects on gene expression. Therefore the same drug may produce estrogenic actions in one tissue while acting as a partial agonist or even an estrogen antagonist at other sites. This is why raloxifene (discussed in Chapter 63) produces typical estrogenic effects to increase bone density in postmenopausal women but does not cause unwanted estrogenic stimulation of breast tissue or the uterus. The pharmacology of tamoxifen and toremifene and the use of these drugs in the treatment of breast cancer is covered in detail in Chapter 37.

DRUG CLASS • Progestins

desogestrel*

ethynodiol*

hydroxyprogesterone (Gesterol LA, Hy/Gestrone, Hylutin, Prodrox)

levonorgestrel (Norplant, Norplant II, Plan B, Mirena)

medroxyprogesterone (Cycrin, Provera, Amen, Curretab, Depo-Provera)

megestrol (Megace)

norethindrone (Micronor, Nor-QD, Aygestin)

norgestimate*

norgestrel (Ovrette)

progesterone (Prometrium, Gesterol, Crinone)

MECHANISM OF ACTION

Progestins used as drugs promote all of the actions of the naturally occurring progestins. Some preparations are most effective as progestational drugs, whereas others have significant effects in other areas. For example, some progestins have detectable androgenic effects. Megestrol has medically useful antianorectic and anticachetic actions in patients undergoing antineoplastic therapy (see Chapter 37). These actions and others all arise as the progestin interacts with the steroid receptors inside target cells to alter gene expression.

USES

Progestins are used clinically for their effects on the endometrium and also as contraceptive agents. High dosages suppress bleeding of the endometrium, and withdrawal induces sloughing of the tissue; thus they may be useful to treat secondary amenorrhea, to treat dysfunctional uterine bleeding, and to induce menses. Progestins are also used to treat endometriosis, a painful condition caused when endometrial tissue becomes implanted in the abdominal cavity outside of the uterus.

Although progestins are most commonly employed in combination with estrogens when used as contraceptives (see later section), they are also used alone for this purpose. Progestins can be taken orally just as combi-

*Used only in combination with estrogens.

nation birth control pills are, but they are also used in slow-release devices implanted subdermally or placed in the uterus to produce localized effects (Table 59-4). Levonorgestrel is available as a relatively high-dose formulation specifically indicated for postcoital contraception (see later section).

PHARMACOKINETICS

Progestins available for medical use include the natural steroid hormone progesterone and synthetic derivatives of that compound. Progesterone itself has very low bioavailability if given orally (although oral formulations are available) and is rapidly biotransformed by the liver (having a plasma half-life of only a few minutes). Hydroxyprogesterone has a somewhat longer half-life but is only given in an oil-based preparation by injection and is slowly absorbed to provide an extended duration of action. Medroxyprogesterone given orally has a half-life of more than a day, but injectable depot preparations of the drug used as a contraceptive can be effective for 3 months (see later section). All the remaining drugs listed above are synthetics with good oral bioavailability and relatively long durations of action (having plasma half-lives of 8 to 20 hours). One of these, levonorgestrel, is employed as a contraceptive in Norplant, a slow-release subdermal implant effective for 5 years.

ADVERSE REACTIONS AND CONTRAINDICATIONS

The most common adverse reaction to systemic progestins is moderate to heavy breakthrough menstrual bleeding or bleeding between regular monthly periods. In some patients, menstrual cycling ceases altogether. Adverse reactions to progestins may involve several organ systems other than reproductive organs. Some of these reactions are similar to those seen with estrogens, including edema, breast tenderness and swelling, GI

disturbances, depression, and weight change. Other reactions include cholestatic jaundice and rashes. Levonorgestrel implants (Norplant) are associated with a relatively high incidence rate of headache and mood changes, usually in the first few months. Return to fertility may be delayed after withdrawal of treatment with medroxyprogesterone. Megestrol is said to produce hyperglycemia in as many as 16% of treated patients. Injections of progesterone are painful and may result in local inflammation.

Progestins should be avoided during pregnancy because many of them have some androgenic activity and may cause masculinization of female fetuses. Norgestrel and levonorgestrel have the most androgenic activity, whereas norgestimate and desogestrel have the least. This activity is also responsible for the excessive hair growth or loss sometimes caused by combination oral contraceptives (see later section).

Patients with a history of thromboembolic disorders or thrombophlebitis should not be treated with progestins. These drugs are also not normally given to patients with breast tumors or hepatic disease because these conditions may be worsened by progestins.

TOXICITY

High dosages of progestins are associated with greater risks of thromboembolic disease. If blood clots form, patients may note sudden, sharp pains; sudden, severe headaches; or sudden changes in speech, vision, or coordination. Any of these signs are reason to seek medical attention immediately. Fatalities have occurred.

INTERACTIONS

Aminoglutethimide reduces the serum concentration of medroxyprogesterone. Drugs such as carbamazepine, phenobarbital, phenytoin, rifabutin, and rifampin may induce enzymes in the liver that biotransform progestins; this action reduces the effect of progestins.

TABLE 59-4

Progestin-Only Contraceptives

Progestin	Brand Name	Route of Administration
levonorgestrel	Plan B	Oral (postcoital)
	Norplant, Norplant II	Subdermal implant (slow-release)
	Mirena	Intrauterine device (slow-release)
medroxyprogesterone	Depo-Provera	Intramuscular injection (depot)
norethindrone	Micronor, Nor-Q.D.	Oral
norgestrel	Ovrette	Oral
progesterone	Progestasert	Intrauterine device (slow-release)

DRUG CLASS • Progesterone Antagonists

mifepristone (RU-486, Mifeprex)

MECHANISM OF ACTION

Mifepristone binds to receptors for progesterone in the cytoplasm of cells in tissues where the hormone acts. The drug thus prevents the action of progesterone (or any other progestin) in target tissues such as the endometrium.

USES

Because the actions of progesterone on the endometrium are required for maintenance of a pregnancy, mifepristone may be used to terminate an intrauterine pregnancy within the first 49 days. It is administered along with misoprostol, a prostaglandin, to stimulate uterine contraction and thus aid in expulsion of the dislodged tissue.

PHARMACOKINETICS

Mifepristone is orally effective (bioavailability is about 70%) and has a half-life of 18 hours. Its action is terminated by hepatic biotransformation.

ADVERSE REACTIONS AND CONTRAINDICATIONS

The vaginal bleeding that accompanies the use of mifepristone is sometimes severe and on rare occasions may require transfusions. The drug often produces abdominal pain or uterine cramping, fatigue, nausea and vomiting. The GI effects accompanying a medical abortion induced by mifepristone may be caused, at least in part, by misoprostol.

Mifepristone should not be used in cases of ectopic pregnancy or in patients with clotting disorders. Because the drug is also a glucocorticoid antagonist, it is also generally contraindicated for patients suffering from adrenal failure or chronic adrenal insufficiency.

INTERACTIONS

Candidates for treatment with mifepristone should not be taking anticoagulants.

DRUG CLASS • Oral Contraceptives

See Tables 59-1 and 59-4.

MECHANISM OF ACTION

Reversible sterility induced by drugs has been possible since the late 1950s, when oral contraceptives first became available. The most common so-called birth control pills contain a combination of estrogen and a progestin, whereas others employ a progestin alone. The effectiveness of oral contraceptives is very high: most reports estimate a 0% to 6% failure rate per year of use for the combined estrogen-progestin drugs and rates almost as low for progestin-only preparations. This failure rate is in contrast to rates of 2% to 27% per year for mechanical devices such as diaphragms, sponges, and condoms.

Estrogen-progestin combinations work primarily by suppressing ovulation. In addition, these drugs change the cervical mucus, making it difficult for sperm to enter the uterus. Changes also occur in the endometrium, making implantation difficult even if fertilization occurs. The formulations containing progestins alone alter the cervical mucus and the endometrium as the combination products do, but they do not always suppress ovulation. Largely for this reason, progestins alone are slightly less effective than the combined preparations.

To achieve contraception and to simulate normal menstrual cycles, combination oral contraceptives usually are taken for 21 consecutive days, followed by 7 days of taking either nothing or a so-called dummy pill containing no active ingredients. The increased estrogen and progestin levels during the 21 days of treatment suppress the hypothalamus and the anterior pituitary so that the secretion of FSH is inhibited and no LH is released at the time when ovulation would normally occur. This is the mechanism by which ovulation is suppressed. During the 7 days when hormones are not administered, the endometrium involutes and sloughs off, primarily as a result of loss of progestin activity. This withdrawal period prevents excessive endometrial proliferation.

In recent years, more complex dosing schemes have been introduced with the intent of lowering the total dose of the hormones administered in a given cycle while still maintaining complete suppression of ovulation. In different versions of these formulations, the dose of one or both components may change either once (biphasic combination oral contraceptives) or twice (triphasic combination oral contraceptives) in the course of the 21-day treatment period.

USES

Regular use of oral contraceptives provides a reliable, convenient, and reversible means of preventing unwanted pregnancy in otherwise healthy women. More recently, several formulations of oral contraceptives have been approved for use as postcoital contraceptives, an approach that involves ingestion of two or four pills as soon after unprotected sex as possible and repeated 12 hours later.

The combination oral contraceptives provide additional benefits that have led to their use for purposes other than prevention of pregnancy. Thus other indications include the treatment of acne and endometriosis as well as the normalization of irregular menses.

PHARMACOKINETICS

The pharmacokinetics of oral contraceptives are the same as previously noted for the individual estrogen or progestin components. As discussed above, synthetic forms of estrogens and progestins are used in oral contraceptives because oral bioavailability of these synthetic forms is better and plasma half-lives are longer than for the natural hormone.

ADVERSE REACTIONS AND CONTRAINDICATIONS

Adverse reactions produced by oral contraceptives may come from either the estrogen or the progestin component. The most troublesome of these are thought to be caused by estrogens and include nausea, bloating, breast fullness, edema, hypertension, and cervical discharge. Patients who report these symptoms may be given a preparation with lower estrogen levels.

Adverse effects associated with progestins include hair loss, excessive hair growth, oily scalp, acne, increased appetite, weight gain, fatigue, depression, breast regression, and reduced menstrual blood flow. Oral contraceptives fall into pregnancy category X.

Oral contraceptives are used by millions of women to prevent pregnancy. Although these drugs are highly effective, questions about their safety are raised from time to time. In particular, the incidence of unexpected serious or fatal medical conditions has been studied in the relatively healthy women who take oral contraceptives. Risk of certain serious medical conditions is now shown to be increased in those who use oral contraceptive compared with similar women who do not take these drugs (see Table 59-3).

As with any drug, oral contraceptives must be considered in terms of the risk-to-benefit ratio. Of primary importance may be how much value the patient places on almost complete protection against unwanted pregnancy. Women who desire this high level of control should then consider the safety factors of the drug. Many of the dangerous complications (e.g., stroke, thromboembolic diseases) are rare even among those who use oral contraceptives. The risk of these complications is greater than the risk among women not taking oral contraceptives but much lower than the risk of these complications during pregnancy. Women should also consider other predisposing risk factors such as cigarette smoking, obesity, and hypertension. The combination of oral contraceptives with these conditions leads to unacceptable risk for many patients, particularly in women over the age of 35. All women who take oral contraceptives should be urged to stop smoking (Table 59-5).

Some medical conditions are improved or the symptoms are lessened by oral contraceptives. Many patients report a reduction in menstrual disorders and especially in dysmenorrhea. Menstrual blood flow usually is reduced, and anemia is prevented or lessened in many women. Benign breast tumors may be improved over time by oral contraceptive therapy, but patients with carcinoma of the breast, cervix, liver, uterus, or vagina should not take these drugs because these cancers may be stimulated by estrogens.

Current medical data suggest that oral contraceptives are safe in young women in whom other risk factors are minimized. Women with a history of hypertension or thromboembolic disease probably should not receive the drugs. Women who choose to take oral contraceptives should undergo thorough physical examinations yearly. The dosage of estrogen and progestin should be the lowest dosage that achieves contraception and prevents unwanted adverse reactions such as breakthrough bleeding.

Taking a careful history may reveal symptoms the patient has not linked to oral contraceptive use. Migraine headaches, dizziness, and visual disturbances often are not related by the patient to oral contraceptive use and may not be mentioned spontaneously. Breakthrough bleeding, excessive cervical mucus formation, and other changes in the reproductive tract as well as breast tenderness usually are quickly connected to oral contraceptive use by patients. These symptoms may be more annoying than serious. Severe headaches or visual disturbances are

TABLE 59-5	

Contraindications to the Use of Contraceptives

Absolute Contraindications	*Relative Contraindications*
Short-Acting Contraceptives	
History of DVT or pulmonary embolus	Migraine headaches
Antiphospholipid antibody syndrome	Severe depression
Protein C deficiency	Oligomenorrhea/amenorrhea
Protein S deficiency	Diabetes mellitus with retinopathy or nephropathy
Concurrent use of rifampin	Symptomatic mitral valve prolapse
Antithrombin III deficiency	History of jaundice or pruritus of pregnancy
Estrogen-dependent breast cancer	Family history of thromboembolic disease
History of heart disease, CVA, uncontrolled hypertension	Family history of elevated triglycerides
Smoking in patients over 35 years	Epilepsy
Pregnancy	Sickle cell disease
Active liver disease	Gallbladder disease
Intestinal malabsorption syndrome	Elective surgery
Long-Acting Contraceptives	
Active thrombophlebitis	Smoking (>15 daily) in patient over 35 years
Thromboembolic disease	History of ectopic pregnancy
Undiagnosed genital bleeding	Diabetes mellitus
Benign or malignant liver tumors	Hypercholesterolemia
Known or suspected breast cancer	Severe acne
Active liver disease	Hypertension
	History of cardiovascular disease
	Gallbladder disease
	Severe vascular or migraine headaches
	Severe depression
	Compromised immune system
	Concomitant use of phenytoin, phenobarbital, carbamazepine, or rifampin

often early signs of impending stroke and may be sufficient cause to discontinue the medications.

The first oral contraceptives contained more estrogens than the drugs available today. These lower estrogen combinations are usually as effective as the older drugs and may be associated with a lower incidence rate of adverse reactions.

TOXICITY

Acute overdoses with oral contraceptives often cause nausea and vomiting. Vaginal bleeding may also occur upon withdrawal from these drugs. These effects are relatively common when oral contraceptives are used at high doses for postcoital contraception (see earlier section on uses).

Higher dosages over longer periods are associated with greater risk of thromboembolic complications.

INTERACTIONS

Oral contraceptives are subject to the same interactions as the individual estrogen and progestin components. Antibiotics may destroy the intestinal flora responsible for enterohepatic cycling and thus reduce the efficacy of oral contraceptives. Hepatic enzyme inducers may also impair effectiveness of oral contraceptives. Either of these interactions may lead to unexpected pregnancy. Hepatotoxic drugs should be avoided. Oral contraceptives interfere with the activity of bromocriptine and anticoagulants as well as increase the toxicity of tricyclic antidepressants.

DRUG CLASS • Contraceptive Implants, Depot Injections, and Intrauterine Devices

When long-term pharmacologic contraception is desired, systemic absorption can be achieved without the need for daily oral dosing. Because most forms of the steroid hormones such as estrogens and progestins are relatively insoluble in water, they are slowly absorbed from tissue sites when injected. This property can be used to advantage by confining the drugs to insoluble polymers that can then be implanted under the skin. Small amounts of drug are continuously released over very long periods. One example of such an application is the contraceptive Norplant (see Table 59-4). Six slender capsules, each containing the synthetic progestin levonorgestrel, are implanted subdermally. This application affords contraceptive protection for up to 5 years. Depot injections of medroxyprogesterone acetate give protection for up to 3 months (Box 59-1).

Long-term contraception can also be achieved with intrauterine devices (IUDs) that release active drug directly to the target tissues. For example, the natural progestin progesterone is used in an IUD (Progestasert) in this way. The very small amounts of progesterone released are retained within the reproductive tract rather than being systemically absorbed. The effectiveness of this device depends on its mechanical effects and on the pharmacologic effects of progesterone. This device provides contraception for up to 12 months. IUDs that release copper are also available. These devices tend to cause local inflammatory responses that affect the ability of an ovum to implant. The copper released by the devices may also affect viability of the sperm and mobility of the ovum. These copper-releasing IUDs provide contraception for 24 months (Copper-T 200), 30 months (Copper-T 200 Ag, Copper-T 380S), or 10 years (Copper-T 380A).

BOX 59-1	Women's Responses to Depo-Provera

Purpose

Depot medroxyprogesterone acetate (abbreviated DMPA; trade name Depo-Provera) is a long-acting method of birth control available in the United States. This drug is administered as an intramuscular injection every 3 months and has a contraceptive efficacy of 99.7%. The purpose of the exploratory study was to have women who had received DMPA answer questions about their experience with the drug so that health care providers could gain a better understanding of typical problems and develop appropriate teaching materials.

Methods

All women in the study had received DMPA at an inner-city health care facility. There were 72 subjects: 63% Hispanic, 29% African American, and 8% white. The mean age was 27.7 years, and the mean educational level was 11.4 years of completed schooling. Each subject was asked 14 questions in a semistructured interview format.

Results

Subjects in the study had chosen DMPA for the following reasons: they forgot to take their birth control pills (25%), they disliked the pills (20%), a doctor or midwife advised them to do so (18%), the method was perceived as easy and safe (18%), and they liked that the drug is administered every 3 months versus daily dosing (12%). A total of 78% expressed satisfaction with the method. The 22% who were dissatisfied cited the following adverse reactions: heavy bleeding, bad headaches, pimples, hair loss, and weight gain. Despite dissatisfaction by some, 65% planned to have another injection. When asked what they would tell a friend about the drug, common answers included "easy," "safe," "don't have to think about it for 3 months," and "don't get periods all the time." However, 6% stated that "you don't have to use condoms," and 18% replied with some variation of "it prevents sex diseases," which are incorrect responses. Adverse reactions reported by 65% of the respondents included amenorrhea (31%), headaches (27%), hair loss (27%), irregular periods (22%), and heavy bleeding (19%). Most women (93%) were satisfied with the information they received before beginning the drug.

Implications

Most of the subjects in this study considered this a safe drug to use, with minimal or tolerable adverse effects. An area of concern was the misunderstanding regarding the need to use condoms to prevent sexually transmitted diseases. This study emphasizes the need to verify the patient's understanding about drug actions and implications so that additional areas of teaching can be identified.

Freda MC, Abruzzo-Fogarassy M, Adams NV, et al: Women's responses to Depo-Provera, *MCN Am J Matern Child Nurs* 21(4):183-186, 1996.

APPLICATION TO PRACTICE

ASSSESSMENT
History of Present Illness

The first step in assessing the patient with a menstrual cycle disorder or for contraceptive counseling is to obtain the reason for the visit. Information should be obtained as to age, drugs or contraceptives used, and a description of complaints. A complete menstrual history, including age of menarche as well as usual interval and duration of menses should be obtained.

Questions about the presence or absence of premenstrual symptoms, such as breast tenderness, bloating, or abdominal pain that occurs midway between menstrual periods (the Mittelschmerz sign), should be included. Signs and symptoms such as the amount and duration of abnormal bleeding, pain associated with bleeding or intercourse, headaches, presence or absence of abdominal pain, hirsutism, vasomotor symptoms, vaginal dryness, mastalgia, breast discharge, and infertility should all be explored. If the patient reports heavy menses, the health care provider should determine if it is associated with periods of dizziness, fainting, or lightheadedness. The extent to which the menstrual disorder is interfering with the woman's activities of daily living should also be established.

Health History

In addition to a menstrual history, information should be gathered regarding past illnesses, hospitalizations, and surgeries. Any chronic diseases—particularly hepatic, renal, thyroid, or other endocrine disorders—should be noted. The health care provider should ask about a history of coagulopathies, excessive bruising, varicose veins, or thrombophlebitis. Previous gynecologic surgery or treatment for gynecologic disorders, such as an abnormal Papanicolaou smear, endometriosis, or leiomyoma, is important to note.

An obstetric history—details of past pregnancies, ectopic pregnancy, abortions (spontaneous or therapeutic)—should be obtained. Inquire about postpartum hemorrhage or infection.

Drugs the patient is currently taking or has recently taken may affect the diagnosis and management of menstrual cycle disorders or contraceptive choices. The use of tobacco, alcohol, antibiotics, or illicit drugs should be explored. Other lifestyle habits that are important include recent or extreme weight loss or gain, exercise level, stress reduction strategies, and sexual practices.

Lifespan Considerations

Perinatal. For the patient of childbearing age with menstrual cycle or gynecologic disorders, the past gynecologic and obstetric history as well as plans for future childbearing are crucial to diagnosis. The possibility of pregnancy as a source of complaints should always be pursued. The health care provider's first encounter with patients of this age group is often for pregnancy care or for contraception. It may be helpful to elicit the chief complaint, history of present illness, and medical history from the patient before having her change into a gown. Women usually do not appreciate meeting their health care provider for the first time after they have changed into an examining gown and placed their legs in stirrups for a pelvic examination.

Pediatric. Examination of the pediatric patient must be adapted to the individual's developmental needs. The usual dorsal lithotomy examination position is not always appropriate. Very young children may be examined in the frog-leg position or in the mother's arms. Adequate visualization of the prepubertal female genitalia can usually be accomplished by gently retracting the labia majora and applying traction downward on the vagina. Pelvic anatomy can be palpated through the rectum. If invasive instruments are required, they must be small.

Foreign bodies inserted into the vagina are common sources of bleeding, discharge, or odor in the pediatric patient. Other gynecologic problems in pediatric patients may be the result of abuse, molestation, or trauma.

It takes approximately 2 years from the onset of puberty for the hypothalamic-pituitary-ovarian axis to fully mature. As a result, adolescent menstrual cycles are frequently anovulatory. Irregular menstrual bleeding and dysmenorrhea are common complaints of the adolescent female. In obtaining a sexual history from an adolescent, ask about the onset of secondary sexual characteristics and about sexual activity, including the number of partners and use of condoms. Unless bleeding is heavy, a bimanual examination or ultrasound is usually sufficient to adequately assess the patient. A Papanicolaou smear should be obtained if the patient is sexually active. Management depends on the signs and symptoms, history, physical examination, and the need for contraception.

Older Adults. Management of patients during perimenopause or menopause depends on symptoms and individual needs. Past and current medical history is essential. After pathologic causes of abnormal bleeding or pain are eliminated, the patient can be managed with various drugs, depending on the patient's lifestyle, medical condition, and personal preferences. At this time, she should be assessed for the likelihood of age-related complications, such as osteoporosis, urogenital atrophy, cancer of the genital tract, and cardiovascular disease.

Cultural/Social Considerations

Human sexuality is a complex phenomenon encompassing biologic, psychologic, cultural, and social aspects. Biologic aspects include the anatomy and physiology of sexual development and sexual activities, and psychologic aspects consist of gender identity, sexual self-concept, and valuing oneself as a male or female. Cultural and social aspects include sexual orientation learned from the value systems of the family, peers, and community. All of these aspects are interrelated and interdependent.

Changing social norms have made discussion of menstrual cycle concerns more acceptable. However, some patients continue to feel extremely uncomfortable discussing issues of menstrual function. For these reasons, the health care provider should be prepared to deal with this aspect of care. Knowledge about sexuality and sexual norms helps in understanding the patient's behavior and reactions to sexuality in health and illness. The health care provider must be aware of differences in individual and cultural attitudes and perspectives regarding sexuality and the menstrual cycle. Pay attention to the attitudes and words used by the patient to describe the symptoms. Begin the interview with a discussion of other issues, and then move to questions about menarche, age of onset of sexual development, and so on. The discussion should focus on the patient's general knowledge and expectations of the visit before moving to specific concerns.

Ask about the patient's knowledge of hormonal therapies, where appropriate. Compliance with hormonal therapy involves the willingness to take the drugs as prescribed, to have breast and pelvic exams, and to arrange for blood pressure measurements every 6 to 12 months.

Physical Examination

After a thorough history is obtained, a complete head-to-toe physical examination should be performed. The health care provider should note general body habitus, development of secondary sexual characteristics, distribution of body fat, distribution and texture of hair, any bruises, and color of mucous membranes. Baseline vital signs, including height and weight, should be evaluated.

The presence of hirsutism, acne, and exophthalmos as well as the color of the sclera should be noted. Extraocular eye movements and the patient's visual field should be tested. The thyroid should be examined for nodules or enlargement, and any lymphadenopathy noted. The breasts should be examined for dimpling or retraction of tissue, masses, and discharge. The health care provider should use this opportunity to counsel the patient concerning breast self-examination.

The external genitalia should be examined for lesions, erythema, and any obstruction such as an imperforate hymen or septum. Clitoromegaly and the pres-

ence of vaginal discharge, erythema, or vaginal or cervical lesions or polyps should be noted. The color of mucous membranes of the vagina and signs of estrogen deficiency, such as absence of rugae or atrophy, should be included. A bimanual examination should be performed to determine uterine size and any tenderness. The adnexa should be palpated for masses or tenderness. The abdomen should be examined for any masses, organomegaly, hernias, or tenderness.

Laboratory Testing

Women of childbearing age who complain of abnormal menstrual bleeding or who come for contraception should have a pregnancy test. Urine testing for pregnancy is usually sufficient. A Papanicolaou smear and complete blood cell count are basic tests for any female patient. Thyroid function tests (thyroxine and TSH) are useful in evaluating amenorrhea. If the patient's history or examination findings suggest, liver function tests, coagulation tests, a progesterone level test, and cervical cultures for chlamydial infection and gonorrhea may be ordered. If a pituitary tumor is suspected, a prolactin measurement is recommended. If the prolactin level is high, computed tomography or magnetic resonance imaging will be needed to rule out pituitary adenoma.

Transvaginal ultrasonography may be useful in evaluating the patient who complains of pelvic pain. This procedure can provide evidence of uterine size, endometrial thickening, presence of ovarian cysts, presence of leiomyoma, and the suspicion or likelihood of an ectopic pregnancy.

In the perimenopausal or menopausal patient with intermenstrual bleeding, an FSH level higher than 40 IU/mL indicates ovarian failure (5 to 20 IU/mL is normal). An endometrial biopsy evaluates for uterine proliferation or hyperplasia. Office hysteroscopy is practical to visualize the endometrium and obtain directed sampling in the patient who is not actively bleeding. Dilation and curettage may be required if an adequate sample cannot be obtained by biopsy or hysteroscopy or if treatment is unsuccessful.

GOALS OF THERAPY

Treatment goals for the patient with menstrual cycle disorders consist of accurate diagnosis followed by amelioration or elimination, when possible, of the symptoms. A primary management goal should be to choose the intervention that carries the fewest risks and adverse effects, is least invasive, and is appropriate for the patient's age and circumstances.

For the patient seeking contraception, the goals are similar to those noted previously. The patient should be provided with effective and reversible contraception that carries a minimum risk for adverse effects.

For the perimenopausal woman, the goals are relief of menopausal symptoms and reduction of the risks for osteoporosis.

INTERVENTION
Administration

In general, multiphasic oral contraceptives are started on day 1 of the menses to ensure first-cycle inhibition of ovulation. Monophasic oral contraceptives are started on day 5 or 6 of the menses. Ovulation is inhibited as long as the drug is started on one of these days.

Alternative dosing schedules have been effectively used by some patients. For example, if the timing of the menstrual flow is problematic, such as for honeymoon, holidays, or athletics, skipping a period is possible. To cause a change in cycle, a new 21-day package is started as soon as the previous one has been completed. The patient should be advised that breakthrough bleeding may occur with this regimen. For women taking a triphasic formulation with significant increase in the progestin component, a new package may be started. This regimen minimizes the chance of spotting as a result of a relative fall in the progesterone level. For the patient taking a monophasic product who experiences headaches or migraines during the week she is off her contraceptive, consideration may be given to changing to a different oral contraceptive. Be sure to contact the health care provider before attempting alternative dosing schedules.

There are several regimens for perimenopausal or menopausal women that assist in controlling signs and symptoms. These regimens are identified in Table 59-2.

For the patient taking an estrogen, assess vital signs, blood pressure, and weight at every office visit. Assess for dependent edema. Monitor liver function test results and serum lipid profile. Patients with metastatic bone disease who are taking estrogens may develop severe hypercalcemia. Monitor serum electrolyte levels (see Chapter 64).

For the patient taking progestins, assess vital signs, blood pressure, vision, menstrual history, weight, and history of weight gain or loss. Assess dependent areas for edema. Assess the skin for acne, and the hair for loss or changes in growth. Perform a mental status examination. Monitor liver function test results.

Monitor the blood pressure, pulse, weight, and skin for the patient taking oral contraceptives. Assess for signs of depression, including withdrawal, insomnia, anorexia, and lack of interest in personal appearance. Tactfully ask about changes in libido; the patient may be reluctant to discuss the problem. Ask specifically about the appearance of any leg pain, sudden onset of chest pain, shortness of breath, hematemesis, dizziness, changes in vision or speech, or weakness or numbness of an arm or leg. These signs and symptoms may indicate pulmonary embolism or other thromboembolic problem. Monitor the blood cell count and liver function test results.

Education

For many women, a gynecologic examination is the most likely time to seek medical care. Therefore it is a valuable time to educate the patient about her body and its function as well as illness prevention and health maintenance. The woman should be taught about the benefits of regular check-ups accompanied by an annual pelvic examination, Papanicolaou smear, clinical breast examination, as well as the value of regular breast self-examinations. The important roles that diet, exercise, recreation, and smoking cessation play in current and future health, including prevention of osteoporosis, should be included in the teaching. Many women are interested in hormone supplements. Be prepared to discuss the benefits and risks of self-treatment with these products (Box 59-2). Emphasize the importance of regular follow-up visits to monitor for adverse effects.

BOX 59-2 | **Phytoestrogens as Sources of Estrogenic Activity**

Whether or not to take estrogen replacement therapy is a difficult decision for many women to make because it involves weighing relative risks of several possible effects. For many women, the fear of increased risk of uterine or breast cancer persuades them to avoid the powerful synthetic or animal-derived estrogens used in replacement therapy. Some of these women seek to lessen symptoms of menopause with phytoestrogens, which are plant-derived chemicals that have mild estrogenic effects. Soy products have been best studied for this effect. At least three servings daily of soy-derived foods are needed for an effect, but more concentrated powders are also available. A concentrate of red clover is available that contains the same type of phytoestrogens, which may reduce the hot flashes associated with menopause. If these weaker phytoestrogens are used with the stronger, prescription estrogens, the phytoestrogens will block some of the effects of the stronger drugs.

Several other plant-derived products are promoted for their estrogenic effects, but these products are less well studied and may produce other, unwanted actions. For example, a product containing black cohosh has sedative and antihypertensive effects that may interfere with drug therapy for hypertension. Some products combine black cohosh, kava, and soy, but these products can produce sedation. A Chinese herbal product, dong quai, is purported to treat symptoms of menopause, but this effect has not been documented and the herb does induce photosensitivity and may be carcinogenic.

Estrogens. Advise the patient to take the drug as ordered even if she is not feeling well. Nausea may develop during the first few weeks of therapy but should diminish with regular use. Instruct the patient to take doses with or just after meals or food to lessen the risk of GI irritation.

Advise the patient using a transdermal hormonal formulation to wash and dry hands before and after handling patches. Apply the patch to a clean, dry, nonoily area of the abdomen or buttocks. Avoid areas with excess hair, the breast, and areas that are irritated. Avoid the waist and other areas that may be rubbed by clothing. Tell the patient to apply the patch firmly for about 10 seconds. If the patch falls off or comes loose, reapply or apply a new patch. Apply each new patch to a different area, allowing at least a week to pass before an area is used again.

Advise the patient using an estrogen vaginal cream to use the drug at bedtime. Tampons should be avoided, but a sanitary napkin may be worn to protect clothing. Instruct the patient not to use the drug as a lubricant during sexual intercourse; regular absorption by the male partner through the skin of the penis may cause adverse effects. Estrogen may also weaken diaphragms, cervical caps, or condoms. Check with the health care provider or pharmacist for guidance.

Teach the proper injection technique if the patient is to administer intramuscular estrogen formulations at home.

Instruct the patient to notify the health care provider if any of the following develop: breast pain, lumps, or nipple discharge; changes in vaginal bleeding such as breakthrough bleeding or amenorrhea; anorexia, nausea, vomiting, or cramps; or headache or jaundice. For men taking estrogens for breast or prostate cancer, review symptoms of possible thromboembolism: severe or sudden headache, shortness of breath, sudden slurred speech, changes in vision, or weakness or numbness in the arm or leg.

Progestins. Advise the patient taking medroxyprogesterone or conjugated estrogens to take doses with meals to limit nausea. Such nausea should pass in a few weeks. Menstrual bleeding may begin again but should stop in 10 months with continued therapy. Breakthrough bleeding may occur for up to 3 months when the progestin is used continuously as a contraceptive (not a combination estrogen-progestin). Instruct the patient to notify the health care provider if excessive or persistent bleeding occurs.

Women who are fertile and sexually active should be advised to use a birth control method while taking this drug, unless the drug is used daily as a contraceptive. Advise the patient to notify the health care provider immediately if pregnancy is suspected or if 45 days have elapsed since the last menstrual period.

Instruct the patient to notify the health care provider of sudden or severe headache; changes in vision; pain in the chest, leg, or groin; shortness of breath; slurred speech; an increase or decrease in weight of more than 2 pounds per day or 5 pounds per week; nipple discharge; depression; GI distress; swelling of the feet or legs; acne; or thinning of the hair.

Review proper insertion technique for the patient using a vaginal suppository. Instruct patients taking a medroxyprogesterone injection formulation to return at 3-month intervals for administration of this contraceptive. Full contraceptive protection begins immediately if the patient receives the injection within the first 5 days of the menstrual period or within 5 days of delivering a baby if the woman is not breast-feeding. Emphasize the importance of returning on schedule for subsequent injections.

Levonorgestrel implant capsules (Norplant) are inserted under the skin of the upper arm by the health care provider. Instruct the patient to keep gauze in place over the insertion site for 24 hours, then remove it. Leave strips of tape in place for 3 days. Full contraceptive protection begins within 24 hours if the insertion is performed within 7 days of the beginning of the menstrual period. Contraceptive protection should last for 5 years, after which the implants are removed and replaced if desired. Counsel the patient concerning signs of infection and tell her to return to the health care provider if symptoms occur.

Progestins may cause tenderness, swelling, or bleeding of the gums. Encourage the patient to brush and floss teeth carefully and regularly as well as to see a dentist regularly for cleanings and examination.

Oral Contraceptives. Teach the patient that oral contraceptives, IUDs, subdermal implants, and contraceptive injections do not provide protection against HIV or other sexually transmitted diseases. Any patient using hormonal contraceptives should be counseled about smoking and the risk for deep vein thrombosis.

Discuss with the patient when to begin the first dose of an oral contraceptive (usually the first Sunday after menses begins) and to take subsequent doses in order and at the same time of the day. It may take up to 1 week for full contraceptive benefits to develop. Oral contraceptives are available in 21- or 28-day packs. The last seven pills of a 28-day pack are placebos only. Some health care providers recommend that an alternative form of birth control be used during the first cycle of oral contraceptive pills to prevent pregnancy. Tell the patient to take doses with meals or a snack to lessen nausea; it usually lessens with continued use.

Check the instruction leaflet supplied with the drug regarding missed doses of oral contraceptives. Guidelines vary somewhat depending on the product being used, but in general, if one dose of an oral contraceptive is missed, it should be taken as soon as it is remembered. If two doses are missed, the patient should take two tablets of the drug each of the next 2 days and should use a supplemental birth control method also for the rest of the pill cycle while continuing to take the oral contraceptive. If more than two consecutive doses are missed, contraception for that cycle is questionable, and a new package of pills should be started after pregnancy has been ruled out and menses begins.

Remind the patient to inform all health care providers of all drugs being taken. It may take several months for these drugs to be completely eliminated even when the patient has stopped taking them. This is also important when diagnostic blood work is performed; recent or current use of oral contraceptives may influence test results.

Warn the patient to avoid driving or operating hazardous equipment if changes in vision occur and to notify the health care provider. Counsel or refer the patient as needed about smoking cessation, weight-loss programs, and modification of diet to decrease the risk of hyperlipidemia. Warn patients who have diabetes to monitor blood glucose levels carefully because oral contraceptives may alter glucose levels. Instruct the patient to report vaginal bleeding or menstrual irregularities and to notify the health care provider immediately if pregnancy is suspected.

The woman using an IUD birth control method should be taught to check for the presence of the IUD strings in the vagina after each period, because the IUD can be expelled during menstruation without the patient's being aware. She should also be counseled to return to the health care provider if signs of infection appear, such as fever, pelvic pain, severe cramping, or increased bleeding. If she misses a period, she should contact the health care provider immediately to evaluate for the possibility of pregnancy.

If the patient discontinues the oral contraceptive to become pregnant, suggest that she use an alternative form of birth control (i.e., condoms) for 2 months after stopping the pills to ensure more complete excretion of the hormones before conceiving. This strategy reduces the potential effects of the hormones on the fetus.

Postcoital Contraception.   Advise the patient that postcoital contraception is required within 72 hours of unprotected sex. Because this form of contraception has a 3-day window of effectiveness and requires multiple doses of pills, the popular term "morning-after pill" is misleading.

A number of oral contraceptives can be used for postcoital contraception. Almost every woman who needs this type of contraception can safely use this intervention, even women with contraindications to the ongoing use of oral contraceptives. However, postcoital contraception may not prevent ectopic pregnancy. Ectopic pregnancies, left untreated, will cause complications that can cause death. Women should seek medical attention if they have signs of ectopic pregnancy: severe pain on one or both sides of the pelvis; abdominal pain and spotting, especially after a very light or missed menstrual period; and feeling faint or dizzy.

Combination hormone postcoital contraception induces nausea in 30% to 50% of women and vomiting in 15% to 25%. Eating a snack with the pills may be helpful. Antiemetic drugs taken 1 hour before the prescribed regimen may reduce these adverse effects. The patient should be taught about the warning signs of estrogen excess: severe leg pain, severe abdominal pain, chest pain or shortness of breath, severe headaches or dizziness, blurred or loss of vision, and jaundice.

The woman should be told that her next menstrual period may not occur at the usual time and to return for a pregnancy test if menses does not occur within 4 weeks. She should also receive counseling about appropriate forms of birth control for regular use.

EVALUATION

Evaluation of a patient with menstrual cycle disorders involves accurate diagnosis followed by successful amelioration or elimination, when possible, of the symptoms. The treatment regimen chosen should cause few risks and adverse effects, should be the least invasive, and should be appropriate for the patient's age and circumstances.

For the patient seeking contraception, the risk of pregnancy should be reduced and the patient should achieve effective and reversible contraception that carries a minimum risk for adverse effects.

The female patient should be seen by a health care provider annually for routine gynecologic follow-up, regardless of whether she receives hormonal therapy. The first return visit should take place after completion of three cycles of hormone treatment.

Bibliography

Drew S: HRT: an easy reference guide for practice nurses: facts at your fingertips, *Pract Nurse* 22(5):36, 2001.

Ferrara LR, Ligniti E: Pharmacotherapeutics. Hormone replacement therapy, *Clin Lett Nurse Pract* 5(3):7-8, insert 2p, 2001.

Goolsby MJ: Clinical practice guidelines: management of menopause, *J Am Acad Nurse Pract* 13(4):147-151, 2001.

Kessenich CR, Cichon MJ: Progesterone cream as a complementary therapy in menopause, *Clin Lett Nurse Pract* 5(3):5-7, insert 2p, 2001.

Overdorf J, Pachuki-Hyde L, Kressenich C, et al: Osteoporosis: there's so much we can do, *RN* 64(12):30-36, 2001.

Penckofer S, Schwertz D: Hormone replacement therapy: primary and secondary prevention, *J Cardiovasc Nurs* 15(3):1-25, 109-110, 2001.

Pennachio DL: New approaches to emergency contraception, *Pat Care Nurse Pract* 4(3):44-45, 49-50, 62-64, 2001.

Saunders CS: Caring for the postmenopausal woman: decisions in prescribing HRT, *Pat Care Nurse Pract* 4(5):45-46, 49-52, 55-56 passim, 2001.

Sherif K: Considerations in drug therapy: the effects of hormone replacement therapy and oral contraceptive pills on blood pressure, *Prog Cardiovasc Nurs* 15(1):21-23, 28, 2000.

Snyder GM, Sielsch EC, Reville B: The controversy of hormone-replacement therapy in breast cancer survivors, *Oncol Nurs Forum* 25(4):699-708, 1998.

Vega V: Cardioprotective benefits of hormone replacement therapy, *J Am Acad Nurse Pract* 13(2):69-79, 2001.

Internet Resources

http://www.arhp.org/clinical/mar99contents.htm.
http://www.endocrineweb.com/osteoporosis/estrogen.html.
http://www.estronaut.com/a/oral_contraceptives_perimenopause.htm.
http://www.health.nih.gov/
http://www.nau.edu/~ronske/bcp.html.
http://www.nlm.nih.gov/medlineplus/druginfo/estrogensandprogestinsovarianh500070.html.
http://www.nlm.nih.gov/medlineplus/druginfo/estrogensandprogestinsoralcont202228.html.
http://www.nlm.nih.gov/medlineplus/druginfo/estrogenssystemic202226.html.

Drugs Affecting Uterine Motility

JOSEPH A. DiMICCO • KATHLEEN GUTIERREZ

 Visit **http://evolve.elsevier.com/Gutierrez/** for additional information.

KEY TERMS

Myometrium, p. 995

Oxytocin, p. 996

Parturition, p. 996

Postpartum bleeding, p. 996

Prostaglandins, p. 995

Tocolytic, p. 999

OBJECTIVES

- Compare the actions and uses of the three different types of oxytocic drugs.
- Explain how ritodrine may control premature labor.
- Discuss prostaglandins and describe their role and use in labor and delivery.
- Develop a nursing care plan for a patient receiving a drug discussed in this chapter.

 PHYSIOLOGY • Labor and Delivery

The pharmacologic management of labor and delivery is best understood when put into the context of the physiologic processes involved. During pregnancy, high progesterone levels aid in maintaining the pregnancy by suppressing contractions of the myometrium, the powerful muscle layer in the uterine wall. As the pregnancy comes to term, progesterone levels begin to decrease, allowing the uterus to begin to produce prostaglandins. Prostaglandins are involved in regulating myometrial activity. These derivatives of fatty acids are readily formed in their target tissues and are rapidly degraded without persisting in blood for any appreciable time. In the uterus, these hormones induce very powerful myometrial contractions. Prostaglandins, especially prostaglandin E_2 and prostaglandin F_2 alpha, may play a role in the natural induction of labor. Prostaglandin levels rise in the amniotic fluid and other pelvic reproductive tissues as term approaches. This increasing concentration of prostaglandins has been suggested to be the stimulus causing Braxton-Hicks contractions, the mild myometrial contractions occurring during the final few weeks of pregnancy. **Oxytocin**, a hormone produced by the posterior pituitary, is also capable of inducing uterine contractions. In fact, the term *oxytocic* has come to mean any drug that enhances or causes uterine motility or contractions. The uterus increases its sensitivity to oxytocin at term and during the puerperium (period immediately after birth).

Parturition, the process of giving birth, is divided into three phases. During stage I, uterine contractions begin to increase in frequency and intensity, and the cervix begins to dilate. The second stage begins when dilation of the cervix is complete and ends with the delivery of the infant. Stage III begins with the delivery of the infant and ends with the delivery of the placenta. Uterine contractions continue for hours to days, with the frequency and intensity of the contractions diminishing with time.

When contractions occur during labor and delivery, the myometrium compresses major blood vessels supplying oxygen to the fetus. The result is that during a contraction the fetus is relatively anoxic (starved for oxygen). When the uterus relaxes between contractions, oxygenated blood quickly returns to the fetus. If the uterus is overstimulated and fails to relax sufficiently between contractions, the prolonged anoxia can harm the fetus. Induction of labor with one of the oxytocic drugs carries with it the risk of producing this condition. Therefore all patients in whom labor is being induced should receive continuous care, and fetal monitoring should be done when possible. Oxytocin is the drug of choice to induce or stimulate labor because it seems to allow the uterus to relax between contractions. The ergot alkaloids and other oxytocic drugs tend to increase the overall tone of the myometrium and the strength of contractions; therefore they carry a greater risk of producing fetal anoxia. Prostaglandins and prostaglandin analogs have been used to produce or facilitate therapeutic abortions and are becoming increasingly popular as another more natural means of enhancing uterine contractility in labor and delivery.

Uterine contractions that occur after delivery have two beneficial effects on the mother. First, they are responsible for expulsion of the afterbirth and produce a general cleansing of the uterus. Second, these contractions aid in controlling **postpartum bleeding** by clamping the vessels that were ruptured by the birth process. If bleeding is a problem at this stage, the physician may use an agent with a longer and more continuous action such as methylergonovine.

DRUG CLASS • Oxytocic Drugs

oxytocin (Syntocinon, Pitocin)

MECHANISM OF ACTION

Oxytocin interacts with specific receptors in the myometrium and raises the level of calcium inside these smooth muscle cells; this action induces contraction of the myometrium. The uterus is relatively insensitive to the action of oxytocin until labor has started.

Oxytocin also acts on breast tissue; it stimulates the myoepithelium of the breast and promotes milk letdown. Suckling by the infant sets off a reflex action in which oxytocin release is stimulated. The central nervous system controls this process; the sight of the infant is sufficient in some women to induce oxytocin release and milk letdown. Oxytocin action is responsible for the improved uterine muscle tone in nursing mothers and for the more rapid return of the uterus to the pregravid (before birth) size in these women.

USES

Oxytocin is the preferred drug to induce or augment labor. In addition, it may be used to control postpartum bleeding by inducing contraction of the myometrium. The intranasal route is used to promote milk letdown and facilitate breast-feeding. Oxytocin has been used to induce or complete an abortion, but mifepristone is now the drug of choice for this purpose (see Chapter 59).

PHARMACOKINETICS

Oxytocin is a peptide and is therefore ineffective orally and quickly broken down by enzymes in target tissues and in plasma. Oxytocin has a quick onset of action by intranasal, intramuscular, or intravenous routes, but the effect disappears within 3 hours. Effects of intranasal doses on milk letdown are lost within 20 minutes.

ADVERSE REACTIONS AND CONTRAINDICATIONS

Maternal adverse reactions include both those related to the drug and those caused by contractions. Adverse reactions to oxytocin are rare but include nausea and vomiting. Oxytocin is known to cause water intoxication and death with prolonged use. Excessive contractions, or increased strength of contractions, can cause blood loss, uterine rupture, and pelvic hematoma. Oxytocin should be avoided in patients with a history of allergy to the drug. It should not be used to augment or induce labor in a patient with abnormal fetal presentation, pronounced cephalopelvic disproportion, placenta previa, fetal distress, or hypertonic uterine contractions.

TOXICITY

At very high doses, oxytocin may cause hypotension with a rebound of hypertension. Reflexive tachycardia and other arrhythmias have also been noted. In rare cases, the intensity of the uterine contractions or a high uterine resting tone can rupture the uterus, an event with potentially fatal consequences for the mother. Other rare but potentially fatal adverse reactions include afibrinogenemia, anaphylaxis, subarachnoid hemorrhoid, coma, and death.

Potentially severe fetal reactions to oxytocin include abruptio placenta, bradycardia, arrhythmias, fetal trauma, brain damage, and fetal death secondary to asphyxia.

INTERACTIONS

Oxytocin may cause excessively strong uterine contractions if combined with other oxytocic drugs or with intraamniotic urea or sodium chloride. Vasoconstricting drugs given concurrently with oxytocin have been linked to severe hypertension. Cyclopropane anesthesia is known to cause tachycardia and hypotension or bradycardia with atrioventricular rhythms. Similarly, thiopental given with oxytocin has been associated with a delay in anesthesia induction.

 DRUG CLASS • **Ergot Alkaloids Used as Oxytocics**

methylergonovine (Methergine)

MECHANISM OF ACTION

Methylergonovine is one of the ergot alkaloids, a compound synthesized by certain types of fungus. Ergot alkaloids were known as poisons since the Middle Ages, when it was noted that dry gangrene developed in people who consumed grain contaminated by fungus. This extreme reaction is caused by the potent vasoconstrictive effect of ergot alkaloids. Blood flow to the limbs may be reduced so severely that the tissues die, causing the limbs to fall away eventually with little bleeding. In addition, pregnant women who ate the affected grain entered an abrupt and devastating labor that expelled fetuses at any stage of development. Methylergonovine has somewhat less vasoconstrictive activity than other ergot alkaloids (which are used to prevent or treat migraine, as discussed in Chapter 15) but acts directly on the uterus to increase the force and frequency of myometrial contractions.

USES

Methylergonovine is indicated for postpartum hemorrhage after delivery of the placenta.

PHARMACOKINETICS

Oral doses of methylergonovine produce effects on uterine contractions within 5 to 10 minutes. The drug can also be given by intramuscular or intravenous injection; when given intramuscularly the onset of uterine contractions occurs within 2 to 5 minutes. Intravenous usage of the drug is limited to life-threatening situations only. Effects are maintained for about 3 hours after administration by any route. Methylergonovine is inactivated in the liver, and the metabolites are excreted in urine.

ADVERSE REACTIONS AND CONTRAINDICATIONS

Methylergonovine may produce bradycardia and coronary vasospasm and has the potential to cause anginal attacks, arrhythmias, and myocardial infarction, although these are rare at clinically used doses. Acute allergic reactions may also occur, but these, too, are very infrequent. More common effects include nausea and uterine cramping.

Any of the ergot alkaloids are avoided in patients with significant cardiovascular disease, peripheral vascular disease, hypertension, eclampsia, or preeclampsia. These conditions are worsened by the vasoconstrictive effects of the drugs.

TOXICITY

At high doses, methylergonovine may produce peripheral vasospasm or vasoconstriction, angina, miosis, confusion, respiratory depression, seizures, or unconsciousness. Uterine tetany may also occur.

INTERACTIONS

Vasoconstrictors may be more potent in the presence of the ergot alkaloids, which are themselves vasoconstrictors.

DRUG CLASS • Prostaglandins

alprostadil (Edex, Muse, Caverject)

bimatoprost (Lumigan)

carboprost (Hemabate, Prostin/15M✽)

dinoprostone (Prepidil,✽ Cervidil, Prostin E$_2$)

epoprostenol (Flolan)

latanoprost (Xalatan)

misoprostol (Cytotec)

travoprost (Travatan)

unoprostone (Rescula)

MECHANISM OF ACTION

Prostaglandins are a family of related naturally occurring compounds derived from arachidonic acid that play important roles in diverse functions of the body (see Chapter 14). Many prostaglandins are potent stimulators of the myometrium and have been successfully used to induce abortion during the second trimester, when the uterus is resistant to oxytocin. Dinoprostone is identical to the naturally occurring prostaglandin E$_2$. Misoprostol is a synthetic analog of prostaglandin E$_1$, whereas carboprost is more closely related to prostaglandin F$_2$ alpha. All three drugs also facilitate delivery by promoting dilation and softening of the cervix (called "ripening"), an effect usually seen at lower doses than those that are required for stimulating uterine motility.

Carboprost and, to a lesser degree, misoprostol may stimulate vascular smooth muscle to cause vasoconstriction as well, while dinoprostone can produce vasodilation.

Several other prostaglandins or analogs are used for effects on other tissues and organs. These include alprostadil (identical to prostaglandin E$_1$), epoprostenol (prostaglandin I$_2$), the prostaglandin F$_2$ alpha analogs latanoprost and travoprost, bimatoprost, and unoprostone (Table 60-1).

TABLE 60-1

Clinical Uses of Prostaglandins and Prostaglandin Analogs

Drug	Identity and Action	Clinical Uses
alprostadil	Identical to prostaglandin E$_1$; causes vasodilation	*Systemic:* Maintenance of patent ductus arteriosus in neonates with congenital heart defects *Local:* Facilitation of penile erection in males with erectile dysfunction or in diagnostic imaging of penile vasculature
bimatoprost	Synthetic prostaglandin analog (a prostamide); enhances drainage of intraocular fluid	*Local:* treatment of glaucoma or ocular hypertension (see Chapter 65)
carboprost	Synthetic analog of prostaglandin F$_2$ alpha; stimulates smooth muscle of uterus and arterioles; facilitates cervical dilation and softening	*Systemic:* Induction of labor or therapeutic abortion; treatment of postpartum hemorrhage
dinoprostone	Identical to prostaglandin E$_2$; stimulates smooth muscle of uterus; facilitates cervical dilation and softening	*Local:* Induction of labor or therapeutic abortion; treatment of postpartum hemorrhage; treatment of benign hydatiform mole
epoprostenol	Identical to prostaglandin I$_2$; vasodilates systemic and pulmonary vasculature and inhibits platelet aggregation	*Systemic:* Treatment of pulmonary hypertension
latanoprost	Synthetic analog of prostaglandin F$_2$ alpha; enhances drainage of intraocular fluid	*Local:* Treatment of glaucoma or ocular hypertension (see Chapter 65)
misoprostol	Synthetic analog of prostaglandin E$_1$; enhances natural defense mechanisms in gastric mucosa and inhibits stimulus-induced gastric acid secretion; enhances or evokes uterine contractions	*Systemic:* Prevention and treatment of NSAID-induced gastric ulcers; therapeutic abortion (with mifepristone); induction of labor (see Chapter 14)
travoprost	Synthetic analog of prostaglandin F$_2$ alpha; enhances drainage of intraocular fluid	*Local:* Treatment of glaucoma or ocular hypertension (see Chapter 65)
unoprostone	Synthetic prostaglandin analog; enhances drainage of intraocular fluid	*Local:* Treatment of glaucoma or ocular hypertension (see Chapter 65)

USES

Carboprost and dinoprostone have been used to induce abortion. However, mifepristone, a progestin antagonist (see Chapter 59), is more reliably effective as an abortifacient and causes fewer adverse effects. In this context, misoprostol is commonly used along with mifepristone to aid in expulsion. Carboprost, because of its vasoconstrictive properties, has also been used to treat postpartum bleeding.

Dinoprostone administered as an intravaginal gel can be employed to induce labor, although oxytocin is usually preferred and has been used in the treatment of hydatidiform (uterine) moles. Dinoprostone or misoprostol can also be used to ripen the cervix to facilitate vaginal delivery. Recently, misoprostol has gained popularity for the induction of labor as well.

The uses of the other drugs in this class illustrate the many roles of prostaglandins in the body. Epoprostenol produces a pattern of changes in cardiovascular function that make it useful in the treatment of pulmonary hypertension. Alprostadil is employed in the treatment of a specific birth defect affecting the heart called patent ductus arteriosus. Alprostadil has also been used in the treatment of erectile dysfunction in males. However, because the drug must be given for this purpose by injection directly into the penis or by a suppository inserted into the urethra, alprostadil has been largely replaced by sildenafil (Viagra; see Chapter 39). Bimatoprost, latanoprost, travoprost, and unoprostone are all used topically in the eye in the treatment of glaucoma (see Chapter 65).

PHARMACOKINETICS

Prostaglandins tend to be rapidly degraded in the blood and unstable in gastric acid. Only misoprostol is given orally for effects related to labor and delivery. The drug is rapidly absorbed and converted in the liver to an active metabolite, misoprostol acid. This metabolite, which is primarily responsible for the action of the drug, is eliminated by the kidneys and has a plasma half-life of 20 to 40 minutes. Thus, the duration of action of an oral dose is about 3 hours.

Dinoprostone is administered as a gel or suppository directly into the vagina. Intravaginal delivery keeps the drug at the site of action and avoids rapid degradation carried out in maternal lung and liver. It also minimizes adverse systemic effects (see later in this chapter). Carboprost can be given by deep intramuscular injection.

ADVERSE REACTIONS AND CONTRAINDICATIONS

These drugs frequently cause significant adverse effects, many of which are related directly to the known actions and roles of prostaglandins in the body (see Chapter 14). Among these reactions are gastrointestinal (GI) adverse effects, including diarrhea, nausea, vomiting, and stomach cramps. Fever, chills, and flushing are also noted.

Less common but more serious reactions include anaphylaxis, arrhythmias, bronchoconstriction, chest pain, hypertension, and peripheral vasoconstriction. Because of these potential problems, these drugs are usually avoided in patients with significant cardiovascular disease or those with a history of asthma or pulmonary disease. All of these adverse effects can be minimized or avoided entirely by localized administration of dinoprostone.

TOXICITY

Overdose of prostaglandins may cause the exaggerated responses already noted as well as uterine cramping or tetany.

INTERACTIONS

Prostaglandins are usually not combined with oxytocin because the risk of uterine tetany or uterine laceration increases.

DRUG CLASS • Uterine Relaxants (Tocolytics)

ritodrine (Yutopar)
terbutaline (Bricanyl, Brethine)

MECHANISM OF ACTION

Premature labor is sometimes treated with drugs that stimulate beta$_2$ receptors because stimulation of these receptors in the uterus causes relaxation of the myometrium, also called a tocolytic effect. Agonists of beta$_2$ receptors cause adverse effects throughout the body, however, as a result of beta receptor stimulation in other tissues. Ritodrine is the beta$_2$ agonist usually used in halting premature labor. This drug effectively relaxes the myometrium but also affects the peripheral vasculature and other tissues. Oral terbutaline, a beta$_2$ receptor agonist is commonly employed as a bronchodilator (see Chapter 12) but is also used in the management of premature labor. Terbutaline is less expensive than ritodrine.

The pharmacology of beta$_2$ receptor agonists in general is discussed in detail in Chapter 12.

USES

Ritodrine is used to halt spontaneous labor when it appears after the twentieth week of pregnancy and before the thirty-sixth week. Spontaneous labor beginning before the twentieth week often is associated with irreversible problems in fetal development and may not be interrupted.

PHARMACOKINETICS

Ritodrine is administered intravenously as soon after premature labor begins as possible. Intravenous administration produces effects within 5 minutes. After intravenous administration, the drug has a distribution plasma half-life of only 6 to 9 minutes, although its elimination half-life may be 2 to 5 hours.

An oral preparation is available in Canada, but bioavailability is low (about 30%), and oral efficacy has not been convincingly demonstrated for the drug. Ritodrine is inactivated in the liver and eliminated by the kidneys.

Terbutaline may be administered orally or subcutaneously. Intravenous administration produces effects within 6 to 15 minutes with peak action reached in 15 to 30 minutes. The duration of action is 1.5 to 4 hours. Elimination of terbutaline is partially achieved through biotransformation in the liver to inactive conjugates that are then excreted in the urine.

ADVERSE REACTIONS AND CONTRAINDICATIONS

The major adverse reactions noted with these drugs are associated with beta stimulation and include anxiety, tachycardia, palpitations, nausea and vomiting, trembling, flushing, and headache. However, these effects appear to be transient and rarely warrant termination of therapy. Patients should be observed for undue tachycardia or signs of cardiac distress such as ST-wave depression and T-wave inversion, particularly with terbutaline. The fetal heart may also be stimulated. Ritodrine increases the workload of the mother's heart and is contraindicated in patients with preexisting cardiac disease.

Ritodrine and terbutaline can cause marked hyperglycemia. Although treatment is usually not required, persistent hyperglycemia can result in fetal tachycardia, hyperinsulinemia, and reactive hypoglycemia in the fetus should partuition proceed. The use of beta agonists in patients with diabetes is hazardous and is usually contraindicated.

Hypokalemia is another consequence of ritodrine administration. This state reflects the movement of potassium into the intracellular compartment. Total body stores are not reduced, and treatment is usually not indicated.

TOXICITY

Overdoses of ritodrine may produce signs of excessive beta stimulation, especially noticed as cardiac stimulation. There is also decreased renal elimination of sodium, potassium, and water with the use of these drugs. This is presumably due to the enhanced secretion of renin. If hydration during $beta_2$ agonist therapy is overly vigorous, pulmonary edema may result, with or without evidence of myocardial failure. Pulmonary edema may occur in up to 15% of patients.

INTERACTIONS

Beta blockers inhibit the effects of ritodrine, whereas beta adrenergic agonists may increase the risk of cardiovascular adverse effects. Corticosteroids increase the risk of pulmonary edema because of their effects on fluid balance.

DRUG CLASS • Other Tocolytic Drugs

CNS depressants may halt premature labor. For example, ethanol, which is an inhibitor of oxytocin release and a CNS depressant, has been used to halt premature labor. The levels required to relax the uterus are sufficient to produce acute alcohol intoxication. Controlled clinical trials have suggested ritodrine is more effective and less toxic than ethanol.

General anesthetics may also relax the uterus. Enflurane and halothane are the preferred drugs. In addition to CNS effects, these drugs may act directly on the myometrium and may also slow catecholamine release from the adrenal gland, thus reducing endogenous stimulators of myometrial activity.

Progesterone is the natural steroid that normally functions as a uterine relaxant. The use of this or other progestins is not recommended in cases of uterine hypertonicity during delivery because the hormone may not reach the uterus in sufficient quantities to relax the uterus quickly and effectively. Use of progesterone during earlier stages of pregnancy may cause undesirable effects on the developing fetus.

Because prostaglandins are now thought to play a role in the natural increase in uterine contractions seen in labor, attempts have been made to suppress premature labor using drugs that inhibit the synthesis of prostaglandins (see Chapter 14). Although some data suggest that the NSAID indomethacin may be somewhat effective in this regard, any effect appears to be relatively modest and more study is needed.

Magnesium sulfate has been used in the past to inhibit preterm labor. Presumably, magnesium acts to decrease uterine contractions by inhibiting the entry of calcium into myometrial muscle cells. Accordingly, recent studies suggest that calcium channel blockers may be highly effective in the treatment of premature labor. Nifedipine and nicardipine have been used most often. Some believe these drugs to be as effective as beta agonists or magnesium in suppressing uterine motility while causing fewer undesirable adverse effects.

 APPLICATION TO PRACTICE

ASSESSMENT
History of Present Illness

The assessment of the patient requiring drugs to induce, augment, or stop labor begins with a detailed nursing history and physical. Ask about the patient's perception of what brought her to the health care provider or hospital. It is exceedingly important to determine the gestational age of the fetus, because the type of drug therapy may differ considerably based on this information. Other questions to ask include whether the last menstrual period was normal, the length of her cycles, whether an ultrasound was done early in the pregnancy, if the ultrasound results changed her due dates, and if the health care provider ever questioned the dates. If the patient is experiencing contractions, the assessment includes time of onset, duration, frequency, and the perceived strength of the contraction. Has the patient noted leaking of vaginal fluid? If the answer is yes, it is important to ascertain the quantity, color, and odor of the fluid.

A complete assessment of the current pregnancy includes reviewing the first, second, and third trimester of the pregnancy for any problems or complications. It is important to determine whether the mother has had previous contractions or bleeding episodes. If the answer is yes, query the patient as to what treatment was initiated and if it was effective. Reviewing the prenatal records, when available, is an essential part of assessing the current pregnancy. The fetus is also a patient; therefore the mother should be asked about fetal movement.

A patient in preterm labor should be asked about recent sexual intercourse. Recent sexual intercourse, because of the release of prostaglandins from the cervix and prostaglandins in the semen, may cause the onset of contractions.

Health History

Important information is gained through the assessment of the medical and surgical history. As part of the drug history, allergies to both food and drugs, including physiologic responses, need to be documented. Document current and previous drug use including prescription drugs, over-the-counter drugs, illicit drugs, and alcohol intake.

The patient's obstetric history can often be insightful. The outcome of all previous pregnancies should be identified. This includes information about any abortions (spontaneous or elective), and previous term or preterm deliveries. The length of labor, type of delivery, the gestational age at delivery, weight of the infant, and any complications are important to ascertain. The past use of drugs to prevent delivery or to induce delivery is important to note.

Lifespan Considerations

Pregnancy is a developmental challenge and a pivotal point in life that is accompanied by stress and anxiety, whether the pregnancy is desired or not. Pregnancy can be viewed as a developmental stage, with its own distinct developmental tasks. If a pregnancy terminates in the birth of a child, the couple enters a new stage of life together. However, the couple must face the realities of labor and birth before parenthood can be achieved.

Assessment of how the woman's pregnancy alters her body image and necessitates a reordering of social relationships and role change should be determined. There may be ambivalence, acceptance, introversion, and mood swings as the woman undertakes to maintain her soundness and that of her family, and at the same time, incorporate new life into the family system. The partner is often viewed as a bystander or observer of the pregnancy. Evaluation of the partner's perception of the pregnancy should be performed. Continued reevaluation will need to be accomplished as the pregnancy progresses.

Cultural/Social Considerations

Cultural assessment is an important aspect of history taking. The health care provider should identify the primary beliefs, values, and behaviors that relate to pregnancy and childbearing. This includes information about ethnicity, degree of affiliation with the ethnic group, patterns of decision-making, religious preferences, language and communication styles, and common etiquette practices. An exploration of the couple's expectation of the health care system should also be noted. The degree to which these variables are in concert with the woman's personal values, beliefs, and behaviors is important when planning care. Discrepancies should be considered and a determination made as to whether the patient's system is supportive, neutral, or harmful in relation to possible interventions. The health care provider then faces two considerations: identifying ways of persuading the patient to accept the proposed therapy, or accepting her rationale for refusing therapy if she is not willing to change her belief system.

Assessing the patient and her partner's views of labor, induction, and use of drugs is an important factor. Couples may have prepared a birth plan. Reading this plan may provide some insight into their views about the laboring and delivery process. Some women perceive the use of any drug during labor as a failure; others are terrified at the thought of labor without some type of pain relief drug or anesthesia. Previous sexual abuse or rape can affect the course of the labor and the amount of discomfort the patient experiences during vaginal examinations and subsequent labor.

Society as a whole tends to view labor as a natural process. "Women have been dropping babies in the fields for years" is a persuasive attitude that has been quoted many times. Therefore, women who require induction of labor or who are in preterm labor may believe that they have failed or that their body has failed them. Added to this problem is anxiety and fear the patient and family have about the survival of the infant. Parents often experience tremendous apprehension about the survival and quality of life of their unborn child. Compounding this issue is the feeling of powerlessness the patient and partner often experience. In America's multicultural society, understanding the patient's cultural views of the labor experience influences how the health care provider perceives the patient's attitudes and influences the plan of care.

Physical Examination

The physical examination should include evaluation of vital signs, along with the assessment of fetal heart tones. A sterile vaginal examination or sterile speculum examination is performed, depending on the status of the fetal membranes and gestational age of the fetus. Before the thirty-seventh week or if it must be determined whether the patient is leaking amniotic fluid, a sterile speculum examination should be done in place of the sterile vaginal examination. The speculum examination eliminates cervical stimulation, which can cause the release of prostaglandins, thus initiating contractions. The speculum examination also decreases the chance of vertical transmission of bacteria that can occur with a vaginal examination. Deep tendon reflexes should be evaluated on all patients.

Laboratory Testing

An initial external fetal monitor strip evaluation yields a wealth of information. The baseline fetal heart rate, the variability, and the presence of periodic changes are evaluated. The monitor strip also informs the health care provider of the timing and duration of uterine contractions. The strength of contractions cannot be truly assessed without an internal uterine pressure catheter.

The patient's urine should be assessed for evidence of dehydration, urinary tract infection, and preeclampsia. The urine should also be checked for glucose, ketones, nitrates, leukocyte esterase, and protein.

Routine blood work for a laboring patient is a complete blood count (CBC) and blood drawn and placed on hold in the event the patient needs a transfusion. The patient in preterm labor is evaluated for infection through blood work and amniocentesis.

GOALS OF THERAPY

The goal of therapy with a uterine stimulant is to establish regular contractions that occur every 3 to 5 minutes and last for 60 to 90 seconds. To affect cervical effacement and dilation, a rate that mimics normal spontaneous labor (approximately 1 cm/hour) is desired to deliver a fetus vaginally without increasing the risk to the mother or the fetus.

Labor augmentation may be warranted when nondrug measures such as amniotomy (artificial rupture of membranes) and nipple stimulation are unsuccessful. It may also be appropriate in cases in which prolongation of pregnancy is dangerous to the fetus or the mother (e.g., hypertension, diabetes). Oxytocin is considered the initial treatment if Bishop's score is 5 or more or in patients who are gravida one or two. However, induction of labor without cervical softening has a high failure rate. Oxytocin should not be used to induce labor for any reason other than medical necessity. The convenience of the health care provider or patient is an unacceptable reason for induction.

The use of prostaglandins produces effective preinduction cervical ripening. When prostaglandins are administered locally, they decrease the duration of labor, shorten the induction to delivery period, decrease the dosage of oxytocin, and reduce the overall failure of induction. Furthermore, uterine response to oxytocin is enhanced in the presence of PGE_2. However, the time to induction and duration of labor are longer with prostaglandin gel, although patient acceptance is greater.

The goal in abortifacient treatment is to cause evacuation of uterine contents with increasing maternal risk for complications. Selection of a uterine stimulant to be used as an abortifacient depends on gestational age. During weeks 1 to 12, suction dilatation and curettage is the procedure of choice. Mifepristone (RU486) may also be used in some instances. Other drugs are generally ineffective during this time. During weeks 13 to 20, dilation plus evacuation is generally preferred. Oxytocin is less effective during this time but may be used as an adjunct, if necessary. Hypertonic solutions (e.g., saline, urea) behave as poisons to the placenta and fetus, thus acting as an abortifacient.

When used, mifepristone is employed in combination with prostaglandins (i.e., misoprostol) for termination of early pregnancy. It is given first, and the prostaglandin is administered 48 hours later. The combination of the two drugs stimulates uterine contractions and the expulsion of uterine contents. The oral formulations of both drugs make the procedure more convenient and less expensive than intramuscular prostaglandins.

The treatment goal in tocolysis is to stop uterine contractions and prevent progression of cervical effacement and dilation. Additionally, it is desired to delay delivery of the fetus long enough (24 to 48 hours) to permit acceleration of fetal lung maturity if the gestation is less than 32 weeks.

Tocolytics stop contractions for 24 to 48 hours, but there is debate about whether they improve perinatal outcomes or reduce the overall rate of preterm birth. There is a trend that suggests tocolytics decrease infant mortality in gestations of 24 to 27 weeks only. Because perinatal morbidity and mortality are not altered, the indication for tocolysis is to delay delivery long enough to administer corticosteroids to the mother. The corticosteroids hasten fetal lung maturity and reduce the incidence of respiratory distress in the premature newborn.

In general, tocolysis is indicated if the onset of labor is between 24 and 32 weeks' gestation, with documented cervical dilation and uterine contractions that occur every 7 to 10 minutes and lasting 30 seconds. Therapy is used only if there are no contraindications to stopping PTL; when major maternal illness cannot be controlled; in the presence of preeclampsia, abruptio placentae, chorioamnionitis, and severe fetal anomalies that are incompatible with life; or in the case of fetal demise.

When the decision to use a tocolytic drug is made, treatment is likely to be successful if cervical dilation is less than 4 cm and cervical effacement is less than 80%. Tocolysis is usually not attempted if the membranes have ruptured because there is a risk of infection. Subcutaneous terbutaline is the drug of choice if the cervix is less than 3 cm dilated. Intravenous magnesium sulfate or a beta$_2$-agonist is used for women with cervical dilation over 3 cm. After 48 hours, indomethacin, a nonsteroidal antiinflammatory drug, may be added if intravenous tocolysis is not slowing uterine contractions.

INTERVENTION
Administration

Uterine Stimulants. Fetal maturity, presentation, and pelvic adequacy should be assessed before administration of oxytocin. Furthermore, the character, frequency, and duration of uterine contractions, resting uterine tone, and fetal heart rate should be monitored during therapy. A Y-connection should be used when preparing the intravenous infusion so that the oxytocin solution can be discontinued if necessary while access to a vein is maintained. Oxytocin should not be administered by more than one route simultaneously, and infusion should be stopped if any of the following conditions exist:
- Contractions are less than 2 minutes apart.
- Contractions are stronger than 50 to 65 mm Hg on the uterine pressure monitor.
- Resting uterine pressure is greater than 15 to 20 mm Hg.
- Contractions that last longer than 60 to 90 seconds.
- A significant change in fetal heart rate occurs.

Should any of these conditions occur, the oxytocin should be discontinued, the patient turned onto the left side (to prevent fetal anoxia) and given oxygen, and the health care provider notified immediately. Terbutaline can be used for fetal distress. Magnesium sulfate should be available if excessive stimulation of the myometrium occurs and the patient has a known cardiac defect. Additionally, the patient should be monitored for signs and symptoms of water intoxication (drowsiness, listlessness, confusion, headache, anuria). The health care provider should be notified if the patient's condition suggests intoxication.

As with oxytocin use, the frequency, duration, force of contractions, and uterine resting tone should be monitored during prostaglandin therapy. Dinoprostone-induced adverse effects can be minimized by pretreatment with an antidiarrheal, antiemetic, and antipyretic (e.g., acetaminophen) drug before the use of high-dose prostaglandin.

For cervical ripening, the degree of effacement should be determined before the insertion of the prostaglandin. Use caution to prevent contact of the prostaglandin with the skin. The patient should be in a dorsal recumbent position, and the cervix visualized by the examiner. Sterile technique is used when inserting the prostaglandin gel or suppository. The patient should remain supine for 15 to 30 minutes to minimize leakage from the cervical canal. During low-dose prostaglandin use, the fetus should be monitored for 2 hours after the drug is administered. Patients with hypertension should not receive an ergot alkaloid.

Tocolytics. Before administration of a tocolytic drug, the patient's blood pressure, heart rate, blood glucose levels, and fluid status should be evaluated, as well as the fetal heart rate. The patient should be placed on the left side to minimize blood pressure changes during the infusion. Intravenous administration of a beta$_2$-agonist or magnesium sulfate should be accomplished with the use of an infusion pump in order to accomplish titration better. The use of sodium chloride for infusion should be avoided due to the risk of pulmonary edema. Ritodrine is incompatible with any other drug in solution or in the syringe.

When used, magnesium sulfate infusions should always be administered via intravenous pumps due to the serious consequences of extremely high magnesium levels. The patient's respiratory rate and patellar reflex should be monitored before and throughout therapy. Patient reports that reflect excessive dosage should be managed by decreasing or shutting off the intravenous infusion and by closely observing the patient until lab results are available. Calcium gluconate, the reversal agent for magnesium sulfate, should be on hand. Serum magnesium levels and renal function should be monitored periodically throughout administration of parenteral magnesium sulfate.

There are many drug interactions associated with parenteral administration of magnesium. A drug interaction reference should be consulted before mixing magnesium sulfate in either Y connectors, piggyback containers, or syringes.

Education

Uterine Stimulants. Patients receiving oxytocin infusions should be taught to expect contractions similar to menstrual cramps. They should be advised of the goal of therapy and informed that the infusion rate will be adjusted based on their response. Women receiving prostaglandins at high doses should be forewarned of frequent adverse effects, including nausea, vomiting, diarrhea, and high temperatures, for which they will be premedicated.

Inform the patient who is to receive a prostaglandin that she may note a warm feeling in her vagina during drug administration. When a prostaglandin is used as an abortifacient, the patient should be advised to notify the health care provider if fever, chills, foul-smelling vaginal discharge, lower abdominal pain, or increased bleeding occurs. Once expulsion of uterine contents and placenta has occurred, the patient is thoroughly examined for trauma (cervical or uterine lacerations).

Tocolytics. Educational needs of the patient at risk for preterm labor include reinforcement of preterm birth prevention principles and warning signs of early labor. Even with tocolytic therapy, contractions may resume; instruct the patient to contact her health care provider for reinstitution of intravenous therapy if signs of labor reappear. Women who are receiving beta$_2$-agonists should be taught about the drug's common adverse effects.

Patients on magnesium sulfate should be informed that this drug may cause nausea and vomiting, especially with the loading dose. Additionally, a flushed feeling, burning at the intravenous site, lethargy, blurred vision, and dry mouth may occur.

Patients at risk for preterm delivery should be educated about the drugs that may be used to promote fetal lung maturity and the reasons for their use. Emotional support is vital during therapy.

EVALUATION

The effectiveness of uterine stimulants such as oxytocin can be demonstrated by the onset of effective contractions and an increase in uterine tone without indications of fluid volume excess. The effectiveness of prostaglandins can be demonstrated by the presence of cervical ripening and the induction of labor. If therapy is not successful in 10 to 12 hours, oxytocin is usually discontinued and the patient allowed to rest. The infusion may be restarted the following day.

The effectiveness of tocolysis is demonstrated by the quieting of uterine contractions and a lack of progression of cervical effacement and dilation. Additionally, tocolysis is considered a success if delivery of the fetus has been delayed long enough (24 to 48 hours) to permit acceleration of fetal lung maturity.

Bibliography

Brucker MC: Management of the third stage of labor: an evidence-based approach, *J Midwifery Women's Health* 46(6):347-351, 381-392, 2001.

Kelly AJ, Tan B: Selected Cochrane systematic reviews: intravenous oxytocin alone for cervical ripening and induction of labour, *Birth* 28(4):280-281, 2001.

Ruiz RJ: Mechanisms of full-term and preterm labor: factors influencing uterine activity, *J Obstet Gynecol Neonatal Nurs* 27(6):652-660, 1998.

Internet Resources

http://192.215.104.222/obgyn/cobra/cobra/TEXT/PROTOCOL/7.htm.

http://pregnancy.about.com/cs/inductionoflabor/index_2.htm.

http://www.druginfozone.org/Publications/OSRS/OSRS_chapter_7/osrs_chapter_7.html.

http://www.spensershope.org/Tocolytic%20Medications.htm.

Fertility Drugs

SHERRY F. QUEENER • KATHLEEN GUTIERREZ

 Visit http://evolve.elsevier.com/Gutierrez/ for additional information.

KEY TERMS

Follicle-stimulating hormone (FSH), p. 1006

Gonadotropin-releasing hormone (GnRH), p. 1005

Gonadotropins, p. 1006

Infertility, p. 1005

Luteinizing hormone (LH), p. 1006

Ovarian hyperstimulation syndrome (OHSS), p. 1010

OBJECTIVES

- Identify the most common causes of infertility in men and women.
- Explain the therapeutic rationale for drugs used for infertility.
- Describe the expected adverse reactions to fertility drugs.
- Create a nursing care plan for a man or a woman undergoing drug treatment for infertility.

 PATHOPHYSIOLOGY • Infertility

Infertility is defined as an inability to conceive after 1 year of unprotected coitus or an inability to carry a fetus to term. It is estimated that 40% of infertility results solely from male factors, 40% solely from female factors, and 20% from both. In general, infertility rates increase with age, but infertility has many causes and the treatment is therefore complex.

DISORDERS OF FEMALE FERTILITY

A failure to ovulate, which accounts for about 25% of female infertility, may arise in several ways (Table 61-1). Gonadotropin-releasing hormone (GnRH) is normally released from the hypothalamus and sets off a cascade of events that support fertility in both men and women (see Chapter 55). If the hypothalamus fails such that

TABLE 61-1

Disorders of Fertility

Disorders of Female Fertility

Ovulation Disorders

Hypothalamic amenorrhea	Birth control pills
Idiopathic hypothalamic dysfunction	Stress, weight loss, anorexia

Pituitary Disorders

Hyperprolactinemia	Sheehan's syndrome
Hypogonadotropic hypogonadism	

Ovarian Disorders

Disorders of sexual development	Gonadotropin-resistant ovary syndrome
Polycystic ovary syndrome	Premature ovarian failure
Luteinized unruptured follicle syndrome	

Uterine, Tubal, and Pelvic Disorders

Structural anomalies	Endometriosis or endometritis
Unfavorable cervical mucus	Uterine leiomyomas

Luteal Phase Defects

Lack of progesterone from corpus luteum	

Other Disorders

Radiation	Complications of pregnancy (abortion, cesarean section, postpartum infection, ectopic pregnancy)
Chemical exposure	
Endocrine disorders	

Disorders of Male Fertility

Pretesticular Disorders

Hypogonadotropic hypogonadism	Isolated gonadotropin deficiency
Pituitary failure	Hyperprolactinemia
Chronic disease	

Testicular Disorders

Dysfunctional spermatogenesis	Toxins
Infection	Varicocele
Klinefelter's syndrome	

Post-testicular Disorders

Obstructions	Vasectomy
Retrograde ejaculation	Physiologic/psychogenic dysfunction
Spinal cord injury	Sperm autoimmunity
Hypospadias	Absence of vas deferens

GnRH is not released in the normal way, the pituitary gland, lacking stimulation from GnRH, fails to produce adequate amounts of gonadotropins (follicle-stimulating hormone [FSH] and luteinizing hormone [LH]). Without adequate FSH, the ovaries fail to develop mature follicles. Without LH as a trigger, ovulation does not occur. Because of this sequential relationship, what is observed clinically as a failure to ovulate may in fact be a failure of the hypothalamus, the pituitary, or the ovaries. Adequate therapy depends on an accurate diagnosis.

Pituitary disorders other than failure to produce gonadotropins can affect fertility. One relatively common condition is hyperprolactinemia, in which excessive prolactin acts on the gonads or the hypothalamus to inhibit gonadotropin secretion. In women, this disorder is associated with amenorrhea. The most common cause of hyperprolactinemia is the presence of a prolactin-secreting adenoma in the pituitary.

Dopamine receptor antagonists can cause an excess amount of circulating prolactin because dopamine is the inhibitory factor that regulates prolactin release by the pituitary (see Chapter 55). Primary hypothyroidism with elevated thyrotropin-releasing hormone (TRH) may also increase prolactin levels. Breast-feeding can induce hyperprolactinemia, leading to anovulation. This action is the basis for the belief that breast-feeding may serve as contraception, although breast-feeding alone as a postpartum contraceptive is unreliable.

Primary defects of the ovaries arise from many causes. Gonadal dysgenesis may occur as an embryonic developmental defect. Gonadotropin-resistant ovary syndrome seems to be an autoimmune disease because ovarian antigonadotropin receptor antibodies in these patients block response to gonadotropins and therefore prevent pregnancy. In polycystic ovary syndrome, a condition where androgenic hormone levels are high, the follicular cysts in the ovaries do not mature fully. Premature ovarian failure affects a group of patients with a history of menstrual infrequency or irregularity who have ceased menstruating before the age of 40 and who have no apparent genetic abnormalities. Their symptoms usually include amenorrhea, elevated gonadotropins, and decreased estrogens. Varying profiles of gonadotropins and steroid hormones are found, many of which are typical of postmenopausal women. It is thought that oocytes are prematurely depleted, a deficient number were developed prenatally, or excessive gonadotropic stimulation has occurred. Autoimmune response to gonadotropins or their receptors is also suspect.

Luteal phase defects are diagnosed in 3% to 4% of infertile women. In women who have a history of habitual abortion, the incidence rate may be higher. An inadequate luteal phase is the result of a deficient secretion of progesterone by the corpus luteum after normal, spontaneous ovulation. Without adequate progesterone the endometrium is inadequately stimulated, blocking conception or preventing maintenance of pregnancy. Luteal phase deficiency consistently accompanies follicular-phase FSH deficiency.

Damaged fallopian tubes are another common cause of female infertility and may require surgical repair. A history of pelvic inflammatory disease, septic abortion, use of intrauterine devices, ruptured appendix, or ectopic pregnancy should alert the health care provider to the possibility of tubal damage. The fallopian tubes consist of three muscular layers and are lined with ciliated cells that wave in the direction of the uterus. Their secretory and contractile functions are vital to the transport of both the sperm and ovum, as well as the ultimate delivery of the embryo to the uterus after fertilization. The secretory activity of the fallopian tubes, which is mainly under the influence of estrogen, varies in response to the hormonal fluctuations of the menstrual cycle. As ovulation approaches and estrogen production increases, secretions accumulate in the tubal lumen to assist in sperm transport. After fertilization, because of the effects of progesterone, the secretions decrease and the fluid becomes clear, enabling the cilia to move the embryo through the tubes to the uterus. However, this transport process is impaired if the cilia are destroyed or the tubes are twisted, scarred, or blocked.

Endometriosis, one of the most common gynecologic disorders, is defined as the presence of hormonally responsive endometrial tissue found implanted outside the endometrial cavity. Although the etiology and pathogenesis are not clear, it is postulated that during menstruation, endometrial cells reflux through the tubes and attach to the pelvic structures. Endometrial fragments are most commonly found in dependent pelvic structures but may also be carried by the lymph and vasculature to distant sites.

Ectopic endometrial tissue contains receptors for estrogen, progesterone, and androgens. They respond to the fluctuating serum levels of these hormones much the same as normal endometrium does, with monthly bleeding that results in inflammation and peritoneal scarring. When the ovaries and tubes are involved, ovum transport is often obstructed by adhesions and the distortion of the anatomic structures in relation to each other. Drugs to control swelling and inflammation of the ectopic tissues may restore fertility or may be used along with surgery to restore fertility.

Uterine leiomyomas, or fibroids, are benign pelvic tumors that affect approximately 20% of American women. Interference with the proliferation of the endometrium may prevent normal expansion of the uterus as pregnancy progresses. Fibroids may cause habitual abortion or abnormalities of implantation, predisposing the pregnancy to placenta previa and premature labor. Fibroids occur more often in later reproductive years and are three to nine times more prevalent in African Americans than in whites.

Intrauterine adhesions, or Asherman's syndrome, cause the destruction of a large area of the endometrium, usually as a result of postpartum curettage, curettage after missed abortion, or infection. A woman who has been exposed to diethylstilbestrol can exhibit a wide range of aberrations of fertility from cervical incompetencies to uterine cavity anomalies.

Cervical factors also contribute to infertility. In some cases, there is a lack of cervical mucus or stenosis. These conditions can be seen in women who were exposed to diethylstilbestrol in utero and women whose cervical glands have been destroyed by cervical cautery or conization.

DISORDERS OF MALE FERTILITY

Pretesticular disorders include hypothalamic and pituitary disorders such as hypogonadotropic hypogonadism (Kallman's syndrome and isolated gonadotropin deficiency), pituitary failure, delayed or premature sexual development, and congenital adrenal hyperplasia. These patients have defects of the hypothalamic-pituitary axis that are either acquired or hereditary. In most of these patients, hypothalamic dysfunction causes GnRH to be low or absent. Both sexual development and spermatogenesis depend on the quantity of gonadotropins secreted. Treatment with various hormones usually promotes sexual maturation and, hence, the restoration of fertility.

Prolactin plays a role in male fertility, much as it does in females. Almost all men with prolactin-producing pituitary tumors are impotent and infertile, regardless of their testosterone level.

Chronic disease can be another source of pretesticular infertility. Diabetes mellitus can cause a lack of emission or retrograde ejaculation. Cystic fibrosis or recurrent upper respiratory infections may cause abnormalities of the seminal vesicles, vas deferens, and epididymis, or they can cause immotile cilia syndrome, which interferes with the transport of sperm through the ductal system.

Testicular disorders include dysfunctional spermatogenesis resulting from genetic or abnormal development or causes such as varicocele; exposure to toxins, drugs, and radiation; or infections. Drugs that affect spermatogenesis include alcohol, amebicides, anabolic steroids, cimetidine, nicotine, nitrofurantoin, sulfonamide drugs, and sulfasalazine.

Infection may cause epididymitis and orchitis. Common causative organisms include *Escherichia coli*, streptococci, staphylococci, *Neisseria gonorrhoeae*, and chlamydiae. Infertility may result from a recurrent or chronic infection that causes mechanical obstruction from scarring. The mumps virus can cause acute orchitis and, in pubertal or adult males, may result in damage to the seminiferous tubules and Leydig's cells, creating testosterone deficiency, hypogonadism, and infertility.

Varicocele is an abnormal dilatation or varicosity of the veins that drain the testicle. Varicoceles are found in up to 15% of the male population. Of these, approximately 50% have poor semen quality. Some studies have shown improved pregnancy rates in partners of men who have undergone surgery.

Posttesticular causes of infertility include a congenital absence of the vas deferens, obstructive problems, vasectomy, retrograde ejaculation, or spinal cord injuries. Sperm autoimmunity can occur in men if their immune system identifies the spermatozoa as foreign when they first appear at puberty. If this problem occurs, there is a decrease in sperm motility and viability because of agglutination, or clumping, and immobilization.

DRUG CLASS • Gonadotropin-Releasing Hormone and Analogs

⚕ gonadorelin (Factrel, Lutrepulse✱)

goserelin (Zoladex)

leuprolide acetate (Lupron, Lupron Depot)

nafarelin (Synarel)

MECHANISM OF ACTION

Gonadotropin-releasing hormone (GnRH) is naturally released in a pulsatile fashion from the hypothalamus to stimulate the release of gonadotropins (FSH and LH) from the pituitary. The frequency and amplitude of the pulses are critical to the stimulatory effects of GnRH. Single-dose injections of gonadorelin, which is synthetic GnRH, elevate plasma levels of gonadotropins for the first 2 to 4 weeks of therapy. With longer therapy, gonadorelin sensitizes receptor sites on the pituitary and suppresses gonadotropin release. Pulsatile administration of synthetic gonadorelin mimics the natural pattern of regulation and causes sustained FSH and LH secretion. As a result, the natural sequence of follicular maturation and ovulation occurs.

Leuprolide, goserelin, and nafarelin are GnRH analogs that can bind to GnRH receptor sites in the pituitary. Initially, the drugs cause a rise in the LH and FSH levels. After approximately 2 to 4 weeks, there is a suppression of the secretion of LH and FSH.

USES

Gonadorelin acetate (GnRH) is useful in treating infertility caused by inadequate secretion of GnRH from the hypothalamus. Multiple pregnancy is possible. Some women with polycystic ovaries may respond to gonadorelin, but they may be hypersensitive; lower doses must then be used.

Leuprolide, nafarelin, and goserelin stimulate release of FSH and particularly LH when used for short-term treatment. Short cycles are beginning to gain popularity as ovulation inducers, being used in much the same way as chorionic gonadotropin.

Long-term regimens are instituted when there is concern about controlling the maturation process of the follicles in assisted reproductive technology. The use of these GnRH analogs to suppress endogenous gonadotropins is also useful in controlling endometriosis by withdrawing hormone support from the ectopic tissue.

PHARMACOKINETICS

Gonadorelin is poorly absorbed by the GI tract and therefore must be administered subcutaneously or intravenously. It is supplied for use in the Lutrepulse pump to be given continuously over 24 hours in preprogrammed doses at a set frequency. It is widely distributed in the extracellular space and has a short elimination half-life (Table 61-2). It is mainly biotransformed and eliminated by the kidneys.

Leuprolide, goserelin, and nafarelin are proteins that are hydrolyzed if given orally and therefore must be administered by different routes (see Table 61-2). These drugs are biotransformed by conversion to peptides, which are removed primarily by renal mechanisms.

ADVERSE REACTIONS AND CONTRAINDICATIONS

Infection at the site of gonadorelin injection may occur. Allergic reactions are also possible.

Hot flashes, sweats, and headache may occur with leuprolide, goserelin, or nafarelin. Alterations of menstrual cycles are also common. For injected drugs, reactions at the site of injection are common. Long-term use may be associated with loss of calcium from bones for nafarelin.

INTERACTIONS

Gonadorelin should not be administered in conjunction with ovulation stimulators such as clomiphene to avoid the risk of overstimulating the ovaries.

TABLE 61-2							

Pharmacokinetics of Selected Fertility Drugs

Drug	Route	Onset	Peak	Duration	PB (%)	$t_{1/2}$	BioA (%)
Gonadotropin-Releasing Hormones							
gonadorelin acetate	IV/SC	Variable	2-6 hr	3-5 hr	UA	2-8 min	100
goserelin	implant	2-4 wk*	8-22 days	until implant removed	27	2-4 hr	UA
leuprolide acetate	SC	1-2 wk*	2-4 hr	3-4 wk	7-15	3 hr	94
nafarelin	IM	4 wk*	10-45 min	3-6 mo	78-84	3 hr	3
Gonadotropins							
chorionic gonadotropin	IM	2 hr	6 hr	36-72 hr	UA	23 hr	UA
follitropin	IM†	UA	UA	UA	UA	27-44 hr	77
FSH	IM	UA	6-18 hr	UA	UA	2.9 hr	UA
menotropin	IM	UA	F: 18 hr M: 4 mo	UA	UA	LH: 4 hr FSH: 70 hr	UA
Others							
bromocriptine	po	30-90 min	1-2 hr	8-12 hr‡	90-96	3-4.5 hr 45-50 hr§	UA
clomiphene citrate	po	5-14 days	UA	UA	UA	5 days	UA

BioA, Bioavailability; *FSH*, follicle-stimulating hormone; *PB*, protein binding; *SC*, subcutaneously; $t_{1/2}$, elimination half-life; *UA*, unavailable.
*Onset of action follows a transient increase during the first week of therapy; depot formulation.
†For women only.
‡The therapeutic effects of bromocriptine when used in hyperprolactinemia are seen after 4 weeks of therapy.
§Initial-phase half-life of bromocriptine is 3 to 4.5 hours, whereas terminal phase is 45 to 50 hours.

DRUG CLASS • Gonadotropins

chorionic gonadotropin (A.P.L., Pregnyl)
follitropin (Follistim, Gonal-F)
menotropins (Pergonal, Repronex)
urofollitropin (Fertinex)

MECHANISM OF ACTION

Three gonadotropins are currently used for fertility disorders: chorionic gonadotropin, FSH, and LH. Both FSH and LH activity are found in menotropins. Urofollitropin contains primarily FSH because the LH has been removed during purification. Follitropin is purified FSH produced by recombinant DNA technology. Chorionic gonadotropin is a polypeptide hormone produced by the placenta and obtained from the urine of pregnant women. Chorionic gonadotropin mimics the action of LH in most circumstances.

In men gonadotropins are used to induce spermatogenesis. Typically treatment would start with chorionic gonadotropin to stimulate the interstitial cells. When steroid production in the testes is established, menotropins would be added to complete the induction of spermatogenesis. The entire process may take months.

In women with normal ovarian function, FSH stimulates the maturation of a cohort of follicles. In the normal menstrual cycle, as the follicular phase progresses, one follicle matures more rapidly and becomes dominant. When the FSH level begins to fall during the mid- to late follicular phase, the less mature follicles begin to atrophy, whereas the dominant follicle continues to mature in spite of a decreasing level of FSH. When exogenous FSH is administered, the nondominant follicles receive the additional stimulation they need to continue to mature; thus a larger cohort of mature follicles are recruited per ovulation cycle, increasing the fertilization potential.

Ovulation, the release of the mature ovum, requires LH. If the endogenous LH level is insufficient to induce rupture of the follicles, treatment with a single large dose of chorionic gonadotropin, which has activity similar to LH, is administered.

Uses

Chorionic gonadotropin is used to treat both male and female infertility. For male hypogonadism, chorionic gonadotropin may be used alone or with either menotropins or clomiphene when pituitary deficiency is the cause of the disorder. For female infertility, chorionic gonadotropin may be used with menotropins, urofollitropin, or clomiphene. The primary use is to induce ovulation by taking advantage of the LH-like activity of chorionic gonadotropin.

Follitropin is used to treat cases of female infertility where ovarian failure has been ruled out as a cause. The drug is also used to stimulate the development of multiple follicles to allow harvesting of many ova for assisted reproductive technology. In men, follitropin can be used to induce spermatogenesis in patients where primary testicular failure has been ruled out as a cause of the infertility.

Menotropins, usually chorionic gonadotropin, are used to treat both female and male infertility. Urofollitropin is used along with chorionic gonadotropin to treat female infertility, especially for cases where polycystic ovarian disease is the cause of infertility, but the drug is ineffective for primary ovarian failure.

PHARMACOKINETICS

The drugs in this class are all proteins and thus are subject to proteolysis in the body. The range of half-lives produced is broad (see Table 61-2). The full pharmacologic effects of the drugs take longer than the pharmacokinetics would suggest. For example, although the peak level of chorionic gonadotropin is achieved within a few hours of dosing, ovulation does not occur for 24 to 40 hours. Breakdown products of these drugs are eliminated primarily by liver and renal mechanisms.

ADVERSE EFFECTS AND CONTRAINDICATIONS

The likelihood of ovulation with chorionic gonadotropin is dose related, as are the complications. Hot flashes are a common adverse reaction. Ovarian enlargement may be mild to moderate with the same complaints as that of clomiphene, but the incidence of the severe ovarian hyperstimulation syndrome is more frequent. **Ovarian hyperstimulation syndrome (OHSS)** develops in about 1% of patients and can be life threatening. As the ovaries are hyperstimulated, mild enlargement can progress to a critical condition with ascites, pleural effusion, hypovolemia, hypotension, oliguria, and electrolyte imbalance. The ovaries may rupture because of their excessive size from the development of multiple follicular cysts, corpora lutea, and stromal edema. Increased coagulability and decreased renal perfusion are the major complications. Androgen secretion induced by chorionic gonadotropin may cause fluid retention. Chorionic gonadotropin should be given with caution to patients with asthma, seizure disorders, migraines, and cardiac or renal problems. Safe use during pregnancy has not been established; chorionic gonadotropin may cause fetal toxicity.

Menotropins are contraindicated for women with primary ovarian failure, thyroid or adrenal dysfunction, intracranial lesions, pituitary insufficiency, or genital bleeding of unknown cause. In men, contraindications include normal pituitary function, primary testicular failure, or infertility from causes other than hypogonadotropic hypogonadism.

Adverse reactions to FSH are similar to those found with menotropin use, the most prominent being OHSS. Other adverse reactions occur infrequently and include ovarian cysts, ovarian enlargement, pelvic or abdominal discomfort, headache, pain or swelling at the injection site, and breast tenderness. As with all gonadotropins, the risk of multiple births is associated with FSH use. FSH is contraindicated for women with primary ovarian failure, ovarian cysts, or enlargement unrelated to polycystic ovary syndrome; abnormal uterine bleeding; uncontrolled thyroid or adrenal dysfunction; or pituitary tumor.

INTERACTIONS

Few interactions are noted, because the drugs are used for very specific purposes over limited time frames.

DRUG CLASS • Antiprolactin Drugs

bromocriptine (Parlodel)

MECHANISM OF ACTION

Bromocriptine resembles the neurotransmitter dopamine in structure and is able to bind to dopamine receptors in the pituitary gland. Prolactin secretion from the pituitary gland is then inhibited, reducing prolactin levels. By substantially reducing elevated prolactin levels, bromocriptine can restore ovulation and ovarian function in amenorrheic women. This appears to be accomplished by direct suppression of pituitary secretion or by stimulating dopamine receptors in the hypothalamus to release prolactin-inhibiting factor. Bromocriptine may also act on dopaminergic receptors in the ovary to restore ovulation. The drug may also stimulate ovulation in women whose prolactin level is not elevated, indicating it may have an effect on hypothalamic release of LH-releasing hormone.

Bromocriptine also suppresses galactorrhea and prolactin levels in men. In most patients with hyperprolactinemia, if bromocriptine is discontinued, prolactin returns to pretreatment levels within 1 to 6 weeks. Amenorrhea returns in 4 to 24 weeks, and galactorrhea returns in 2 to 12 weeks.

USES

Bromocriptine is indicated for patients with infertility associated with hyperprolactinemia, pituitary adenomas, and galactorrhea. It is also used for the restoration of menstrual function in patients who desire it or for those for whom restoration of ovarian function is necessary to prevent bone loss.

Oligospermia, if caused by elevated prolactin levels, may also be treated with bromocriptine. Men show an increased sperm count when elevated prolactin levels are corrected.

PHARMACOKINETICS

Bromocriptine is rapidly and completely absorbed in the GI tract. A single dose has been found to decrease serum prolactin levels within 2 hours; maximal suppression occurs within 8 hours (see Table 61-2). The most therapeutic effects in hyperprolactinemic patients are seen after 4 weeks of therapy. Bromocriptine is biotransformed in the liver and eliminated in the feces through biliary elimination. A small portion is eliminated in the urine.

ADVERSE EFFECTS AND CONTRAINDICATIONS

The most frequently experienced adverse effects of bromocriptine are nausea and vomiting related to GI intolerance. These symptoms usually resolve spontaneously within a few days and may be avoided by a slow increase of the dosage to achieve the desired effects. Some patients experience severe postural hypotension and syncope on initiation of therapy. Hypertension, although rare, occurs usually after about 2 weeks of therapy. Treatment should be discontinued if hypertension or severe, progressive, or unremitting headache results or if signs of CNS toxicity are present.

Patients wishing to breast-feed should avoid bromocriptine because of its suppressive effects on lactation. Prolactin levels in the fetus of a pregnant woman treated with bromocriptine are decreased in utero but return to normal after birth. Bromocriptine is routinely discontinued when conception is verified.

INTERACTIONS

The effectiveness of bromocriptine in decreasing prolactin levels is antagonized by drugs known to elevate prolactin such as amitriptyline, imipramine, phenothiazines, and methyldopa. Additive neurologic effects may occur with levodopa, as well as additive hypotensive effects when the drug is used with antihypertensives. Severe hypertension may occur when bromocriptine is given concomitantly with certain ergot alkaloids, which may lead to severe cardiovascular and CNS complications.

Sulfites contained in some commercial food preparations may cause an allergic reaction in susceptible patients. Consumption of alcohol is contraindicated.

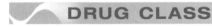

DRUG CLASS • Antiestrogen

clomiphene citrate (Clomid, Milophene, Serophene)

MECHANISM OF ACTION

Clomiphene's precise mechanism of action is unknown. It appears to compete with estradiol for estrogen-binding sites in the hypothalamus, where it increases the release of GnRH to stimulate the pituitary to increase FSH and LH secretion. Clomiphene stimulates the events of the normal cycle that lead to ovulation.

Clomiphene has no progestational, androgenic, corticotropic, or antiandrogenic effects. It does not appear to interfere with normal adrenal or thyroid function.

USES

Use of clomiphene citrate is indicated in the treatment of ovulatory failure. Patients with polycystic ovary syndrome may benefit from treatment with clomiphene because the drug competes for the estrone-binding sites and inhibits negative feedback. If the high level of estrogen is not inhibited, gonadotropin secretion continues to be inhibited, suppressing ovulation.

Clomiphene has been used in a limited number of patients for menstrual disorders, endometrial anaplasia or hyperplasia, persistent lactation, oligospermia, and fibrocystic breast disease. However, it is not approved for these purposes. It is also used for the treatment of male infertility.

PHARMACOKINETICS

Clomiphene citrate is taken orally and is readily absorbed in the GI tract. Biotransformation appears to take place in the liver, and the drug metabolites are eliminated in the feces. There is evidence that some of the drug may be stored in body fat or undergo entero-hepatic circulation to be slowly released from the body.

ADVERSE REACTIONS AND CONTRAINDICATIONS

The most common adverse reaction to clomiphene citrate is the occurrence of menopause-like hot flashes. The hot flashes are related to the antiestrogenic properties of the medication, which causes vasomotor flushing. Abdominal bloating, distension, and discomfort have also been reported as well as breast tenderness, nausea and vomiting, headache, and visual disturbances. Other adverse effects include hair loss or dryness, urinary frequency, increased appetite, weight gain, skin rash, tension, fatigue, insomnia, dizziness, and mood swings.

Clomiphene is contraindicated for women with pre-existing ovarian cysts and those with persistent ovarian enlargement after treatment has begun. The ovary may increase in size for several days after the drug is discontinued. Normally, the enlargement spontaneously subsides without any intervention or sequela. If ovarian en-

largement does occur, the treatment should be stopped and the dosage of the next cycle decreased.

Some patients with polycystic ovary syndrome are unusually sensitive to the gonadotropin levels induced by normal doses of clomiphene and may have an exaggerated response. Again, discontinuation of the medication is recommended, and the condition is expected to resolve spontaneously.

Clomiphene citrate is contraindicated for patients who are hypersensitive to gonadotropins or those who have liver disease, a history of liver dysfunction, abnormal uterine bleeding of unknown cause, or endometriosis. This drug is also contraindicated for those with pituitary tumors as well as thyroid and adrenal dysfunction. The patient and her partner should be warned about the risk of multiple gestation, especially with higher doses, and about the risks inherent in a multiple-gestation pregnancy.

INTERACTIONS

Clomiphene is usually not given with other ovarian stimulators, so that the risk of overstimulating the ovaries is avoided.

DRUG CLASS   •   Male or Female Steroid Hormones

progesterone gel (Crinone)

testolactone (Teslac)

testosterone

Testosterone is used mainly for replacement of endogenous hormone when there is deficient endocrine function of the testes (see Chapter 62).

Testolactone is an antineoplastic drug with antiestrogenic effects (see Chapter 37). It prevents the conver-

sion of androgens to estrogens. When testolactone is used with GnRH in men with hypothalamic GnRH deficiency, it enhances the release of LH and FSH and stimulates testicular maturation and spermatogenesis.

Progesterone is used for luteal phase support in patients with luteal phase defects because the supplemental progesterone enhances endometrial development. Progesterone for this purpose is administered intravaginally.

APPLICATION TO PRACTICE

ASSESSMENT

Assessment of the couple desiring treatment for infertility requires a thorough assessment of both the woman and her male partner. A primary assessment, including a comprehensive history and physical examination, should be performed before an expensive, time-consuming, and emotionally arduous investigation is initiated.

History of Present Illness

Pretreatment assessment is essential before starting treatment for infertility and should include a thorough history that will identify potential medical or drug-induced

causes. Patients usually report an inability to conceive after an extended period of time of unprotected sexual relations. In other cases, an inability to carry a fetus to term is the chief complaint. A thorough sexual history is obtained from both partners, and it is essential to begin formation of a database. The sexual history should include information on the frequency as well as the timing of coitus and the use of drugs that may decrease fertility. The use of lubricants, positions used, and douching practices should also be noted.

Elicit information regarding the male partner's history of groin injury, mumps after adolescence, and acute viral illnesses in the past 3 months. A surgical history should be noted, including hernia repair, vasectomy, reversal of a vasectomy, or varicocele repair.

Health History

Obtain a complete reproductive and menstrual history, including specific information related to premenstrual syndrome, the Mittelschmerz sign (midcycle ovulation pain), dysmenorrhea, amenorrhea, or intermenstrual spotting. History of pelvic disease, ovarian cysts, endometriosis, hormone-dependent tumors, sexually transmitted diseases (STDs), and pelvic inflammatory disease (PID) should be noted. Prior exposure to radiation or diethylstilbestrol and a history of tobacco and alcohol use should be noted. The past use of contraceptive measures (type, duration, and complications of use) and when they were used should be elicited.

Exposure to potentially toxic substances, sitting for extended hours, strenuous exercise, and the use of hot baths after exercise should be noted, particularly in the case of the male partner. Furthermore, a genetic history, a history of birth defects, and any reproductive problems in family members should be included in the interview.

Lifespan Considerations

For many couples, treatment for infertility represents a final chance to have biologic children before resorting to adoption. A waiting period of up to 7 years is not uncommon for couples attempting to adopt a child. Couples who choose to remain childless need as much support for their decision as does the couple who chooses to accept fertility treatment. Answers to questions that address the couple's self-image, guilt and blame, and sexuality are important data to obtain.

Receiving the diagnosis of infertility is often a life-altering event. Patients may demonstrate an array of reactions ranging from denial to anger and grief. There may be repercussions of this diagnosis such as low self-esteem, marital discord, and divorce as well as parenting difficulties when treatment is successful. Ethical and religious issues often further complicate the course of treatment. Counseling, referrals, and individualized support as well as follow-up are important aspects of the care provided by the fertility specialists and the perinatal team.

Cultural/Social Considerations

Drug treatment of infertility is a very costly, often complicated, and emotionally as well as physically draining endeavor. When a multiple pregnancy is the outcome of treatment for infertility, the cost of prolonged hospital bed rest is enormous. When the multiple pregnancy culminates in premature delivery with the potential for neonatal death, the daily costs increase exponentially.

Before beginning treatment, the couple must be made fully aware of the costs, the amount they can expect to be reimbursed by their insurance if they are covered, and the expense that can be incurred if complications ensue. In other words, they need to understand the economic implications of multiple births. Hospitalization costs for the antepartum mother and the potential cost of multiple premature infants can be devastating (see the Case Study: Infertility).

Clomiphene citrate is usually the first drug given to patients requiring ovulation induction. It is relatively inexpensive and requires fewer office visits and interventions when compared with other drugs used for this purpose.

Menotropin (hMG) is significantly more expensive than clomiphene citrate. An ampule is estimated to cost approximately $45; therefore the cost of treatment can run up to $1000 for one cycle of the medication alone. FSH is as expensive as menotropin. The average cost of one dose of human chorionic gonadotropin (hCG) is approximately $50. Leuprolide and progesterone, commonly used adjuvant treatments, add to the expense. Their use requires consideration of the motivation and willingness of the participants in this type of intervention.

Physical Examination

The infertile female patient should have a baseline pelvic examination. Attention is paid to the size, shape, position, and mobility of the uterus; the presence of congenital anomalies; and the possibility of endometriosis. Evaluation of the adnexa, ovary size, fixations, and tumors should be noted. A rectovaginal examination should be performed, noting the presence of a retroflexed or retroverted uterus or a rectouterine pouch mass.

During examination of the male patient, note the presence or absence of phimosis, location of the urethral meatus, and size and consistency of each testis, vas deferens, and epididymis. The presence of a varicocele should be noted. A rectal examination is used to identify the size and consistency of the seminal vesicles and prostate; microscopic evaluation of prostatic fluid should be used to gather evidence of infection.

Vital signs including blood pressure, temperature, height, and weight should be noted in both partners. The female patient should also be examined for evidence of thyroid dysfunction (e.g., exophthalmos, lid lag, tremor, or palpable gland).

Laboratory Testing

All patients with infertility problems need a thorough laboratory workup before drug therapy. Basal body temperature charts are used to assess for biphasic elevations and evidence of ovulation. A semen analysis is also performed during early diagnostic testing. Routine laboratory tests include LH, FSH, and estradiol levels; thyroid studies (T_3, T_4, T_7, and TSH); and prolactin levels. Other evaluation methods include cervical mucus studies, hysterosalpingogram, laparoscopy, laparotomy, endometrial biopsy, and postcoital semen analysis. For the male partner, assessment also includes an evaluation of endocrine functioning.

GOALS OF THERAPY

The general goal in the treatment of infertility is to determine the cause of the infertility and to correct, if possible, endocrinopathies, infections, anatomic aberrations, and hormonal imbalances or deficiencies. The use of assisted reproductive technology (ART) is very common in the field of infertility (Box 61-1).

The goal of achieving pregnancy with minimal adverse reactions takes skill and timing to achieve. Studies have shown that up to 90% of patients taking hMG ovulate and that 50% to 70% achieve pregnancy after an average of three treatment cycles. Some have noted improved cervical mucus with hMG that may be therapeutic in itself, making coitus more natural and efficient. Multiple pregnancy rates range from 10% to 30% and mostly result in twins; 5% of pregnancies result in three or more fetuses. The spontaneous abortion rate is 20% to 25%, which is slightly higher than the general norm.

Although clomiphene is a first-line drug, in the case of an anatomic abnormality such as nonpatent fallopian tubes, ovulation induction followed by coitus and normal fertilization, conception, and implantation is not an option. In this case, the health care provider moves straight to ART with drugs such as hMG, FSH, and hCG. The particular regimen is largely based on the preference of the health care provider. Different providers routinely use drugs they are most familiar with and in which they have the most confidence to bring about the best results.

INTERVENTION
Administration

Clomiphene citrate should be taken exactly as directed at the same time each day. Missed doses should be taken as soon as they are remembered. The dose should be doubled if it is not remembered until the next dose

---

BOX 61-1 The Ethics of Using Fertility Drugs

Reproductive health presents one of the thorniest moral questions faced by health care providers. The topic of promoting fertility by drug administration may produce less ardent political arguments than does abortion, but it does contain clear conflicts and difficult choices.

Couples who want children but cannot conceive experience a unique type of emotional suffering. They live in a world where abortion is easily available, the adoption process is difficult and lengthy, and abuse of children is the fodder of daily news. Every new tale of child abuse appears as an affront to justice, particularly to couples who are bitter about their continued infertility. Surely one can argue that they deserve relief.

Other participants in the area of fertility promotion may hold complementary if differing viewpoints. The issue of justice is easy to assert. However, how many pregnancies come to disaster because prenatal care is lacking? How much prenatal care could be purchased for the price of a single in vitro fertilization or artificial insemination? Do numbers win out, or does the claim of the individual person?

The hazards of fertility treatments also demand a hearing. Preparation for harvesting ova requires painful and lengthy hormonal treatment. Aside from the cost and short-term adverse effects, are long-term adverse health effects also possible? The use of ovulation-stimulating drugs can produce showers of ova, contributing to multiple births that may be complicated by their prematurity. Do parents have the right to demand neonatal intensive care for quadruplets once infertility is overcome? Is it ethical to advocate abortion for some fetuses in a multiple pregnancy to improve the odds for one or two others? The entire issue of fertility treatment remains morally unacceptable when one's beliefs forbid any intervention in conception.

Critical Thinking Discussion

- What alternatives should be available to a couple who cannot conceive children?
- What increases in insurance premiums in your own plan are acceptable to ensure that all infertile participants have access to fertility treatment?
- Does a single woman who desires to bear children have the same right to treatment of infertility as a married couple?
- Is surrogacy a proper resource for an infertile couple when the woman cannot carry a pregnancy to successful termination?
- What considerations would you have a patient reflect on before consenting to infertility treatment?

Courtesy of Jonathan J. Wolfe, Pharm D.

is due. The health care provider should be notified if more than one dose is missed. Monitor liver function tests as well as hCG and urinary LH levels.

A typical regimen for clomiphene is to count the first day of the menstrual cycle as day 1. Begin clomiphene in the dose ordered on day 5 and continue daily until the prescribed number of doses is completed. Review instructions with the patient and ensure that she understands the dosing schedule. In addition, the health care provider may want the patient to use an ovulation prediction kit; review the manufacturer's instructions with the patient. Advise the couple to have frequent inter-

course at or around the time ovulation is anticipated. The drug may also be prescribed for men; review the prescription with the patient.

Because hCG is destroyed in the GI tract, it is necessary to administer it via a painful intramuscular injection. The intramuscular formulation requires reconstitution using normal saline provided by the manufacturer. Steps should be taken to relieve the discomfort of the injection as much as possible. The reconstituted drug is stable for 90 days when refrigerated.

Read the health care provider's orders carefully; there is an injectable subcutaneous form and an intramuscular

---

CASE STUDY  *Infertility*

ASSESSMENT

HISTORY OF PRESENT ILLNESS

DJ is a 35-year-old nullipara who has been unable to become pregnant after 5 years of unprotected intercourse. She visits today, accompanied by her partner, for follow-up and to discuss treatment of infertility.

HEALTH HISTORY

DJ's history is benign for contributing factors to infertility. Her menses started at age 12 with 28- to 29-day cycles and periods lasting 4 to 5 days. She reports no unusual discomfort, bleeding, or symptoms of PMS. History is negative for STDs and PID. No family history of infertility. Mother had four spontaneous term pregnancies without complications.

LIFESPAN CONSIDERATIONS

DJ is considered to be of advanced maternal age. In light of diagnosis, she is an immediate candidate for ART. Possibility of multiple embryo development would satisfy the couple's desire for family in one pregnancy. DJ and partner have experienced a wide range of emotions from denial to anger and grief. They have experienced low self-esteem and marital discord for a time. Counseling provided needed support while waiting for diagnosis. Relationship now stable and supportive. Couple willing and capable of doing whatever is necessary for DJ to conceive, including in vitro fertilization (IVF).

CULTURAL/SOCIAL CONSIDERATIONS

DJ and partner are gainfully employed, and have financial stability and a large savings account from which they can draw funds if required to pay for one cycle of ovulation induction (approximately $10,000) and IVF procedure. Cost of laboratory and ultrasound monitoring covered by health insurance.

PHYSICAL EXAMINATION

DJ is 5'9" tall and weighs 130 pounds. Manual pelvic examination reveals slightly retroverted uterus with ovaries of normal size and location. Speculum examination reveals nulliparous cervix with no unusual findings. Remainder of physical examination unremarkable.

LABORATORY TESTING

LH, FSH, estradiol, thyroid function studies, prolactin levels, cervical mucus, hysterosalpingogram, and laparoscopy are within normal limits. Pregnancy test negative.

PATIENT PROBLEM(S)

Primary infertility.

GOALS OF THERAPY

Foster follicle stimulation for ART. Achieve and maintain pregnancy.

CRITICAL THINKING QUESTIONS

1. The health care provider orders the following drug regimen: *Step 1:* Leuprolide acetate 0.5 mg SC bid initially, to start in midluteal phase of previous cycle until FSH started, then single 0.5 mg doses SC daily. *Step 2:* Follicle-stimulating hormone 150 IU IM qd for 7 to 12 days to start on day 3 of cycle. *Step 3:* hCG 10,000 units IM 24 hours after last dose of leuprolide acetate and FSH. What is the mechanism of action of these drugs?
2. Of which adverse effects should DJ be aware?
3. What is the primary health care concern regarding the use of fertility drugs?
4. DJ asks what percentage of couples diagnosed with infertility achieve pregnancy and carry the fetus to term. What is the appropriate response?
5. DJ is worried about the risk of ovarian hyperstimulation syndrome. What should she be told?

depot form of leuprolide. Leuprolide acetate is only for intramuscular injection. The depot form should be administered by the health care provider. If the patient is to self-administer the drug at home, review the patient instruction leaflet supplied with the subcutaneous form. The patient should be instructed to store the drug at room temperature.

When hMG is used, the reconstituted formulation should be used immediately and any unused portion discarded.

Education

Compliance with the complex regimen of fertility treatment requires a firm understanding of the plan of care with attention to timing of drug administration and coital activities. Teach the patient to keep a record of basal body temperature, consistency of cervical mucus, and a 24-hour urine specimen as prescribed by the health care provider. Ensure that the patient understands the best time of the month to have intercourse on the basis of the drugs being used. An understanding of the couple's relationship and commitment to a treatment regimen is vital to treatment success.

When treatment is initiated, the couple should be taught to self-administer the subcutaneous injections. Information on aseptic technique and how to recognize infection at the injection site should be included. Warnings about the importance of compliance should be provided. The patient should be instructed to report signs and symptoms of ovarian hyperstimulation to the health care provider as soon as identified. Instruct the patient to notify the health care provider immediately if pregnancy is suspected, because these drugs should not be continued during pregnancy.

Review the anticipated benefits and possible adverse effects of therapy. Encourage the patient to notify the health care provider if adverse or unexplained events develop. Warn the patient to avoid driving or operating hazardous equipment if changes in vision, dizziness, or light-headedness occur.

EVALUATION

The effectiveness of bromocriptine therapy can be demonstrated by the resumption of normal ovulatory menstrual cycles and restoration of fertility. Clomiphene citrate effectiveness is demonstrated by the occurrence of ovulation as measured by estrogen elimination, biphasic body temperature elevations, and endometrial histologic changes. If conception is not achieved after three to four treatment cycles, the original diagnosis should be reevaluated.

Effectiveness of hMG is evaluated by the maturation of follicles. hMG therapy is followed by hCG, which should lead to ovulation. If ovulation does not occur after three to six menstrual cycles, therapy may be discontinued. For the male patient, effectiveness is evident by increased spermatogenesis after 4 months of therapy. Treatment effectiveness of hCG can be noted by an increase in spermatogenesis in men.

Although the couple may believe that the only successful outcome of treatment is a pregnancy, that outcome cannot and should not be guaranteed. However, when pregnancy has been detected and the embryonic sac and heart rate can be detected by ultrasound, treatment with fertility drugs is considered successful.

Bibliography

Adamson D, Chang RJ, DeCherney AH, et al: A model for initial care of the infertile couple, *J Reprod Med* 46(suppl 4):409-426, 2001.

Aronson DD: Defining infertility . . . "Infertility: from a personal to a public health problem," *Public Health Rep* 115(1):6, 2000.

Kainz K: The role of the psychologist in the evaluation and treatment of infertility, *Women's Health Issues* 11(6):481-485, 2001.

McConnell EA: Research reviews: social and ethical aspects of in vitro fertilization, *AORN J* 71(5):1071, 2000.

Roupa Z, Sapountzi-Krepia D, Salakos N, et al: Health counseling and in-vitro fertilization, *Icus Nurs Web J* (9):13p, 2002.

Sandlow JI: Shattering the myths about male infertility: treatment of male factors may be more successful and cost-effective than you think, *Postgrad Med* 107(2):235-239, 242, 245, 2000.

Wootton JC: Webwatch: women's health and gender-based medicine. Infertility, *J Women's Health Gend Based Med* 9(3):329-331, 2000.

Internet Resources

http://www.ihr.com/infertility/.
http://www.nlm.nih.gov/medlineplus/infertility.html.
http://www.womens-health.com/health_center/infertility/.

Androgens, Anabolic Steroids, and Related Drugs

JOSEPH A. DiMICCO • KATHLEEN GUTIERREZ

 Visit **http://evolve.elsevier.com/Gutierrez/** for additional information.

KEY TERMS

5-alpha-reductase, p. 1018

Anabolic, p. 1018

Androgens, p. 1017

Angioedema, p. 1020

Aromatase, p. 1018

Benign prostatic hyperplasia (BPH), p. 1022

Dihydrotestosterone, p. 1018

Leydig's cells, p. 1017

Male pattern baldness, p. 1022

Seminiferous tubules, p. 1017

Testosterone, p. 1017

OBJECTIVES

- Describe the uses of androgens and anabolic steroids.
- Describe the use of antiandrogens.
- Explain the roles of dihydrotestosterone and 5-alpha-reductase.
- Describe the uses of 5-alpha-reductase inhibitors.
- Create a nursing care plan for a patient receiving androgens.

 ## PHYSIOLOGY

The major reproductive hormones in men are **androgens**. These steroids are synthesized primarily in the testes and, to a lesser extent, in the adrenal glands. Within the testes, the status of interstitial or **Leydig's cells** and of the cells comprising the **seminiferous tubules** are most important for determining male sexual potential. Leydig's cells synthesize **testosterone**, the primary masculinizing steroid

hormone. The seminiferous tubules contain the germ cells that produce functional sperm in adult males.

Sexual function in adult males depends on the proper interaction of the hypothalamus, anterior pituitary, and the testes. Regulation of testicular function is by a negative feedback loop (see Chapter 55). The primary hormones in this cycle are testosterone, from the testes; luteinizing hormone (LH) and follicle-stimulating hormone (FSH), from the anterior pituitary; and gonadotropin-releasing hormone (GnRH), from the hypothalamus. When testosterone levels in the blood are low, GnRH is released from the hypothalamus to enter the anterior pituitary through a portal venous system. Under the influence of GnRH, both LH and FSH are released from the pituitary into general circulation and act on testicular tissues in males to stimulate production of androgens.

The effects of these regulatory hormones differ depending on the stage of life. During fetal development, Leydig's cells develop in the embryonic testes as a result of stimulation with the maternal hormone human chorionic gonadotropin (hCG). These embryonic cells produce the small amounts of testosterone necessary for development of the male external genitalia; without testosterone, genetically male infants are born with female genitalia. After birth, Leydig's cells regress because the stimulus of hCG is no longer available.

The second stage when these regulatory processes are most important is puberty. In childhood, very low concentrations of gonadotropins are found in blood. With the onset of puberty the anterior pituitary begins to synthesize and release greater quantities of LH and FSH. The targets for LH in males are Leydig's cells (i.e., the site where LH stimulates testosterone production). FSH acts directly on cells in seminiferous tubules to prepare that tissue for spermatogenesis. This process cannot be completed unless testosterone from Leydig's cells is also present. With FSH and testosterone acting on the seminiferous tubules, mature sperm can be produced. Testosterone acts not only within the testes but also throughout the body at this stage of life. These actions are discussed in the next section.

The third period of life to be considered is sexual maturity. During this time LH is important in the maintenance of sexual function because it is still required for the synthesis of testosterone, which maintains spermatogenesis.

The major steroid affecting male sexual function is testosterone. This hormone is synthesized in the Leydig's cells and in the adrenal cortex. Testosterone is a potent androgen and therefore stimulates growth of the organs of the male reproductive tract. Testosterone is responsible for the enlargement and maturation of the penis, scrotum, seminal vesicles, prostate gland, and other accessory tissues of the male reproductive tract.

These actions constitute the primary sexual effects on the male.

Testosterone is also responsible for development of secondary sexual characteristics. The increased testosterone level during puberty stimulates growth of facial and pubic hair as well as hair on the chest and armpits. Sustained levels of testosterone trigger the onset of baldness in genetically predisposed males. The other dramatic changes that occur in the pubertal male are also related to the increased testosterone levels and include lowering of the voice caused by thickening of the vocal cords, stimulation of sebaceous glands, and stimulation of libido. Psychologists who work with primates other than humans have related aggression to high testosterone levels.

In addition to these primary and secondary sexual effects, testosterone also has profound effects on metabolism. Androgens are **anabolic** (i.e., they stimulate synthetic rather than degradative processes). This anabolic action is responsible for the increase in muscle mass associated with puberty and the distribution of this mass in the male pattern. Testosterone increases nitrogen retention, protein formation, and overall metabolic rate. In addition, calcium is retained, and the size and strength of bone are enhanced. Blood-forming cells are also affected so that more red blood cells may be formed.

Although testosterone is the major circulating androgen in human males, it is not the only metabolically important androgen. Some target tissues for testosterone contain an enzyme called **5-alpha-reductase**. This enzyme transforms testosterone to **dihydrotestosterone**, which is a more potent androgen than testosterone and is thought to be primarily responsible for certain effects of testosterone (including effects on hair follicles). Small amounts of another androgen, androstenedione, may also affect various tissues of the body.

Testosterone and androstenedione are close chemical relatives of the estrogens, steroid hormones that have feminizing effects. Some tissues in the brain, breasts, and testes can convert androgens to estrogens through an enzyme called **aromatase**. Therefore low estrogen concentrations are normally found in the blood of healthy adult men. These estrogens are now thought to play a physiologic role in males in the closure of epiphyses to terminate the growth of long bones and in maintenance of normal bone density. Under certain circumstances, these normal low estrogen concentrations may increase and produce pathologic signs such as breast development.

PATHOPHYSIOLOGY • Hypogonadism

Hypogonadism is caused by deficient secretion of testosterone by the testes. Hypogonadism, whether a result of chromosomal, pituitary, or testicular disorders, involves the nondevelopment or regression of secondary male characteristics along with a fragile libido and waning potency. It may be classified as disease in the testes themselves (primary hypogonadism) or as insufficient gonadotropin secretion by the pituitary (secondary hypogonadism). The distinction and differential diagnosis between the two disorders are essential to the choice of drug therapy.

Both primary and secondary hypogonadism may occur in the prepubertal or postpubertal male. Hypogonadism is commonly seen in primary care. It generally has significant effects on the psychosocial as well as the physical well-being of the male patient.

In prepubertal hypogonadism, more commonly known as delayed puberty, androgenic stimulation of undifferentiated embryonic tissues is deficient or absent. Lack of stimulation results in undeveloped and immature male sex accessory organs.

Prepubertal hypogonadism can be caused by deficient production of testicular steroids (congenital and acquired), insensitivity syndrome of target organs (e.g., receptor defects, 5-alpha-reductase deficiency), deficient secretion of pituitary gonadotropin, deficient hypothal-amic secretion of gonadotropin-releasing hormone, hyperprolactinemia, or other unknown factors. Onset of normal pubertal development is delayed. Male secondary sexual characteristics and behavior, accelerated growth, and the initiation of spermatogenesis do not occur.

Postpubertal hypogonadism is classified as either hypergonadotropic primary or hypogonadotropic secondary hypogonadism. Hypergonadotropic hypogonadism occurs as a result of testicular destruction (e.g., castration, radiation, mumps, orchitis). Defects in testicular response to gonadotropin release lead to decreased secretion of testosterone and, as a result of normal feedback mechanisms, high levels of circulating gonadotropins. In the absence of adequate testosterone levels, spermatogenesis is impaired.

Hypogonadotropic testicular failure, secondary to hypopituitarism in the adult, is usually associated with complete destruction or removal of the pituitary gland. In this situation, gonadotropin levels are low because of feedback inhibition. In the absence of adequate gonadotropin secretion, Leydig's cells are not stimulated to secrete testosterone, and sperm maturation is not promoted in Sertoli's cells. Spermatogenesis depends not only on appropriate stimulation by gonadotropins but also on an appropriate response by the testes.

DRUG CLASS • Androgens and "Anabolic Steroids"

⚛ testosterone (Testoderm, Androderm, Androgel, Delatestryl, Depo-Testosterone, Malogen✳)

danazol (Danocrine, Cyclomen)

fluoxymesterone (Halotestin, Android-F)

methyltestosterone (Testred, Virilon, Android 10, Android 25, Metandren✳)

nandrolone (Deca-Durobolin)

oxandrolone (Oxandrin, Anapolon)

oxymetholone (Anadrol 50)

stanozolol (Winstrol)

MECHANISM OF ACTION

The androgens are steroids that, like other steroid hormones, diffuse into cells and bind to specific receptors found in the cytoplasm of target tissues. The bound drug- or hormone-receptor complex then moves to the nucleus of the cell and changes gene expression, which in turn alters cell function. The effects on the body are as described previously for naturally produced androgens.

It was once thought that certain synthetic steroids (nandrolone, oxandrolone, oxymetholone, and stanozolol) had significantly greater anabolic than androgenic activity and so these were called "anabolic steroids." However, these drugs produce typical androgenic effects in humans and, therefore, differ significantly from testosterone only with regard to their pharmacokinetics and profile of adverse reactions.

USES

Testosterone and its derivatives are primarily used in replacement therapy for patients who have abnormally low production of endogenous androgens. For some patients the loss of androgens occurs early and prevents the normal changes of puberty. Androgen loss after puberty may cause a reduction in libido or sexual desire, or may even cause mild feminizing tendencies. Aging males produce less testosterone than younger men and may experience a loss of sexual drive. Some older men have more severe symptoms suggestive of a male climacteric or male menopause. These conditions and others related to specific malfunctions of the male sexual organs may be treated with testosterone or one of the other androgenic compounds. For patients with reduced natural testosterone production, this treatment constitutes replacement therapy.

Androgens may be employed for the treatment of conditions involving hormone-dependent tissues in women. These are sometimes used for the treatment (usually palliative) of advanced or metastatic breast cancer in postmenopausal women. The high dosages used for this purpose exceed those required for replacement therapy and may be expected to cause masculinization. The synthetic androgen danazol has been used for various conditions in females, such as relief of dysmenorrhea, menopausal symptoms, and postpartum breast engorgement, but other agents are now preferred. Danazol is still occasionally employed in the treatment of endometriosis and in fibrocystic breast disease. The mechanisms responsible for the beneficial effects of androgenic stimulation in these states are not clear, but they may involve inhibition of the release of gonadotropins from the pituitary.

The so-called anabolic steroids are sometimes used to treat conditions for which increased nitrogen retention and protein formation are desirable. Accordingly, these drugs may alleviate the catabolic state produced by severe trauma. Patients who have extensive burns or have had surgery may benefit from the action of the anabolic steroids. The effects of anabolic/androgenic steroids on red blood cell formation also make these drugs valuable in the treatment of certain forms of anemia.

The orally active anabolic steroids are also used in the treatment of **angioedema**. An autosomal dominant disorder, angioedema results from a genetic deficiency of functional C1 esterase inhibitor. This deficiency allows unopposed activation of the first component of complement. With this deficiency, there is a local release of vasoactive peptides and greater vascular permeability. The anabolic steroids are effective because they promote the hepatic synthesis of C1 esterase inhibitor; this action tends to reverse the genetically induced deficiency.

Anabolic steroids are inappropriate for use in athletes who seek to increase muscle mass. In healthy young men, the effects on muscle strength and performance are statistically significant but minimal, whereas the adverse effects can be serious (altered liver function, reduced gonadotropin levels, lowered testosterone synthesis, changes in serum lipid profiles, and depressed spermatogenesis). In healthy young women, bone and muscle mass may be increased more dramatically but at the cost of virilization and menstrual disturbances.

PHARMACOKINETICS

As with other endogenous steroids, testosterone in its natural form is not water-soluble and therefore is used as an aqueous suspension suitable only for intramuscular injection. In this form the drug has a short duration of action and produces somewhat erratic clinical responses. Testosterone can be absorbed from the gastrointestinal tract; however, this route of administration does not produce clinically useful testosterone concentrations in blood because the steroid absorbed from the intestine passes directly into portal circulation to the liver, where it is subject to inactivation before it circulates to the rest of the body. To circumvent this problem, several formulations of testosterone have been devised to provide slow parenteral release and a prolonged androgenic effect. These include transdermal delivery through a gel (AndroGel) or patch (Androderm or Testoderm) applied to the skin daily, as well as subcutaneous pellets (Testopel) that may produce therapeutic effects for as long as 6 months. Two different types of transdermal patch systems are currently available. One is specifically designed to be placed on the skin of the scrotum and the other is designed to be used elsewhere.

Prior to these new transdermal and subcutaneous delivery systems, testosterone esters (cypionate, enanthate, and propionate) were employed instead of testosterone to produce more sustained androgenic effects. These derivatives are supplied in forms that are slowly absorbed into the bloodstream from intramuscular injection sites. Once they reach the circulation, the esters break down and testosterone is released. These preparations may be effective for 2 to 4 weeks, but during this time plasma testosterone levels may vary markedly from relatively high early in this period to low later on. None of the testosterone esters available in the United States are effective orally; however, testosterone undecanoate, an ester that is unusually resistant to breakdown, is an effective oral preparation (Andriol) available only in Canada.

Because testosterone and testosterone esters were relatively ineffective as oral preparations, synthetic androgens were developed. These synthetic compounds are resistant to the action of liver enzymes that degrade testosterone and thus have good oral bioavailability in addition to a relatively long duration of action. For example, methyltestosterone and fluoxymesterone have biological half-lives of about 3 hours and 9 hours, respectively; whereas the half-life of testosterone in circulation is only minutes.

ADVERSE REACTIONS AND CONTRAINDICATIONS

The reactions experienced with androgens differ in men and women. Men often report urinary tract infections and bladder irritation. Women, who generally receive higher doses than men, experience menstrual irregularities, hypercalcemia, or virilization (see later section this chapter). Precocious virilization may also be seen in boys who receive androgens.

Less common symptoms in men and women include edema, erythrocytosis, liver dysfunction, nausea, or vomiting. Acne, diarrhea, and changes in libido are also possible. Men may also experience pain in the scrotum or groin, and difficulty in urination may signal changes in the prostate gland. Androgens are usually avoided in men with known prostatic or breast carcinoma, because androgens often stimulate growth of these tumors.

As discussed previously, all anabolic steroids possess androgenic properties. These androgenic effects may become obvious, especially when the compounds are used to treat women or children. Patients receiving these compounds may develop increased libido. Men may develop priapism (continuous erection). Women may show androgen-induced changes, such as inappropriate hair development, voice changes, or personality alterations. Children should be watched closely for precocious sexual development. These compounds, while promoting bone growth in children, also promote fusion of the epiphyses, which permanently halts skeletal growth. Therefore full adult height may be reduced in spite of a growth spurt when the drugs are first given.

For this reason and because of the effects on sexual development, these drugs are less than ideal for therapy in children.

In men, high doses of testosterone (or any other androgenic steroid) may suppress gonadotropin release from the pituitary, resulting in reduced spermatogenesis and sterility. Paradoxically, at very high doses, testosterone may produce signs of feminization in men. These effects, which may include tender breasts and gynecomastia, result primarily from the biotransformation of circulating testosterone to estrogen by aromatase.

TOXICITY

The most important toxicity of androgens is directed to the liver. The orally effective synthetic drugs are associated with liver toxicity of various types, including cholestatic jaundice.

INTERACTIONS

Androgens increase the effects of anticoagulants; therefore dosages must be adjusted. Hepatotoxic drugs are avoided with androgens because of the risk of additive damage to the liver.

 DRUG CLASS • Antiandrogens

bicalutamide (Casodex)

flutamide (Evlexin)

nilutamide (Nilandron)

MECHANISM OF ACTION

Antiandrogens occupy androgen receptors, thereby blocking the actions of these receptors. However, their usefulness in this regard is limited because they also cause marked increases in gonadotropin release from the pituitary, resulting in greatly elevated circulating levels of testosterone.

USES

The antiandrogens are indicated for the treatment of advanced or metastatic prostate cancer. Because these agents given alone would greatly increase circulating testosterone levels in the presence of a normally functioning pituitary-gonadal axis, antiandrogens are used only in conjunction with a GnRH analog such as leuprolide (see Chapter 37) or given to patients who have been surgically castrated.

Some evidence also suggests that flutamide may be effective in the treatment of hirsutism in females.

PHARMACOKINETICS

The antiandrogens are all rapidly and nearly completely absorbed. They are highly protein bound and subject to hepatic metabolism; nilutamide and flutamide are biotransformed to products that are also active. One of the metabolites of flutamide may cause hepatic damage, hemolytic anemia, and methemoglobinemia in certain individuals. Nilutamide and bicalutamide have plasma half-lives of 40 to 60 hours and 5 to 7 days, respectively. For flutamide the half-life of the parent compound is only 6 to 10 hours, but its duration of action is significantly prolonged because of its active metabolite.

ADVERSE REACTIONS AND CONTRAINDICATIONS

Some data suggests an association between the use of flutamide and malignant breast cancer in men, but a causal link is not clear. Any of these agents may cause reduced sperm counts and infertility. Flutamide may cause severe hepatotoxicity and should not be given to patients with impaired liver function. Nilutamide has been reported to cause interstitial pneumonitis and should not be given to patients with severe respiratory problems. Other adverse effects that have been reported include anemia, nausea, diarrhea or constipation, hot flashes, and upper respiratory tract infections.

INTERACTIONS

Nilutamide inhibits hepatic cytochrome P450 enzymes responsible for metabolizing many other drugs and also causes facial flushing, malaise, and hypotension in some patients when combined with alcohol. Flutamide appears to increase clotting time in patients stabilized on warfarin.

 DRUG CLASS • 5-Alpha-Reductase Inhibitors

dutasteride (Dutasteride)
finasteride (Propecia, Proscar)

MECHANISM OF ACTION

Both of these drugs are specific inhibitors of 5-alpha-reductase, the enzyme responsible for biotransformation of testosterone to dihydrotestosterone in certain target tissues (including the skin and the prostate gland). Because dihydrotestosterone is much more effective when it interacts with androgen receptors, the effect of inhibiting this enzyme is a reduction in androgenic stimulation at these sites. This inhibition prevents androgen-induced overgrowth and enlargement in the prostate, and it also reduces the androgenic overstimulation of hair follicles in the skin. Dutasteride, a relatively new drug, may be more effective than finasteride.

USES

Finasteride and dutasteride are both indicated for the treatment of **benign prostatic hyperplasia (BPH)** in men. Many men are also using saw palmetto, an herbal remedy available OTC (Box 62-1). Finasteride is also approved for the treatment of **male pattern baldness**. (Dutasteride is currently in clinical trials for this application.) However, to maintain increased hair growth, the drug must be taken continuously.

PHARMACOKINETICS

Both drugs are well absorbed orally and have good bioavailability. Finasteride is biotransformed by hepatic metabolism to products that have much less activity than the parent compound and has a plasma half-life of about 6 hours. The plasma half-life of dutasteride is highly dependent on the dose, ranging from as long as 5 weeks at high plasma concentrations to as short as 3 days.

ADVERSE REACTIONS
AND CONTRAINDICATIONS

Finasteride has been reported to cause breast tenderness and gynecomastia, as well as skin rashes in some patients. Preliminary data suggest that the drug may also cause a slight increase in the risk of prostate can-

---

BOX 62-1 | **Alternative Therapies for Prostate Disorders**

Saw Palmetto

The drug consists of the dried fruits of *Serenoa repens*. The plant is a member of the palm family and it grows wild in Georgia and Florida.

Saw palmetto fruits and their preparations are used widely in Germany, France, and Italy to treat symptoms associated with benign prostatic hyperplasia (BPH). Liposterolic extracts of the fruit have been shown to exert antiandrogenic and antiinflammatory effects. Its effectiveness against BPH is supported by results of placebo-controlled, double-blind studies in more than 2000 BPH patients in Germany. Stomach upset has been reported as an adverse effect of saw palmetto extract.

Preparations of saw palmetto are available without prescription in the United States, but health care providers should caution against its unsupervised use and urge anyone who thinks they may have BPH to consult with their health care provider before using.

Saw palmetto is also promoted for female breast enlargement. There is, however, no evidence to support this claim.

---

cer. Decreased libido and impotence may occur early in therapy with finasteride but usually subsides with continued use of the drug. Experience with dutasteride is limited, but a similar profile of adverse effects is anticipated.

Inhibitors of 5-alpha-reductase pose special risks with regard to pregnant women. Dihydrotestosterone is necessary for normal development of the genitalia in male fetuses. Therefore, women who are pregnant or may become pregnant should not even handle tablets containing these drugs.

INTERACTIONS

No significant specific drug interactions have been reported for these drugs.

APPLICATION TO PRACTICE

ASSESSMENT
History of Present Illness

A principal aim in assessment of the patient with hypogonadism is to determine the patient's perception of the illness or health problem. It is important to understand what concerns or symptoms caused the patient to seek health care. Eliciting information about the symptoms, their onset, and duration is critical.

The man with primary hypogonadism may report a history of infertility, reduced libido and potency, alterations in behavior (e.g., loss of motivation or irritability), and perhaps some loss of secondary sexual characteristics. He may note decreases in axillary and pubic hair, muscle mass, testicular and penile size, as well as changes in body shape that reflect a more "female-like" fat distribution.

Patients with angioedema may report swelling of the face and extremities lasting 2 to 3 days with no known precipitating factor. Occasionally, patients have cramping, abdominal pain accompanied by watery diarrhea and, in extreme cases, partial to complete airway obstruction.

Health History

A thorough health history is needed because some chronic diseases and conditions may prohibit the use of androgens. For example, androgens are contraindicated in males with a history of cancer of the breast or prostate, prostatic hypertrophy, or hypercalcemia. A history of hepatic, cardiac, and renal disease may also preclude the use of these drugs.

Information concerning current drug usage should be obtained, because androgens alter the effectiveness of certain drugs. Allergy or sensitivity to mercury compounds contraindicates the use of testosterone as well.

The clinical history of the patient with angioedema varies greatly, which makes diagnosis difficult. Ask about a family history of the disease, when the disease first appeared, the frequency of attacks, and if there is any history of unexplained swelling or abdominal colic. In most patients the initial episode occurred in early childhood; however, a few patients with angioedema have their first attack between 50 and 70 years of age. Some patients have weekly attacks, whereas others have occasional attacks spread over several decades.

Lifespan Considerations

Perinatal. Androgens and anabolic steroids are not used during pregnancy because of the teratogenic risk. Because danazol may be effective in the treatment of immune thrombocytopenic purpura, classic hemophilia, and alpha$_1$-antitrypsin deficiency, it is conceivable that health care providers will encounter more patients who began taking this drug while unknowingly pregnant.

Pediatric. Hypogonadism in the adolescent male is usually not diagnosed until the patient reaches 16 or 17 years of age, when delayed puberty can be ascertained. At that time, diagnostic testing would include an endocrine evaluation to determine the specific cause of the dysfunction.

The adolescent male can benefit from androgen therapy; however, caution must be exercised, because androgens accelerate epiphyseal closure and may affect linear growth. X-ray studies of the epiphyseal area of the hand and wrist should be performed on a regular basis, usually every 6 months, during androgen therapy.

Generally, in the prepubertal male with delayed onset of puberty, androgen therapy with testosterone is likely to be only one part of the drug regimen. Other drugs that may be used are hormones that release LH, hCG, and GnRH.

The adverse effects of giving anabolic steroids to young children are not fully understood. The risk-to-benefit ratio needs to be evaluated carefully before anabolic steroids are prescribed. Anabolic steroid use in children may accelerate epiphyseal maturation more quickly than linear growth, thus compromising adult height. The drug action may continue for up to 6 months after the drug has been discontinued.

Older Adults. Older adults often have hypertension or other cardiovascular disorders that may be aggravated by the sodium and water retention associated with anabolic steroids. In men the drugs may increase prostate size and interfere with urination, raise the risk of prostate cancer, and cause excessive sexual stimulation and priapism.

Cultural/Social Considerations
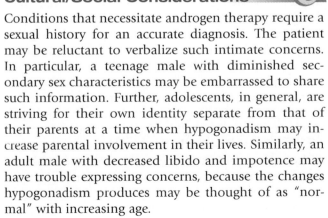

Conditions that necessitate androgen therapy require a sexual history for an accurate diagnosis. The patient may be reluctant to verbalize such intimate concerns. In particular, a teenage male with diminished secondary sex characteristics may be embarrassed to share such information. Further, adolescents, in general, are striving for their own identity separate from that of their parents at a time when hypogonadism may increase parental involvement in their lives. Similarly, an adult male with decreased libido and impotence may have trouble expressing concerns, because the changes hypogonadism produces may be thought of as "normal" with increasing age.

During androgen therapy, virilizing and masculinizing effects are seen in both males and females. The changes in body image may be unwanted and may lead to lowered self-esteem and possible noncompliance with drug therapy. However, some of the adverse effects are reversible if the drug dosage can be reduced (see the Case Study: Primary Hypogonadism).

Some patients may be concerned about taking anabolic steroids because of an awareness of their reputation for abuse. The health care provider must be sensitive to the patient's concerns and explain the different uses of the drugs.

Adherence to a drug regimen is important in prevention or control of any disease process. In anabolic steroid therapy the presence of masculinizing and virilizing adverse effects could lead to noncompliance with the drug regimen. Although these adverse effects would be more tolerable for men, women may discontinue the drug if such effects occur.

Physical Examination

Physical examination findings of primary hypogonadism in an adult male may include feminization in physical appearance and atrophy of external genitalia. Reduced muscle mass and decreased axillary and pubic hair may also be evident.

During an acute attack of angioedema, facial and extremity swelling may be observed. Occasionally, abdominal palpation reveals a tender abdomen with cramps and pain.

Laboratory Testing

Endocrine studies are used to determine whether the suspected hypogonadal state exists because of a testicular, pituitary, or hypothalamic dysfunction. Evaluation and monitoring of hypogonadism consists of serum testosterone measurements. Testosterone levels fluctuate and are generally elevated in the morning; therefore more than one assay may be necessary for careful evaluation. A low serum testosterone level is further evaluated in light of serum levels of luteinizing hormone and follicle-stimulating hormone. Luteinizing hormone and follicle-stimulating hormone levels tend to be high in patients with primary hypogonadism but low or inappropriately normal in men with hypogonadotropic hypogonadism. Patients with low gonadotropin levels may undergo further evaluation for other pituitary abnormalities, such as hyperprolactinemia. Hemoglobin and hematocrit values may be slightly below the normal male range because of hypogonadism. The laboratory workup should include both urine and blood tests. Additionally, sper-

matogenesis may be impaired, which will be reflected in sperm counts.

In patients with angioedema, the complement system reflects a low level of C4 in the presence of normal C1 and C3 levels and a low level of C1 INH in about 80% to 85% of patients. It is usually recommended that a C4 evaluation be performed as a simple screening test for angioedema and the diagnosis confirmed by measurement of C1 INH levels. In 20% of patients this inhibitor protein may be present in normal or even increased amounts, but its function is abnormal.

GOALS OF THERAPY

The treatment goal for the adult male with primary hypogonadism caused by testicular dysfunction is to restore sexual function, normalize behavior, and promote virilization. In prepubertal males who are androgen deficient, treatment interventions are directed at reestablishing and maintaining masculine characteristics and functions.

The primary treatment objective in angioedema is to decrease the frequency and severity of attacks. Further, the patient must avoid overuse or abuse of these drugs because of their "body building" effects.

INTERVENTION
Administration

Androgens and anabolic steroids are available in tablets for oral use, in solution for injection, and in a transdermal formulation. Oral androgen formulations should be administered with food to decrease the possibility of gastric distress. Intramuscular injections should be given deep into the gluteal muscle using a Z-track technique.

The transdermal formulation of testosterone should be worn on a shaved area of the scrotum 22 hours a day with a new patch applied daily. Chemical depilatories should not be used to remove hair from the scrotal surface before application of the transdermal patch. There is a potential for transfer of testosterone from the scrotal patch to a female sexual partner, who may be affected by mild virilization.

Education

Because of the virilizing and masculinizing effects of androgens, patients should be taught about the potential changes in secondary sex characteristics that may accompany therapy. The changes that do occur should be monitored, because certain changes require a reduction in dosage or discontinuation of the drug. Instruct patients that if they miss a dose, they should not double up on the next dose but should continue with the original dosage regimen.

CASE STUDY  *Primary Hypogonadism*

ASSESSMENT

HISTORY OF PRESENT ILLNESS

AB is a 62-year-old man with vague complaints of decreased motivation and an inability to perform sexually for the last several months. He believes that his scrotum and penis have gotten smaller. He thinks this may be due to his age but wants verification.

HEALTH HISTORY

AB denies having a history of renal disease, hepatic disease, prostate disease, or carcinoma. He takes warfarin for atrial fibrillation and reports no recent weight loss or gain. He exercises sporadically and takes no prescription or OTC drugs.

LIFESPAN CONSIDERATIONS

AB may be at risk for benign prostatic hypertrophy. AB is concerned about what he describes as symptoms of "aging." He is reluctant to verbalize specific concerns about sexual performance, but states he feels like "less of a man." His adult children live in the same community.

CULTURAL/SOCIAL CONSIDERATIONS

AB belongs to an HMO with pharmacy privileges. His primary income is derived from a job in the construction industry.

PHYSICAL EXAMINATION

VSS. Decreased muscle mass relative to visit of 5 years ago. Relative atrophy of genitalia with loss of pubic and axillary hair. Prostate examination reveals 25 to 30 g bilobular organ. Other organ systems examination unremarkable.

LABORATORY TESTING

Electrolytes, liver function values, blood urea nitrogen, creatinine, lipid panel, and hemoglobin are within normal limits. Serum calcium levels 8.5 mg/dL. Testosterone level 220 mcg/mL (normal, 300-900 mcg/mL). Twenty-four-hour urine for LH, 25 IU/24 hr (normal, 5-20 IU/24 hr). Twenty-four-hour urine for FSH, 30 IU/24 hr (normal, 1-20 IU/24 hr).

PATIENT PROBLEM(S)

Primary hypogonadism.

GOALS OF THERAPY

Restore sexual function, normalize behavior, and promote virilization.

CRITICAL THINKING QUESTIONS

1. The health care provider orders testosterone intramuscularly every 3 weeks until a therapeutic response is noted. Why do you think the intramuscular formulation was ordered rather than an oral formulation?
2. What is the mechanism of action of testosterone?
3. What adverse effects does AB need to be aware of?
4. AB comes to the clinic for his every-third-week injection. What technique will the nurse use to administer the testosterone?
5. What intervention will most likely be required when taking into account the interaction of AB's warfarin and testosterone?

Health care providers should be sensitive to the emotional responses of both male and female patients to therapy. Encourage the patient to discuss his or her concerns and emotional responses to a changing body image.

Inform the patient about the importance of regular medical supervision. Periodic laboratory tests to monitor liver function, lipids, hemoglobin, and hematocrit are needed. Because anabolic steroids cause sodium, chloride, water, potassium, phosphate, and calcium imbalances, electrolytes should be closely monitored. Ankle swelling or a weight gain of more than 2 pounds per week should be reported to the health care provider. Restriction of dietary sodium and the use of diuretics may be indicated.

EVALUATION

The efficacy of androgen replacement therapy is assessed primarily by monitoring the patient's clinical response. Although there is variability in response, most men experience an awakening of libido, resumption of sexual activity, and improved sense of well-being 1 to 2 months after androgen therapy is started. Whether therapy continues depends on the patient's symptoms.

The effectiveness of anabolic steroids in the management of angioedema is evidenced by reductions in the frequency and severity of attacks. Comparing the frequency of attacks before and after a trial period of anabolic steroids is necessary.

Bibliography

Korkia P: Anabolic-androgenic steroid series: part I. Adverse effects of anabolic-androgenic steroids: a review, *J Subst Misuse Nurs Health Soc Care* 3(1):34-41, 1998.

Morley JE, Perry HM III: Androgen deficiency in aging men: role of testosterone replacement therapy, *J Lab Clin Med* 135(5):370-378, 2000.

Internet Resources

Moul JW, Lipo DR: Prostate cancer in the late 1990s: hormone refractory disease options. Urology Nurses Online. Available online at http://www.duj.com/moul.html.

http://www.healthcentral.com/mhc/top/001866.cfm.
http://www.nlm.nih.gov/medlineplus/druginfo/androgenssystemic202036.html.
http://www.nlm.nih.gov/medlineplus/druginfo/antiandrogensnonsteroidalsyste203418.html.
http://www.nlm.nih.gov/medlineplus/druginfo/finasteridesystemic202649.html.
http://www.phoenix5.org/Infolink/advanced/antiandrogens.html.
http://www.rxlist.com/cgi/generic/finas.htm.

CHAPTER

63

Vitamins and Minerals

SHERRY F. QUEENER • SUSAN SCIACCA

 Visit **http://evolve.elsevier.com/Gutierrez/** for additional information.

KEY TERMS

Fat-soluble vitamins, p. 1033

Macrominerals, p. 1039

Microminerals, p. 1041

Osteomalacia, p. 1030

Osteoporosis, p. 1030

Recommended dietary allowance (RDA), p. 1035

Retinol, p. 1033

Vitamin D, p. 1028

Vitamins, p. 1027

Water-soluble vitamins, p. 1036

Xerophthalmia, p. 1033

OBJECTIVES

- Learn the classes of vitamins and minerals.
- Identify the medical uses of essential vitamins and minerals.
- Discuss the risks from deficiencies of vitamins and minerals.
- Compare and contrast the adverse reactions from overdoses of vitamins.
- Establish a reliable source of information about dietary supplements.
- Develop a nursing care plan, including a teaching plan, for a patient receiving vitamin or mineral therapy.

 PHYSIOLOGY • **Vitamins and Minerals**

Thirteen vitamins and 17 minerals are considered essential for human health (Table 63-1). Vitamins are compounds that indirectly assist other nutrients through the processes of digestion, absorption, biotransformation, and elimination. The study of vitamins and minerals is an important part of the field of nutrition, and references to that literature are given in the bibliography. The coverage in this text focuses on the pharmacology of clinically important vitamins and minerals. The important terminology concerning nutritional requirements for vitamins and minerals is explained in Box 63-1.

BOX 63-1

BOX 63-1 **Who Sets the Standards for Vitamin and Mineral Intake?**

The basic standard for nutrition in the United States for the last 20 years has been the Recommended Dietary Allowance (RDA). The RDA was defined as "the levels of intake of essential nutrients that, on the basis of scientific knowledge, are judged by the Food and Nutrition Board to be adequate to meet the known nutrient needs of practically all healthy persons." The RDA is now being replaced by Dietary Reference Intakes (DRI). The old RDA was designed to prevent nutrient deficiencies. The DRI are designed to help prevent chronic diseases that are now known to have a dietary component.

The RDA was a single value, but the DRI has four components. The **estimated average requirement (EAR)** is the intake that meets the nutrient needs of half the individuals within a specific age group or other category. The new **Recommended dietary allowance (RDA)** is the intake that meets the nutrient needs of most healthy persons in a specific age or gender group. The RDA is set at two standard deviations above the EAR to afford adequate intake to about 97% of the population within a specific group. **Adequate intake (AI)** was defined when there was insufficient data to estimate an average requirement. For example, the AI for calcium is now 1000 to 1300 mg of calcium daily, which observation suggests is adequate to prevent osteoporosis for most otherwise healthy persons. **Tolerable upper intake level (UL)** has been defined as the maximum intake that a normal healthy person could maintain without the risk of significant adverse effects.

These new standards are being established by the Standing Committee on the Scientific Evaluation of Dietary Reference Intakes of the Food and Nutrition Board, Institute of Medicine, National Academy of Sciences. Health Canada is contributing so that standards may be used by both countries.

TABLE 63-1

Classification of Vitamins and Minerals

Fat-Soluble Vitamins

Vitamin A	Vitamin D
Vitamin E	Vitamin K

Water-Soluble Vitamins

Biotin	Cyanocobalamin (vitamin B_{12})
Folic acid (vitamin B_9)	Niacin (vitamin B_3)
Pantothenic acid (vitamin B_5)	Pyridoxine (vitamin B_6)
Riboflavin (vitamin B_2)	Thiamin (vitamin B_1)
Vitamin B complex	Vitamin C

Macrominerals

Calcium	Chloride
Magnesium	Phosphorus
Potassium	Sodium
Selenium	Silicon
Zinc	

Microminerals

Chromium	Cobalt
Copper	Fluoride
Iodine	Iron
Manganese	Vanadium

Regulation of Calcium Metabolism

Calcium is needed for the proper function of all cells and tissues. Close control of calcium levels is required because very small changes in blood calcium levels can profoundly alter many cellular functions, with effects on most body systems. Because of this fundamental role in maintaining function, calcium uptake, distribution, and elimination are very tightly controlled in the body to maintain a constant concentration of 4.7 to 5.6 mEq/L in plasma or serum.

The term vitamin D refers to a group of related lipid-soluble substances. Cholecalciferol, or vitamin D_3, is formed from cholesterol in skin when it is exposed to sunlight. The vitamin may also be acquired through diet (Box 63-2). Depending on what form of the vitamin is ingested, various biotransformations are possible. The liver converts vitamin D_3 to the more active 25-hydroxyvitamin D_3. The kidney converts 25-hydroxyvitamin D_3 to calcitriol, the most active metabolite of vitamin D.

Vitamin D acts like a hormone in the body, regulating calcium concentrations in concert with parathyroid hormone and calcitonin (see Chapter 56). Specifically, vitamin D promotes release of calcium and phosphate from bone, blocks renal excretion of these materials, and promotes their absorption from the GI tract. All of these actions increase calcium concentration in blood. Vitamin D interacts with receptors in target cells throughout the body to produce these effects. The vitamin D receptor, like the receptors for corticosteroids and thyroid hormones, is found in the cytoplasm of cells and moves to cell nuclei where the hormone-receptor complex influences gene expression.

Synthesis of vitamin D_3 in skin occurs continuously, so long as exposure to sunlight is adequate. Formation of the most active form of vitamin D, calcitriol, is promoted by relative deficiencies of calcium, phosphate, or vitamin D. Active stimulation of the process occurs with parathyroid hormone, whereas very high vitamin D intake can inhibit conversion to the more active metabolite.

Dietary Considerations for
WHERE DO I GET MY VITAMINS?

Vitamins are among the essential nutrients. If the patient's diet is varied and plentiful, vitamin deficiencies are rare. Good sources of major vitamins are listed in the following examples.

Vitamin A (Retinol)

Preformed vitamin A occurs only in foods of animal origin, either in storage areas such as the liver or in association with fat. Rich sources of vitamin A include liver, kidney, fish liver oils, cream, butter, whole milk, whole-milk cheese, fortified margarine, skim milk, and skim-milk products. Vitamin A precursors (carotenoids) are found in dark green, leafy vegetables, and red-yellow-orange fruits and vegetables. Deeper colors are associated with higher levels of carotenoids.

Vitamin D

Cholecalciferol (vitamin D_3) is found in animal products (e.g., herring, salmon, sardines, shrimp, and fish liver oils). Cholecalciferol is also formed in the body, when the skin is exposed to sunlight. Vitamin D is found in variable amounts in butter, cream, egg yolks, and liver. Most milk is fortified with 10 mcg/quart (400 IU/quart) of irradiated ergosterol (vitamin D_2). Powdered milk and evaporated milk are also fortified, as well as some margarines, butter, certain cereals, and infant formulas. Milk used to make cheese or yogurt may not be fortified.

Vitamin E

Seed oils (e.g., wheat germ oil, corn oil, soybean oil, sunflower oil) are the richest source of vitamin E. Smaller amounts are present in fruits, vegetables, and animal fats. Peanut, olive, coconut, and fish oils are poor sources of vitamin E.

Vitamin K

Dietary sources of large quantities of vitamin K include dark green or leafy vegetables (kale, turnip greens, spinach, broccoli, cabbage, lettuce). Cauliflower, tomatoes, fruits, cereals, wheat bran, cheese, egg yolks, and liver contain smaller amounts. Significant amounts of vitamin K are formed by the bacterial flora in the GI tract.

Vitamin C (Ascorbic Acid)

The best dietary sources of ascorbic acid are fresh citrus fruits, leafy vegetables eaten raw, tomatoes, strawberries, cantaloupe, cabbage, green peppers, and potatoes. The ascorbic acid content of fruits and vegetables varies with the conditions in which they are grown and the degree of ripeness when harvested. Refrigeration and quick freezing help retain the vitamin.

Thiamine (Vitamin B_1)

Dietary sources of thiamine include organ meats, legumes, nuts, whole or enriched grain products, wheat germ, and brewer's yeast.

Riboflavin (Vitamin B_2)

Good sources for riboflavin are milk and milk products, cheddar cheese, cottage cheese, organ meats, eggs, and leafy green vegetables. Sixty percent of riboflavin is lost when flour is milled; thus most breads and cereals are enriched with riboflavin.

Niacin (Vitamin B_3)

Niacin is found in meats, legumes, nuts, peanut butter, and whole-grain and enriched-grain products. Tryptophan, a niacin precursor, is also found in protein foods of animal origin.

Pantothenic Acid (Vitamin B_5)

Liver, kidney, salmon, eggs, legumes and peanuts, whole grains, milk, fruits, vegetables, molasses, and yeast are good sources of pantothenic acid. Much of the pantothenate in meat is lost during thawing and cooking. Approximately half of the pantothenic acid contained in flour is lost in the milling process.

Pyridoxine (Vitamin B_6)

Pyridoxine is found in meat (especially liver), fish, egg yolks, legumes, nuts, potatoes, whole grains, wheat germ, yeast, prunes, raisins, and bananas.

Biotin (Vitamin B_7)

Liver, kidneys, egg yolk, soybeans, yeast, milk, fish, nuts, and oatmeal are good sources of biotin. Biotin is also synthesized in considerable amounts by intestinal bacteria.

Cobalamin (Vitamin B_{12})

Cobalamin is found in liver, kidney, milk, eggs, fish, cheese, and muscle meats. Some cooked sea vegetables contain cobalamin in the same concentration as beef liver. Well over half of the cobalamin (40% to 90%) is lost during pasteurization and evaporation.

Folic Acid

Good sources of folic acid include liver; kidney beans; lima beans; fresh, dark green, leafy vegetables; broccoli; asparagus; spinach; orange juice; white bread; dried beans; and ready-to-eat cereals. Small quantities of folic acid are found in milk, eggs, fruits (except oranges), root vegetables, and most meats. Only 25% to 50% of dietary folic acid is nutritionally available, but intestinal bacteria synthesize large amounts, which add to the daily intake.

PATHOPHYSIOLOGY • Calcium and Vitamin D Metabolism

An adult human has two sources of calcium that may be used to meet the daily needs of the body: dietary calcium and calcium deposited in bones. Adults require 1000 to 1200 mg/daily, and pregnant or lactating women require more. These large amounts of calcium can be obtained in a diet rich in dark green, leafy vegetables, seafood, and milk products, but the diets of many Americans do not contain adequate amounts of calcium. If dietary calcium is insufficient, the body will begin to resorb calcium from bones to meet metabolic needs for the element.

Vitamin D deficiency can occur in persons who are not adequately exposed to sunlight and who ingest a diet poor in the vitamin. Vitamin D deficiency limits the amount of dietary calcium and phosphorus that can be absorbed. In children, vitamin D deficiency leads to a condition called rickets, in which the calcium that would normally be used to build bones is robbed to serve other life-supporting needs; the result is softened bones that are deformed by bearing weight. In adults, vitamin D deficiency can contribute to **osteoporosis** (localized weakening of the bones) because the inadequate absorption of calcium from the diet leads to bone resorption to supply the necessary element. Osteoporosis is most commonly found in postmenopausal women or those with sedentary life styles. **Osteomalacia** is a related condition characterized by decreased bone density and strength.

Vitamin D excess can produce hypercalcemia (see Chapter 56, Table 56-4). The most common cause of vitamin D excess is overdosage with dietary supplements.

DRUG CLASS • Calcium Supplements

MECHANISM OF ACTION

Calcium present in the diet or in dietary supplements replaces calcium that would otherwise be mobilized from bone to supply the body's metabolic needs. Maintaining an adequate intake of calcium helps prevent loss of calcium from bones and maintains their strength. Because the uptake of calcium is regulated by vitamin D, maximum benefit from dietary calcium supplements is seen when adequate vitamin D uptake is also maintained.

USES

Oral calcium supplements (Table 63-2) are designed primarily to prevent calcium deficiency and maintain bone strength. These preparations are also often used as antacids.

TABLE 63-2

Selected Calcium Supplements

Generic Name	Brand Name	Comments
calcium carbonate	BioCal, Caltrate 600, Rolaids, Tums	625-mg tablets contain 250 mg calcium; 1500-mg tablets contain 600 mg calcium
	Vivactiv	Vivactiv 20 calorie chew contains 500 mg calcium, 100 IU vitamin D, 40 mcg vitamin K
calcium carbonate, oyster-shell derived	Os-Cal 500, Oysco, Oyst-Cal	625-mg tablets contain 250 mg calcium; 1500-mg tablets contain 600 mg calcium
calcium citrate	Citracal	950-mg tablets contain 200 mg calcium
calcium glubionate	Calcionate, Neo-Calglucon	Syrup contains 115 mg calcium in 5 mL
calcium gluconate	generic	1000-mg tablets contain 90 mg calcium
calcium lactate	generic	650-mg tablets contain 84 mg calcium
dibasic calcium phosphate	generic	500-mg tablets contain 115 mg calcium
tribasic calcium phosphate	Posture	1600-mg tablets contain 600 mg calcium

PHARMACOKINETICS

Calcium is primarily absorbed in the upper part of the duodenum where an acid medium prevails. Absorption is greatly reduced in the lower part of the GI tract, where the contents are alkaline. Ordinarily, only about 20% to 30% of calcium taken by mouth, either as foods or supplements, is absorbed. Calcium is absorbed through the action of calcitriol. Calcitriol increases calcium uptake at the brush border of the intestinal mucosa by stimulating production of a calcium-binding protein. Certain fiber-rich foods can diminish absorption. Calcium elimination from the body is regulated by the kidneys, under the influence of parathyroid hormone and other factors (see Chapter 56).

ADVERSE REACTIONS AND CONTRAINDICATIONS

Systemic reactions are uncommon with oral calcium preparations, but constipation and loss of appetite may occur. Calcium supplements should not be used in patients with symptoms of hypercalcemia, including those with sarcoidosis or renal calculi. Patients with renal impairment should not receive calcium phosphate because the excess phosphate is not easily handled without adequate renal function.

TOXICITY

High dosages of calcium supplements can produce signs of hypercalcemia (see Chapter 56, Table 56-4).

INTERACTIONS

Calcium preparations diminish the absorption of several drugs, including etidronate, phenytoin, and tetracyclines. Calcium also directly antagonizes the effects of drugs such as gallium nitrate and magnesium sulfate. Iron-containing preparations interfere with the absorption of calcium.

DRUG CLASS • Vitamin D

alfacalcidol (One-Alpha✲)

calcifediol (Calderol)

calcitriol (Calcijex, Rocaltrol)

ergocalciferol (Drisdol, Ostoforte, Radiostol)

MECHANISM OF ACTION

Vitamin D is required for proper absorption of calcium. Vitamin D, taken as a supplement, has the same action as the vitamin D normally produced in the body.

USES

Vitamin D derivatives are used to control hypocalcemia caused by hypoparathyroidism (see Chapter 56). Ergocalciferol is the drug of choice for vitamin D deficiency, unless renal failure is present. For vitamin D deficiency in patients with renal failure, calcitriol is used to replace the calcitriol normally formed in the kidneys but missing in these patients; another strategy is to use alfacalcidol, which is converted to calcitriol by the liver.

PHARMACOKINETICS

Vitamin D is a highly lipid-soluble material that is readily absorbed orally. Once in the blood, vitamin D is bound to specific alpha-globulins for transport to target tissues. This fat-soluble vitamin is concentrated in liver and other fat stores. The metabolic fate of vitamin D depends on which form is taken. Vitamin D_3 (cholecalciferol) and vitamin D_2 (ergocalciferol) are both converted to calcifediol by the liver. Calcifediol and alfacalcidol are both converted by renal tissue to calcitriol, the most active vitamin D derivative. Most vitamin D metabolites are excreted in bile.

ADVERSE REACTIONS AND CONTRAINDICATIONS

Excess of vitamin D produces symptoms that are primarily those expected with high blood calcium concentrations (see Chapter 56, Table 56-4).

TOXICITY

Large overdosages of vitamin D may be fatal because cardiovascular and renal function is impaired. Chronic overdosage can cause deposits of calcium in blood vessels, kidneys, and other tissues.

INTERACTIONS

Antacids or other preparations containing magnesium may be more dangerous when given with vitamin D because high magnesium concentrations in blood may occur.

DRUG CLASS • **Biphosphonates**

alendronate (Fosamax)

etidronate (Didronel)

pamidronate (Aredia)

risedronate (Actonel)

tiludronate (Skelid)

MECHANISM OF ACTION

The biphosphonates are synthetic analogs of inorganic pyrophosphate that block removal of calcium from bone. These drugs act on osteoclasts, the cells that remove calcium from bone to supply metabolic needs and to remodel bone. Alendronate and risedronate inhibit activity of the osteoclasts, but the cells remain bound to remodeling sites in bone. Etidronate lowers the number of osteoclasts. Pamidronate blocks attachment of osteoclasts to bone. Tiludronate causes osteoclasts to detach from bone. All of these drugs slow bone resorption and allow calcium to be retained in bone.

USES

Biphosphonates are used to control Paget's disease (see Chapter 56), as well as to treat osteoporosis. In addition, etidronate or pamidronate may be used to control hypercalcemia, especially when the condition arises from malignancies of the bone. Etidronate has also been used for heterotropic ossification, a nonmalignant overgrowth of bone that may follow hip replacement surgery. Alendronate is used for prophylaxis of postmenopausal osteoporosis.

PHARMACOKINETICS

These drugs have a low oral bioavailability that is further impaired by food or beverages other than water. Absorbed drug binds to bone, concentrating at sites where bone is being remodeled. The effects on serum calcium levels develop slowly with oral doses. Therapeutic effects on bone remodeling may persist for months after therapy is stopped because of the long persistence of drug in bone.

ADVERSE REACTIONS AND CONTRAINDICATIONS

Nausea, diarrhea, and allergic reactions are common with these drugs. Many patients with Paget's disease suffer tenderness or pain weeks or months after therapy is started. Alendronate is often associated with abdominal pain, pain and erosion of the esophagus, and with muscle pain. Risedronate also causes abdominal pain, as well as arthralgia, chest pain, headache and dizziness. Tiludronate often causes back or generalized body pain, as well as symptoms of upper respiratory infection or congestion.

Biphosphonates are avoided in patients with impaired renal function (creatinine clearance below 35 ml/min) because the drugs may accumulate. Several of the drugs are also contraindicated in patients with preexisting esophagitis.

TOXICITY

Higher dosages of the drug may cause more severe GI tract symptoms and possibly hypocalcemia.

INTERACTIONS

Foods or drugs that have a high content of metal ions impair the oral absorption of bisphosphonates, preventing their action. Antacids, mineral supplements, multivitamins with added minerals, calcium salts, and calcium-rich dairy products may all be involved.

 DRUG CLASS • **Selective Estrogen Receptor Modulator**

raloxifene (Evista)

MECHANISM OF ACTION

Raloxifene interacts with estrogen receptors in bone and causes an estrogen-like increase in the accumulation of calcium in bone. Unlike true estrogens, raloxifene causes no proliferation of reproductive tissues and does not block hot flashes and other symptoms of estrogen deficiency.

USES

Raloxifene is indicated for the prevention of osteoporosis in postmenopausal women. Controlled trials with raloxifene and an anticancer agent tamoxifen showed that raloxifene may have a protective effect against breast cancer in women, a possibility that is still under study.

PHARMACOKINETICS

Raloxifene is adequately absorbed orally, but the drug is rapidly converted to the glucuronide by a first-pass effect (see Chapter 1). The drug is eliminated primarily in bile.

ADVERSE REACTIONS AND CONTRAINDICATIONS

A variety of symptoms, including joint or muscle pain, leg cramps, rash, vaginitis, sore throat, painful urination, insomnia, and depression, appear in 3% to 6% of treated patients. About 25% of women treated with raloxifene report hot flashes, which are caused by the antiestrogen effects of the drug. Raloxifene should be avoided in women with a history of thromboembolic disorders.

TOXICITY

Many of the adverse effects of raloxifene may be dose related and would be expected to worsen at higher dosages.

INTERACTIONS

Cholestyramine should be avoided because it reduces the absorption of raloxifene and interferes with enterohepatic recirculation. Estrogens should also be avoided. Warfarin effectiveness is increased by raloxifene, which may lead to bleeding episodes.

PATHOPHYSIOLOGY • Fat-Soluble Vitamins

Fat-soluble vitamins are chemically related to fats and thus are absorbed from the diet along with other lipids. Efficient absorption requires the presence of bile and pancreatic juice. The fat-soluble vitamins are then transported to the liver via the lymph system as a part of lipoproteins and stored in various tissues. The fat-soluble vitamins are not normally eliminated in urine but are stored in body fat. The fat-soluble vitamins include vitamin D (discussed earlier in this chapter), as well as vitamins A, E, and K. These vitamins have very different functions, which are revealed partly through the symptoms of their deficiency states.

Vitamin A deficiency causes night blindness, xerophthalmia (abnormal dryness of the conjunctiva and cornea), and corneal scarring. Without vitamin A, the protective barrier of mucous membranes is lost. There is a progressive deterioration of epithelial tissues and reduced resistance to invasion by bacteria, viruses, or parasites. The number of circulating T cells as well as their response may be reduced. The skin becomes dry, scaly, and rough.

Vitamin E deficiencies are uncommon. When present, they are usually related to malabsorption or lipid transport abnormalities (e.g., abetalipoproteinemia). Deficiency of vitamin E is associated with symptoms of peripheral neuropathy. A deficiency of vitamin E also lowers host resistance by depressing the proliferation of lymphocytes, lowering the antibody response to pathogens, and lowering delayed hypersensitivity reactions.

Vitamin K deficiency is common in newborns because their diet is low in vitamin K and they lack intestinal synthesis of the vitamin during the first week of life. After infancy, deficiency usually results from diseases that interfere with the absorption (biliary tract, GI disorders) or function of vitamin K (cirrhosis, hepatitis). The signs and symptoms of severe vitamin K deficiency include petechiae, ecchymosis, signs of internal bleeding, asthenia, and hypovolemic shock.

DRUG CLASS • Vitamin A Family

vitamin A (Aquasol A, generic)

MECHANISM OF ACTION

The term vitamin A refers to a group of retinoids that maintain function of the retina, influence embryonic development, and support growth and differentiation of epithelial cells. Forms of vitamin A with the most activity in the body are retinol, retinal, and retinoic acid. Retinal is a component of the visual pigment rhodopsin and, as such, is essential to the integrity of photoreception in the rods and cones of the retina. Retinoic acid binds to nuclear receptors that alter gene transcription and thus affect differentiation and function of epithelial cells. Basal epithelial cells are prompted to produce mucin by the action of vitamin A, or retinol, which protects the cornea and other tissues from losing function and becoming open to infection. Vitamin A is also thought to have an anticancer effect and to promote function of the immune system, but the mechanisms for these actions are not yet fully understood.

USES

Vitamin A is used as a dietary supplement to reverse vitamin A deficiency states. Vitamin A deficiency may occur in generally malnourished patients or in patients with malabsorption syndrome. Vitamin A deficiency does not occur in persons who eat a normal balanced diet.

Tretinoin (all-trans-retinoic acid) is used to treat a specific form of leukemia (see Chapter 37). Isotretinoin and other retinoids are also used to treat severe acne (see Chapter 67).

PHARMACOKINETICS

Most of the retinol in the diet (see Box 63-2) exists as an ester with a fatty acid such as palmitic acid. Cells within the intestine have very efficient mechanisms to remove nearly all retinol from the intestinal contents. The absorbed retinol is incorporated into chylomicrons, under normal conditions, and transported to the liver where the chylomicron is taken up and the retinol is added to the liver stores. Approximately 90% of vitamin A is stored in the liver, with the remainder deposited in fat, the lungs, and kidneys. Normal blood levels of vitamin A can be maintained for months, in the face of restricted dietary intake, by using these liver stores of vitamin A.

Dietary beta-carotene can be used by the body and coverted to retinol. The newest estimates are that 12 mcg of beta-carotene must be absorbed in order to produce one microgram of retinol. Other dietary carotenes are less efficiently converted; thus 24 mcg are required to produce one microgram of retinol. Using the older system of international units (IU), one IU of vitamin A is equivalent to 0.3 mcg of all-trans-retinol, 3.6 mcg of all-trans-beta-carotene, and 7.2 mcg of other provitamin A carotenes.

Transport of retinol to tissues is mediated by retinol-binding protein, a specific carrier that also complexes with the thyroxine carrier protein transthyretin. This complex delivers retinol to cellular retinol-binding proteins that exist on all cell surfaces. These cellular receptors facilitate biotransformation of retinol to more bioactive forms and the movement of the activated vitamin to the nucleus, where gene expression is altered.

The effects of beta-carotene are somewhat different from that of vitamin A. Beta-carotene inactivates single oxygen molecules, which is what makes it an antioxidant. It is believed that the protective antioxidant function is performed by the intact beta-carotene molecule rather than vitamin A.

ADVERSE REACTIONS AND CONTRAINDICATIONS

Administration of 700 to 900 mcg of retinol to healthy adults is adequate to reverse or prevent signs of vitamin A deficiency. These doses usually cause no adverse reactions.

TOXICITY

Acute toxicity is associated with single doses of retinol of more than 15,000 mcg in adults; lower dosages produce toxicity in children. Symptoms include headache, fatigue, weakness, anorexia, nausea, and vomiting. Cerebrospinal fluid pressure increases and may contribute to vertigo, blurred vision, and muscular incoordination. A bulging fontanelle may be seen in infants.

Chronic hypervitaminosis A in adults occurs when intake exceeds 30,000 mcg daily for several months. Symptoms often include liver toxicity, GI discomfort, vomiting, seizures, dry skin, increased intracranial pressure, bone pain, and yellow patches on skin. Symptoms disappear weeks or months after the supplement is discontinued. Patients with liver disease, children, and pregnant women are most prone to hypervitaminosis A. Vitamin A is teratogenic; congenital malformations are likely to develop in fetuses exposed to high levels.

 DRUG CLASS • Vitamin E

vitamin E (alpha tocopherol; Aquasol E, E-200, E-400, E-1000, E-Complex-600, E-Vitamin, Vita-Plus E, Webber Vitamin E)

MECHANISM OF ACTION

Vitamin E is an antioxidant with actions on muscles, nerves, and the immune system. Vitamin E protects cellular membranes from oxygen-containing free radicals. By scavenging free radicals, vitamin E prevents destructive peroxidation of polyunsaturated fatty acids that maintain structure and function of cell membranes.

USES

Vitamin E is an accepted supplement to treat or prevent vitamin E deficiency. This condition is unlikely to occur in normal adults who eat a varied diet (see Box 63-2) but is more likely in situations that impair fat absorption, during total parenteral nutrition, or in infants receiving formula without adequate vitamin E.

Vitamin E is not accepted as effective to prevent cancer, skin conditions, arthritis, or other conditions.

PHARMACOKINETICS

Vitamin E resides inside low-density lipoprotein particles to prevent renal elimination of vitamin molecules. The absorption of vitamin E is variable, ranging between 20% and 80%. Vitamin E is stored in the liver and to a larger extent in fatty tissues. It is metabolized in the liver, entering the enterohepatic circulation. The metabolites are eventually eliminated in both the urine and feces.

Newborns have low tissue concentrations of vitamin E because little vitamin E is transferred across placental membranes. Breast milk contains enough vitamin E to meet the needs of a breast-feeding infant.

ADVERSE REACTIONS AND CONTRAINDICATIONS

Vitamin E activity is expressed in milligrams of alpha-tocopherol equivalents (α-TE). The average American's intake of α-TE is estimated to be 7.4 to 9 mg α-TE daily. Supplements at or near these levels have few adverse reactions.

TOXICITY

The risk of vitamin E toxicity is low, even at relatively high levels. Signs and symptoms of toxicity may be noted when intake approaches 2000 to 4000 IU/day. Signs and symptoms of excess include headache, fatigue, blurred vision, and diarrhea. Vitamin E toxicity in preterm infants is characterized by respiratory distress, renal failure, liver disease, ascites, and thrombocytopenia.

DRUG CLASS • Vitamin K

phytonadione (Aquamephyton, Mephyton)

MECHANISM OF ACTION

Vitamin K functions as a lipid cofactor for membrane-bound peptide carboxylase. The cofactor is essential for the formation of prothrombin (factor II), proconvertin (factor VII), plasma thromboplastin component (factor IX), and Stuart factor (factor X) in the liver. The cascade theory of blood coagulation is discussed in Chapter 43. Vitamin K may also participate in energy production through oxidative phosphorylation.

USES

Vitamin K is used for treatment and prevention of hypoprothrombinemia and may be used to prevent or treat hemorrhagic disease in newborns. It is also used as an adjunct to patients who have had too much warfarin and who may be bleeding. Supplements are also used to prevent or reverse deficiencies of the vitamin.

PHARMACOKINETICS

Vitamin K occurs naturally in two forms: phytonadione (phylloquinone, or vitamin K_1), which is found in green plant foods, and menaquinone (vitamin K_2), which is formed by bacteria in the intestinal tract. The fat-soluble synthetic formulation menadione (vitamin K_3) is twice as potent as primary food sources for vitamin K_3.

Vitamin K is primarily absorbed from the upper intestine in the presence of bile and dietary fats. It is incorporated into chylomicrons and lipoproteins, and carried to the liver but is not stored in large quantities. Vitamin K is metabolized in the liver and eliminated in urine and feces.

ADVERSE REACTIONS AND CONTRAINDICATIONS

Although the recommended dietary allowance (RDA) for vitamin K is 65 to 70 mcg daily, dosages of up to 25 mg phytonadione are usually well tolerated. Possible reactions include hemolytic anemia, jaundice, flushing of the face, hypotension, or anaphylaxis.

TOXICITY

An excess of vitamin K is unlikely to occur from dietary intake. It may occur when vitamin K is used as an antagonist to oral anticoagulants, although clinical manifestations of excess vitamin K rarely develop. Excessive doses of synthetic vitamin K have produced kernicterus in an infant. The forms of vitamin K that can be mixed with water have a much wider margin of safety.

INTERACTIONS

Vitamin K antagonizes the effects of oral anticoagulants. Coadministration of vitamin K with hemolytic drugs such as quinidine, procainamide, or sulfonylureas may increase the risk of this dangerous adverse reaction.

PATHOPHYSIOLOGY • Water-Soluble Vitamins

Water-soluble vitamins are ingredients of essential enzyme systems and are soluble in plasma and other aqueous fluids. Many water-soluble vitamins support energy biotransformation. The water-soluble vitamins include vitamin C and the extensive family of B vitamins (see Table 63-1). Water-soluble vitamins are not stored in appreciable amounts and are normally eliminated in small quantities in the urine. The water-soluble vitamins tend to be easily depleted from the body and thus must be replaced regularly by adequate dietary intakes (see Box 63-2).

The occurrence of frank vitamin C deficiency (scurvy) is rare, but marginal deficiencies may occur in people whose diets are devoid of fruits and vegetables, people who consume excess quantities of alcohol, older adults with very limited diets, critically ill people under chronic stress, and infants fed exclusively cow's milk. Mild deficiency of ascorbic acid is reflected as irritability, malaise, arthralgia, and an increased tendency to bleed. More severe deficiencies involve most body tissues, as collagen defects cause breakdown of skin and other tissues. Symptoms include bleeding of the gums, loosening of teeth, disturbances of bone growth, anemia, loss of hair, and dry, itchy skin.

Biotin deficiency in adults may cause dermatitis, glossitis, lassitude, depression, hyperesthesia, pallor, anorexia, loss of sleep, depression, muscle pains, and hypercholesterolemia. In infants younger than 6 months of age, biotin deficiency appears as seborrheic dermatitis and alopecia. Biotin deficiency is a common disorder in patients receiving total parenteral nutrition, but there is an inherited form of biotin deficiency (i.e., biotin-dependent multiple carboxylase deficiency syndrome).

Cobalamin deficiency produces megaloblastic or pernicious anemia. Megaloblastic anemia is associated with glossitis, hypospermia, GI disorders, decreased numbers of abnormally large red blood cells, fatigue, and dyspnea. With severe deficiency, leukopenia, thrombocytopenia, arrhythmias, heart failure, and infections may occur. Neurologic changes may cause numbness, tingling, and burning of the feet, as well as stiffness and generalized weakness of the legs.

Folate deficiency may be the most common vitamin deficiency in humans. Deficiency causes poor growth, megaloblastic anemia and other blood disorders, elevated blood levels of homocysteine (an amino acid linked to atherosclerosis), glossitis, and GI tract disturbances. Folic acid deficiency may be an independent risk factor for heart disease, unrelated to cholesterol levels, hypertension, or diabetes. Neural tube defects (e.g., spina bifida, anencephaly) have been associated with folic acid deficiency.

Niacin deficiency may occur in persons who have severely inadequate diets low in protein. Early niacin deficiency manifests as muscular weakness, anorexia, indigestion, and skin eruptions. Severe niacin deficiency leads to pellagra, which is characterized by skin eruptions, dementia, diarrhea, tremors, sore tongue, and impairment of peripheral motor and sensory nerves.

Pyridoxine deficiency is rare. Signs and symptoms include skin and mucous membrane lesions, malaise, depression, and glucose intolerance. Extreme deficiency leads to CNS abnormalities in infants whose formulas do not contain pyridoxine. A deficiency syndrome has been noted in children with an inborn error of pyridoxine biotransformation. Seizures and mental retardation occur unless pyrixodine supplementation is started in the neonatal period.

Riboflavin deficiencies usually occur in combination with deficiencies of other water-soluble vitamins. Signs such as photophobia, lacrimation, burning and itching of the eyes, capillary overgrowth around the cornea, glossitis, angular stomatitis (cracks in the corners of the mouth), and cheilosis (fissuring of the lips) usually occur after long periods of riboflavin deficiency.

Thiamine deficiencies are rare unless the diet is severely restricted. Alcohol-related thiamine deficiency (Wernicke-Korsakoff syndrome) is the third most common cause of dementia in the United States. Thiamine deficiency (beriberi) may cause confusion, tachycardia, pulmonary edema, and an enlarged heart. Muscular wasting, energy deprivation, inactivity, and peripheral neuropathy with paralysis of the lower extremities may also occur. Infantile beriberi, although rare, has occurred in infants fed unusual formulas without adequate thiamine supplementation. Deterioration of the infant occurs suddenly with cardiac failure and cyanosis.

DRUG CLASS • Water-Soluble Vitamins

ascorbic acid (Apo-C,✲ Ascorbicap, Cebid, Cecon, Cemill, Cenolate, Cetane, Cevi-Bid, Flavorcee, Sunkist Vitamin C, Kamu-Jay✲)

cyanocobalamin (Anacobin,✲ Bedoz,✲ Cobex, Cobolin-M, Crystamine, Crysti 1000, Cyanoject, Cyomin, Neuroforte, Nascobal, Primabalt, Vibal, Vitabee12, Rubion✲)

folic acid (Apo-Folic,✲ Folvite, Novo-Folacid, Novo-Folacid✲)

hydroxocobalamin (Hydrobexan, Hydro Cobex, Hydro-Crysti 12, Hydroxy-Cobal, LA-12, Vibal LA)

niacin (Endur-Acin, Nia-Bid, Niac, Niacor, Nico-400, Nicobid, Nicolar, Nicotinex, Novo-Niacin,✲ Slo-Niacin)

pantothenic acid

pyridoxine (Beesix, Doxine, Nestrex, Pyri, Rodex, Hexa-Betalin)

riboflavin

thiamine (Betaxin,✲ Bewon,✲ Biamine)

MECHANISM OF ACTION

Ascorbic acid (vitamin C) is essential as either a coenzyme or cofactor for collagen formation and thus is required for wound healing and tissue repair. Ascorbic acid plays a part in the synthesis of fats and proteins, the preservation of blood vessel integrity, and resistance to infection. It blocks the degradation of ferritin to hemosiderin, from which iron is poorly mobilized, thus ensuring a more available supply in the form of ferritin. Ascorbic acid is essential in the oxidation of phenylalanine and tyrosine, the conversion of folic acid to tetrahydrofolic acid, and the formation of serotonin and norepinephrine. The role of ascorbic acid as an antioxidant is under investigation.

Biotin is required in the synthesis of fatty acids, generation of the tricarboxylic acid cycle, and the formation of purines. Biotin is metabolically related to folic acid, pantothenic acid, and cobalamin.

Cobalamin along with folic acid, choline, and methionine participates in the synthesis of nucleic acids, purine, and pyrimidines. It is also vital to DNA synthesis, and it affects myelin formation.

Folic acid (also called folate) forms coenzymes known as tetrahydrofolates needed for one-carbon transfers in biotransformation. Folic acid is essential for the synthesis of the bases necessary for DNA and RNA synthesis. Folate and cobalamin regulate the formation of red blood cells in the bone marrow.

Niacin is the generic term for nicotinamide (niacinamide) and nicotinic acid. Niacin is obtained from food and by endogenous synthesis from tryptophan. Nicotinamide is an essential coenzyme used in glycolysis, fat synthesis, and tissue respiration. Large doses of niacin decrease hepatic lipoprotein and triglyceride synthesis and inhibit the release of free fatty acids from adipose tissue (see Chapter 42).

Pantothenic acid is needed to form acetyl coenzyme A, which is involved in the release of energy from carbohydrates via the citric acid cycle, in the degradation and biotransformation of fatty acids, and in the synthesis of cholesterol, phospholipids, steroid hormones, and orphyrin for hemoglobin and choline.

Pyridoxine has three interchangeable forms (pyridoxine, pyridoxal, and pyridoxamine) that may convert to the coenzyme pyridoxal phosphate. Pyridoxine is required for glycogenolysis. The synthesis of hemoglobin, antibodies, prostaglandins, and neurotransmitters (e.g., epinephrine, norepinephrine, tyramine, dopamine, serotonin, and gamma-aminobutyric acid) are all dependent upon pyridoxine. The formation of sphingolipids involved in the development of the myelin sheath surrounding nerve cells is also pyridoxine-dependent.

Riboflavin is a constituent of two coenzymes (flavin mononucleotide and flavin adenine dinucleotide) that are essential for the production of adenosine triphosphate (ATP). Riboflavin is also a component of amino acid oxidases and xanthine oxidase and may also function in the production of corticosteroids and red blood cells, as well as in gluconeogenesis.

Thiamine, in either its pyrophosphate or triphosphate form, is a coenzyme vital in the Krebs cycle. Thiamine is thus essential for biotransformation of carbohydrates, as well as fats, proteins, and nucleic acids.

USES

Ascorbic acid is used to treat or prevent vitamin C deficiency. The RDA of 60 mg prevents the onset of symptoms of scurvy for 4 weeks and provides a margin of safety. The value of ascorbic acid in the prevention and treatment of the common cold has not been supported.

Most B vitamins are indicated only for treatment or prevention of specific deficiencies.

Folic acid supplementation is especially important during periods of increased need for the vitamin, which includes pregnancy. It has been estimated that 75% of abnormalities related to neural tube defects in fetuses could be prevented by the use of folic acid supplements during pregnancy.

Niacin is used to treat or prevent vitamin deficiencies. It is also used to treat lipidemias (see Chapter 42).

PHARMACOKINETICS

Ascorbic acid is readily absorbed from the small intestine by an active mechanism and by diffusion. Ninety percent of ascorbic acid from foods is bioavailable to the body when taken in quantities between 20 and 120 mg. At very high dosages, bioavailability falls to only 16%. Diets high in zinc and pectin may decrease absorption, whereas absorption may be increased in the presence of natural citrus extract. Ascorbic acid is readily taken up by the tissues. Amounts in excess of those needed by the body are exhaled as carbon dioxide or eliminated in the urine as oxalic acid or ascorbic acid.

Biocytin, a natural provitamin, is readily absorbed and hydrolyzed to biotin, which is taken up by muscle, the liver, and the kidneys. It is protein bound in most natural foods. A vegetarian diet may alter the normal flora of the bowel to enhance synthesis of biotin or promote its absorption, or both.

Stomach acids release cobalamin from peptide bonds in food. Intrinsic factor from the stomach binds cobalamin and this complex is absorbed in the ileum. Once absorbed, cobalamin circulates bound to plasma proteins. The highest concentrations of cobalamin are found in the liver and kidneys. Enterohepatic circulation recycles cobalamin from bile and other intestinal secretions; thus it may take 5 or 6 years for a cobalamin deficiency to appear. Excess cobalamin is eliminated in urine.

Folic acid is broken down to a monoglutamate form by enzymes from the pancreas and the intestinal mucosa. This form of folate is then absorbed by carrier-mediated active transport. A small percentage of folic acid is absorbed by pH-sensitive passive diffusion. During or after absorption, the monoglutamate form of folic acid is changed to methyltetrahydrofolic acid and is stored.

The absorption of niacin takes place in the small intestine. Only a small amount of niacin is stored in the body. Excess niacin is eliminated through the kidneys in the urine. Patient response to nicotinamide becomes observable within 24 hours, with cessation of diarrhea and less redness of the tongue.

Pantothenic acid is readily absorbed from the GI tract and distributed to all tissues. Pantothenic acid is apparently not degraded in the body because the intake and elimination of the vitamin are nearly equal. Approximately 70% of the absorbed pantothenic acid is eliminated in urine.

All three forms of pyridoxine are absorbed by mucosal cells of the upper small intestine and phosphorylated to form pyridoxal phosphate and pyridoxamine phosphate. Pyridoxal phosphate is distributed bound to plasma albumin. Some pyridoxine is stored in the body, but a large percentage is eliminated in urine. Fifty percent of the total body content of pyridoxine is stored in muscle. Pyridoxine levels in breast milk correlate with the adequate intake in the maternal diet.

Riboflavin is well absorbed from the proximal small intestine in the presence of food. Riboflavin is stored in small amounts in the liver and kidneys, but the quantities stored are not sufficient to meet all of the body's needs. Thus, riboflavin must be regularly supplied in the diet. Riboflavin is biotransformed in the liver to variable degrees and eliminated in urine.

Thiamine is well absorbed orally and widely distributed to body tissues. It crosses the intestinal membranes by active transport in specific areas of the small intestine. Thiamine is stored in variable degrees in the liver and eliminated through the kidneys. Additional intake is required during pregnancy and during lactation to allow for increased energy needs and the elimination of thiamine in breast milk.

ADVERSE REACTIONS AND CONTRAINDICATIONS

At normal doses, few reactions are noted for most water-soluble vitamins.

The timed-release form of niacin helps reduce hypoglycemic symptoms, especially during withdrawal from sugar. It can also lower blood pressure and improve circulation by dilating blood vessels. Because of this action, some individuals experience flushing of the skin similar to that produced by an allergic reaction. This flushing is not harmful and usually disappears within 15 to 20 minutes. However, timed-release niacin must be used with caution because it can sometimes cause elevation of liver enzymes, and on rare occasions, it can cause hepatitis in sensitive individuals.

TOXICITY

Excessive intake of ascorbic acid may cause diarrhea from the osmotic effect of the unabsorbed vitamin passing through the intestinal tract. Megadoses of ascorbic acid may produce excessive amounts of oxalate and urate in the urine, leading to renal calculi. Excessive ascorbic acid may also cause retention of iron stores, particularly in blacks who are sensitive to iron.

Antioxidants in foods combat the effects of harmful free radicals in physiologic amounts, but ascorbic acid and other antioxidants taken in excess of physiologic needs may be pro-oxidants in some populations. Rebound scurvy may be seen when massive doses of ascorbic acid are taken and then suddenly discontinued. For this reason, high-dose ascorbic acid therapy should be withdrawn slowly.

The large doses of niacin (2 to 6 g daily) that are used to treat hyperlipidemia (types I and II) result in transient flushing, headache, cramps, and nausea and vomiting as well as increased blood sugar and uric acid levels. Liver function tests reflect hepatic response to excess niacin.

The risk of toxicity to pyridoxine is low; however, prolonged ingestion of high doses has resulted in severe ataxia and sensory neuropathy. Discontinuation of the drug has resulted in complete recovery within 6 months.

INTERACTIONS

The elimination of ascorbic acid is increased when the patient is under stress and when the patient has received adrenocorticotrophic hormone by injection. Persons who smoke have lower serum concentrations of ascorbic acid, and may need to increase their intake of ascorbic acid to at least 100 mg/day.

The anticonvulsant drugs primidone and carbamazepine inhibit biotin transport in the intestine, leading to biotin deficiency.

Oral contraceptives, sulfasalazine, phenytoin, and barbiturates impair the utilization of folic acid. Excessive alcohol intake either impairs the absorption of folic acid or increases its elimination.

PATHOPHYSIOLOGY • Macrominerals

Among the essential minerals required to maintain health are the so-called **macrominerals**, which are defined as those requiring an intake of at least 100 mg/day. The macrominerals are primarily electrolytes and include calcium, magnesium, potassium, sodium, phosphorus, chloride, zinc, and sulfur (see Table 63-1).

Sodium, potassium, and chloride are primary electrolytes that are discussed in Chapter 64. Calcium, a key mineral with both structural and biochemical functions, is discussed at the beginning of this chapter, along with vitamin D. The use of intravenous solutions containing calcium or magnesium is also discussed in Chapter 64.

Magnesium deficiency may be caused by conditions in which there is decreased intake or increased loss. Increased calcium or phosphorus intake can decrease magnesium absorption from the intestines. Magnesium deficiency is also possible in patients with renal disease, malabsorption syndrome, hyperthyroidism, pancreatitis, diabetes, parathyroid gland disorders, postsurgical stress, or vitamin D–resistant rickets. Deficiency of magnesium may cause muscle spasm, personality changes, anorexia, nausea, vomiting, seizures, and coma.

Phosphorus deficiency is unlikely because the element is widely available in a variety of foods. Clinical hypophosphatemia most often results from total parenteral nutrition without added phosphorus, excessive use of phosphate-binding drugs, hyperparathyroidism, the treatment of diabetic ketoacidosis, alcoholism, or the long-term administration of intravenous glucose. Premature infants can also develop clinical hypophosphatemia if they are fed unfortified human milk. Symptoms of hypophosphatemia include muscular weakness, hemolytic anemia, encephalopathy, cardiomyopathy with congestion, ventilatory collapse, and GI and skin hemorrhages.

Acquired zinc deficiency may develop from malabsorption, starvation, or increased loss in body fluids. Patients abusing alcohol and those receiving total parenteral nutrition have developed signs of clinical zinc deficiency. The first sign of zinc deficiency may be hypogeusia (decreased taste acuity). Prolonged zinc deficiency causes hypogonadism, growth retardation, mental disturbances, anemia, lethargy, skin lesions, delayed wound healing, alopecia, and susceptibility to frequent infections.

DRUG CLASS • Macrominerals (Selected)

magnesium chloride (Chloromag, Mag-L-100, Slow-Mag)

magnesium citrate (Citroma, Citro-Mag✳)

magnesium gluceptate (Magnesium-Rougier✳)

magnesium gluconate (Almora, Maglucate,✳ Magonate, Magtrate, MGP)

magnesium hydroxide (Phillips' Chewable Tablets, Phillips' Magnesia Tablets,✳ Phillips' Milk of Magnesia)

magnesium lactate (Mag-Tab Sr)

magnesium oxide (Mag-200, Mag-Ox 400, Maox, Uro-Mag)

magnesium pidolate (Mag-2✳)

magnesium sulfate (Epsom salt)

potassium phosphates (K-Phos, Neutra-Phos-K)

potassium and sodium phosphates (K-Phos-Neutral, K-Phos No. 2, Neutra-Phos, Uro-KP-Neutral)

zinc gluconate and zinc sulfate (Orazinc)

zinc sulfate (PMS-Egozinc,✳ Verazinc, Zinc-220, Zincate)

MECHANISM OF ACTION

Calcium and magnesium have complementary roles. Calcium gives bones their strength, whereas magnesium helps them maintain their elasticity to prevent injury. More than half of the body's magnesium is found in bones. Along with calcium, magnesium also modulates the transmission of impulses to nerves and the contraction of all muscle. Magnesium promotes transport of sodium and potassium across cell membranes and the synthesis and release of parathyroid hormone. Magnesium is necessary for the conversion of adenosine triphosphate (ATP) to adenosine diphosphate (ADP) and thus the release of energy from carbohydrates, proteins, and fats. Magnesium also promotes vasodilation of peripheral arteries and arterioles.

Phosphorus aids in bone growth and mineralization of teeth. Approximately 80% of phosphorus contained in the body is in the form of calcium phosphate crystals. Phosphorus is also a component of molecules such as ATP and cyclic adenosine monophosphate (cAMP), which are essential for energy biotransformation and cellular regulation. Phosphate is a buffer in intracellular fluids and the kidneys.

Zinc stabilizes cell membranes, supports functions of the immune system, increases sperm counts in males, and supports proper cell growth and division. It may help protect the heart from cardiomyopathy and angiopathy. Zinc supplements help with burn and wound healing, as well as in the treatment of acne and skin disorders. Zinc is an essential component of many enzymes (e.g., alcohol dehydrogenase, DNA polymerase, retinol dehydrogenase), and is a component of the hormone insulin.

USES

Magnesium salts administered intravenously are used to correct electrolyte imbalances or treat seizures associated with preeclampsia (see Chapter 64). Oral forms of magnesium are used as antacids (see Chapter 48), as laxatives (see Chapter 49), and to prevent or treat hypomagnesemia.

Phosphates may be given to acidify the urine to aid in dissolving uric acid stones in the urinary tract. Phosphates may also be given as an electrolyte replenisher.

Zinc supplements are used to prevent or treat zinc deficiency. Increased intake may be necessary to help support healing in patients with burns or extensive trauma.

PHARMACOKINETICS

Magnesium is absorbed from the small intestine at the same site as calcium, but absorption is not influenced by vitamin D. Most absorption occurs through simple and facilitated diffusion. The efficiency of absorption is usually 35% to 45% but varies with the composition of the diet as a whole, the magnesium status of the individual, and the amount of magnesium consumed in the diet. Magnesium in plasma exists as free ions or as a complex with phosphate, citrate, or protein. The kidneys conserve magnesium; reabsorption tends to vary inversely with that of calcium.

Various food components are hydrolyzed in the intestinal lumen by alkaline phosphatase to release inorganic phosphate. The acidic environment of the proximal duodenum maintains the solubility of phosphorus and thus the bioavailability. Phosphorus is eliminated through the kidneys.

A positive zinc balance is attained with intakes of 112.5 mg/day from a mixed diet, based on a 20% efficacy of absorption. A protein-rich meal promotes zinc absorption by forming zinc–amino acid chelates that present zinc in a more absorbable form. Zinc is widely distributed usually bound to plasma albumin, but some zinc is transported by transferrin and by alpha-2-macroglobulin. Ninety percent of the mineral is eliminated in the feces, with the remainder lost in urine and sweat.

ADVERSE REACTIONS OR CONTRAINDICATIONS

Oral magnesium supplements rarely cause adverse reactions when used at levels required to prevent magnesium deficiency. Diarrhea is the most common complaint.

Oral forms of phosphate supplements may cause nausea, vomiting, or diarrhea.

Zinc supplements have few adverse reactions when used at doses appropriate to reverse zinc deficiency. Large doses may cause GI distress.

TOXICITY

Toxic levels of magnesium produce flaccid paralysis, CNS depression, anesthesia, and even paralysis, especially in patients with renal insufficiency. Cardiac arrest is possible. Magnesium crosses the placenta and may produce serious reactions in the fetus at high doses.

Phosphorus excess is rare, but when it is present, it may cause tachycardia, nausea and diarrhea, abdominal cramps, muscle weakness, and hyperreflexia.

Excess oral ingestion of zinc to the point of toxicity is rare, but continued supplementation in excess of the RDA interferes with copper absorption and may promote anemia. The most serious form of zinc toxicity is seen in patients with renal failure who are on hemodialysis. The signs and symptoms of overdose include nausea, vomiting, hypotension, or pulmonary edema.

INTERACTIONS

Many drugs increase the risk of magnesium deficiency. Excessive amounts of phosphorus (from overuse of antacids) inhibits oral absorption of magnesium. Diuretics and antibiotics (e.g., carbenicillin, aminoglycosides, amphotericin B) interfere with renal handling of magnesium as either a primary action or an adverse effect. Cisplatin, corticosteroids, and digoxin may also affect magnesium elimination.

Oral contraceptives may alter zinc distribution; however, there is no evidence available showing that these changes alter the dietary requirement. Tetracylines may interfere with absorption of zinc.

PATHOPHYSIOLOGY • Microminerals

Microminerals are those needed in quantities of less than 100 mg/day to maintain normal function. Because so little is needed, deficiencies of most of these minerals are seldom noted. Iron is an exception to that rule.

Iron deficiency is the most common cause of anemia among women and children worldwide. Groups at most risk for iron deficiency include infants younger than 2 years of age, adolescents (particularly girls), pregnant women, and older adults. Iron deficiency is most often caused by chronic blood loss but can be aggravated by a diet insufficient in iron, protein, folic acid, vitamin B_{12}, pyridoxine, and ascorbic acid. Menstruation is the most common cause of iron deficiency in women. Iron deficiency as well as iron overload can alter the immune response and result in an infection. T cell and natural killer cell concentrations are reduced with iron deficiency, and the mitogenic response is muted.

Copper deficiency is manifested in adults as microcytic hemochromic anemia, but the best early indicators of copper deficiency are neutropenia and leukopenia. Bone changes include osteoporosis, metaphyseal spur formation, and soft tissue calcification noted in infants on prolonged total parenteral nutrition. Copper deficiency is also possible as a result of a sex-linked recessive gene that causes Menkes' disease. Infants affected with this disorder experience growth retardation; defective keratinization and pigmentation of the hair; hypothermia; degenerative changes in aortic elastin; abnormalities of the metaphyses of long bones; and progressive mental deterioration.

Chromium deficiency may cause insulin resistance, with impaired function in the presence of normal insulin concentrations. Ninety percent of diets are deficient in chromium as a result of modern agricultural techniques and the consumption of refined foods. Signs and symptoms of deficiency include anxiety; fatigue; elevated serum cholesterol and triglyceride concentrations; an increased incidence of aortic plaque; corneal lesions; decreased fertility and sperm counts; and glucose intolerance.

Despite a wide range of intake, selenium deficiency is rare in humans. Cardiomyopathy in patients on long-term total parenteral nutrition has been associated with selenium deficiency. A deficiency of selenium reduces glutathione peroxidase activity, causing jaundice in neonates. Deficiency of selenium can also lead to seborrheic dermatitis, dandruff, macular degeneration, low thryoid function, inflammation of the heart muscle, high cholesterol levels, and pancreatic insufficiency.

Fluoride deficiency is indicated by dental caries and a greater increase in the severity of osteoporosis.

True deficiency states for other trace minerals have been difficult to define.

DRUG CLASS • Micronutrients

chromium (Chroma-Pak)

cupric sulfate (Cupri-Pak)

ferrous fumarate (Femiron, Feostat, Ferretts, Fumasorb, Fumerin, Hemocyte, Ircon, Neo-Fer,✽ Nephro-Fer, Novo-Fumar,✽ Palafer,✽ Span-FF)

ferrous gluconate (Apo-Ferrous Gluconate, Fergon, Ferralet, Fertinic, Novo-Ferrogluc, Simron)

ferrous sulfate (Apo-Ferrous Sulfate,✽ Feosol, Feratab, Fer-gen-sol, Fer-In-Sol, Fero-Gradumet, Ferospace, Ferralyn, Ferra-TD, Mol-Iron, Novo-Ferrosulfate,✽ PMS-Ferrous Sulfate, Slow FE)

iron dextran (Dexferrum, DexIron,✽ InFed)

iron polysaccharide (Hytinic, Niferex, Nu-Iron)

iron sorbitol (Jectofer✽)

iron sucrose (Venofer)

selenious acid (Sele-Pak, Selepen)

sodium ferric gluconate (Ferrlecit)

MECHANISM OF ACTION

Nearly three fourths of body iron is in hemoglobin in red blood cells. About one fourth is stored in the liver, bone marrow, and spleen as ferritin and hemosiderin. Ferritin is a good indication of iron storage status. Hemosiderin is similar to ferritin but contains more iron and is very insoluble. The remaining small amount of iron is in myoglobin and enzymes or bound to transferrin in the plasma. Transferrin is a transport protein and along with beta-globulin regulates iron absorption. Myoglobin aids oxygen transport and use by the muscles. High levels of ferritin are required for proper function of the immune system. Iron is also critical for normal brain development and function at all ages.

Copper is necessary for the function of the antioxidant enzyme superoxide dismutase as well as for maintenance of connective tissue and immune function. Copper is also vital for production of red blood cells, apparently by regulating storage and release of iron for hemoglobin. Copper is essential for correct functioning of the central nervous, cardiovascular, and skeletal systems.

Selenium forms part of the structure of the antioxidant enzyme glutathione peroxidase. Selenium may protect the body from toxic effects of mercury and cadmium and protects cell and organelle membranes from free-radical lipid peroxidase damage by combining with tocopherol. Selenium also aids in immunoglobulin and ubiquinone (coenzyme Q) synthesis.

Chromium potentiates insulin action and, as such, influences carbohydrate, protein, and fat metabolism. It is a part of glucose tolerance factor, a biologically active substance manufactured in the body that regulates sugar metabolism. Glucose tolerance factor is a hormone-like compound that helps insulin move glucose out of the blood and into cells.

USES

Supplemental iron is used to increase available iron in the blood. Dosage is calculated in terms of elemental iron. Iron preparations vary greatly in how much elemental iron they contain. Ferrous sulfate, for example, contains 20% iron. Thus, each 300-mg tablet provides about 60 mg of elemental iron.

Copper, chromium, or selenium supplements are used to correct or prevent deficiencies, which may be more common with total parenteral nutrition or severe malnutrition.

PHARMACOKINETICS

The absorption of iron from food varies widely but is normally about 10%. The acidity of gastric fluids increases solubility of dietary iron. Iron absorption is increased in the presence of dietary ascorbic acid. Calcium combines with phosphate, oxalate, and phytate, preventing iron from binding to them and becoming unabsorbable. Periods of increased blood formation such as pregnancy and growth increase iron absorption. Less than 1 mg of iron is eliminated daily in urine, sweat, bile, and feces, and from the skin in desquamated cells. The average woman loses another 0.5 mg of iron daily and 15 mg monthly during menses.

Copper is absorbed from the stomach, but maximal absorption takes place in the small intestine. It is transported bound to plasma albumin. Some copper is stored in the liver, with elimination via the bile into the intestines and feces. Small amounts of copper are present in urine, sweat, and menstrual blood.

ADVERSE REACTIONS AND CONTRAINDICATIONS

Iron supplements taken orally may cause GI distress and constipation. Injection of iron supplements may cause headache, sweating, flushing, hypotension, rash, difficulty breathing, or numbness.

Adverse reactions are rare with copper or zinc supplements, but large doses of zinc may cause heartburn, indigestion, nausea, sore throat, and tiredness or weakness.

TOXICITY

Iron overload can be caused by hereditary hemochromatosis and transfusion overload. Iron overload in African Americans may be linked to a combination of dietary iron intake and the presence of a predisposing gene.

Copper toxicity damages the liver, kidneys, and other organs. Symptoms may include anorexia, blood in vomitus or urine, coma, diarrhea, dizziness, fainting, headache, jaundice, and taste abnormalities.

Zinc toxicity may cause chest pain and shortness of breath, dizziness or fainting, signs of jaundice, or vomiting.

INTERACTIONS

Supplements containing copper, iron, phosphorus or zinc must not be taken at the same time; doses should be spaced at least two hours apart in order to avoid interfering with uptake of one or more of the supplements. Fiber-rich foods and dairy products can also impair uptake of iron or zinc. Antacids and calcium supplements should not be taken with iron supplements because of decreased iron uptake.

APPLICATION TO PRACTICE

ASSESSMENT
History of Present Illness

A nutritional assessment should be conducted for all patients in a health care system. The information obtained in a nutritional assessment is usually used as the basis for designing the nutritional care plan. The patient's typical daily nutritional intake should be assessed to determine the sufficiency of vitamin and mineral requirements. Obtain information about current weight; usual weight; and if weight has been gained or lost in the past month, 6 months, last year, and over the last 2 years. Ask if there has been a change in appetite, if the patient takes vitamin and mineral supplements, and if a special diet is followed at home. Have there been changes in taste and smell? Ask about any anorexia, ageusia (absence or impairment of the sense of taste), dysgeusia (distortion of the sense of taste), anosmia (absence of the sense of smell), chewing or swallowing problems, frequent meals away from home, an inability to eat for more than 7 to 10 days, and maintenance of intravenous fluids for more than 5 days. Inquire if the patient has problems with heartburn, bloating, flatus, diarrhea, constipation, or abdominal distention. Determine the frequency of the problem and if home remedies are used to treat the complaint. Assess for allergies and determine if the female patient might be pregnant.

Health History

Inquire about any recent major surgery of the GI tract and about the patient's past history of alcohol use, using care to present this line of questioning in a tactful manner. Ask if the patient has chronic health problems and how they are managed. Determine if a dietary modification is required for the chronic illness, and identify any drugs used in its treatment.

Lifespan Considerations

Perinatal. During pregnancy, there should be an increase in all nutrients to meet the physiologic demands of maternal changes and fetal growth. The amount of increase in essential nutrients depends on a number of factors. These factors include the woman's general nutritional status before pregnancy; current health status; age and parity; amount of time between pregnancies; height and bone structure; weight; and activity level. If the woman's nutritional status is poor before she becomes pregnant, the additional demands of pregnancy on her body may further compromise her nutritional status.

Adolescent pregnancies have been associated with low birthweight, short gestational periods, and perinatal mortality. High parity or conceptions that occur more often than 12 months apart deplete the woman's nutritional reserves. Low pre-pregnancy weight and insufficient weight gain during pregnancy may result in low-birthweight infants and other complications of pregnancy.

Despite these issues, health care providers do not agree on the use of vitamin and mineral supplements in pregnancy. Some believe that if the woman has a well-balanced diet, supplementation other than iron and folic acid is usually unnecessary. However, accepted practice in antepartum care today is the routine prescription of prenatal vitamins. In general, the pregnant women needs additional folic acid, pyridoxine, ascorbic acid, calcium, phosphorus, iron, zinc, copper, magnesium, iodine, and vitamins A, D, and E. These nutrients may be supplied using a prenatal vitamin.

Pediatric. Premature infants require the same vitamins and minerals as full-term infants. Poor body stores, physiologic immaturity, illness, and rapid growth increase the need for supplementation. Weight is a more sensitive measure of growth and an earlier clue to nutritional inadequacy than length or height. Head circumference for an infant is not useful as a nutritional screening tool. Head size increases so slowly after age 3 that malnutrition has little effect on it. Head circumference is useful primarily as an indicator of nonnutritional abnormalities. Check the fontanelle in children.

The American Academy of Pediatrics does not support routine use of vitamin and mineral supplements for normal, healthy children. The exception is fluoride in unfluoridated areas. Parents who desire to give a vitamin and mineral supplement need not be concerned. The quantities of vitamins and minerals contained in supplements do not exceed those of the RDA; however, megadoses should be avoided.

Nutrients likely to be low or deficient in children's diets include calcium, iron, zinc, pyridoxine, magnesium, and vitamin A. Clinical signs of malnutrition in American children, however, are rare. Children at nutritional risk include those from deprived families; those from the inner city; homeless children; children with anorexia, poor appetite, and poor eating habits; children with chronic disease (e.g., cystic fibrosis) or liver disease; and those on dietary programs for obesity or who are vegetarians.

Adolescents incorporate two times the amount of calcium, iron, zinc, and magnesium during growth spurts. Forty-five percent of bone growth occurs during these growth spurts. Adolescents are thus in need of additional supplementation. Their need for vitamins A and E, ascorbic acid, pyridoxine, and folic acid are the same as for an adult, but they need additional thiamine, riboflavin, niacin, vitamin B complex, and vitamin D.

Older Adults. As lean body mass declines with age, perhaps so does the need for trace elements required for muscle metabolism. Glucose intolerance associated with aging may indicate the need for additional chromium. Increased calcium is needed owing to bone loss from osteoporosis, hypochlorhydria, and decreased intestinal absorption of calcium. Zinc requirements decline in the older adult, but these patients are in need of additional beta-carotene, vitamin D, vitamin E, ascorbic acid, and cyanocobalamin caused by loss of intrinsic factor. Pyridoxine (vitamin B_6), cyanocobalamin, and folic acid protect against certain neurologic deficits and elevated homocysteine levels, an independent factor for cardiovascular disease.

Lack of transportation, loss of functional ability, immobility, and a limited income may lead to social isolation. Additionally, older adults living alone may be deprived of stimulating interaction with others and thus lack incentive to cook and eat meals. Depression frequently accompanies social isolation, the loss of a spouse or friend, retirement, changes in body appearance, impaired vision, and poor physical fitness. Anorexia and lack of interest in eating, which are common symptoms of depression, result in limited food intake and increased risk of nutrient deficiency. There is growing concern that the elderly are particularly deficient in vitamin B_{12}, vitamin B_6, and folate.

Cultural/Social Considerations

Poor dietary intake is often associated with low-income status. Limited access to food and food choices plus inadequate facilities for food storage and preparation has a significant impact on both the quantity and quality of food intake. Inquire as to who does the shopping and cooking. Ask also about the impact of cultural beliefs on dietary habits.

Physical Examination

Physical signs and symptoms of poor nutrition provide vital supporting evidence for a diagnosis of a nutritional problem. Assess patient for physical signs of malnutrition indicative of a deficiency of a particular vitamin or mineral (Table 63-3). The physical examination can also identify chronic medical conditions that may be related to nutritional deficiencies.

Anthropometry, including measurements of height, weight, certain body circumferences (e.g., calf measurement, midarm), and skin-fold thickness, are useful because body growth is related to nutrition. A body mass index should be calculated based on height and weight measurements. If the patient is in a balanced state of nutrition, height, weight, skin-fold thickness, and body circumferences should fall within normal limits on standardized tables.

Because dental caries are preventable to some extent and are partially caused by poor nutritional practices, a dental examinations should be part of the total assessment. This factor is particularly true with older adults, who may eat poorly because of loosely fitting dentures or missing teeth.

Table 63-3 provides an overview of the signs and causes of malnutrition. Findings of concern that indicate the need for an in-depth assessment include the following:

- Sudden or unexplained weight loss of 10% or more of body weight
- Rapid weight loss of more than 2 pounds per week
- Significant change in weight after age 25
- Height for age is above 10th percentile, but weight for height is less than 5th percentile in children
- Excess weight for height (greater than the 95th percentile) in children

Laboratory Testing

Many biochemical tests are the most objective measures of nutritional status, but not all are appropriate, nor is a single test diagnostic of a nutritional status. Laboratory tests can be helpful in detecting subclinical or marginal deficiencies, such as anemia, when clinical signs are not yet evident. They are also helpful in confirming a suspicion of a deficiency based on dietary or clinical evaluation. However, caution must be used in interpreting results, because they can be dependent on the disease state and the various treatment modalities. The most common laboratory testing includes hemoglobin and hematocrit, complete blood count with differential, serum albumin, total protein, serum glucose, folate levels, and urinalysis; this group of tests is recommended as a minimum evaluation data set.

Bisphosphonate therapy requires monitoring of renal function, electrolyte levels, CBC and differential, hematocrit, and hemoglobin levels, before and during therapy, as ordered. Serum calcium levels should be monitored during calcium therapy as ordered (see the Case Study: Pernicious Anemia).

Vitamin B_{12} therapy requires monitoring of serum potassium levels during the first 48 hours. Hepatic function should be monitored during niacin therapy as ordered.

Renal function and serum potassium levels should be monitored during potassium therapy as ordered. Magnesium levels should be rechecked after repeated doses of magnesium.

Hemoglobin, hematocrit, and reticulocyte count should be monitored during ferrous fumarate and sodium ferric gluconate complex therapy as ordered. Additionally, sodium ferric gluconate complex therapy requires monitoring of serum ferritin and iron saturation levels.

GOALS OF THERAPY

Many people take vitamin and mineral supplements in an effort to promote health and prevent deficiencies. Treatment goals should center on ingesting appropriate amounts of dietary vitamins and minerals from viable sources, avoiding megadoses of vitamin supplements and minerals unless recommended by the health care provider, and avoiding symptoms of vitamin or mineral deficiency or excess. The need for vitamin and mineral supplementation is based on the following considerations:

- Daily requirements of the nutrient for healthy individuals
- The nature of the deficiency, disease, or injury
- Body storage of the specific nutrient
- Normal and abnormal losses of the nutrient through the skin, urinary tract, and GI tract
- Possible nutrient-drug interactions

INTERVENTION
Administration

Vitamins prescribed by health care providers to prevent or treat deficiencies exert the same physiologic effects as those obtained from foods. Synthetic vitamins have the

TABLE 63-3

Physical Signs and Causes of Malnutrition

Body Part	Signs of Malnutrition	Deficient Nutrient
Hair	Lacks natural shine, dull, sparse, straight, color changes, easily plucked	Multiple nutrient deficiencies
Face	Malar and supraorbital pigmentation, nasolabial seborrhea, moon face	Riboflavin, niacin, pyridoxine
Eyes	Pale conjunctiva, conjunctiva and corneal xerosis, keratomalacia, redness and fissuring of eyelid corners	Vitamin A, iron
Lips	Cheilosis, angular fissure, and scars	Niacin, riboflavin
Tongue	Glossitis	Folic acid, niacin, cyanocobalamin, pyridoxine
	Magenta color	Riboflavin
	Pale, atrophic	Iron
	Filiform papillary atrophy	Niacin, folic acid, cyanocobalamin, iron
Teeth	Mottled enamel	Excess fluoride
Gingiva	Spongy, bleeding, receding	Ascorbic acid
Glands	Thyroid enlargement (goiter)	Iodine
Skin	Follicular hyperkeratosis, xerosis with flaking	Vitamin A, insufficient unsaturated and essential fatty acids
	Hyperpigmentation	Folic acid, niacin, cyanocobalamin
	Petechiae	Ascorbic acid
	Pellagrous dermatitis	Niacin
	Scrotal and vulval dermatosis	Riboflavin
Nails	Koilonychia (spoon nails), brittle, ridged	Iron
Musculoskeletal system	Frontal and parietal bossing, epiphyseal swelling, craniotabes (soft, thin skull bones in infants), persistently open anterior fontanelle, knock knees or bowlegs, beading of ribs (rachitic rosary)	Vitamin D
Gastrointestinal tract	Hepatomegaly	Multiple deficiencies
Nervous system	Mental confusion and irritability	Thiamine, niacin
	Sensory loss, motor weakness, loss of position sense, loss of vibratory sense, loss of ankle and knee jerks, calf tenderness	Thiamine
Heart	Cardiac enlargement, tachycardia	Thiamine

same structure and function as natural vitamins derived from animal and plant sources. There is no evidence to suggest that natural vitamins are superior to synthetic vitamins. Furthermore, natural vitamins are usually more expensive. Vitamin formulations available OTC cannot and should not be used interchangeably or indiscriminately without concern for safety.

For deficiency states, oral vitamin preparations are preferred when possible. They are usually effective, safe, convenient, and relatively inexpensive. If the deficiency involves a single vitamin, that vitamin alone should be taken rather than using a multivitamin. However, a multivitamin product may be used because one vitamin deficiency usually does not occur in isolation. Dosages should be titrated as near as possible to the amount needed by the body.

Many OTC products promoted for use as dietary supplements contain 50% of the RDA. In patients who consume a reasonably well-balanced diet, nutrient needs may be exceeded if these supplements are used. Products used for the treatment of deficiencies may contain as much as 300% to 500% above the RDA. These products should not contain more than the recommended amounts of vitamin A, vitamin D, and folic acid. Furthermore, combination products (i.e., multivitamins) often contain minerals as well, although the quantities are ordinarily much smaller than those recommended for the average adult's daily needs.

Multivitamins for treating deficiencies should be used only for therapeutic purposes and for limited periods. When fat-soluble vitamins are given to correct deficiency, there is a risk of producing excess states. When water-soluble vitamins are used, excesses are less likely but may still occur with large doses.

Monitor the patient taking high dosages of a vitamin or mineral for adverse reactions. Watch for chronic or acute toxicity.

Most vitamin and mineral supplements are taken on a once-daily basis. Oral vitamin products should not be taken at the same time as mineral oil because the oil absorbs fat-soluble vitamins and thus prevents their systemic absorption. Orally administered supplements should be taken with a full glass of water.

Parenterally administered vitamins should be given with care to avoid tissue damage. Manufacturers' instructions should be reviewed before administering the drug. Careful aspiration of intramuscular or subcutaneous injections should be done to avoid inadvertent intravenous administration.

Calcium products should be administered with extreme caution to patients with renal or cardiac disease. The intramuscular route should be used only when the oral or intravenous routes are not available. Be aware that calcium salts are not interchangeable. Verify the formulation before use. Intravenous solutions should be warmed to body temperature before administration. Intravenous calcium therapy requires monitoring of the ECG. The patient should remain recumbent for 15 minutes after the end of the intravenous infusion. The infusion should be stopped and the health care provider notified if the patient complains of chest discomfort.

Ergocalciferol should be used with extreme caution in patients with heart disease, renal disease, or arteriosclerosis. Raloxifene should be used cautiously in patients with severe hepatic impairment. Monitor the patient for signs of blood clots during raloxifene therapy. Additionally, the drug should be discontinued at least 72 hours before prolonged immobilization and resumed only after the patient is fully mobilized. Monitor the patient taking raloxifene for unexplained uterine bleeding and breast pain or enlargement. Adverse reactions should be reported to the health care provider.

Etidronate and tiludronate should be administered 2 hours before or 2 hours after meals to maximize drug absorption and should not be given with antacids or mineral supplements. Tiludronate and alendronate should be administered with 8 ounces of water. Instruct the patient not to lie down for at least 30 minutes after administering alendronate to reduce the risk of esophageal irritation and to facilitate delivery of drug to the stomach.

Etidronate for intravenous administration should be diluted in at least 250 mL of normal saline or 5% dextrose solution (D_5W) and infused over a minimum of 2 hours. Intravenous administration of pamidronate requires reconstitution of the drug with 10 mL sterile water. After the drug is completely dissolved, add to 1000 mL of half-normal saline, normal saline, or D_5W. The solution should be inspected for precipitate before administration and given only by infusion. Nephropathy may occur when the drug is given as a bolus.

Monitor the patient for signs and symptoms of hypercalcemia during vitamin D therapy (headache, irritability, weakness, fatigue, thirst, nausea, anorexia, and constipation) and notify the health care provider if hypercalcemia is suspected. Monitor the patient for signs and symptoms of hypocalcemia during bisphosphonate therapy (muscle spasms, paresthesias, confusion, abdominal cramping, and difficulty breathing), and notify the health care provider if hypocalcemia is suspected.

To intravenously administer phytonadione (vitamin K), dilute with normal saline solution, D_5W, or D_5W in normal saline. Give by slow infusion not to exceed 1 mg/minute.

Oral niacin preparations (except for time-release forms) should be taken with meals, after meals, or at bedtime. The patient should be instructed to sit or lie down for about 30 minutes after administration to reduce the risk of falls caused by drug-related vasodilation, dizziness, and hypotension. The vasodilation occurs within a few minutes but may last up to 1 hour. A single adult aspirin tablet given 30 minutes before the niacin dose, as ordered, reduces the flushing response to niacin.

Intramuscular or intravenous administration of niacin should be reserved for patients in whom oral administration is not feasible. Niacin may cause a rise in glucose intolerance, particularly when given in large doses. Therefore blood glucose should be monitored closely in diabetic patients.

Because sensitivity reactions have occurred with thiamine, an intradermal test dose is recommended. Thiamine must be diluted before intravenous administration and the drug given cautiously. Have epinephrine available in case of anaphylaxis.

Check the manufacturer's instructions for the infusion rate of intravenous magnesium. The patient should be monitored for respiratory depression and heart block during infusion. Emergency equipment should be available to support respiration. Intramuscular administration should be given by deep intramuscular injection.

Fifty percent solutions of magnesium chloride may be given undiluted to adults, however they must be diluted to a 20% or less solution for use in children.

Parenteral magnesium chloride should be used with extreme caution in patients with impaired renal function. Have intravenous calcium available to reverse magnesium intoxication. Deep tendon reflexes should be tested before each dose. If reflexes are absent, the health care provider should be notified and the magnesium held until reflexes return. Additionally, the nurse should monitor fluid intake and output. If given to a pregnant woman within 24 hours before delivery, the neonate should be observed for signs and symptoms of magnesium toxicity including neuromuscular and respiratory depression.

Potassium should be used cautiously in patients with cardiac or renal impairment. The nurse should monitor ECG and fluid intake and output during potassium therapy. Potassium bicarbonate tablets should be dissolved in 4 to 8 ounces of water and taken with meals. Potassium supplements should not be administered postoperatively until urine flow has been established. The intravenous route should be used only for life-threatening hypokalemia or when the oral route is not possible. Administration is by slow intravenous infusion. Potassium should never be given intravenous push or by the intramuscular route. Emergency treatment of potassium overdose includes intravenous sodium bicarbonate and calcium gluconate.

Oral iron preparations should be administered between meals for optimum absorption. Monitor for constipation and be alert that black stools could mask the presence of blood. The stool should be tested for the presence of blood if there is a possibility of GI bleeding.

Z-track technique should be used for intramuscular injections of iron sorbitol and iron dextran. After drawing up the drug a new sterile needle should be used to administer injection. The drug should be injected deeply into the upper outer quadrant of the buttock, never into the arm or other exposed areas. Gentle pressure should be applied to the site after administration.

Sodium ferric gluconate complex is administered intravenously. Monitor the patient closely for potentially life-threatening hypersensitivity reactions (cardiovascular collapse, cardiac arrest, bronchospasm, oral or pharygeal edema, dyspnea, angioedema, urticaria, and pruritus) during infusion. Supportive measures should be available to treat anaphylactic reactions. Vital signs should be monitored during administration and for 30 minutes after the end of the infusion. A test dose of 2 mL (25 mg of elemental iron) should be given diluted in 50 mL of normal saline and given over 1 hour. The therapeutic dose should be diluted in 100 mL of normal saline and given over 1 hour. A period of at least 1 hour is appro-

priate between administration of the test dose and the therapeutic dose.

Education

Patients should be taught that taking a vitamin and mineral supplement each day does not preclude the importance of eating a well-balanced diet because vitamins in their natural form are often better than those synthesized in the laboratory. Teach the patient about good food sources containing the vitamin or mineral the patient is lacking.

All vitamins and minerals should be kept out of the reach of young children and should never be referred to as candy. Vitamins containing iron can cause poisoning in children if taken in excess of the recommended dose. There is no known health benefit to ingesting more mineral nutrients than the body needs. It is important to counsel the patient about the advisability of taking megadoses of vitamins and minerals because some vitamins and minerals are toxic if they are taken in more than the recommended doses. Acute toxicity may result from a single dose if taken in a large quantity. The patient should be taught the signs of overdose and to notify the health care provider should he or she develop signs of overdose.

Teach the patient not to share prescribed vitamins with others. Generally, vitamin and mineral preparations should be protected from light and stored at room temperature. Extended-release forms should be taken whole and not chewed or crushed. Counsel the patient on the importance of follow-up visits and laboratory studies, if ordered.

Instruct the patient to take oral calcium 1 hour after meals if GI upset occurs. Counsel the patient to avoid eating foods containing oxalic acid (rhubarb and spinach), phytic acid (bran and whole-grain cereals), or phosphorus (milk and dairy products) within 2 hours of taking calcium because these foods interfere with calcium absorption.

Counsel the patient taking raloxifene to avoid long periods of restricted movement, such as during travelling, because of the risk for developing blood clots. Advise the patient to report unexplained uterine bleeding or breast abnormalities to the health care provider.

Teach the patient to restrict intake of magnesium-containing antacids while taking vitamin D. Instruct them to report signs and symptoms of hypercalcemia (headache, irritability, weakness, fatigue, thirst, nausea, anorexia, and constipation) during vitamin D therapy.

Additionally, teach the patient taking vitamin B_{12} or vitamin B_6 to avoid alcohol use. Stress the need for the patient with pernicious anemia to return for monthly vitamin B_{12} injections.

Teach the patient receiving bisphosphonate therapy the signs and symptoms of hypocalcemia (muscle spasms, paresthesias, confusion, abdominal cramping, and difficulty breathing) and the importance of reporting these to the prescriber. Instruct the patient to take etidronate and tiludronate 2 hours before or 2 hours after meals. Antacids, mineral supplements, or multivitamins with added minerals should not be taken with etidronate and tiludronate. Stress the importance of taking alendronate and tiludronate with 8 ounces of water at least 30 minutes before food or other beverages. Warn the patient not to lie down for at least 30 minutes after taking alendronate to facilitate delivery of the drug to the stomach and to reduce the risk of esophageal irritation.

Instruct the patient to take riboflavin with meals because food increases drug absorption. Additionally, inform the patient that riboflavin causes the urine to be bright yellow or orange.

Teach the patient that niacin is a potent drug that may cause serious adverse reactions. Explain that while flushing is a harmless adverse effect of niacin therapy, concurrent use of alcohol may increase flushing. Advise the diabetic patient taking niacin supplements to monitor blood glucose levels closely because niacin may cause an increase in glucose intolerance.

Instruct the patient to dissolve potassium tablets in 4 to 8 ounces of cold water and to take the drug with meals. Liquid potassium should be slowly sipped to minimize GI irritation. Teach the patient to report signs of hyperkalemia (nausea, vomiting, muscle weakness) to the health care provider. Advise the patient not to use salt substitutes without first talking with the health care provider.

Teach the patient taking copper, iron, phosphorus, or zinc supplements to avoid concurrent use by spacing doses at least 2 hours apart to maximize the therapeutic effects of each element. Advise patients that although hemoglobin levels return to normal after about 2 months of iron therapy, an additional 6 months of therapy is recommended to restore the body's iron stores. Tell the

---

CASE STUDY — *Pernicious Anemia*

ASSESSMENT

HISTORY OF PRESENT ILLNESS

TW is a 66-year-old woman who complains of fatigue, weakness, and "pins and needles" sensations in her hands and feet. She states that she occasionally loses her balance while walking. TW reports a weight loss of 6 pounds during the last 3 months. Previously, she had maintained a weight of 122 pounds.

HEALTH HISTORY

TW gives no significant past medical history. She denies alcohol use and substance abuse. She is not currently taking any prescription drugs. The only OTC drug currently taken is a multivitamin with iron. TW reports eating a well-balanced diet and her husband concurs.

LIFESPAN CONSIDERATIONS

TW may have decreased hepatic and renal function because of age-related physiologic changes.

CULTURAL/SOCIAL CONSIDERATIONS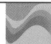

TW is retired from working as an accountant. She lives with her husband and has two married children who live within a 15-minute drive. TW's children visit her at home and, along with her husband, help with household duties and preparation of meals. Fatigue and weakness have prevented TW from caring for her 4-year-old grandson in the last several months.

PHYSICAL EXAMINATION

TW's vital signs are stable. Her temperature is 99.8° F oral; she is 5'1" tall and weighs 116 pounds.

LABORATORY TESTING

Decreased reticulocyte count, decreased vitamin B_{12} and folic acid levels, decreased RBC count, decreased hematocrit, hemoglobin, and platelet counts, with hypersegmentation of neutrophils with no band cells.

PATIENT PROBLEM(S)

Pernicious anemia.

GOALS OF THERAPY

A resolution of the symptoms of the deficiency of vitamin B_{12}.

CRITICAL THINKING QUESTIONS

1. The health care provider orders 100 mcg cyanocobalamin intramuscularly qd × 7 days initially; then 100 mcg intramuscularly once monthly. What is the mechanism of action of this drug?
2. TW asks what pernicious anemia is. As her nurse, how do you explain this disorder to TW?
3. What education is appropriate regarding the need for TW to continue to receive monthly intramuscular injections of cyanocobalamin for the rest of her life?
4. What laboratory tests might be ordered before instituting cyanocobalamin therapy?

patient taking liquid iron preparations to dilute and sip the formula through a straw to avoid staining the teeth. Patients should be aware that iron preparations turn the stools dark green or black.

EVALUATION

Treatment effectiveness can be demonstrated through resolution of symptoms of deficiency with no evidence of overdosage.

Bibliography

ADA reports: Position of the American Dietetic Association: food fortification and dietary supplements, *J Am Diet Assoc* 101(1):115-125, 2001.

Anderson J, Kessenich C: Cardiovascular disease and micronutrient therapies, *Top Adv Pract Nurs eJournal* 1(2):1-6, 2001.

Buck M: Vitamin K for the prevention of bleeding in newborns, *Pediatr Pharmacol* 7(10),1-4, 2001.

Centers for Disease Control and Prevention: Vitamin A deficiency among children—Federated States of Micronesia, 2000, *Morb Mortality Wkly Rep* 50(24), 2001.

Christen WG, Gaziano JM, Hennekens CH: Study methods and design. Design of Physicians' Health Study II—a randomized trial of beta-carotene, vitamins E and C, and multivitamins, in prevention of cancer, cardiovascular disease, and eye disease, and review of results of completed trials, *Ann Epidemiol* 10(2):125-134, 2000.

Cohen S, Paeglow R: Scurvy: an unusual cause of anemia, *J Am Board Fam Pract* 14(4):314-316, 2001.

Fishman SM, Christian P, West KP, Jr: The role of vitamins in the prevention and control of anaemia, *Public Health Nutr* 3(2):125-150, 2000.

Fleischauer A, Olson S, Mignone L, et al: Dietary antioxidants, supplements, and risk of epithelial ovarian cancer, *Nutr Cancer* 40(2):92-98, 2002.

Healthy news. Sink your teeth into new RDA guidelines, *Health (San Francisco)* 15(3):25, 2001.

Hooper L: Dietetic guidelines: diet in secondary prevention of cardiovascular disease, *J Hum Nutr Diet* 14(4):297-305, 2001.

Johansson S, Melhus H: Vitamin A antagonizes calcium response to vitamin D in man, *J Bone Miner Res* 10(16):1899-1905, 2001.

Johnson S: Gradual micronutrient accumulation and depletion in Alzheimer's disease, *Med Hypotheses* 56:595-597, 2001.

Jones G, Riley M, Whiting S: Association between urinary potassium, urinary sodium, current diet, and bone density in prepubertal children, *Am J Clin Nutr* 73(4):839-844, 2001.

Keenan DP, AbuSabha R, Robinson NG: Consumers' understanding of the Dietary Guidelines for Americans: insights into the future, *Health Educ Behav* 29(1):124-135, 2002.

Kontush A, Mann U, Arlt S, et al: Influence of vitamin E and C supplementation on lipoprotein oxidation in patients with Alzheimer's disease, *Free Radic Biol Med* 31:345-354, 2001.

Lindsey A, Ott C, Gross G, et al: Postmenopausal survivors of breast cancer at risk for osteoporosis: nutritional intake and body size, *Cancer Nurs* 25(1):50-56, 2002.

Lips P, Duong T, Oleksik A, et al: A global study of vitamin D status and parathyroid function in postmenopausal women with osteoporosis: baseline data from the multiple outcomes of raloxifene evaluation clinical trial, *J Clin Endocrinol Metab* 86(3):1212-1221, 2001.

More C, Bettembuk P, Bhattoa H, et al: The effects of pregnancy and lactation on bone mineral density, *Osteoporos Int* 12(9):732-737, 2001.

Robinson RF, Nahata MC: Pediatric pharmacology. Prevention and treatment of osteoporosis in the cystic fibrosis population, *J Pediatr Health Care* 15(6):308-317, 2001.

Schünemann HJ, Freudenheim JL, Grant BJB: Epidemiologic evidence linking antioxidant vitamins to pulmonary function and airway obstruction, *Epidemiol Rev* 23(2):248-267, 2001.

Shaw AM, Escobar AJ, Davis CA: Reassessing the food guide pyramid: decision-making framework, *J Nutr Educ* 32(2):111-118, 2000.

Smart about supplements? Test yourself with our not-so-easy questions about vitamins, herbs, and other dietary supplements, *Consum Rep Health* 12(2):7-10, 2000.

Southern Medical Association: NIH consensus development panel on osteoporosis prevention, diagnosis, and therapy. March 7-29, 2000: highlights of the conference, *South Med J* 94(6):569-573, 2001.

Wang H, Wahlin A, Basun H, et al: Vitamin B(12) and folate in relation to the development of Alzheimer's disease, *Neurology* 56:1188-1194, 2001.

Ward D: The role of nutrition in the prevention of infection, *Nurs Stand* 16(18):47-52, 2002.

Warren C: Emergent cardiovascular risk factor: homocysteine, *Prog Cardiovasc Nurs* 17(1):35-41.

Willett WC, Stampfer MJ: What vitamins should I be taking, Doctor? *N Engl J Med* 345(25):1819-1824, 2001.

Internet Resources

http://ods.od.nih.gov/index.asp.

http://www.cdc.gov/nchs/fastats/vitamins.htm.

http://www.nap.edu/books/.

http://www.nlm.nih.gov/medlineplus/druginfo/.

Fluids, Electrolytes, and Acid-Base Balance

LYNN ROGER WILLIS • SHERRY F. QUEENER • KATHLEEN GUTIERREZ

 Visit http://evolve.elsevier.com/Gutierrez/ for additional information.

KEY TERMS

Buffer, p. 1056

Diffusion, p. 1054

Extracellular fluid (ECF), p. 1052

Hydrostatic pressure, p. 1053

Hyperkalemia, p. 1055

Hypernatremia, p. 1055

Hypokalemia, p. 1055

Hyponatremia, p. 1055

Interstitial fluid, p. 1052

Intracellular fluid, p. 1052

Isotonic, p. 1053

Metabolic acidosis, p. 1057

Metabolic alkalosis, p. 1056

Oncotic pressure, p. 1053

Osmosis, p. 1052

pH, p. 1055

Respiratory acidosis, p. 1057

Respiratory alkalosis, p. 1056

OBJECTIVES

- Explain what forces control the movement of water between body compartments.
- Describe the causes and signs of dehydration and suggest fluids to reverse dehydration.
- Describe the causes and signs of fluid excess and suggest ways to control it.
- Explain the principles of acid-base balance.
- Describe the appropriate nursing actions in response to common problems encountered with intravenous fluids.

PATHOPHYSIOLOGY • Fluid or Electrolyte Imbalances

REGULATION OF SALT AND WATER BALANCE
Fluid Compartments

Water comprises 50% to 60% of an average person's weight. Although water passes easily through most tissues, certain physical and permeability barriers allow the body to be divided into compartments in which water content may be independently regulated. For example, a 70-kg man contains 42 L of water, of which 28 L are inside cells (Figure 64-1). This water, along with its dissolved solutes, is called **intracellular fluid**. **Interstitial fluid** bathes the outside of cells and allows them to excrete waste products and receive nutrients. Plasma constitutes an important separate fluid compartment similar to interstitial fluid, but it is more accessible to manipulation and testing. **Extracellular fluid (ECF)** primarily includes interstitial fluid and plasma but also other fluids such as lymph and cerebrospinal fluid.

Composition of Body Fluids

The fluid compartments in the body differ in the concentration of important ions and other solutes. In plasma, the major solute is sodium chloride (Figure 64-2). The primary buffers maintaining the pH of blood at 7.4 are bicarbonate (HCO_3^{-1}, 27 mEq/L) and protein (16 mEq/L). Interstitial fluid is similar to plasma but has a much lower protein concentration.

Inside the cell, high concentrations of protein and potassium are found, but the sodium ion concentration is much lower. Phosphate, the major buffer for intracellular fluid, is shown in Figure 64-2 as PO_4^{-3} but is actually present as a mixture of HPO_3^{-2} and $H_2PO_3^{-1}$. Magnesium ions, important components of critical enzyme systems, are also significant constituents of intracellular fluid.

Movement of Fluid and Electrolytes between Compartments

Water moves freely through the vascular walls separating plasma from interstitial fluid and through the cell membranes separating intracellular fluid from interstitial fluid. However, movement of ions and other solutes is rigidly controlled so that optimum concentration differences are maintained between compartments. The concentrations of these solutes influence the disposition of water among the compartments. To understand the distribution of water and the various solutes, certain concepts from chemistry and physiology must be recalled.

Osmosis describes the movement of water across a semipermeable membrane (a membrane that selectively limits passage of some chemicals). For example, a cell membrane is semipermeable. The direction of movement is determined by the concentration of solutes in the water on either side of the membrane. Water moves toward the solution having the higher concentration. Osmosis reduces the difference in concentration of the solutions on either side of a semipermeable membrane.

The movement of water by osmosis across semipermeable membranes creates osmotic pressure. For ex-

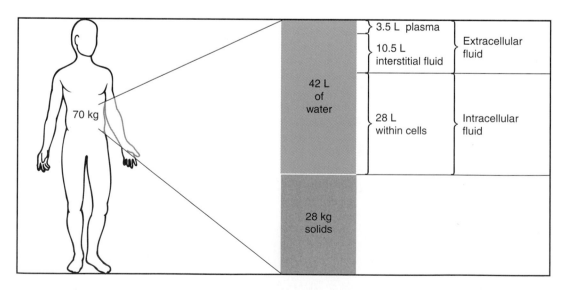

FIGURE 64-1   Distribution of water in men. In women, about 50% of body weight is found as water, but the proportion of intracellular to extracellular fluid is the same as for men.

ample, if a glucose solution is enclosed in a synthetic membrane that allows water but not glucose to pass through the membrane and the sealed sac is submerged in pure water, two things will happen. Water will enter the sac at a greater rate than it leaves the sac. As water enters the solution-filled sac, pressure inside the sac increases and opposes the entry of more water. The pressure required to completely prevent the net movement of water into the sac is a measure of the osmotic pressure of the solution.

The osmotic properties of a solution relate to the concentration of solute, but the number of particles (ions, atoms, or molecules) is important, not the mass of the solute. For example, a 0.5 molar solution of glucose contains 90 g/L of glucose and has a potential osmotic pressure of 9650 mm Hg. In contrast, a 0.5 molar solution of sodium chloride contains 29 g/L of sodium chloride and has a potential osmotic pressure of 19,300 mm Hg. The greater potential osmotic pressure of the sodium chloride solution results from the ionization of sodium chloride to release two particles for every molecule of salt: a sodium ion and a chloride ion. Glucose does not ionize, and each molecule of the glucose remains a single particle.

Osmolarity of the ECF is determined mainly by the concentration of sodium chloride. Solutions that have the same osmolarity as plasma are called **isotonic**.

Isotonic solutions include 5% dextrose (D_5W) and 0.9% sodium chloride (NaCl) solutions. Hypertonic solutions have a higher osmolarity than plasma (greater than 310 mOsm/L) and therefore tend to draw water out of cells. Hypotonic solutions have lower osmolarity than plasma and thus cause water to move into cells.

Oncotic pressure regulates the movement of water between plasma and interstitial fluid. This pressure is generated by the difference in protein concentration between plasma and interstitial fluid. Although most solutes in plasma pass freely through pores of the vascular walls that separate plasma from interstitial fluid, proteins cannot leave plasma by that route. Proteins retained in plasma act like other solutes to promote the movement of water from interstitial fluid toward plasma.

Without a balancing force, oncotic pressure tends to dilute the protein in plasma and increase pressure in the plasma compartment. Oncotic pressure is balanced by **hydrostatic pressure** generated by the force of contraction of the heart. In arterioles where blood pressure is high, hydrostatic pressure exceeds oncotic pressure. In the arteriolar side of capillaries, water, along with dissolved nutrients and other solutes, moves from plasma into the interstitial fluid, where it is available to cells. Pressure on the venous side of the capillaries is lower and is not sufficient to fully block the movement

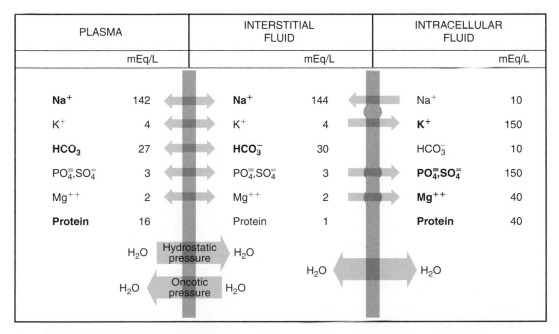

PLASMA		INTERSTITIAL FLUID		INTRACELLULAR FLUID	
mEq/L		mEq/L		mEq/L	
Na^+	142	Na^+	144	Na^+	10
K^+	4	K^+	4	K^+	150
HCO_3	27	HCO_3^-	30	HCO_3^-	10
$PO_4^=, SO_4^=$	3	$PO_4^=, SO_4^=$	3	$PO_4^=, SO_4^=$	150
Mg^{++}	2	Mg^{++}	2	Mg^{++}	40
Protein	16	Protein	1	Protein	40
H_2O　Hydrostatic pressure	H_2O				
H_2O　Oncotic pressure	H_2O	H_2O	H_2O		

FIGURE 64-2　Movement of water and solutes between body compartments. Double-headed arrows represent simple diffusion; straight arrows indicate pressure-regulated processes. Arrows passing through or in contact with circles represent active transport of solutes.

of water. Oncotic pressure thus predominates on the venous side of capillaries, allowing water, solutes, and waste products to move back into plasma and be carried away.

Diffusion describes the movement of solutes across semipermeable membranes. The direction of movement is toward the less concentrated solution. As with osmosis, this process lowers the difference in concentration between the two solutions. Free diffusion of most ions and solutes takes place between plasma and interstitial fluid, but the cell membrane is not normally permeable to most solutes found in ECF. Sensitive control of uptake and release of solutes is maintained by active transport systems on the cell membrane. For example, the high intracellular concentration of potassium is maintained by Na^+-K^+-ATPase, an active transport system that hydrolyzes a molecule of adenosine triphosphate (ATP) to exchange three sodium ions for two potassium ions. Other active transport systems maintain the high intracellular concentrations of phosphate and magnesium ions.

CLINICAL INDICATIONS FOR FLUID THERAPY
Loss of Extracellular Fluid Volume (Fluid Volume Deficit)

Several clinical conditions can cause water and solutes to be lost from ECF. For example, sudden hemorrhage, prolonged vomiting, excessive diarrhea, or plasma loss through large areas of burned skin may cause fluid and salt loss, but the fluid remaining in the extracellular compartment may for a time stay essentially normal in composition. If the fluid loss is excessive and uncompensated, the patient may develop hypovolemic shock, in which the blood volume becomes so depleted that organ perfusion is compromised. The symptoms of this condition include lowered blood pressure, increased heart rate, rapid respiration, restlessness, pale and clammy skin, and decreased urine output. Without adequate perfusion, the kidneys may fail completely. Hypovolemic shock is potentially life threatening and requires rapid replacement of fluid and electrolytes.

In certain conditions, ECF volume may be decreased primarily by water loss. For example, patients who fail to take in adequate water may dehydrate. This condition is common in older adults who may have inefficient thirst centers in the brain. Unconscious patients lose between 1000 and 1700 mL of water through breath, urine, and imperceptible perspiration each day; this water must be replaced daily to avoid dehydration. In certain circumstances watery diarrhea and high-volume renal failure may cause loss of water in excess of salt loss (Box 64-1). All these circumstances may require replacement of lost volume and restoration of the proper proportion of solutes in the ECF.

Fluid Volume Excess

In certain conditions ECF volume is expanded to a degree that may impair cardiovascular functioning, in part by increasing venous pressure. Fluid excess may arise from conditions impairing the body's ability to eliminate fluid such as heart failure or renal impairment. Alternatively, fluid excess can arise from the improper administration of intravenous fluids. The main route for elimination of excess fluid is through the kidneys. Treatment aims to prevent further overload and, if necessary, to assist the kidneys by pharmacologic means. For example, digoxin given to strengthen contraction of the heart in heart failure improves perfusion of the kidneys and assists in mobilizing and eliminating excess fluid. Diuretics also enhance urine production.

BOX 64-1 | **Diarrhea in Infants**

In most cases diarrhea is mild and self-limiting, but infants and young children may be thrown into dangerous states of dehydration and electrolyte imbalance if diarrhea is severe or prolonged. Hypotension and coma can arise when fluid losses equal 5% of body weight; losses of 10% can cause shock, and death ensues at higher losses.

Associated or Contributing Factors

In underdeveloped nations diarrhea is a significant cause of mortality in infants and children, with death resulting from dehydration and electrolyte imbalance. Poor sanitation may expose children and adults to infectious agents that cause diarrhea. Even if the diarrhea is caused by bacterial contamination of food or water, treatment is often successful if salt and water balance are maintained. Intravenous replacement of fluids is expensive, unavailable to many people, and unnecessary in the majority of cases. Aggressive oral replacement with properly balanced solutions is first-line treatment.
- Oral rehydration therapy (ORT) should begin early in the course of the disease.
- In the United States preparations are available under the trade names Lytren, Pedialyte, Rehydralyte, and Resol.
- In Canada, Lytren and Pedialyte are available.
- In other countries the World Health Organization (WHO) Diarrheal Disease Control Program supplies ORS-bicarbonate or ORS-citrate in premeasured packets that are mixed with 1 L of potable water before use.

Electrolyte Imbalances

The proper concentrations of ions and solutes in the extracellular compartment can be disrupted by diseases or medical interventions (Table 64-1). Sodium is the major determinant of osmolarity in plasma and interstitial fluid.

Hypernatremia (excessive sodium ion concentration in plasma) can arise when a patient loses water but retains salt. Alternatively, hypernatremia may arise when excessive sodium has been administered with fluids or drugs. In hypernatremia, water moves from cells into the ECF in an attempt to reduce the sodium ion concentration and restore equal osmolarity between the fluid compartments.

Hyponatremia (plasma sodium concentrations less than 130 mEq/L) arises most commonly in patients who are losing water and electrolytes but are receiving water without adequate electrolyte replacement. In an extreme case this condition is called water intoxication. The low sodium ion concentration of the ECF causes water to move into cells in an attempt to restore equal osmolarity between the two compartments.

Hyperkalemia (excessive potassium ion concentration in plasma) causes less osmotic disturbance than sodium ion imbalance, but potassium ion imbalances can be life threatening because cardiac function may be affected. Potassium-induced arrhythmia appears in the electrocardiogram (ECG) as depressed ST segments, widened QRS complexes, and peaked T waves. Hyperkalemia may result from massive tissue injury (e.g., a crushing injury) when large numbers of cells die, releasing their high intracellular concentrations of potassium into the ECF. Renal failure may also cause retention of potassium, as may the potassium-sparing diuretics discussed in Chapter 46.

Hypokalemia (low potassium ion concentration in the plasma) can be caused by the use of loop or thiazide diuretics (see Chapter 46). Poor nutrition or poor GI tract absorption may also cause hypokalemia. Vomiting depletes the body of potassium, along with fluid and other salts. Replacement of potassium is necessary to restore normal function, but the replacement should be spread out over several days to avoid excessive cardiac stress.

Regulation of calcium ion concentrations in the body is discussed in Chapters 56 and 63.

Acid-Base Balance. The acid-base status of the body fluids is normally expressed in terms of **pH**, which is an indicator of the hydrogen ion concentration. The term pH is calculated as the negative logarithm of the hydrogen ion concentration, which means the lower the pH of a solution, the higher the concentration of hydrogen ions, or acid, in the solution, and vice versa.

The pH of blood normally ranges from 7.35 to 7.45. The body maintains careful control of the pH of the blood and acts quickly to adjust the retention or elimination of hydrogen ions whenever conditions threaten to take the pH outside of the ideal range. Control of the acid-base system is maintained so tightly because even slight deviations in hydrogen ion concentration may profoundly affect the rate of important metabolic processes. However, despite the day-to-day reliability of the body's pH-regulating processes, alkalinizing or acidifying drugs are sometimes needed to correct imbalances, particularly if the systems responsible for regulating acid-base balance lose their effectiveness.

TABLE 64-1

Common Electrolyte Imbalances

Solute	Normal Concentration in Plasma	Signs of Deficiency	Signs of Excess
Bicarbonate ion	24-31 mEq/L (pH 7.35-7.45)	Metabolic acidosis (pH <7.35); weakness; deep, rapid breathing (Kussmaul respirations); stupor or unconsciousness	Metabolic alkalosis (pH >7.45); hypertonicity of muscles; depressed respirations; tetany
Calcium ion	4.7-5.6 mEq/L	Tetany; prolonged QT interval on electrocardiogram	Weakness, fatigue, thirst; nausea, anorexia, muscle cramping
Magnesium ion	1.3-2.3 mEq/L	Flushing, hypertension; neuromuscular irritability	Nausea, vomiting; diarrhea, colic
Potassium ion	3.5-5 mEq/L	Muscle weakness; diminished tendon reflexes; paralytic ileus; cardiac arrhythmia	Nausea and vomiting; muscle weakness; electrocardiographic changes
Sodium ion	136-145 mEq/L	Anorexia, nausea, vomiting; increased intracranial pressure; oliguria leading to anuria	Dry, sticky membranes; fever; weakness and disorientation; oliguria

The body maintains three major lines of defense against unwanted changes in acid-base balance: natural buffers in the body, the lungs, and the kidneys.

A **buffer** is any chemical that prevents dramatic changes in pH even when acid or base is added to the system. The main buffer in the blood is the bicarbonate/carbonic acid buffer system. Phosphate, sulfate, and ammonium ions also act as buffers. A buffer behaves somewhat like a sponge. The buffer either soaks up hydrogen ions from the blood when they are in excess, or returns them to the blood when they come into short supply. Buffers react instantaneously when the hydrogen ion concentration changes. This quick action prevents abrupt changes in the pH of the blood.

The respiratory system influences pH by regulating the exhalation of carbon dioxide, which connects to the acid-base system by the scheme illustrated in Figure 64-3. For example, if the pH of the blood were suddenly to become acidic, the respiratory system would readjust the concentration of hydrogen ions in the blood within a couple of minutes by increasing the respiratory rate, which in turn increases the rate at which carbon dioxide is exhaled. By eliminating carbon dioxide, the lungs therefore eliminate carbonic acid from the blood and move the pH of the blood toward normal. If the pH of the blood were to become alkaline, the respiratory response would be opposite that when the blood became acidic.

Whereas the buffer systems adjust immediately to changes in the pH of the blood and the lungs restore acid-base balance within a matter of minutes, the kidneys have the responsibility for the long-term management of acid-base balance. The kidneys help regulate the pH of the blood by adjusting the urinary retention and excretion of hydrogen and bicarbonate ions. Although the kidneys are the most powerful regulators of acid-base balance, they are also the slowest, requiring hours to days to correct an imbalance. Together, the buffers, lungs, and kidneys share responsibility for maintaining normal acid-base balance, but disease, drugs, and other influences can overpower them. When that happens, drug therapy to restore the balance is required.

An acid-base imbalance results in respiratory or metabolic alkalosis or respiratory or metabolic acidosis (Table 64-2). These imbalances can occur as primary, mixed, or compensated forms. Primary imbalances originate from an acute condition such as respiratory alkalosis caused by hyperventilation. Mixed imbalances occur when there is more than one cause of the imbalance. Compensated imbalances involve the body's attempt to bring the pH back to normal after a primary imbalance has occurred. The body compensates for a primary imbalance by pushing the balance in the opposite direction. Compensated imbalances are usually found with chronic disorders (e.g., chronic airway limitation). In essence, respiratory imbalances are compensated for by the kidneys; metabolic imbalances are compensated for by the lungs.

Alkalosis is defined as a decrease in hydrogen ion concentration of the blood and is reflected by an arterial pH above 7.45. It is not a disease as such but a consequence of a pathologic process. Alkalosis results from an actual or relative increase in the concentration or strength of base in the blood. Alkalosis causes disturbances in metabolism and pulmonary respiration with serious and potentially life-threatening results. The most common manifestations of alkalosis include stimulation of the neuromuscular, cardiovascular, and central nervous systems.

Respiratory alkalosis, occurring as a result of alveolar hyperventilation, results in decreased serum carbon dioxide levels (hypocapnia) resulting from excessive exhalation of carbon dioxide. As described previously, the removal of carbon dioxide from the blood by exhalation decreases the concentration of carbonic acid, which in turn decreases the hydrogen ion concentration in the blood. Consequently, the pH of the blood increases. The kidney attempts to compensate for the alkalosis by increasing the excretion of bicarbonate.

Metabolic alkalosis results from excessive accumulation of a base or excessive loss of acid. Excessive vomiting or gastric suctioning that cause large losses of stomach acid (hydrochloric acid) may bring on metabolic alkalosis. Diuretics are another major cause of metabolic alkalosis mediated through excessive urinary losses of chloride ions and the relative accumulation of bicarbonate ions in the blood (see Chapter 46).

$$H^+ + HCO_3^- \longleftrightarrow H_2CO_3 \longleftrightarrow CO_2 + H_2O$$

FIGURE 64-3 The bicarbonate/carbonic acid buffer system. An increase in the acidity of the blood raises the hydrogen ion concentration (H^+), which combines with bicarbonate ions (HCO_3^-) to produce carbonic acid (H_2CO_3). The enzyme carbonic anhydrase quickly converts the carbonic acid to carbon dioxide (CO_2) and water (H_2O). The CO_2 is then exhaled through the lungs. Impaired respiration will cause CO_2 to accumulate and drive the reaction in the other direction. The kidneys will then excrete the accumulated hydrogen ions to restore acid-base balance.

Overuse of antacids, such as sodium bicarbonate, can also produce metabolic alkalosis.

Acidosis is defined as an arterial blood pH below 7.35. Like alkalosis, acidosis is not a specific disease but rather a symptom of a disease or pathologic process. Acidosis results from an actual or relative increase in the concentration of acids.

Respiratory acidosis results from retention of carbon dioxide because of hypoventilation. Abnormally slow or shallow respirations, or poor alveolar ventilation resulting in inadequate gas exchange causes carbon dioxide to accumulate in the lungs and the blood, increasing carbonic acid levels in the blood and lowering pH (see Figure 64-3). Respiratory acidosis can be acute in onset, as in sudden ventilatory failure, or chronic, as in emphysema. The body attempts to compensate by increasing the renal reabsorption of bicarbonate.

Metabolic acidosis results from excessive accumulation of acids or loss of base in body fluids. Acids are produced by metabolism or can be ingested and absorbed into the blood. The body's immediate response to an accumulation or overload of acid is to increase respiration. The kidneys begin to compensate as well by excreting more hydrogen ions and conserving bicarbonate. However, as discussed previously, this process, though very effective, is slow.

TABLE 64-2

Overview of Acid-Base Imbalances

Condition/Mechanism	Contributing Conditions
Respiratory Acidosis	
Retention of CO_2 increases carbonic acid and H^+	Airway obstruction, bronchospasm or laryngospasm, foreign body or tumor
	CNS conditions that may suppress respiration: cerebral edema, drugs (alcohol, benzodiazepines, opioids), spinal cord injury
	Conditions that weaken chest muscles or prevent chest expansion: crush injury, Guillain-Barré syndrome, hypokalemia, muscular dystrophy, myasthenia gravis, skeletal deformities
	Pulmonary disease: adult respiratory distress syndrome, emphysema, pneumonia, pulmonary edema, tuberculosis
Respiratory Alkalosis	
Excessive loss of CO_2	Conditions causing hyperventilation: anxiety or fear, improper mechanical ventilation
	Organ system impairment: CNS infection, stroke, or tumor; hyperthyroidism; liver failure
	Pulmonary disorders or other conditions producing hypoxia: asthma, high altitudes, pneumonia, pulmonary emboli, or pulmonary edema
	Toxicity: carbon monoxide poisoning, drugs (aminophylline, catecholamines, progesterone), salicylate overdose
Metabolic Acidosis	
Overproduction of H^+ ions	Excess of organic acids: diabetic ketoacidosis, excessive exercise, fever, lactic acidosis (anoxia or other causes), seizure, starvation
	Toxicity: ethanol intoxication, methanol or ethylene glycol poisoning, salicylate intoxication
Reduced elimination of H^+ ions or lower production of HCO_3	Organ failure: kidney failure, liver failure lowers production of HCO_3, pancreatitis lowers production of HCO_3
Increased loss of HCO_3	Fluid or electrolyte imbalance: dehydration, diarrhea, excessive organic acid buffering
Metabolic Alkalosis	
Excess base accumulated	Excess intake of organic bases: antacid or sodium bicarbonate intake high over long period, blood transfusion, milk-alkali syndrome, parenteral nutrition
	Excess loss of acids: gastric suctioning, hyperaldosteronism, thiazide diuretics, prolonged vomiting

CNS, Central nervous system.

DRUG CLASS • Hydrating Solutions

⚠ dextrose in water

   lactated Ringer's solution

   Ringer's solution

⚠ sodium chloride in water

See Table 64-3.

MECHANISM OF ACTION

Conditions such as hemorrhage or shock, in which plasma volume is suddenly reduced, require replacement of fluid as initial therapy. Replacement of lost fluid volume allows maintenance of kidney function, preventing further development of dangerous electrolyte imbalances. Perfusion of other vital organs is also maintained by this strategy.

USES

Isotonic saline replaces ECF volume and treats sodium depletion and metabolic alkalosis. Ringer's solution and lactated Ringer's solution are used to replace fluid, sodium, and other electrolytes. Often called balanced or maintenance solutions, these preparations are appropriate to replace volume if renal function is normal. Ringer's solution is appropriate replacement therapy for patients who have lost fluid and electrolytes through the GI tract, for burn patients, for postoperative patients, and for patients with dehydration or sodium depletion. Lactated Ringer's solution is most appropriate for patients who, along with other electrolyte imbalances, have acidosis. The lactate in this solution, converted to bicarbonate by the liver, elevates blood pH and provides

---

TABLE 64-3

Hydrating and Electrolyte Replacement Solutions

Principal Electrolyte	*Comments*
Bicarbonate	
Sodium bicarbonate in water (4.2%, 5%, 7.5%, 8.4%)	Individualized to reverse acidosis. May be diluted; 1 L of 1.4% sodium bicarbonate contains 167 mEq/L of sodium ion.
Calcium	
Calcium acetate (0.5 mEq Ca^{++}/mL)	Rate of infusion should not exceed 1.8 mEq Ca^{++} per minute.
Calcium chloride (1.36 mEq Ca^{++}/mL)	
Calcium gluceptate (0.9 mEq Ca^{++}/mL)	
Calcium gluconate (0.47 mEq Ca^{++}/mL)	
Magnesium	
Magnesium sulfate (10%, 12.5%, 20%, 50%)	Infuse 10% solution at <1.5 mL/min; 10% solution nearly isotonic
Potassium	
KCl in water (0.1, 0.2, 0.3, 0.4, 1.5, or 2 mEq K^+/mL)	Dilute before use to 0.04 mEq/mL; infuse at 20 mEq/hr; higher rates occasionally are used for emergencies; monitor ECG when infusion rates exceed 20 mEq/hr.
KCl in 5% dextrose (10, 20, 30, or 40 mEq K^+/L)	
KCl in 0.9% saline (20 or 40 mEq K^+/L)	
Sodium	
NaCl in water (0.45%, 0.9%, 3%, 5%)	Isotonic (0.9%) or hypotonic (0.45%) infused at 90-125 mL/hr or higher for initial therapy; 3% saline infused at <80 mL/hr; 5% saline infused at <50 mL/hr.
NaCl concentrate (2.5 or 4 mEq Na^+/L) NaCl in 2.5%, 5%, or 10% dextrose (0.11%, 0.2%, 0.225%, 0.3%, 0.33%, 0.45%, or 0.9% in NaCl)	Isotonic saline supplies 154 mEq/L Na^+ and 154 mEq/L of Cl^-.
NaCl in 5% dextrose with KCl (0.2%, 0.225%, 0.33%, 0.45%, or 0.9% NaCl with 0.075%, 0.15%, 0.224%, or 0.3% KCl)	NaCl concentrate used for mixing with other intravenous solutions. Monitor for potassium overload when using NaCl in dextrose with KCl.
Multiple Electrolytes	
Ringer's solution (0.86% NaCl, 0.03% KCl, 0.033% $CaCl_2$)	Balanced salt solution supplies, in mEq/L, the following ions: Na^+ 147, K^+ 4, Ca^{++} 4.5, Cl^- 156.
Lactated Ringer's solution (0.6% NaCl, 0.03% KCl, 0.02% $CaCl_2$, 0.31% Na lactate)	Balanced salt solution supplies, in mEq/L, the following ions: Na^+ 130, K^+ 4, Ca^{++} 3, Cl^- 109.
Electrolytes in 5% dextrose (Electrolyte No. 48, No. 75, Ionosol Isolyte, Normosol, Plasmalyte)	Complex mixtures are used in special circumstances to correct massive electrolyte imbalances

ECG, Electrocardiogram.

stronger basic cations in the blood than simple inorganic salt solutions.

Dextrose, or glucose, in an isotonic solution (5%) is appropriate for most situations in which rehydration is needed. In addition to fluid, the solution supplies about 170 cal/L or 560 kJ/L. Electrolytes are not supplied in this solution. Hypertonic dextrose solutions may be used to shift fluid from the interstitial space into the plasma. Isotonic dextrose solutions may be infused through peripheral veins to hydrate patients and to replace sodium loss, but hypertonic dextrose solutions should be infused through a central vein to avoid excessive irritation. Five percent dextrose in 0.45% saline may be used to shift fluid from plasma into the interstitial space, which may cause difficulty for patients with cardiac, renal, or liver disease, who also have edema and poor venous return.

PHARMACOKINETICS

All these intravenous fluids readily distribute through the body via osmosis and diffusion.

ADVERSE REACTIONS AND CONTRAINDICATIONS

Dangers associated with sodium chloride infusion include circulatory overload and hypernatremia. Metabolic acidosis may arise when excess chloride ion in blood promotes bicarbonate ion loss in the kidneys. Hypokalemia may occur if excess sodium ion forces potassium ion excretion by the kidneys. Hypertonic saline solutions should be used in small volumes and administered carefully to correct severe hyponatremia. Use of sodium chloride solutions that contain preservative requires special precautions (Box 64-2).

The potassium found in Ringer's and lactated Ringer's solutions cannot be eliminated and may accumulate to dangerous levels if renal function is impaired. Therefore renal function must be established before these fluids are administered.

Hypertonic glucose solutions are given slowly to avoid tissue damage.

INTERACTIONS

Dextrose solutions may have other components added for infusion, but not all additives are compatible. For example, dextrose solutions are never used in the same intravenous line with whole blood because the glucose causes hemolysis (rupture of red blood cells). The pharmacist or a standard reference such as the *Handbook on Injectable Drugs** can provide information about compatibilities of intravenous fluids.

| BOX **64-2** | **Benzyl Alcohol** |

Benzyl alcohol is a bacteriostatic agent commonly used in solutions of sodium chloride and other drugs. Neonates are especially sensitive to this agent, and deaths have occurred when solutions containing benzyl alcohol were used in children in this age group.
- Avoid administration of bacteriostatic saline (with benzyl alcohol) to newborns.
- Do not dilute drug with bacteriostatic saline if the drug is to be used in newborns.
- With newborns, do not flush intravenous lines with bacteriostatic saline.

DRUG CLASS • Alkalinizing Drugs

acetazolamide (Diamox✱)

sodium acetate

sodium bicarbonate (Neut)

sodium citrate/citric acid (Shohl Solution, Bicitra, Oracit)

sodium lactate

tromethamine (Tham)

MECHANISM OF ACTION

Sodium bicarbonate dissociates in the blood to increase bicarbonate concentration, which decreases hydrogen concentration by shifting the equilibrium to the right, as shown in Figure 64-3. The kidneys then increase the urinary excretion of bicarbonate ions, which increases the urinary pH. Sodium acetate, lactate, and citrate are converted metabolically to bicarbonate and then act on systemic pH in the same fashion as sodium bicarbonate.

Tromethamine binds the hydrogen ions of carbonic acid, releasing bicarbonate and raising the pH of the blood. The tromethamine molecule is neither metabolized nor reabsorbed by the renal tubule and therefore also acts as an osmotic diuretic (see Chapter 46 for an explanation of osmotic diuresis).

---

*Trissel LA: *Handbook on injectable drugs,* ed 11, Bethesda, Md, 2000, American Society of Health-System Pharmacists, Inc.

Acetazolamide inhibits carbonic anhydrase, which promotes the urinary excretion of bicarbonate ions. Accordingly, the pH of the urine becomes alkaline. However, since the urinary excretion of bicarbonate reduces the bicarbonate concentration in the blood, metabolic acidosis develops systemically under the influence of acetazolamide. In other words, acetazolamide effectively alkalinizes the urine but is not a systemic alkalinizing drug.

USES

Alkalinizing drugs such as sodium bicarbonate, acetate, citrate, lactate, and tromethamine are used to increase blood pH and thus correct metabolic acidosis.

Sodium bicarbonate is also used, as is acetazolamide, to increase urinary pH as a means of treating selected drug overdoses. Alkalinization of the urine enhances the excretion of weak organic acids by causing them to exist more in the ionized (nonreabsorbable) state than in the nonionized state (reabsorbable) state (see Chapter 1).

Tromethamine is also used on a short-term basis to correct acidosis associated with cardiac disease, bypass surgery, or after cardiac arrest. It is also effective against severe respiratory acidosis associated with status asthmaticus or respiratory distress syndrome of the newborn. Because tromethamine is sodium free, it can be used to prevent or correct acidosis in patients for whom sodium retention would be hazardous.

PHARMACOKINETICS

Sodium bicarbonate is 100% bioavailable when administered intravenously. The drug has an immediate onset, with peak drug action reached in 15 minutes. It is widely distributed to extracellular fluid.

At a pH of 7.4, 30% of tromethamine is nonionized and therefore is capable of reaching equilibrium with body water. The drug penetrates cells and neutralizes acidic anions of intracellular fluid. Elevation in pH has been noted 1 hour after administration. Tromethamine is eliminated unchanged in the urine.

ADVERSE REACTIONS AND CONTRAINDICATIONS

The adverse reactions associated with alkalinizing drugs are usually associated with large dosages. Excessive sodium bicarbonate causes metabolic alkalosis that manifests as hyperirritability, tetany, or both. When administered too rapidly to correct diabetic ketoacidosis, bicarbonate causes tissue hypoxia, cerebral dysfunction, and lactic acidosis. The high sodium content (276 mg of sodium/g) causes water retention and edema in some patients. Thus sodium bicarbonate should be used cautiously in patients with heart failure, renal failure, or other disorders of fluid balance. Sodium bicarbonate is contraindicated in patients with chloride losses or hypocalcemia. Oral administration of sodium bicarbonate produces gastric distention and flatus when it combines with hydrochloric acid in the stomach and releases carbon dioxide.

Sodium citrate produces fewer adverse effects than sodium bicarbonate, but in excess, it can also cause metabolic alkalosis or tetany, or may aggravate existing cardiovascular disease by increasing calcium levels. Orally administered sodium citrate produces a laxative-like effect.

Sodium lactate also produces fewer adverse effects than sodium bicarbonate but in excess can cause metabolic acidosis (rather than alkalosis). Because the sodium content is high (204 mg/g), water retention and edema may develop.

The adverse reactions to tromethamine range from irritation at the intravenous site to hypoglycemia, respiratory depression, and hyperkalemia. Tromethamine can accumulate to toxic levels in patients with impaired re-

---

TABLE 64-4

Drug Interactions of Selected Alkalinizing and Acidifying Drugs

Drug	Action	Interacting Drugs
sodium bicarbonate	Increases renal reabsorption of:	Amphetamines, ephedrine, flecainide, methadone, pseudoephedrine, quinidine, quinine
sodium bicarbonate salicylates	Increases renal elimination of:	Aspirin and other salicylates, chlorpropamide, lithium, phenobarbital, tetracycline
sodium bicarbonate	Causes excessive sodium retention with:	Glucocorticoids
arginine HCl	Reduces the response to: Increases the risk of hyperkalemia with:	Glucagon, insulin, sulfonylureas Potassium-sparing diuretics

nal function. The drug is contraindicated in patients with uremia or anuria.

Acetazolamide produces a wide range of adverse effects. CNS reactions include headache, sedation, confusion, and paresthesias. In a patient with severe liver disease, acetazolamide can raise the blood sugar, decrease uric acid elimination, produce metabolic acidosis, and precipitate hepatic coma. Hypersensitivity reactions and bone marrow depression can lead to aplastic anemia.

INTERACTIONS

Drug interactions for alkalinizing drugs are identified in Table 64-4. The most common interactions are related to their ability to increase the renal tubular reabsorption or urinary excretion of interacting drugs.

 DRUG CLASS • Acidifying Drugs

ammonium chloride

arginine hydrochloride

ascorbic acid (Ascorbicap)

hydrochloric acid

MECHANISM OF ACTION

Ammonium chloride ionizes to the fixed chloride ion and the labile ammonium ion. In the blood, ammonium ions dissociate into ammonia (uncharged) and hydrogen ions. The hydrogen ions acidify the blood. The liver subsequently converts ammonia to urea, which is excreted in urine. The resulting urine is also acidified because the kidneys will increase the excretion of hydrogen ions in response to the acidosis produced by ammonium chloride.

Arginine provides hydrogen ions via the normal metabolic utilization of the amino acid. The hydrogen ions acidify the blood. Ascorbic acid directly acidifies the blood by dissociating to ascorbate and free hydrogen ions. The resulting urine is also acidified.

USES

Acidifying drugs are used to correct metabolic alkalosis and to acidify the urine in order to increase or delay the elimination of certain drugs.

PHARMACOKINETICS

Ammonium chloride taken orally is completely absorbed in 3 to 6 hours. Drug action peaks 1 to 3 hours after intravenous administration.

Arginine has an immediate onset when it is given intravenously, with peak drug action noted in 20 to 30 minutes. The duration of action of arginine is 1 hour. Arginine is incorporated into many biochemical pathways in the liver, filtered at the glomerulus, and almost completely reabsorbed by the renal tubules.

Sodium bicarbonate has a peak effect within 15 minutes of intravenous administration and the effect persists for 1 to 2 hours. In contrast, ascorbic acid takes days to produce its acidifying effects.

ADVERSE REACTIONS AND CONTRAINDICATIONS

The adverse reactions to acidifying drugs are usually mild. Ammonium chloride can cause anorexia, nausea, vomiting, and thirst when taken orally. Large doses of ammonium chloride can cause metabolic acidosis secondary to hyperchloremia, especially in patients with impaired renal function. Other adverse reactions to large doses of ammonium chloride include rash, headache, hyperventilation, bradycardia, progressive drowsiness, confusion, and excitement alternating with coma. Calcium-deficient tetany, hyperglycemia, glucosuria, twitching, hyperreflexia, and electroencephalogram changes have also been reported. Most of these adverse effects are related to ammonia toxicity resulting from inability of the liver to convert ammonium ions to urea. Because the acidifying action of ammonium chloride depends on hepatic conversion to urea, the drug is contraindicated in patients with liver disease. Safe use in perinatal and pediatric populations has not been established.

Arginine hydrochloride has a low incidence of adverse reactions; however, rapid intravenous infusion may produce flushing, nausea, vomiting, numbness, headache, and local venous irritation. Extravasation from an intravenous site causes superficial phlebitis and necrosis. Nasal obstruction and discharge, choking, sweating, and tachycardia have also been reported during intravenous administration of arginine. These effects may represent an allergic response to the drug. Abdominal pain and bloating have been reported following oral administration.

High doses of ascorbic acid can produce nausea, vomiting, diarrhea, abdominal cramps, flushing, headache, and insomnia. In patients with glucose 6-phosphate dehydrogenase deficiency, hemolytic anemia can develop after the administration of high doses of ascorbic acid.

INTERACTIONS

Drug interactions of acidifying drugs are identified in Table 64-4. Severe, potentially fatal hyperkalemia has occurred following arginine therapy. The patients affected were those with hepatic disease who had taken spironolactone 2 or 3 days before receiving arginine.

The combined use of potassium-sparing diuretics and arginine should thus be avoided.

   DRUG CLASS • **Parenteral Nutrition Formulations**

MECHANISM OF ACTION

Parenteral nutrition fluids are designed to supply calories and required nutrients to patients unable to take adequate amounts enterally. Patients require maintenance with intravenous nutrients for many reasons (Box 64-3). Many choices are available, allowing some tailoring of the regimen for individual patient needs. Dextrose solutions supply some calories, but only about 3 L of fluid can be administered daily without overloading the circulatory system. Therefore about 500 calories can be supplied each day from isotonic dextrose solutions. For longer-term therapy, more calories from different sources are required. Total parenteral nutrition (TPN) is possible using synthetic amino acids, dextrose, and fat emulsions (Table 64-5).

USES

Hypertonic dextrose is required for TPN. Amino acids used in TPN prevent negative nitrogen balance and breakdown of protein in the body. Pure amino acid solutions, rather than protein hydrolysates, are preferred. At 3.5% concentrations, the amino acid solutions offer about 140 cal/L and a variety of electrolytes. Extra potassium is often required by patients receiving amino acid solutions because potassium is depleted by amino acid metabolism.

Fat emulsions may be administered intravenously during TPN to prevent essential fatty acid deficiency. Because fats have a high caloric content, these preparations may supply a significant proportion (up to 60%) of the daily caloric requirement.

BOX 64-3   **Conditions Warranting Parenteral Nutrition**

- Inability to use the alimentary tract for enteral feedings
- Intolerance of long-term enteral feedings or inability to provide sufficient nutrition by enteral feeding alone
- Illness that is sustained and debilitating
- Impaired absorption of protein from the GI tract
- Long-term wound infection, abscess, or fistula resulting in extreme nitrogen loss
- Bowel rest required for longer than 1 week secondary to GI surgery, injury, or inflammatory GI disorders
- Hypoproteinemia as a result of loss of protein or substantial increase in protein requirements
- Chronic diarrhea or vomiting
- Persistent weight loss in excess of 10% of body weight
- Liver and renal failure resulting in altered amino acid requirements

---

TABLE 64-5

Parenteral Nutrition Fluids

Preparation	Trade Names	Comments
Amino acids, crystalline	Aminosyn, BranchAmin, FreAmine, HepatAmine, NephrAmine, Novamine, ProcalAmine, RenAmine, Travasol, TrophAmine	Solutions contain various mixtures of essential and nonessential amino acids as well as appreciable amounts of sodium and other electrolytes. Adults need about 1 g/kg body weight per day to prevent protein breakdown. A 3% solution is nearly isotonic and may be administered via a peripheral vein. Higher concentrations must be administered via a central IV line. Aminosyn and TrophAmine contain taurine, an amino acid required by neonates.
Dextrose (2.5% to 70%)		Adults need about 150 g/day of dextrose. Solutions at higher concentrations are diluted before use. The 5% solution is isotonic.
Fat emulsions (10% or 20%)	Intralipid, Liposyn II, Liposyn III, Soyacal	Soybean oil stabilized with egg yolk phospholipids, with glycerol to adjust isotonicity. Lipids should not supply more than 60% of total calories. Liposyn II contains both safflower and soybean oil, giving more linoleic acid, but less linolenic acid than other preparations.

IV, Intravenous.

PHARMACOKINETICS

Solutions of dextrose for administration are prepared from 50% or 60% stock solutions, but as they are administered, the concentration of dextrose is only 25% to 30%. This hypertonic solution must be administered via a large central vein in which blood flow is sufficient to dilute the strong glucose solution and prevent tissue damage. A 10% dextrose solution is hypertonic but can be given peripherally without damage to veins.

TPN solutions are given by a central intravenous line to provide adequate dilution of the nutrients and prevent damage to veins. The dextrose, amino acids, and fats from these solutions are transported through the body and used by cells in the same way as absorbed nutrients.

ADVERSE REACTIONS AND CONTRAINDICATIONS

The greatest risk with parenteral nutrition is infection. The problem may be restricted to the infusion site, but it is likely that the infection will spread and cause septicemia, which can be life threatening.

Large doses of dextrose (glucose) can cause metabolic imbalances including hyperglycemia and a fatty liver. Abruptly stopping dextrose infusions can also produce rebound hypoglycemia. Large doses of amino acids may lead to ketosis. Electrolyte imbalances are also common. Large doses of fat emulsions can lead to hyperlipidemia. Fat overload syndrome may also be characterized by fever, focal seizures, leukocytosis, hepatomegaly, splenomegaly, spontaneous bleeding, and shock.

INTERACTIONS

In general, no drug should be added to parenteral nutrition solutions. Other interactions occur with drugs administered by different routes. For example, insulin requirements may increase when a diabetic patient is on parenteral nutrition. Tetracycline antibiotics and certain diuretics may cause a negative nitrogen balance and thus antagonize the positive effects of TPN solutions.

DRUG CLASS • Solutions to Correct Specific Electrolyte Imbalances

See Table 64-3.

Calcium salts are used by intravenous infusion to correct acute hypocalcemia and to supply calcium for parenteral nutrition. Calcium salts have also been used to stimulate cardiac function, to treat hyperkalemia, to treat magnesium intoxication, and to replace calcium in patients receiving large volumes of citrated blood (see also Chapter 56 and 63).

Magnesium sulfate is used to correct severe magnesium deficiencies and to control seizures in women with pregnancy-induced hypertension. The 10% solution is

nearly isotonic and may be used intravenously, but the 50% solution is strongly hypertonic and is used intramuscularly. Magnesium sulfate may be added to parenteral nutrition solutions for maintenance.

Potassium chloride may be added to intravenous fluids to replace potassium lost from the GI tract or through the kidneys. Replacement must be undertaken carefully to avoid causing hyperkalemia and its dangerous adverse effects. Dosage is calculated based on the estimated loss for the individual patient.

APPLICATION TO PRACTICE

ASSESSMENT
History of Present Illness

The patient who has a fluid, electrolyte, or acid-base imbalance may note a variety of signs and symptoms. Inquire specifically about signs and symptoms of fluid volume excess and deficits, and electrolyte or acid-base imbalances (see Tables 64-1 and 64-2). Family members can be a source of information because some alterations in fluid or acid-base balance cause changes in the patient's cognitive function or emotional status.

Health History

Ask if the patient has a recent history of vomiting or diarrhea, a history of heart or renal failure, cirrhosis, diabetes mellitus, chronic airway limitation, or recent surgery. In the case of ongoing medical problems, access to previous charts or data is helpful in planning individualized interventions.

A drug history is important to elicit because drugs can cause or contribute to fluid, electrolyte, and acid-base imbalance. Ask about the use of OTC drugs and herbs but pay particular attention to cardiac drugs and diuretics. Many of these drugs alter acid-base, fluid, or electrolyte balance.

Lifespan Considerations

Perinatal. Physiologic changes during pregnancy affect fluid, electrolyte, and acid-base balance (see Chapter 2). In the first trimester, human chorionic gonadotropin secretion can cause nausea and vomiting, alter carbohydrate metabolism, and result in changes in smell and taste. Intravenous therapy may be required if hyperemesis gravidarum (severe vomiting in early pregnancy) occurs. In rare but severe cases, TPN may be required until vomiting subsides.

Because pregnancy increases cell numbers and additional oxygen is required, hormonal and anatomic changes are directed at facilitating oxygen availability. Progesterone stimulates the respiratory rate. Additionally, pregnancy induces a small degree of hyperventilation as tidal volume (amount of air breathed with ordinary respiration) decreases steadily throughout pregnancy. In the process, excess carbon dioxide is blown off. The resulting decrease in carbonic acid creates a pH difference during pregnancy. Although the normal pH range is from 7.35 to 7.45, in pregnancy the pH tends toward the upper range of 7.42 to 7.45. Thus there may be a slight degree of respiratory alkalosis throughout pregnancy.

Pediatric. As discussed in Chapter 3, infants and small children have a proportionately higher percentage of total body water than adults. The distribution of fluid is also different. Extracellular fluid leaves the body through the lungs, GI tract, and kidneys. For this reason, infants are more susceptible to fluid volume deficits because their daily water turnover is greater than older children and adults.

Acid-base buffering systems are less well developed in infants and children than in adults, and they tend to develop acid-base imbalances more easily. Common conditions that predispose an infant to acid-base imbalances include fevers, upper respiratory infections, vomiting, and diarrhea. Furthermore, infants and small children are less able to describe symptoms such as thirst or changes in sensation (e.g., paresthesias). Therefore, a careful evaluation of early changes in acid-base balance should be performed.

Older Adults. The physical changes of aging predispose the patient to iatrogenic fluid and electrolyte imbalances (see Chapter 4). The normal aging process is accompanied by a decrease in the efficiency of the body's compensatory mechanisms. This results in a narrow margin of safety and a longer recovery time once homeostasis has been interrupted. Fluid, electrolyte, and acid-base imbalances are common problems among older adults. Imbalances often increase the frequency and length of hospital stays and may threaten the patient's ability to return to an independent lifestyle.

Because of decreased chest wall compliance, elasticity of lung tissues, number of alveoli, and respiratory muscle strength, the older adult cannot eliminate carbon dioxide as readily. This limits the ability to compensate for metabolic alterations and predisposes the patient to respiratory acidosis.

The physical changes of aging also result in a decreased number of nephrons. By returning some substances to body fluids and eliminating others, the kidneys compensate for even large deviations from the normal range. However, as aging continues, compensatory abilities decline. As a result the older adult may take 18 to 48 hours to reestablish homeostasis after an acid-base upset, whereas a younger adult may need only 6 to 10 hours.

Cultural/Social Considerations

An awareness of the patient's cultural, ethnic, and religious background is important. The patient and family should be made aware of what intravenous therapy involves and what solution is used. Additionally, any concerns they may have should be addressed. Sodium chloride is required in most cases for the administration of blood and blood products. If the patient's religious beliefs preclude the use of blood products, the health care provider should be notified and the information documented in the patient's record. Alternative intravenous solutions may be available for this patient, or a court order may be obtained if a blood transfusion is the only proper therapy.

Physical Examination

A head-to-toe physical examination should be completed and documented before the initiation of therapy if the patient's condition permits (Table 64-6). Critical assessments of fluid, electrolyte, or nutritional imbalances include general appearance and mental status, vital signs, accurate daily weights, and intake and output. The skin turgor and temperature, as well as the condition of the mucous membranes, the lips, the hair, and the nails, should be noted. In infants, head circumference and the integrity of the fontanelles should be noted. Jugular venous distention, the presence of crackles or wheezes, edema, and arrhythmias give the health care provider a sense of cardiovascular integrity. Involuntary neuromuscular activity, altered deep tendon reflexes, or changes in sensation may suggest electrolyte imbalances as well.

Clinical manifestations of alkalosis are the result of the related hypocalcemia or hypokalemia. The presence of Trousseau's and Chvostek's signs, carpopedal spasms,

TABLE 64-6		
Comparison of Fluid Volume Excess and Deficit		
Parameter	*Fluid Volume Excess*	*Fluid Volume Deficit*
General survey	Confusion, irritability Weight gain Bounding pulse Increased blood pressure Venous distention Growth and development delay	Lethargy Weight loss Weak or thready pulse Decreased blood pressure and pulse pressure Tachycardia Orthostatic hypotension Temperature low (depends on cause) Growth and developmental delay Decreased activity*
Integumentary	Warm, moist, supple skin Tight, shiny skin Edema with possible pitting	Dry skin Decreased skin turgor Possible tenting of skin
Head, face, neck	Taut fontanelles* Increased head circumference*	Sunken fontanelles* Dry, cracked lips Furrowed tongue Lack of tears* Dry mucous membranes, thick secretions
Respiratory	Inspiratory crackles Increased respiratory rate Shortness of breath Dyspnea on exertion Paroxysmal nocturnal dyspnea Pulmonary edema	Normal breath sounds
Cardiovascular	Elevated central venous pressure Chest pain in patients with heart disease	Decreased central venous pressure Decreased cardiac output Decreased tissue perfusion Arrhythmias
Elimination	Intake exceeds output Urine has low specific gravity	Decreased output Urine has high specific gravity
Neuromuscular	Decreased level of consciousness Seizure activity Irritability	Lethargy, disorientation Seizure activity Confusion
Laboratory data	Hemoglobin and hematocrit normal or low Electrolyte values increased	Hemoglobin and hematocrit elevated Electrolytes values decreased

*Pediatric findings.

tetany, hyperactive deep tendon reflexes, skeletal muscle weakness, and muscle cramping and twitching are evident in patients with hypocalcemia. Syncopal episodes, seizures, and coma are possible. Although skeletal muscles contract as a result of overstimulation, the muscles themselves become weaker because of the alkalosis and hypokalemia. Hand-grasp strength is reduced, and the patient may be unable to support body weight or walk. Respiratory efforts become less effective as the skeletal muscles of respiration become weaker. Because alkalosis produces increased myocardial irritability, especially in the presence of an accompanying hypokalemia, the heart rate increases and the pulse becomes thready. The blood pressure may be normal or low.

Clinical manifestations of acidosis are similar whether the cause is respiratory or metabolic. Depressed CNS function is common in patients with acidosis and may be manifested as lethargy progressing to confusion, especially in the older adult. The patient becomes stuporous as acidosis worsens or if it is accompanied by hyperkalemia. The acidotic state and accompanying hyperkalemia cause a decrease in muscle tone and deep tendon reflexes. The muscle weakness is bilateral and can progress to flaccid paralysis.

If the acidosis is of respiratory origin, breathing effectiveness is greatly diminished, with rapid but shallow respirations. If the acidosis has a metabolic origin, the rate and depth of respirations increase in proportion to the increase in hydrogen ion concentration. The respirations are rapid, deep, and regular and are not under voluntary control (Kussmaul's respirations). The skin and mucous membranes are pale to cyanotic in color because respirations are ineffective.

However, in metabolic acidosis, breathing effectiveness is essentially unaffected and the rate increased, the patient's skin is pink, warm, and dry. Cardiovascular manifestations of acidosis include tachycardia. As acidosis worsens or is accompanied by hyperkalemia, electrical activity through the heart is reduced and bradycardia results. As a result of changes in heart activity, peripheral pulses can be difficult to locate and are easily obliterated with light pressure. Hypotension is the result of vasodilation.

Laboratory Testing

The rapidity with which a patient's condition can change magnifies the need for careful monitoring of laboratory values. Baseline studies that are appropriate before and throughout intravenous therapy include a complete blood count, electrolytes, platelet count, prothrombin time, blood urea nitrogen (BUN), and creatinine, as well as glucose, total protein, uric acid, liver function tests, cholesterol, triglyceride levels, and arterial blood gases (Table 64-7).

Daily monitoring of laboratory data varies based on the solution used. Once the patient is stabilized, less frequent routine monitoring is needed. With all parenteral nutrition, daily, if not more frequent, monitoring of glucose, in addition to intake, output, and weight, is necessary. Liver function, electrolytes, BUN, and creatinine are checked two to three times weekly. Acid-base balance is diagnosed and monitored via determinations of electrolytes and arterial blood gases.

GOALS OF THERAPY

The major goals with intravenous therapy include maintenance of daily requirements, replacement of existing deficits, restoration of ongoing or concurrent losses, and prevention of complications in patients at risk.

Treatment goals for the patient with alkalosis are directed at increasing the levels of hydrogen ions; preventing further hydrogen, potassium, calcium, and chloride losses; and restoring fluid balance. Treatment goals for the patient with acidosis are directed at cor-

---

TABLE 64-7

Laboratory Findings in Acid-Base Imbalances

		Gas Parameters*			Electrolytes†		
Imbalance	Compensation	pH	$PaCO_2$	HCO_3	K	Ca	Cl
Respiratory alkalosis	Uncompensated	↑7.45	↓35		N		
	Partially compensated	↑7.45	↓35	↓22			
	Compensated	N	↓35	↓22	↓	↓	↑
Respiratory acidosis	Uncompensated	↓7.35	↑46		N		
	Partially compensated	↓7.35	↑46	↑26			
	Compensated	N	↑46	↑26	↑	N	↑↓
Metabolic alkalosis	Uncompensated	↑7.45	N	↑26			
	Partially compensated	↑7.45	↑46	↑26			
	Compensated	N	↑46	↑26	↓	↓	↓
Metabolic acidosis	Uncompensated	↓7.35	N	↓22			
	Partially compensated	N or ↓7.35	↓35	↓22			
	Compensated	N	↓35	↓22	↑	N	↑

↑,Value above normal range; ↓, Value below normal range; *N*, normal.
*Arterial blood gas values at sea level:
  pH   7.35-7.45
  $PaCO_2$ 35-46 mm Hg
  HCO_3 22-26 mEq/L
†Electrolyte levels relative to sodium values. Normal electrolyte values:
  Potassium 3.5-5.0 mEq/L
  Chloride   98-106 mmol/L
  Calcium   8.8-10.0 mg/dL

recting the underlying cause of the acidosis and normalizing acid-base balance. It should be evident that overtreating one type of imbalance may upset the balance in the opposite direction.

INTERVENTION
Administration

Become familiar with agency or institutional policies and procedures regarding intravenous administration. Policies may specify who may start intravenous fluids and add electrolyte solutions or drugs to infusions. There may also be procedures specified for routinely changing the tubing or insertion site, or for redressing central line insertion sites. Inspect intravenous solutions carefully before using. Do not use solutions that are leaking, discolored, or contain particulate matter.

Venous Access Devices. How fluids are administered is an important part of intravenous therapy. Administration decisions include not only what solution is used but also which venous access device is appropriate and what delivery system is indicated. Become familiar with the intravenous equipment used in the agency. Read the package inserts and attend in-service programs about new equipment. Venous access devices are selected based on the quality of the patient's veins, age, clinical condition, anticipated duration of treatment, and the solution type and amount to be delivered.

Choose a needle or catheter, administration set, and tubing length appropriate for the patient and the drug. Peripherally inserted needles or catheters work well for most forms of intravenous therapy. Small sizes are usually sufficient unless large amounts of fluid must be given rapidly or if the fluid is viscous. Centrally placed catheters, implanted infusion ports, and peripherally inserted central catheters are used for patients who require long-term therapy. These access devices have greater longevity and also make it possible to deliver solutions that are irritating to smaller veins. Intravenous therapy should be discontinued as early as possible to prevent infusion-related complications.

For example, the larger the diameter of the needle or catheter, the faster the fluid will infuse, but the larger the diameter, the more difficult it is to insert the needle or catheter into the chosen vein and the greater the risk of phlebitis. The higher the fluid reservoir (bag or bottle) is above the patient, the faster the rate of infusion; generally, the reservoir should be about 36 inches above the insertion site. The viscosity of the fluid also influences the rate of flow; for example, blood infuses more slowly than normal saline or 5% dextrose solutions.

The longer the tubing from the fluid reservoir to the patient, the slower the rate of flow. Choose a tubing long enough to allow safe movement by the patient but

short enough to ensure that the tubing will not get tangled in the siderails or significantly restrict flow. Finally, choose an administration set appropriate to the ordered rate of flow. Use a minidrip set and volume control devices for infants or small children, when a keep-open or slow rate is in use, or when a drug dosage is measured according to patient response, such as when an intravenous drug (e.g., dopamine) is adjusted based on the patient's blood pressure.

Fluid Reservoirs. Label all fluid reservoirs as directed by agency procedure. A common method is to place a length of adhesive tape along the side of the bag or bottle next to the volume markers on the container. The correct fluid level per hour is marked on the tape. For example, if 1000 mL of fluid is started at 8 AM and the fluid is to infuse at 100 ml/hr, there should be 900 mL remaining at 9 AM and 800 mL at 10 AM. Thus any nurse on duty can determine at a glance whether the infusion is running at the correct rate. If an infusion is slow, do not try to catch up by doubling or increasing the rate for the next hour or two. Assess the situation and, if necessary, restart the infusion at another site. If the solution is infusing too rapidly, slow the rate and assess the patient for signs of fluid overload (see Table 64-6). If the extra volume infused was minimal and the patient's condition is satisfactory, resume the prescribed rate. If the volume is excessive or signs of fluid overload are present, maintain the intravenous unit at the keep-open rate and notify the health care provider.

Label all intravenous solutions carefully, especially when additives such as potassium, vitamins, heparin, insulin, and other drugs have been included.

Volume Control Devices. Intravenous pumps and controllers are widely used today. These electronic devices help maintain a constant rate of flow. Because they contain alarms, they warn the health care provider when a problem occurs. The intravenous pump delivers the intravenous fluid with pressure, whereas the intravenous controller adjusts the rate of fluids infusing via gravity. Become familiar with devices used at your site. Electronic devices do not replace careful patient assessment and care but can assist in managing intravenous therapy.

Use volume control devices to limit the volume a patient could receive in a specified time. The volume control device is filled with a specified volume of fluid and the flow rate adjusted. The patient can receive only the volume contained in the device until it is refilled. For example, consider an infant requiring intravenous fluids. Even if a 500-mL reservoir bag were hung instead of a 1000-mL bag, the danger of fluid overload would be significant if all 500 mL were to infuse rapidly. The volume control device can be filled with the amount ordered for 1 hour (e.g., 30 mL for this patient) and the flow rate adjusted. Even if all of the fluid in the device infuses rapidly, the danger of fluid overload is much less than with 500 mL. Volume control devices permit the addition of drugs to the fluid in the chamber while decreasing the risk of intravenous fluid overload.

Infusion Pumps. Although the use of an infusion pump results in an additional charge to the patient, it is a necessary piece of safety equipment in many clinical situations. These electronic devices help maintain a constant rate of flow. Because they contain alarms, they warn when a problem occurs. The intravenous pump delivers the fluid with pressure, whereas the intravenous controller adjusts the rate of fluids infusing by gravity. Become familiar with devices used in your agency. Electronic devices do not take the place of careful patient assessment and care but can assist is managing intravenous therapy.

Parenteral nutrition fluids, lipids, and the administration of intravenous potassium formulations require the use of an infusion pump. An accurate infusion rate is extremely important in children and for patients with renal, cardiovascular, endocrine, or neurologic disorders.

Use measures to prevent complications of intravenous administration, in addition to assessing for the patient's development and subsequent treatment. For example, cleanse insertion sites thoroughly before initiating intravenous therapy and wear sterile gloves when starting the intravenous line. Clean injection ports well with an alcohol or povidone-iodine swab before puncturing them. Use a Luer-Lok type of connection to prevent accidental pulling apart of intravenous tubing. Choose insertion sites where catheters are less likely to be dislodged by patient movement and tape catheters securely. Wear gloves also when discontinuing an intravenous line.

In-Line Intravenous Filters. The use of in-line intravenous filters for all drugs and solutions is not universally accepted. Nevertheless, many agencies require them. Become familiar with the advantages of the filters in use in your agency. For example, some filters remove only particulate matter, and some do not have air-eliminating capability. The 0.22-mm filter can remove particulate matter, fungi, bacteria, and air but cannot filter TPN solutions because it is too small. Tubing for blood administration is equipped with a filter. Fat emulsions cannot be filtered.

Monitoring the Infusion. Maintain vigilance whenever working with intravenous fluids or drugs because the administration of any substance directly into the vascular system can cause serious and rapid consequences.

Assess the patient receiving intravenous fluids at least hourly, noting the correct infusion rate. Inspect the bag or bottle, tubing, monitoring devices, and area surrounding the insertion site. Assess for signs of fluid overload and observe for any of the common problems associated with intravenous fluid therapy. Monitor skin turgor, intake and output, and weight and inspect dependent areas for edema. Check vital signs, auscultate for heart and lung sounds, and monitor central venous pressure and pulmonary capillary wedge pressures if required. See Table 64-8 for a summary of common intravenous problems and suggested nursing actions. Record the administration of all intravenous solutions carefully.

Hydrating and Replacement Solutions. Dextrose solutions require monitoring of the blood glucose level at a frequency based on the patient's condition and the concentration of solution. The hypotonic and isotonic solutions have little effect on blood glucose levels of patients who are not glucose intolerant. Hypertonic glucose solutions and centrally administered TPN requires frequent monitoring of blood glucose levels in all patients.

Potassium. Potassium chloride is the most common electrolyte added to intravenous fluids. Potassium chloride is most often added to the intravenous fluid by the nurse or pharmacy. Determine that the patient has adequate kidney function before administering intravenous potassium. Always check the dose of potassium chloride and dilute the drug before administration. Carefully label containers to which potassium has been added.

Monitor the patient's ECG changes, serum potassium level, and infusion rate. See Table 64-1 for signs of common electrolyte imbalances. The classic ECG changes seen with hypokalemia include ST depression, flattened T waves, the presence of U waves, and ventricular arrhythmias. The classic ECG changes with hyperkalemia include tall thin T waves, prolonged PR interval, ST depression, widened QRS complex, and loss of P waves.

To treat hyperkalemia, discontinue potassium replacements (intravenous or oral) and limit potassium-rich foods. Emergency treatment includes intravenous sodium bicarbonate, calcium gluconate (if not contraindicated by existing cardiac conditions), and intravenous glucose and insulin (which help shift potassium into the cell). Dialysis may also be used. Subacute hyperkalemia is treated with cation exchange resins such as sodium polystyrene sulfonate (e.g., Kayexalate, SPS suspension), which exchanges sodium for potassium in the intestine. The effect is not evident for several hours to 1 day after administration. The resin is given orally, via nasogastric tube, or as a retention enema.

TABLE 64-8

Intravenous Infusion: Problems, Signs and Symptoms, and Suggested Nursing Actions

Problem	Signs and Symptoms	Nursing Actions
Pain during infusion	Patient discomfort	Slow rate of infusion to prevent drugs from irritating veins. Warm IV fluids to room temperature before hanging. Rule out phlebitis.
Occluded infusion	Decreased rate of infusion or no infusion Backup of blood into tubing Possible discomfort	Verify that clamp is open or electronic device is turned on. Inspect tubing for kinks. Remove dressing over IV site using aseptic technique; check for kinks, replace dressing, and retape insertion site. If fluid level in bag is low, raise level of bag or replace it with full bag. With some infusion deveices or with multilumen central catheters, use thrombolytics such as urokinase to dissove clots occluding IV flow; follow agency policies. If all else fails, restart IV.
Extravasation (leaking of fluid or drug into tissue surrounding vein, caused by tear in vein)	Decreased rate of infusion or no infusion Patient discomfort Puffiness, edema of extremity or insertion site Coolness distal to insertion site No blood return when bag lowered below level of insertion site	Assess pulse. Elevate extremity. Discontinue IV; restart IV line at another site. Apply ice or warm soaks (follow agency policy). If drug is known to be caustic, carry out any specific measures, including infiltration of area with steroids or drug antidote; consult health care provider or agency policies.
Phlebitis (irritation or inflammation of the vein)	Patient discomfort Site may be tender to touch Red streak coursing up arm Site warm to touch; may be edematous	Slow rate of infusion while assessing. If phlebitis is confirmed, discontinue IV and restart line at another site. Apply warm soaks (follow agency procedures). To prevent recurrence, consider one or more of the following: slow IV rate, use smaller-diameter catheter, add in-line filter, or dilute drug in larger volume.
Septicemia (systemic infection)	Fever, chills, malaise Symptoms of shock, hypotension Normal-looking IV insertion site Nausea, vomitting, headache	Notify health care provider. Monitor vital signs. Rule out other causes (e.g., wound infection, urinary tract infection, respiratory tract infection). Discontinue IV line, culture catheter tip and fluid (or as agency procedure directs), and restart IV line at another site.
Fluid overload	Noisy, rapid respiration, crackles Distended neck veins Increased pulse rate or blood pressure Distress Puffiness, edema of dependent areas Weight gain	Slow infusion rate to keep line open. Raise head of bed. Notify health care provider. Remain calm to reassure patient.
Embolism	Shortness of breath Chest and shoulder pain Unequal breath sounds Cyanosis Hypotension, weak pulse Loss of consciousness	Stop infusion and notify health care provider. Place patient on left side, in Trendelenburg position. Remain with patient, monitoring vital signs.

IV, Intravenous.

Monitor for the adverse effects of cation exchange resin, which includes hypokalemia, hypocalcemia, anorexia, nausea, vomiting, and constipation. Monitor electrolyte levels. When the resin is given orally or via nasogastric tube, constipation is common, so a mild laxative may be administered concurrently. For oral administration, dilute the drug in water, syrup, fruit juice, or soft drink.

Monitor potassium levels carefully in patients with cardiac conditions because hypokalemia potentiates the effects of cardiac glycosides. Do not administer potassium to patients receiving potassium-sparing diuretics.

Work with patients to find an acceptable form of oral potassium. Oral preparations are often unpalatable or difficult to swallow. Enteric-coated tablets have been implicated in small bowel ulceration. Effervescent preparations are often unpalatable, and patients soon stop taking them. Oral solutions work well but often have a bitter, salty taste. Dilute oral solutions in juice or milk if acceptable to the patient. Avoid tomato juice if the patient is on a low-sodium diet. Instruct patients to take potassium with meals to reduce gastric irritation.

Dissolve the soluble powders, granules, or tablets in at least 4 ounces of juice or water. Allow fizzing to stop before the patient drinks the solution. Extended-release tablets and capsules should be swallowed whole without being chewed or crushed. A few tablets may be crushed or broken and a few capsules may be opened, but most should not be; check with the pharmacist.

Calcium. Oral calcium compounds are used as antacids (see Chapters 56 and 63). Read the physician's orders carefully. Intravenous calcium compounds should be warmed to body temperature before administering when possible. The intravenous route is preferred in infants, but scalp veins should be avoided because extravasation may cause tissue necrosis. Monitor ECG changes during intravenous administration. Keep patient recumbent for 30 minutes after intravenous administration; monitor blood pressure and serum calcium levels.

If intravenous administration is not possible, calcium gluceptate, calcium gluconate, or a combination of calcium glycerophosphate and calcium lactate may be administered intramuscularly. (Do not give calcium chloride intramuscularly.) Use a large muscle mass and rotate injection sites. If more than 5 mL is to be administered intramuscularly to an adult, divide the dose in half and administer via two injections. With children, determine whether the dose should be divided.

Severe hypocalcemia manifests as tetany; Chvostek's sign and Trousseau's sign may be positive. Pad the siderails. Have resuscitation equipment readily available.

Magnesium. Magnesium sulfate is administered orally to promote defecation and parenterally to treat or prevent hypomagnesemia. It is also available as an anticonvulsant, especially in pregnancy-induced hypertension (PIH). Table 64-1 identifies signs and symptoms of magnesium imbalance. If magnesium imbalance is suspected, monitor the serum magnesium level.

Intramuscular administration of magnesium is painful. Use large muscle masses and rotate sites. Inject the drug slowly. Have equipment available for resuscitation in settings where parenteral magnesium sulfate is administered. Have available calcium gluconate and calcium gluceptate as specific antidotes for magnesium overdose.

The goal in treating pregnancy-induced hypertension with magnesium is to obtain a serum level that inhibits seizures but does not cause respiratory or cardiac paralysis. Several dosage regimens are followed for this purpose; most are initiated with a loading dose and followed by a maintenance dose. Assess the deep tendon reflexes, respiratory rate, ECG changes, and urinary output. If reflexes diminish or cease, if the respiratory rate decreases, or if the urinary output falls below 30 to 100 mL/hr, the dose of magnesium sulfate may require reduction. ECG changes caused by increasing magnesium levels include prolonged PQ interval and widened QRS complex. Monitor vital signs, intake and output, serum magnesium levels, and fetal heart sounds. In severe cases, monitor maternal ECG changes and attach a fetal monitor to assess infant status. Newborns of mothers who received magnesium sulfate should be monitored for several hours after delivery for signs of hypermagnesemia (see Table 64-1).

Total Parenteral Nutrition. Hypertonic dextrose, amino acids, and fat emulsions are the mainstay of TPN therapy. The flow, additives (vitamins, minerals, and electrolytes), and their concentrations must be specifically ordered by the health care provider. TPN solutions for adults are based on age, weight, laboratory values, and heart and renal function. A slow infusion rate allows for microsomal proteins within the body to use the TPN products. Additionally, the pancreas is slowly stimulated, thereby increasing its release of insulin. The infusion rate is increased over a 24-hour period until the desired maximum rate is reached.

A thorough investigation of alternatives is warranted before a decision is made to use TPN. The cost of TPN in the United States varies from one hospital to another, as well as from one geographic region to another. The estimated daily cost of inpatient TPN therapy varies from $75 to $500, with a median cost of approximately $200 daily. Outpatient costs exceed $50,000/year. On the other hand, the use of TPN is cost effective compared with the cost of malnutrition. For example, the cost of healing a single decubitus ulcer, which is one complication of malnutrition, ranges from $5000 to $40,000 and may take several months.

Once the patient is stabilized on TPN, the infusion may be interrupted for a short period (e.g., 2 hours) each day. The period that TPN is interrupted may be gradually increased to 8 hours. A 5% to 10% dextrose solution may be hung during the 2-hour period. It is thought that periodic interruption of TPN infusions promotes better use of nutrients and fats that have accumulated in the liver.

Hypoglycemic reactions may occur if a TPN solution with greater than 20% glucose is suddenly discontinued. A 10% glucose in water solution should be administered at the same rate as the previous solution until the TPN can be restarted. Any TPN solution that has been interrupted must be discarded.

Patients receiving TPN solutions with high concentrations of glucose must be monitored for hyperglycemia. Supplemental administration of insulin may be required. TPN solutions containing less than 25% dextrose generally do not require supplemental insulin after the first day or two of therapy. Experience has shown that a sliding scale insulin dose is used for a day or two to learn daily requirements, then regular insulin is added to the TPN bag with sliding scale insulin used as a backup. Regardless of the regimen that is used, patients with diabetes are carefully monitored throughout TPN therapy, and insulin adjustments are made accordingly.

To avoid the possibility of contamination and degradation of additives (e.g., vitamins), TPN solution containers should be changed every 24 hours. TPN tubing is also changed every 24 to 72 hours, depending on agency policy. TPN bags, tubing, and filters are changed daily without exception. Filters prevent problems (e.g., phlebitis) caused by particulate contaminants. They are also life saving in cases of precipitates. It is thought that the filters assist in preventing infection, although their effectiveness has not been substantiated. Blood, drugs, and other intravenous fluids that are needed are administered through a separate intravenous line to avoid contamination of the TPN catheter.

Because intravenous therapy is invasive, the potential for infection and sepsis increases. The patient receiving TPN who complains of sudden chills, fever, or chest or back pain should be evaluated right away for septicemia. If infection at the insertion site is suspected, all lines should be removed and the TPN solution and catheter tips cultured. Peripheral blood cultures may also be needed. Other sources of infection should also be ruled out.

Most agencies have a protocol for monitoring the patient, including the frequency of blood work such as serum electrolyte levels, albumin levels, BUN levels, liver function studies, and blood glucose levels; the frequency of vitamin and mineral infusions; the procedures for culturing the catheter tip and fluid if infection develops; and the frequency of weighing the patient.

Do not add drugs to the solution or administer drugs via the TPN line unless specifically permitted by agency protocol or the pharmacist. Vitamins, electrolytes, trace elements, heparin, and insulin may be administered via a TPN line, but other drugs should not. Do not premix these drugs with TPN; administer via a Y connector.

Maintain the infusion at a steady rate. Erratic infusion rates cause fluctuations in blood glucose levels, which contribute to the risk of hyperglycemia and hypoglycemia. If the infusion stops or must be discontinued abruptly, standing orders (at most facilities) are to begin a peripheral infusion of 10% dextrose to prevent hypoglycemia. When the need for TPN therapy has resolved, gradually slow the rate of infusion to prevent hypoglycemia.

Prepare TPN solutions in a laminar flow hood, where risk of contamination is low. Follow aseptic technique when manipulating the TPN infusion. These fluids provide favorable conditions for growth of harmful bacteria. It is essential to prevent infection. Follow agency procedures for maintenance of TPN. Procedures usually specify how often to dress the insertion site, what method to use for dressing, what agent is used to clean injection sites (e.g., povidone-iodine or alcohol), and how often to change tubing.

Monitor vital signs and assess for fluid overload. Monitor the patient's temperature every 4 hours in the hospital. Assess the patient for appearance of dry, flaky skin; hair loss; and rashes. These signs may indicate essential fatty acid or zinc deficiency.

Fat Emulsions. Assess for a history of allergy to eggs, legumes, soybeans, or previous fat emulsion use before administration. Inspect the fat emulsion before using but do not shake. If the emulsion has cracked (if the oil has separated from the other products), it should not be used.

Administer fat emulsions via a central or peripheral intravenous line. Read the manufacturer's information supplied with the bottle of fat emulsion. The fat emulsion tubing may be piggybacked into the Y connector of the TPN tubing closest to the intravenous insertion site. By piggybacking the emulsion at this site, the length of time the emulsion is in contact with TPN solution is reduced. Because fat emulsion particles are very large, a 1.2-micron in-line filter is used. Be sure to check agency policy and manufacturer's instructions for safe use of TPN and fat emulsions.

Begin the infusion slowly and observe the patient. Assess for adverse effects including thrombophlebitis, vomiting, chest pain, back pain, and allergic reactions.

If no adverse effects have appeared after 15 to 30 minutes, increase the rate of infusion to the desired rate. In general, fat emulsions are administered over an 8- to 12-hour period.

Blood, some drugs, and other intravenous fluids should be administered through a separate intravenous line to avoid contamination of the fat emulsion. Routine blood work should be delayed until 2 to 6 hours after the infusion of a fat emulsion so that the extra fat in the bloodstream will not distort results. In addition, as much as possible, the patient should not be transported anywhere, because this causes agitation of the bottle.

Fat emulsion should comprise no more than 60% of the total daily caloric intake. Monitor serum triglyceride levels. Fat emulsions can cause hyperlipidemia, which should clear between infusions; if not, withhold the next dose and notify the physician.

Fat emulsions are less expensive than TPN but are relatively expensive compared to the cost of dextrose solutions and are therefore not used routinely in adults on short-term (less than 3 weeks) parenteral nutrition therapy. Again, the cost of combined TPN and fat emulsion therapy remains less than the cost of managing complications of nutritional deficiencies. The expenses incurred during intravenous therapy include not only the cost of the solutions but also the cost of the access devices, tubing, and infusion pumps. The requirement for sterility and frequent equipment changes increases the expense. It is important to be conscious of cost of therapy. Each time a decision is made to change intravenous fluids before a hanging bag is completed the cost to the patient increases. Furthermore, an infusion pump is necessary for patients with compromised renal, cardiac, or neurologic function, or if the specific solution infused warrants a pump for safety.

Alkalinizing and Acidifying Drugs. Orally administered drugs should be taken as ordered with a full glass of water. A missed dose should be taken as soon as remembered unless it is almost time for the next dose. Doses should not be doubled if missed.

Intravenous alkalinizing and acidifying drugs should be given in a patent, free-flowing intravenous line. Attention should be paid to the intravenous site for evidence of extravasation, phlebitis, or irritation. Extravasation of an alkalinizing drug is treated by elevating the extremity, applying warm compresses, and administering hyaluronidase, lidocaine, or both, as indicated to minimize tissue damage.

To prevent incompatibilities, the intravenous line should be flushed before and after drug administration. Syringe, Y-connector compatibilities, additive compatibilities, and potential drug-drug interactions should also be noted. Infusion rates should be carefully monitored.

Sodium bicarbonate should not be taken concurrently with milk products. Renal calculi or hypercalcemia may result. Check manufacturer's guidelines for intravenous administration guidelines. For intravenous administration the drug is diluted and administered at the identified rate. During resuscitation efforts, sodium bicarbonate may be given by direct intravenous push to help correct metabolic acidosis. The drug is packaged in labeled, prefilled syringes that are usually included in the emergency drug box or on the resuscitation cart. Signs of overdose include metabolic alkalosis and hypernatremia (see Table 64-2). Monitor serum electrolyte and arterial blood gas levels regularly.

Sodium citrate/citric acid is more palatable when diluted with 60 to 90 mL of water and refrigerated before use. It should be administered 30 minutes after meals or bedtime snack to minimize its saline laxative effects. Tromethamine should not be used for more than 24 hours to minimize severe adverse effects.

Monitor for signs and symptoms of overdose in the patient receiving alkalinizing or acidifying drugs. Respiratory rate, volume, patterns, breath sounds, and ABGs should be monitored. The patient should be observed and attended to as necessary to ensure safety. Restraints may be needed in some cases. Skin color, temperature, peripheral pulses, and capillary refill should be assessed. If signs of overdosage appear (CNS irritability or depression), the drug should be withheld and the health care provider notified.

Education

Education of the patient who is to receive intravenous therapy is determined by the patient's needs and the delivery setting. An awareness of the patient's cultural, ethnic, and religious background may be important when considering intravenous therapy. Intravenous therapy is especially threatening to those who have not experienced it before. The patient and family should be told what the procedure involves and what solution is being used. If there are concerns about the procedure or the fluid being administered, it is important to address those concerns before starting the infusion.

In acute care settings with extremely ill patients, in which intravenous therapy orders may change rapidly, information is given to the patient and family in small amounts and at a very basic level. However, intravenous therapy is often administered in settings in which a health care provider is not present. In this situation, education of the patient and any other home-based caregivers is important.

The patient or caregivers need to understand why the intravenous therapy is required and how the infusion delivery system works. Teach the techniques needed for assessment and care of the access site. Basic information about the fluid being administered, storage precautions, potential complications, and adverse effects should be discussed. Help them to identify what information to document and how and when to seek help from the health care provider.

Fluid and electrolyte imbalances may cause mental status changes, restlessness, and irritability in the patient. Confused patients may play with the intravenous tubing, change the rate, or dislodge the venous access device. Caregivers should be instructed how to manage the infusion in such a situation. Repeated explanations, as well as protection from injury during the infusion, are important.

Home Intravenous Therapy. A patient's desire to stay at home and minimize the cost of care, coupled with reimbursement concerns focused on shorter lengths of hospital stays, make home intravenous therapy an increasingly popular option. Home intravenous therapy may be suitable for patients requiring hydration, TPN, intravenous drugs for pain control, antibiotics, or antineoplastic drugs. However, home intravenous therapy presents some concerns and implications that are unique. The most significant concern is that of educating the patient and caregivers. The assessment, plan, and interventions for intravenous therapy are not different in the home, but the need for patient and family education far exceeds that required for an inpatient setting. In particular, perinatal, pediatric, and older adult patients may require more intensive assessment, education, and care depending on their physical, mental, and emotional status. The education content includes the following:

- Signs and symptoms of fluid volume excess and deficit
- Aseptic technique and signs and symptoms of infection
- Mechanics of intravenous therapy and how to troubleshoot the infusion pump
- Infusion schedule and rate
- Documentation of response to therapy
- Documentation for reimbursement purposes
- Emergency care information
- Contact names and numbers

Providing education in verbal and written form with clear, concise, and specific guidelines makes intravenous therapy in the home a safe, viable option. It should be noted that pharmacists cannot dispense home intravenous drugs without written documentation stating that the patient or caregiver has been properly educated.

Home care services must be coordinated to prevent home therapy from becoming fragmented, duplicated, or unsafe. Coordination requires communication with the patient and caregiver, but also with pharmacists, health care providers, equipment companies, and insurance companies. The home care nurse, social worker, and discharge planner play central roles in the process because they are familiar with the rules and regulations governing home care and can provide answers to questions regarding reimbursement for home care services.

Patients should be advised of the importance of regular follow-up examinations to monitor fluid, serum electrolytes, and acid-base balance. Refer the patient to a social services agency and to a community-based nursing care service.

Review with patients the importance of taking potassium preparations as ordered. Some patients will be able to maintain potassium levels through dietary intake of potassium-rich foods. Instruct patients to avoid salt substitutes, low-sodium foods, and milk unless this is first discussed with the health care provider.

Instruct patients to take missed doses if remembered within 2 hours of the scheduled time; otherwise omit the missed dose and resume regular dosing schedule. Do not double up for missed doses.

EVALUATION

The criteria used for evaluation of fluid, electrolytes, and acid-base therapy is based on the goals of therapy. If the original purpose of therapy was to correct an existing fluid or electrolyte imbalance or nutritional problem, evaluation determines whether the problem has been corrected or alleviated. Skin turgor, the absence of thirst, edema, growth (in infants), changes in body weight and urine characteristics, and certain conditions of mucous membranes (i.e., dry, moist, pink) indicate changes in hydration levels. The patient's psychological response to intravenous therapy should also be evaluated. Did the patient accept the therapy? Are the patient and caregivers able to cope with the prescribed therapy? The resolution of the signs and symptoms of the acid-base imbalances should occur without the appearance of the opposite disorder.

Bibliography

Karadag A, Gorgulu S: Devising an intravenous fluid therapy protocol and compliance of nurses with the protocol, *J Intraven Nurs* 24(4):232-238, 2000.

Tokars JI, Cookson ST, McArthur MA, et al: Prospective evaluation of risk factors for bloodstream infection in patients receiving home infusion therapy. A peek at the past—a look at the future, *Cina* 16:66-72, 2000.

White SA: Peripheral intravenous therapy-related phlebitis rates in an adult population, *J Intraven Nurs* 24(1):19-24, 2001.

Internet Resources

http://jama.ama-assn.org/issues/v280n23/abs/jce80032.html.
http://www.globalrph.com/tpn.htm.
http://www.lite.org./
http://www.nursefriendly.com/nursing/linksections/intravenoustherapylinks.htm.

CHAPTER

65

Ophthalmic Drugs

SHERRY F. QUEENER • KATHLEEN GUTIERREZ

 Visit http://evolve.elsevier.com/Gutierrez/ for additional information.

KEY TERMS

Acute (closed-angle) glaucoma, p. 1078

Aqueous humor, p. 1078

Cycloplegia, p. 1076

Intraocular pressure (IOP), p. 1079

Miosis, p. 1076

Mydriasis, p. 1076

Open-angle glaucoma, p. 1078

OBJECTIVES

- Define miosis, mydriasis, and cycloplegia, and give examples of when they are therapeutically produced.
- Discuss the use of anticholinergic drugs for the eye.
- Explain the differences between chronic and acute glaucoma.
- Discuss the categories of drugs used to treat glaucoma.
- Discuss the categories of drugs used specifically for eye infections or inflammation.
- From a list of drugs used to treat glaucoma, develop a teaching plan to prepare patients for discharge.

PHYSIOLOGY • **Preparing the Eye for Examination**

The amount of light penetrating the eye is controlled by the size of the pigmented iris, which contains two sets of muscles—the sphincter and dilator muscles. The sphincter muscles, which form a circular band around the iris, contain muscarinic receptors innervated by the parasympathetic nervous system. As shown in Figure 65-1, the pupil is constricted when the sphincter muscles contract so that only a small surface on the eye transmits light. The dilator muscles contain alpha receptors innervated by the sympathetic nervous system. **Miosis** refers to a constricted pupil and is achieved primarily by stimulating the muscarinic receptors of the sphincter muscles. **Mydriasis** refers to a dilated pupil and is achieved by blocking muscarinic receptors of the sphincter muscles or by stimulating alpha receptors of the dilator muscles.

The cornea and the lens determine the focus of images onto the retina. The cornea accomplishes the coarse focusing, but the fine focusing for sharp images and near vision is accomplished by the lens. The shape of the lens is controlled by muscarinic receptors of the parasympathetic nervous system. As diagrammed in Figure 65-1, the accommodation for near vision requires the contraction of ciliary muscles to change the shape of the lens. Ligaments normally pull the lens to keep it relatively flat. Contraction of the ciliary muscles relaxes the ligaments so that the lens becomes more round as required for near vision. **Cycloplegia** refers to paralysis of the ciliary muscles by drugs that block muscarinic receptors. Cycloplegia causes blurred vision, because the shape of the lens can no longer be adjusted to near vision.

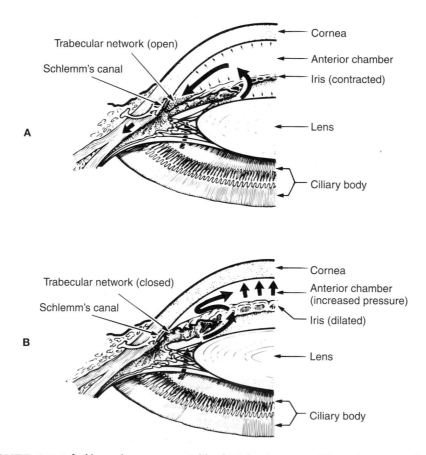

FIGURE 65-1 A, Normal eye or eye with chronic glaucoma. Flow of aqueous humor is shown from ciliary body and around iris. Aqueous humor is normally absorbed into body through trabecular network into Schlemm's canal. In chronic glaucoma, aqueous humor accumulates because trabecular network degenerates. **B,** Eye in acute glaucoma. Flow of aqueous humor is stopped because iris has blocked trabecular network and Schlemm's canal. Aqueous humor can accumulate quickly to cause a significant rise in ocular pressure that may damage optic nerve.

DRUG CLASS • Muscarinic Antagonists

⚠ atropine (Atropair, Atropine Care, Atropisol, Atrosulf, Isopto Antropine, Minims Atropine, ✳ Ocu-Tropine)

cyclopentolate (Akpentolate, Cyclogyl, Pentolair)

cyclopentolate + phenylephrine (Cyclomydril)

homatropine (AK-Homatropine, I-Homatrine, Isopto Homatropine, Spectro-Homatropine)

scopolamine (Isopto Hyoscine)

tropicamide (Mydriacyl, Tropicacyl)

MECHANISM OF ACTION

Classic anticholinergic actions include dilated pupils (mydriasis) and blurred vision caused by cycloplegia (see Chapter 11). Anticholinergic drugs block the muscarinic receptors of the sphincter muscles so the pupil cannot contract (see Figure 65-1), producing mydriasis. The ciliary muscles controlling the shape of the lens are also paralyzed; thus the eye can no longer accommodate and produce focused images.

USES

The major use of the anticholinergic drugs is to induce mydriasis and cycloplegia for examination of the eye. Accurate measurement of lens refraction requires both actions. Some anticholinergics are used in the treatment of inflammation of the eye (uveitis). The relaxation of sphincter and ciliary muscles hastens healing of inflammatory conditions, especially after eye surgery. Adhesions (synechia) are also reduced.

Atropine is the drug of choice for children, because it is potent and long acting, and children have an active accommodation. Atropine is also used before surgery and for other conditions requiring prolonged mydriasis. Cyclopentolate is used to aid refraction, for ophthalmoscopy, and for preoperative mydriasis. A combination of cyclopentolate and phenylephrine is useful to produce rapid onset of mydriasis without noticeable cycloplegia. Tropicamide is commonly used for routine eye examinations.

PHARMACOKINETICS

These drugs are instilled as solutions or ointments in the eye and are gradually removed through systemic circulation. Atropine has a very long duration of action (Table 65-1), because the drug is tightly bound to pigment cells in the iris and slowly released to act on the muscles in the eye. Mydriasis occurs more rapidly in blue eyes, because less pigment is present to bind the drug as it is instilled.

The other drugs in this class act more rapidly and have a shorter duration of action compared to atropine (see Table 65-1). Recovery from homatropine and scopolamine usually takes 2 to 3 days instead of 6 days. Recovery from cyclopentolate occurs within a day. Because tropicamide has the fastest onset of action and the shortest duration, it is most useful for routine eye examinations.

TABLE 65-1

Topical Drugs for Mydriasis and Cycloplegia

Generic Name	Onset	Peak	Duration
Muscarinic Antagonists for Mydriasis and Cycloplegia			
atropine			
Cycloplegia	30-40 min	30-40 min	6 days
Mydriasis	1-3 hr	1-3 hr	12 days
cyclopentolate	15-60 min	25-75 min	24 hr
homatropine	10-90 min	10-90 min	2-3 days
scopolamine	20-60 min	20-60 min	3-7 days
tropicamide	15-30 min	20-40 min	3-8 hr
Adrenergic Drugs For Mydriasis Only			
phenylephrine	15-60 min	60-90 min	6 hr
phenylephrine + cyclopentolate	15 min	30 min	<24 hr
Alpha Blocker (Reverses Mydriasis Caused by Phenylephrine)			
dapiprazole	Rapid	NA	NA

ADVERSE REACTIONS AND CONTRAINDICATIONS

The most common reactions are photosensitivity because of the dilated pupil and blurred vision because of the cycloplegia.

Systemic reactions may occur when anticholinergic drugs are absorbed into the body; these reactions are particularly likely with atropine. Systemic reactions are typical anticholinergic effects such as dry mouth and dry skin, fever, thirst, confusion, and hyperactivity (see Chapter 11). Children are the most prone to systemic toxicity from ophthalmic drugs. Systemic effects are rare with tropicamide.

Acute (closed-angle) glaucoma may occur in certain patients when the iris crowds the anterior chamber (an effect of mydriasis). The combination of phenylephrine and cyclopentolate is contraindicated for patients with glaucoma because of the rapid onset of profound mydriasis. Patients with protrusion of the central cornea or with Down's syndrome are also especially sensitive to the mydriatic effect of anticholinergic drugs.

Atropine may cause contact dermatitis of the eyelids. Scopolamine can be given to patients who are allergic to atropine.

INTERACTIONS

Tropicamide interferes with the lowering of intraocular pressure caused by carbachol, pilocarpine, or anticholinesterase inhibitors used in the eye.

 DRUG CLASS • **Alpha-Adrenergic Drugs**

dapiprazole (Rev-Eyes)

phenylephrine (AK-Dilate, Dilatair, Mydfrin, Ocu-Phrin)

phenylephrine + cyclopentolate (Cyclomydril)

MECHANISM OF ACTION

Phenylephrine acts as an agonist on the alpha receptors of the dilator muscles to produce mydriasis without cycloplegia. Dapiprazole is an alpha blocker.

USES

Phenylephrine is used as a mydriatic when only the interior structures of the eye are examined and cycloplegia is not required. Cyclomydril, a combination of cyclopentolate and phenylephrine, is used when maximal dilation is required. The alpha-adrenergic blocker dapiprazole is used only to reverse mydriasis produced by phenylephrine.

Phenylephrine is also used in the treatment of uveitis and postoperative inflammation. Dilute solutions of phenylephrine are used to bring temporary relief of redness caused by minor eye irritations.

PHARMACOKINETICS

Drugs in this class act promptly (see Table 65-1). Dapiprazole acts rapidly but is slower in more heavily pigmented brown eyes than in blue or green eyes. Some systemic uptake can occur with these drugs. Systemic uptake of cyclomydril should be blocked by compressing the lacrimal sac for 2 to 3 minutes after instillation of the drops.

ADVERSE REACTIONS AND CONTRAINDICATIONS

When dapiprazole drops are used, about 50% of patients experience a burning sensation and about 80% experience redness in the eyes (conjunctival injection) lasting about 20 minutes.

INTERACTIONS

Using dapiprazole (an alpha-adrenergic blocking drug) to reverse mydriasis produced by the alpha agonist phenylephrine is an example of a therapeutically useful interaction.

 PATHOPHYSIOLOGY • **Glaucoma**

Glaucoma is a common cause of visual impairment and blindness. About 3 million people in the United States have glaucoma, and as many as half are unaware of their condition. An estimated 150,000 people in the United States are blind as a consequence of glaucoma. The risk factors for glaucoma are indicated in Box 65-1.

Primary **open-angle glaucoma**, also called chronic glaucoma, is the most common form of the disease. The defect results in a slow degeneration of the anterior chamber that impairs the uptake of aqueous humor. **Aqueous humor**, the fluid that fills the anterior chamber, is formed by the ciliary body. As illustrated in Figure 65-1, this fluid is normally reabsorbed through the trabecular spaces into Schlemm's canal. If the aqueous humor cannot be reabsorbed through the anterior chamber, the fluid accumulates and intraocular pressure (IOP) increases above the normal range of 12 to 15 mm Hg. If the intraocular pressure is not relieved the optic nerve may be damaged, resulting in blindness. Therapy is aimed at reducing fluid production with drugs or improving fluid outflow with either drugs or surgery.

Acute (closed-angle) glaucoma is characterized by the iris bulging up to shut off access of the aqueous hu-mor to the anterior chamber (see Figure 65-1). This creates an emergency because the buildup of intraocular pressure may rapidly become severe, damaging the optic nerve and causing blindness. Emergency treatment may include a cholinomimetic drug, a carbonic anhydrase inhibitor, epinephrine, and an osmotic diuretic. This drug regimen provides transient treatment while the patient is being prepared for eye surgery in which the iris is cut to restore fluid access to the anterior chamber.

Either of these types of glaucoma may be triggered by certain drugs (e.g., steroids) or diseases (e.g., diabetes). In addition, other forms of glaucoma are known. For example, some patients with normal intraocular pressure may develop what is called normal-tension glaucoma. In this condition, damage to the optic nerve progresses similarly to the cases in which intraocular pressure is elevated. These patients also benefit from having intraocular pressure lowered, suggesting that the optic nerve is exceptionally sensitive in this condition. Another form of glaucoma arises when the iris releases pigment granules into the aqueous humor. These granules may plug the channels for fluid outflow and thus raise intraocular pressure.

Therapy for glaucoma is not curative but is aimed at lowering intraocular pressure to slow the onset or limit the damage of the disease.

DRUG CLASS • Adrenergic Agonists Used to Treat Glaucoma

apraclonidine (Iopidine)

brimonidine (Alphagan)

 dipivefrin (Akpro, Propine)

MECHANISM OF ACTION

Tissues of the eye contain alpha$_1$, alpha$_2$, and beta$_2$ receptors, but the relationship of these receptors to the function of the eye is not completely understood. Apraclonidine and brimonidine, the newest antiglaucoma drugs of this class, are alpha$_2$-adrenergic agonists. Dipivefrin is a prodrug (dipivalyl epinephrine) for epinephrine, which acts on both alpha- and beta-adrenergic receptors. These drugs all decrease the production of aqueous humor, thus decreasing intraocular pressure.

USES

Apraclonidine can be added to glaucoma therapy short term to reduce elevated intraocular pressure, but the drug will not add any benefit to a combination of a beta blocker and a carbonic anhydrase inhibitor. Apraclonidine is also used to prevent acute, transient spikes in in-traocular pressure after laser surgery. The drug is administered 1 hour before surgery and again just before surgery. Brimonidine and dipivefrin are used to treat chronic glaucoma.

PHARMACOKINETICS

Dipivefrin is inactive but is converted to epinephrine—its active form—by esterases in the cornea and anterior chamber of the eye. Dipivefrin is more lipid-soluble than epinephrine and, therefore, concentrates in the eye more readily than epinephrine. Adrenergic agonists may be systemically absorbed from the eye, primarily through the nasolacrimal system. These drugs all have similar time courses of action (Table 65-2).

ADVERSE REACTIONS AND CONTRAINDICATIONS

Adverse reactions include reddening of the eye, blurred vision, headache, hypersensitivity, and photosensitivity. In addition, when these drugs are absorbed systemically from the eye they may cause any of the adverse effects noted for this drug class in Chapter 12. The most

---

TABLE 65-2

Drugs for Lowering Intraocular Pressure and Treating Glaucoma

Generic Name	Route	Onset	Peak	Duration
Adrenergic Agonists (Sympathomimetics) (lower aqueous humor production; lower resistance to outflow)				
apraclonidine	Topical	1 hr	3-5 hr	ca. 8 hr
brimonidine	Topical	1 hr	2 hr	8-12 hr
dipivefrin	Topical	30 min	1 hr	12 hr
Beta Blockers (lower aqueous humor production)				
betaxolol	Topical	30 min	2 hr	12 hr
carteolol	Topical	0.5-1 hr	1-2 hr	6-8 hr
levobetaxolol	Topical	30 min	2 hr	12 hr
levobunolol	Topical	<1 hr	2-6 hr	24 hr
metipranolol	Topical	<30 min	2 hr	24 hr
timolol	Topical	30 min	1-2 hr	12-24 hr
Direct-Acting Cholinergics (increase aqueous humor outflow)				
carbachol	Topical	20 min*	4 hr	8 hr
pilocarpine	Topical	30 min*	75 min	4-14 hr
	Insert	NA	1.5-2 hr	7 days
Cholinesterase Inhibitors (Indirect-Acting) (increase aqueous humor outflow)				
demecarium	Topical	4 hr	24 hr	1-28 days
echothiophate	Topical	4 hr	24 hr	1-28 days
isofluorophate	Topical	4 hr	24 hr	1-28 days
Carbonic Anhydrase Inhibitors (lower aqueous humor production)				
acetazolamide	Oral	2 hr	2 hr	12 hr†
brinzolamide	Topical	2 hr	NA	12 hr
dorzolamide	Topical	2 hr	NA	>8 hr
methazolamide	Oral	2-4 hr	NA	10-18 hr
Prostaglandin Analogs (increase aqueous humor outflow)				
latanoprost	Topical	NA	NA	NA
unoprostone	Topical	NA	NA	NA
Osmotic Agents (remove fluid from eye)				
glycerin	Oral	10 min	1 hr	6-8 hr
mannitol	IV	15 min	30-60 min	4-8 hr
urea	IV	10 min	1-2 hr	5-6 hr

IV, Intravenous; *NA,* not available.
*Onset of miosis; lower pressure would follow.
†Extended release formulation.

---

common systemic adverse effects of apraclonidine include a sensation of dry mouth or nose. This occurs more often in patients treated with the 1% solution than with the 0.25% or 0.125% solutions.

These drugs may be contraindicated for patients before iridectomy in closed-angle glaucoma, because they may precipitate an acute attack.

INTERACTIONS

Concurrent use of atropine and these ophthalmic adrenergic agonists may increase the risk of hypertension or tachycardia if the ophthalmic drugs are systemically absorbed.

DRUG CLASS • Beta-Adrenergic Blockers Used to Treat Glaucoma

betaxolol (Betoptic)

betaxolol + pilocarpine (Betoptic Pilo)

carteolol (Ocupress)

levobetaxolol (Akbeta, Betaxon)

levobunolol (Betagan)

metipranolol (Optipranolol)

⚕ timolol (Timpotic)

timolol + dorzolamide (Cosopt)

MECHANISM OF ACTION

Beta-adrenergic blockers act in the eye to decrease the production of aqueous humor, thus reducing intraocular pressure. This action is shared by both selective and nonselective beta-blockers.

USES

An ophthalmic preparation of one of the beta blockers is the drug of choice for the initial treatment of chronic glaucoma. The major advantage of beta blockers is that neither pupil size nor reactivity to light is altered. This selectivity is particularly beneficial for young patients with active accommodation and for older adult patients who have opaque lenses and cannot tolerate miotics.

Betaxolol and levobetaxolol are selective $beta_1$-blockers and are thought to be less likely to cause pulmonary problems (especially asthma) than nonselective drugs such as timolol.

PHARMACOKINETICS

The beta blockers are applied as ophthalmic solutions directly to the eye. The onset of action is 30 to 60 minutes, and the duration of action varies with the beta blocker used (see Table 65-1). The drug is removed by gradual systemic uptake and excretion. Some systemic absorption can occur through the nasolacrimal system.

ADVERSE REACTIONS AND CONTRAINDICATIONS

Beta blockers applied to the eye may cause ocular pain, dizziness, or headaches. The eyes may be red, and occasionally, the irritation can be severe. Other occasional adverse effects include blurred vision, different size of pupils, discoloration of pupils, and double vision. These reactions may disappear even with continued administration. The ophthalmic suspension form of betaxolol appears to be less irritating than the ophthalmic solution form but, in general, betaxolol produces more eye irritation than the other beta blockers. Decreased night vision has been reported for carteolol.

Systemic concentrations of beta blockers administered to the eye are seldom significant. Nevertheless, patients with severe cardiovascular disease or severe asthma should not take these drugs. The systemic absorption of beta blockers may worsen asthma, or may mask signs of hyperthyroidism or hypoglycemia in diabetic patients taking insulin.

INTERACTIONS

Beta blockers provide an additive reduction in intraocular pressure when administered with topical miotics or systemically administered carbonic anhydrase inhibitors.

DRUG CLASS • Cholinomimetics Used to Treat Glaucoma

carbachol (Carbastat, Miostat)

⚕ pilocarpine (Ocusert Pilo-20, Ocusert Pilo-40, Pilopine, Salagen)

pilocarpine + betaxolol (Betoptic Pilo)

MECHANISM OF ACTION

Pilocarpine and carbachol are direct-acting cholinomimetic drugs formulated for ophthalmic application in treating glaucoma. Pilocarpine and carbachol mimic the action of the neurotransmitter acetylcholine (see Chapter 11). Cholinomimetic drugs produce contraction of the sphincter (circular) muscles in the eye, which constricts the pupil (a process called miosis). Therapeutic ef-

fectiveness results from the spread of the trabecular spaces of the anterior chamber when the sphincter muscles contract. The larger area allows improved uptake of the aqueous humor, which relieves intraocular pressure.

USES

Pilocarpine is widely used alone or in combination with beta blockers and other drugs to control glaucoma, although beta blockers alone are now more commonly prescribed for the initial therapy. Pilocarpine is also used in emergency treatment of acute-angle glaucoma, both before and after surgery. The drug also counteracts the effects of cycloplegics and mydriatics after ophthalmoscopic examinations.

Carbachol is used as a replacement drug when the eyes have become resistant or intolerant to pilocarpine. Carbachol is also used to induce miosis during ocular surgery.

PHARMACOKINETICS

Pilocarpine administered as drops of a 1% or 2% solution produces miosis in 15 to 30 minutes and lasts for 2 to 4 hours. To increase the duration of action, pilocarpine may also be administered as a gel, which lasts 18 to 24 hours. A more sophisticated delivery system is the Ocusert (Figure 65-2). This drug delivery system is placed in the upper or lower cul-de-sac of the eye and allows pilocarpine to slowly diffuse out. The system is designed to deliver pilocarpine over 7 days, but the duration varies with the individual.

Carbachol is more potent and slightly longer acting than pilocarpine.

ADVERSE REACTIONS AND CONTRAINDICATIONS

Pilocarpine is well tolerated. Because it is applied in small amounts directly to the eye, systemic effects are uncommon. The most common reactions are some stinging and local irritation. Ciliary spasm and miosis may be troublesome when starting therapy. Miosis makes vision in dim light poor, so patients should be cautioned against driving at night.

The Ocusert system may migrate and produce pain, but this is uncommon. Patients with loose lids may be unable to retain the system and may need to check for its presence each morning.

Patients with acute iritis or other conditions in which pupillary constriction is undesirable should not take pilocarpine or carbachol.

INTERACTIONS

Pilocarpine can be administered with carbonic anhydrase inhibitors, epinephrine, or beta blockers to con-

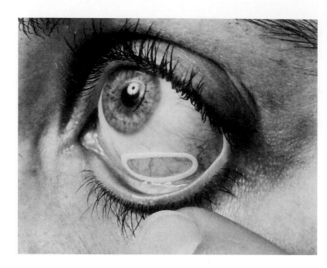

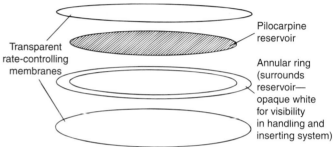

FIGURE 65-2 Ocusert ocular therapeutic system for delivery of pilocarpine for treatment of glaucoma. Flexible wafer is placed under eyelid and provides drug for 1 week. Eyelid is shown displaced to expose device. Expanded view denotes purpose of each component. (Courtesy ALZA Corp.)

trol glaucoma, because the mechanisms of action vary and are therefore synergistic when combined. Pilocarpine and carbachol counteract the anticholinergic effects of atropine and other anticholinergics.

DRUG CLASS • Anticholinesterase Miotics

demecarium (Humorsol)

echothiophate (Phospholine)

isoflurophate (Floropryl)

MECHANISM OF ACTION

Demecarium, echothiophate, and isoflurophate inhibit degradation of acetylcholine. The increased amount of acetylcholine then causes miosis. As with the direct-acting miotic pilocarpine, therapeutic effectiveness results from

the spread of the trabecular spaces of the anterior chamber when the sphincter muscles contract. The larger area allows improved uptake of the aqueous humor, which relieves intraocular pressure.

USES

Demecarium, echothiophate, and isoflurophate are potent miotics. They are generally used only for patients with chronic glaucoma that is not well controlled by other agents.

PHARMACOKINETICS

The anticholinesterase miotics are applied directly to the eye and are very long acting. Miosis begins in about 1 hour and lasts for up to 1 month after the drug is discontinued. Reduction in intraocular pressure begins in 4 hours and lasts about 1 to 2 days after the drug is discontinued.

ADVERSE REACTIONS AND CONTRAINDICATIONS

Miotics inhibit accommodation, so patients taking these drugs have poor vision in dim light. Other common local effects can include brow ache, ocular pain, ciliary and conjunctival congestions, tearing, and twitching of the eyebrows. In patients older than 60 years, the development of cataracts can be accelerated.

Anticholinesterase inhibitors, especially echothiophate and demecarium, occasionally cause systemic cholinergic effects, including muscle weakness, hypersalivation, sweating, nausea, vomiting, abdominal pain, urinary incontinence, diarrhea, bradycardia, severe hypotension, and bronchospasm.

Anticholinesterase inhibitors are contraindicated during pregnancy. They are contraindicated for patients with retinal detachment or uveitis and those with glaucoma associated with iridocyclitis. Patients with myasthenia gravis should not receive anticholinesterase miotics.

TOXICITY

Symptoms of systemic toxicity include ataxia, confusion, seizures, coma, and muscle paralysis. The most common symptoms in children are abdominal cramps and diarrhea with a runny nose and tearing.

INTERACTIONS

Other agents with anticholinesterase activity should be avoided when an anticholinesterase miotic is taken, because of the additive toxicity. Drugs to avoid include atropine, anticholinesterases for treatment of myasthenia gravis, and pesticides with anticholinesterase activity.

Demecarium, echothiophate, and isoflurophate can decrease plasma concentrations of plasma cholinesterases, thereby enhancing the neuromuscular blockade of succinylcholine. This effect can be present for several weeks or months after the anticholinesterase has been discontinued.

 DRUG CLASS • Carbonic Anhydrase Inhibitors Used to Treat Glaucoma

acetazolamide (Diamox)

brinzolamide (Azopt)

dorzolamide (Trusopt)

dorzolamide + timolol (Cosopt)

methazolamide (Neptazane)

MECHANISM OF ACTION

Carbonic anhydrase inhibitors decrease the formation of aqueous humor by 50% to 60% by blocking ocular carbonic anhydrase. A significant fall in intraocular pressure is seen only in individuals with glaucoma.

USES

Acetazolamide or methazolamide is used principally as an adjunct in the treatment of chronic glaucoma when other drugs alone do not control intraocular pressure. Acetazolamide may be used with osmotic agents, miotics, and beta blockers for the emergency treatment of acute (closed-angle) glaucoma on a short-term basis only. Acetazolamide is also used as an anticonvulsant and in the treatment of altitude sickness. Brinzolamide and dorzolamide are used only in the treatment of glaucoma.

PHARMACOKINETICS

Acetazolamide is given orally and distributed throughout the body. The bioavailability of acetazolamide varies significantly with some brands. The preferred formulation is an extended-release preparation. Methazolamide and acetazolamide have similar kinetics (see Table 65-2).

Brinzolamide and dorzolamide are formulated for direct application into the eye to treat glaucoma. Effects are seen quickly but may also build over time as the drugs saturate carbonic anhydrase in the eye. Both drugs are absorbed systemically from the eye and bind to carbonic anhydrase in red blood cells. Because of this binding, the drugs tend to have very long half-lives in the body. Brinzolamide has a half-life of 111 days; the drug is eliminated primarily unchanged in urine.

ADVERSE REACTIONS AND CONTRAINDICATIONS

Acetazolamide is generally not well tolerated for prolonged therapy. Malaise, weight loss, fatigue, headache, nervousness, loss of libido, impotence, and tingling sensations are all common adverse effects. Infants show a failure to thrive. Occasionally, acetazolamide causes confusion, ataxia, tremor, and tinnitus. Diuresis is common initially but usually subsides. Hypokalemia is a problem if acetazolamide is used in combination with other drugs that lower body potassium.

Acetazolamide may precipitate acute pulmonary failure in patients with chronic obstructive lung disease. Gout may also be precipitated in patients with a history of this disease. Acetazolamide is also teratogenic and should not be given to pregnant patients. Patients with renal failure develop excessively high concentrations of the drug.

Brinzolamide is related to sulfonamides and can cause the same types of adverse effects; special concern should yield to allergies, skin reactions, blood dyscrasias and Stevens-Johnson syndrome (see Chapter 30).

Dorzolamide and brinzolamide commonly cause a bitter taste, blurred vision, and eye discomfort or pain. The systemic concentration is considered too low to affect renal or pulmonary function. However, patients with a history of kidney stones should not be given dorzolamide.

INTERACTIONS

Acetazolamide is highly bound to plasma protein. Diflunisal, a nonsteroidal antiinflammatory drug, has been reported to displace bound acetazolamide, thereby increasing adverse effects.

DRUG CLASS • Prostaglandin Analogs

latanoprost (Xalatan)

unoprostone (Rescula)

MECHANISM OF ACTION

Latanoprost is an analog of prostaglandin $F_{2\alpha}$. It increases the outflow of aqueous humor, perhaps by promoting some breakdown of the extracellular matrix that can obstruct fluid outflow.

USES

Prostaglandin analogs are used topically for glaucoma and often in combination with other drugs.

PHARMACOKINETICS

Latanoprost is applied once a day, in the evening. Unoprostone is applied twice daily. The pharmacokinetics

of these drugs are not fully known, but unoprostone is cleared from plasma within 1 hour of application to the eye.

ADVERSE REACTIONS AND CONTRAINDICATIONS

A few patients have gradual changes in eye color as a result of an increased amount of brown pigment in the iris. Other local effects can include stinging, blurred vision, redness, and the feeling of having a foreign body in the eye. Lashes and hair adjacent to the eye may thicken.

INTERACTIONS

No interactions have been documented for either systemic or local effects, but the drops should be administered at least 5 minutes before or after other eye medications, as a precaution.

DRUG CLASS • Specific Osmotic Agents Used to Treat Glaucoma

glycerin (Glyrol, Osmoglyn)

mannitol (Osmitrol)

urea (Ureaphil)

MECHANISM OF ACTION

These drugs remain in the vascular compartment and cause fluid to move from tissues into the vascular compartment. This fluid movement in the eye reduces ocular pressure.

USES

The osmotic agents are used as a short-term treatment only to lower the intraocular pressure of glaucoma be-

fore surgery or as an emergency treatment of acute (closed-angle) glaucoma.

PHARMACOKINETICS

Glycerin is administered orally, whereas mannitol and urea are administered intravenously. These drugs all have a rapid onset of action, making them useful in emergencies.

ADVERSE REACTIONS AND CONTRAINDICATIONS

Because glycerin is metabolized, it does not cause diuresis; however, glycerin can cause hyperglycemia in diabetic patients. Headache, nausea, and vomiting are additional adverse effects of glycerin. Mannitol produces a pronounced diuresis and often causes headache, nausea and vomiting, and dehydration.

Urea is less satisfactory than mannitol, because it can penetrate the eye and cause a rebound increase in intraocular pressure when the systemic osmotic effect is over, 8 to 12 hours after administration. Urea is also highly irritating on injection.

INTERACTIONS

Mannitol may increase the risk of digitalis toxicity.

 ## PATHOPHYSIOLOGY • Inflammation and Infection of the Eyes

Red eye is a physical manifestation of inflammation caused by vasodilation of the conjunctival, episcleral, and scleral vessels. The common diagnoses associated with red eye include bacterial, viral, fungal, allergic, and irritative conjunctivitis; corneal abrasions and foreign bodies; subconjunctival hemorrhage; episcleritis or scleritis; keratitis; iritis; and acute (closed-angle) glaucoma.

Of all ambulatory patients, 2% to 3% have symptoms of one of the aforementioned ocular disorders. Viral conjunctivitis and allergic reactions are more common than bacterial conjunctivitis. Viral conjunctivitis occurs in epidemics and is most common in young adults. In contrast, bacterial conjunctivitis is seen in patients of all ages at any time of the year. It may occur in an epidemic form known as pink eye. Allergic conjunctivitis is sporadic and seasonal, occurring frequently in patients with a history of allergies, during times of high pollen counts. Irritative conjunctivitis is most often caused by exposure to dust or smoke.

Corneal abrasions and foreign bodies occur most often in patients who spend time outdoors or in debris-filled environments, such as metal shops or lumber mills. Subconjunctival hemorrhage can occur as a result of trauma, recurrent Valsalva maneuvers (such as coughing), or during labor and delivery. Episcleritis and scleritis occur in patients with systemic autoimmune and connective tissue disorders. Immunocompromised patients may also be at risk for keratitis. Approximately 50% of patients with iritis are positive for the HLA-type B27 antigen, suggesting there is a genetic predisposition to the disorder.

The classic description of acute inflammation includes rubor (redness), tumor (edema), calor (warmth), and dolor (pain, discomfort). The manifestations can be divided into two categories—vascular and cellular responses. (See Chapter 14 for more thorough explanation of inflammation.)

The vascular response begins almost immediately after injury or exposure to microorganisms. A momentary period of vasoconstriction is followed immediately by vasodilation of the arterioles and venules that supply the area. As a result the area becomes congested, red, and warm. An increase in capillary permeability allows fluid to escape into tissues and causes edema. Pain ensues as the result of tissue swelling and the release of chemical mediators.

The cellular response is marked by the movement of white blood cells into the injured area. As fluid leaves the capillaries, blood viscosity increases and white blood cells move to the periphery of the vessel. White blood cells migrate into tissue spaces because they are attracted to microorganisms and cellular debris. They engulf and degrade the organisms and cellular debris from the area of inflammation.

Untreated infections can cause permanent eye damage. Untreated inflammation causes unnecessary pain and may also lead to eye damage. The treatment strategy is to remove the cause of inflammation, which may require antimicrobial agents, and to control the symptoms of inflammation to aid healing and patient comfort.

DRUG CLASS • Antibacterial Drugs Used to Treat Ophthalmic Diseases

bacitracin (Bacitracin)

bacitracin zinc + polymyxin B sulfate
(Polysporin)

bacitracin zinc + polymyxin B sulfate +
neomycin sulfate (Neosporin)

chloramphenicol (Chloromycetin, Chloroptic)

chlortetracycline (Aureomycin)

erythromycin (Ilotycin)

gramicidin + neomycin sulfate + polymyxin B
sulfate (Neosporin)

neomycin sulfate + polymyxin B sulfate
(Statrol)

oxytetracycline + polymyxin B sulfate
(Terramycin W/Polymyxin B)

sulfacetamide (Bleph-10, Bleph-30, Cetamide,
Isopto Cetamide, Ocusulf-10, Sulf-10, Sulf-
15, Sulfacel-15)

tobramycin (Aktob, Tobrex)

MECHANISM OF ACTION

Antibiotics for use in the eye come from many of the same families used to treat systemic infections and have the same mechanisms of action. Bacterial protein synthesis inhibitors previously covered include chloramphenicol and tetracyclines (see Chapter 28), erythromycin (see Chapter 26), and tobramycin (see Chapter 29).

Other antibiotics used are too toxic to be used at full systemic doses but are effective for localized topical use. Examples include bacitracin (a bacterial cell wall inhibitor), neomycin and gramicidin (inhibitors of bacterial protein synthesis), and polymyxin B sulfate (produces a detergent-like action on bacterial membranes).

USES

These drugs are intended for short-term use to treat eye infections.

PHARMACOKINETICS

These drugs remain for varying periods in the eye, and most pass to some degree through the nasolacrimal pathway into systemic circulation. The amounts absorbed tend to be very small and are usually quickly eliminated by liver or renal mechanisms.

ADVERSE REACTIONS AND CONTRAINDICATIONS

Adverse reactions to these drugs may include stinging or burning, irritation, tearing, or blurred vision. On rare occasions, the drugs may precipitate more serious allergic reactions if the patient has a history of prior allergy to the drug or the drug class.

INTERACTIONS

Few interactions have been noted, because these drugs do not enter systemic circulation in significant amounts.

DRUG CLASS • Antifungal Drug Used to Treat Ophthalmic Diseases

natamycin (Natacyn)

MECHANISM OF ACTION

Natamycin is related to the polyene antifungal agents (see Chapter 32). All polyenes interfere with membrane function in fungi, causing necessary internal components to be lost.

USES

Natamycin is the only antifungal agent formulated for use directly in the eyes. It is the drug of choice for fungal keratitis. When fungal infections are deep-seated or when the patient is immunosuppressed, systemic antifungal drugs may be required to protect vision.

PHARMACOKINETICS

Natamycin uptake from the eye is possible, but the doses are small enough to make systemic effects unlikely. Natamycin also fails to penetrate into deeper corneal layers unless epithelial defects are present.

ADVERSE REACTIONS AND CONTRAINDICATIONS

Natamycin may cause additional eye irritation, redness, or swelling unrelated to the infection.

INTERACTIONS

Few interactions have been noted because of the low absorption of natamycin into systemic circulation.

DRUG CLASS • Antiviral Drugs Used to Treat Ophthalmic Diseases

cidofovir (Vistide)

foscarnet (Foscavir)

ganciclovir (Cytovene, Vitrasert)

idoxuridine (Dendrid, Herplex)

trifluridine (Viroptic)

valganciclovir (Valcyte)

vidarabine (Vira-A)

MECHANISM OF ACTION

Ganciclovir acts similarly to acyclovir; both drugs are readily activated within virus-infected cells to a form that inhibits virus reproduction (see Chapter 31). Unlike acyclovir, ganciclovir is also activated, to a limited degree, by normal cells. Cidofovir is activated by phosphorylation to a form that selectively inhibits viral DNA polymerase. Thus viral replication can be blocked at concentrations of cidofovir that do not normally affect human DNA polymerase. Foscarnet inhibits viral DNA polymerases and reverse transcriptases. Because foscarnet is a chemical relative of inorganic phosphate, it does not require activation within cells.

Idoxuridine, trifluridine, and vidarabine are cytotoxic drugs that are too toxic to be used systemically but they can interfere with DNA synthesis in viruses when used for localized infections. Idoxuridine is incorporated into DNA in place of thymidine, thus preventing normal DNA replication and halting virus formation. Trifluridine, like idoxuridine, is activated by viral and host-cell thymidine kinase to a form of drug that inhibits DNA polymerase. Vidarabine inhibits viral DNA synthesis in a variety of DNA viruses. Vidarabine is activated by host-cell enzymes to ara-ATP, a potent and selective inhibitor of viral DNA polymerase. Clinically important selectivity of action is achieved against herpesvirus-infected cells.

USES

Ganciclovir is indicated only for treatment of cytomegalovirus (CMV) retinitis in immunocompromised patients. Cidofovir is used only to treat CMV retinitis in AIDS patients. Foscarnet has shown activity against HIV, herpes viruses, and hepatitis B, but is presently indicated only for control of CMV retinitis in HIV-infected patients.

The topical antivirals (idoxuridine, trifluridine, and vidarabine) are indicated primarily for keratitis caused by herpes simplex virus. These drugs are too toxic for systemic use.

PHARMACOKINETICS

Ganciclovir is poorly absorbed orally with a bioavailability of less than 5%. Therefore administration is by intravenous infusion. The drug distributes widely into tissues, including the eye. Ganciclovir is not biotransformed and is excreted unchanged in urine. An implantation form for insertion into the vitreous humor has recently been developed. This form releases the drug directly into the eye for 5 to 8 months before it must be surgically replaced.

Cidofovir is given only by intravenous infusion and is sometimes combined with probenecid. It is rapidly cleared by renal excretion if given alone but, if combined with probenecid, renal excretion is slowed.

Foscarnet is poorly absorbed orally and therefore must be given by intravenous injection or infusion. The drug distributes to tissues, including brain tissues, although levels are variable. As an analog of inorganic phosphate, foscarnet seems to be incorporated into bone. Most of the remainder of the drug is excreted unchanged in urine.

Topical antiviral drugs are not well absorbed from the eye.

ADVERSE REACTIONS AND CONTRAINDICATIONS

Ganciclovir causes granulocytopenia, marked by sore throat and fever, in about 40% of patients. It also causes thrombocytopenia, marked by bruising and unusual bleeding, in 20% of patients. These reactions are usually reversible. Anemia, allergies, and signs of CNS irritability have also been reported, though less often. Ganciclovir is used cautiously, if at all, in patients with low neutrophil or platelet counts. Dosages must be reduced in patients with renal failure.

Nephrotoxicity is a common adverse reaction to cidofovir and is usually dose limiting. Neutropenia, GI upset, and headache also occur.

Renal toxicity is the major concern with foscarnet. Signs of serious renal toxicity may occur in up to 25% of patients. Some protection may be afforded by ensuring adequate hydration before administering foscarnet. Its other adverse effects include nausea, headache, dizziness, and anemia. Nephrotoxicity may include acute renal tubular necrosis.

When used topically in the eye, little idoxuridine enters the systemic circulation. The drug can produce local reactions in the eye, the most serious being corneal defects. It may also interfere with corneal epithelial regeneration and healing. Idoxuridine is potentially mutagenic and carcinogenic. Herpes simplex infections of the cornea, conjunctiva, and eyelids tend to recur. Idoxuridine does not prevent reappearance of infection, nor does it prevent scarring and resultant loss of sight in serious cases. Vidarabine use is not usually associated with serious adverse effects, but local eye irritation and sensitivity to light may occur. It is potentially mutagenic and carcinogenic. Trifluridine may be less damaging to the cornea than idoxuridine or vidarabine; nevertheless, conjunctival or corneal burning can occur when the drug is placed in the eye. Swelling of the eyelids (palpebral edema) has also been noted. Trifluridine is potentially mutagenic and carcinogenic.

TOXICITY

Subcutaneous or intramuscular injection leads to severe tissue damage, because ganciclovir preparations have a very high pH. Thus care must be taken with intravenous administration to avoid infiltration into surrounding tissues.

INTERACTIONS

Ganciclovir may cause dangerous blood dyscrasias when combined with zidovudine. Other bone marrow depressants may lead to unacceptable adverse effects with ganciclovir.

Neither cidofovir nor foscarnet should be used with other nephrotoxic drugs.

DRUG CLASS • Antiinflammatory Drugs

Single Formulations

dexamethasone (Decadron, Maxidex)

diclofenac (Voltaren Ophthalmic)

fluorometholone (Flarex, FML)

flurbiprofen (Ocufen)

hydrocortisone acetate (generic)

prednisolone (Econopred, Inflamase, Pred)

rimexolone (Vexol)

suprofen (Profenal)

Antibiotics + Antiinflammatory Drugs

bacitracin zinc + polymyxin B sulfate + neomycin sulfate + hydrocortisone (Cortisporin)

chloramphenicol + hydrocortisone acetate (Chloromycetin Hydrocortisone)

gentamicin + prednisolone (Pred-G)

neomycin sulfate + dexamethasone sodium phosphate (Neodecadron)

neomycin sulfate + polymyxin B sulfate + dexamethasone (Dexacidin, Dexasporin, Maxitrol)

neomycin sulfate + polymyxin B sulfate + hydrocortisone (Cortisporin)

neomycin sulfate + polymyxin B sulfate + prednisolone acetate (Poly-Pred)

oxytetracycline + hydrocortisone (Terra-Cortril)

sulfacetamide + fluorometholone (FML-S)

sulfacetamide + prednisolone (Blephamide, Cetapred, Isopto Cetapred, Metimyd, Vasocidin)

tetracycline + hydrocortisone (Achromycin)

tobramycin + dexamethasone (Tobradex)

tobramycin + fluorometholone (Tobrasone)

Flurbiprofen and suprofen are nonsteroidal antiinflammatory drugs (NSAIDs) specifically for ophthalmic use. Diclofenac (Voltaren Ophthalmic) is an NSAID used ophthalmically to treat inflammation after cataract surgery. Ophthalmic surgery may stimulate the synthesis of prostaglandins (chemical transmitters synthesized in response to local tissue stimulation), causing a miosis that resists the mydriatic action of atropine. The locally applied NSAIDs therefore prevent miosis during surgery by blocking synthesis of prostaglandins (see Chapter 14).

Steroidal antiinflammatory drugs are covered in Chapter 57. These powerful agents are useful in the short term but should be avoided if infection is present, because they mask signs of infection and limit the normal defense mechanisms to infection. Many formulations are available that include an antiinflammatory drug along with an antibacterial drug.

Corticosteroid use has been associated with the development of posterior subcapsular cataract (PSC). Patients who use 10 to 16 mg/day of oral prednisone or its equivalent for 1 year or more are at highest risk. At doses above 16 mg/day for 1 year, the incidence of PSC is 70%. Any patient receiving long-term oral corticosteroids should have routine eye examinations. Patients should be instructed not to rub the eyes because ocular corticosteroids increase the possibility of bruising the delicate eye tissues.

DRUG CLASS • Ocular Antihistamines and Decongestants

cromolyn sodium (Crolom, Cromoptic)

levocabastine (Livostin)

Iodoxamide (Alomide)

naphazoline (Albalon, Nafazair, Vasocon)

olopatadine (Patanol)

Ocular antihistamines such as levocabastine, Iodoxamide, and olopatadine are used in the management of seasonal allergic conjunctivitis. These drugs block histamine receptors in the eye and prevent some of the reactions to irritants (e.g., pollen). The most common adverse effects include headache and burning or stinging in the eye. Cromolyn sodium is discussed in Chapter 53.

Decongestants such as naphazoline are alpha-receptor agonists. They cause vasoconstriction in the eye, which reduces the redness and congestion that may accompany allergies. The most common adverse effects include transient burning or stinging, dryness, blurred vision, or mydriasis. Rebound congestion and eye redness may occur if the drug is overused. The onset of action is within 10 minutes, and the duration is 2 to 6 hours. Some systemic uptake can occur, which may produce headache, nervousness, dizziness, weakness, hypertension, or cardiovascular effects in some patients.

APPLICATION TO PRACTICE

ASSESSMENT
History of Present Illness

The most common eye complaint is often a change or loss of vision, but the effects may also be less specific (e.g., headache, eyestrain). Symptoms can often be divided into problems that affect appearance, vision, and sensation. It is not unusual for the patient to be unable to verbalize a specific complaint. Therefore it is important to elicit information from the patient regarding the onset, location, duration, and characteristics (such as frequency and severity) of the symptoms. Determine whether there have been abnormal sensations such as itching, burning, or pain. The circumstances surrounding the onset of symptoms are important, as well as the patient's response to any treatment.

The most common ocular disorder is a red eye. It may be caused by minor irritation, inflammatory disorders or infection, allergy, vascular congestion, subconjunctival hemorrhage, and trauma. Changes in the external appearance may include abnormal positioning, lesions, redness, and edema.

Visual changes may be related to eye abnormalities and problems along the visual pathway. Patient complaints often include glare or halos resulting from scratches on the lens of glasses, uncorrected refractive errors, dilated pupils, corneal edema, or cataracts. "Floaters" in the field of vision may represent inflammatory cells, blood cells, pigment, or strands in the vitreous. The patient may complain of double vision in one or both eyes that may be caused by refractive errors, muscle imbalance, or neuromuscular disorders.

Patient descriptions of abnormal sensations include eyestrain, pressure, or fullness; a pulling; or generalized headache. The location of the abnormal sensation may be described as behind the eye (retrobulbar), within the eye, or surrounding the eye (periocular). Deep internal aching may suggest inflammation or infection, muscle spasm, or glaucoma. Spasm of the ciliary muscle and the sphincter of the iris appear with inflammation and result in brow ache and photophobia or miosis. Itching is ordinarily a sign of allergy. Dryness, burning, or sensation of a foreign object in the eye can occur with mild corneal irritation or dry eyes. Tearing can be caused by irritation or an abnormality of the lacrimal ducts. Infections, noninfectious irritations, and allergic reactions may manifest as complaints of increased ocular secretions.

Health History

Health history focuses on the patient's general state of health. Ask the patient specifically about chronic, systemic disorders that are commonly associated with eye disorders (e.g., diabetes, arthritis, hypertension, thyroid disease) and inquire about childhood illnesses and immunizations, particularly about rubella (measles).

If glasses or contact lenses are currently worn, ask the patient when the last eye examination was performed and when the last prescription was changed. Determine whether the patient has had eye (e.g. laser treatments) or brain surgery.

Many eye disorders have a familial predisposition; thus it is important to inquire specifically about myopia (nearsightedness, near vision better than distant vision), hyperopia (farsightedness, distant vision better than near vision), glaucoma, and strabismus. Other common familial disorders affecting the eyes include macular degeneration, migraine headaches, sickle cell anemia, retinitis pigmentosa, and retinoblastoma.

The drug history should include the current use of any drugs, because many systemically administered drugs affect the eyes (see Table 65-2). Ask if the patient uses eye drops or ointments, and note the name, dose, and dosage frequency. Determine whether OTC eye preparations that may dry the eyes (e.g., antihistamines, decongestants) are used. Determine if the patient has ever had an allergic reaction to ophthalmic drugs or experienced other reactions that affected the eyes.

Lifespan Considerations

Perinatal. Pregnant women may have visual disorders that require drug therapy. However, the normal changes of pregnancy may alter visual acuity in some cases. Systemic absorption of ocular drugs should be considered when assessing the patient's signs and symptoms. The woman should be questioned about visual blurring, vision changes, or scotomata. The results of the funduscopic examination should be recorded on the patient's record.

The elevated blood sugar level that accompanies gestational diabetes may cause alterations in vision. The woman's blood sugar should be checked at the appropriate time during the three gestational periods. A hypertensive crisis can also alter vision; thus, the woman's blood pressure should be monitored regularly and recorded.

Pediatric. Few studies of ophthalmic drug use in children have been reported. Further, the conditions for which adults need therapy (e.g., glaucoma, cataracts) rarely occur in children. Glaucoma may be present at birth, although 50% of affected infants have symptoms that may not be readily apparent. Symptoms usually develop during the first year of life. In about 40% of cases, the IOP is elevated in the fetus and the infant is born with ocular enlargement. Both eyes are affected in about 75% of those infants though the severity of the disorder varies.

Older Adults. The incidence of cataracts, dry eye, retinal detachment, glaucoma, entropion, and ectropion increases with age. Ptosis may occur with aging but also results from edema, disorders of the third cranial nerve, and neuromuscular disorders. Older adults are at risk for ocular disorders, especially glaucoma and cataracts. They are also more likely to have cardiovascular disorders that can be aggravated by systemic absorption of topical eye drugs. The principles of drug therapy are the same as those for young adults, however.

Cultural/Social Considerations

When assessing the patient with an eye disorder, factors that influence ocular health should be noted as well as health management behaviors. Questions about the nature of the patient's work include information about exposure to irritating fumes, smoke, or airborne particles. The use of safety goggles or protective eyewear when engaging in sports activities (e.g., racquetball, baseball, contact sports), a problem of sufficient lighting, or glare in the workplace should be noted. If contact lenses are worn, are they cared for correctly and regularly, and are they stored as recommended? If the patient has a chronic disease, does the patient actively manage the disease?

Because the level of independence varies with the individual eye disorder, information supplied by the patient or family helps to determine how much help may be needed with activities of daily living. Referrals to home health care or social services for assistance with rehabilitation or finances may be needed in some cases. Planning for housekeeping and meal preparation, safety in the home environment (because of altered vision), transportation, and assistance with the eyes should be explored and documented.

It is important to note how the patient is coping with chronic alterations in vision. Although people adapt differently, patients usually experience stages of grief and loss and may be at any stage of the process. Loneliness may be a significant finding. Patients may be understandably anxious during physical examinations, because vision has not improved, or has worsened (see Case Study this chapter: Glaucoma).

Physical Examination

Assess the patient for redness, swelling, tearing, discharge, and decreased visual acuity. The external examination includes the eyebrows, lashes, lids, lacrimal apparatus, and anterior portion of the eyes, pupils, sclera, conjunctiva, cornea, and irises. Symmetry and alignment should be noted. Hair loss over the lateral aspects of the eyebrows occurs with aging and is considered normal. Also, in the older adult, a thin, white ring around the edge of the cornea may be seen (arcus senilis) and is also considered a normal change of aging.

Tests for ocular motility, corneal light reflex (Hirschberg's test), cover-uncover test, visual acuity, and visual fields should be completed. It is important to remember that, while an abnormal acuity suggests an uncorrected refractive error or pathologic process, normal acuity does not exclude disease or disorder of the visual system. Further, patients who wear contact lenses may not respond to the corneal reflex test to the same degree as patients who do not wear them, because they become somewhat insensitive to the stimulus. Internal eye structures are visible only through direct and indirect funduscopic examinations.

The patient's physical features should be observed for age and any obvious deformities. For example, hand deformities and abnormal gait may provide a clue in diagnosing associated eye disorders such as Sjögren's syndrome (i.e., rheumatoid arthritis, xerostomia, and keratoconjunctivitis sicca).

Laboratory Testing

For the patient with glaucoma, a tonometry reading reflects increased IOP. Aqueous humor maintains the shape of the eye while keeping a relatively uniform pressure within the globe. As pressure increases, the eye becomes firmer, and a greater force is required to cause the same amount of indentation with the tonometer. Normal pressure is considered to be 15 +/- 2.5 mm Hg. The IOP should be measured at different times of day, because variations of as much as 10 mm Hg or more may occur over a 24-hour period. The use of fluorescein staining and special lighting (Wood's lamp) can help identify corneal or conjunctival damage, as well as the presence of a foreign body.

GOALS OF THERAPY

The primary goal in the treatment of glaucoma is to facilitate the outflow of aqueous humor through the outflow channels, thus preventing damage to the ganglion cells and optic nerve fibers as well as preventing loss of visual field. The main treatment goals in the management of infection and inflammation are to reduce symptoms and prevent recurrence of the disorder while minimizing adverse effects.

Ocular solutions are sterile, easily administered, and usually do not interfere with vision. Yet the solutions are in contact with the eye for only a short time, whereas ointments are comfortable on administration and stay in contact with the eye for longer periods. Ointments can interfere with vision, though, because a film or haze tends to form over the eye. They may also cause a higher incidence of contact dermatitis than solutions, and most are not sterile formulations. Ocular gels and ocuserts, the newer delivery systems, were developed to overcome the problems associated with conventional eyedrops and ointments. The major advantage to using ocuserts is their longer duration of action, which, in turn, increases patient compliance. Ocusert use also avoids the peak-and-valley responses that have been associated with solutions and ointments.

Treatment of glaucoma varies with the type and the presence of comorbid conditions. Most patients are treated first with ocular beta blockers; then with epinephrine, pilocarpine, and anticholinesterase miotics; and finally with carbonic anhydrase inhibitors. However, drug selection for the patient with primary open-angle glaucoma depends largely on how well the patient tolerates adverse effects. If the first topical drug fails to reduce pressure sufficiently and noncompliance has been ruled out as a cause of treatment failure, substitution of an-

other drug may be done before proceeding to combination therapy. Laser trabeculoplasty is usually reserved for patients whose IOP has not been sufficiently reduced, despite maximally tolerated therapy with an ocular miotic, beta blocker, epinephrine, and orally administered carbonic anhydrase inhibitor.

INTERVENTION
Administration

Assess the patient for redness, swelling or other irritation, and systemic effects that were not present before treatment was started. Otic and ocular drug containers are often similar in appearance, but only ocular formulations should be used. Otic and dermatologic drug formulations should not be used in the eye. Eye drops that have changed color or become cloudy should be discarded. Further, the use of an eyecup is discouraged because of the potential for contamination and risk of spreading disease.

The normal, healthy eye holds about 10 microliters of fluid. The average eyedropper delivers 25 to 50 microliters per drop; thus more than a dropperful is not useful. When more than one drop is to be administered, it is best to wait 5 minutes between drops. The wait ensures that the original drop is not rinsed away by the second; or that the second drop is not diluted by the first.

Wash hands thoroughly before administering ocular drugs. Instruct the patient to tilt the head backward or assume a lying position with the eye gazing upward. The lower lid is gently pulled down and, holding the dropper above the eye, the drop is placed inside the lower lid. The lid is released slowly. Instruct the patient not to blink or rub the eye for approximately 30 seconds.

For adults with a strong blink reflex or for pediatric patients, the closed-eye technique can be used to administer eyedrops. Have the patient lie down, and place the drop on the inner canthus of the eyelid. Opening the lid causes the drops to fall into the eye by gravity.

Systemic absorption of eyedrops can cause adverse reactions. Nasolacrimal occlusion is effective in decreasing drug loss through the nasolacrimal system into the posterior nasopharynx. The occlusion is accomplished by placing a finger over the inner canthus for a period of 3 to 5 minutes. This permits maximal drug effects while using lower concentrations and less frequent administrations.

When ointments are used for the first time, the first one-fourth inch should be squeezed out and discarded. To facilitate ointment flow, warm the container for a few minutes by holding it in the hand. Gently pull down the lower lid and place one-fourth to one-half inch of ointment inside the lower lid by gently squeezing the tube. Instruct the patient to close the eye for 1 to 2 minutes and roll the eye in all directions. The patient should be advised that temporary blurring might occur with the use of ointments; remove excess ointment around the eye or ointment tube with tissue. Wait at least 5 minutes for drops and 10 minutes before using another drug if the patient is using more than one ocular agent.

Cholinergic Miotics and Anticholinesterase Miotics. Cholinergic and anticholinesterase miotic solutions and ointments require frequent instillation. However, the need for frequent instillation decreases patient compliance. When possible, miotic solutions should be administered at bedtime to minimize blurring and interference with vision. The adverse effects of cholinergics are less severe, however, and occur less often than those produced by anticholinesterase drugs.

Carbonic Anhydrase Inhibitors. When oral liquid acetazolamide is needed, crush and mix the tablets with a highly flavored carbohydrate syrup (such as raspberry, cherry, or chocolate). Tablets can also be softened in hot water and added to honey or syrup. Sustained-release capsules should not be opened or crushed.

Osmotics. Topical osmotic solutions such as glycerin may cause pain and eye irritation. A topical, local anesthetic is usually instilled shortly before administration of the topical osmotic. Do not give the patient hypotonic fluids following administration of an osmotic solution, because these fluids will cancel the osmotic effect of the osmotic.

Education

Patients with eye conditions (particularly glaucoma) that put them at risk for blindness often have high levels of anxiety. As a result, they may be unable to comprehend simple verbal administration instructions; written instructions are helpful to ensure compliance. Patients should be encouraged to continue regular use of their drugs for effective treatment of glaucoma. Because chronic glaucoma is a silent disease, much like hypertension, there is little positive reinforcement to continue therapy. The only noticeable effects are the drug's adverse effects.

Patients who require ocular drugs should be taught how to store and administer the preparation properly. The label should be checked to be sure that the correct drug and concentration is used. Solutions that become cloudy or darkened should be discarded. Particular attention should be given to storage information on the label, because some ophthalmic drugs require refrigeration. Most formulations have a 3-month shelf life once they are opened or should be discarded at the end of the current illness. If the drug is stored past these times, it may become contaminated.

The patient should be taught to maintain the sterility of the drug as well as the dropper. The tube tip or dropper should not come in contact with anything, including skin. A dropper should be held with the tip pointing downward to prevent the drug from flowing into the dropper bulb. The container should be closed when it is not in use.

The patient should also be taught what adverse effects indicate a worsening of the condition, as well as the signs of improvement. Specific instructions about what to do and whom to contact should be provided if adverse effects appear. Patients should be instructed when to contact the health care provider for follow-up and to avoid sharing their eye drugs with others. Other individuals requiring eye drugs should have their own supply. Ocular drugs should not be stopped without first consulting the health care provider.

Cholinergic Miotics and Anticholinesterase Miotics. Patients taking cholinergic miotics or anticholinesterase miotics should be advised that they may have difficulty adjusting to changes in lighting. This problem can be particularly serious for older adults, because their adaptation abilities and visual acuity are often reduced. Nighttime can be especially dangerous. Advise patients to use the drug at bedtime to minimize interference caused by blurring.

Because blurring and difficulty in focusing may occur, instruct patients to avoid potentially hazardous activities (e.g., driving, operating machinery). Anticholinesterase miotics can cause spasm of the blink reflex, which can be particularly annoying to some patients.

Ocular Beta Blockers. A fall in blood pressure and pulse can be caused by concomitant blockade of beta receptors in the heart and vascular system. Therefore all other beta-blocking drugs should be discontinued before using an ocular beta blocker, such as timolol. Frequent checks of blood pressure and pulse during the initial phase of therapy and later during maintenance are usually necessary. Further, a tendency toward tolerance has been noted with long-term beta blocker therapy; therefore periodic measurements of IOP are warranted.

Adrenergics. Patients taking adrenergic eye drugs should be advised to remove soft contact lenses before administering a miotic drug because of the possibility of staining.

Contact Lens Products. Many adverse effects have been reported when patients who wear contact lenses ingest or topically apply certain drugs. The effects of certain topically administered ophthalmic drugs may be enhanced when soft lenses are in place. The soft lens absorbs the drug and releases it over time, creating a sustained-release dosage form. Drug effects may be decreased, because the lens absorbs the drug and binds it so that it is slowly released into the eye. Further, contact time of the drug with the eye is increased regardless of the type of contact lens. Increased drug absorption may occur secondary to compromised corneal epithelium that is present during contact lens wear. Further, the preservatives, vehicles, tonicity, and pH of the solution could alter the lenses. For example, hypertonic solutions such as 10% sodium sulfacetamide or 8% pilocarpine may cause soft lens dehydration and lens disfigurement.

Topical drugs that have an acidic pH promote lens dehydration and steepening, whereas alkaline drugs promote hydration and flattening. Topical suspensions can cause a buildup of particulate matter, leading to discomfort and lens intolerance. Gel and oil formulations alter the relationship between the contact lens and the surface of the cornea.

Some systemic drugs are secreted into the tears and may interact with contact lenses. For example, the antimicrobial drug rifampin stains the lenses and tears orange. Gold salts are secreted into the tears and may cause ocular irritation. The active ingredient of certain topical products (such as epinephrine) may discolor lenses. Other drugs may affect tear production, the refractive properties of the eye, the shape of the cornea, or the actual lens of the eye.

In general, patients should be advised not to wear contact lenses when any ocular solution or ointment is required. The only exceptions to this rule are products that are specifically formulated to be used with contact lenses.

CASE STUDY   *Glaucoma*

ASSESSMENT

HISTORY OF PRESENT ILLNESS

LH is a 65-year-old black man who comes to the ophthalmologist today on referral from his primary care nurse practitioner. He has been complaining of eye pain; reduced visual acuity, particularly peripheral vision; and persistent headaches. He denies having inflammation, itching, or discharge. He reports that the vision changes started about 6 weeks ago and have become progressively worse. He reports taking an OTC nonsteroidal antiinflammatory drug for occasional arthritis pain and has no known drug allergies.

HEALTH HISTORY

LH's history is unremarkable for cardiovascular, respiratory, or renal disease. His last eye examination was about 6 months ago, when he had his last eyeglass prescription filled.

LIFESPAN CONSIDERATIONS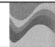

Although a widower, LH is active in his church and drives the van for church activities.

CULTURAL/SOCIAL CONSIDERATIONS

LH states he is "one of the luckies" who does not have a problem with systemic hypertension. He participates in his community to increase awareness in his culture: "My vision just can't go now. I have too much to do." LH receives a small retirement check and is covered by both Medicare and FHP insurance. He wants his care to be cost effective and yet therapeutic without "draining the insurance."

PHYSICAL EXAMINATION

Physical examination reveals white sclera and pink conjunctiva without inflammation or discharge. Visual acuity is 20/80 (large Snellen). Funduscopic examination is unremarkable at this time. No AV nicking, papilledema, or exudates found.

LABORATORY TESTING

Schiøtz tonometry value 21 mm Hg (normal: 15 +/– 2.5).

PATIENT PROBLEM(S)

Chronic open-angle glaucoma.

GOALS OF THERAPY

Facilitate outflow of aqueous humor, thus preventing damage to optic nerve and loss of visual field.

CRITICAL THINKING QUESTIONS

1. The health care provider orders a timolol 0.25% solution into the lower conjunctival sac bid. What other classes of drugs could have been used for LH?
2. What class of drugs is the standard of care for treatment of chronic open-angle glaucoma?
3. What is the major advantage for using beta blockers rather than other classes of drugs when taking into consideration post-administration adverse effects?
4. What disease or conditions contraindicate the use (or at least require cautious use) of a beta blocker for LH?
5. How can systemic absorption of ophthalmic drugs be reduced or prevented?

EVALUATION

When evaluating the effectiveness of IOP-lowering drugs the IOP should be measured at different times during the day, because variations of as much as 10 mm Hg or more may occur over a 24-hour period. In addition, the condition of the optic nerve and visual field status must be determined at least twice a year (or more frequently when indicated). Close monitoring is necessary to ensure there is no progressive damage to the eye from persistently elevated IOP, intermittent noncompliance, or other causes.

A reduction in inflammation, discharge, and discomfort should be noted. In some cases, the use of the drug (e.g., ocular antivirals) may need to continue for 5 to 7 days to prevent recurrence of the infection.

Bibliography

Anonymous: New drugs for allergic conjunctivitis, *Med Lett Drugs Ther* 42(1077):39-40, 2000.

Berardinelli C, Kupecz D: Drug news. Keeping up with recent ophthalmic drug approvals, *Nurs Pract* 26(4):61-62, 64, 67, 2001.

Deblinger L: Evaluation and management of red eye, *Patient Care* 35(24):36-44, 2001.

DeGrezia MG, Robinson M: Ophthalmic manifestations of HIV: an update, *J Assoc Nurses AIDS Care* 12(3):22-32, 2001.

Derrington D: Eye conditions affecting the elderly, *Nurs Resid Care* 4(1):32-34, 46-47, 2002.

Kamoun L: The red eye, *Top Emerg Med* 22(4):37-51, 2000.

LoBuono C: Clinical clips. Is glaucoma undertreated in African Americans? *Pat Care Nurse Pract* 3(5):91, 2000.

Noecker RJ: Changing the paradigm for first-line treatment may result in healthier, happier patients, *J Ophthalmic Nurs Technol* 19(2):96-98, 2000.

Ritch R: Directed therapy for specific glaucomas, *Ophthalmol Clin North Am* 13(3):429-441, 2000.

Shields SR: Managing eye disease in primary care. Part 2: how to recognize and treat common eye problems, *Postgraduate Medicine* 108(5):83-86, 91-94, 96, 2000.

Tanna AP, Jampel HD: Normal-tension glaucoma, *Ophthalmol Clin North Am* 13(3):455-464, 2000.

Turkoski BB: Pharmacology. Glaucoma and glaucoma medications, *Orthop Nurs* 19(5):71-76, 2000.

Internet Resources

http://www.glaucoma.org/.
http://www.glaucoma-foundation.org/.
http://www.iga.org.uk/home.htm.
http://www.nei.nih.gov/publications/glauc-pat.htm.
http://www.nlm.nih.gov/medlineplus/glaucoma.html.

Otic Drugs

MICHAEL R. VASKO • KATHLEEN GUTIERREZ

 Visit **http://evolve.elsevier.com/Gutierrez/** for additional information.

KEY TERMS

Cerumen, p. 1096
Otitis externa, p. 1095
Otitis media, p. 1095
Ototoxicity, p. 1100

OBJECTIVES

- Describe the various treatments for otic disorders that require the use of topical drugs.
- Identify the factors that contribute to external ear canal infections.
- Describe the symptoms that arise with external otic infections.
- Discuss the importance of treating cerumen impaction and the consequences of lack of treatment.
- Describe the uses and adverse effects of the various classes of drugs used to treat external ear infections.
- Identify drug therapies associated with a significant risk for ototoxicity.
- Develop a nursing care plan for the patient using an otic drug.

 PATHOPHYSIOLOGY • Ear Infections

Treatment of middle and inner ear disease often requires oral or parenteral medications. External ear pathologies, however, depend on topical otic drugs administered locally to prevent or treat disorders. These infections include those of the external ear (otitis externa) and those of the middle ear (otitis media). Otic drugs instilled directly into the external meatus of the ear include antibiotics, antiinfective drugs, antiinflammatory drugs, anesthetics, drying agents, and cerumen solvents. These drugs are used exclusively for their local actions, and direct administration allows distribution to all surface areas of the external canal. Many otic drugs are combinations of two or more drugs and are primarily used to treat external ear infections, inflammation, pain, and the removal of excessive or impacted cerumen (Table 66-1). It is important to note that in many instances ear infections are treated by systemic administration of antibiotics. As with other infections the choice of drug depends on the infecting bacteria. These antibiotics are covered in detail in Chapters 24 through 30 and will not be discussed here.

Infection of the external ear is common when the integrity of the external canal is compromised, allowing invasion of pathogenic organisms into the tissue. Patients whose ears are frequently exposed to water from swimming, bathing, or environmental factors are at greatest risk for alterations in the integrity of the skin tis-

---

TABLE 66-1

Selected Drug Preparations for Otic Administration

Generic Name	Brand Name	Comment
Anesthetics		
benzocaine	Americaine Otic Topical Anesthetic Ear Drops	Used for analgesia in acute otitis media
benzocaine + antipyrine	Auralgan	Used for analgesia in acute otitis media and as an adjunct for cerumen removal
Antibacterial and Drying Drugs		
acetic acid	Acetasol, VoSol	For superficial infections of the external ear canal; not to be used for extended periods
acetic acid + aluminum acetate	Domeboro	For superficial infections of the external ear canal; not to be used for extended periods
isopropyl alcohol + glycerin	Auro-Dry, Star-Otic, others	Used to dry external ear canal
Antibiotics		
chloramphenicol 0.5% otic solution	Chloramycetin	For use in the superficial external ear canal; not to be used longer than 10 days
ofloxacin 0.3% otic solution	Floxin	For treatment of otitis externa and otitis media
Antibiotic and Steroid Combinations		
acetic acid + hydrocortisone	Acetasol HC, VoSol HC	For the treatment of superficial infections complicated by inflammation
acetic acid + hydrocortisone + neomycin	Neo-Cort-Dome	Used for susceptible infections of the external auditory canal, fenestration cavities, or mastoidectomy
ciprofloxacin + hydrocortisone	Cipro HC	Used for otitis externa in children and adults
colistin + hydrocortisone + neomycin + thonzonium	Coly-Mycin S, Cortisporin TC	Used for susceptible infections of the external auditory canal, fenestration cavities, or mastoidectomy
hydrocortisone + neomycin + polymixin B	Cortisporin, Oticair, Pediotic, others	Used for infections of external auditory canal; not to be used longer than 10 days
hydrocortisone + polymixin B	Otobiotic	Used for infections of external auditory canal
Ceruminolytics		
carbamide peroxide	Auro Ear Drops, Otix drop, others	Used for cerumen removal; sold in OTC preparations
trolamine-polypeptide + oleate-condensate	Cerumenex	Used for cerumen removal; irrigate repeatedly with warm water
Steroids		
betamethasone	Betnesol✱	For use in inflammation of the external canal; not available in the United States
dexamethasone	Decadron	For use in inflammation of the external canal

✱ Available only in Canada.

sue of the external ear. Additionally, patients who traumatize the skin with cotton swabs or other foreign objects inserted into the canal are at risk for developing an external ear infection. The usual pathogens causing external ear infections include *P. aeruginosa, S. aureus, E. coli, Proteus* species, and anaerobes.

Infection results in inflammation and pain. With inflammation, blood flow to the area increases, capillary permeability increases, and fluid flows into the affected tissues, producing edema and erythema. The ear contains many sensory nerve fibers that, when inflamed, produce

significant pain. External canal structures become red, edematous, and painful even to slight touch. Extensive swelling leads to a conductive type of hearing loss resulting from obstruction of the canal. Fever, malaise, anorexia, and fatigue are signs of systemic involvement and require systemic therapy rather than topical preparations. Drug therapy is designed to alleviate pain through either the reduction of inflammation or direct anesthetic effects. Acute otitis media and infections of the inner ear require systemic antibiotic therapy to combat the organism effectively (see Chapters 24 through 30).

 DRUG CLASS • **Antibiotics Used to Treat Ear Infections**

chloramphenicol otic (Chloromycetin Otic, Sopamycetin✴)

ofloxacin otic (Floxin Otic)

MECHANISM OF ACTION

Otic antibiotics work through direct contact with the microorganism on the skin. They are not designed for systemic absorption. As a broad-spectrum antibiotic, chloramphenicol acts on both gram-negative and gram-positive organisms such as *S. aureus, E. coli, Haemophilus influenzae, P. aeruginosa, Aerobacter aerogenes, Klebsiella pneumoniae,* and *Proteus* species. Ofloxacin is used primarily for *S. aureus, P. aeruginosa, S. pneumoniae, H. influenzae,* and *Moraxella catarrhalis.* Chloramphenicol produces primarily bacteriostatic effects by inhibiting protein synthesis, whereas the bactericidal effects of ofloxacin result from inhibition of DNA gyrase.

USES

Otic antibiotics are used in the treatment of external otitis, a superficial infection of the ear. Other antibiotics, including ciprofloxacin, colistin, and neomycin, are also used in combination with steroids (see later section and Table 66-1). In addition, otic antibiotics are sometimes prescribed in the treatment of chronic suppurative otitis media and otorrhea following tympanotomy tube insertion. Systemic antibiotics are used when the infection is extensive or resistant to antibiotic therapy.

Pharmacokinetics

Typical pharmacokinetic properties do not apply to topical otic antibiotics. These drugs are not absorbed, biotransformed, or eliminated systemically. Absorption of otic antibiotics only occurs superficially through otic tissues. The otic antibiotic must remain in direct contact with the infected otic tissue long enough to be effective.

If possible, before administration of the otic antibiotic, all exudate, cerumen, debris, and other secretions should be removed from the canal via warm water irrigation (Figure 66-1). Elimination occurs through evaporation, normal physiologic ear cleaning, or water irrigation.

ADVERSE REACTIONS AND CONTRAINDICATIONS

Contact dermatitis is the most common adverse reaction to topical antibiotics. Itching, burning, angioedema (e.g., local wheals accompanied by swelling of subcutaneous tissue), urticaria, vesicular lesions, and maculopapular dermatitis are symptoms associated with contact

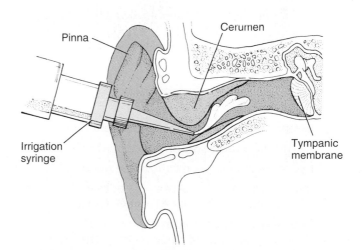

FIGURE 66-1 Irrigation of the external canal. A stream of warm water is directed above or below the blockage. This allows back pressure to push out cerumen and other debris rather than to further impact the external canal. (From Ignatavicius DD, Workman ML, Mishler MS: *Medical-surgical nursing: a nursing process approach,* ed 4, Philadelphia, 2002, Saunders. Used with permission.)

dermatitis. Prolonged use can lead to an overgrowth of nonsusceptible organisms, including fungi.

Otic antibiotics are contraindicated for patients with a perforated tympanic membrane. Chloramphenicol otic is ototoxic if it enters the inner ear. Patients with known adverse reactions to kanamycin, paromomycin, streptomycin, or gentamicin should use chloramphenicol with caution. Allergies to preservatives such as benzethonium chloride, sulfites, and thiomersal need to be

considered because many otic preparations contain these products.

INTERACTIONS

Given the topical nature of otic preparations, the likelihood of drug interaction is rare. Topical otic antiinflammatory and analgesic drugs are often used concurrently with antibiotics to alleviate ear discomfort.

 DRUG CLASS • Antibacterial and Drying Drugs

acetic acid (VoSol)

acetic acid + aluminum acetate (Otic Domeboro)

acetic acid + hydrocortisone (VoSol HC)

isopropyl alcohol + glycerin (Auro-Dri, Star-Otic, others)

MECHANISM OF ACTION

Antibacterial and drying formulations used for the ear can contain acetic acid, astringents, steroids, and isopropyl alcohol as drying agents. The actions of acetic acid eliminate and prevent susceptible organisms from accumulating in the external ear canal via weak antimicrobial action.

USES

Antibacterial otic drops are used to treat superficial infections of the external ear caused by susceptible organisms. Drying agents suppress the growth of organisms and help prevent recurrent ear canal infection. Drying

agents are used frequently by swimmers, who have a higher incidence rate of repeated ear infections than the general population.

PHARMACOKINETICS

Antibacterial and drying agents are designed to be effective through direct contact with external ear canal tissue. Normal pharmacokinetic principles do not apply to otic antibacterial and drying drugs because they are not designed for absorption, distribution, or biotransformation. Elimination of these drugs takes place through evaporation, normal physiologic ear cleaning, or water irrigation.

ADVERSE REACTIONS AND CONTRAINDICATIONS

Adverse reactions include local irritation and contact dermatitis with burning, stinging, pruritus, tenderness, erythema, rash, urticaria, and edema. Antibacterial and drying drugs should not be used when the tympanic membrane has been perforated.

 DRUG CLASS • Steroids and Steroid-Antibiotic Combinations

betamethasone (Betnesol, Garasone✳)

dexamethasone sodium phosphate (Decadron)

hydrocortisone + ciprofloxacin (Cipro HC)

hydrocortisone + colistin + neomycin sulfate + thonzonium (Coly-Mycin S, Cortisporin TC)

hydrocortisone + neomycin sulfate + polymyxin B (Cortisporin Otic, Oticair, Pediotic, Cortisporin,✳ others)

hydrocortisone and polymyxin B (Otobiotic Otic)

MECHANISM OF ACTION

Steroid and steroid-antibiotic combinations are given to reduce inflammation, edema, pruritus, and pain. Similar to other topical steroids, they act to decrease inflammation by suppressing the immune response. They require direct contact with the skin and are given for their local topical effect. Detailed discussion of the actions and adverse effects of steroids is found in Chapter 57.

USES

Inflammation of the external canal from infection or trauma leads to severe pain. Corticosteroids are given only to reduce inflammation and control pain. Corticosteroid-antibiotic combinations have a dual effect: the corticosteroid helps alleviate discomfort, and the antibiotic treats the infection. Hydrocortisone and dexamethasone are the most common corticosteroids used as otic drugs. Betamethasone is available in Canada for the same use. The broad-spectrum antibiotic neomycin sulfate is used in combination with corticosteroids because of its bactericidal effect.

PHARMACOKINETICS

Normal pharmacokinetics do not apply to steroids and steroid-antibiotic combinations, because they are not designed for absorption, distribution, or biotransformation. Some of a given drug may be absorbed unintentionally through the skin, depending on the dosage, integrity of the skin, the length of use, and whether an occlusive dressing was used. These drugs are eliminated through evaporation, normal physiologic ear cleaning, or water irrigation.

ADVERSE REACTIONS AND CONTRAINDICATIONS

The most common adverse effects of steroid and steroid-antibiotic combinations are overgrowth of organisms, delayed healing, and contact dermatitis. Limiting the length of treatment to no more than 4 days helps prevent problems. Steroid and steroid-antibiotic combinations are contraindicated for patients with a perforated tympanic membrane, herpes simplex, vaccinia, and varicella. Allergies to preservatives such as benzethonium chloride, sulfites, and thiomersal need to be considered because many otic preparations contain these products.

INTERACTIONS

Little fear of interactions among otic steroids and other drugs exists unless the otic steroid is systemically absorbed (see Chapter 57 for interactions with systemic steroids).

 DRUG CLASS • Otic Anesthetics

benzocaine (Americaine Otic, Otocain)

benzocaine-antipyrine (Allergen Ear Drops, Auralgan Otic, Auralgan✷)

MECHANISM OF ACTION

Otic anesthetics temporarily stabilize neuronal membranes by blocking activation of voltage-gated sodium channels. Depolarization of the neuronal membrane is inhibited, thereby blocking the initiation and conduction of nerve impulses and sensitivity to pain.

USES

Otic anesthetics contain benzocaine and are used for the relief of pain and pruritus associated with the acute congestion of serous and external otitis. Otic anesthetics have no effect on microorganisms or inflammation.

PHARMACOKINETICS

Much like the other otic drugs, topical anesthetics must come in direct contact with ear tissue to be effective. Normal pharmacokinetics do not apply to topical local anesthetics because they are not designed for absorption, distribution, or biotransformation.

ADVERSE EFFECTS AND CONTRAINDICATIONS

Benzocaine may mask the symptoms of fulminating infection of the middle ear if it is used indiscriminately. Rarely, methemoglobinemia may result from the use of otic benzocaine. This condition causes respiratory distress and cyanosis. As with other otic drugs, anesthetics are not given to patients who have a perforated tympanic membrane.

INTERACTIONS

Benzocaine antagonizes the antibacterial activity of sulfonamides; therefore these drugs should not be administered together. When both benzocaine and sulfonamides must be used, the potential drug interaction is prevented if benzocaine preparations are instilled in the ear to achieve anesthesia first. The benzocaine is then removed before the administration of the sulfonamide.

PATHOPHYSIOLOGY • Cerumen Impaction

Cerumen, or earwax, is a normal sebaceous gland secretion functioning to protect and lubricate the canal. The primary purpose for cerumen is to gather bacteria and debris for removal. Normally, when the external ear canal gets wet and drains, cerumen is eliminated. Various factors lead to insufficient elimination of cerumen, which may cause the cerumen to become impacted in the canal.

Patients with cerumen impaction may have no symptoms or may complain of a sensation of fullness in the ear with or without associated conductive hearing loss. Complaints of pain, itching, or bleeding from the ear are also common. Treatment requires removal of the impacted cerumen by irrigation with warm water. If the impaction is resistant to irrigation, commercially prepared ceruminolytics can be used to soften the cerumen for ease of removal.

DRUG CLASS • Ceruminolytics

carbamide peroxide (Auro Ear Drops, Otix Drops, others)

trolamine, polypeptide oleate, and condensate (Cerumenex)

MECHANISM OF ACTION

Ceruminolytics contain glycerin to soften cerumen and carbamide peroxide to loosen debris by effervescence of oxygen. These agents emulsify and disperse excess or impacted cerumen.

USES

Ceruminolytic drugs help soften cerumen for removal to avoid painful instrumentation with a metal curette. Cerumen removal may be necessary for otoscopic examination, audiometry, and tympanometry as well as when the patient experiences discomfort or hearing loss caused by excessive or dry cerumen. Additionally, cerumen solvents provide antiseptic protection.

PHARMACOKINETICS

Normal pharmacokinetics do not apply to cerumen solvents, because they are not designed for absorption, distribution, or biotransformation. The drug is placed directly on the affected tissue and is then mechanically removed using warm water irrigation.

ADVERSE REACTIONS AND CONTRAINDICATIONS

Ceruminolytics are irritating and may cause allergic reactions, especially with prolonged exposure. If the patient has excessive irritation, adequate softening of cerumen may often be achieved with plain anhydrous glycerin followed by flushing with plain warm water. The friability of older skin, especially of the external canal, may contribute to a greater likelihood of contact dermatitis in older adults. Ceruminolytics are not used in patients with a perforated tympanic membrane.

PATHOPHYSIOLOGY • Ototoxicity

When inner ear structures or the auditory nerve (cranial nerve VIII) are damaged by drug therapies, the drugs are considered ototoxic. Damage occurs as different structures are affected. A variety of mechanisms, including toxic levels of drugs in the perilymphatic fluid, may damage the hair cells in the organ of Corti. Additionally, drug therapy can change enzymatic activity in the inner ear, causing damage.

Topical or systemic drugs have the potential to produce ototoxicity. This toxicity occurs primarily when a given drug comes into direct contact with the inner ear structures. Therefore the chance of ototoxicity is lessened if the tympanic membrane is intact, preventing direct contact with the inner ear. Categories of systemically administered drugs known to be ototoxic include the aminoglycosides and other antibiotics, loop diuretics, antimalarial drugs, nonsteroidal antiinflammatory drugs, and some antineoplastic drugs (Table 66-2).

Symptoms of ototoxicity depend on the inner ear structure most affected. Tinnitus and sensorineural hearing loss are present with damage to the cochlea. Damage to the vestibular apparatus produces vertigo, ataxia, lightheadedness, headache, giddiness, inability to focus or fixate on images, nausea, vomiting, and cold sweats. Factors such as dosage, renal function, concomitant use of other ototoxic drugs or chemicals, inherent

TABLE 66-2

Impact of Ototoxic Substances on Auditory and Vestibular Function

Drug	Auditory Problems	Vestibular Problems	Drug	Auditory Problems	Vestibular Problems
Antibiotics			**Nonsteroidal Antiinflammatory Drugs**		
amikacin	XX	X	ibuprofen	X	X
chloramphenicol	X	X	indomethacin	X	None
erythromycin	X to XX	X	Salicylates	XX	None
gentamicin	XX	X	**Other Drugs**		
			alcohol	None	XX
kanamycin	XX	X	cisplatin	X	X
neomycin	XX	X	quinine	X	XX
streptomycin	XX	X			
tobramycin	XX	X			
Diuretics					
ethacrynic acid	XX	X			
furosemide	XX	X			

Adapted from Ignatavicius DD, Workman ML, Mishler MS: *Medical-surgical nursing: a nursing process approach*, ed 4, Philadelphia, 2002, Saunders.
X, Slight; *XX*, significant.

susceptibility, age, and exposure to high-intensity noise affect the ototoxicity of various drugs.

Hearing loss resulting from ototoxic drugs can be transient or permanent, unilateral or bilateral, and related or unrelated to dosage. In addition to auditory function tests, monitoring of renal function is essential for patients treated with ototoxic drugs that are eliminated unchanged in the urine (e.g., aminoglycosides). With these drugs, renal function tests are indicators of drug clearance, and ototoxicity increases with decreased renal function. Older patients are especially prone to developing ototoxicity because of a normal age-related decline in renal function.

APPLICATION TO PRACTICE

ASSESSMENT
History of Present Illness

Patients with ear disorders require a comprehensive nursing history to determine problems, goals, and interventions appropriate for treatment. Ask the patient about bathing and swimming behaviors, recent trauma to the ear or head, and any changes in hygiene activities or products used in or around the ears (e.g., cotton swabs and bobby pins). Complaints of malaise, anorexia, and fatigue should be noted.

Health History

A health history summarizing the patient's overall physical condition should be completed. Elicit from the patient the dates and results of any audiometric or tympanography testing.

Ask specifically about the use of OTC or prescription drugs. Explore with the patient the use of any substances that may cause irritation to the skin. Allergies to drugs, foods, preservatives (e.g., benzethonium chloride, thimerosal, and sulfites), and hygiene products used in or near the ear should be elicited from the patient.

Concomitant diseases such as upper respiratory tract infections, head injury, and neurologic disorders should be identified. Otic disorders and cerumen impaction may cause hearing loss, dizziness, and ataxia similar to those caused by some severe neurologic disorders. Determine if the patient is pregnant or lactating. Few otic preparations have been studied in this population and are used only with caution.

Lifespan Considerations

Perinatal. As a general rule, the risk of otic disorders in the pregnant woman is no greater than that of the general population. However, systemic antibiotics should be used with caution because some are known to be teratogenic. For example, chloramphenicol readily crosses the placental membranes and may produce gray baby syndrome (i.e., fetal abdominal distention, drowsiness, low body temperature, cyanosis, hypotension, and respiratory distress). Any otic drug absorbed systemically has teratogenic potential.

Pediatrics. Children are more susceptible to disorders of the middle ear than to external otitis because of their relatively straight and short eustachian tubes. The eustachian tube can easily be blocked by the adenoid tissue in the nasopharynx, especially in conjunction with upper respiratory tract infections. The straight, short external canal of childhood makes children less susceptible to cerumen impaction than adults.

Generally, children diagnosed with otitis media are treated with systemic antibiotics. Most otic preparations are not recommended for infants younger than 1 year because of the danger of potential systemic absorption, which may hinder normal development.

In addition, infants who feed from a bottle while lying down are more likely to have pooling of fluids in their nasopharynx and eustachian tubes, resulting in a greater risk of serous otitis and otitis media. The most common use of otic drops in infants and children with serous otitis and otitis media is for the treatment of ear pain. Systemic antibiotic drugs are necessary to treat the otitis media.

Older Adults. The friability of older skin, especially of the ear canal, may contribute to a greater risk of contact dermatitis and systemic absorption of otic drugs. Stiffening of ear cilia combined with a higher keratin content of cerumen causes the cerumen to become impacted easily, decreasing the ability to hear. In addition, physiologic changes of aging may alter the manifestation of an otic disorder, causing the disorder to be overlooked.

Cultural/Social Considerations

Cerumen is naturally removed when the ear canal is washed out during showering. People who shower or wash their hair infrequently are more prone to cerumen impaction. Patients living in humid environments are more susceptible to ear infections. Prior diagnosis of external otitis increases the risk of recurrence. Sleeping patterns are often disrupted by ear disorders. Appropriate use of otic preparations just before bedtime may relieve discomfort and enhance sleeping patterns.

Physical Examination

The ear examination begins with an inspection and palpation of the external ear and mastoid, followed by an otoscopic visualization. Finally, signs of systemic infection such as fever are noted. Cerumen impaction is evident when the entire length of the external canal and the tympanic membrane cannot be visualized.

Laboratory Testing

Discharge from the external ear is rarely cultured. However, a culture and sensitivity test is performed in cases where initial therapy fails to produce a response. Additionally, audiometry testing with tympanometry may be performed to assess hearing and to determine movement potential of the tympanic membrane before long-term use of aminoglycosides or furosemide.

Should the health care provider suspect that inflammation and pain are associated with a systemic disorder, laboratory testing may include a complete blood count and sedimentation rate. Allergy testing can be performed to identify substances irritating to particular patients.

GOALS OF THERAPY

Treatment goals include relieving ear pain, reducing inflammation, and curing infection. To prevent further episodes of external otitis, the patient should use otic drying drugs to keep the external canal dry and to make it less likely to support organism growth. When cerumen impaction is the problem, the treatment goals are to soften and remove excess cerumen from the external canal, decrease conductive hearing loss, and improve comfort.

INTERVENTION
Administration

Otic drugs are instilled directly into the external canal. In cases where the external auditory canal is obstructed with edema, an earwick can be devised from a small piece of gauze and inserted beyond the edematous portion of the canal toward the tympanic membrane (Figure 66-2). Otic drops are applied to the outside portion of the gauze wick and are absorbed by the ear along the gauze in the depths of the canal. Because of the discomfort involved with insertion of an earwick, the gauze may be changed every 2 days. Generally, edema in the canal has subsided after 2 days, and the otic drug can then be administered directly to the ear canal. Following administration, a cotton pledget can be inserted into the canal to keep the solution from draining out.

Antibacterial and drying drugs are instilled in the external canal in a manner similar to that used for other otic

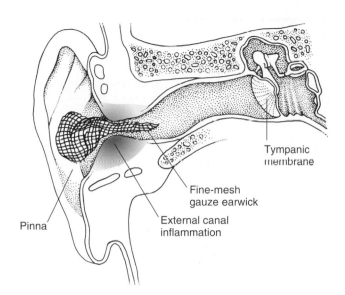

FIGURE 66-2   Earwick for instillation of antibiotics into the external canal. Otic solutions are placed on the external portion of the earwick to be absorbed through the canal. This is particularly helpful when the canal is blocked by edema. (From Ignatavicius DD, Workman ML, Mishler MS: *Medical-surgical nursing: a nursing process approach*, ed 4, Philadelphia, 2002, Saunders. Used with permission.)

drugs. Following use of these drugs, the ear canal is carefully dried with compressed air or a hair dryer on the cool or low-heat setting. The canal is not dried with a cotton swab. If cerumen has accumulated in the external canal, it is removed before applying the antibacterial solution.

Prolonged use of anesthetics may mask the signs and symptoms of a fulminating infection.

In the case of ceruminolytics, the ear canal is filled liberally and the solution allowed to remain in place for 15 to 30 minutes. The patient then repeatedly irrigates the external canal with warm water using an ear syringe (see Figure 66-2). The irrigation displaces and evacuates the cerumen from the external canal. The whole procedure can be repeated daily until the canal is cleared. In cases where cerumen is resistant to removal, the ceruminolytic agent is instilled in the evening and a cotton pledget is inserted, allowing the drug to remain in place overnight. The ear is then irrigated the next morning. Once the impaction has been cleared, the procedure may be repeated weekly to remove loose cerumen and to prevent development of future impaction.

Education

Handwashing and proper disposal of contaminated ear drainage may prevent spread to others. If the patient wears some form of ear device for employment (e.g., telephone earpiece or earplugs), the devices should be kept clean and free of debris. Ear devices should not be shared with other workers.

Teach patients the general principles of otic drug storage and administration. Solutions are kept tightly closed and are stored at 59° to 86° F. Administration of cold otic drugs causes nausea, vomiting, and ataxia. The patient is instructed to warm the container to body temperature passively by holding it in the hands for 5 to 10 minutes. Eardrops should never be warmed in a microwave oven.

Otic drugs are more easily administered by someone other than the patient. Family members or friends can be taught how to administer the drug. The person administering the eardrops should wash his or her hands thoroughly. Using one hand, straighten the ear canal by gently pulling the auricle down and back for children under 3 years of age, or upward and outward for children over 3 years and adults. Rest the hand holding the dropper about ½ inch above the ear canal. Instill the drops on the side of the ear canal, allowing them to flow in without falling directly on the tympanic membrane. Have the patient maintain a side-lying position for 2 to 3 minutes. Apply gentle pressure or massage the tragus with your finger. If drops are ordered for the other ear as well, wait 5 minutes and repeat this procedure. A cotton pledget may be inserted in the external canal to prevent the drug from leaking out.

If the dropper accidentally touches the ear, the dropper is wiped clean with a tissue before being replaced in the bottle. To prevent cross-contamination and infection, patients are cautioned not to share otic drugs with others. Proper disposal of contaminated ear drainage and soiled cotton pledgets prevents spread of infection to others. The patient and caregiver should be cautioned not to use otic solutions in the eyes.

Special teaching needs with regard to steroid and steroid-antibiotic combinations as well as anesthetics include advising the patient to limit the use of pain-controlling drugs only to when ear pain is present. Furthermore, patients are also cautioned against keeping drugs from previous illnesses and self-treating for recurrent ear problems. Patients should be advised that a change in the treatment regimen may be required if pain continues after 2 or 3 days of use.

Advise patients to monitor symptoms and to contact the health care provider if symptoms persist or worsen. It is not uncommon for ear discomfort to disrupt sleeping patterns. Appropriate use of otic drugs before retiring for the night may enhance sleeping patterns. Significant improvement is noted after 1 or 2 days of antibiotic therapy.

Patients should be instructed to avoid activities that might dilute or wash out an otic drug from the ear. Such activities include showering without proper ear protection and swimming with the head exposed to water. Ideally,

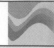

CASE STUDY   *Bilateral Otitis Media*

ASSESSMENT

HISTORY OF PRESENT ILLNESS

CC is 3 years old. She comes to the clinic today accompanied by her mother with complaints of fever, congestion with runny eyes and nose, noisy breathing at night, and irritable behavior.

HEALTH HISTORY

CC was born 5 weeks prematurely, weighing 6 pounds, 14 ounces. Her APGAR scores were 8 and 9. She was transferred to a special care nursery 12 hours after birth and placed on a ventilator for 2 days for episodes of apnea and bradycardia; she was also given a course of antibiotics (mother does not remember the name of the drug). CC was discharged home with an apnea monitor, which she used for 5 months. She had several colds the first 6 months after birth and began to have multiple episodes of otitis media when placed in a day care situation. She was seen seven times between the ages of 6 and 18 months for ear infections and used six different antibiotics (amoxicillin, cefaclor, cefixime, Augmentin, cefprozil, and Bactrim). At age 2½ years, she had bilateral myringotomy tubes placed and has had two documented cases of otitis media since that time. CC continues to have frequent colds and congestion, and the question of allergies has been raised. The family practice doctor has referred CC to an ear, nose, and throat (ENT) doctor for possible tonsillectomy and adenoidectomy.

CC's father and mother are in good health. The father has a history of "sensitive skin" and has recurrent boils and dry skin conditions. He is allergic to bromide in swimming pools. The paternal grandfather has a history of cerebrovascular accident, hypertension, and colorectal cancer. The maternal grandmother has a history of diabetes, emphysema, and depression.

LIFESPAN CONSIDERATIONS

CC is in preschool. Her school has a full-time nurse.

CULTURAL/SOCIAL CONSIDERATIONS

CC lives with her parents, two cats, and one dog. Both parents smoke, as do several of their close friends. CC also vis-

its her maternal aunt and uncle frequently, and they both smoke. CC goes to a day care center because both parents work. The father is a house painter, and the mother manages a liquor store. The parents own their own home, and CC has her own room.

PHYSICAL EXAMINATION

CC's blood pressure is 78/40 mm Hg; temperature 100.8° F; respirations 26; pulse 96. Cervical lymphadenopathy is present. Tonsils 3+, no exudate; clear nasal discharge, mouth breathing. Tympanic membranes red, tubes in place bilaterally draining pus; tympanogram flat. No other significant findings.

LABORATORY TESTING

Consider audiometric testing and repeat tympanometry if problem persists.

PATIENT PROBLEM(S)

Bilateral otitis media.

GOALS OF THERAPY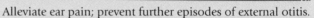

Alleviate ear pain; prevent further episodes of external otitis.

CRITICAL THINKING QUESTIONS

1. What additional information should you gather in planning care for this child?
2. What is the likely bacterium or virus causing CC's otitis media?
3. What elements in CC's history and physical examination might explain her apparent susceptibility to ear infections?
4. What problems can you identify that need nursing intervention?
5. What antibiotic would be warranted to treat CC's otitis media? Why is this the appropriate drug?
6. What other pharmacologic and nonpharmacologic interventions might be ordered?
7. What points need to be covered in the education plan for the parents? What reasons should be cited for following up on CC's treatment?

antibacterial and drying drugs are used upon rising, at bedtime, and after bathing, swimming, or circumstances when the ear has been exposed to added moisture.

Patients having problems with cerumen should be taught about the normal production, function, and elimination of cerumen. Teach also about nonpharmacologic means for the removal of cerumen from the canal. Allowing warm water from a shower to run in the ear and using a clean towel to wipe out the larger ear structures daily is effective.

Teach patients about the potential for hearing loss associated with impaction. If there has been a recent change in hearing associated with the impaction, the patient can expect hearing to improve markedly with removal of the impacted cerumen. If hearing does not return, the patient is instructed to contact a health care provider to have additional hearing testing and tympanometry conducted.

Several commercial preparations are available to soften cerumen. Advise patients with known sensitivity to any topical drug to use ceruminolytics with caution to avoid possible irritation. Thorough teaching about alternate methods for cerumen removal and ways to prevent impaction is important. Anhydrous glycerin is very inexpensive and when used over several days can be as effective as other ceruminolytic products. The cost of different products varies but all are relatively inexpensive.

EVALUATION

Evaluation involves determining the efficacy of the otic preparation. When the drugs are effective, the patient no longer complains of pain, edema, itching, or sensorial or perceptual alterations. Effectiveness of antibacterial and drying drugs is noted when external otitis does not recur.

The effectiveness of ceruminolytics is demonstrated when there are no further complaints of discomfort or hearing loss and when removal of cerumen has been successful. When hearing loss persists after other signs and symptoms are resolved, audiology testing with tympanometry may be performed. Decreased movement of the tympanic membrane indicates conductive hearing loss, which requires additional diagnosis and corrective measures to restore hearing.

Bibliography

Bates DE, Beaumont SJ, Baylis BW: Ototoxicity induced by gentamicin and furosemide, *Ann Pharmacother* 36(3):446-451, 2002.

Fitzgerald MA: Acute otitis media in an era of drug resistance: implications for NP practice, *Nurse Pract* 24(suppl 10):10-14, 1999.

Kujdych N: Prescribing trends in the treatment of acute otitis media. Reining in resistant bacteria, *Adv Nurse Pract* 7(10): 30-35, 1999.

La Rosa S: Primary care management of otitis externa, *Nurse Pract* 23(6):125-128, 131-133, 1998.

Melnyk BM, Herendeen PM: Inside and out. The latest on otitis media and otitis externa, *Adv Nurse Pract* 6(8):36-38, 43-45, 1998.

Montville NH, White MA: Diagnosis and pharmacological management of acute otitis media. *Pediatr Nurs* 24(5):423-429, 1998.

Newell P, Churchill E: Chronic otitis media in children. Helping families cope, *Adv Nurse Pract* 8(1):55-56, 80, 2000.

Palomar GV, Abdulghani MF, Bodet AE, et al: AV: Drug-induced ototoxicity: current status, *Acta Otolaryngol* 121(5):569-572, 2001.

Tigges BB: Acute otitis media and pneumococcal resistance: making judicious management decisions, *Nurse Pract* 25(1): 69, 73-80, 85, 2000.

Internet Resource

http://www.kidshealth.org/parent/common/otitis_media.html.

Dermatologic Drugs

SHERRY F. QUEENER • ELIZABETH KISSELL

 Visit http://evolve.elsevier.com/Gutierrez/ for additional information.

KEY TERMS

OBJECTIVES

- Discuss the structure of skin and its physiologic role.
- Identify the goal of acne therapy.
- Explain the uses and limitations of antimicrobial drugs used topically.
- Summarize points about topical treatment of genital warts that the nurse should discuss with the patient.
- Develop a nursing care plan for a patient using a topical dermatologic drug.

The skin has been described as the largest organ in the body. It covers the body's surface and acts as a shield from the environment. Skin diseases are one of the most common concerns that arise in the health care setting.

For most diseases, drugs are administered at a site that is distant from the target organ; however, in dermatology, drugs can be directly applied to the site. Topical therapy can be used to restore skin hydration, reduce inflammation, protect the skin, reduce scales and calluses, cleanse and debride, and eradicate microorganisms. Some skin problems, such as burns and decubitus ulcers, take extensive, aggressive intervention to resolve.

PHYSIOLOGY • Structure and Function of Skin

The skin is composed of three distinct layers: the epidermis, the dermis, and subcutaneous tissue (Figure 67-1). Skin appendages such as the hair and nails make up a fourth component.

The **epidermis**, the outer layer of the skin, is composed almost entirely of closely packed cells. Its primary function is to retard the loss of fluids from the inner body to the outside environment. It also acts as a barrier against the entry of foreign substances.

Four distinct cellular layers make up the epidermis: the basal layer, stratum spinosum, stratum granulosum, and the stratum corneum. Cell division occurs in the basal layer, the deepest layer, which is the only place where epidermal cells are mitotically active. All

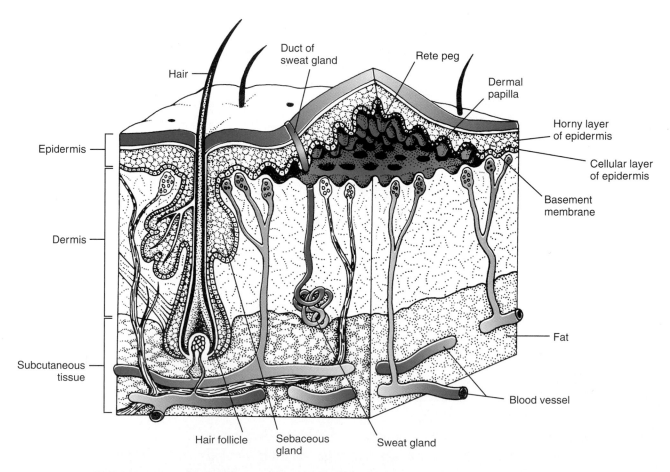

FIGURE 67-1 The anatomy of the skin includes the three growth layers of the epidermis and other structures. (From Ignatavicius DD, Workman ML, and Mishler MS: *Medical-surgical nursing: a nursing process approach,* ed 4, Philadelphia, 2002, Saunders. Used with permission.)

cells of the epidermis arise from this layer. The epidermis has no direct blood supply of its own, relying on diffusion for its nutrition. It normally takes 3 to 4 weeks for the epidermis to produce new cells and push older cells outward.

Above the basal layer is the stratum spinosum. This cellular layer is called spinous because of the delicate spinelike processes projecting from its surfaces. The stratum spinosum absorbs water. Water absorption is readily seen when the skin of the palms and the soles become white and swollen during bathing.

During the ascent upward through the epidermal layers, the **keratinocytes** (the cells of the epidermis that synthesize **keratin**, a protein with strong mechanical properties) become smaller and flatter. As they near the skin surface, they die. In the granular cell layer, the stratum granulosum and keratinocytes differentiate to cornified cells.

Cells of the **stratum corneum**, the fourth layer, are large, flattened, polyhedron-shaped cells filled with keratin. They are stacked vertically, producing a tightly packed, semi-impermeable layer that forms the major physical barrier of the skin. Through a process that is not completely understood, the stratum corneum undergoes continuous exfoliation (i.e., shedding), whereby dead cells on the surface are lost.

The skin has the lowest water permeability of any biologic membrane, but the skin is not an absolute barrier to all transport. Thus, transdermal absorption of certain lipid-soluble compounds is possible; this route is used for several important drugs (Box 67-1).

Three other important cell types are located in the epidermis: melanocytes, Langerhans cells, and Merkel cells. **Melanocytes**, found primarily in the basal layer, produce melanin and transfer it to keratinocytes, where it is deposited over the surface of the nucleus on the side of the cell facing the sun. The difference in skin pigmentation depends mostly on the activity level of the melanocytes rather than on the number, size, and dispersion of the cells in the skin.

Langerhans cells serve as the first-line immunologic defense, protecting against environmental antigens by migrating to lymph nodes, where they contribute to the uptake, processing, and presentation of a foreign substance to T lymphocytes.

Merkel cells are considered touch receptors. They are thought to detect mechanical deformities of the epidermis and to regulate epithelial proliferation. Unlike melanocytes and Langerhans cells, Merkel cells do not shed under normal circumstances.

The **dermis** lies beneath the epidermis, is composed largely of collagen, and is approximately 40 times thicker than the epidermis. Collagen fibers, the most abundant protein in the body, constitute about 70% of the dry weight of the whole dermis. Most importantly, this layer contributes to the support and nourishment of the epidermis. The basement membrane links the epidermis with the dermis. This membrane along with elastic and reticular fibers comprises the dermal matrix. Reticular fibers are overabundant in certain pathologic conditions such as granulomas and tumors.

BOX 67-1   **Factors Influencing Absorption of Drugs through the Skin**

Several factors influence transdermal absorption of drugs. Drug penetration and absorption are increased by as much as 10% with hydration of the stratum corneum. Hydration causes the cells to swell, decreasing their density and thus their resistance to diffusion. High ambient humidity increases hydration of the skin, as do certain drug formulations. Occlusion under impermeable plastic film enhances drug absorption by preventing transepidermal water loss and increasing epidermal hydration. Furthermore, the more occlusive the formulation (e.g., emulsions, ointments) the greater the permeability. The low solubility of some formulations limits drug concentration and reduces the rate of absorption.

Because absorption of topical drugs occurs by passive diffusion, higher drug concentrations increase the amount of the drug absorbed. Absorption from abraded or damaged skin surfaces is also much greater than that from intact skin and when drugs are left in place for prolonged periods.

Mucous membranes, facial skin, and intertriginous areas are sites of enhanced drug penetration and often toxicity because of the thinness of the stratum corneum at these sites. In addition, hair follicles and sweat ducts provide epidermal fenestrations that provide limited but low-resistance pathways for drug penetration.

Topical absorption from areas with thick skin (e.g., the palms of the hand and the soles of the feet) is relatively slow. Peak rates are not achieved for 12 to 24 hours. However, large fluctuations in plasma concentrations and increased first-pass effects commonly seen with some orally administered drugs can sometimes be avoided with transdermal administration. The use of topical rather than systemic drugs also may improve the therapeutic index of many compounds and enhance patient compliance.

Three groups of mesodermal cells exist in the dermis. Of these, the reticulohistiocytic group, consisting of histiocytes and mast cells, are linked to many skin diseases such as atopic and contact dermatitis as well as lichen planus. The myeloid groups of cells are the origin of various dermatoses, especially those caused by allergies. The cells of the lymphoid group contribute to inflammatory lesions of the skin. Myeloid and lymphoid groups of cells also exist in specific neoplasms of the skin.

Other structures found in the dermis include nerves, blood vessels, the sebaceous glands, and hair follicles (also called the pilosebaceous apparatus), and the eccrine and apocrine glands. Apocrine glands open into hair follicles and are found in the axillae, breast areas, and genital organs. Bacteria grow on their secretions and yield characteristic body odors. Fungal infections are the most common disorders of the pilosebaceous apparatus. Eccrine glands (sweat glands) are widely distributed over much of the body but are found predominantly on the palms of the hands and the soles of the feet. The eccrine glands help regulate body temperature and protect against excessive dryness.

Sebaceous glands are large fat-containing cells that produce sebum. Sebum is an oily substance that lubricates and protects the skin so that the skin is not only water repellent but also antiseptic. Normal skin pH is 4.5 to 5.5. This acid pH provides a protective mechanism because microorganisms grow best at a pH of 6 to 7.5. Stimulation of the sebaceous glands by a surge of androgenic hormones is a contributing factor in the development of acne.

Sensory nerves direct tactile sensations such as heat, touch, pressure, and pain from the skin to the brain. Motor nerves, part of the involuntary sympathetic nervous system, control the sweat glands, smooth muscles of the skin, and arterioles.

The arterioles help control temperature and provide nutrition to the skin. Temperature regulation is achieved via pathways located in the papillary dermis. By conducting heat from internal structures to the skin surface, heat is removed from the body. Arteriolar circulation carries nutrients to the skin.

A layer of **subcutaneous** tissue, largely made up of fat, lies beneath the dermis. This layer insulates the body from cold, cushions deep tissues from trauma, and serves as a reserve source of calories.

PATHOPHYSIOLOGY • Skin Disorders

NONINFECTIOUS INFLAMMATORY DERMATOSES

Dermatitis and eczema are noninfectious inflammatory dermatoses. Dermatitis is a general term denoting an inflammation of the skin caused by exogenous irritants, allergens, or trauma. The term eczema is often used as a synonym for endogenous dermatitis. Regardless of the cause, erythema, vesicle formation, edema, oozing, excoriation, crusting, and scaling usually characterize dermatitis. With chronic scratching, the tissues become thickened (a process called lichenification).

Atopic dermatitis, also called atopic eczema, is a pruritic dermatosis. People with atopy tend to develop pruritus under stress. Among patients with this disease, 40% to 65% have a family history of hay fever or asthma with a hereditary predisposition to a lowered cutaneous threshold to pruritus. Most react to common food and inhaled allergens by producing immunoglobin E (IgE) antibodies. In adults, the dermatitis may be a response to harsh chemicals or scratching; lesions are most often noted on the forehead, wrists, feet, and sides of the neck. There may be lichenification on flexor surfaces with continued scratching and rubbing. Lesions in infants and children are found primarily on the cheeks and extensor surfaces of the antecubital or popliteal surfaces.

Contact dermatitis is a rash resulting from contact between an allergen and the skin. It is a form of allergic, exogenous dermatitis and may be caused by chemical or mechanical irritation. Common substances that produce contact dermatitis include plants (e.g., poison ivy), jewelry that contains nickel, adhesive tape, shoe leather, elastic, rubber, cosmetics, and perfumes. Contact dermatitis has clinical symptoms that include red, thick, crusty, fissured, suppurating areas in various stages. The affected areas are those in direct contact with the offending substance.

Seborrheic dermatitis affects hairy areas, often appearing on the scalp, eyebrows, ears, or sternum. The skin becomes red, scaly, and greasy in appearance, and it often itches. Untreated patients may excoriate the skin by scratching, thus allowing a secondary infection to develop. In babies, scalp seborrhea is often called cradle cap. In the adult, mild seborrhea may appear as dandruff. Patients with AIDS or parkinsonism may develop especially prominent seborrhea.

Urticaria (hives) is an IgE-mediated allergic response to external agents (e.g., insect bites) or to internal allergens (i.e., food allergies) that reach the skin through the bloodstream. The characteristic lesion of urticaria is itchy and edematous and has an erythematous wheal with a pallid center. The lesions typically blanch with pressure. Urticaria occurs in about 15% to 20% of the population. It is usually self-limiting but may also become chronic. Chronic urticaria appears as a large hive without the sensation of itching. It is often accompanied by angioedema.

Psoriasis is a chronic, papulosquamous disorder that alters the appearance of the epidermis by increasing its thickness. It follows an erratic course. The primary defect is an accelerated maturation of the epidermis. Instead of turning over every 26 to 28 days, epidermal cells complete their growth cycle in less than 7 days. Symmetric patches appear on extensor surfaces, knees, elbows, buttocks, or on the scalp. Initial papules coalesce into red plaques. Both papules and plaques are covered with silvery scales that may be pruritic. The nails often become thick, irregular, and exhibit pits of 1 mm or less. Removal of the scales frequently leaves fine bleeding points called Auspitz's sign.

Pityriasis rosea is also a papulosquamous disease but is self-limited. It initially appears as a single oval salmon-colored patch (called a herald patch) covered with scales 2 to 10 cm in diameter. The major patches appear on the trunk, following the cleavage lines of the skin. Smaller patches appear on peripheral areas. It occurs predominantly in female patients between the ages of 10 to 35 years. Seasonal onset is typical during fall and spring.

Lichen planus, another papulosquamous disease, produces lesions that are 2 to 8 mm in size, are flat and purple, and have borders that are polygonal. The surface of the lesions is crisscrossed with white or silver lines called Wickham's striae. The lesions first appear on the flexor surfaces of the wrists and forearm, the legs above the ankles, the sacral area, the penis, or the mucous membranes. The onset of the disease occurs between the ages of 30 and 70 years.

INFECTIOUS INFLAMMATORY DERMATOSES

Bacterial infections of the skin are most often caused by streptococcal or staphylococcal invasion of the skin where the barrier function has been compromised by trauma or inflammation. Organisms may be introduced below the epidermis by wounds or disturbances in normal anatomy (e.g., hair follicle or hangnail). Virulence of the organisms and host immune factors combine to determine the occurrence and extent of an infection.

Cellulitis is characterized by tenderness, edema, and erythema that spread to subcutaneous tissues. Erysipelas is a form of cellulitis caused by group A *Streptococcus pyogenes*. The visible signs include round or oval patches on the skin that promptly enlarge and spread, becoming swollen, tender, and red. The affected skin is hot to the touch, and the adjacent skin occasionally blisters. Sys-

temic manifestations such as headache, malaise, fever, chills, vomiting, and complete prostration can occur.

Folliculitis is an infection of hair follicles. It most often occurs on the scalp or the bearded areas of the face.

Furuncles (boils) and carbuncles (clusters of boils) are usually caused by *Staphylococcus aureus*. They are often a symptom of poor health. Furuncles tend to recur, resulting from infection of hair follicles. They usually appear on the neck, face, axillae, buttocks, thighs, and perineum. Carbuncles involve multiple hair follicles with pustules. Similar to furuncles, carbuncles are caused by pus-forming bacteria. Systemic manifestations may include malaise, fever, leukocytosis, and bacteremia. Scar tissue is formed with healing.

Acne vulgaris is a skin disorder commonly found in 30% to 85% of adolescents and young adults. The lesions usually appear on the face, neck, chest, shoulders, and back. Open comedones are the most common lesions of mild acne. A comedo forms when sebum combines with keratin to form a plug within a skin pore. Oxidation causes the exposed surface of the sebum plug to turn black, hence the term blackhead. Closed comedones, known often as whiteheads, develop when pores fill below the skin surface with sebum and scales. In its most severe form, acne is characterized by abscesses and inflammatory cysts (Box 67-2).

Acne is stimulated by the increased production of androgens during adolescence. Under their influence, sebum production and the turnover of follicular epithelial cells increase, leading to plugging of the pores. Symptoms are exacerbated by the activity of *Propionibacterium acnes*, an organism that converts sebum into irritating fatty acids. The bacterium releases chemotactic factors that promote inflammation. Oily skin, hormonal changes, and a genetic predisposition are additional contributing factors.

Impetigo is a superficial skin infection that is highly contagious and usually found on exposed skin surfaces in children. It is caused by group A *Streptococcus pyogenes*, *Staphylococcus aureus*, or both. It is common to find the disease in adolescents who are involved in wrestling activities because the microorganisms seem to reside on the wrestling mats. The lesions appear as rapidly crusting clear vesicles 2 or 3 mm to 2 cm in diameter. The honey-colored crusts are moist and oozing. If the crusts are removed, the base is red and eroded.

Fungal infections of the hair, skin, and nails are a major source of morbidity throughout the world. It has been estimated that fungal infections account for 5% of new outpatient referrals to dermatologists in temperate climates and as much as 20% in tropical climates. Most of the infections are caused by either dermatophytes or yeasts, most commonly the *Candida* species.

Tinea (ringworm) is a superficial infection in which the fungus lives on the dead, horny layer of the skin. It

BOX 67-2   **Acne Vulgaris**

Acne vulgaris is classified as follows: grade I acne includes primarily sparse comedones; grade II acne is characterized by comedones, papules, and occasional pustules; in grade III acne, there is a predominance of papules and pustules with small cysts; and with grade IV acne, there are overt signs of cystic acne. Treatment regimens vary with the grade.

Treatment of Grade I Acne

Treatment of grade I acne consists of removing excess sebum from the skin by washing and promoting the production and turnover of new skin to prevent closure of the pilosebaceous orifices of the hair follicle. The skin should be washed with warm water, mild soap, and a soft washcloth, no more than three times daily. The washing and rubbing produce some drying and peeling of the skin. Closure of the pilosebaceous orifices can be prevented by the topical application of mildly irritating agents, which promote desquamation (peeling) and stimulate growth of new skin cells.

Desquamating drugs available in OTC form include sulfur (2% to 10%), resorcinol (1% to 4%), and salicylic acid (0.5% to 2%). Resorcinol and salicylic acid often appear in alcoholic solutions that dry quickly and do not leave a visible film. Some products contain all three drugs. Dosage forms of these drugs include creams, lotions, gels, and liquids. Ointment bases tend to be greasy and messy. Some soaps include desquamating agents, but this formulation is irrational because rinsing and drying remove the agents from the skin.

Benzoyl peroxide is a stronger irritant and desquamating agent than is sulfur, resorcinol, or salicylic acid. Used in concentrations of 5% to 10%, it generally produces mild stinging and warming of the skin. For mild acne, benzoyl peroxide is probably no more effective than the OTC desquamating drugs and should be used only after the milder irritants and faithful adherence to a regular skin-washing schedule have been unsuccessful. Benzoyl peroxide is highly irritating and should not contact the eyelids, neck, or lips. Its use should be discontinued if severe and prolonged stinging or irritation occurs.

Alternative therapy is tretinoin (Retin-A) or adapalene (Differin) applied topically after washing the skin.

Treatment of Grade II and Grade III Acne

Treatment may include those drugs used for grade I acne. In addition, topical clindamycin (Cleocin T), topical erythromycin (Akne-Mycin, Emgel, Erycette, Erygel), or topical erythromycin with benzoyl peroxide (Benzamycin) may be indicated. If the condition continues to worsen, oral antibiotics such as tetracycline, minocycline, doxycycline, or erythromycin may be used.

Treatment of Grade IV Acne

All strategies noted for grade III acne should be tried before moving to oral isotretinoin (Accutane). Although often effective, this drug carries significant adverse reactions common with retinoids (see Chapter 63) and is extremely teratogenic.

---

causes the skin to scale and disintegrate, the nails to crumble, and hair to break off. Lesions often appear as scaly, erythematous, circular lesions. Tinea pedis refers to fungal infection of the feet (athlete's foot). It is transmitted through shared bathing facilities where warm, moist feet enhance fungal growth. Men are more commonly affected than women.

Tinea unguium (onychomycosis) is a fungal infection of toenails often seen in persons who have long-standing tinea pedis. The affected nails appear dull and thick. The distal edge becomes separated from the nail bed (onycholysis), causing a misshapen appearance. Fingernails may also become infected.

Tinea capitis is ringworm of the scalp. This highly contagious infection is common in children. A consistent sign is the broken-off hair "stub" that leads to patches of partial baldness.

Tinea cruris is a fungal infection of the groin; tinea corporis, infection of the body; tinea barbae, the beard;

and tinea manus, the hand. Tinea versicolor appears as a brown discoloration.

Candidiasis is an infection caused by the yeast *Candida albicans*. Predisposition to this infection occurs in people treated with antibiotics, women taking oral contraceptives, those who are on corticosteroid or antineoplastic therapies, babies and adults in diapers, and those who have weakened immune systems (e.g., diabetes mellitus, AIDS). *Candida* organisms have a predilection for warm, moist sites; thus intertriginous sites (skin folds), the mouth, and the vagina are common sites for infection. With candidal growth, the skin may be denuded, leaving a raw, glistening base. Red papules (satellite lesions) are scattered away from the margins of the raw areas. The presence of the scattered papules is useful in distinguishing candidiasis from tinea. The most prominent symptom of vaginal candidiasis is severe itching.

Viral infections commonly cause skin lesions. The symptoms may be caused by replication of the virus in the skin, by immune responses of the host, or both. Viral infections of the skin include herpes simplex, herpes zoster, varicella (chicken pox), verrucae, and other dermatoses.

Herpes simplex lesions appear as vesicles with an inflamed base. Primary infections have an incubation period of up to 2 weeks. Type I herpes infections involve the skin and oral cavity. Type II herpes infections most often involve the skin of neonates, which can lead to encephalitis. The genital mucosa is a common site for herpes infections. Herpes infections can also spread to the lungs and brain in immunocompromised individuals. Recurrent infection is due to either a reactivation of an older infection or a new infection.

Herpes zoster (shingles) is caused by reactivation of the chicken pox virus, varicella. The virus survives in a latent form in dorsal root ganglia. Unknown stimuli allow the virus to traverse down the axon to the skin, where vesicles appear in a dermatome distribution pattern. Pain, itching, or irritation precedes the skin eruption by 48 to 72 hours. The lesions begin with a red base, on which appears a small but enlarging clear vesicle. The vesicle becomes white and then yellow before rupturing. Fluid oozes to form a crust that may take 7 to 10 days to heal. Systemic symptoms may be present.

Verrucae (warts) are of various types. Verruca vulgaris is a viral infection of the hands and fingers. Verruca plantaris (plantar wart) is an inward growth on the sole of the foot. It may be covered by a callus or hyperkeratosis. Verrucae plana are flat warts located on the dorsum of the hands and face.

Condyloma acuminata (genital warts) are soft, skin-colored, fleshy warts caused by the human papilloma virus (HPV). There are at least 70 known types of HPV; only a handful are associated with condyloma acuminata. This virus affects a minimum of 10% to 20% of sexually active women. Studies in men suggest a similar prevalence. The incubation period may be from 1 to 6 months.

SKIN TRAUMA

Trauma can contribute to an infection when physical injury disrupts the integrity of the skin surface. Common wounds include lacerations (cuts or tears), abrasions (shearing or scraping of the skin), puncture wounds, surgical avulsions, traumatic amputations, incisions, and burns.

Burns are classified according to the depth of destruction. Superficial partial-thickness (first-degree) burns involve only the epidermis, are painful, and appear red or pink and dry. There are no blisters. An example of a superficial, partial-thickness burn is a mild sunburn.

Deeper partial-thickness (second-degree) burns involve the epidermis and parts of the dermis. These burns are red, moist, blistered, and painful. Mottling is often present with pink or red to waxy white areas with blisters

and edema. The entire epidermal and dermal layers are affected in a deep second-degree or partial-thickness burn. Sweat glands and hair follicles remain intact.

Full-thickness (third-degree) burn injuries are painless because nerve fibers are destroyed. The burns vary in color with much edema noted. The eschar is hard, dry, and leathery, but the wound leaks fluid from the underlying tissues.

A blackened, depressed, full-thickness burn involving muscle, fascia, and bone is classified as a fourth degree burn. Exposure of bones and ligaments is common. When bone is involved, the wound appears dull and dry.

DRUG REACTIONS

Drug reactions take on many forms and are caused by a variety of mechanisms. A rather common form is a fine, reddish, papular rash located over the trunk (or any part of the body). Among hospitalized patients, 10% experience at least one adverse drug reaction, and 5% must have an extended hospital stay as a result. Allergic manifestations to drugs may or may not result in specific antibody formation or sensitized lymphocytes. For this reason, the recognition of clinical manifestations of a drug reaction is of utmost importance. Adverse drug reactions that produce dermatologic signs are noted in Table 67-1.

STINGS, BITES, AND INFESTATIONS

The stings of bees, wasps, hornets, and yellow jackets are potential causes of skin lesions, and they are responsible for approximately 50 to 100 reported deaths per year. Most victims are younger than 20 years. Reactions are more frequent when stings occur around the head and neck, but reactions can occur from stings in other areas as well. Severe edema of the pharynx, epiglottis, and trachea is the major cause of death in hypersensitive individuals. Reactions may range in severity from transient redness, edema, and pain to acute anaphylactic shock (usually within 15 minutes). The peak reaction usually appears within 48 to 72 hours and lasts up to 7 days. Neurologic or vascular reactions as well as immune complex disease may also be seen.

Bites of mosquitoes, flies, and midges may cause local irritation and discomfort but are not usually directly life-threatening unless the insect is a disease vector, such as the *Aedes* mosquito, which carries malaria (see Chapter 34).

Ectoparasites are insects that live on the outer surface of the body. Strictly speaking, the term encompasses fungal infections of the skin as well as infestations by mites and lice. In practice, it refers only to mites and lice.

Scabies is a highly communicable disease caused by the itch mite, *Sarcoptes scabiei*. It is transmitted from one person to another by close contact. Transmission between bed partners is common and does not require body con-

TABLE 67-1		

Adverse Drug Reactions that Produce Dermatologic Symptoms

Common Drug-Induced Dermatologic Reactions		
Acneiform reactions	ACTH, androgens, bromides, corticosteroids, hydantoins, iodides, lithium, oral contraceptives, trimethadione	
Alopecia	Alkylating drugs, allopurinol, anticoagulants, antimetabolites, antithyroid drugs, colchicine, indomethacin, levodopa, norethindrone acetate, oral contraceptives, retinoids, trimethadione, vitamin A	
Contact dermatitis	bacitracin, benzocaine, benzoyl peroxide, chloramphenicol, chlorpromazine, ephedrine, formaldehyde, iodine, isoniazid, lanolin, meprobamate, neomycin, nitrofurazone, PABA, penicillin, phenol, streptomycin, sulfonamides, thiamine, thimerosol	
Photosensitivity	acetohexamide, amitriptyline, antimalarials, barbiturates, carbamazepine, doxycycline, gold salts, haloperidol, nortriptyline, oral contraceptives, phenytoin, phenothiazines, salicylates, sulfonamides, tetracyclines, thiazides, topical steroids, tricyclic antidepressants	
Purpura	ACTH, allopurinol, amitriptyline, anticoagulants, barbiturates, chloral hydrate, chlorpropamide, chlorpromazine, corticosteroids, gold salts, griseofulvin, iodides, meprobamate, penicillin, quinidine, rifampin, sulfonamides, thiazides, trifluoperazine	
Urticaria	ACTH, amitryptyline, barbiturates, beta-lactam antibiotics, chloramphenicol, dextran, erythromycin, griseofulvin, hydantoins, iodides, meperidine, meprobamate, nitrofurantoin, opioids, pentazocine, phenothiazines, salicylates, serums, streptomycin, sulfonamides, tetracyclines, thiouracil	
Life-Threatening, Drug-Induced Skin Eruptions		
Stevens-Johnson syndrome	barbiturates, beta-lactam antibiotics, carbamazepine, chloramphenicol, clindamycin, codeine, pentazocine, phenobarbital, phenytoin, sulfonamides, tetracyclines	
Exfoliative dermatitis	PAS, barbiturates, carbamazepine, chlorpropamide, demeclocycline, diphtheria vaccine, furosemide, gold salts, griseofulvin, isoniazid, isosorbide, measles vaccine, nitroglycerine, oral hypoglycemics, penicillins, phenothiazines, phenytoin, sulfonamides	
Lupus erythematosus	PAS, chlorpromazine, digitalis, ethosuximide, gold salts, griseofulvin, hydantoins, hydralazine, isoniazid, methyldopa, methysergide, oral contraceptives, phenobarbital, phenothiazines, primidone, prophylthiouracil, rifampin, thiazides, trimethadione	

ACTH, Adrenocorticotropic hormone; *PABA,* para-aminobenzoic acid; *PASA,* para-aminosalicylic acid.

tact. Infestation occurs most often in the sides of the fingers, interdigital webs, flexor surfaces of wrists, elbows, skin around the nipples, and penis. Other lesions, including erythematous papules, lichenified patches, and pustules, can occur on the abdomen, thighs, and buttocks. In infants and young children, the mites burrow in the palms and soles, and papular lesions may be seen on the scalp, face, and neck.

Pediculosis is an infestation of the body with lice. The incidence rate of infestation has been increasing in North America and Western Europe. It was once thought that overcrowding, poor hygiene, lack of laundry and bathing facilities, and general uncleanliness promoted the infestation. This assumption, however, has proven to be untrue. The infestation is transmitted from one person to another by close contact or through sharing of combs, clothing, or towels.

There are three varieties of infestation. Observation of nits or lice in the hair and scalp confirms the diagnosis of head lice (pediculosis capitis). They are found most often over the postauricular and occipital regions of the head. Nits attached to the seams of clothing, often in undergarments, indicate the presence of body lice (pediculosis corporis). Body lice are usually not found directly on the body. Nits or lice attached to pubic hairs indicate pubic lice (crabs; pediculosis pubis). Pubic infestations are found only in postpubertal individuals. Less commonly, lice are found on axillary hair, beards, mustaches, eyebrows, and eyelashes. Common signs and symptoms are pruritus with occasional sky-blue macules on the inner thighs or lower abdomen.

ULCERATIONS

An ulceration of the skin and subcutaneous tissue over or near a bony prominence is referred to as a **decubitus ulcer** (bedsore). Decubitus ulcers are caused by sustained pressure or friction of a body part resting against an external object. Other factors such as poor nutritional status, inadequate hydration, and a compromised immune response increase the risk of ulcer formation.

A decubitus ulcer reflects several pathophysiologic tissue changes. Obstruction of capillary blood flow by externally applied pressure causes tissue hypoxia (lack of oxygen to the tissue). An early sign of pressure is blanching erythema, an area of redness to the skin that turns white when pressed with a finger. Nonblanching erythema is a more serious sign of impaired blood supply to the tissues. Deeper, irreversible tissue damage is likely when hyperemia persists. Muscle damage can occur if ischemia persists for long periods. A cycle of cellular death and release of metabolic wastes into the surrounding tissues accompanies ischemia. Edema encroaches on interstitial spaces, slowing tissue perfusion and increasing hypoxia.

Decubitus ulcers are categorized by stages. A stage I ulcer involves only the superficial layer of skin. There is visible erythema that does not resolve within 30 minutes of pressure relief. Stage II ulcers involve loss of epidermis with possible penetration into, but not through, the dermis. The wound base is moist, pink, and painful. A stage III ulcer involves subcutaneous tissue, making a shallow crater. Deep tissue destruction extends through subcutaneous tissue to fascia, muscle layers, joints, or bone. Eschar, necrotic tissue, tunneling, exudate, and infection appear with stage III ulcers, but there is usually no pain. Stasis dermatitis often precedes a venous stasis ulcer and is found on the lower legs. There is a brown, eczematous appearance. Stasis ulcerations are often secondary to poor vasculature and venous stasis but may be confused with viral rashes.

DRUG CLASS • Antiseptics

benzoyl peroxide

chlorhexidine gluconate (Hibiclens)

hexachlorophene (pHisoHex)

hydrogen peroxide

isopropyl alcohol

povidone iodine (Betadine)

silver nitrate

zinc oxide

MECHANISM OF ACTION

Antiseptics are organic or inorganic preparations that kill or inhibit the growth of bacteria, fungi, and viruses; however, antiseptics are used primarily to prevent infections rather than to treat them. The term antiseptic generally refers to a preparation used on skin or mucous membranes. Disinfectants, in contrast, are preparations designed to kill microorganisms on equipment, surfaces, and other inanimate objects.

Vegetative forms of bacteria are most sensitive to antiseptics, followed by fungi, lipophilic viruses, tubercle bacilli, and hydrophilic viruses. Bacterial and fungal spores are resistant to most antiseptics. Peroxides act through oxidation-reduction processes to alter surface tension, thus increasing the permeability of the organism's cell wall and leakage of cell contents. These agents liberate oxygen when in contact with pus or organic substances.

Hexachlorophene is bacteriostatic against gram-positive bacteria but is relatively ineffective against gram-negative bacteria and fungi. Fungal and gram-negative organisms may actually increase in number with the chronic use of hexachlorophene preparations.

USES

The therapeutic index of an antiseptic is a crucial consideration because the drug must be considerably more toxic to surface pathogens than to adjacent living tissues. The chemicals used as antiseptics are in general too toxic to be used systemically and can only be used topically.

Alcohols may be used for cleansing intact skin before injections or surgical incisions. They are bactericidal to common bacteria but are less effective against viruses and fungi. When applied to the skin, alcohol kills approximately 90% of bacteria within 2 minutes if the area is kept moist for that period. When applied as a single swipe and left to evaporate, about 75% of bacteria are killed.

Peroxides are used for wound cleansing, cleansing of tracheostomy tubes; to remove cerumen from the external ear; as a mouthwash diluted with equal parts of water, saline, and commercial mouthwash; and in the treatment of acne vulgaris. Hydrogen peroxide is more effective as a debriding and cleansing agent than as an antiseptic. It is of doubtful value on intact skin. Benzoyl peroxide is bactericidal for anaerobic bacteria (e.g., *Corynebacterium*) and is often used in the treatment of acne vulgaris.

Chlorhexidine is used primarily as a skin cleanser to prevent the spread of microorganisms. It is generally effective against both gram-positive and gram-negative organisms. Some gram-negative organisms are resistant to this type of antiseptic.

Povidone-iodine is used in the prevention and treatment of infections of the skin, scalp, and mucous membranes of the mouth and vagina. It is effective against most bacteria, fungi, and viruses, but antiseptic activity depends on the concentration of iodine. When applied to the skin, a 1% solution kills approximately 90% of bacteria within 90 seconds.

Metallics are most often used in the treatment of burn wounds and for cauterizing warts or wounds. Zinc preparations may be used in the treatment of eczema, impetigo, tinea infections, venous stasis ulcers, pruritus, psoriasis, and seborrhea. In fact, zinc pyrithione is a common ingredient in OTC dandruff shampoos. Silver nitrate was once the drug of choice for preventing eye infections in newborns, but it has been generally replaced by a 0.5% erythromycin ointment (see Chapter 26).

Sulfur has fungicidal and keratolytic properties, and it may be used alone or in combination with other keratolytic drugs (e.g., coal tar, resorcinol, or salicylic acid). It is widely used in dermatology for the treatment of psoriasis, seborrhea, and dermatitis.

PHARMACOKINETICS

Antiseptics are not intended to be absorbed through the skin, although some (e.g., hexachlorophene) may be,

especially if used repeatedly. The intent of use of an antiseptic is to let it remain on the skin and rid the skin of potential pathogenic microorganisms.

ADVERSE REACTIONS AND CONTRAINDICATIONS

Adverse reactions to antiseptics vary with the specific drug; however, most are irritating to skin surfaces. In some cases, they interfere with the body's natural healing processes. Furthermore, most antiseptics are drying to the skin.

The American Medical Association recommends that hexachlorophene not be used routinely to bathe infants. It is heavily absorbed through broken skin or when applied excessively and has been shown to cause neurotoxicity.

 DRUG CLASS • Topical Antibacterial Drugs

bacitracin (Baci-IM, Baci-RX)

bacitracin zinc + polymyxin B sulfate (Polysporin)

bacitracin zinc + neomycin sulfate + polymyxin B sulfate (Neosporin)

benzoyl peroxide + clindamycin (BenzaClin)

benzoyl peroxide + erythromycin (Benzamycin)

mupirocin (Bactroban)

silver sulfadiazine (Thermazene, Silvadene, SSD)

MECHANISM OF ACTION

Bacitracin interferes with bacterial cell wall biosynthesis, but the drug is too toxic to be used systemically. Polymyxin B interferes with bacterial membrane integrity, and neomycin inhibits bacterial protein synthesis; these drugs are also too toxic for systemic use. Several drugs that have systemic applications can occasionally be used topically, e.g. clindamycin (see Chapter 30), erythromycin (see Chapter 26), and sulfadiazine (see Chapter 30). Benzoyl peroxide may be added for an additional antiseptic action; silver adds antibacterial action.

Mupirocin has a unique mechanism of action in that it binds bacterial isoleucyl-tRNA synthetase, the enzyme responsible for linking a required amino acid to a spe-

cific tRNA. Without isoleucyl-tRNA, bacterial protein synthesis halts or proceeds slowly, producing fatal errors.

USES

Mupirocin is used in infection control programs to eradicate the carrier state for methicillin-resistant *S. aureus*. By eliminating the organism from the nasal passages of healthy adult patients or health care workers in a health care facility, transmission to new patients can be interrupted. It is also used to treat impetigo caused by *S. aureus*, beta-hemolytic streptococci, and *S. pyogenes*. Mupirocin has been used to treat superficial skin infections, although it is not approved by the FDA for such use at this time.

The preparations containing bacitracin are used primarily to treat superficial skin infections. Formulations containing benzoyl peroxide are primarily used to treat acne. Silver sulfadiazine is an important topical drug to control infections in burns, including serious or deep burns. It penetrates burn eschar to exert antibacterial action against pseudomonads and many other organisms.

PHARMACOKINETICS

None of these drugs is intended to be systemically absorbed. In adults, only about 3% of the intranasal dose of mupirocin is absorbed systemically, but the drug cannot be used in neonates or premature infants, because they may absorb much more of the drug. Prolonged use of these drugs over extensive areas of heavily damaged skin may increase the risk of systemic absorption.

ADVERSE REACTIONS AND CONTRAINDICATIONS

Nearly all of the adverse reactions to mupirocin are local effects such as rhinitis, burning, stinging, and taste perversion. Headache, pharyngitis, and cough are also reported, but the incidence rate of all adverse reactions is less than 10%. The other preparations in this group commonly only cause local reactions.

INTERACTIONS

Mupirocin is incompatible with salicylic acid and should not be mixed in hydrophilic vehicles (e.g., Aquaphor) or coal tar solutions. Chloramphenicol may interfere with the bactericidal action of mupirocin.

 DRUG CLASS • Topical Antifungal Drugs

See Table 67-2.

Drugs for fungal infections are covered in Chapter 32. Some of the same drugs and their chemical relatives are also used topically for superficial fungal infections. These drugs are rarely absorbed through the skin and cause few adverse reactions other than local irritation (Table 67-2).

TABLE 67-2

Drugs to Treat Topical Fungal Infections

Generic Name	Brand Name	Comments
butenafine	Mentax	For athlete's foot. Avoid contact with eyes.
ciclopirox olamine	Loprox,* Penlac	For tinea infections. Avoid contact with eyes. Do not use occlusive dressing.
clotrimazole	Canesten, ✽ Lotrimin, Mycelex	For tinea or candidiasis. Avoid contact with eyes.
econazole	Ecostatin, ✽ Spectrazole	For mucocutaneous candidal or tinea infections. Avoid eyes; do not use occlusive dressing.
griseofulvin	Fulvicin,* Grifulvin, Grisactin	Oral medication for tinea infections. Side effects include headaches and gastrointestinal disturbances.
ketoconazole	Nizoral	For tinea and cutaneous candidal infections. Avoid contact with eyes.
miconazole nitrate	Micatin*	For dermatophytoses. Local irritation occurs. Avoid contact with eyes
naftitine	Naftin*	For tinea infections. Local irritation may occur. Avoid contact with eyes or mucous membranes.
natamycin	Natacyn	For fungal blepharitis, conjunctivitis, or keratitis. Eye irritation may occur with this chemical relative of amphotericin B.
nystatin	Mycostatin,* Nilstat,* Nystex	For candidal infections of skin. Skin irritation may occur.
oxiconazole	Oxistat	For tinea infections. Rash or burning may occur.
sulconazole	Exelderm	For tinea infections. May not be effective for athlete's foot.
terbinafine	Lamisil	For tinea infections. Rarely causes irritation or sensitization.

*Available in Canada and the United States.
✽Available only in Canada.

DRUG CLASS   •   Systemic Antifungals for Fungal Skin Infections

griseofulvin (Fulvicin, Grisactin)

terbinafine (Lamisil)

MECHANISM OF ACTION

Griseofulvin interferes with mitotic spindle formation in fungal cells, causing arrest of cell growth. Terbinafine inhibits ergosterol biosynthesis by a different mechanism than the azole antifungal drugs, but the effect is the same: the drug disrupts fungal cell membranes and kills affected fungi.

USES

Griseofulvin is effective against several types of dermatophytic infections, including infections of the scalp. Terbinafine is used orally for fungal infections of the nails and nail beds.

PHARMACOKINETICS

Griseofulvin is used orally rather than topically. The usefulness of this drug as an oral agent depends on its ability to localize in the skin after oral absorption. Skin cells containing high concentrations of griseofulvin are resistant to infection by dermatophytes. Ultimately, all infected cells are lost through the natural sloughing off of skin cells, and the disease is cured. This process takes considerable time, and thus griseofulvin therapy may need to be continued for several weeks or months, depending on the site and severity of the infection.

Terbinafine is well absorbed orally with or without food. Because it is highly lipophilic, terbinafine distributes well to tissues, especially to the skin, hair follicles, and nail beds. The drug is readily biotransformed in the liver to inactive forms eliminated primarily in urine. Despite relatively effective elimination processes, terbinafine persists in tissues for prolonged periods as a result of its high lipid solubility.

ADVERSE REACTIONS AND CONTRAINDICATIONS

Griseofulvin may cause headache or, less commonly, GI distress, insomnia, and fatigue.

Terbinafine commonly causes anorexia, diarrhea, nausea, stomach pain, and vomiting. The drug may also change the sensation of taste. Allergies are possible, and these may rarely be severe, including life-threatening conditions such as Stevens-Johnson syndrome. Terbinafine should be used cautiously, if at all, in patients with a history of alcoholism or hepatic impairment. These patients may be at increased risk of terbinafine-induced hepatotoxicity. Patients with renal impairment may require reduced dosage of the drug.

INTERACTIONS

Griseofulvin may stimulate biotransformation of anticoagulants such as warfarin or of oral contraceptives; the effects of these drugs is then diminished.

Terbinafine should not be used along with other hepatotoxic drugs. Therefore patients taking terbinafine should avoid the use of alcohol or high dosages of vitamin A or niacin. Other drugs to avoid include steroids, sulfonamides, phenothiazines, or zidovudine.

DRUG CLASS   •   Topical Antiviral Drugs

acyclovir (Zovirax)

imiquimod (Aldara)

podofilox (Condylox)

Imiquimod and podofilox are new drugs intended for use topically against genital warts, a sexually transmitted disease caused by papillomaviruses. Podofilox is a potent inhibitor of mitosis and tends to cause the infected cells and surrounding tissues to undergo necrosis as a result of treatment. In contrast, imiquimod seems to induce cytokines, which may aid normal immune processes to destroy the infected tissue, but is not itself cytotoxic.

These topically applied drugs cause few systemic effects but are likely to cause redness, peeling, itching, or swelling at the site of application. It is also important to avoid spreading these drugs to unaffected tissues or to the eyes.

DRUG CLASS • Scabicides and Pediculicides

crotamiton (Crotan, Eurax)

lindane

malathion (Ovide)

permethrin (Elimite)

MECHANISM OF ACTION

An organophosphate pediculicide, malathion has been shown to destroy lindane-resistant lice by inhibiting cholinesterase. Permethrin has a high cure rate (up to 90%) in treating head lice after only a single application. It acts on the louse's nerve cell membranes to disrupt the sodium channel, thereby delaying repolarization and paralyzing the parasite. Lindane is a chlorinated hydrocarbon insecticide related to the banned DDT. Malathion is an organophosphorous insecticide that inhibits cholinesterases. Permethrin is related to natural insecticides found in chrysanthemums. These compounds affect neuronal membrane function. The mechanism of action of crotamiton is unknown.

USES

The drug of choice for treatment of scabies is crotamiton. The other drugs in this category can be used as general-purpose insecticides as well as for treating scabies or lice. The drug of choice for lice is lindane, although malathion and permethrin are being used more commonly because of their ovicidal effect.

PHARMACOKINETICS

These drugs are used topically to control infestations of the skin and hair; systemic absorption is undesirable, although it has been noted especially with lindane.

Crotamiton is massaged into the skin from the chin down, with attention to body creases and folds. It is reapplied in 24 and 48 hours and then washed from the body surface (crotamiton requires two applications for one treatment). Two applications usually eradicate most infestations. In resistant cases, it may be applied again 1 week later. Permethrin in a single-dose regimen of 8 to 14 hours has been used with success. For adults, 1% lindane cream or lotion is often used in an 8- to 12-hour treatment, followed by thorough washing.

ADVERSE REACTIONS AND CONTRAINDICATIONS

The patient should be advised that the pruritus and dermatitis might persist for days after adequate treatment with lindane. This drug is contraindicated for infants and pregnant women. Chrysanthemum sensitivity must be assessed if permethrin is prescribed, because patients allergic to the flower are much more likely to be allergic to the drug. Crotamiton may also cause skin irritation or rashes.

TOXICITIES

Most of these drugs can cause serious reactions if they are used at high doses or absorbed unusually well. Permethrin is the least toxic of the group. Poisoning with lindane may cause tremors, ataxis, convulsions, and collapse. Malathion has been linked to chromosomal breaks or other changes in genetic structure, following prolonged high exposure.

INTERACTIONS

Interactions are unlikely with these externally applied drugs. However, if lindane is absorbed through the skin, it can induce drug-biotransforming enzymes in the liver, which can affect the persistence of other drugs in the body.

DRUG CLASS • Proteolytic Enzymes

collagenase (Santyl)

fibrinolysin + deoxyribonuclease (Elase✱)

fibrinolysin + deoxyribonuclease and chloramphenicol (Elase-Chloromycetin)

papain + urea (Accuzyme)

streptokinase-streptodornase (Varidase✱)

MECHANISM OF ACTION

The proteolytic enzymes are all capable of digesting available proteins found in sloughing or necrotic tissue in decubitus ulcers and other wounds. Collagenase specifically attacks collagen, which is an abundant structural protein in cells. As cells die, the collagen may remain to hold the dead or dying cells to the living cells within the wound. Dissolving the collagen makes sloughing of necrotic tissue easier and creates a better surface within the wound for healing to occur. Maximum activity occurs at a pH of 6 to 8.

Papain is a protease capable of digesting a variety of proteins. Combining the papain with urea increases the action of papain by making the substrate proteins more accessible. This preparation is active over a wide pH range.

Fibrinolysin specifically digests fibrin. Some products of this breakdown may stimulate release of growth factors by macrophages, thus improving wound healing. Deoxyribonuclease is included to destroy the nucleic acid released by dying cells. This product is no longer used in the United States, because the actions against fibrin may impair early wound-healing steps. The preparation that also includes chloramphenicol is still available in the United States.

Streptokinase and streptodornase are enzymes that digests fibrin and proteins associated with nucleic acids. There is no action on collagen. This preparation is no longer available in the United States.

USES

Proteolytic enzymes are used to chemically debride burn wounds, decubitus ulcers, and venous stasis ulcers. Enzymatic debridement removes sloughing tissue and helps facilitate granulation of the wound. To prevent delayed healing, the proteolytic enzyme should be discontinued when the wound is clean with healthy, pink granulation tissue present. Surgical debridement may be required if a decubitus ulcer is very serious or if complications such as osteomyelitis are present. Surgical skin closure or grafting may be required after chemical debridement has taken place.

PHARMACOKINETICS

These drugs are proteins applied to wounds and surrounding skin; they are not expected to be absorbed systemically.

ADVERSE REACTIONS AND CONTRAINDICATIONS

Adverse reactions to proteolytic enzymes consist of a mild, transient pain, paresthesias, bleeding, and transient dermatitis. Even with high concentrations, adverse effects are minimal, primarily consisting of local hyperemia. Adverse effects severe enough to warrant discontinuation of therapy have occasionally occurred. No systemic toxicity has been observed as a result of topical application of proteolytic enzymes.

Because papain is a component of pineapple, patients who are allergic to pineapple may suffer a reaction to this component.

INTERACTIONS

No significant interactions are known for these drugs.

 DRUG CLASS • Antiinflammatory Drugs

See Chapter 57, Table 57-3.

Many inflammatory skin conditions respond to topical or intralesional administration of adrenal corticosteroids. Although most often applied topically, they may also be administered systemically for severe disorders. Topical corticosteroids are used in the treatment of disorders such as psoriasis because of their antiinflammatory, antipruritic, and vasoconstrictive actions. They also have an ability to decrease cellular proliferation. When high-potency topical corticosteroids are used, the patient should be switched to less potent drugs before treatment is stopped to minimize the risk of rebound flare of the disease.

Most topically administered dermatologic drugs have limited distribution. However, the skin functions as a reservoir for some drugs. For example, a topical corticosteroid under occlusion for 24 hours establishes a drug reservoir in the stratum corneum that can persist for as long as 2 weeks. Most drugs that pass through the stratum corneum to the epidermis are biotransformed there. Drugs that are not biotransformed in the epidermis pass unchanged into the systemic circulation. Drugs reaching the systemic circulation are eliminated through the kidneys, much like orally administered drugs.

The highly potent corticosteroids such as betamethasone or dexamethasone are the most likely to cause atrophy, telangiectasia, purpura, striae, and acneiform eruptions. Thin-skinned areas are particularly susceptible to the development of atrophy. Purpura is seen on the dorsal aspect of the forearms and hands with long-term use of potent corticosteroids. Allergic contact dermatitis, burning sensations, dryness, itching, hypopigmentation, facial hirsutism, folliculitis, moon facies, and alopecia (usually of the scalp) are also possible. Other adverse effects include overgrowth of bacteria, fungi, and virus, and immunosuppression. Topical steroids may cause rosacea if they are used on the face. Infants may have more severe symptoms of rosacea because of a relative increase in body surface area.

A wide variety of combinations including corticosteroids are available. For example, antibiotics or other antimicrobial drugs are often combined with corticosteroids. The rationale is that the antimicrobial drug should treat or prevent infection while the corticosteroid relieves symptoms caused by inflammation. One problem with this rationale is that corticosteroids also may mask signs of a worsening infection.

DRUG CLASS • Melanizing and Demelanizing Drugs

trioxsalen (Trisoralen)

methoxsalen (Oxsoralen, Uvadex)

monobenzone (Benoquin)

Melanizing drugs are used to stimulate deposition of melanin in vitiligo, a disorder characterized by a loss of pigmentation. Two closely related drugs of the psoralen family, trioxsalen and methoxsalen, are the major melanizing drugs. Exposure to ultraviolet light is an integral part of the treatment protocol because the psoralens are effective in stimulating melanocytes only after photoactivation.

Demelanizing preparations include hydroquinone and monobenzone, which are occasionally used to bleach blemishes such as freckles, old-age spots, and the melasma of pregnancy or oral contraception. Some preparations of hydroquinone are formulated in an opaque base that shields ultraviolet light. Protecting the affected area from ultraviolet light significantly hastens the response. Hydroquinone is contraindicated for patients with malaria, sunburn, or skin irritation as well as when depilatory agents are used.

Adverse reactions associated with melanizing drugs are minimal, but some patients experience nausea, GI irritation, protoporphyria, and an exacerbation of lupus erythematosus. The only adverse effect of demelanizing drugs is a skin rash.

 DRUG CLASS • Sunscreens

The sun emits principally two types of ultraviolet radiation, UVA and UVB. UVA radiation causes tanning of the skin. UVB radiation causes sunburn. Sunburn occurs when UVB radiation damages small blood vessels in the skin, causing them to become leaky and congested. Many people incorrectly consider sunburn a harmless, although painful, price to pay for a seasonal tan.

UVA radiation tans the skin by stimulating production of the dark pigment melanin. The darkness of the tan depends on how much melanin is produced. People who do not tan easily do not produce enough melanin. Melanin absorbs UVA and UVB radiation and protects the skin from harmful effects of ultraviolet radiation. Naturally dark skin contains more melanin than pale skin and is correspondingly better protected.

The harmful effects of ultraviolet radiation can be serious, permanent, and potentially life threatening. These effects, including premature aging and wrinkling of the skin as well as skin cancer, occur after years of repeated exposure and may occur without significant episodes of sunburn. Sunscreens diminish the harmful consequences of ultraviolet radiation by absorbing or reflecting it. Used correctly, they prevent sunburn and premature aging of the skin and reduce the risk of skin cancer. Chemical sunscreens selectively absorb and screen out most of the harmful burning radiation but permit tanning radiation to reach the skin. Physical sunscreens scatter and reflect all ultraviolet radiation. They prevent sunburn well, but they also prevent tanning.

The FDA has approved 21 chemical sunscreens. Those most commonly available include aminobenzoic acid, cinoxate, homosalate, menthyl anthranilate, oxybenzone, and padimate O. Sunscreen products may contain one or several of these agents. Physical sunscreens include titanium oxide and zinc oxide in ointments and creams. They are intended for complete coverage of small areas of sunburn-prone skin such as the nose and lips.

Not all suntan products contain sunscreens. Some contain cosmetically appealing but otherwise inactive ingredients such as cocoa butter, mineral oil, and lanolin. None of these ingredients prevents sunburn or promotes tanning.

Some drugs, cosmetics, and soaps sensitize the skin to ultraviolet radiation and cause it to burn more easily than usual. Examples of such photosensitizing drugs include tetracycline antibiotics (see Chapter 28) and diuretics (see Chapter 46). Photosensitivity reactions are triggered by UVA radiation. Most sunscreens absorb little if any of this radiation and will not prevent it. Those that do block UVA radiation include menthyl anthranilate and oxybenzone.

APPLICATION TO PRACTICE

ASSESSMENT
History of Present Illness

Initial questions to a patient with a dermatologic complaint should include time of onset and body part affected. Establishing the time of onset helps determine whether the problem is acute or chronic or whether relapse has occurred. The patient's description of the initial lesion is essential. The distribution, development, and progression of individual lesions is often characteristic. Information regarding any changes in the lesions should be elicited. Gaining information on other symptoms assists in determining whether the skin changes relate to a systemic or localized disease. Questioning the patient about treatments that have been implemented is important, since some lesions may be altered by these therapies favorably or unfavorably.

Questioning the patient about exposure to others with a similar skin condition may indicate the presence of a contagious illness. Asking the patient what he or she thinks may be causing the problem may provide some insight into the cause.

Other factors to be considered are the patient's occupational, home, and workplace environments. It is important to understand what the patient comes in contact with and to what extent. For example, does the patient work around chemicals or dyes? What agents are used in the home? Do hobbies require contact with chemicals or other topical solutions? Are there pets, plants, or flowers in the home or workplace? Additionally, patient-determined or health care provider–prescribed factors that may have alleviated the condition should be noted. The patient's psychologic response to the skin condition is important to ascertain. A travel history can also be helpful, particularly if the travel included hiking or exposure to a variety of outdoor plants, shrubs, and trees. Does the patient engage in recreational activities that involve prolonged exposure to the sun or unusual cold? Inquire about the use of tanning salons.

Question the patient regarding self-care behaviors. Determine the types of soaps, lotions, abrasives, and cosmetics used as well as the frequency of their use. Record the brand names of any products used. Ask if there have been new purchases of bedding or clothing and how these items are cleaned. Inquire about exercise and sleep patterns because these factors affect circulation, nourishment, and wound healing.

Health History

Ask if the patient has had a similar problem in the past. This question may help reveal a recurrent skin condition. Obtain an allergy history. Determine if there are other skin lesions or rashes. Inquire about chronic illnesses or immunocompromised states that may leave a patient vulnerable to delayed or prolonged healing.

It is important to gather a thorough family history; genetically transmitted dermatologic conditions include alopecia (loss of patches of hair), ichthyosis, atopic dermatitis (eczema), and psoriasis. Other conditions that have familial tendencies include asthma, hay fever, and allergies. Systemic diseases with dermatologic complications include diabetes, blood dyscrasias, and connective tissue diseases such as lupus erythematosus.

A thorough drug history should also be compiled, since a vast number of dermatologic reactions to drugs are possible. Note the type of reaction. Question the patient on any photosensitivity reaction he or she may have experienced. Information about the use of products obtained from health food stores should also be elicited. Some products may be life threatening. The most common drugs involved in life-threatening, drug-induced skin eruptions are identified in Chapter 64, Table 64-1.

Lifespan Considerations

Perinatal. For the pregnant woman, increased estrogen levels and possibly increased progesterone levels are responsible for chloasma, the so-called mask of pregnancy. It appears as a blotchy, brownish tone to the skin over the cheek, forehead, and nose of some women. Striae gravidarum (stretch marks) may also appear. Vascular spider nevi may be caused by increased blood flow to the subcutaneous area in response to increased estrogen levels. Oily skin, hirsutism, and fingernail changes are other skin alterations seen during pregnancy.

Pediatric. Providing drug therapy for children with dermatologic conditions presents a unique set of challenges. Children undergo profound physiologic changes during their growth and development, and failure to understand these changes and their effects can lead to incorrectly determining the drug dosage. The potential for failure of therapy, for severe adverse reactions, or for fatal toxicity must be considered when treating children.

Additionally, children have an increased risk of systemic toxicity from topically applied drugs for two reasons. First, because of greater surface area–to–weight ratio, a given amount of applied drug represents a greater dose (in milligrams per kilogram) for children than for adults. Secondly, because of the greater body surface area and skin permeability in relation to total body mass, more of the drug is absorbed (see Chapter 3).

For the adolescent, the most common skin condition is acne, which can be psychologically devastating. Hormonal changes in adolescents with the development of

EVIDENCE-BASED PRACTICE
Topical Negative Pressure for Treating Chronic Wounds

Setting

Chronic wounds primarily involve older adults and those with multiple health problems. Despite the use of modern drugs and dressings, some of these wounds take a long time to heal, fail to heal, or recur, causing significant pain and discomfort as well as increased cost of health care services. Topical negative pressure (TNP) using suction is applied to promote healing of surgical wounds by draining excess fluid from wounds.

Objective of Literature Review

To assess the effectiveness of TNP (e.g., Wound-Vac) in treating patients who have chronic wounds and to identify an optimum treatment regimen.

Criteria for Inclusion of Studies in Review of Literature

Two investigators reviewed all available randomized, controlled studies in which the effectiveness of TNP in treating chronic wounds was evaluated. Eligibility for inclusion in the studies, extraction of data, and details of the studies were reviewed independently and a narrative synthesis of the results compiled.

Data Extraction and Analysis

The Cochrane Wounds Group Specialized Trials Registry was searched. Investigators also contacted relevant companies requesting information about ongoing and recently completed trials. In addition, reference lists from relevant articles were reviewed for additional studies.

Results of Review

Only two small studies with a total of 34 subjects fulfilled the selection criteria, but each had different outcome measures. The first study included subjects with any type of chronic wound. The second study looked at subjects who had diabetic foot ulcers only. The studies compared TNP (as open-cell foam dressing with continuous suction) with saline gauze dressings for the first 48 hours. The first study reported a statistically significant reduction in wound volume at 6 weeks with use of TNP. The results of the second study, which used TNP as continuous suction for the first 48 hours followed by intermittent suction after 48 hours, reported a reduction in the number of days to healing and a reduction in wound surface area at 2 weeks with use of TNP. However, no statistical analyses were given, and there were no reports regarding the effect of TNP on cost, quality of life, pain, and comfort level.

Investigators' Conclusions

The findings of these two studies must be interpreted with caution, given the small sample sizes and the limitations of methodology. The two studies provided weak support for TNP being superior to saline gauze dressings in healing chronic human wounds.

Evans D, Land L: *Topical negative pressure for treating chronic wounds* (Cochrane Review). In *The Cochrane Library*, Issue 2, Oxford, 2002, Update Software.

acne may be accompanied by low self-esteem and poor body image. When dealing with an adolescent with skin conditions, body image considerations need to be addressed in the treatment plan.

The predominant age for the development of genital warts is between the ages of 15 and 30 years. These ages are when adolescents and young adults are most sexually active. The risk factors for genital warts include adolescence and young adults who are sexually active but who do not use condoms. A white ethnic background, pregnancy, smoking, and poor hygiene may be associated with this disorder, which affects men and women equally.

Older Adults. Physiologic changes in the aging population affect the condition of the skin. Progressive impair-ment of the peripheral vascular circulation alters the cutaneous response to physical trauma, changes in temperature, and infection. In contrast to pediatric patients, the skin of older adults is less permeable to drugs, perhaps because of the loss of subcutaneous tissue (see Chapter 4). The ability to sense pressure and pain and to differentiate temperatures are diminished in the older adult.

Cultural/Social Considerations

Alternations in skin integrity are visible to others and may have a profound psychologic effect on the patient who perceives a given skin condition as an abnormality. Considering cultural influences and assessing the patient's response to his or her skin condition allows an individualized approach to their care.

It is important to assess the patient's diet history and eating habits when evaluating a skin condition. Some foods may contribute to skin disorders. Other foods are known to provoke an allergic response with resulting urticaria.

Socioeconomic considerations cannot be ignored, since many topical therapies are expensive. Compliance with a treatment plan and returning for follow-up care are influenced by social expectations or ability to pay for prescribed drugs and treatments.

Physical Examination

A differential diagnosis of a dermatologic condition is based on one feature: the appearance of the skin lesion. Therefore inspection and palpation are essential when evaluating skin lesions. Bilateral comparison should be accomplished using a good light source.

Lesions should be inspected for the following characteristics: location and distribution (localized or generalized), size (using the metric system), shape, margin characteristics, arrangement (clustered, linear, annular, or dermatomal), types (macules, papules, vesicles), texture, temperature, odor, presence of drainage, evidence of healing, and whether the lesions are primary or secondary. Documentation of the lesions needs to be specific.

Palpation of lesions is important, particularly for patients with dark skin. For example, erythema may not be noticeable, but warmth and edema of the involved area can be identified through palpation. The effect of pressure on or near the lesion and any pulsatility should also be identified.

Primary lesions develop without any preceding skin changes. In many cases, the health care provider does not see these lesions and must depend on the patient to describe them when they first appear. Primary lesions include macules, papules, patches, plaques, nodules, wheals, vesicles, bullae, and pustules. Accuracy of diagnosis relies heavily on the description of these primary lesions.

Secondary lesions result from changes in primary lesions. These lesions often occur in the epidermal layer of the skin and can be influenced by patient scratching or infection. Secondary lesions include scales, crusts, erosion, keloids, ulcers, and fissures.

The use of the Norton Scale or the Braden Scale for Predicting Pressure Sore Risk can help identify at-risk patients and the specific factors that place them at risk for pressure ulcers. All patients at risk should undergo a systematic skin inspection at least daily. Particular attention should be paid to bony prominences.

Watch for genital warts during the examination. Genital warts are highly contagious, appearing singly or in groups. They can be large or small. They are noted most often in the vagina, on the cervix, around the external genitalia, in the urethra, and around the anus and rectum. Perianal lesions are usually rough and cauliflower-like in appearance. There may be multiple finger-like projections. Penile lesions are often smooth and papular, occurring in groups of 3 or 4 on the frenulum, corona, glans, prepuce, meatus, shaft, or scrotum. In women, the warts may be identified during a pelvic examination and Pap smear. These warts can also appear on the conjunctiva and the nasal, oral, laryngeal, and pharyngeal areas.

Laboratory Testing

Skin testing is conducted for three major reasons: to detect a person's sensitivity to allergens such as dust or pollen, to determine sensitivity to organisms believed to cause disease, and to determine if cell-mediated immune functioning is normal. There are three types of skin tests: scratch tests, patch tests, and intradermal testing.

For scratch tests, extremely small quantities of allergens are introduced into small scratches made on the patient's back or forearm. Swelling or redness at the site within 30 minutes indicates a positive reaction. A patch test requires that a small gauze square be impregnated with the substance in question and applied to the skin of the forearm. Swollen or reddened skin at the site of the patch after a short time indicates a positive reaction. Intradermal testing is performed by injecting the substance into the epidermis (e.g., the Mantoux test for tuberculosis).

Other special tests important in the field of dermatology include fungus examinations, biopsies, and cytodiagnosis. Fungal cultures are performed to identify the specific type of fungus. Scraping the affected skin area or mucous membrane and viewing it under a microscope constitutes one form of examination. Potassium hydroxide (KOH) testing determines the presence of mycelial fragments, arthrospores, and budding yeast cells. When potassium hydroxide is used in a darkened room, infected hair will fluoresce a bright yellow-green. The use of a Wood's lamp assists in determining the presence of a fungus.

Biopsy is an important tool in ruling out malignancies of skin nodules when the cause is unknown. A small sample of skin tissue is excised from the patient, stained, and examined under the microscope.

The Tzank test is the microscopic assessment of fluids and cells from vesicles and bullae. A smear of cells is collected from the affected area and prepared for microscopic observation. A cytologic assessment is then performed. The Tzank test is useful in diagnosing some viral infections. The presence of HPV is often reported along with the Pap smear results.

GOALS OF THERAPY

Patient education with the resulting prevention is the key goal in controlling dermatologic disorders. Primary treatment goals include identifying and removing the cause (when possible) as well as restoring, protecting, and maintaining normal structure and function of the skin. Additional objectives include reducing inflammation, reducing scales and calluses, cleansing and debriding, eradicating microorganisms, and providing symptom relief.

INTERVENTION

There are many dermatologic drugs and formulations that can be used to prevent or manage skin conditions. The choice of drugs is based on the condition of the lesion, signs and symptoms of infection, the presence of pruritus, any infectious agent, and the location and distribution of the lesion(s). In general, the health care provider becomes familiar with a few dermatologic drugs in each category rather than attempting to learn about numerous drugs.

It is impossible to discuss all of the vast number of preparations and formulations available in the United States and Canada. Furthermore, not all generic topical drugs are equivalent to their brand name counterparts, either in potency or in the presence of ingredients that may cause irritation or allergy. When in doubt about the appropriate plan of care, it is generally considered prudent to undertreat rather than overtreat the disorder.

Many patients use OTC skin care products, such as moisturizers, cleansers, and sunscreens. These products are not always compatible with the patient's skin type or prescribed drugs. For example, oily moisturizers used by patients with acne are likely to undermine the beneficial effect that would be obtained from drying agents. Although the effectiveness of the drying agent could still be achieved without taking this factor into consideration, a better effect can be achieved when the use of both products are coordinated with the patient's skin type.

Furthermore, the most effective results are obtained when the degree of moisturizing or drying associated with a specific drug is tailored to the patient's skin type. The most effective topical drug is one that produces just enough moisture or dryness to meet the patient's needs. A description of the various vehicles and formulations can be found in Table 67-3.

The quantity of the topical drug required for a planned treatment regimen is an important factor when ordering one. For example, a 10- to 14-day course of treatment applied two to three times daily requires 30 g for the face, 45 g for the hands or feet, 60 g for arms or legs, and 60 to 90 g for the trunk. Coverage for the entire body requires 120 to 150 g or more.

Administration

Standard precautions are recommended when caring for the patient with altered skin integrity. Careful handwashing by the health care provider and the patient pre-

vents self-inoculation of other body parts and minimizes the possibility of spreading the condition to others. Manufacturers' instructions for application should be followed. Applying one drug on top of another should be avoided unless specifically ordered. Before applying antiseptics, ensure that dirt, soil, organic matter, or other contaminants are removed from the skin surface. Such materials not only harbor organisms but also provide a physical barrier that restricts access of the antiseptic and may chemically inactivate specific antiseptics.

Emollients are greasier than creams and are best reserved for thick, scaling, or keratotic lesions. Emollients are very moisturizing because of a thick barrier that prevents water loss and exerts prolonged protective action when applied at night. When using emollients, application should begin at the midline of the lesion using long, even strokes outward and in the direction of hair growth. This technique reduces the risk of follicle irritation and skin inflammation.

Lotions are best suited for hairy areas or for wet, oozing lesions and are more drying than creams. Creams are good for daytime use and should be rubbed in until they disappear. They are particularly effective when rubbed into oozing, denuded areas.

Ointments and pastes are not suited for hairy areas or on oozing surfaces. Pastes are applied with a tongue depressor. Pastes are porous enough to permit heat to escape from the skin. To remove the paste, use a cloth soaked with mineral oil or vegetable oil.

Paints have a drying effect on moist areas where two skin surfaces are in contact. They sometimes stain the skin and clothing and are messy to apply.

Before applying topical proteolytic enzymes, the wound should be thoroughly cleansed with water or saline. Antiseptics such as hexachlorophene, heavy metal compounds, benzalkonium chloride, nitrofurazone, and iodides should not be used before or during the use of proteolytic enzymes, because they have the potential for inactivating the enzyme. Any previously applied ointment should be removed before fresh application of the enzyme. Proteolytic enzymes are applied directly to the wound tissue and then covered with a thin layer of moist gauze or other nonadhering dressing. Enzyme activity depends on adequate moisture; therefore the dressings are kept moist at all times and changed one to three times daily. Care should be taken not to allow the enzyme to contact healthy skin.

Keratolytics are for external use only. They should not be applied over moles, birthmarks, warts with hair growing from them, or warts on the face or mucous membranes

Occlusive dressings should be applied over small surface areas only. Such dressings increase the risk of adverse systemic effects because of enhanced absorption

TABLE 67-3

Vehicles and Formulations

Vehicle/Formulation	Physical Characteristics	Advantages and Disadvantages	Examples
Ointments	Up to 10% of active ingredients in a fatty base	*Advantages:* Very moisturizing because of thick barrier that prevents water loss *Disadvantages:* Greasier than creams; not suitable for use on hairy areas or oozing surfaces	betamethasone, acyclovir, combination antibiotics
Emollients	Base preparations of fixed oils such as olive oil, cotton seed, or flaxseed	*Advantages:* Keeps skin soft; prevents evaporation of water and development of dryness *Disadvantages:* Cannot use if patient is allergic to wool	lanolin, petrolatum, vitamins A and D creams, vitamin E oil, cream, liquid, or ointment
Creams (solid emulsions)	Active ingredients put into emulsion-type hydrophobic base that vanishes when rubbed in	*Advantages:* Good for daytime use particularly with potent active ingredients that are effective when rubbed onto oozing, denuded surfaces	hydrocortisone cream
Lotions (liquid emulsions)	Powder suspended in oil or water with active ingredients; requires shaking to disperse ingredients	*Advantages:* Best for hairy areas or for lesions that are wet and oozing; protects and cools acutely inflamed areas on face and on hairy body surfaces *Disadvantages:* More drying than creams	calamine lotion
Aqueous solutions	Active ingredients put into a liquid that contains water as the solvent	*Advantages:* Only mildly drying due to slow evaporation of water *Disadvantages:* Alcohol solutions are very drying because ethanol and other low molecular weight alcohols rapidly evaporate	aluminum acetate, potassium permanganate, zinc stearate, boric acid
Pastes	Ointments into which powders are mixed (e.g., zinc oxide, starch, talc, tars, salicylic acid)	*Advantages:* Prolonged protective and occlusive action; porous enough to permit heat to escape from skin *Disadvantages:* Not suited for hairy or oozing surfaces	zinc oxide paste, anthralin paste
Paints	Liquids used to touch up small localized areas or intertriginous surfaces	*Advantages:* Desirable drying effect on moist areas where two skin surfaces meet *Disadvantages:* Sometimes stain and are messy	gentian violet, salicylic acid
Powders	Materials in fine particles for dusting on surfaces	*Advantages:* Absorb moisture and reduces friction from large areas; exert cooling or protective effects *Disadvantages:* May cause irritation of respiratory tract in susceptible people and small children	talcum powder
Gels	Semisolid oil-based product of precipitated or coagulated colloid; contains large amounts of water; deposits film of active ingredients on skin	*Advantages:* Used in hairy areas as well as on smooth skin *Disadvantages:* Somewhat drying when used on nonhairy areas	betamethasone, coal tar gel, Sea Breeze Facial Cleansing Gel

TABLE 67-3

Vehicles and Formulations—cont'd

Vehicle/Formulation	Physical Characteristics	Advantages and Disadvantages	Examples
Rubs/liniments	Higher proportions of oil than ordinary lotions; include counterirritants such as methyl salicylates, camphor, oil of cloves, capsaicin	*Advantages:* Used for pain relief on intact skin; may include antiseptic, analgesic, anesthetic additives; can be formulated as gel, cream, lotion, or ointment *Disadvantages:* Irritating to abraded skin; some formulations are greasy	Vicks VapoRub, Ben-Gay
Colloidal and emollient baths	Decrease the drying effect of water	*Advantages:* Is soothing to irritated skin and helps relieve itching. *Disadvantages:* May cause bathtub to be slippery, increasing the risk for falls	Alpha Keri Bath Oil, Aveeno Regular Bath
Soaps	Sodium salts, palmitic, oleic, and stearic fatty acids; prepared by saponifying fats or oils with alkalies; consistency depends on the acid and alkali used	*Advantages:* Some contain antiseptics but only work to the degree that they mechanically clean the skin *Disadvantages:* Dry and irritating if used excessively	Yardley Aloe-Vera Soap, Boraxo
Cleansers	Contains emollient substance with pH adjusted to be neutral or slightly acidic	*Advantages:* Recommended for persons with sensitive, dry, or irritated skin or who may have had a previous reaction to a soap product *Disadvantages:* May contain soaps	Aveeno Cleansing Bar, Phisoderm
Hydrocolloid dressings	Made of hydrophilic granules embedded in a polymer base; absorbs water from wound to form protective gel	*Advantages:* Stimulates tissue granulation; excludes bacteria; waterproof; easy application; reduces pain	DuoDerm, Restore, Ultec
Transparent	Thin, polyurethane adhesive dressing; permeable to vapor and gas; supports cellular regeneration	*Advantages:* Wound is visible; waterproof; good adhesion; cost effective *Disadvantages:* Nonabsorbent; difficult to apply; limited to superficial tissues	Tegaderm, Opsite

of the topically administered drug. Large body areas should not be wrapped.

For the patient with a parasite or infection, all household and intimate contacts should be treated to prevent recurrence or continued transmission. Clothing (especially undergarments), bedding, and towels should be laundered in hot water. As with other parasitic diseases, the patient should be advised regarding strategies to minimize exposure.

One effective treatment regimen for head lice is a shampoo with permethrin cream rinse. A 5-minute lindane shampoo of the pubic area can be used for pubic in-

festations. After treatment, lice and nits can be removed using a metal comb with teeth 0.1 mm apart. Moisture or oil rinses may make this easier. Wet hair should not be exposed to open flame or to hair dryers on high setting. Mechanical removal is recommended for facial and pubic louse infestations. Lindane should be used with caution in infants, children, and pregnant women.

Preventing recurrence of lice involves treatment of human contacts and materials. Pillowcases, hats, scarves, and other items should be washed or dry-cleaned. Infested combs and brushes should be cleaned and boiled or soaked for 1 hour in 1% lindane or 2% Lysol. Away from the body, head and body lice survive only about 3 days, 10 days maximum.

Sexual partners of persons with pubic lice should also be treated, and their bedding, towels, and clothing should be washed or dry-cleaned. Pubic lice do not survive longer than 24 hours away from the body. Transmission via toilet seats is unlikely. Fumigation is generally unnecessary, although vacuuming is helpful to remove stray lice and shed hairs with affixed nits. As with other parasitic diseases, the patient should be advised about strategies to minimize exposure.

Education

The patient must understand the importance of handwashing each time the affected skin area is touched. Good hygiene of the unaffected areas of the body should be maintained and the affected area cleansed only in the pre-

scribed fashion. The patient should avoiding touching the affected areas as much as possible and to dress in a manner that will minimize contact with the involved area.

Teach patients that soaps should be used only in the axillae, groin, and on the feet by persons with dry or irritated skin. Unless the patient's occupation exposes him or her to excessive soiling, most patients need not use soap on all body surfaces. When informed, most patients often comply with this restriction rather than to a total ban on soap. Baths containing a small amount of bath oil may be used but are less effective than application of oils to the skin after bathing.

The patient should be taught how to apply the prescribed drug appropriately and to continue its use for the recommended time period, even if results are not immediate or the symptoms are slow in subsiding. They should be informed that acute skin disorders do not clear up in

---

CASE STUDY   *Scabies*

ASSESSMENT

HISTORY OF PRESENT ILLNESS

GB, a 76-year-old immunocompromised man, is a debilitated, dehydrated resident of a long-term care facility. He is now being admitted to the hospital for physical evaluation and hydration. He is complaining of a rash and severe nighttime itching of hands, arms, trunk, and perineal area. It is unknown how long the rash has been present. GB is incontinent of stool and has a sheath catheter in place for urine drainage. No treatment for rash has been recorded.

HEALTH HISTORY

Documented war trauma was found in old records. No other health history is available. He suspects his HIV infection may have been through heterosexual transmission. Records indicate GB has no known drug allergies but is allergic to chrysanthemums. He is taking no drugs at this time except for an occasional aspirin for leg aches.

LIFESPAN CONSIDERATIONS

None specific, although GB is going through the known physiologic changes of aging.

CULTURAL/SOCIAL CONSIDERATIONS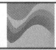

GB has been a long-time resident of the long-term care facility. He has been divorced for 5 years, and has no family in this area. He receives a Veterans' Administration pension.

PHYSICAL EXAMINATION

GB weighs 110 pounds. Temperature is 99° F, pulse 66, respirations 22, blood pressure 124/82 mm Hg with orthosta-

tic changes. Oral cavity is dry and sticky. Breath sounds with wheezes and crackles are present. Cachexia with poor muscle tone and skin turgor. Stage II decubiti on left ischial crest and sacrum. Fresh dressings in place. Soft fleece pads on elbows, heels. Patient lying on sheepskin. Urine scant, foul-smelling, and dark. Skin examination reveals burrows in finger webs and along the sides of his fingers. His perineum is excoriated, as are his axillary folds, waistline, and buttocks.

LABORATORY TESTING

Skin and hair scrapings identified the presence of mites, eggs, and cases.

PATIENT PROBLEM(S)

Active infestation of scabies.

GOALS OF THERAPY

Clear the infestation of scabies.

CRITICAL THINKING QUESTIONS

1. What risk factors does GB have for contracting scabies?
2. The health care provider orders crotamiton for GB. What is the mechanism of action of this drug?
3. How is crotamiton applied?
4. Why do you think the health care provider did not use lindane instead of crotamiton?
5. What precautions should nursing personnel take when caring for GB?

3 to 4 days. In some cases, it can take several weeks or months before significant improvement is noted. However, if the condition worsens, lesion characteristics change, or the lesion shows signs and symptoms of infection, the patient should contact the health care provider.

Burns. Prevention is the key to avoiding burns. Parents and childcare providers must be taught to keep matches out of the reach of children, and children need to be taught the dangers of fire. Handles on pots and pans should be turned to the inside of the stove. A fire extinguisher should be close at hand, and a smoke alarm should be installed in the home.

Sunburns are potentially dangerous and can lead to extensive skin damage. Skin damage is caused by excessive exposure to the sun's ultraviolet rays. Damage can be minimized by avoiding long periods of time in the sun; wearing loose, light clothing that covers exposed body parts; and using a sunscreen.

Explain to the patient that the effectiveness of sunscreens is rated by the sun protection factor (SPF), which is listed on the product label. The SPF relates the amount of time it takes a person to get mild sunburn without sunscreen protection to the time required after a given sunscreen has been applied to the exposed skin. The higher the SPF value, the greater the protection. For example, skin that ordinarily burns after 30 minutes of exposure to the sun will, if treated with a sunscreen with an SPF of 4, be able to stay in the sun for 2 hours (4 times as long) before it burns to the same degree. A sunscreen

---

CASE STUDY   *Contact Dermatitis*

ASSESSMENT

HISTORY OF PRESENT ILLNESS

SM is a 66-year-old retired horticulturist who comes to the health care provider with complaints of itching as well as weeping lesions on his neck, forearms, and hands that have been present for about 2 weeks. He denies exposure to known environmental irritants, ophthalmic medications, or the use of new skin care products. He had one other episode with similar characteristics about 2 months ago that "went away on its own" while he was on vacation. Character of lesions and distribution have not changed since onset of symptoms.

HEALTH HISTORY

SM denies history of drug or food allergies. He has mild seasonal hay fever and has a brother with asthma. Current drugs include hydrochlorothiazide 25 mg po qd for mild hypertension.

LIFESPAN CONSIDERATIONS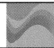

SM spends Sunday afternoons leading children's tours of the local botanical gardens. He is in the stage of older adulthood, where adaptation to retirement and changing physical abilities is often necessary.

CULTURAL/SOCIAL CONSIDERATIONS

SM works occasionally during busy seasonal periods, fills in when other employees are on vacation, and conducts tours at the local botanical gardens on a weekly basis. He enjoys woodworking in his shop at home, making and refinishing furniture. SM lives on a fixed retirement income. He is enrolled in Medicare parts A and B and carries a secondary insurance that covers any additional charges and pharmacy needs.

PHYSICAL EXAMINATION

SM has diffuse, erythematous, vesicular lesions over his neck, forearms, and hands. There is no evidence of secondary lesions at this time. He is afebrile, and no evidence of systemic involvement has been found

LABORATORY TESTING

Patch test of 2 years ago evidences contact allergy to common herbicide used at nursery.

PATIENT PROBLEM(S)

Contact dermatitis.

GOALS OF THERAPY

Remove or avoid underlying allergen; reduce severity of pruritus; reduce inflammatory process; prevent infection of affected areas.

CRITICAL THINKING QUESTIONS

1. The health care provider orders include a thick layer of triamcinolone lotion to the affected areas twice daily for 10 to 14 days along with the concomitant use of a moisturizer cream. What is the mechanism of action of the triamcinolone cream?
2. Which other formulation of triamcinolone might be more moisturizing for SM?
3. Of which adverse effects should SM be made aware?
4. SM wants to be able to cover the affected areas with an occlusive dressing. What is the appropriate response to this request?
5. What is the most important point to teach SM about prevention of contact dermatitis?

with an SPF of 8 protects 8 times as long (4 hours). Products with SPFs greater than 8 (some go as high as 50) screen out nearly all tanning and burning radiation. These products offer approximately equal protection from the radiation and differ only in the length of time that they allow a person to stay exposed to the sun. However, in some cases the higher SPF is of marginal value. For example, a sunscreen with an SPF of 15 would let someone who normally burns in 60 minutes to stay in the sun for 15 hours. This would extend the time of protection into the night.

The choice of SPF depends on how easily the person burns or tans, the length of time spent in the sun, the usual intensity of the sun in the patient's geographic area, and the formulation preferred. The intensity of sunlight at 5000 feet is about 20% greater than that at sea level and is at its highest between the hours of 10 AM and 2 PM in most areas. Snow and white sand are reflectors that intensify the brilliance of sunlight. The FDA recommends products with an SPF of 8 or more for people who always burn and never tan, 6 to 7 for those who always burn and seldom tan, 4 to 5 for those who burn moderately and tan gradually, 2 to 3 for those who burn minimally and always tan well, and 2 for those who rarely burn and tan profusely.

Inform the patient that sunscreens should be applied at least 30 minutes before each exposure to the sun to allow the chemicals time to penetrate the skin. The sunscreen should be reapplied every 2 hours, after swimming, or during heavy perspiration. Even sunscreens that are labeled waterproof or water-resistant are removed by toweling and perspiration. No sunscreen or suntan product will promote a deeper tan than a person's skin can naturally produce. If skin does not readily produce melanin, it will never tan as well as skin that readily produces the pigment.

Pressure (Decubitus) Ulcers. Prevention is also the key to the development of a pressure ulcer. Skin care must be individualized, and the skin should be cleaned at least at the time of soiling and at routine intervals throughout the day. Turning the immobile patient every 2 hours minimizes the development of pressure ulcers. Education of the patient needs to focus on environmental factors that lead to skin breakdown, including dry skin from low humidity and exposure to cold. Exposure to moisture from incontinence, perspiration, or wound drainage should be prevented. Gently massaging the skin around the pressure sites will increase the circulation to the area. The use of protective positioning, proper transfer, and turning

techniques minimizes skin injury from friction and shearing forces. Adequate protein and calorie intake are necessary to promote skin integrity and healing. Nutritional supplements or support needs to be available when required. Rehabilitation efforts must be initiated early in the treatment regimen.

EVALUATION

Acute skin lesions should decrease in size and eventually disappear when treatment has been successful. It should be noted, however, that acute skin lesions do not resolve in a few days. They require time and frequent observation. Chronic skin conditions, some pressure ulcers, and severe burns may take weeks to months or even years to heal. Documentation of the assessment of skin lesions and unaffected areas helps determine progress toward achieving the desired outcome or resolution of the skin disorder.

Bibliography

Ebling AM: Evidence-based practice. Effectiveness of oral antibiotics and topical retinoid therapy in the treatment of acne in adolescents, *Pediatr Nurs* 27(4):410-411, 421, 2001.

Gradwell C, Haynes M: Dermatology problems, *Pract Nurse* 22(11):32, 34, 36 passim, 2001.

Johnson BA, Nunley JR: Use of systemic agents in the treatment of acne vulgaris, *Am Fam Physician* 62(8):1823-1830, 1835-1836, 2000.

Laude TA: Acne in childhood and adolescence: update on treatment choices, *Consultant* 40(3):457-462, 464, 466 passim, 2000.

O'Donnell JA, Hofmann MT: Skin and soft tissues: management of four common infections in the nursing home patient, *Geriatrics* 56(10):33-38, 41, 2001.

Perlman S, Leach E, Dominguez L, Ruszkowski AM, Rudy SJ: "Be smart, be safe, be sure": the revised pregnancy prevention program for women on isotretinoin, *J Reprod Med* 46(suppl 2):179-185, 2001.

Russell JJ: Topical therapy for acne, *Am Fam Physician* 61(2):357-366, 2000.

Savage AI: Nurse-managed clinic improves care for acne patients, *Viewpoint* 22(6):1, 8-10, 2000.

Venna S, Fleischer AB Jr, Feldman SR: Scabies and lice: review of the clinical features and management principles, *Dermatol Nurs* 13(4):257-262, 265-266, 2001.

Webster GF: Acne vulgaris and rosacea: evaluation and management. *Clin Cornerstone* 4(1):15-22, 48-56, 2001.

Internet Resources

http://quickcare.org/skin/acne.html.
http://www.woundcarenet.com/.

Dietary Considerations

ADULT IDEAL BODY WEIGHT CALCULATION

IBW of men in kg =
$\qquad$ 50 kg + (2.3 kg for each inch in height over 5 feet)

IBW of women in kg =
$\qquad$ 45.5 kg + (2.3 kg for each inch in height over 5 feet)

CHILD IDEAL BODY WEIGHT CALCULATION (IBW is in kg; height is in cm)

Ages 1 to 18 years:

$$IBW \text{ in kg} = \frac{(\text{height [in cm]}^2 \times 1.65)}{1000}$$

Over 5 feet:

IBW of boy in kg =
$\qquad$ 39 kg + (2.27 kg for each inch in height over 5 feet)

IBW of girl in kg =
$\qquad$ 42.2 kg + (2.27 kg for each inch in height over 5 feet)

CALCULATION OF BODY MASS INDEX

$$BMI = \frac{\text{weight in kg}}{\text{height in m}^2}$$

CALCULATION OF BODY SURFACE AREA

$$BSA \ (\text{m}^2) = \frac{\text{square root of height in cm} \times \text{weight in kg}}{3600}$$

ESTIMATED NITROGEN BALANCE (ENB)

$$ENB = \frac{\text{protein intake in g}}{6.25} - (\text{24-hr urine urea nitrogen [UUN] in g} + 4)$$

ESTIMATING KILOCALORIES IN PARENTERAL SOLUTIONS

Glucose in amino acid solutions:

concentration of solution × g of glucose in solution =
$\qquad$ physiologic amino acid infused × fuel factor

Example: To determine kcal/g in 3000 mL of D_5W:

$$\frac{3000 \text{ mL} \times 5 \text{ mg glucose}}{100 \text{ mL}} + \frac{150 \text{ g glucose} \times 3.4 \text{ kcal}}{1 \text{ g}} = 510 \text{ kcal}$$

To determine the amount of protein in 2000 mL of 3.5% amino acid solution:

$$\frac{2000 \text{ mL} \times 3.5 \text{ g amino acid}}{1000 \text{ mL}} + 70 \text{ g amino acids/protein}$$

FAT EMULSIONS

$\qquad$ 1 mL of 10% fat emulsion = 1.1 kcal/mL

thus:

$\qquad$ Number of mL × 1.1 = kcal of fat

$\qquad$ 1 mL of 20% fat emulsion = 2.0 kcal/mL

thus:

$\qquad$ Number of mL × 2 = kcal of fat

Example:
500 mL of a 20% fat emulsion = 500 mL × 2 kcal/mL = 1000 kcal

FOODS THAT ACIDIFY THE URINE

Breads
Cereals
Cheeses
Cranberries
Eggs
Fish
Meats
Plums
Poultry
Prunes
Tomato sauce
Tomatoes

FOODS THAT ALKALINIZE THE URINE

All fruits (except cranberries, plums, and prunes)
All vegetables (except corn and lentils)
Buttermilk
Chestnuts
Coconuts
Cream
Milk

FOOD HIGH IN DOPAMINE

Broad (fava) beans

FOODS HIGH IN FOLIC ACID

Cantaloupe
Dark green, leafy vegetables
Liver
Navy beans
Nuts
Oranges
Whole-wheat products
Yeast

FOODS HIGH IN OXALIC ACID

Beets
Chard
Cranberries
Gooseberries
Rhubarb
Spinach

FOODS HIGH IN PURINES

Anchovies
Broth
Consommé
Mincemeat
Organ meats
Roe
Sardines
Scallops

FOODS HIGH IN CALCIUM

Blackstrap molasses
Bok choy
Broccoli
Canned salmon/sardines
Clams
Cream soups
Milk and dairy products
Oysters
Spinach
Tofu

FOODS HIGH IN IRON

Cereals
Dried beans, peas
Dried fruit
Leafy green vegetables
Lean red meats
Organ meats

FOODS HIGH IN VITAMIN D

Breads
Cereals
Fish and fish liver oils
Fortified milk

FOODS HIGH IN POTASSIUM

Apricots
Artichokes
Avocado
Bananas
Broccoli
Brussels sprouts
Cantaloupe
Carrots
Chard
Chicken
Dried fruit
Garbanzo beans
Grapefruit
Honeydew melon
Ketchup
Kidney beans
Lima beans
Navy beans
Orange juice
Oranges
Pears
Pinto beans
Potatoes
Prune juice
Prunes
Pumpkin

Rhubarb
Soybeans
Spinach
Tomato juice
Tomatoes
Turkey
Vegetable juice
Watermelon
Whole milk

FOODS HIGH IN PHYTATES

Brans
Whole-grain cereals

FOODS CONTAINING SULFITES

Acidic juices
Avocados
Beer
Dried fruits
Dried vegetables
Instant potatoes
Processed foods
Shrimp
Wine

FOODS HIGH IN SODIUM

Baking mixes
Barbecue sauce
Butter/margarine
Buttermilk
Canned chili
Canned seafood
Canned soup
Canned/bottled sauces
Cold cuts
Cured meats
Dried soup mixes
Fast foods
Ham
Ketchup
Macaroni and cheese
Most Chinese food
Pickles
Potato chips
Potato salad
Pretzels
Relish
Salted nuts
Sauerkraut
Soy sauce

FOODS HIGH IN VITAMIN K

Asparagus spears
Avocado

Broccoli, raw or cooked
Canola oil
Cole slaw
Collard greens
Dill pickles
Dry soybeans
Green, cooked peas
Head, Bibb, red leaf lettuce
Margarine
Mayonnaise
Olive oil
Raw bean pods
Raw cucumber peel
Raw endive
Raw green scallions
Raw parsley
Raw red cabbage
Sauerkraut

CAFFEINE SOURCES
Coffee (150 mL)

Brewed coffee (115 mg)
Brewed, decaffeinated
  coffee (3 mg)
Instant coffee (65 mg)
Instant, decaffeinated
  coffee (2 mg)
Percolated coffee (80 mg)

Tea (150 mL)

Brewed, U.S. brand (40 mg)
Brewed, imported (60 mg)
Iced tea (35 mg)
Instant tea (30 mg)

Carbonated Beverages (360 mL)

Citrus drinks (0-54 mg)
Coca-Cola (45 mg)
Diet Pepsi (38 mg)
Dr. Pepper (40 mg)
Ginger ale (0 mg)
Mellow Yellow (40 mg)
Mountain Dew (53 mg)
Mr. Pibb (54 mg)
Orange drinks (0 mg)
Other soft drinks (0-43 mg)
Pepsi-Cola (41 mg)
Root beer (0 mg)
Soda, seltzer (0 mg)
Tab (47 mg)

Foods

Baker's chocolate (26 mg/30 mL)
Chocolate cake/frosting (15.8 mg/one-twelfth of cake)
Chocolate milk (5 mg/240 mL)
Chocolate syrup (4 mg/30 mL)
Cocoa (4 mg/150 mL)
Dark, semi-sweet chocolate (20 mg/oz)
Milk chocolate (6 mg per ounce)

TYRAMINE-RESTRICTED DIETS
General Information

- Tyramine-restricted diets are designed for patients taking monoamine oxidase (MAO) inhibitors, drugs that have been reported to cause hypertensive crisis when taken concurrently with tyramine-rich foods. These include foods in which aging, protein breakdown, and putrefaction is used to increase flavor. As little as 5 to 6 mg of tyramine can produce a response, and 25 mg is a dangerous amount.
- Food sources of other pressor amines, such as histamine, dihydroxyphenylalanine, and hydroxytyramine, should also be avoided.
- Avoid over-the-counter (OTC) drugs such as decongestants, cold remedies, and antihistamines.

Tyramine-Containing Foods to Be Avoided

Cheeses: New York State Cheddar, Gruyère, Stilton, Emmentaler, Brie, Camembert, processed American

Other Aged Cheeses: Blue, Boursault, brick, cheddars, Gouda, mozzarella, Parmesan, Romano, Roquefort

Wines, Beers, and Ales: All tap beer, Chianti, domestic nonalcoholic beer, Riesling, sauterne, sherry, vermouth

Yeast and Yeast Products: Homemade bread, yeast extracts such as soup cubes, canned meats, marmite

Meat: Aged game, beef, and chicken liver; canned meats with yeast extracts; any meats marinated over 24 hours

Fish (salted dried): Anchovies, cod, herring, pickled herring

Other: Broad bean pods, chocolate, (especially sour) cream, dates, dried figs, eggplant, nuts, overripe fruit, raisins, salad dressing, sauerkraut, soy sauce, vanilla, yogurt

Tyramine-Containing Foods That Should Be Cautiously Consumed by Persons Taking MAO Inhibitors

Avocado (fresh)—maximum 1 per day

Aspartame-containing foods and beverages—not more than 3 servings per day

Chocolate candy—up to 4 ounces per day

Cottage cheese or cream cheese, fresh—up to 4 ounces per day of each

Monosodium glutamate in prepared foods, snack foods, Chinese foods—minimize use

Processed American cheese, fresh—up to 2 ounces per day

Raspberries—not more than 1½ ounces per day

Sour cream—up to 4 ounces per day

Soybean paste or tofu—not more than ½ ounce per day

Yogurt—8 ounces fresh, refrigerated, or frozen

TABLE A-1

Effects of Foods on Drug Absorption

Drug Absorption Reduced or Delayed
acetaminophen, alcohol, amoxicillin, ampicillin, aspirin, atenolol, cefaclor, cephalexin, diclofenac, digoxin, doxycycline, erythromycin stearate, hydrocortisone, hydrochlorothiazide, ibuprofen, isoniazid, levodopa, nafcillin, oxacillin, oxytetracycline, penicillins G and VK, phenobarbital, propantheline, rifampin, sotalol, sulfonamides, tetracycline

Drug Absorption Enhanced
carbamazepine, chlorothiazide, diazepam, dicumarol, erythromycin estolate, erythromycin ethylsuccinate, griseofulvin, hydralazine, labetalol, metoprolol, nitrofurantoin, phenytoin, propranolol, spironolactone

TABLE A-2

Selected Drugs Causing Primary Nutrient Malabsorption

Drug	Use/Class	Nutrient	Mechanism
Antacids	Hyperacidity	Calcium, iron, magnesium, zinc	Raises gastric pH and chelates the minerals
aspirin	Analgesia, antipyretic	Calcium, iron	Damages gastric villi and microvilli; inhibits brush border enzymes and intestinal transport systems
cimetidine	Hyperacidity	Vitamin B_{12}	Reduces cleavage from its dietary sources, reduces secretion of intrinsic factor
cholestyramine	Hypercholesterolemia	Fat, iron, vitamins A, E, K, B_{12}	Binding agent for bile salts, nutrients
colchicine	Gout	Fat, vitamin B_{12}, sodium, potassium, carotene, lactose	Enzyme damage, inhibits cell division
coumarin	Anticoagulant	Vitamin K	Antagonizes vitamin K activity
cephalosporins	Antibiotic	Vitamin K	Depletes vitamin K
cisplatin	Antineoplastic	Magnesium	Depletes magnesium
Diuretics	Diuresis	Sodium, potassium, magnesium, zinc	Increases elimination of nutrients
D penicillamine	DMARD	Pyridoxine (vitamin B_6), zinc	Interferes with pyridoxine metabolism, chelates heavy metals
furosemide	Diuresis	Calcium	Reduces calcium absorption
hydralazine	Hypertension	Pyridoxine (B_6)	Interferes with pyridoxine metabolism
isoniazid, cycloserine	Tuberculosis	Pyridoxine (B_6)	Interferes with pyridoxine metabolism
levodopa	Parkinson's disease	Pyridoxine (B_6)	Interferes with pyridoxine metabolism
methyldopa	Hypertension	Vitamin B_{12}, folic acid, iron	Unclear, possible autoimmune action
methotrexate	DMARD, antineoplastic	Folate	Inhibits synthesis of specific enzymes by competing with vitamin or vitamin metabolites
Mineral oil	Laxative	Vitamins D, K, beta-carotene	Nutrients dissolve in oil, excreted in stool
neomycin	Antibacterial	Fat, vitamin B_{12}, sodium, potassium, iron, calcium, lactose, sucrose	Binds bile salts, lowers pancreatic lipase
para-aminosalicylic acid	Antimycobacterial	Vitamin B_{12}	Enzyme damage, inhibits cell division
potassium chloride	Potassium replacement	Vitamin B_{12}	Lowers ileal pH
pyrimethamine	Malaria, ocular toxoplasmosis	Folate	Inhibits synthesis of specific enzymes by competing with vitamin or vitamin metabolites
sulfasalazine	Ulcerative colitis	Folic acid	Blocks mucosal uptake of folic acid
trimethoprim	Antibacterial	Folic acid	Competitively inhibits folate transport mechanisms

TABLE A-3

Selected Drugs Affecting Taste and Smell

Drug Class	Drugs	Drug Class	Drugs
Amebicides, antihelminthics	metronidazole, niridazole	CNS stimulants	amphetamines (bitter taste), psilocybin
Analgesics	codeine, hydromorphone, morphine	Corticosteroids	cortisone, prednisone
Anesthetics (local)	amylocaine, benzocaine, cocaine, procaine, tetracaine	Diuretics	diazide, diazoxide, furosemide (peculiar sweet taste)
Anticoagulants	phenindione	Hypoglycemia drugs	glipizide, phenformin (metallic taste)
Anticonvulsants	phenytoin	Immunosuppressive drugs	D-penicillamine, doxorubicin, methotrexate, azathioprine
Antifungal drugs	griseofulvin	NSAIDs, DMARDs	allopurinol, colchicine, gold, levamisole, phenylbutazone
Antihistamines	chlorpheniramine, cycloheptadine	Psychoactive drugs	amitriptyline, carbamazepine, chlordiazepoxide, chlorpromazine, meprobamate, diazepam, flurazepam, lithium carbonate (metallic taste), phenytoin, triazolam, trifluoperazine
Antihypertensives	captopril	Skeletal muscle relaxants	baclofen, chlormezanone, levodopa
Antilipemics	clofibrate		
Antimicrobial drugs	methicillin		
Antineoplastic drugs	5-fluorouracil		
Antiparkinson drugs	baclofen, chlormezanone, levodopa		
Antithyroid drugs	methimazole, thiouracil, methylthiouracil, propylthiouracil		

TABLE A-4

Selected Drug-Food Interactions

Class	Drug	Foods	Interaction
Antibiotics	erythromycin, penicillin	Acidic fruit juices, carbonated beverages	Decreases drug's effect
	tetracycline	Dairy products, iron	Impairs absorption
Anticoagulants	warfarin sodium	Fatty fish; foods high in vitamin K, avocado, green leafy vegetables, broccoli	Potential bleeding; can reverse or reduce drug effects
Anticonvulsants	phenytoin	Foods high in folic acid; supplements high in calcium	Decreases seizure threshold
Antidepressants	amitriptyline	Crackers, cookies, Brazil nuts, walnuts, eggs, pasta, meat, fowl, fish, cheese, cranberries, bread, plums prunes, corn, lentils, peanuts	Interferes with benefit of drug
Antihistamines	pseudoephedrine, nifedipine	Alkaline foods, grapefruit	Increases risk of adverse reactions
Cardiac glycosides	digoxin	Bran	Decreases absorption of glycoside
Diuretics	furosemide, bumetanide, ethacrynic acid, triamterene, spironolactone, amiloride	High-sodium foods or antacids	Increases body fluids and blood pressure, alters electrolyte balance
Bronchodilators	theophylline	Charcoal-broiled foods	Reduces effectiveness
Antihypertensives	felodipine hydralazine	Grapefruit juice Nutritional supplements (e.g., Ensure, Sustacal, Meritine)	Increases serum level of drug
Acne drugs	isotretinoin	Fats, vitamin A supplements	Increases triglycerides; increases risk of toxicity and adverse reactions
Antiparkinson drugs	levodopa, carbidopa	Vitamin B_6, meat or meat extracts, liquid nutritional supplements	Reduces effectiveness of drug

Selected Drug-Induced Adverse Reactions*

ANTIMUSCARINIC (ANTICHOLINERGIC)

Antidepressants, including MAO inhibitors and tricyclics

Antihistamines (H_1-receptor blockers only)

carbamazepine

disopyramide

meclizine

Phenothiazines

procainamide

quinidine

BLOOD DYSCRASIAS (DOSE-RELATED MYELOTOXICITY)

Anticancer drugs (some exceptions exist, e.g., bleomycin)

amphotericin B (all formulations)

chloramphenicol

ganciclovir

Interferons

zidovudine

CNS DEPRESSION

Anesthetics, general or parenteral-local

Antidepressants, including MAO inhibitors and tricyclics

Antihistamines (first-generation H_1-receptor blockers)

Barbiturates

Benzodiazepines

Beta-adrenergic blockers

droperidol

ethanol

haloperidol

meclizine

methyldopa

Opioid analgesics

Phenothiazines

scopolamine

KIDNEY TOXICITY

acetaminophen (very high doses)

acyclovir

Aminoglycoside antibiotics

amphotericin B

cisplatin

cyclosporine

ifosfamide

lithium

methotrexate

Nonsteroidal antiinflammatory drugs

pentamidine

Sulfonamides

Tetracyclines (exceptions: doxycycline, minocycline)

tretinoin

vancomycin

LIVER TOXICITY

acetaminophen

Anabolic steroids

Androgens

ACE inhibitors

---

*These lists should not be taken as inclusive; they simply give representative drugs and drug classes known to cause adverse reactions in a significant number of patients.

Azole antifungal drugs (e.g., ketoconazole, itraconazole)
Estrogens
ethanol
HMG-CoA reductase inhibitors
nevirapine
nilutamide
Nonsteroidal antiinflammatory drugs
Phenothiazines
phenytoin
rifampin
Sulfonamides
tretinoin
valproic acid
zidovudine

OTOTOXICITY

Aminoglycoside antibiotics
carboplatin
chloroquine
cisplatin
ethacrynic acid
furosemide
Nonsteroidal antiinflammatory drugs
quinidine
Salicylates
vancomycin

PANCREATITIS

ACE inhibitors
acetaminophen
cisplatin
Corticosteroids
cyclosporin
didanosine
Estrogens

ethacrynic acid
Furosemide
HMG-CoA reductase inhibitors
methyldopa
metronidazole
Opioids
pentamidine
procainamide
propoxyphene
Thiazide diuretics
valproic acid
Vinca alkaloids (vincristine, vinblastine)
zalcitabine

PERIPHERAL NEUROPATHY

altretamine
Aminoglycoside antibiotics
Anticonvulsants, hydantoin
carboplatin
chloramphenicol
ciprofloxacin
cisplatin
cyclosporine
didanosine
ethambutol
ethionamide
fludarabine
imipenem
Interferons
isoniazid
lithium
metronidazole
quinidine
vincristine
zalcitabine

Answer Guidelines for Critical Thinking Questions

CHAPTER 1

PHARMACOKINETICS

1. It takes about four half-lives for a plateau to be reached, which in this case would be about 48 hours.

2. The adverse effects that James complained of are typical for antihistamines and may indicate that his plateau level of drug is too high. The daily dosage was cut in half by dosing every 24 hours instead of every 12 hours.

3. The plateau concentration of drug in blood will fall to a new plateau, which will be achieved in about 48 hours (four half-lives).

4. The recurrence of James' allergic symptoms near the time for his next dose on the 24-hour dosing schedule suggests that the drug concentration in his blood is falling to subtherapeutic levels. By taking a smaller dose at 12-hour intervals, it is hoped that James will have control of his allergies for the full 24 hours.

5. After the second dose change, the plateau did not shift, because the amount of drug given in a day did not change. What did change was the fluctuation of the blood level around the plateau. More fluctuation around a plateau occurs with once-daily dosing than if the same total daily dose is given in smaller, equally spaced doses. Thus with 1.34 mg taken every 12 hours the blood level should not fall as low as with 2.68 mg taken every 24 hours, and control of the symptoms may be maintained around the clock.

CHAPTER 9

SUBSTANCE ABUSE MASQUERADING AS HYPERTENSION

1. Diagnostic criteria involve one or more of the following: (a) failure to fulfill major role obligations at work, school, or home; (b) use in physically hazardous situations; (c) recurrent substance-related legal problems; or (d) use despite persistent or recurrent social or interpersonal problems as a result of use.

2. Two teenagers at home, work problems, spending more and more time away from home, recent displays of unpredictable behavior that have in turn created problems at work and at home, past experimentation with marijuana and cocaine, concerns about meeting college expenses for children.

3. Elevated GGT, AST:ALT ratio; depressed magnesium, calcium, phosphorous, albumin, total protein levels.

4. Nicotine.

5. Tolerance is the repeated use of a substance, resulting in a loss of its effectiveness at the dose used, thus requiring increasing amounts of the drug to achieve the same physiologic or psychologic effect of the drug; dependence is drug use that manifests itself as either psychologic or physical reliance on a drug and is associated with detrimental effects on the individual or society; withdrawal is the result of sufficient chronic exposure to a drug, so that a series of physiologic signs and symptoms occurs with diminishment or discontinuation of the drug.

6. Alcoholics Anonymous (Al-Anon), Alateen, behavior approaches, marital and family counseling, hypnosis, and drug therapy with disulfiram.

CHAPTER 13

POSTOPERATIVE ANALGESIA

1. Perception and interpretation. Perception is affected by opioids.

2. Hourly rate, lockout time, and bolus dose, if any.

3. Depressed respirations, constipation, urinary retention, orthostatic hypotension, and mental state.

4. Naloxone; it acts by displacing the opioid from the receptor. Naloxone produces no pharmacologic effects of its own.

5. Ambulation, increased fluids and fiber, prune juice, and laxatives, if needed.

6. 30 mg morphine given po around the clock q3-4h; pentazocine 150 mg po q3-4h; hydromorphone 7.5 mg po q3-4h; methadone 20 mg po q6-8h.

7. Can be given orally; maintains the "kick" of an opioid while protecting against withdrawal symptoms, and its long half-life reduces withdrawal symptoms to a tolerable level.

CHAPTER 14

RHEUMATOID ARTHRITIS

1. Analgesic, antipyretic, and antiinflammatory. Age, urinary pH, kidney function, liver function, and how drug is formulated.
2. Methotrexate is a folic acid antagonist that inhibits DNA, RNA, and protein synthesis and thereby slows rapidly growing cells; it also reduces leukotrienes, suppresses cell-mediated immunity, inhibits gene suppression for collagenase, and reduces proliferation of synovial fibroblasts and endothelial cells.
3. Level 2. It will take 2 to 6 weeks to notice improvement, with a plateau at about 6 months.
4. Glucosamine sulfate and chondroitin sulfate, warmth, rest, splinting of hands during an acute phase, paraffin baths, imaging, biofeedback, and physical therapy.
5. Ibuprofen-methotrexate, increased risk of methotrexate toxicity; methotrexate-glipizide, increased risk of methotrexate toxicity.
6. Laboratory tests necessary before therapy is started include baseline blood chemistry, renal and liver function tests, and chest x-ray; these should be repeated periodically throughout therapy, based on patient signs, symptoms, and response to therapy. The nadir of leukopenia and thrombocytopenia occurs in 7 to 14 days. These low counts usually recover 7 days after the nadir.

CHAPTER 15

HEADACHE

1. Stimulation of 5-HT$_{1B}$ receptors produces vasoconstriction. Activation of the 5-HT$_{1D}$ receptor reduces the release of neuropeptides from small-diameter sensory neurons. The decreased quantity of neuropeptides reduces inflammation in the area of the blood vessels surrounding the brain and reduces pain signals in the trigeminal system.
2. Blood pressure and pulse should be assessed; sumatriptan raises the blood pressure and heart rate, resulting in increased workload on the heart. Monitoring helps prevent inadvertent use in a patient with undiagnosed hypertension or someone at risk for stroke or myocardial ischemia.
3. Help SB examine her lifestyle, recognize stressful situations, and plan effective coping strategies. Identify precipitating factors. Suggest daily exercise, relaxation periods, socialization, relaxation, meditation, yoga, self-hypnosis, massage, and moist hot packs to the neck and head.
4. SB should take the rizatriptan sublingually with the onset of the aura and lie down in a darkened room immediately after taking the drug. She should limit noise in the environment, turn off the lights, and apply a cold compress. Emphasize the importance of taking the drug as ordered for best effect, but not increasing the dose or frequency of administration unless approved by the health care provider. The drug should be kept out of the reach of children and should not be shared with others. Caution the patient to avoid driving or engaging in potentially

dangerous activities until the effects of the drug are known. Remind SB not to use alcohol or any other CNS depressant. She should contact the health care provider if the drug is ineffective in relieving her headache rather than increasing the dose.
5. Salami sandwiches on homemade rye bread.

CHAPTER 17

PANIC DISORDER

1. Paroxetine, an antidepressant, is approved for panic disorders because of its mild sedating effects. Alprazolam, a benzodiazepine, is used for short-term relief of anxiety associated with depression. Cognitive-behavioral therapy is a form of psychotherapy that provides a context for learning alternative patterns of behavioral and emotional responses.
2. Therapeutic level should be achieved in 2 to 5 days.
3. Alprazolam increases the action of the inhibitory neurotransmitted GABA and opens a chloride channel in the postsynaptic membrane to reduce the neuron's excitability.
4. Daytime sedation initially, ataxia, dizziness, and headaches. Reassure RD that these adverse effects will go away relatively quickly. Other possible adverse effects include blurred or double vision, hypotension, tremor, amnesia, slurred speech, urinary incontinence, and constipation.
5. Over a period of 2 to 16 weeks.
6. Teach RD to avoid alcohol and substances of abuse, other CNS depressant drugs, and antihistamines without first checking with the health care provider. Take the drug with food or fluids to reduce gastric distress. Have prescriptions consistently filled by the same pharmacy. Use caution while driving or operating dangerous machinery until the effects of the antidepressant and anxiolytic drug are known. Take the drugs as prescribed. Store the drugs away from the bedside.

CHAPTER 18

MAJOR DEPRESSION

1. History of mild depression, declining health status, loss of husband, loss of social status, and declining financial and transportation independence.
2. All antidepressant classes are effective in treatment of major depression. All have roughly equal response with similar efficacy rates.
3. Lack of lethality in overdose is an important advantage for newer drugs, especially in light of MG's vague suicidal ideations.
4. Sertraline may displace phenytoin from its binding sites, thus increasing the risk of phenytoin toxicity. Obtain serum phenytoin levels periodically.
5. Inform MG's daughter that the effects of sertraline are usually seen in 2 to 4 weeks.
6. Common adverse effects: nausea, nervousness, insomnia. Less common adverse effects: headache, tremor, anxiety, drowsiness, dry mouth, sweating, diarrhea.

RAPID-CYCLE BIPOLAR DISORDER

1. Divalproex is recognized as the most effective drug for the treatment of rapid-cycle bipolar disorder.

2. Divalproex is a complex of valproic acid and its sodium salt. Valproate increases the concentration of the inhibitory neurotransmitter GABA.

3. SN's impulsivity, poor judgment, and history of a suicide attempt may indicate that a drug with a wide therapeutic index is safer.

4. All drug regimens require laboratory monitoring. Valproate monitoring is less frequent and extensive. However, because of SN's rapid cycling, she may not initially comply with the need for monitoring.

5. Divalproex has the most rapid onset of action, compared with lithium or carbamazepine.

CHAPTER 19

SCHIZOPHRENIA

1. Clozapine produces some sedation and muscle relaxation but few extrapyramidal symptoms. Because of its potential life-threatening effects, patients taking it must be registered with the manufacturer and weekly blood counts monitored closely. Clozapine is not known to cause tardive dyskinesia and may in high doses attenuate it. Fatal agranulocytosis has been reported. Risperidone increases the tendency to cause extrapyramidal symptoms (EPS) and tardive dyskinesia (TD), although all antipsychotic drugs have the potential to cause TD and to lower the seizure threshold. They should be used with caution in patients with a seizure disorder.

2. Risperidone binds primarily to the 5-HT$_2$ and dopamine receptors in the CNS and periphery. It is thought to block the positive symptoms and improve the negative symptoms of psychoses.

3. Resperidone is more likely than other atypical antipsychotic drugs to cause extrapyramidal effects. It also raises prolactin levels. Other adverse effects include dizziness, sexual dysfunction, and mood or mental changes. Monitor for acute dystonia, akathisia, pseudoparkinsonism, and tardive dyskinesia.

4. Antipsychotic effects arise from receptor blockade in the limbic system. Antiemetic effect arises from blockade of receptors in the chemoreceptor trigger zone. Extrapyramidal effects arise from blockade in the corpus striatum of neurons from the basal ganglia. Endocrine effects result from blockade in the pituitary gland.

5. Functional psychoses and toxic psychoses. Organic psychoses are not as successfully treated with antipsychotic drugs as other types of psychoses.

CHAPTER 20

ATTENTION-DEFICIT HYPERACTIVITY DISORDER (ADHD)

1. Exact mechanism of action is unknown, but methylphenidate is thought to block the reuptake of dopamine into dopaminergic neurons.

2. Anorexia, nausea, abdominal pain, nervousness, insomnia, tachycardia, a risk of psychologic dependency on the drug, a temporary slowing of growth in prepubertal children that probably results from appetite suppression.

3. Very high dosages of methylphenidate can cause agitation, confusion, palpitations, arrhythmia, hypertension, delirium, seizures, and coma. Symptoms of withdrawal seen after prolonged use at high dosages include bizarre behavior, depression, and unusual tiredness or weakness.

4. Dantrolene (Dantrium).

5. Review periodic CBC counts (with differential) and platelet counts to monitor for anemia and leukopenia. Check urine catecholamines before and during methylphenidate therapy to determine any increase in the level of dopamine.

6. Improvement in the signs and symptoms identified in Box 20-1.

CHAPTER 21

MULTIPLE SCLEROSIS

1. Although the exact mechanism of action is unknown, observations of CNS neurons suggest that baclofen inhibits neurotransmitters at the spinal level. It also reduces pain in patients with spasticity by inhibiting the release of substance P in the spinal cord.

2. Dantrolene also relieves spasticity.

3. Common adverse effects of baclofen therapy include transient drowsiness, vertigo, confusion, sleepiness, increased weakness, and nausea. Less common effects include headache, fatigue, nasal congestion, abdominal pain, anorexia, diarrhea or constipation, dysuria, urgency, urinary incontinence, and sexual dysfunction in men. Ataxia, insomnia, slurred speech, muscle stiffness, increased excitability, ankle edema, hypotension, tachycardia, and weight gain are also possible adverse effects. Severe adverse effects of baclofen rarely occur but include syncope, chest pain, dark urine, auditory and visual hallucinations, and tinnitus.

4. Concurrent use of dantrolene in women more than 35 years old who are receiving estrogen replacement therapy increases the potential for hepatotoxicity.

LOW BACK PAIN WITH SPASM

1. Cyclobenzaprine acts at the level of the brainstem to reduce muscle tone and hyperactivity.

2. Per manufacturer's recommendations, maximal treatment time with cyclobenzaprine is from 2 to 3 weeks.

3. SK has a history of intermittent porphyria. Carisoprodol is contraindicated in patients with a history of porphyria.

4. Common adverse effects of therapy with cyclobenzaprine include headaches, sleepiness, visual disturbances, and dry mouth. Less common effects include nausea, vomiting, constipation, diarrhea, and urine retention.

CHAPTER 22

EPILEPSY

1. Although the mechanism of action of phenytoin is not clearly understood, calcium and sodium transport is altered and cell membranes are stabilized. The site of action is the motor cortex and the brainstem, where the tonic phase of tonic-clonic seizures originates.

2. The most common adverse effects of phenytoin include dizziness, ataxia, sensory neuropathies, nausea, vomiting, nystagmus, and diplopia. Less common adverse effects include gingival hyperplasia, hypertrichosis and exfoliative dermatitis, coarsened facial features, impaired cognition, dyskinesia, urinary incontinence, and thyroid disorders. The most serious adverse effects include agranulocytosis, encephalopathy, and coma.

3. Breast-feeding is not appropriate during therapy with phenytoin because the drug enters breast milk.

4. Monitoring the serum blood level of phenytoin will indicate whether the blood level values are therapeutic, subtherapeutic, or toxic.

CHAPTER 23

MYASTHENIA GRAVIS

1. Improvement in muscle strength after administration of a test dose of edrophonium is suggestive of the diagnosis of myasthenia gravis.

2. Pyridostigmine inhibits the enzyme acetylcholinesterase, thereby reducing the degradation of acetylcholine. Because acetylcholinesterase is present throughout the neuromuscular junction, inhibition of the enzyme allows acetylcholine to accumulate at the neuromuscular junction, ensuring that available receptors are activated.

3. Common adverse effects of pyridostigmine therapy include nausea, vomiting, excessive salivation, perspiration, muscle cramps, fasciculations, and weakness.

4. Although the mechanism of action of corticosteroids is not clearly understood, prednisone is thought to protect acetylcholine receptor sites from immunologic attack by immunoglobulin G, thus increasing the amount of acetylcholine available at the site. Another hypothesis is that the drug reduces the total number of circulating antibodies and the degradation of the receptor sites, thereby increasing the effectiveness of acetylcholine. Overall, the corticosteroids suppress the patient's immune response.

5. The adverse effects of prednisone therapy are many and include: euphoria, insomnia, psychosis, pseudotumor cerebri, vertigo, headache, seizures, heart failure, hypertension, arrhythmia, thrombophlebitis, thromboembolism, cataracts, glaucoma, peptic ulceration, GI irritation, increased appetite, pancreatitis, nausea, vomiting, menstrual irregularities, hypokalemia, hyperglycemia, carbohydrate intolerance, hypercholesterolemia, hypocalcemia, growth suppression in children, muscle weakness, osteoporosis, hirsutism, delayed wound healing, acne, cushingoid state, increased susceptibility to infections, and acute adrenal insufficiency. Furthermore, sudden withdrawal may be fatal after long-term therapy.

ALZHEIMER'S DISEASE

1. Donepezil permits elevated acetylcholine level in the cerebral cortex, thereby slowing the neuronal degradation that occurs with Alzheimer's disease.

2. Common adverse effects of donepezil include insomnia, fatigue, dizziness, confusion, ataxia, somnolence, tremor, agitation, depression, difficulty in problem solving, anorexia,

nausea, vomiting, dyspepsia, abdominal pain, and diarrhea. Although less common, hepatotoxicity is possible.

3. Teach the patient diagnosed with Alzheimer's disease and the family that donepezil does not alter the underlying degenerative disease but rather slows the progression of the disease and alleviates symptoms.

4. It is important to include the family and significant others when obtaining a health history of a patient with suspected Alzheimer's disease and when providing education, because patient memory deficits and judgment impairments may not allow for a complete and accurate history or independent patient management of drug therapy.

PARKINSON'S DISEASE

1. Levodopa crosses the blood-brain barrier and is converted to dopamine. It is believed that dopamine restores the normal balance between inhibition and excitation in the caudate nucleus and putamen. Carbidopa allows a greater concentration of levodopa to reach the brain and decreases its peripheral adverse effects.

2. The nurse should monitor the patient for dystonia, dyskinesias, nausea, vomiting, dry mouth, dysphagia, ataxia, increased hand tremors, numbness, weakness, faintness, agitation, and anxiety.

3. The nurse should explain to the patient that abrupt withdrawal of the drug could cause a drastic increase in parkinsonian symptoms, deterioration of control, or precipitation of a serious hyperpyretic state similar to neuroleptic malignant syndrome.

4. The so-called on-off phenomenon is the decline in patient response after an improvement in clinical status. The loss of therapeutic effect manifests as an abrupt onset of akinesia. The phenomenon is most often associated with long-term therapy.

CHAPTER 25

SOFT TISSUE INFECTION

1. Ceftriaxone acts by inhibiting the action of transpeptidase enzymes that cross-link the bacterial cell wall peptidoglycan, which in turn weakens and ruptures the cell wall, leading to death of the organism.

2. History of noncompliance, unstable status of his diabetes mellitus, status postoperative total hip replacement increases the risk of infection of the joint, status post–myocardial infarction on anticoagulant therapy.

3. Pain, phlebitis, or thrombophlebitis at intravenous administration site, superinfection. Consider also the need to adequately control and monitor LM for hyperglycemia, because the hyperglycemic environment is more conducive to microbial proliferation.

4. Declining hepatic and renal functions.

5. There are no drug-drug interactions among warfarin, insulin, and ceftriaxone.

6. According to the Advisory Committee on Immunization Practices, Td should be given if there is an unknown history of vaccination or if the patient received less than three of the vaccinations in the series. Tetanus immune globulin (TIG) is

also used if the wound is infected or contaminated with dirt, feces, or saliva. See Chapter 35 for more information regarding vaccinations.

CHAPTER 26

CHLAMYDIA INFECTION

1. Erythromycin base binds to bacterial ribosomes, thus preventing bacterial protein synthesis. At a low concentration the drug is bacteriostatic; at a high concentration it is bacteriocidal.
2. Nausea, vomiting, diarrhea, and cramping are most common. Headache and dizziness possible.
3. An effective serum concentration of the drug may not be achieved.
4. The liver.
5. The esters of erythromycin and many tissues and bacteria cause the release of free erythromycin, thus increasing tissue and blood concentrations of the drug.
6. Cholestatic hepatitis.

CHAPTER 27

COMMUNITY-ACQUIRED PNEUMONIA

1. Yes; her renal function is within normal limits.
2. Fluoroquinolones interfere with DNA replication in bacteria by inhibiting the functioning of topoisomerases.
3. To reduce the risk of nephrotoxicity.
4. Yes; she is taking warfarin sodium, a drug whose effects may be enhanced by the levofloxacin, and a multivitamin, which may reduce the absorption of levofloxacin.
5. A patient with preexisting CNS disease, such as previous seizure activity.
6. Drug-drug interactions include decreased absorption of the levofloxacin in the presence of iron, aluminum-, zinc-, magnesium-, and calcium-containing products (e.g. multivitamins, antacids, sucralfate). Yes, the drug should be taken on an empty stomach.
7. About 48 hours. Have the patient return for reevaluation and possible hospitalization.

CHAPTER 28

LYME DISEASE

1. Doxycycline blocks bacterial growth by preventing ribosomes from binding messenger RNA, thereby preventing the start of protein synthesis; bacteriostatic; broad spectrum.
2. Nausea, vomiting, diarrhea, superinfection, dizziness, unsteadiness, rash, and urticaria.
3. Hepatotoxicity, metabolic derangement in older adults, and staining of teeth in children under age 8.
4. It is better absorbed. All tetracyclines are acid labile except for doxycycline and are partly destroyed by stomach acid. Tetracyclines are not highly water-soluble, and solubility is further reduced when the drug binds with metal ions or with solid material in the intestines. Insoluble forms of tetracyclines are not absorbed but remain in the intestine to be excreted.
5. Kidneys, biliary excretion, and intestines.

6. Mutations that confer resistance travel via plasmids that are transmitted from bacterium to bacterium, therefore spreading rapidly throughout bacterial populations. Resistant bacteria lose the ability to take in tetracyclines.
7. Absorption from intramuscular sites of administration is poor. Local tissue irritation and pain at injection site limit its use.
8. Fanconi syndrome manifests as polyuria, polydipsia, acidosis, nausea and vomiting, as well as a loss of amino acids, proteins, and glucose in the urine.
9. Contact health care provider for permission to obtain a urine pregnancy test before starting doxycycline therapy.

CHAPTER 29

SEPSIS

1. This dosage is within the safe dosage range as long as the patient's peak serum level is not exceeded.
2. Amikacin binds to the (30s) bacterial ribosome; the defective proteins that form damage the bacterial cell. Bacteriocidal; narrow-spectrum.
3. Rash, fever, headache, paresthesias, tremor, nausea, vomiting, anemia, hypotension, eosinophilia, arthralgias. Serious reactions include neuromuscular blockade as well as renal and auditory toxicities.
4. Trough: <5 mcg/mL; peak not to exceed 35 mcg/mL.
5. Renal.
6. At least 30 minutes of slow intravenous drip. To reduce the risk of neuromuscular blockade.
7. Impairs nerve transmission at the neuromuscular junction.
8. Urinalysis, BUN, creatinine, creatinine clearance, liver function (AST, ALT, serum alkaline phosphatase, bilirubin, and LDH concentrations), serum calcium, magnesium, potassium, and sodium.
9. The very young and the older adult.

CHAPTER 30

URINARY TRACT INFECTION

1. Sulfamethoxazole competitively inhibits dihydropteroate synthase, which converts paraaminobenzoic acid (PABA) and other small molecules to dihydropteroate. Sulfonamides are thus selectively toxic to organisms that must form folic acid from PABA. Trimethoprim inhibits bacterial dihydrofolic acid reductase, thus preventing THFA formation in bacteria. The combined effects are synergistic.
2. Bacteriostatic. Broad spectrum.
3. The most common adverse reactions are skin rashes and itching, photosensitivity, and periorbital edema, but drug fever and other more serious reactions such as Stevens-Johnson syndrome may occur.
4. Phenazopyridine exerts an analgesic effect on the mucosa of the urinary tract and relieves the dysuria, frequency, and urgency associated with the UTI.
5. Make regular urination a habit (i.e., at 3- to 4-hour intervals); avoid long waits. Practice good hygiene, including wiping from front to back after urination and bowel movements.

Take a shower rather than a bath. Avoid bubble bath, perfumed soap, feminine hygiene sprays, or products containing hexachlorophene. Increase fluid intake, especially water, to a minimum of six to eight glasses daily. Drink cranberry, blueberry, or prune juice or other foods and take vitamin C to help acidify the urine and relieve symptoms. Urinate before and after intercourse to empty the bladder and cleanse the urethra. Consider changing from a diaphragm and spermicide for birth control to another method if prone to UTIs. Complete prescribed drug regimens even though symptoms are diminished. Do not use drugs left over from previous infections.

CHAPTER 31

HIV INFECTION AND *PNEUMOCYSTIS CARINII* PNEUMONIA (PCP)

1. The combination of efavirenz, lamivudine, and ritonavir during early-stage disease produces significant and sustained reduction of the viral load as well as an increase in CD4 cell count. The same combination in late-stage disease with CD4 counts of less than 50 cells/mm^3 usually reduces mortality. Sulfamethoxazole/trimethoprim blocks bacterial synthesis of essential nucleic acids, producing bacteriocidal action against the *Pneumocystis carinii* organism. Efavirenz is a nonnucleoside reverse transcriptase inhibitor (NNRTI) and lamivudine is a nucleoside reverse transcriptase inhibitor (NRTI); both interfere with HIV-dependent polymerase reverse transcriptase (RT). Ritonavir interferes with the formation of the HIV precursor protein into the active enzymes the virus needs to mature fully.
2. Sulfamethoxazole/trimethoprim: Rash, GI upset, diarrhea caused by *Clostridium difficile*, leukopenia, neutropenia, anemia, ataxia, hyperkalemia. Efavirenz; skin rash, diarrhea, headache, nausea, bizarre dreams, dizziness, sleep disorders, aggression, depression, paranoia, suicidal thoughts. Lamivudine: lipodystrophy, lactic acidosis, hepatotoxicity, granulocytopenia, anemia. Ritonavir: abdominal pain, diarrhea, nausea, vomiting, weakness, paresthesia. CBC, CD4 counts, K, BUN, creatinine, liver function test, viral loads. Every 3 months.
3. Teach the patient to take the drugs exactly as prescribed, adhering to dietary considerations. Report adverse effects to the health care provider, and avoid exposure to persons who are ill. Assist patient in finding and utilizing community resources for emotional as well as financial support for drug therapy.
4. Treatment failure is defined as a failure of viral loads to drop tenfold within the first 4 weeks of treatment; the viral load fails to drop to undetectable levels within the first 4 to 6 months of treatment; the viral load rebounds after falling to an undetectable level; CD4 counts continue to drop despite antiretroviral therapy; or clinical symptoms continue to progress in the presence of drug therapy.
5, 6, 7. Open discussion with colleagues. No definitive answer.

CHAPTER 32

VAGINAL CANDIDIASIS DURING PREGNANCY

1. Given MR's lifestyle, it may be safer to use a one-time dose versus the common 7-day regimen. She needs to be encour-

aged to seek prenatal care as soon as possible, perhaps from the local health department.
2. Explain that although fluconazole is a one-time-dose drug, it is a category C drug that may cause harm to her unborn child. Clotrimazole is a pregnancy category B drug.
3. Clotrimazole inhibits the synthesis of ergosterol, an essential component of the fungal cytoplasmic membrane; leakage of cellular contents results.
4. Erythema, burning, pruritus, vaginal irritation.
5. See Box 32-2.

CHAPTER 33

ACTIVE TUBERCULOSIS

1. Multidrug therapy reduces probability of organism resistance but also makes compliance difficult, given the length of time that therapy is required. Per the American Thoracic Society, Centers for Disease Control and Prevention, and manufacturer's recommendations, minimum duration of therapy is 6 months, most often 6 to 9 months. The variety of adverse effects associated with multidrug therapy requires close monitoring.
2. LR's alcohol intake may be a contraindication to isoniazid and pyrazinamide.
3. Failure either of a health care provider to prescribe adequate drug therapy for an infection or of the patient to take all the drugs as prescribed. Acquired resistance represents a genetic change that converts previously drug-sensitive bacteria to a drug-resistant type.
4. CBC count; liver function tests; blood urea nitrogen (BUN), creatinine, uric acid; and urinalysis before initiating drug therapy and every 1 to 2 months thereafter. Serum drug levels every 1 to 2 months.

CHAPTER 34

MALARIA

1. Protozoa transmitted to bloodstream of humans by the bite of anopheline mosquitoes. Sporozoites enter human blood and travel directly to the liver, persisting there for prolonged periods. Merozoites, the plasmodial form produced in liver cells, attack red blood cells, causing them to rupture, thus producing the fever, chills, and sweating characteristic of malaria. Gametocytes cause a mosquito to become infectious and capable of transmitting the disease. Thus patients at this stage of the disease can transmit parasites to mosquitoes and thence to other human hosts.
2. Proguanil interferes with folic acid metabolism in malaria parasites. Atovaquone blocks energy production.
3. Because *P. falciparum* is often resistant to chloroquine.
4. Abdominal pain, headache, nausea, and vomiting.
5. Atovaquone, feces; proguanil, urine.

CHAPTER 38

CHRONIC HEART FAILURE

1. MB has a dilated heart, low ejection fraction, an S$_3$ gallop, and a history of coronary artery disease. Adding digoxin may help to relieve symptoms through different mechanisms. He remains symptomatic in spite of ACE inhibitors

and diuretics. Digoxin is most effective in patients with these symptoms.

2. Digoxin: slows ventricular rate through AV node. Benazepril: causes mixed preload and afterload reduction by decreasing conversion of angiotensin I to angiotensin II; improves coronary artery blood flow by inhibiting the breakdown of bradykinin. Furosemide: decreases plasma volume and increases elimination of sodium and water.

3. Digoxin and furosemide: electrolyte abnormalities, increased risk of toxicity related to hypokalemia (serum potassium level below 3.5 mEq/L, skeletal muscle weakness, ileus, constipation, polyuria and nocturia caused by impaired concentrating ability of the kidneys, hyperglycemia, ventricular arrhythmia, hypotension, cardiac arrest). Benazepril: benign cough most common but may also note hypotension.

4. No. Despite the fact that MB is taking a potassium-losing diuretic (furosemide), potassium supplementation is not ordinarily needed in patients taking an ACE inhibitor and in fact can be potentially dangerous because these drugs may increase the risk for hyperkalemia. Potassium-containing supplements, low-salt milk, salt substitutes.

5. Apical pulse, blood pressure lying and standing. Evaluate intake, output, skin turgor, and the presence of edema.

6. Name of the drugs, dosage, reason for use; radial pulse and to do so at least once daily; take the drug at the same time each day; if a dose is missed, it should be taken as soon as remembered, although the dose should not be doubled; contact the health care provider if dosages for 2 or more days are missed; avoid concurrent use of other drugs including antacids and antidiarrheal drugs and foods high in sodium and potassium; check with health care provider before using salt substitutes.

CHAPTER 39

ANGINA PECTORIS

1. Nitroglycerin preferentially causes dilation of veins over arterioles, resulting in a pooling of blood in the periphery which in turn reduces venous return to the heart, left end diastolic pressure, and left end–diastolic volume (preload).

2. Cautious use of beta blockers is warranted because of JS's history of reactive airway disease.

3. The common adverse effects include headache and flushing, hypotension, orthostatic hypotension, transient episodes of syncope if standing still, blurred vision, and dry mouth.

4. In angina pectoris, calcium channel blockers reduce myocardial oxygen demand by reducing afterload, increasing coronary blood flow, and by reducing myocardial contractility and heart rate.

5. Stop smoking, lose weight, reduce stress, exercise regularly, take drug as directed, identify and avoid factors that precipitate anginal attacks, notify health care provider if angina episodes worsen in frequency, intensity, duration, location of pain, or response to antianginal drugs.

CHAPTER 40

ATRIAL FIBRILLATION

1. Digoxin: increases the activity of the vagus nerve resulting in decreased automaticity of pacemakers in the SA node and slows conduction through the AV node; protects the ventricles from a high atrial rate. Furosemide: inhibits the Na^+-K^+-Cl^- pump in the ascending limb of the loop of Henle, thus increasing amount of sodium chloride remaining in tubular fluid and excreted in urine with the osmotic equivalent of water. Diltiazem: blocks calcium channels in the SA node and AV node to reduce heart rate. Warfarin: inhibits vitamin K-dependent clotting factors in the liver, thus reducing the risk of thrombus formation related to alterations in blood flow through the heart.

2. Warfarin sodium.

3. Heart rate and rhythm, breath sounds, digoxin and electrolyte levels, weight gain or loss, intake and output, note any unexplained bruising or bleeding, complaints of shortness of breath, dependent edema, vision changes, appetite.

4. Therapeutic serum digoxin level is 0.8 to 2 mcg/mL. Yes, monitor the PT/INR for the warfarin. Furosemide requires monitoring serum K levels. Diltiazem does not require laboratory testing.

5. Low amplitude fibrillatory waves without clear P waves and irregular pattern of QRS complexes. Improved amplitude with clear P waves and a regular pattern of QRS complexes; normal sinus rhythm.

CHAPTER 41

HYPERTENSION

1. Check blood pressure readings again to determine if they have remained high. Contact the health care provider immediately. Arrange for patient to rest in a quiet environment.

2. Clonidine reduces activity of sympathetic nervous system by stimulating alpha$_2$ receptors in the region of the medulla. Losartan binds tightly to AT1 subtype of AII receptors. By blocking effects of the peptide at this receptor, losartan relaxes vascular smooth muscle, resulting in vasodilation and a reduction in blood pressure. It also reduces salt and water retention, which in turn reduces plasma volume.

3. Take blood pressure and pulse before administering the drug and then 15 and 30 minutes later. Monitor the patient for adverse reactions such as drowsiness and dizziness. Have the patient change position slowly.

4. Losartan is an effective ACE inhibitor, has an improved adverse reaction profile, allows monotherapy and once-daily dosing.

5. Diet: obtain thorough diet history. Encourage patient to eliminate or decrease consumption of processed foods, eliminate salt when cooking, decrease intake of fried or fast foods, and minimize consumption of alcoholic beverages. Exercise: obtain thorough exercise history, identify activities that are enjoyable for the patient, obtain a history of daily activities to work in acceptable forms of exercise, especially walking. Stress reduction: encourage the patient to express feelings related to her children's move out of the home; ascertain the positives and negatives about these moves; review which stress reduction techniques have been used with success in the past; review activities that are pleasurable for the patient; encourage sharing her concerns with her husband; and encourage involvement and support from the husband based on the patient's needs and desires. Involvement of the patient in plan of care is essential.

6. Explore the possibility that a naturopathic intervention may be contributing to the patient's hypertension. Advise MD that her blood pressure is too high not to treat urgently with drug therapy. Once her blood pressure is under control, it may be possible for her to return to naturopathy.

CHAPTER 42

HYPERLIPOPROTEINEMIA

1. Nicotinic acid lowers triglyceride levels by 20% to 50%, LDL by 5% to 25%, and raises HDL by 15% to 35%; atorvastatin lowers total plasma cholesterol by 20% to 45%, LDL by 18% to 55%, triglycerides by 7% to 30%, and increases HDL by 5% to 15%.

2. Nicotinic acid has a tendency to cause intense flushing and pruritus of the trunk, face, and arms. A slow titration helps MM tolerate the drug. The daily aspirin helps control the flushing and pruritus.

3. Age over 45, ethnicity, blood pressure over 140/90 mm Hg, smoker, father with MI before age 55, noncompliance with diet and exercise regimen, HDL less than 40; total cholesterol, LDL, and triglycerides above normal range.

4. Headache, GI distress, hepatotoxicity.

5. Myalgias that progress to rhabdomyolysis and acute renal failure.

6. Drug action and adverse effects; importance of dietary modification (reduced intake of saturated fat, increased intake of polyunsaturated fats); weight reduction; increased physical activity; importance of regular follow-up with health care provider and laboratory testing of liver function tests.

CHAPTER 43

DEEP VEIN THROMBOSIS

1. In general, clot formation is hindered by the inhibition of specific clotting factors. Enoxaparin specifically inhibits thrombus formation by blocking factors Xa and IIa. Warfarin suppresses coagulation activity by interfering with the production of vitamin K–dependent clotting factors in the liver. By reducing the amount of available vitamin K, clotting factors II, VII, IX, and X are reduced.

2. PT is the abbreviation for prothrombin time. INR is the abbreviation for international normalized ratio. These values are used to monitor warfarin therapy and assist in determining therapeutic drug dosage. The thromboplastin preparation used to perform PT tests varied from laboratory to laboratory, leading to difficulty in interpretation of test results. This problem led to the development of the INR as the monitoring standard. The INR is derived by multiplying the PT ratio by a correction factor specific to the thromboplastin preparation being used to perform the test.

3. The nurse should look for signs of bleeding or bruising during enoxaparin or warfarin therapy. Other adverse effects the nurse should look for during therapy include GI disturbances, skin necrosis, dermatitis, hair loss, urticaria, fever, and orange-red urine discoloration.

4. Large variances in the daily consumption of foods high in vitamin K alter the anticoagulant effects of warfarin. Foods with a high vitamin K content include dark green leafy vegetables, broccoli, Brussels sprouts, liver, and avocados.

5. To avoid unnecessary bruising, aspiration does not precede drug injection when administering enoxaparin.

CHAPTER 44

ACUTE MYOCARDIAL INFARCTION

1. Thrombolytic drugs dissolve thrombi after formation. Alteplase binds to fibrin in a thrombus and converts the trapped plasminogen to plasma, initiating local fibrinolysis in clots.

2. Overall, bleeding represents the most common complication of thrombolytic therapy, occurring in 8% to 16% of patients. Other adverse effects include hypotension, reperfusion arrhythmia, an increase in temperature, nausea and vomiting, and hypersensitivity reactions including anaphylaxis.

3. JH's history of strep throat infections places him at risk for an allergic reaction and anaphylactic shock during therapy with alteplase. The window of time for successful treatment of acute MI is 6 hours from the onset of chest pain.

CHAPTER 46

FLUID VOLUME EXCESS

1. What medications are you presently taking and when do you take the medications? Have you noticed any adverse effects? How often are you urinating during the day? During the night? Tell me about your diet for the last 24 hours. What do you add to your foods during cooking, and when you are eating? Do you have any questions or concerns? What does your activity level consist of?

2. Furosemide is a loop diuretic with primary action site in the loop of Henle. Inhibits Na^+-K^+-Cl^- symporter at site. NaCl stays in tubular fluid and is excreted in urine with the osmotic equivalent of water.

3. JR is taking both a loop diuretic (furosemide) and cardiac glycoside (digoxin).

4. Digitalis toxicity: nausea, vomiting, anorexia, bradycardia, arrhythmia, and visual disturbances. Hypokalemia: vertigo, hypotension, arrhythmia, nausea, vomiting, diarrhea, abdominal distention, muscle weakness, and leg cramps.

5. Loop diuretics.

6. Renal dysfunction. JR is at risk because of a history and diagnosis of renal insufficiency and heart failure. Both of these could lead to reduced renal profusion.

CHAPTER 48

GERD WITH *HELICOBACTER PYLORI* INFECTION

1. Lansoprazole acts by blocking the enzyme that pumps hydrogen ion into the secretory side of parietal cells of the stomach in turn blocking the production of stomach acid. Amoxicillin: inhibits *H. pylori* cell wall mucopeptide synthesis. Clarithromycin: inhibits *H. pylori* protein synthesis by binding to the 50S ribosome.

2. Lansoprazole: headache, diarrhea, nausea/vomiting, and abdominal pain. Amoxicillin: diarrhea, yeast infections. Clarithromycin: diarrhea, nausea, headache, and a bad taste in the mouth.

3. NSAID use, smoker, eating before bedtime, stress.

4. Avoid oranges, grapefruit, and their juices; tomato products in all forms; chocolate, alcohol, mint, yellow onions, and heavy, fatty meals; and caffeine.
5. Sleep with the head of the bed frame elevated 4 to 6 inches (not just extra pillows). Avoid lying down within 2 to 3 hours of eating.
6. *H. pylori* organisms identified on blood work.

CHAPTER 49
CONSTIPATION

1. Psyllium hydrophilic muciloid acts by combining with water in the intestine. An emollient gel or viscous solution is formed, which increases peristalsis and reduces transit time. Docusate calcium incorporates water and lipids into the stool, producing an emollient action that reduces surface tension. By incorporating water into the stool, a softer fecal mass results.
2. Psyllium formulations should be diluted at the bedside with 8 ounces of water, milk, or juice and the mixture taken immediately; otherwise it will congeal. Ingestion should be followed by another glass of fluid.
3. Bulk-forming laxatives and stool softeners are acceptable in the treatment of constipation during pregnancy. Castor oil can cause uterine contractions, and mineral oil interferes with absorption of nutrients.
4. The most common adverse effect of stool softeners is diarrhea.
5. Antidiarrheal activity occurs because the drug takes on water within the intestinal lumen.

CHAPTER 50
MOTION SICKNESS

1. Vomiting occurs when the chemoreceptor trigger zone (CTZ) located in the lateral reticular formation of the brain stem is stimulated by various inputs (e.g., emotion, pain, motion sickness, anticipation of sickness), resulting in excitatory inputs to the emesis center. The second pathway arises from peripheral stimuli, causing vomiting related to injury or disease of a body tissue or organ. The third pathway is when the CTZ is sensitive to stimulation by circulating drugs and toxins.
2. Meclizine inhibits stimulation of receptors in the labyrinth of the ear that govern equilibrium. Meclizine also has central anticholinergic, CNS depressant, and antihistaminic properties. Scopolamine is a reversible inhibitor of the actions of acetylcholine at muscarinic receptors. Thus it prevents the actions of acetylcholine in the vestibular system.
3. Blurred vision, sensitivity to light, dry mouth, drowsiness, and urinary retention.
4. Place one patch behind the ear at least 4 hours before travel (patch will release 0.5 mg of scopolamine over 72 hours).
5. Small, frequent meals while avoiding bland, very sweet, fatty, salty, and spicy foods. Sip clear liquids slowly and take food served cool or at room temperature. Visual, auditory, and olfactory stimulation should be minimized and noxious stimuli removed from the environment when possible. Avoid or at least decrease activity during episodes of nausea. To relieve mouth dryness caused by the anticholinergic effects of some antiemetics, frequent rinsing and sugarless gum or candy may be used. A cool, wet washcloth to the face and neck may help the patient feel more comfortable.

CHAPTER 51
HEPATIC ENCEPHALOPATHY

1. Neomycin eliminates many of the bacteria that produce nitrogenous wastes in the bowel, thus reducing ammonia buildup. Lactulose decreases the ammonia level that appears to be associated with biotransformation of the sugar in the bowel. The breakdown of lactulose to organic acids causes a drop in the pH of colon contents from 7 to 5. It also inhibits the diffusion of ammonia from the colon into the blood. In addition, because the contents of the colon are more acidic than blood, ammonia is converted to ammonium ions, thereby preventing absorption of ammonia into the blood.
2. Neomycin: ototoxicity and nephrotoxicity; lactulose: anorexia, nausea, vomiting, abdominal cramping, diarrhea, flatulence, distension, and belching.
3. Serum ammonia level is checked periodically during therapy. BUN, creatinine, and creatinine clearance values are required before and throughout prolonged therapy with neomycin. No specific laboratory tests are required when using lactulose.
4. It is based on the number of daily stools, usually two to three.
5. The usual protein restriction is 20 to 40 g daily.

CHAPTER 52
ACUTE ASTHMA ATTACK

1. Aminophylline acts to increase cellular cAMP concentrations by inhibiting degradation by the enzyme phosphodiasterase, which relaxes bronchial smooth muscle and inhibits mast cell degranulation. In addition, it is thought that the xanthine exerts its effect by blocking adenosine receptors in bronchial smooth muscle.
2. Stimulation of beta$_2$ receptors in bronchial smooth muscle cells causes an increase in intracellular cAMP, which translates into muscle relaxation and bronchodilation with subsequent ventilatory improvement.
3. Palpitations, tachycardia, and arrhythmia; CNS stimulation can cause tremors, headache, nervousness, and hypotension with the metaproterenol. Headache, dizziness, and nervousness are common with aminophylline; agitation, exaggerated reflexes, and mild muscle tremors occur at higher serum levels. The combination increases CNS stimulation and the risk of toxicity.
4. Cromolyn is a prophylactic drug and is not used for acute respiratory disorders.
5. Maintain a calm but efficient attitude. Do not leave the patient unattended for long periods. Keep the call bell within easy reach of the patient. Monitor the patient's pulse, blood pressure, respiratory rate, and pulse oximetry, and obtain arterial blood gas values if indicated. Auscultate for breath sounds. Establish an intravenous line to provide access for drugs and to keep the patient hydrated.
6. Use the beta agonist first, followed by the glucocorticoid, with several minutes' pause in between puffs. Rinse the mouth after using the inhalers. Rinse the actuator device after use. Do not exceed prescribed dosage. The patient should know under which circumstances to return to the health care provider or emergency room if the drugs are ineffective.

CHAPTER 53

SEASONAL RHINITIS WITH SECONDARY RHINITIS MEDICAMENTOSA

1. The oxymetazoline was stopped because it was causing rebound congestion and AR was becoming dependent on the drug, which only worsens nasal congestion.
2. Fexofenadine acts by blocking H_1 receptors in nerve endings and in capillaries; as a result, fluid does not escape from the capillaries, edema does not develop, and redness and itching are prevented.
3. The short-term use of pseudoephedrine may help AR feel less stuffy while she withdraws from the oxymetazoline nasal spray.
4. Headache, dizziness, and possible drowsiness may occur, although it is less commonly seen with second-generation antihistamines.
5. Wipe her face with a cool cloth frequently throughout the day to remove dust and pollen from around facial features. Brush hair thoroughly before going to bed to remove the day's dust and pollens. Wash hands thoroughly. Increase fluids. Use sugarless gum or hard candy if the mouth becomes dry. Use air conditioning during allergy season with limited outside exposure. Instruct as to the best housekeeping tactics for controlling allergens. Discourage household pets. Avoid known allergens as much as possible. Avoid operating machinery until the sedative effects of the antihistamine are known or have worn off. The nurse should also teach AR about the adverse effects of the fexofenadine and pseudoephedrine.

CHAPTER 54

COMMON COLD WITH RHINORRHEA

1. Wrong season for seasonal rhinitis; coworkers and children also ill with similar symptoms.
2. Guaifenesin stimulates the production of airway mucus by irritating the stomach lining and setting off the same neuronal response that promotes mucous flow and salivation. Phenergan is an antihistamine that binds selectively to receptors in airways to block the action of histamine, thus relieving allergy symptoms. Codeine inhibits the area of the medulla that controls cough to suppress cough.
3. Drink plenty of water. Humidity.
4. Follow each dose with a full glass of water (codeine works in the cough center in the medulla, not in the back of the throat); use caution while operating machinery or driving until the sedative effects of the codeine is known; do not share the drug with others; do not take other CNS depressants concurrently.
5. May be used for a dry, hacking cough that keeps the patient awake at night.

CHAPTER 55

DIABETES INSIPIDUS

1. Desmopressin acts by increasing cellular permeability to water, thereby increasing the amount of water absorbed and decreasing urine output.
2. Desmopressin is the only drug on the market at this time.

3. Adverse reactions to desmopressin include rhinitis with rhinorrhea, local congestion, and irritation of nasal passages, in addition to heartburn, headache, and conjunctivitis.
4. JS should have urine specific gravity, urine volume, and serum electrolytes monitored throughout therapy.
5. Desmopressin is administered through a flexible nasal catheter used to measure the drug. Once the drug is drawn into the catheter, one end is placed in the nose and the other end in the mouth. The patient then blows into the catheter to deposit the drug in the nasal passageways.

CHAPTER 56

HYPOTHYROIDISM

1. Basal metabolic rates are increased by actions on nuclear receptors in skeletal muscle as well as in the heart, liver, lungs, intestines, and kidneys. They promote gluconeogenesis, thus increasing the utilization and mobilization of glycogen stores. The drugs also stimulate protein synthesis as well as cell growth and differentiation, and they aid in the development of the CNS.
2. 4 to 6 weeks.
3. There are few adverse reactions to levothyroxine. The most common suggest overdosage with the drug and include irritability, insomnia, nervousness, headache, weight loss, and tachycardia.
4. A few patients may be allergic to the tartrazine dye used in the yellow or green levothyroxine tablets. Although the incidence of tartrazine sensitivity in the general population is low, it is frequently found in patients who have aspirin hypersensitivity.
5. The treatment objective for hyperthyroidism is to reduce the levels of circulating thyroid hormones in anticipation of a spontaneous remission and a euthyroid state. Reducing the uncomfortable signs and symptoms is also important.

HYPOPARATHYROIDISM

1. Maintaining an adequate intake of calcium helps prevent loss of calcium from bones and maintains their strength. Because the uptake of calcium is regulated by vitamin D, maximum benefit from dietary calcium supplements is seen when adequate vitamin D uptake is also maintained. Vitamin D is required for proper absorption of calcium.
2. Calcium is primarily absorbed in the upper part of the duodenum, where an acid medium prevails.
3. Serum calcium, phosphorus, and albumin levels should be monitored before start of therapy and periodically throughout.
4. Constipation and loss of appetite may occur.
5. Chvostek's and Trousseau's signs; muscle cramps; and tingling of the circumoral area, hands, and feet.

CHAPTER 57

ADRENAL INSUFFICIENCY

1. Prednisone: glucocorticoids enter a target cell and bind to specific receptors in the cell cytoplasm. The binding of the glucocorticoid activates the receptor, which allows the

complex to enter the nucleus. In the nucleus, the complex binds to selected DNA sites known as glucocorticoid response elements (GREs). This promotes or inhibits the transcription of specific mRNAs. In turn, the synthesis of the respective proteins is promoted or inhibited. Fludrocortisone: binds to mineralocorticoid receptors in the kidney to promote the reabsorption of sodium and water and the excretion of potassium.

2. ADT lessens HPA-axis suppression.

3. Early adverse effects include weight gain, mood changes, glucose intolerance, potassium and sodium changes, and transient adrenal suppression. Late adverse effects include central obesity, skin fragility, myopathy, osteoporosis, and growth failure.

4. The treatment goal for the patient with adrenal insufficiency is to reduce signs and symptoms to a tolerable level.

5. As a replacement drug, prednisone and fludrocortisone are given between 6 and 9 AM and 4 and 6 PM.

6. Instruct the patient and family to avoid activities likely to cause injury and bruising. A normal exercise regimen is required to prevent excessive muscle wasting and to help maintain bone mass; however, it should be interspersed with adequate rest periods. Avoid contact with individuals with active infections. Avoid contact with anyone who has measles or chicken pox. Wear a medical alert identification tag or bracelet.

CHAPTER 58

INSULIN-DEPENDENT TYPE 2 DIABETES MELLITUS

1. Insulin acts by binding to insulin receptor sites on cells to allow transport of glucose into the cell. Glipizide XL stimulates beta cell release of insulin. VH's pancreas is no longer as functional as before.

2. The potential for hypoglycemia exists for both insulin and oral drugs.

3. VH's blood glucose level remained elevated each morning despite maximum dose of sulfonylurea.

4. Insulin is a protein and would be digested if taken by mouth.

5. Chlorpropamide.

6. There is no clear peak level evident for insulin glargine because of the constant and slow rate of absorption. Extended-release forms of glipizide peak about 12 hours after administration.

7. Patients should be instructed to take at least 15 g of a fast-acting carbohydrate as found in 4 to 6 ounces of fruit juice (without added sugar); ½ cup of regular (not diet) carbonated beverage; six Life Saver candies; two or three squares of graham crackers; 4 teaspoons of granulated sugar; 1 cup of milk; six sugar cubes; or ½ cup of regular gelatin (not diet), followed by a complex carbohydrate and a protein.

CHAPTER 61

INFERTILITY

1. Leuprolide, FSH, and hCG support luteal phase and maintain pregnancy through its first trimester. Leuprolide suppresses endogenous LH and FSH to better control stimulation

process and induces maturation of multiple follicles. hCG causes an LH surge, leading to final maturation of ova so eggs can be retrieved for in vitro fertilization (IVF).

2. Leuprolide: hot flashes, sweats, headache, alterations in menstrual cycle, reactions at the site of injection. FSH and hCG: hot flashes, ovarian hyperstimulation syndrome (OHSS), increased coagulability, decreased renal perfusion, fluid retention.

3. Multiple fetuses.

4. 50% to 60%.

5. About 1% of patients experience this disorder.

CHAPTER 62

PRIMARY HYPOGONADISM

1. Synthetic oral testosterone preparations have a greater tendency to cause adverse effects.

2. The androgens are steroids that diffuse into cells and bind to specific receptors found in the cytoplasm of target tissues. The drug complex moves into the nucleus of the cell and changes gene expression, which in turn alters cell function and stimulates growth of the male reproductive tract organs.

3. Acne, urinary tract infections, bladder irritation, edema, nausea or vomiting, diarrhea, pain in the scrotum or groin, and priapism.

4. Z-track.

5. PT and INR values will need to be monitored with possible dosage adjustment of the warfarin, because androgens increase the effects of the warfarin.

CHAPTER 63

PERNICIOUS ANEMIA

1. Cyanocobalamin, also known as vitamin B_{12}, is a coenzyme that stimulates metabolic function and is needed for cell replication, hematopoiesis, and nucleoprotein and myelin synthesis.

2. Pernicious anemia is a deficiency of vitamin B_{12} that indirectly causes anemia. Persons with pernicious anemia do not properly absorb vitamin B_{12} from the intestinal tract because they lack intrinsic factor. Vitamin B_{12} is necessary for the production of red blood cells and for maintenance of the myelin sheath of nerves.

3. Monthly intramuscular injections of cyanocobalamin will be required for the rest of TW's life because anemia will recur, and irreversible neurologic damage may occur if not treated monthly. Only intramuscular injections are effective for treating pernicious anemia because the intestine is bypassed.

4. Reticulocyte count, hematocrit, vitamin B_{12}, iron, and folate levels are typically ordered before beginning cyanocobalamin therapy and periodically thereafter.

CHAPTER 65

GLAUCOMA

1. Cholinergic miotics, anticholinesterase miotics, anticholinergics, adrenergics, carbonic anhydrase inhibitors, and osmotics are all appropriate for use with primary open-angle

glaucoma. Beta blockers are efficacious, most commonly used, and usually considered the standard of care.

2. Beta blockers.

3. The major advantage of beta blockers is that neither pupil size nor reactivity to light is altered.

4. Patients with severe cardiovascular disease or severe asthma.

5. Occlude the nasolacrimal duct with one finger for 1 to 2 minutes after instilling the drug. This is particularly important when the drugs are given to infants and children.

CHAPTER 66

BILATERAL OTITIS MEDIA

1. Did CC get all of the drug? Did the ears clear? Was this validated by the health care provider with an ear recheck? Did CC's fever respond to an antipyretic? Which one does the mother use? What do the parents know about secondhand smoke?

2. The most common bacteria causing otitis media are *S. pneumoniae*, *H. influenzae*, and *M. catarrhalis*. Any virus can settle in the inner ear.

3. Elements in CC's history include the smoking by the parents, other relatives, and friends; the amount of time spent in day care; and possibly the large tonsils.

4. The potential lack of knowledge concerning secondhand smoke and eustachian tube dysfunction as well as the potential for allergies (e.g., from animal dander).

5. Azithromycin, a macrolide that is indicated for community infections; CC has had a number of penicillins, cephalosporins, and sulfa drugs for previous infections. A danger in prescribing multiple antibiotics is that CC will become resistant to them all.

6. Another pharmacologic preparation to use would be acetaminophen to reduce fever and minimize discomfort. An antihistamine, a decongestant, or a combination of the two may also be ordered. Preferred use is a one-ingredient drug rather than a combination, so a sympathomimetic such as pseudoephedrine HCl (Sudafed) is suggested. However, the parents could try different decongestants and/or antihistamine preparations until they find one that works for the child. Nonpharmacologic interventions include fluids and rest for the child as well as smoking cessation for the parents. Good nutrition and hygiene can be taught as best as possible to a 3-year-old child to enhance the immune system (stopping day care is not an option).

7. Educational points to cover with the parents include the following: the research-supported link between secondhand smoke and recurrent otitis media (see the web site *http://www.kidshealth.org/parent/common/otitis_media.html*); ways to give antibiotics and other drugs if needed; signs and symptoms to watch for; when to call back; and the importance of an office visit for ear recheck, repeat tympanogram for comparison, parents' recall of patient behavior, and administration of all the drug.

CHAPTER 67

SCABIES

1. Advanced age, crowded living conditions, debilitation, and HIV-positive status. Scabies should be suspected in immunocompromised patients.

2. Crotamiton's mechanism of action is unknown.

3. It is massaged into the skin from the chin down, with attention to body creases and folds. It is reapplied in 24 and 48 hours and then washed from the body surface (crotamiton requires two applications for one treatment).

4. Lindane is primarily used for lice. Additionally, lindane is known to be absorbed through the skin with CNS toxicity and is contraindicated for patients with an allergy to chrysanthemums. There is also the potential for greater transdermal absorption because of his age.

5. Universal precautions should be used to prevent spread of the scabies to themselves and others.

CONTACT DERMATITIS

1. Triamcinolone cream acts by reducing the inflammatory response and thus the itching.

2. A cream or ointment.

3. There are minimal to no adverse effects with the short-term use of a topical mild-high corticosteroid.

4. A topical corticosteroid under occlusion for 24 hours establishes a drug reservoir in the stratum corneum that can persist for as long as 2 weeks. This increases the risk of a high serum level of the drug caused by systemic absorption.

5. Avoid the known allergen.

Disorders Index

Comprehensive Index